DRUG THERAPY FOR ASTHMA

LUNG BIOLOGY IN HEALTH AND DISEASE

Executive Editor: **Claude Lenfant**

Director, National Heart, Lung, and Blood Institute
National Institutes of Health
Bethesda, Maryland

Volume 1 IMMUNOLOGIC AND INFECTIOUS REACTIONS IN THE LUNG, *edited by Charles H. Kirkpatrick and Herbert Y. Reynolds*

Volume 2 THE BIOCHEMICAL BASIS OF PULMONARY FUNCTION, *edited by Ronald G. Crystal*

Volume 3 BIOENGINEERING ASPECTS OF THE LUNG, *edited by John B. West*

Volume 4 METABOLIC FUNCTIONS OF THE LUNG, *edited by Y. S. Bakhle and John R. Vane*

Volume 5 RESPIRATORY DEFENSE MECHANISMS (in two parts), *edited by Joseph D. Brain, Donald F. Proctor, and Lynne M. Reid*

Volume 6 DEVELOPMENT OF THE LUNG, *edited by W. Alan Hodson*

Volume 7 LUNG WATER AND SOLUTE EXCHANGE, *edited by Norman C. Staub*

Volume 8 EXTRAPULMONARY MANIFESTATIONS OF RESPIRATORY DISEASE, *edited by Eugene Debs Robin*

Volume 9 CHRONIC OBSTRUCTIVE PULMONARY DISEASE, *edited by Thomas L. Petty*

Volume 10 PATHOGENESIS AND THERAPY OF LUNG CANCER, *edited by Curtis C. Harris*

Volume 11 GENETIC DETERMINANTS OF PULMONARY DISEASE, *edited by Stephen D. Litwin*

Volume 12 THE LUNG IN THE TRANSITION BETWEEN HEALTH AND DISEASE, *edited by Peter T. Macklem and Solbert Permutt*

Volume 13 EVOLUTION OF RESPIRATORY PROCESSES: A COMPARATIVE APPROACH, *edited by Stephen C. Wood and Claude Lenfant*

Volume 14 PULMONARY VASCULAR DISEASES,
edited by Kenneth M. Moser

Volume 15 PHYSIOLOGY AND PHARMACOLOGY OF THE AIRWAYS,
edited by Jay A. Nadel

Volume 16 DIAGNOSTIC TECHNIQUES IN PULMONARY DISEASE (in two parts),
edited by Marvin A. Sackner

Volume 17 REGULATION OF BREATHING (in two parts),
edited by Thomas F. Hornbein

Volume 18 OCCUPATIONAL LUNG DISEASES:
RESEARCH APPROACHES AND METHODS,
edited by Hans Weill and Margaret Turner-Warwick

Volume 19 IMMUNOPHARMACOLOGY OF THE LUNG,
edited by Harold H. Newball

Volume 20 SARCOIDOSIS AND OTHER GRANULOMATOUS
DISEASES OF THE LUNG,
edited by Barry L. Fanburg

Volume 21 SLEEP AND BREATHING,
edited by Nicholas A. Saunders and Colin E. Sullivan

Volume 22 *PNEUMOCYSTIS CARINII* PNEUMONIA:
PATHOGENESIS, DIAGNOSIS, AND TREATMENT,
edited by Lowell S. Young

Volume 23 PULMONARY NUCLEAR MEDICINE:
TECHNIQUES IN DIAGNOSIS OF LUNG DISEASE,
edited by Harold L. Atkins

Volume 24 ACUTE RESPIRATORY FAILURE,
edited by Warren M. Zapol and Konrad J. Falke

Volume 25 GAS MIXING AND DISTRIBUTION IN THE LUNG,
edited by Ludwig A. Engel and Manuel Paiva

Volume 26 HIGH-FREQUENCY VENTILATION IN INTENSIVE CARE
AND DURING SURGERY,
edited by Graziano Carlon and William S. Howland

Volume 27 PULMONARY DEVELOPMENT: TRANSITION
FROM INTRAUTERINE TO EXTRAUTERINE LIFE,
edited by George H. Nelson

Volume 28 CHRONIC OBSTRUCTIVE PULMONARY DISEASE, second edition, revised and expanded
edited by Thomas L. Petty

Volume 29 THE THORAX (in two parts),
edited by Charis Roussos and Peter T. Macklem

Volume 30 THE PLEURA IN HEALTH AND DISEASE,
edited by Jacques Chrétien, Jean Bignon, and Albert Hirsch

Volume 31 DRUG THERAPY FOR ASTHMA: RESEARCH AND CLINICAL PRACTICE
edited by John W. Jenne and Shirley Murphy

Other volumes in preparation

DRUG THERAPY FOR ASTHMA

RESEARCH AND CLINICAL PRACTICE

Edited by

John W. Jenne

Department of Medicine
Loyola-Stritch School of Medicine
Maywood, Illinois
Pulmonary Diseases Section
Edward Hines, Jr. Veterans Administration Hospital
Hines, Illinois

Shirley Murphy

Pediatric Pulmonary Division
Department of Pediatrics
University of New Mexico School of Medicine
Albuquerque, New Mexico

MARCEL DEKKER, INC. New York • Basel

Library of Congress Cataloging-in-Publication Data

Drug therapy for asthma: research
and clinical practice

(Lung biology in health and disease ; v. 31)
Includes bibliographies and indexes.
1. Antiasthmatic agents. 2. Bronchodilator agents.
3. Asthma--Chemotherapy. I. Jenne, J. W. [date]. II. Murphy,
Shirley [date]. III. Series. [DNLM: 1. Asthma--
drug therapy. 2. Bronchodilator Agents. W1 LU62 v. 31 /
QV 120 A853]
RO591.A817 1987 616.2'38061 87-576
ISBN 0-8247-7633-X

MARCEL DEKKER, INC.
270 Madison Avenue, New York, New York 10016

Current printing (last digit):
10 9 8 7 6 5 4 3 2 1

PRINTED IN THE UNITED STATES OF AMERICA

Dedicated to Max Samter, who has provided to so many the wisdom, critical perspective, humor, and encouragement of a great teacher

INTRODUCTION

> The Yellow Emperor said "Man is afflicted when he cannot rest and when his breathing has a sound . . . he may have his rest and his exercise and his breathing is troubled; or he may not get any rest and be unable to walk about and his breathing is troubled. There are those who do not get a rest and those who rest and yet have troubled breathing. . . . I desire to hear about their causes."
>
> Chi Po answered: "If, however, the habits of life are as usual and breathing is noisy; and if one cannot rest, or if one rests there is troubled breathing, then something has temporary residence in the breath; water follows the saliva and moves. The water of the kidneys influences the saliva, disturbs the rest and causes the troubled breathing."
>
> The Emperor said "Excellent!"

This dialogue took place in 2500 BC and was published in the Yellow Emperor's *Classic of Internal Medicine.* Huang Ti, the Yellow Emperor, was said to have ruled China for nearly 100 years!

Whether all modern asthma experts would recognize this dialogue as a description of asthma is uncertain. Personally, I would. This *Classic of Internal Medicine* also discussed the treatment of "troubled breathing" with acupuncture, and it is noteworthy that modern China still uses acupuncture for the treatment of asthma.

Today, asthma is a prevalent disease that constitutes a major public health problem. Moreover, there is some evidence that in some countries the number of deaths due to asthma is increasing. Thus, it is no surprise that over the last two decades we have witnessed a huge investment in research relative to asthma, an investment that is now paying some very handsome dividends. Foremost, our understanding of the pathogenesis and pathophysiology of the disease has remarkably increased and paved the way for new investigations now being actively pursued. Moreover, these investigations are having major spin-offs that benefit other disease entities. The drug industry in the United States and in other countries has also seen the need to search for new therapies. Today, practicing physicians are presented with a large array of drugs and therapeutic regimens that enable them to truly tailor each patient's treatment.

Because of the many advances relative to asthma and its treatment, I was extremely pleased to be able to entice Drs. Jenne and Murphy to edit a monograph on *Drug Therapy for Asthma: Research and Clinical Practice.* This volume is an important and timely addition to the series "Lung Biology in Health and Disease." It presents viewpoints that will provoke researchers and assist practitioners. I am grateful to them and to all the contributors for their efforts. They have many reasons to be proud of this contribution. Certainly, the series of monographs is enhanced by its inclusion.

Claude Lenfant, M.D.

PREFACE

The inspiration behind this book was to provide in one source both the theoretical groundwork and the practice specifics of asthma drug therapy. The book should serve as a starting point and literature framework at the level of the fellow in training or the young researcher. We have covered the major drugs now in common use. Although we have devoted a chapter to drug actions on mediators, we have not attempted to anticipate specific new compounds in that evolving field. Also, we have not included material on expectorants or mucolytics.

The chapter authors will be recognized as among the leaders of their fields. The clinical section was specifically designed to present the variations in adult and pediatric practice, with chapters on the acute and chronic management of each. We are particularly pleased to have a strong section on the approach to the asthmatic in the United Kingdom, contrasting in some respects with the United States. We have emphasized the "how to" specifics that most textbooks and review articles leave out. The appendix contains drug formulas and dosage schedules.

In this endeavor, the editors have been privileged to be exposed to the spirit and dedication of their contributors. We hope our readers will sense and share in this.

John W. Jenne
Shirley Murphy

CONTENTS

CONTRIBUTORS

William M. Abraham, Ph.D. Adjunct Associate Research Professor, Department of Medicine, University of Miami School of Medicine, Miami, and Research Associate, Mt. Sinai Medical Center, Miami Beach, Florida

Richard C. Ahrens, M.D. Assistant Professor of Pediatrics, Division of Pediatric, Allergy, and Pulmonary Diseases, University of Iowa, Iowa City, Iowa

Tahir Ahmed, M.D. Associate Professor, Department of Medicine, University of Miami School of Medicine, Miami, and Associate, Division of Pulmonary Disease, Mt. Sinai Medical Center, Miami Beach, Florida

Peter J. Barnes, D.M., F.R.C.P. Professor and Director, Department of Clinical Pharmacology, Cardiothoracic Institute, Brompton Hospital, London, England

Steven E. Borst, M.D. Professor, Department of Pharmacology, UCLA School of Medicine, Los Angeles, California

Judith Cohn, M.D., Ph.D. Division of Clinical Pulmonary Disease, Rush-Presbyterian Medical Center, Chicago, Illinois

Matthew E. Conolly, M.D. Director, Department of Clinical Pharmacology, UCLA School of Medicine, Los Angeles, California

Howard Eigen, M.D. Professor, Department of Pediatrics and Medical Director, Pediatric Intensive Care Unit, Indiana University School of Medicine, and Director, Section of Pulmonary Diseases, James Whitcomb Riley Hospital for Children, Indianapolis, Indiana

Elliot F. Ellis, M.D. Professor, Department of Pediatrics, and Chief, Department of Pediatrics, Children's Hospital of Buffalo, State University of New York at Buffalo, Buffalo, New York

Roger Ellul-Micallef, M.D., Ph.D. Professor of Pharmacology, Department of Medical Sciences, Faculty of Medicine, University of Malta, Msida, Malta

Nicholas J. Gross, M.D., Ph.D. Professor of Medicine, Department of Medicine, Stritch-Loyola School of Medicine, Maywood, and Section Chief, Medical Services, Edward Hines, Jr. Veterans Administration Hospital, Hines, Illinois

Christopher Hardy, M.D.* Lecturer, Department of Medicine, Southampton General Hospital, University of Southampton, Southampton, England

Stephen T. Holgate, M.D. Professor of Medicine, Department of Medicine, Southampton General Hospital, University of Southampton, Southampton, England

Ka Kit Hui, M.D. Department of Clinical Pharmacology, UCLA School of Medicine, Los Angeles, California

John W. Jenne, M.D. Professor of Medicine, Department of Medicine, Loyola-Stritch School of Medicine, Maywood, and Section Chief, Pulmonary Diseases, Hines, Jr. Veterans Administration Hospital, Hines, Illinois

Jan-Anders Karlsson, Ph.D. Pharmacological Laboratory, AB Draco, Lund, Sweden

H. William Kelly, Pharm. D. Assistant Professor of Pharmacy and Pediatrics, Department of Pediatrics, College of Pharmacy, University of New Mexico School of Medicine, Albuquerque, New Mexico

Wayne Kepron, M.D. Associate Professor, Department of Immunology, Faculty of Medicine, University of Manitoba, Winnipeg, Manitoba, Canada

Siow-Kee Kong, Ph.D. Department of Immunology, Faculty of Medicine, University of Manitoba, Winnipeg, Manitoba, Canada

J. Frederick Krall, Ph.D. Biochemical Pharmacology Laboratory, and the UCLA-SFVP Department of Medicine, Veterans Administration Medical Center, Sepulveda, California

Claes-Göran Lofdahl, M.D. Department of Clinical Pharmacology, Sahlgrenska University Hospital, Gothenburg, Sweden

---

**Present affiliation*: Senior Registrar in Thoracic Medicine, Wythenshawe Hospital, Manchester, England

Bennie Mc Williams, M.D. Assistant Professor, Department of Pediatrics, and Director, Pediatric Pulmonary Physiology Laboratory, University of New Mexico School of Medicine, Albuquerque, New Mexico

Richard W. Mitchell, Ph.D. Department of Physiology and Immunology, Faculty of Medicine, University of Manitoba, Winnipeg, Manitoba, Canada

John Morley Preclinical Research, Sandoz AG, Basel, Switzerland

Shirley Murphy, M.D. Associate Professor, Department of Pediatrics, and Director, Pediatric Pulmonary/Critical Care Division, University of New Mexico School of Medicine, Albuquerque, New Mexico

Virgil Nathaniel, M.Sc. Department of Physiology and Immunology, Faculty of Medicine, University of Manitoba, Winnipeg, Manitoba, Canada

Carl G. A. Persson, Ph.D. Professor, Department of Clinical Pharmacology, University Hospital of Lund, and Research Adviser, Pharmacological Laboratory, AB Draco, Lund, Sweden

Charles E. Reed, M.D. Professor of Internal Medicine, Department of Medicine, Mayo Medical School, and Chairman, Division of Allergic Diseases and Internal Medicine, Allergy Division, Mayo Clinic, Rochester, Minnesota

Charles Scoggin, M.D. Professor, Division of Pulmonary Science, University of Colorado Health Sciences Center, Denver, Colorado

Chun Y. Seow, B. Engrg. Department of Physiology, Faculty of Medicine, University of Manitoba, Winnipeg, Manitoba, Canada

Morton S. Skorodin, M.D. Assistant Professor, Department of Medicine, Stritch-Loyola School of Medicine, Maywood, Medical Director, Respiratory Care Department, and Staff Physician, Ambulatory Care and Medical Service, Edward Hines, Jr. Veterans Administration Hospital, Hines, Illinois

R. Michael Sly, M.D. Director, Department of Allergy and Immunology, Children's Hospital National Medical Center, Washington, D.C.

Sheldon L. Spector, M.D. Professor, Department of Medicine, UCLA School of Medicine, and Allergy Medical Clinic, Los Angeles, California

Newman L. Stephens, M.D., F.R.C.P. Professor, Department of Physiology and Immunology, Faculty of Medicine, University of Manitoba, Winnipeg, Manitoba, Canada

Gerald S. Supinski, M.D. Assistant Professor, Department of Medicine, Case Western Reserve University School of Medicine, Cleveland, Ohio

Nils Svedmyr, M.D. Department of Clinical Pharmacology, Sahlgrenska University Hospital, Gothenburg, Sweden

Stanley J. Szefler, M.D. Director, Pediatric Clinical Pharmacology, National Jewish Center for Immunology and Respiratory Medicine; Associate Professor of Pediatrics and Pharmacology, University of Colorado Health Sciences Center, Denver, Colorado

Donald P. Tashkin, M.D. Professor, Department of Medicine, Division of Pulmonary Diseases, UCLA School of Medicine, Los Angeles, California

John H. Toogood, M.D., F.R.C.P. (C), F.C.C.P. Professor, Department of Medicine, University of Western Ontario, and Director, Allergy Clinic, Victoria Hospital, London, Ontario, Canada

Adam Wanner, M.D. Professor, Department of Medicine, Director, Pulmonary Division, University of Miami School of Medicine, Miami, Florida

Archie Wilson, M.D., Ph.D. Head, Pulmonary Division, Department of Medicine, University of California at Irvine Medical Center, Orange, California

1

Theory

Anatomy and Physiology of Respiratory Smooth Muscle Tone

NEWMAN L. STEPHENS, VIRGIL NATHANIEL, WAYNE KEPRON, RICHARD W. MITCHELL, CHUN Y. SEOW, and SIOW-KEE KONG

University of Manitoba
Winnipeg, Manitoba, Canada

I. Introduction

This chapter discusses the ultrastructure, biophysics, and biochemistry of airway smooth muscle; these in turn subserve bronchodilation. The important role of neural control, and of muscle membrane electrophysiology and pharmacology, is dealt with elsewhere in this book.

Ideally speaking, all the data reported should relate to observations made in human asthmatics. Though some beginnings have been made (Adelstein and Eisenberg, 1980; Akasaka et al., 1975; Antonissen et al., 1979), currently, this is not feasible because of the difficulty in obtaining appropriate surgical or autopsy material. Much of the research conducted in vitro has used airway smooth muscle from dogs (Stephens, 1975; Stephens et al., 1969; Suzuki et al., 1976), guinea pigs (Douglas et al., 1973), cats (Lullich et al., 1976; Bai et al., 1984), cows (Cameron and Kirkpatrick, 1976), sheep (Eyre, 1973), horse (Eyre, 1973; Chand and Eyre, 1978), and rat (Fleisch et al., 1980).

Our mandate is to deal with the anatomy and physiology of respiratory smooth muscle tone. The latter, as we understand it, is the presence of a small amount of active force or tension in airway smooth muscle without any concomitant shortening. Its presence can be demonstrated by appropriate pharmacologic or metabolic blockade. While the question of tone is of some significance we do not believe that it is the most important airway smooth muscle parameter to consider. The important parameter contributing to the respiratory distress of asthma is narrowing of central airways in the acute phase of the attack, and of peripheral airways in the delayed phase; hence for in vitro experiments shortening is the major parameter to study. Increased tone, as we have defined it, can affect air flow to some extent by rendering the airways stiffer, but major control is by regulation of airway cross-sectional area. Another way in which tone may affect the responsiveness of airways is by regulating the appearance of various receptors. It is believed, for example, that the increased intracellular calcium present in a muscle with tone increases the number of α-adrenoceptors presenting at membrane surface and thus increases the muscles' contractile response. All this notwithstanding, we will discuss mainly the shortening properties of both normal and sensitized airway smooth muscle and their ability to shorten at different velocities. The documentation of increased shortening capacity (L_{max}) would provide the explanation for allergic bronchospasm, however, the mechanism of the increased L_{max} would still need to be elucidated. This is discussed below. Increased shortening velocity (V_o or V_{max}) if present in sensitized airway smooth muscle would not, per se, provide a direct explanation for increased shortening. However force-velocity data in all muscles always demonstrate that highest velocities are seen at lowest loads and are associated with largest L_{max} values. Thus there seems to be a relation between the two, and understanding the former may provide insight into the latter. Furthermore, the increased V_o indicates that the actin-activated myosin ATPase of the sensitized airway smooth muscle is increased in activity. This provides insight into alterations in muscle energetics in airway smooth muscle.

It should be pointed out that failure to relax could contribute to bronchospasm just as much as normal contraction. While this is an important area of research, it will be dealt with only briefly in this chapter.

Research in striated muscle has demonstrated the great importance of ultrastructural studies in understanding muscle function. Hence we propose to describe first what is known of smooth muscle structure in general and of airway smooth muscle in particular.

II. Anatomy of Airway Smooth Muscle

The discussion is based on data from canine tracheal smooth muscle which bears, in general, striking similarity to the features of human airway smooth muscle and to muscle in airways lower down the respiratory tree. Admittedly there are differences in innervation and in some pharmacologic features but the general features of the smooth muscle cells themselves do not differ to any great extent.

The gross anatomical features of airways and airway smooth muscle have been well documented by von Hayek (1960) and Krahl (1964) and the reader is referred to these sources for detail.

A. Multiunit, Intermediate, and Single-Unit Types of Smooth Muscle

Smooth muscle has been classified into multiunit and single unit types. Examples of the former are the large and intermediate-sized blood vessels and vas deferens. Such muscles are characterized by no spontaneous rhythmic mechanical activity, no oscillations of the resting membrane potential and no action potentials. Agonists stimulate the muscle by means of graded depolarization. Innervation is quite rich, creating many independent nerve-muscle units—hence the name. By the same token, cell-to-cell communications by way of gap junctions are sparse. Finally, such muscles do not possess a myogenic response; they are termed tonic muscles. Single-unit muscle possesses considerable spontaneous, rhythmic, electrical, and mechanical activity of a phasic type. The resting membrane potential oscillates quite markedly, with the crests of the depolarization being associated with action potentials. Electromechanical coupling is well displayed. Cell-to-cell coupling by way of low-impedance gap junctions is excellent and innervation is correspondingly sparse. Single-unit muscle possesses a strong myogenic response. Examples of such muscles are the taenia coli, the uterus at term, the ureter, and small arteries and arterioles (Burnstock, 1970; Miller and Marshall, 1975). Canine tracheal smooth muscle seems to be of an intermediate variety in terms of Burnstock's classification (Burnstock, 1970) since it does not manifest the typical features of either multiunit or single-unit smooth muscle. In not possessing any spontaneous phasic activity, nor any action potentials, and in possessing a tonic mechanical response, it resembles multiunit muscle. However, in possessing a somewhat sparser innervation than expected it displays features of single unit muscle. The mixture of properties has led to its being placed in the intermediate category.

The classification of airway smooth muscle is not merely an academic exercise. It has been suggested by Macklem (personal communication) that normal airway smooth muscle is of multiunit type but in asthmatics becomes converted to single unit. This is said to be associated with the increased excitability typical of asthmatic subjects. Akasaka et al. (1975) have developed an extracellular electrode (for use in human cases of asthma), that can be introduced into airways via a catheter. Their data show, quite clearly, fairly strong smooth muscle integrated, action-potential type of activity in asthmatics. In normal subjects, where an absence of such activity is expected, examination of their records shows that action potentials are present but are few and far between. Our interpretation is that normal human airway smooth muscle possess single-unit characteristics but that these are expressed in attenuated form. With the development of asthma they become more strongly expressed. Akasaka's report is the only one of its kind and confirmatory evidence is required.

We have reported (Kroeger and Stephens, 1975) that the addition of tetraethylammonium chloride to the bathing solution converts canine tracheal smooth muscle from multiunit type to single unit. This is identified by the development of partial membrane depolarization with oscillation, and compound action potentials carried almost entirely by Ca^{2+}. A strong myogenic response also develops. Electrophysiological measurements also show that the space constant increases by about 30%. These changes can be explained by tetraethylammonium reducing potassium conductance. Kannan and Daniel (1980) have shown a significant increase in number of gap junctions after tetraethylammonium chloride treatment. These develop within 10 min and their appearance is not inhibited by colchicine, which suggests that they are synthesized on an ad hoc basis from preformed materials present in the membrane. Among factors involved in the development of gap junctions are calcium (Lowenstein and Rose, 1978), which leads to functional uncoupling without any detectable change in morphology; cyclic AMP, which has been shown to regulate the size of gap junctions in hepatoma cells (Johnson et al., 1974); steroid hormones; protein synthesis; prostaglandins; and a degradation process.

Similar spontaneous activity has been seen in tracheal smooth muscle after treatment with histamine, or when the tissue has been roughly handled during dissection.

This phenomenon of multiunit to single-unit conversion has generated some interest because of the possibility that such a conversion in human beings results in the development of the hyperexcitable airways of allergic bronchoconstriction.

It must be pointed out that there is a lack of consistently good correlation between the degree of electrical coupling between cells and the presence of nexuses, which has suggested the existence of other structural mechanisms of coupling, in addition to the nexus. Kannan and Daniel (1978) have observed good electrical coupling in smooth muscle in vitro, before the appearance of gap junctions. This makes it difficult to believe that gap junctions are the sites of low-impedance intercellular communications.

More complex junctional structures are seen between muscle cells involving the interdigitation of the ends of two cells, each having divided into numerous lamellar and cylindrical processes (Gabella, 1984). The space (50–100 nm in width) between these processes is filled with microfibrils and a material that appears to be similar to basal lamina. Such fingerlike processes at the cells ends have been described in the guinea pig vas deferens (Merrillees et al., 1963) and as prominent features of the muscle tendon junctions in skeletal muscle fibers. As stated above, these fingerlike invaginations and divisions of the cells ends also

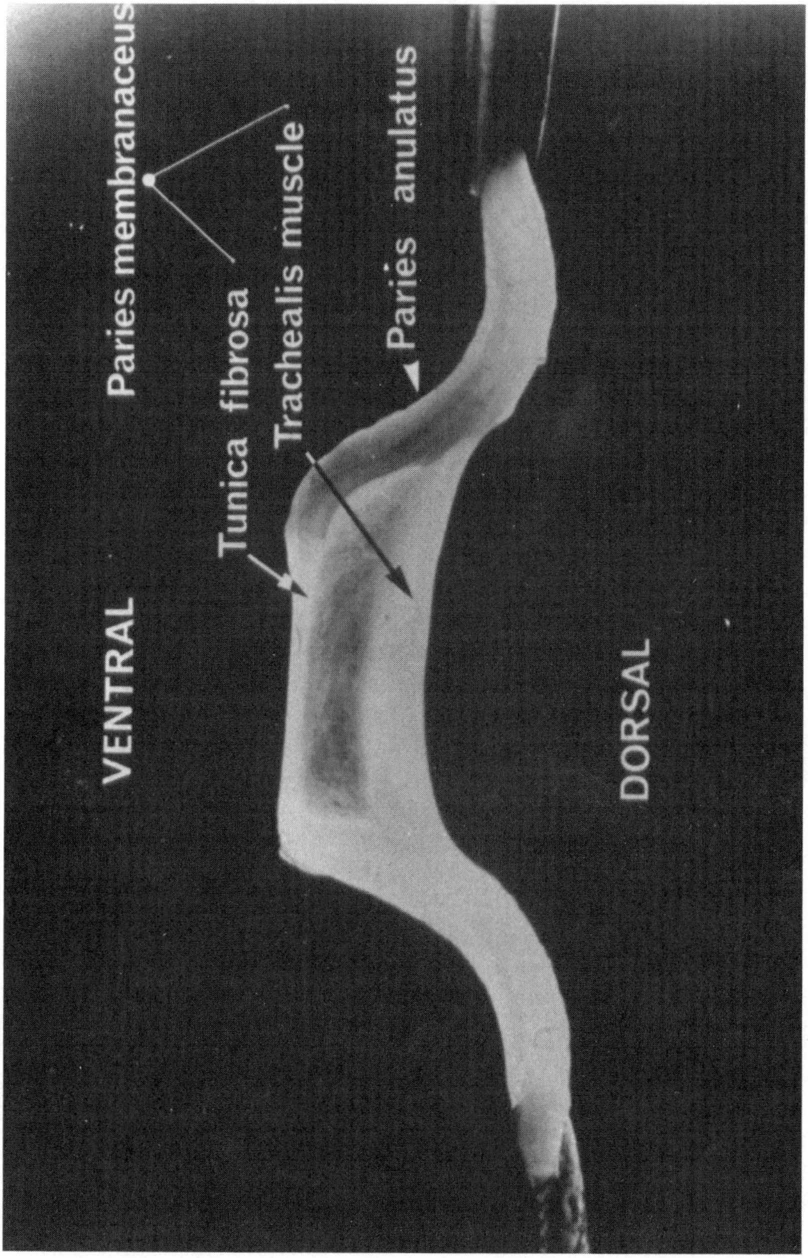

Figure 1 Cut everted canine tracheal ring; separation of tunica and tracheal smooth muscle is well seen (reprinted from Stephens et al., 1969, with permission).

interdigitate between other cells forming end-to-end and end-to-side junctions. These types of coupling have been suggested to be a major form of cell-to-cell mechanical transmission.

Aside from these regularly observed junctions, isolated cell processes and invaginations of the cell surface that partially penetrate into a neighboring cell are sometimes seen. These junctions are of the so-called peg-and-socket variety. The actual contact planes are of the intermediate junction type.

B. Muscle Bundles and Fibers

With respect to structure, our studies have shown that tracheal smooth muscle is arranged in bundles that run parallel to each other. It is worth pointing out that in the dog the posterior membrane joining the ends of the incomplete cartilaginous tracheal rings consists of a muscular layer and a tunica fibrosa (see Fig. 1). The muscle layer is external to the latter. This arrangement varies in different animal species. In some of these (von Hayek, 1960), the muscle layer is situated internal to the tunica propria.

Figure 2 is a low-power electronmicroscopic montage of canine tracheal smooth muscle. It displays bundles of spindle-shaped muscle cells arranged parallel to each other. Those cut in the appropriate plane reveal a central oblong nucleus which in this figure is twisted because of the shortening of the muscle. By planimetry of muscle and nonmuscle structures we have found that 75% of the tissue is made up of muscle (Stephens et al., 1969). Biochemical estimates of collagen and noncollagen protein have confirmed this. The parallel arrangement of the muscle cells make this an excellent model for mechanical studies. The muscle was fixed at its optimal length and in maximal isometric tetanic contraction. In this state the cell outline shows a crenated appearance. A muscle fixed at rest shows a perfectly smooth outline.

Study of such montages has shown that the muscle cells are arranged in bundles of 30-40 cells. The muscle bundles are fastened by elastic tendons to the external perichondrium of the tracheal cartilage (toward the dorsal ends of the cartilage) and the annular ligaments. Luschka (1963) has reported that bundles of muscles extend from the trachealis and insert into the ventral wall of the esophagus. The individual muscle cells are extremely long: length exceeding 1 mm and width being 3.3 μm (Suzuki et al., 1976). The bundles are separated by collagen and elastin.

C. Innervation of Smooth Muscle

In this zone, interfascicular nerve axons are visible (Fig. 2). Mast cells, capillaries, and fibroblasts can also be readily seen. Morphometric studies by Kannan and Daniel (1980) have shown there are 29 smooth muscle cells per nerve terminal. Our own studies demonstrate 10 smooth muscle cells/nerve terminal. This inner-

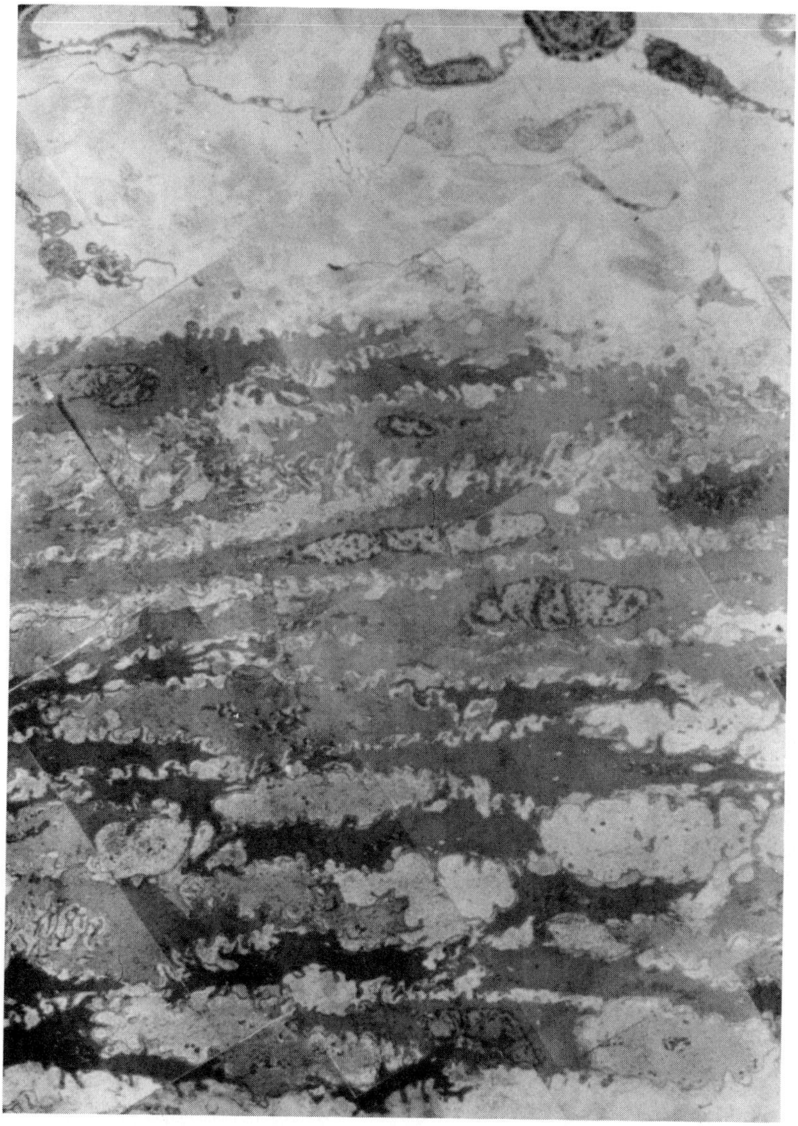

Figure 2 Photograph of a montage constructed from a series of micrographs taken from a portion of longitudinally sectioned canine tracheal smooth muscle. Muscle was in a contracted state isometrically during fixation. Mast cells, capillaries, and fibroblasts can readily be seen lying in the extracellular space alongside the muscle bundles (× 1,920).

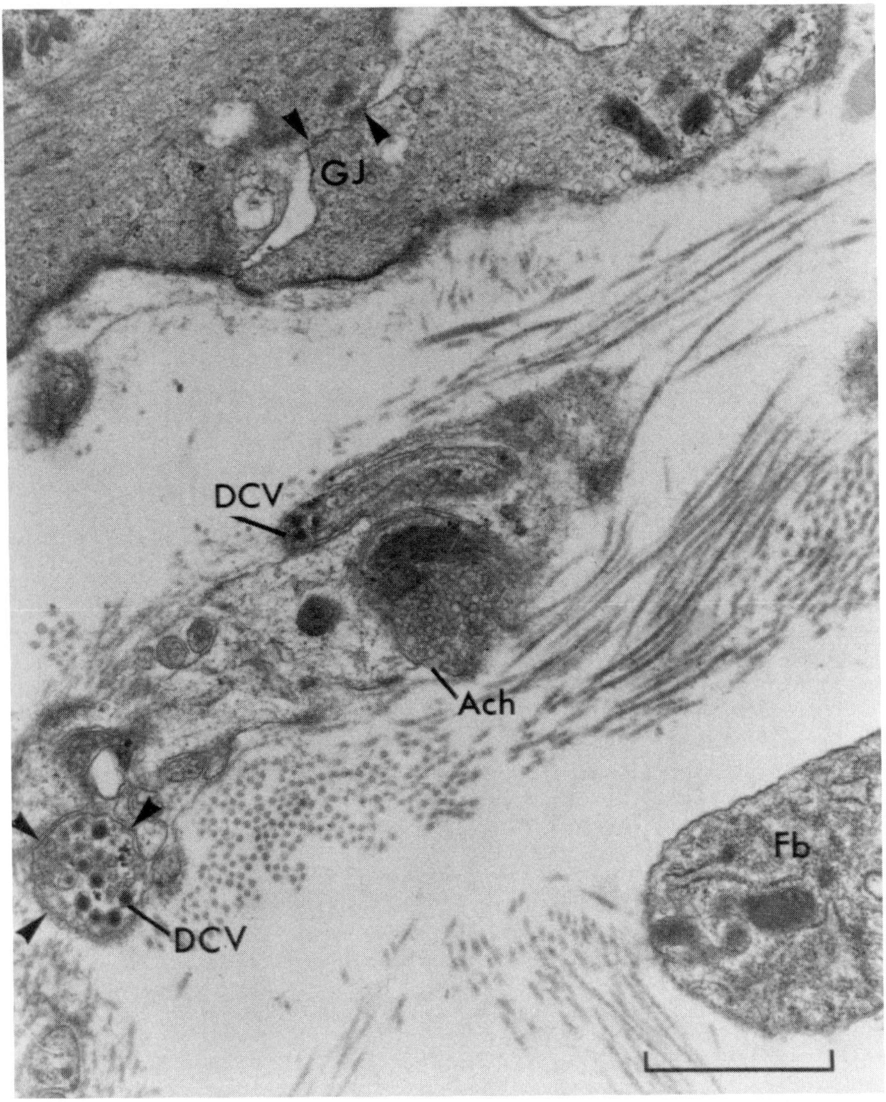

Figure 3 Longitudinal section of tracheal smooth muscle (X 49,760). The muscle cells at the top of the picture show a gap junction (GJ). Slightly above and to the right of this an intermediate junction (zonula adherens) is seen. A nerve terminal with some dense covered vesicles (DCV) and numerous clear (cholinergic) vesicles can be seen (X 28,980).

vation density is between what is seen in single unit and multiunit smooth muscle, and, as stated before, characterizes tracheal smooth muscle as being of Burnstock's (1970) intermediate variety.

Cholinergic System

These nerves are all unmyelinated. Figure 3 shows that the axons contain many clear vesicles, indicating that they are cholinergic. A few axons containing large, dense, cored vesicles are occasionally seen. These are adrenergic. These findings confirm that the major innervation to tracheal smooth muscle is vagal. Others have shown (Russell, 1978b) that vagal innervation becomes sparse as one proceeds to the small bronchi and bronchioles. The motor system to the small airways is histaminergic or utilizes some other neurotransmitter.

Adrenergic System

While it is well known that a considerable number of β-adrenoceptors are present in airway smooth muscle, the status of their neural control is not clear. For example, it has not been shown that the few adrenergic nerves present do in fact regulate airway smooth muscle contraction. It is possible that these nerves are really destined for pulmonary vasculature. Alpha-adrenoceptors are not normally seen in canine or human airway smooth muscle. However, if a small amount of tone is induced, the presence of these receptors can be detected (Bergen and Kroeger, 1980). These, of course, would subserve bronchoconstriction.

Nonadrenergic, Noncholinergic Inhibitory System

In human material, Richardson and Beland (1976) have reported the absence of adrenergic nerves, and that the major system producing relaxation is in fact the nonadrenergic, noncholinergic inhibitory system. It has been speculated that a reduction in the function of this system could be responsible for asthmatic bronchoconstriction. Such nerves possess vesicles containing large, opaque granules (120-160 nm in diameter). While the transmitter has not been clearly identified, current evidence suggests that it is vasoactive intestinal polypeptide (Dey and Said, 1981; Uddman et al., 1978) (VIP). However, there are other contenders.

Nonadrenergic, Noncholinergic Excitatory System

A nonadrenergic, noncholinergic excitatory nerve system has also been reported (Wharton et al., 1979). This is an unmyelinated sensory nervous system. Its transmitter is substance P and the system is capsaicin-sensitive (Dey et al., 1981; Lundberg and Saria, 1983). It produces bronchoconstriction by antidromic activity.

Others

While a host of agonists and antagonists exert their effects on airway smooth muscle, only a few are described here. Histamine (H_1) receptors are also present in airway smooth muscle. However, in the dog, H_2 receptors have not been found.

One peculiarity about the neural control of airway smooth muscle is that while axons are found in the interfascicular spaces, filaments do not penetrate into the depths of muscle fiber bundles. Just how these cells are neurally stimulated presents a problem. One speculation is that these are like denervated muscle cells and may therefore be supersensitive to agonists. Thus, they could respond to the very weak concentrations of neurotransmitters reaching them.

D. Fiber Morphology

Nucleus

A prominent, centrally placed nucleus is present. Mitochondria and Golgi bodies are generally seen close to the nucleus. A nuclear membrane, which contains pores, is present, as are nucleoli.

Golgi Bodies and Lysosomes

Golgi bodies, in common with mitochondria, are usually seen at the poles of the nucleus in tracheal smooth muscle. Lysosomes are also seen, but not with regularity (Burnstock, 1970). We have seen them only in tissues rendered hypoxic for 4-6 hr. Occasional myelin figures are also present.

Mitochondria

Mitochondria are seen primarily at nuclear poles although they are by no means restricted to this zone alone. They are often closely associated with glycogen granules.

Stephens and Wrogemann (1970) have studied the oxidative phosphorylation parameters for isolated canine tracheal smooth muscle mitochondria and found that the ADP/O and respiratory control ratios are similar to those for skeletal muscle. However, the quantity of mitochondrial protein present per gram wet weight of muscle is much less than in skeletal muscle. From these findings they calculated the ATP synthesized oxidatively in smooth muscle is only 10% of that reported for skeletal muscle.

The role of mitochondria in excitation-contraction coupling in smooth muscle is under investigation. Somlyo et al. (1972) have shown that sarcolemmal pinocytotic vesicles and mitochondria are often very close to each other in vascular smooth muscle. They could well act as an excitation-contraction coupling mechanism. We have seen similar arrangements in tracheal smooth muscle. It is believed that mitochondria could act as sinks for calcium but probably not as sources (Verbeke et al., 1977). However, this is probably not true for physiological concentrations of calcium.

The Sarcoplasmic Reticulum

In airway smooth muscle, this appears poorly developed. In Figure 3 (top half), reticular structures are seen between the sarcolemma and the four mitochondria present. The reticular tubules are in contact with pinocytotic vesicles. Their morphology varies from smooth muscle to smooth muscle. Somlyo et al. (1972) have suggested that these structures play a role in excitation coupling. However Sugi and Daimon (1977) have shown, using pyroantimonate as a marker for calcium in electromicrophotographs, that the major portion of the calcium is released from the cytoplasmic face of the sarcolemma.

Rough endoplasmic reticulum is seen in tracheal smooth muscle though in much smaller amounts as compared, for example, to fibroblasts. Yamauchi and Burnstock (1969) have reported that these structures are particularly prominent in developing smooth muscle.

Caveolae or Pinocytotic Vesicles

Caveolae are typically seen in large numbers in smooth muscle cells. They are essentially invaginations of the sarcolemma and it is believed that they always retain this connection, no matter how pedunculated they may become. Their role in airway smooth muscle has not been elucidated. In endothelial cells such vesicles do have true micropinocytotic activity and are involved in active transport across the endothelium (Palade, 1960; Jennings et al., 1962; Bruns and Palade, 1968). The necks of the caveolae are surrounded by intramembranous particles in smooth muscles. Perhaps the most obvious function served by caveolae is in increasing the area of the cell membrane, owing to the fact that the caveolae are basically saccules continuous with the plasma membrane. Gabella and Blundell (1978) have shown that smooth muscle cells contain 170,000 caveolae per cell, producing an increase in the area of the cell membrane by 70%. Beyond this, not much is known about the function of caveolae.

Sarcolemma, Dense Bands, Dense Bodies, and Cell-to-Cell Junctions

The sarcolemma has the usual bimolecular lipid leaflet characteristics of such membranes in other cell types. Its tram line structure is clearly visible in Figure 7. Overlying the sarcolemma a basement membrane is seen. It displays a very loosely knit structure. Well-defined, transversely cut collagen bundles are seen. Study of the serial sections show that they spiral around the muscle bundles.

Elastin is also seen in the interfascicular space, where collections of amorphous and fibrous elastin are present. Collagen and elastin fibers intermesh with each other and also with the basement membrane. The figure also shows a fibroblast. The sarcolemma shows outpouchings, which are commonly seen in contracted cells. The most striking example of these have been reported in supercontracted single stomach muscle cells of *Bufo marinus* (Fay, 1976). Generally these outpouchings are considerably electron-lucent; they do not contain contractile filaments but do contain organelles such as pinocytotic vesicles and sarcoplasmic reticulum. Adjacent to the outpouchings the sarcolemma is relatively free of undulations and is very electron-dense. The overlying basement membrane is also very dark. The increased electron density delineates sarcolemmal dense bands within which are inserted action filaments. Electron-dense structures called dense bodies, are scattered throughout the cytoplasm. Actin filaments are attached to them as are the 10 nm intermediate filaments. The dense bands and bodies are thought to delineate minisarcomeres; it is interesting that the protein structure of these bodies and bands is much like that of the Z bands of striated muscle. Our quantitative measurements revealed that the amount of cell membrane profile occupied by dense bands was roughly 50% at the level of the cell nucleus. However, in the tapering parts of the ends of the cell, the percentage area occupied by dense bands increased, up to 100% in the smallest of profiles.

There appear to be intercellular connections between dense bands on adjacent cells through collagen and elastin interconnections. These may transmit force in a lateral direction between cells. In such areas the cells are very close to each other (30-40 nm apart) and some condensation of basement membrane materials occurs between the two dense areas. Generally a single layer of basement membrane is seen in the center of the separation between the two cells. Intermediate junctions or zonula adherens are much more numerous than gap junctions in tracheal smooth muscle. A good example is seen above and to the left of the gap junction (GJ) in Figure 3. The gap junction or nexus is an area of closer apposition than the intermediate junction, the gap being 2-3 nm. It can be penetrated by small tracers such as lanthanum (Uehara and Burnstock, 1972).

As stated before, gap junctions are said to be areas of low electrical impedance and enable electrical coupling between cells. As expected, single-unit muscle cells show a large number of such junctions. For example, in guinea pig ileum (Gabella and Blundell, 1978) they are quite numerous and occupy roughly 0.2% of the cell surface. In multiunit muscle (Henderson et al., 1971; Gabella and Blundell, 1979) they are very sparse. Gap junctions in tracheal smooth muscle range from 0.07 to 0.09 μm in length.

Contractile Apparatus

This is made up of contractile (actin and myosin) and regulatory (myosin light chain, and tropomyosin) proteins. The contractile myofilaments are made up of thick, myosin (15 nm diameter), and thin, actin, filaments (5 nm diameter). In addition intermediate filaments (10 nm) are present. The orientation of the contractile filaments is reported as either parallel to the long axis of the cell (Small, 1977) or oblique across the cell (Fay, 1976; Bagby, 1983). The correct identification of this orientation is important for correctly carrying out mechanical studies of smooth muscle. If the muscle strip is cut in the wrong axis, the force developed by the muscle will be less than expected. From a functional point of view we have cut the muscle into a number of helical strips of pitch varying from 0° to 90° and mounted them in the isometric myograph. The pitch of the strip developing the greatest muscle stress is identified as optimal (0°).

Thick Filaments

These were impossible to visualize in the early days of smooth muscle research, which led to these muscles being termed smooth. However, Somlyo's group (Somlyo et al., 1973; Somlyo and Somlyo, 1975) has reported that well-defined myosin thick filaments in repeating arrays could be demonstrated, but that this required both the fixation of muscles under "physiological conditions" and an independent means of controlling the state of the contractile apparatus during fixation.

The thick filament has been shown to be 15.0–18.0 nm in diameter and displays relatively regular lateral spacing. (Rice et al., 1971; Somlyo et al., 1973). Cross-bridges just like those in striated muscle are seen to project from the myosin filament. Although classic sarcomeric patterns have not been demonstrated in smooth muscle, the striking similarities between the contractile proteins and in mechanical properties between striated and smooth muscles suggests that sarcomeres do exist but current methods of fixing and staining lead to loss of structure. X-ray diffraction studies (14.3 nm meridional reflections) (Lowy et al., 1970; Shoenberg and Haseltone, 1974) indicate that smooth and striated muscle thick filaments are similar. However, the thick filaments of smooth muscle do not show a central bare zone.

Thin Filaments

The thin filaments (actin) of vertebrate smooth muscle lack any associated troponin and consist of only actin and tropomyosin (Sobieszek and Small, 1976). In all vertebrate smooth muscles, actin has been shown to be the major protein component. Actin:myosin ratios vary considerably and are much larger than in skeletal muscle. In taenia coli the ratio is 10-13:1 (Small, 1977) and 15:1 in vascular smooth muscle (Somlyo et al., 1973). The ratio has not been worked out for airway smooth muscle.

Murphy (personal communication) has recently found that actin isoforms exist in smooth muscle.

Tropomyosin can be extracted in greater amounts from smooth muscle than skeletal. Its orientation in relation to actin thin filaments is believed to be analogous to that in skeletal muscle. Vibert et al. (1972) have adduced x-ray diffraction evidence in support of this. It has been observed that changes in the intensities of these reflections occur upon contraction, akin to those in skeletal muscle. This finding is of interest, since if smooth muscle contraction is myosin-regulated, as currently believed, then tropomyosin would be expected to lie nearer the center of the groove in the actin filament, even in a relaxed muscle (Huxley, 1977). This paradox has yet to be resolved.

Intermediate Filaments

These 10 nm filaments were first recognized in immature striated muscle cells and in certain nonmuscle cells (Ishikawa et al., 1968) and have since been observed as components of virtually all types of animal cells (Gaskin and Shelanski, 1976). They form a cytoplasmic network with connections to cytoplasmic dense bodies and sarcolemmal dense bands (Cooke and Fay, 1972; Cook, 1976; Sobieszek and Small, 1977). Suggested roles for these filaments include intracellular transport (Goldman and Knipe, 1973) interconnection of contractile filaments (Lazarides and Hubbard, 1976), and positioning of the cell nucleus (Small and Celis, 1978). Perhaps the most accepted role is that of providing a cytoskeleton. Somlyo's group has suggested that they may serve to stabilize the recently recognized "minisarcomeres" of smooth muscle. The major polypeptide component of these filaments has been called desmin (Lazarides and Hubbard, 1976) or vimentin depending on the type of smooth muscle. An actinin-like polypeptide may also be an integral component of the intermediate filament.

No data from the study of intermediate filaments in airway smooth muscle have yet been reported.

Minisarcomeres in Smooth Muscle

Though no work of the type to be described has been carried out in airway smooth muscle, because of their importance to the field in understanding smooth muscle function, we will describe other smooth muscles. In recent years, evidence has begun to accumulate to suggest that if tissue fixation and preparation are carried out under appropriate conditions, thick filaments are seen in large numbers and appear highly organized. Somlyo et al. (1973) have demonstrated this in the rabbit portal mesenteric vein preparation. Data from Fay et al. (1983) and Somlyo et al.'s (1984) laboratories have shown that dense bodies and bands are not randomly scattered throughout the cytoplasm but appear organized into repeating patterns. It has been suggested that they are analogous to striated muscle Z bands and their regular arrangement strongly suggests that they act as the limits of sarcomeres or minisarcomeres. Figure 4, from a paper

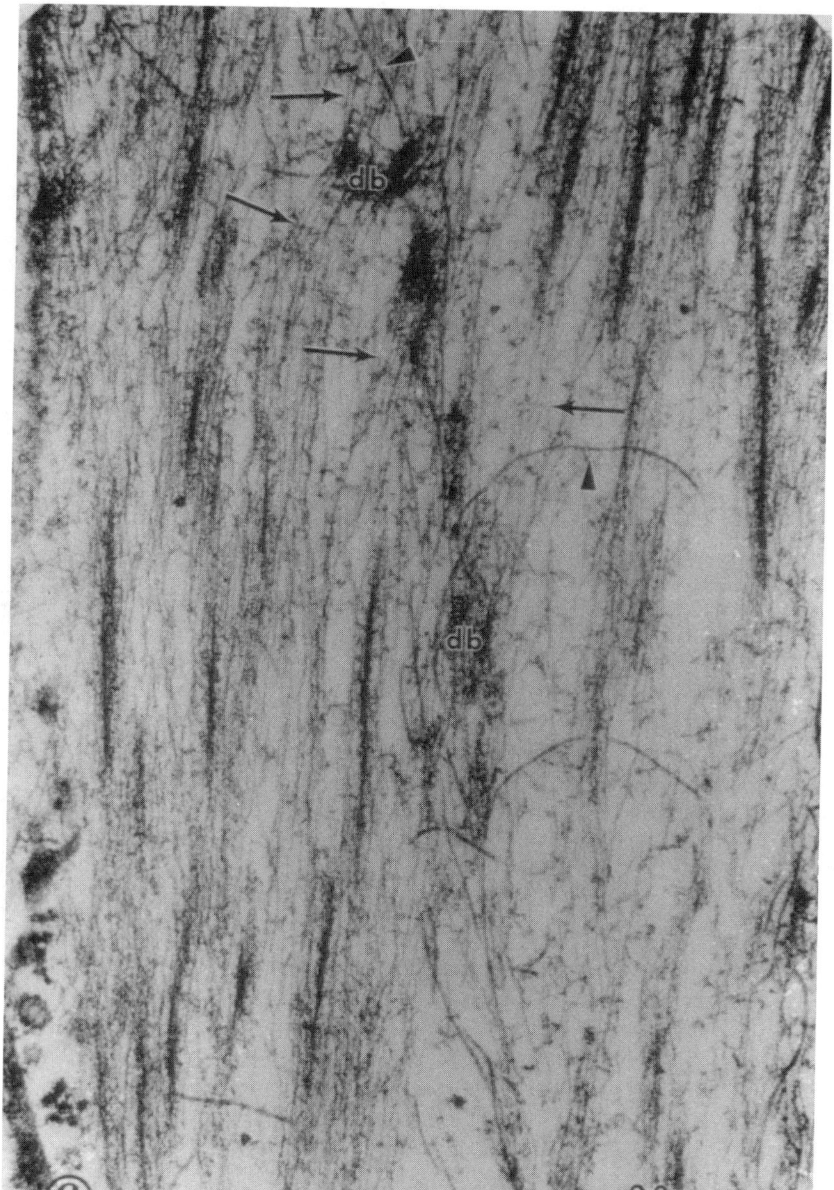

Figure 4 Longitudinal section of a portal vein smooth muscle cell briefly skinned with saponin and fixed in the presence of tannic acid (from Somlyo et al., 1984).

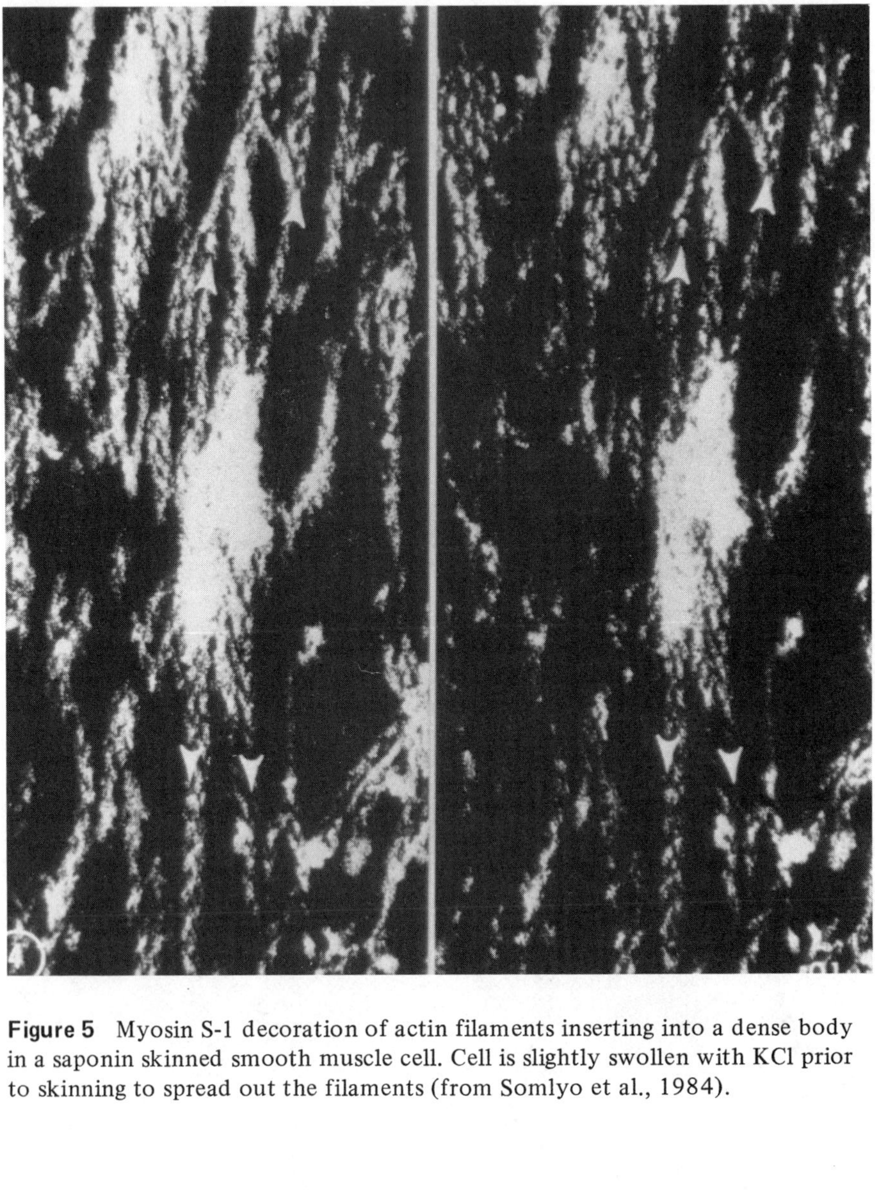

Figure 5 Myosin S-1 decoration of actin filaments inserting into a dense body in a saponin skinned smooth muscle cell. Cell is slightly swollen with KCl prior to skinning to spread out the filaments (from Somlyo et al., 1984).

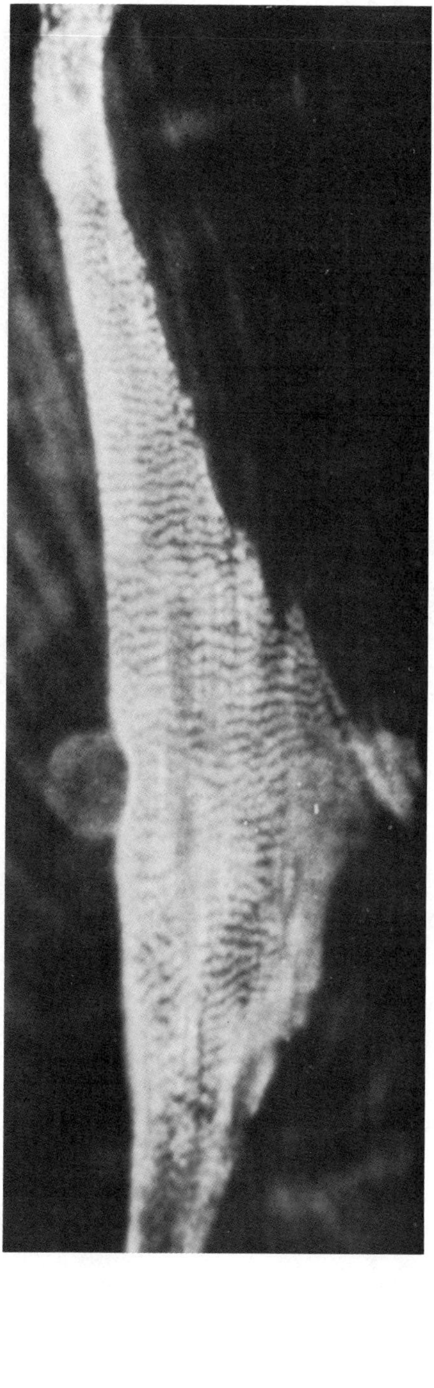

Figure 6 Anti-smooth muscle myosin immunofluorescence of guinea pig vas deferens in culture (X 1,670; from Groschel-Stewart, U., et al: *Histochemistry 43*: 215, 1975).

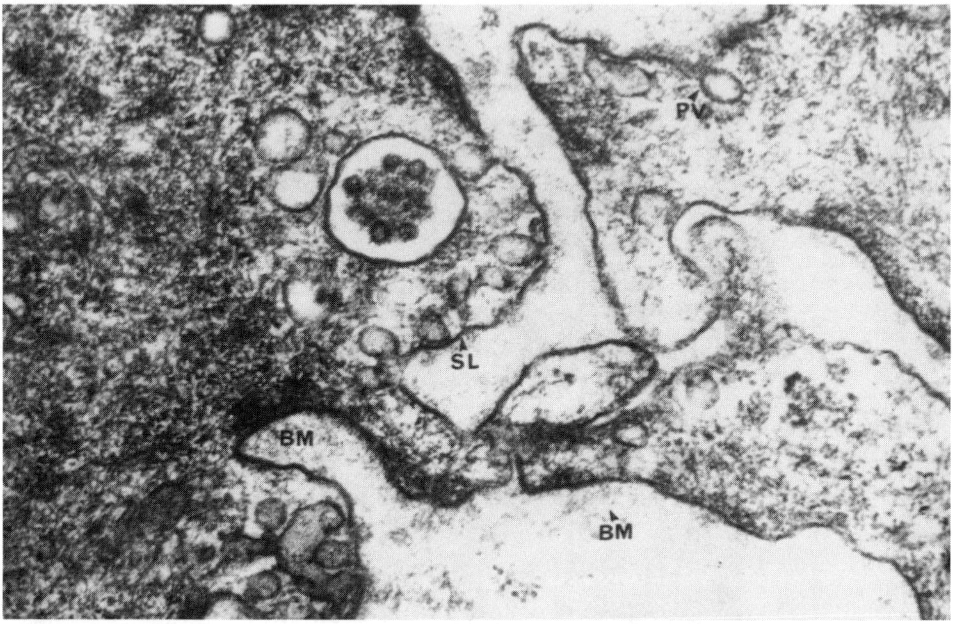

Figure 7 Electron micrograph of transverse section of canine tracheal smooth muscle. The lacy basement membrane (BM) and the "railway track" membrane of the sarcolemma (SL) are clearly seen (X 75,000; from Stephens and Kroeger, 1980).

by Somlyo et al. (1984), shows actin filaments running through the dense body from either side. Intermediate filaments are also seen; they are reported as looping between dense bodies and thus stabilizing the sarcomere. The figure also shows a well-defined myosin filament between two actins; cross-bridges between the two are clearly seen. Using heavy meromyosin decoration of actin and special immunohistochemical techniques, Somlyo has demonstrated reversed polarity of actin filaments on either side of the dense body, thus strengthening the analogy between Z bands and dense bodies (Fig. 5).

Final evidence comes from data published by Groschel-Stewart et al. (1975), shown in Figure 6, which shows light microscopic pictures of smooth muscle cells treated with antimyosin fluorescent antibodies. A very striking cross-striation pattern is seen, indicating that sarcomeres probably exist in smooth muscle, and that forces are transmitted via intercellular connective tissue connections (Fig. 7).

These structural considerations indicate that the skeletal muscle model relating structure to function may be applied to smooth muscle also.

III. Physiology of Airway Smooth Muscle: Biophysical Properties

A. Electrophysiological Characteristics

These have been reviewed before by us (Stephens and Kroeger, 1980) for canine tracheal smooth muscle. Suzuki et al. (1976) have also delineated the electrical properties of the same tissue in detail. Kirkpatrick (1975) has described the electrophysiology of bovine tracheal smooth muscle. We will summarize by saying that in keeping with its intermediate-unit type of muscle properties, canine tracheal smooth muscle possesses a steady membrane potential of about −47 mV ± 2.4 (SE). As stated before, only under abnormal conditions are spontaneous action potentials seen. Agonists produce graded depolarization and the mechanical threshold differs from the equilibrium membrane potential by only 3-4 mV (Suzuki et al., 1976). Current-voltage plots reveal considerable rectification due to increased potassium conductance and this accounts for absence of action potentials. Current injection experiments using an Abe and Tomita type bath system (1968) show that the space constant is about 1.6 mm.

In vascular smooth muscle research one of the most important developments has been the finding that endothelial cells profoundly affect the mechanical responses of the smooth muscle cells (Furchgot and Zawadzki, 1980; Vermeir and Vanhoutte, 1979). We have not found any evidence that epithelial cells affect tracheal smooth muscle function. However Vermeire and Vanhoutte (1979) have shown that bronchial smooth muscle function is affected. Future investigators of bronchial and bronchiole airway smooth muscle function will have to bear this factor in mind.

B. Mechanical Characteristics

Perhaps the most exciting development in the smooth muscle field has been the demonstration that quite unlike what occurs in striated muscle, contraction is subserved by two types of cross-bridges recruited sequentially (Siegman et al., 1977; Dillon et al., 1981). Early in contraction, normally cycling cross-bridges are activated; later, slowly cycling ones are. We have recently found (unpublished observations) that most of the muscle's shortening, under isotonic conditions, is effected by normally cycling bridges while a major part of force development is effected by slowly cycling bridges. All studies of mechanics of smooth muscle in the future will have to analyze their results in terms of these two types of bridges. Evaluation of smooth muscle data will be more complex than in striated muscle. The properties of these bridges will be discussed below.

Stimulus-Response Relationships

In tracheal smooth muscle these are of the graded type and a threshold and maximal voltage or current density can be determined. On the average maximal density is about 400 mA/cm^2. Supramaximal voltage is generally set at 1 or 2 V greater than maximal. The most effective and convenient stimulus to use is 60 Hz; this is best delivered by mass platinum plate discharge so as to activate the whole muscle synchronously and eliminate stray compliance effects stemming from asynchrony. Square wave pulses delivered by a Grass stimulator can also be employed. Generally 100 Hz is satisfactory, with a pulse width of 0.5-1 msec. However the current delivered by the Grass stimulator is inadequate for tracheal smooth muscle and special power boosters have to be used. Biphasic rectangular pulses are best, since they reduce electrodepolarization effects. The 0.5-1-msec pulse width has been chosen since this is optimal for nerves. In canine tracheal smooth muscle, stimulation is predominantly via the nerve terminals present in the tissue. These act by releasing acetylcholine, as proved by the fact that atropine can block 97% of the response to electrical stimulation. To stimulate the muscle directly after nerve block requires extremely high current densities. With these a maximal response can be elicited, but the muscle deteriorates very rapidly.

It is worth pointing out that the contractile response to a maximal stimulus demonstrates a fade in tracheal smooth muscle. The contractile response (incidentally the contraction time is about 10 sec) drops rapidly after 10 sec to about 30% of the maximum value. This has been ascribed to depletion of acetylcholine presynaptically. When contraction is elicited by carbachol, very little fade is seen and the muscle can stay contracted for 2 hr with about a 10% drop in force. Cholinesterase inhibitors such as eserine also eliminate the fade.

It is interesting that marked tachyphylaxis to histamine is present. This has been ascribed to the action of prostaglandins (Szentivanyi, 1968) though Kroeger and Tesarowski dispute this (personal communication).

Stress-Strain Relationships

Conventional-length tension curves can be delineated for resting and maximally stimulated airway smooth muscle. We have published such curves for the canine trachealis and the bronchus (Stephens et al., 1968, 1969).

Figure 8 shows mean curves for the trachealis. The resting stress at the muscle's optimal length (l_o or L_{max}) is very small, indicating the muscle's high compliance. This property of the muscle facilitates studies of its force-velocity properties, since at l_o the preload is low and hence velocities can be elicited over a wide range of loads. The active stress curve (AP_{max}) shows the expected Starling type of configuration and suggests that the same subcellular mechanism of contraction operates in smooth muscle as in striated muscle. The summit of the curve (P_o) is relatively flat and there is no significant difference in active stress over lengths ranging from 0.90 l_o to 1.1 l_o. This is another desideratum for force-velocity studies, for it suggests that at the moment when maximum short-

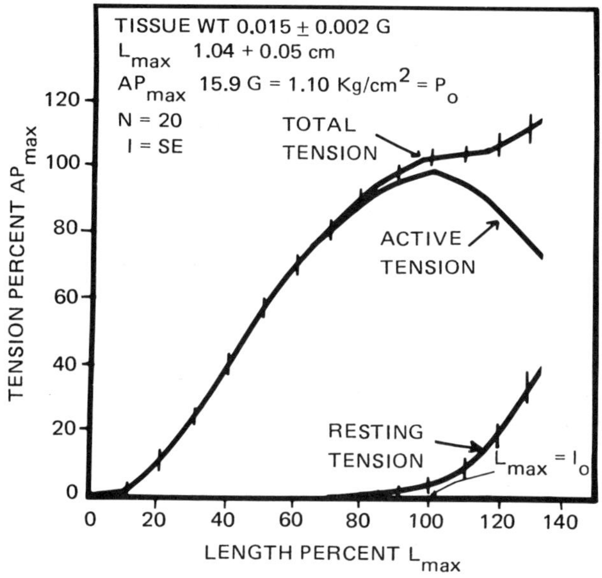

Figure 8 Length-tension curves for canine tracheal smooth muscle (from Stephens et al., 1969).

ening velocity is measured (this usually occurs within 1–1.5 sec of onset of stimulation) for a given load, there is no appreciable alteration in contractility as assessed by P_o.

While the ascending limb of the stress-strain curve is fairly easy to measure, the descending limb is much more difficult when compared to skeletal muscle. The angle of descent of the descending limb in smooth muscle is much steeper than the angle of ascent of the ascending limb. Why this should be so is not understood.

The maximum stress P_o (g/cm^2 or N/mm^2) developed for the trachealis is about the same for other smooth muscles and for skeletal muscle. When it is remembered that smooth muscle contains only one fifth the stress-generating sites, the smooth muscles' ability is noteworthy and is made possible by its considerably greater mechanical efficiency. The latter could, in turn, be due to the fact that at the time when stress is measured (at the peak of the contractile response, which is about 10 sec), latch bridges are operative. It would be interesting to delineate stress-strain curves for normally cycling bridges that operate for the first 2–3 sec of contraction and to compare their efficiency with those of the latch bridges. Measurements of utilization of high-energy phosphates (Siegman et al., 1977), which show that it is almost four times greater in early contraction, indicate that normally cycling bridges are much less efficient than latch bridges.

From the stress-strain curve one can deduce the maximal ability of tracheal smooth muscle to shorten. This is about 80% of l_0 and is in marked contrast to striated muscle, which can only shorten by about 35% of l_0; the smooth muscle has therefore been termed a supercontracter. This factor may be of significance in the pathogenesis of asthma, and will be discussed below.

Stress-strain curves can be elicited by the conventional isometric methods just described. They can also be derived from isotonic, after-loaded, and free-loaded shortening contractions. They should all coincide. However, in tracheal smooth muscle they do not coincide; the isometric curve lies to the left of the others. Presumably, the antecedent shortening prevents the development of full contraction. This leads us to conclude that the stress-strain properties of airway smooth muscle depend crucially on the history of contraction.

Finally we come to consideration of the phenomenon of reduced activation of the muscle at short lengths, that is at $l < l_0$. Taylor (1976) has shown, in single skeletal muscle fibers, that for any length less than l_0, the maximum isometric stress is not the real maximum at that length. In fact, it can be considerably increased by treating the fiber with caffeine and high calcium concentrations (10 mM). From these experiments they concluded that as length diminished, contractility also decreased. Microscopy, using interference optics, showed that central myofibrils of the fiber did not contract but were thrown into passive folds. The explanation was that as the muscle shortened it became wider, with resultant distortion of T-tubules and impairment of excitation-contraction coupling.

We (Kromer and Stephens, 1983) have found (Fig. 9) in strips of trachealis, that at l_0, P_0 can be more than doubled by increasing calcium concentration to 4.75 mM using 127 mM KCl as an agonist. This is unlike single skeletal muscle fibers where P_0 at l_0 is unaffected. However, at $l < l_0$ the contractile response is reduced in the smooth muscle.

Figure 10 shows normalized length-tension plots that adjust for the fact that P_0 at l_0 is increased. The curves demonstrate reduced activation at short lengths. Since the tissue consists of many cells, the skeletal muscle explanation cannot easily be applied. However, Siegman et al. (1985) have recently reported that wavy myosin filaments can be seen in cells of a smooth muscle preparation at $l < l_0$. Our findings of reduced activation at short lengths is of some applied significance. If reduced activation at short lengths prevents the muscle from shortening maximally under normal condition, then perhaps in asthma the increased bronchoconstriction seen is due to elimination of this process. Woolcock's data (personal communication) dealing with histamine aerosol dose-response curves in human asthmatics and controls indicates that asthmatics do in fact superconstrict, and that reduced activation at short lengths is not ocurring.

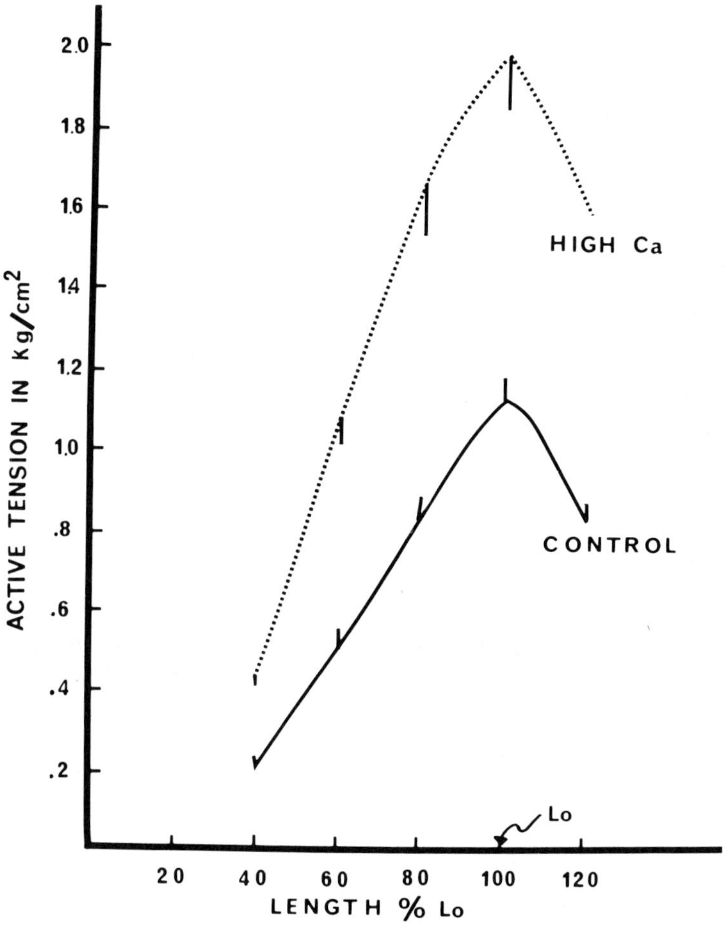

Figure 9 Active tension-length curves for canine trachealis obtained at control (2 mM) and high (4.7 mM) calcium concentrations. Means and SE bars are shown: n = 16. Iso-osmotic KCl solution was used as agonist (from Kromer and Stephens, 1983).

Force-Velocity Relationships

While stress-strain properties of airway smooth muscle tell us about the ability of the muscle to bear a load, they relate to static conditions only. One can deduce from the curves the work done by the muscle in shortening a certain distance. However, this is a theoretical maximum and does not take cognizance of the extra energy consumed by the shortening muscle to overcome viscous and inertial forces. Hence, study of force-velocity curves (and their integrated power

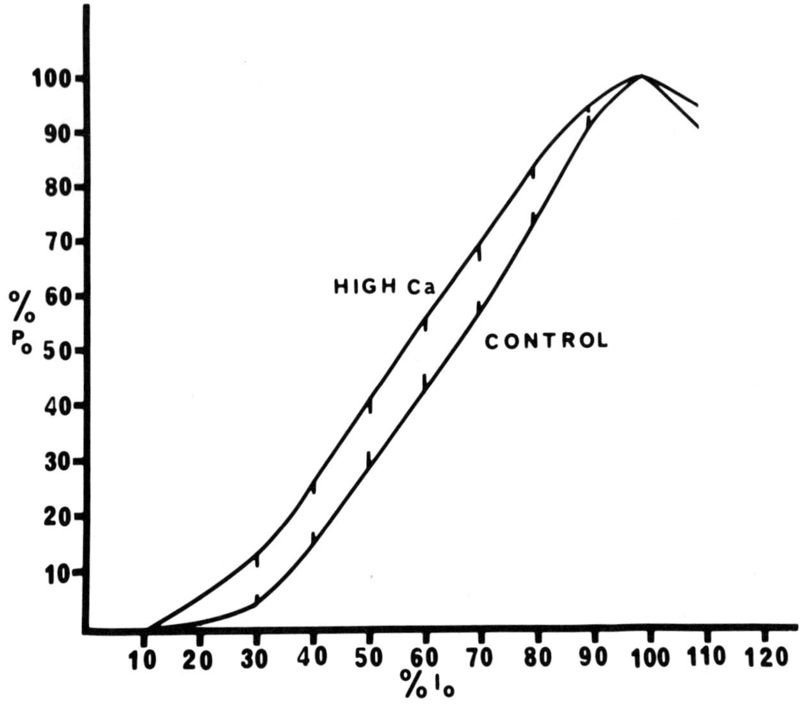

Figure 10 Same data as in Figure 10 expressed in percent optimal muscle length (L_o) is represented by 100% on the abscissa (from Kromer and Stephens, 1983).

curves) is a better way to understand muscle function. Although the point has been made before, it is worth reiterating that in most locations where it exists the main function of smooth muscle is to control flow. Thus whether it is blood flowing through vessels, air down airways, products of digestion down the intestinal tract, or the products of conception down the uterine passageways, the main modality involved is that of narrowing or dilating, that is, in controlling conductance and resistance. Manifestly, smooth muscle shortening or lengthening is of paramount importance. Though stiffness can influence flow to a small extent, shortening exerts the greater influence. By the same token, the meaningful parameter to study in vitro work is isotonic or auxotonic shortening. It is surprising that the vast bulk of research carried out on isolated smooth muscle is of isometric contraction. One can only conclude that this is so because it is technically easier. Unfortunately, it does not tell us anything about the muscle's shortening ability. The argument has been put forward that isometric stress is a good index of muscle contractility and hence shortening ability can be inferred from isometric studies. This is only true if the inotropic substance being studied

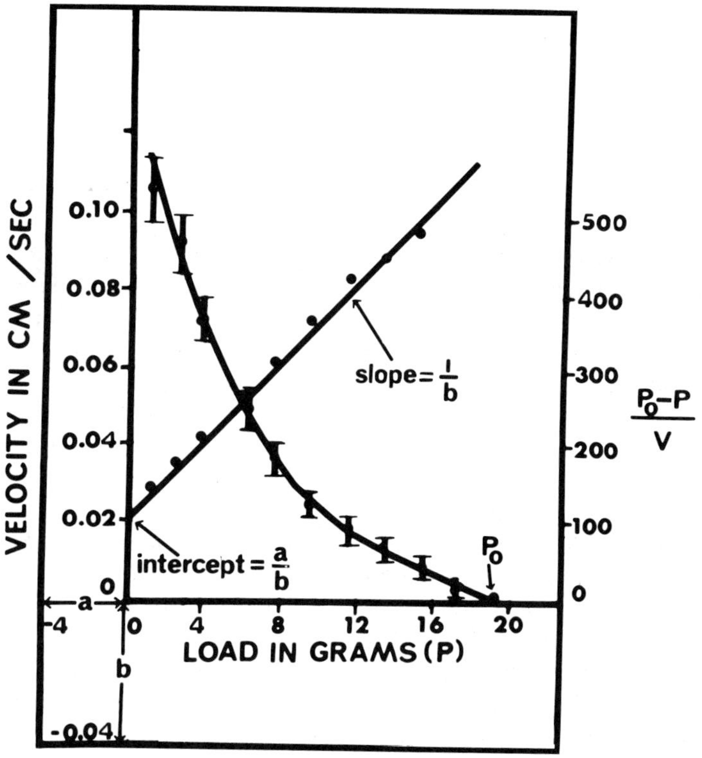

Figure 11 Mean force-velocity curve of canine tracheal smooth muscle, n = 32. P = load on muscle, V = maximum velocity of shortening of that load, P_o = maximum load muscle can support, *a* and *b* are constants with units of force and velocity, respectively. Note the right hand ordinate applies to the linear transform of Hill's equation (from Stephens et al., 1969).

shifts the force-velocity curve parallel to the control. The onus, however, is on the investigator to show that this is so, since there are many situations in both smooth and striated muscle where it is not. For example, in both these muscles the effect of cold is to reduce the maximum velocity of shortening (V_o) considerably without affecting P_o at all (Yeatman et al., 1969; Stephens et al., 1977).

Conventional Force-Velocity Curves in Tracheal Smooth Muscle

These can be elicited using supramaximal electrical stimulation with the muscle held at its optimal length, or l_o. An electromagnetic muscle lever system was adapted by us (Mitchell and Stephens, 1983) from a model developed by Brutsaert et al. (1978) for cardiac muscle. Plots of force and afterloaded isotonic shortening were obtained from which force-velocity data points for given loads were obtained. From these, the force-velocity curve shown in Figure 11 was obtained.

It displays a hyperbolic shape and the Hill equation (1938) can be fitted to it. The equation is as follows:

$$(P + a)(V + b) = (P_o + a) b$$

where P is the given load on muscle; P_o is the load the muscle is just unable to lift; the latter is also equal to the maximum isometric tetanic force developed by the muscle. The constants *a* and *b* define the asymptotes of the rectangular hyperbola: *a* possesses units of force and *b* those of velocity. The only muscle constant undefined so far is that of maximum unloaded velocity of shortening (V_{max} or V_o). This can be obtained by inserting a value of 0 for P and solving the Hill equation. V_o under these conditions equals $P_o b/a$. V_o can also be obtained by graphic extrapolation but the method is prone to error. It can only be used for those muscles where other methods of measuring V_o provide the same answer as the graphical. To obtain a satisfactory fit, the common practice of rejecting the force-velocity points at higher loads is followed. It must be pointed out that generally two such data points immediately preceding P_o have to be rejected to obtain a statistically significant good fit.

Closer scrutiny of the data reveals that at heavier loads the velocity obtained is lower than expected. We have recently elucidated the reason for this behavior. Work in our laboratory has shown us that up to the first 2 sec of contraction, normally cycling cross-bridges are operative, thereafter latch bridges come into action with their fourfold slower shortening velocity. The significance of these findings is that under lower loads maximum velocity of shortening occurs very early in contraction; generally within 2 sec of stimulus onset. At the heavier loads (0.75 P_o, 0.90 P_o) the muscle spends a considerably greater amount of time in isometric mode before it develops a force equal to the load. Shortening follows and the maximum velocity that now develops is at least 3 sec after the onset of stimulation, at which time latch bridges are operative. It is clear, therefore, that quite unlike striated muscle, the conventional smooth muscle force-velocity curve is really made up of two distinct curves. At lighter loads the curve for normally cycling cross-bridges contributes. This curve is characterized by a relatively higher shortening velocity and a lower-load-bearing ability. At heavier loads the force-velocity curve of latch bridges contribute. This curve demonstrates a lower V_o but a higher P_o. These two types of curves are described in greater detail below.

Conventional force-velocity curves obtained from canine tracheal smooth muscle reveal that while the stress developed is almost equal to that of skeletal muscle, the maximum velocity of unloaded shortening (V_o) is almost 100 times

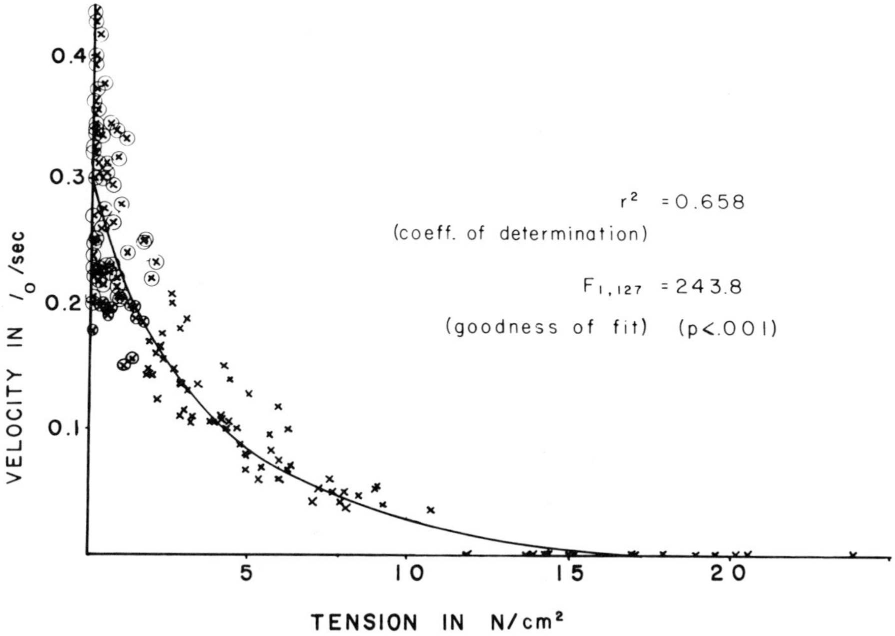

Figure 12 Mean force-velocity curve. Both afterload (greater than preload and denoted by crosses) and load clamped (to loads less than preload including zero load clamp, denoted by circles), force-velocity data points are shown. Linearized transform of Hill equation was fitted to the data with a coefficient of determination (r^2) of o,658, $P < 0.001$. Both afterloaded and load-clamped data fall on the same curve (from Mitchell and Stephens, 1983).

slower. Any inference about the significance of the *a* and *b* constants and of a/P_0 (index of efficiency of contraction) in smooth muscle is clouded by the fact that two types of force-velocity curves exist.

Problems in Measuring V_0

Conventionally V_0, or maximum unloaded isotonic shortening velocity, is obtained by graphic or mathematical extrapolation as mentioned above. This is prone to some degree of error. Using the zero load-clamp technique we have directly measured V_0.

Figure 12 shows data points obtained by the two methods. Fortunately in tracheal smooth muscle the two estimates of V_0 are the same, hence the conventional way of obtaining V_0 (by extrapolation from isotonic, afterloaded curves), is valid.

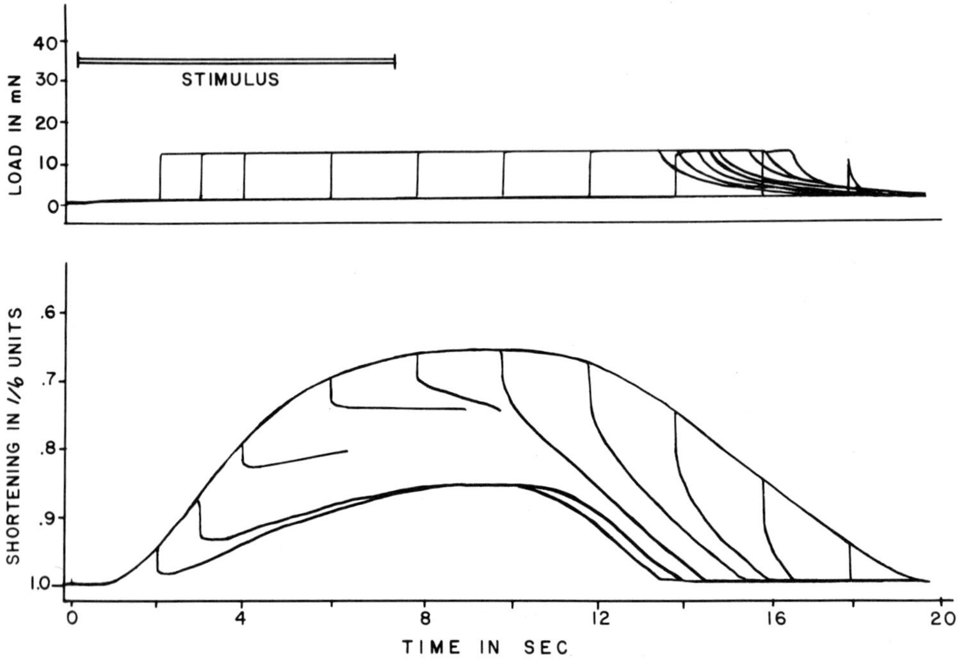

Figure 13 Oscilloscopic records of force and shortening changes vs. time. The muscle was set at its optimal length, l_o. Length is shown in normalized units; note shortening increases in an upward direction (from Stephens et al., 1985).

Two Types of Cross-Bridges in Tracheal Smooth Muscle

Siegman et al. (1977) and Dillon et al. (1981) showed that isotonic shortening velocity is much reduced later in contraction than in the early phase. This is quite different from skeletal muscle where the velocity later in contraction is, if anything, slightly greater than in early phase (Jewell and Wilkie, 1958). Dillon et al. (1981) also showed that myosin light-chain phosphorylation is maximal early in contraction and then rapidly diminishes to baseline levels when load-bearing capacity is considerably increased. They suggested that the ability of bearing load associated with a much reduced shortening velocity was due to dephosphorylation of recently phosphorylated cross-bridges. Chatterjee and Murphy (1983) further showed that the development of latch bridges was also related to intracellular calcium concentration. However, these concentrations were much lower than those involved in early contraction and led them to suggest that latch bridge formation depended not only on dephosphorylation but also on calcium binding to a different locus on the myosin molecule. The role of

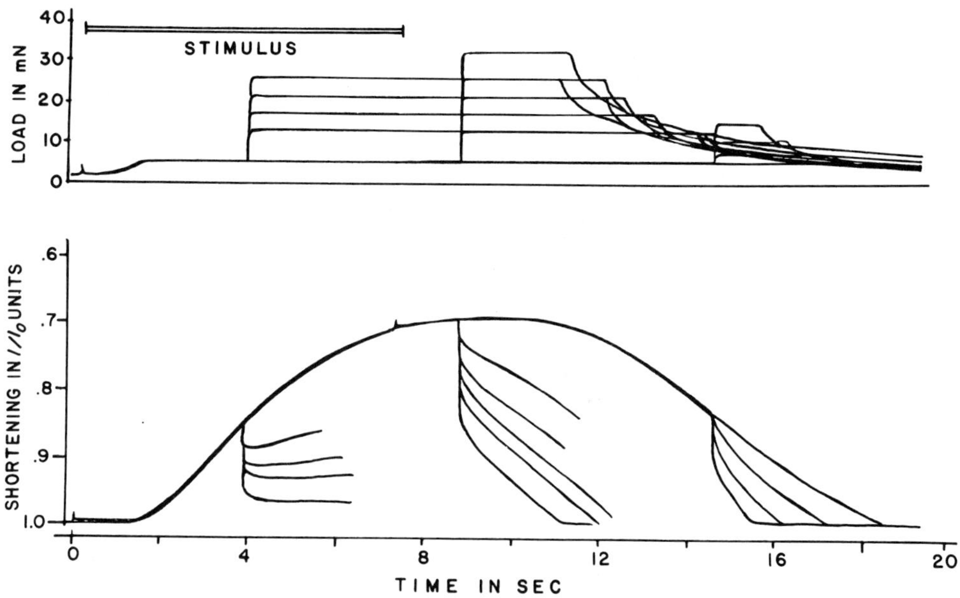

Figure 14 Oscilloscopic records are shown similar to those in Figure 13, except that in place of applying only one load clamp a range of clamps was applied at 4, 9 and 15 sec.

dephosphorylation in the production of latch bridges is currently hotly debated because several investigators do not find that dephosphorylation occurs (Siegman et al., 1977; Hacherk et al., 1985; Barsotti et al., 1985). However, from a mechanical point of view there is no doubt that normally cycling and latch bridges do exist; all workers in the field agree on this point.

Another controversy exists over the explanation for the very slow cycling rates of the bridges recruited later in the contraction. According to Murphy, who coined the term latch bridge, some bridges do form a true noncycling latch. These act as an internal load on the remaining normally cycling bridges, resulting in an overall reduced velocity of shortening. Siegman (personal communication) disagrees. She believes that no latch bridges develop and that the reduced velocity of shortening is due to a reduction in velocity of all the normally cycling cross-bridges. The definitive experiment to resolve the controversy would be to obtain some measure of internal resistance to shortening as a function of time during the contraction.

Using the after-loaded, isotonically shortening canine tracheal smooth muscle preparation to which abrupt load clamps are applied, we have obtained

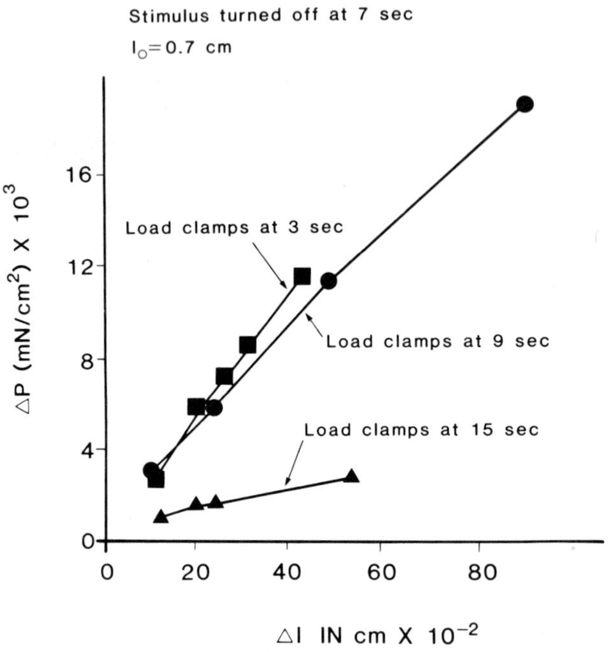

Figure 15 The length-tension data of the rapid transients (series elastic component) are plotted to provide plots of the stiffness of the series elastic component.

data that enable us to analyze the behavior of normally cycling and latch bridges.

Figure 13 (lower panel) shows a record of shortening versus time for a preloaded (5 mN was sufficient to stretch the musle to l_o) muscle. At given moments in the isotonic shortening the load was abruptly (within 3 msec) clamped to 10 mN and the resulting records are shown in the upper panel. A rapid transient was seen, which stemmed from the muscle's series elastic component. This was followed by a slow transient. Up to 5 sec, redevelopment of shortening was evident and thereafter no such redevelopment was seen. The moment at which this occurred was 5.5 sec on the average, and was termed the transition time (t_T). Our interpretation was that at this time the normally cycling bridges were replaced by latch bridges. Another explanation could have been that while the load remained the same the numbers of active cross-bridges was reduced after 5 sec and so the load on the remaining bridges would increase, resulting in an inability to shorten.

To test this a series of load clamps were applied at 4 sec and 9 sec, as shown in Figure 14. Load clamps were also applied at 15 sec, at which time

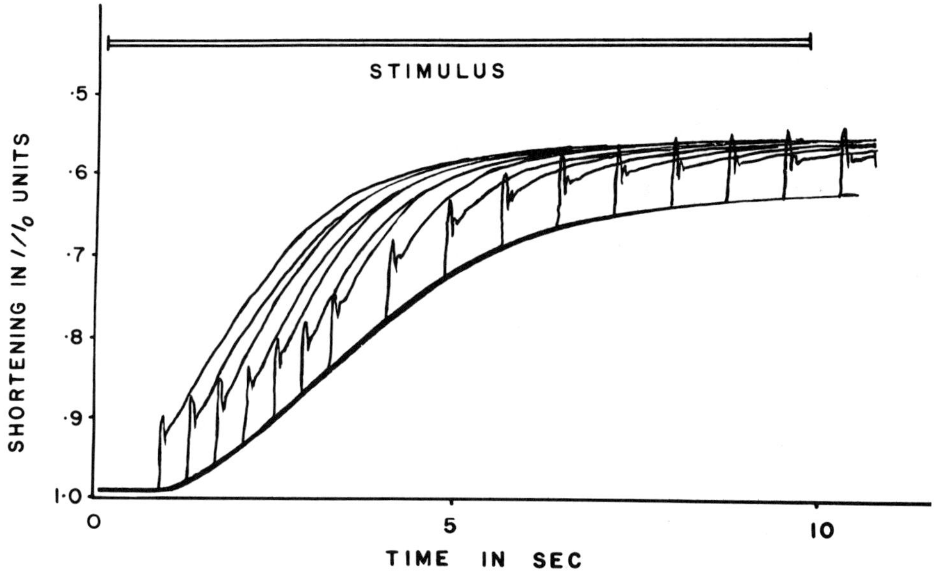

Figure 16 Records from a single typical experiment are shown. Shortening in normalized units is plotted against time in seconds. The lowest, sigmoidal curve represents preloaded isotonic shortening. Load records are not shown but are of the same type as shown in Figure 14. At different times during shortening, zero load clamps (rise time, 3 msec) were applied. For each record, optimal damping was determined. Each zero load clamp record shows two transients: an initial rapid one stemming from recoil of the series elastic component, and a slower one whose maximum slope provide the maximum velocity of shortening (V_0) for that particular instant in time. The progressive diminution of V_0 with time is evident (from Stephens et al., 1985).

the muscle was relaxing and cross-bridges would be undoubtedly reduced in number.

The stress-strain curves for the rapid transients were plotted and are shown in Figure 15. It is clear that the slopes at 4 and 9 sec are the same. Since the stiffness of the series elastic component in striated (Huxley and Simmons, 1971) and smooth muscle (Paul and Peterson, 1975) is an index of numbers of cross-bridges, we concluded that no change had occurred in these numbers at 4 and 9 sec. This in turn led us to conclude that the reduced cycling rate at 9 sec was due to a qualitative change in the nature of the cross-bridges.

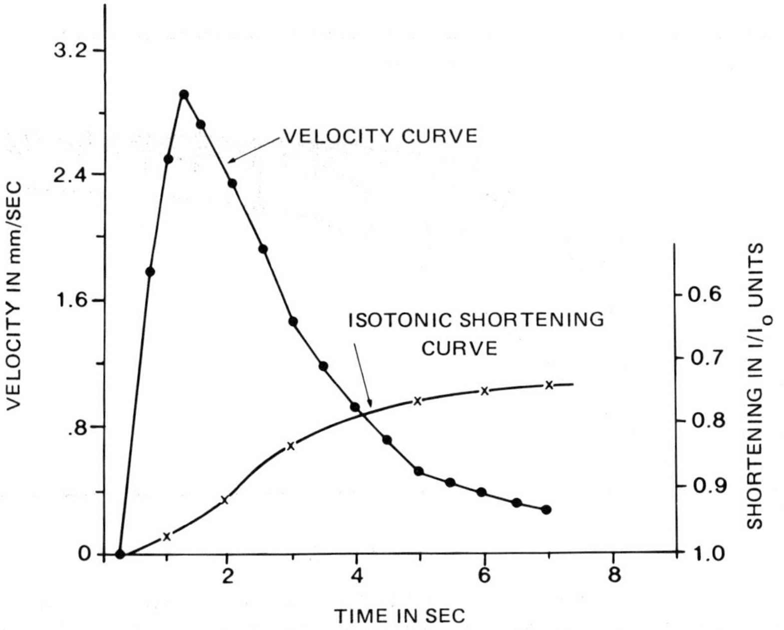

Figure 17 Plot of V_os vs. time. The original preloaded isotonic shortening record is also shown (right hand ordinate) (from Stephens et al., 1985).

Studies with Zero Load Clamps

It was evident that transition time would depend not only on the intrinsic ATPase activities and cycling rates of the two types of crossbridges but also on the load on the muscle. For this reason we repeated our studies using abrupt zero load clamps. Zero load clamps were applied at given intervals during the course of preloaded isotonic shortening.

A representative set of experimental records is shown in Figure 16. Rapid and slow transients are again seen in response to the load clamps. The maximum slope of the slow transient represents V_o.

These velocities are plotted against time in Figure 17. The corresponding isotonic shortening curve is also shown. The velocity plot shows that maximum V_o develops at 1.75 sec in this example; the mean value for 10 experiments was 2.0 s ± 0.31 (SE). The lower values of V_o between onset of stimulus and the 2 sec point must be due to the fact that the active state of the muscle does not develop instantaneously but takes 2 sec to reach a maximum. The cross-bridges operative up to this time are presumably of normally cycling type.

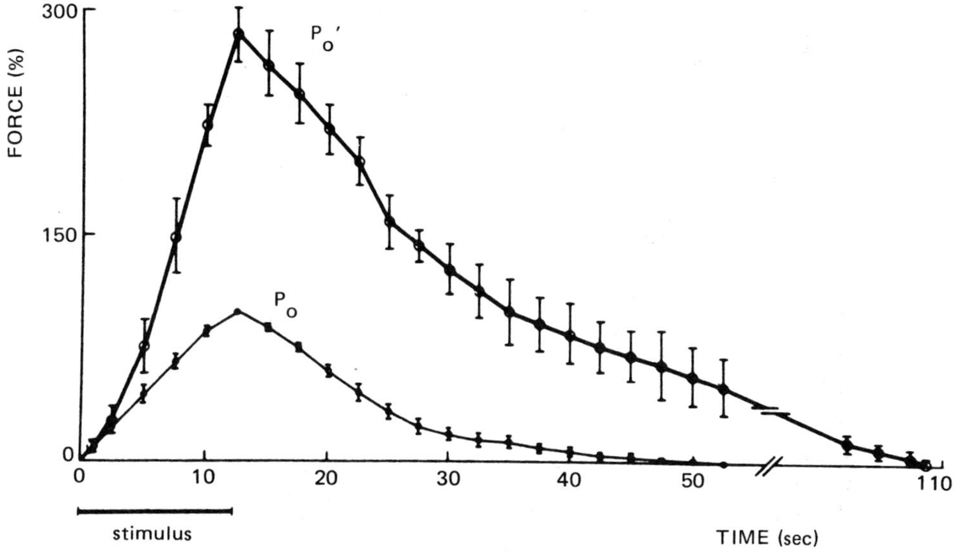

Figure 18 Time course of maximal force potential (P_o) in tetanic isometric contractions of tracheal smooth muscles (mean % ± SE values of force in control isometric contractions (P_o). Values are obtained from highest possible force level, that is, where the clamped load could be sustained for 100 msec, for load clamps at various times during isometric contractions (from Stephens and Brutsaert, 1982).

Some evidence in support of this is provided in Figure 18. The P_o curve depicts a mean isometric myogram, while the P_o curve represents the maximum load-bearing capacity (Stephens and Brutsaert, 1982). It is clear from the figure that between 0 and 2 sec, maximum load-bearing capacity is very poor; this must be due to the fact that since the bridges are cycling relatively rapidly they are unable to withstand the rapid elongation imposed by the load clamps. A second piece of evidence that supports this idea is that oxygen uptake of the muscle strip is three times higher at this time than at the plateau of the contraction (Stephens and Skoog, 1974). Siegman et al. (1977) have also shown that the rate of high-energy phosphate utilization is four times higher during the development phase of contraction than at its plateau.

Analysis of the V_o vs. time curve shows that after 2 sec, V_o decreases in an exponential matter. We have interpreted this as resulting from the progressive recruitment of latch bridges.

Figure 19 shows a compartmental analysis of the descending limb of the curve in Figure 18. An equation of the form $V_o = 105\ e^{-0.49t} + 105\ e^{-0.19t}$

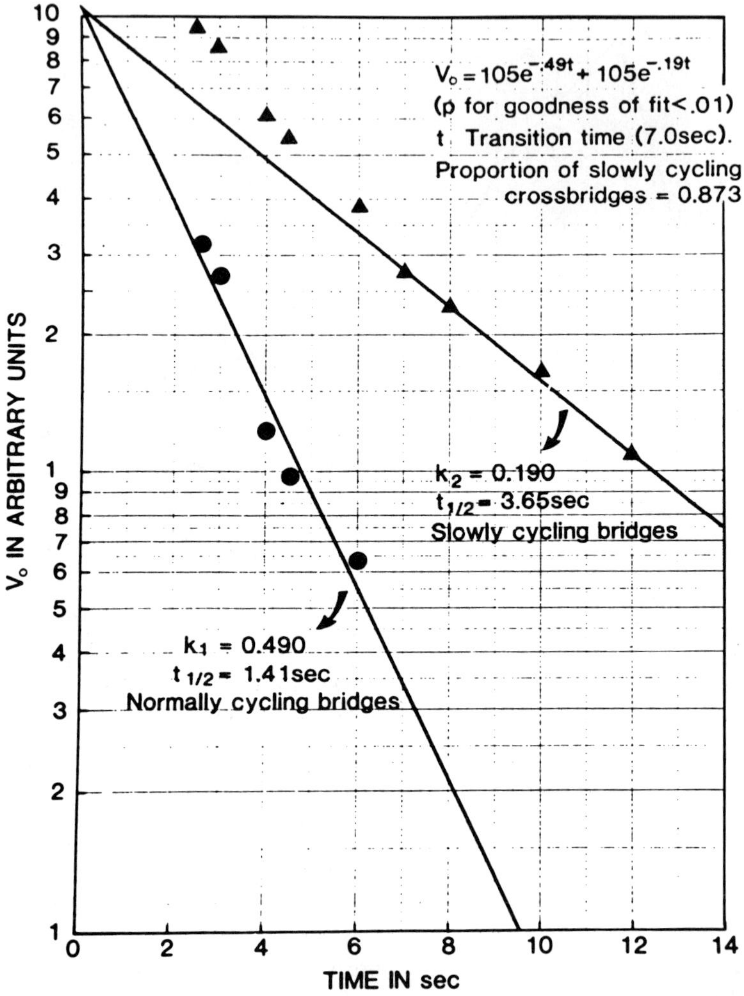

Figure 19 Compartmental analysis of descending limb of curve shown in Figure 17. Solid triangles represent the velocity points. Ordinate values are logarithmic. A straight line was fitted to the last four triangles. Deviations from this line are replotted as solid circles and fitted by a second straight line. From these lines, rate constants and half times were computed.

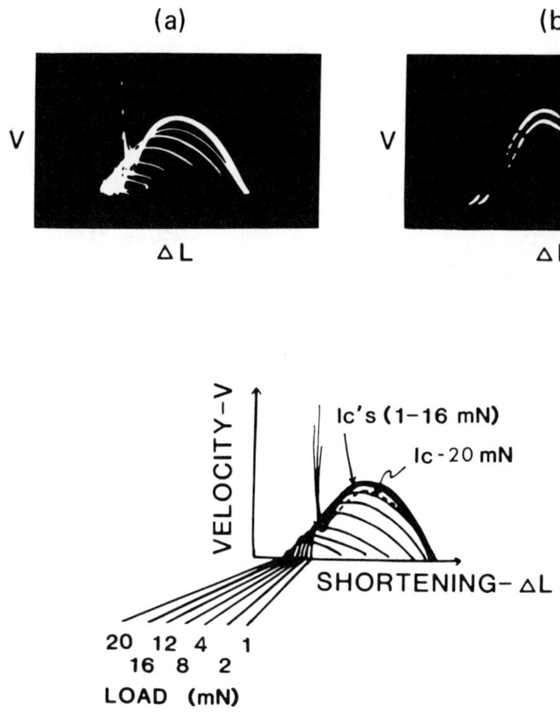

Figure 20 Velocity-length phase planes of tracheal smooth muscle, results from a single typical experiment are shown (from Stephens et al., 1985).

was fitted to the data. Note that arbitrary units were used for the ordinate. However, the equation shows that the first exponential term represents a compartment (presumably the normally cycling cross-bridges) turning over almost three times as fast as that described by the second term (latch bridges). This analysis provides support for the existence of the two types of cross-bridges. Furthermore, using the equation, the proportion of the two types of bridges operative at any given time may be obtained. Calculation shows, for example, that at the transition time (t_T) of 7 sec determined in this particular experiment, about 87% of the bridges are of the latch type.

The zero load clamp data also enabled us to determine the earliest onset of mechanical activation in the tracheal smooth muscle; this is important in elucidating the biochemical mechanisms controlling contraction. It is obvious that such mechanisms should be studied at a time that precedes the onset of mechanical activation. By applying zero load clamps at 100 msec intervals and running the recording chart at high speed, we found that mechanical activation

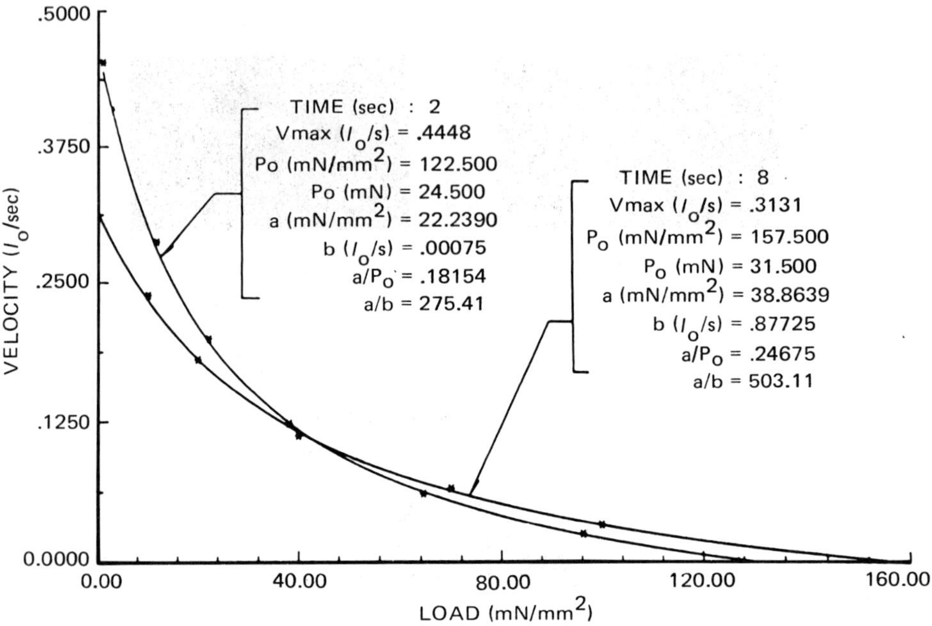

Figure 21 By applying a series of load clamp at 2 and 8 sec during an isometric contraction, force-velocity data were obtained and are shown in the figure.

commences 600 msec after the onset of the electrical stimulus. Hence regulatory biochemical processes must be measured prior to this. This in turn necessitates rapidly freezing the tissues with at least 100 msec resolution.

One factor that could account for the slow velocity of the latch bridges is muscle length. It is possible that at the moment when latch bridge activity is measured the contractile element has shortened to such a length as to reduce contractility. For example Brutsaert et al. (1978) have shown in cardiac muscle that contractility, as measured by V_o is reduced once muscle length changes by about 13%.

Figure 20 shows velocity-length phase planes for canine trachealis. Panels a and b are oscilloscopic records while below them a schematic combining them is shown. Phase planes are shown for the muscle shortening from different initial lengths, which in turn are determined by the preload on the muscle. The after-loaded isotonic shortening phase planes show that as the load increases the peak velocity attained drops. However, it is difficult to determine whether the reduced velocity is due to the length change or the load. To settle this, the contractions were repeated except that 100 msec after the onset of shortening the load was abruptly clamped to zero. The load-clamped contractions are recognizable by their fast transient artifacts. Panel a and the schematic show that for all lengths (set by loads ranging from 1 to 16 mN) the zero load clamp velocity was the same and the trajectories, in fact coincided. Panel b shows two phase planes, the upper for a 16 mN load and the lower for a 20 mN load. The latter is shown in the schematic by a broken line. Calculation showed that for a length change of 25% l_o, velocity was independent of length. For a length change greater than that (i.e., as set by the 20 mN preload), V_o decreased. Hence we were able to conclude that the reduced velocities seen along the descending limb of the curve in Figure 20 were not due to a change in muscle length since at peak isotonic shortening the length change was not greater than 25%.

Since the above analysis indicated that two types of cross-bridges were sequentially recruited during the course of a contraction, experiments were carried out to delineate force-velocity curves for the two. This was achieved by applying a range of abrupt load clamps at 2 sec and 8 sec in the course of an isometric contraction.

Figure 21 shows the two force-velocity curves obtained, with their constants. A least-squares fitting technique was used to fit the data points to hyperbolic functions.

Consider the Hill equation without time dimension; let $(P_o\text{-}P)/V$ be equal to Y; $1/b$ = M, and a/b = C. The equation then becomes of the linear form: Y = mP + C. For n pairs of data points, to minimize the deviation from those calculated from the equation, we partially differentiate $\sum_{i=1}^{n} (mP_i + C - Y_i)^2$ with respect to m and C and obtain

$$nC + m\Sigma P_i = \Sigma Y_i \tag{1}$$

$$C\Sigma P_i + m\Sigma P_i^2 = \Sigma P_i Y_i \tag{2}$$

By solving simultaneously we obtain values for m and C from which a and b may be obtained.

In fitting the data to the equations, the isometric tension, $P_o(t)$, developed at the time when the muscle was released had to be specified. The curve $P_o(t)$ vs. time, obtained from isometric contraction varied slightly but significantly from one contraction to another due to the intrinsic instability of the muscle. Application of load clamps (especially zero load clamps) increased the instability. In practical terms P_o could vary as much as ± 6% from its mean. Due to the nature of the hyperbolic equation, the goodness of fit of the experimental data to the calculated equation is very sensitive to the value of $P_o(t)$ chosen. Thus a trial and error procedure was carried out (within the ± 6% P_o range) to obtain a value of

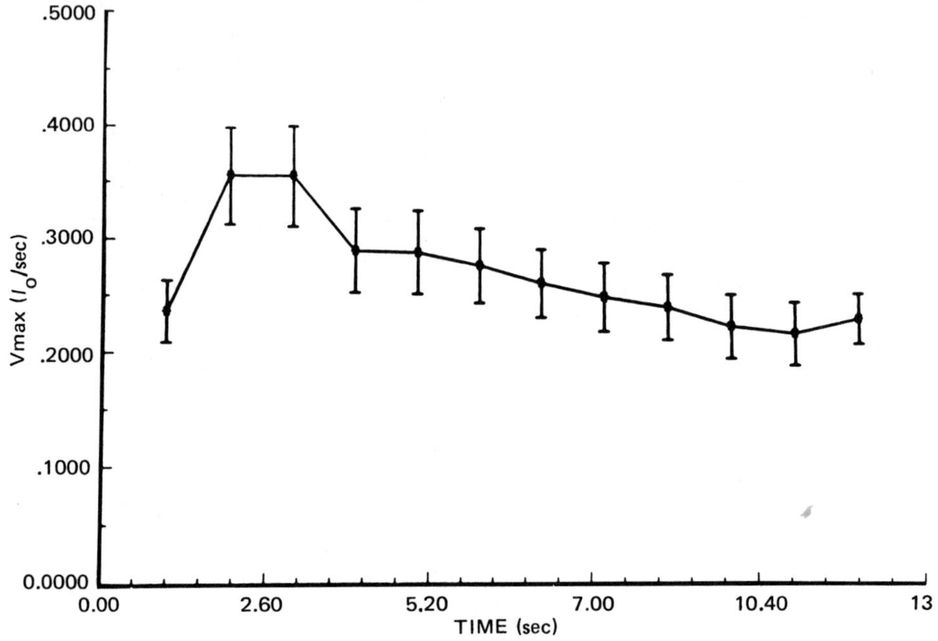

Figure 22 Plot of V_o (obtained during the course of an isometric contraction) vs. time.

$P_o(t)$ that gave the best fit. A computer program was developed using the least-squares best-fit method just described, to fit the data to the equation with a specified value of $P_o(t)$. By varying $P_o(t)$, different curves were obtained and from the best fitting one the constants *a* and *b* were selected. It is evident that the curve elicited at 2 sec, which represents the activity of normally cycling crossbridges, possesses a V_o 1.45-fold greater than that for the 8 sec (latch bridge) curve. As expected the P_o for the 8 sec bridge was 1.25-fold greater than that for the 2 sec bridge.

Force-velocity curves can also be obtained by applying load clamps in the course not of an isometric contraction as just described, but during an isotonic contraction. Such curves were obtained for the 2 sec and 8 sec crossbridges. These were similar to the isometric ones but there was a quantitative difference in that V_o values obtained late in contraction were much lower than those obtained by quick release during an isometric contraction. This is not unexpected since in isotonic contraction the muscle's contractile element shortens more than in the isometric.

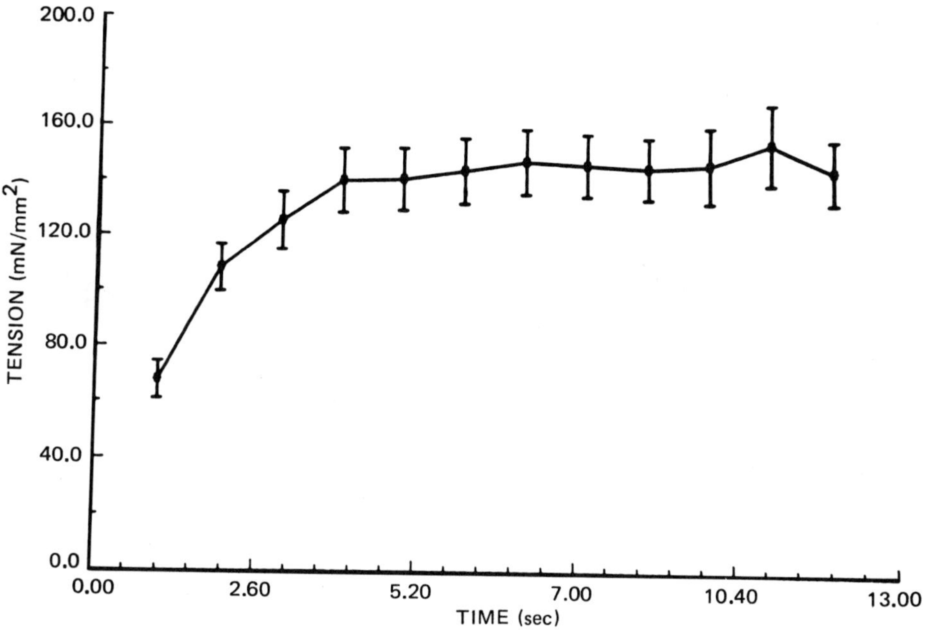

Figure 23 Mean stress plotted as a function of time: an isometric myogram.

These observations are of some importance since they clearly show that we can no longer analyze smooth muscle contraction in terms of homogeneous contractile units. Disturbances in muscle contractility with altered P_os and V_os could be the result of a predominant effect on one or other type of cross-bridge. For example, preliminary unpublished experiments from our laboratory have shown that mild hypoxia affects shortening ability much before any change in P_o is detected. Cross-bridge analysis revealed that the decrease in shortening ability was associated with a decrease in the maximum velocity of shortening of normally cycling cross-bridges; the latch bridge velocities were unaltered. We also found, in ovalbumen-sensitized canine tracheal smooth muscle, and increased capacity (ΔL_{max}) and velocity (V_o) of shortening of normally cycling cross-bridges; latch bridge rates were again unchanged.

To summarize, muscle shortening is the most important modality to study in muscle mechanics. In studying shortening, it is of crucial importance to determine which type of cross-bridge is involved. Most pharmacologic analyses are carried out in the isometric preparation. This could be misleading and incorrect. All these dose-response studies need to be repeated using shortening development (ΔL_{max}) and maximum velocity of shortening at the 2 sec point; the latter describes the activity of normally cycling cross-bridges.

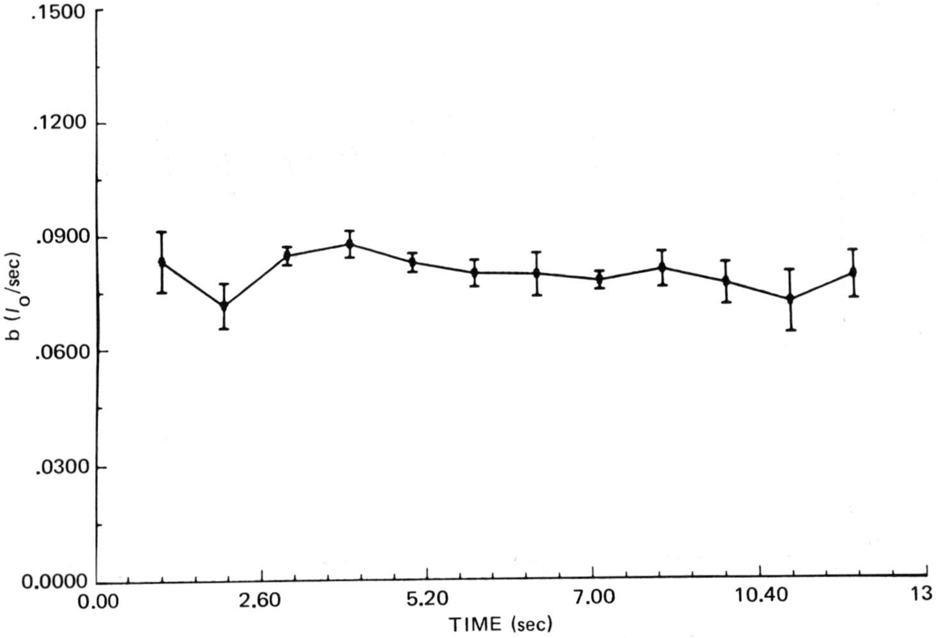

Figure 24 Plot of mean values of constant ± vs. time.

Analysis of Muscle Constants Obtained from Force-Velocity Curves: Delineation of Internal Resistance to Shortening

We have obtained force-velocity curves by applying load clamps at 1 sec intervals throughout the course of an isometric contraction. The experiment is tedious but if handled carefully the muscle's contractility changes less than 15%. From each curve, force-velocity constants akin to those shown in Figure 21 were computed and the time course of each plotted.

Figure 22 shows a plot of V_{max} vs. time. Much as in Figure 17, peak V_o develops at about 2 sec. It must be remembered that the curves of Figure 16 were obtained by applying load clamps throughout the course of an isotonic contraction, while those in Figure 22 were obtained during isometric contractions. The maximum V_o for the former does not differ from that for the latter since it falls within the confidence interval of the latter. The subsequent time course differs, since for the isometric experiments V_o decreases by a strikingly smaller amount than for isotonic experiments. Our calculations show that the greater fall in V_o in the isotonic experiments is due to the increased shortening of the muscle's contractile element.

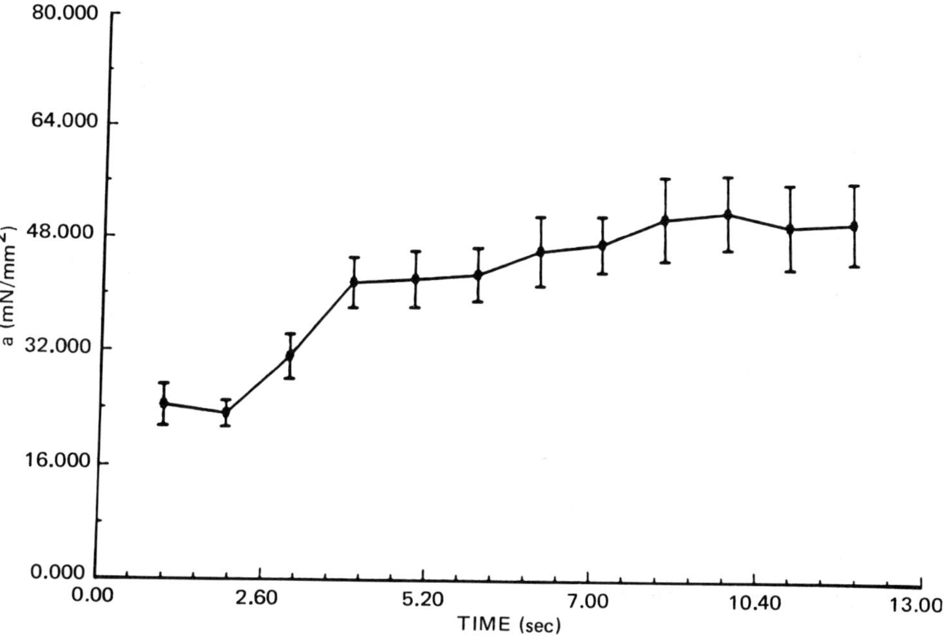

Figure 25 Plot of mean values of constant *a* vs. time.

Figure 23 is a plot of mean stress (tension in mN/mm^2) vs. time and resembles the isometric myogram as expected.

The muscle constant *b* is plotted versus time in Figure 24. This constant is the value of one of the asymptotes of the rectangular force-velocity hyperbola for tracheal smooth muscle and possesses the units of velocity. No significant difference between the various data points was found.

Figure 25 shows a plot of the *a* constant (this has units of force) vs. time. This shows a progressive increase with time.

Figure 26 shows a plot of a/b as a function of time. This parameter a/b, as we shall shortly show, is an index of internal resistance to shortening. The figure indicates that this resistance or viscosity increases with time, which is to say it increases pari passu with the recruitment of latch bridges. We believe that this plot supports the latch bridge idea over the slowly cycling cross-bridge notion, since in the latter a/b should not have increased.

Internal Resistance to Shortening: a(t)/b(t)

If a system is subjected to elastic, viscous, inertial, and external forces as shown in Figure 27, then the force balance equation is:

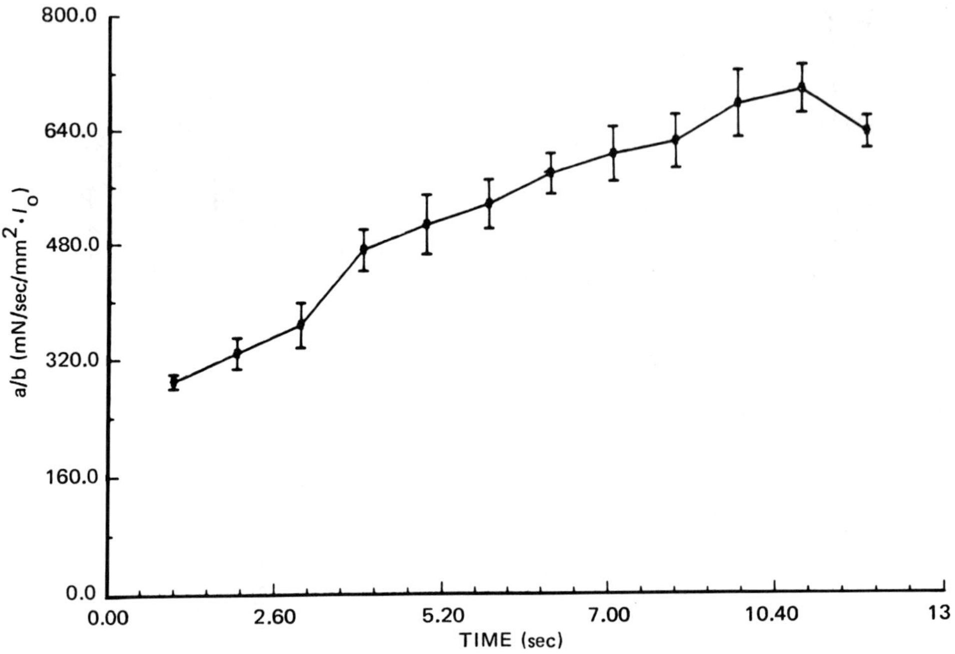

Figure 26 Plot of mean values of constant a/b vs. time.

$$F(t) = kX + \alpha V + mA \tag{3}$$

where F(t) is external force, k is the spring constant, X is displacement from equilibrium; α is the coefficient of viscosity, V is velocity, m is mass, and A is acceleration. If the system is an active muscle, then the force balance equation becomes:

$$P_o(t) = kX + \alpha V + mA \tag{4}$$

In an isotonic contraction under a constant load, the length of the series elastic component in the muscle remains constant during contraction. Hence kX is constant and equals P, the afterload on the muscle. Equation (4) therefore becomes:

$$P_o(t) = P + \alpha V + mA \tag{5}$$

Inertial force is very small in a system involving small mass and acceleration, as in a contracting muscle, hence the last term of Equation (5) may be ignored to give:

$$P_o(t) = P + \alpha V \tag{6}$$

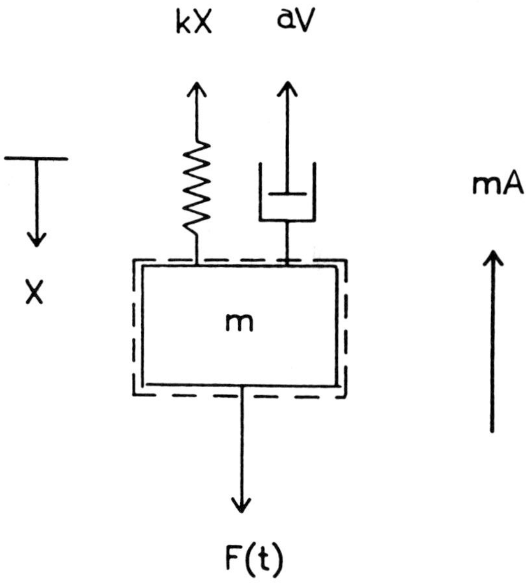

Figure 27 Schematic of a system subjected to elastic, viscous, inertial, and external forces.

Rearranging the Hill equation, we obtain:

$$P_o(t) = P + [P + a)/b]V \quad (7)$$

Comparing Equations (6) and (7) we see than

$$\alpha = (P + a)/b$$

which by dimensional analysis turns out to be [(force x time)/length^3]. Clearly (P + *a*)/*b* is the active "viscosity" or internal resistance of muscle to shortening and it is a function of both load and time. When muscle is shortening under zero load, the internal resistance of the muscle is $a(t)/b(t)$.

The Relaxation Process in Airway Smooth Muscle

Relaxation in muscle is not simply a passive process. It entails the sequential activation of a number of biochemical and biophysical processes. Disturbances in relaxation may be responsible for clinical disease. For example Shibata et al. (1973) reported that in caudal arterial smooth muscle from the spontaneously hypertensive rat, the relaxation process is considerably prolonged; this could contribute to the development of hypertension. It is possible that similar changes

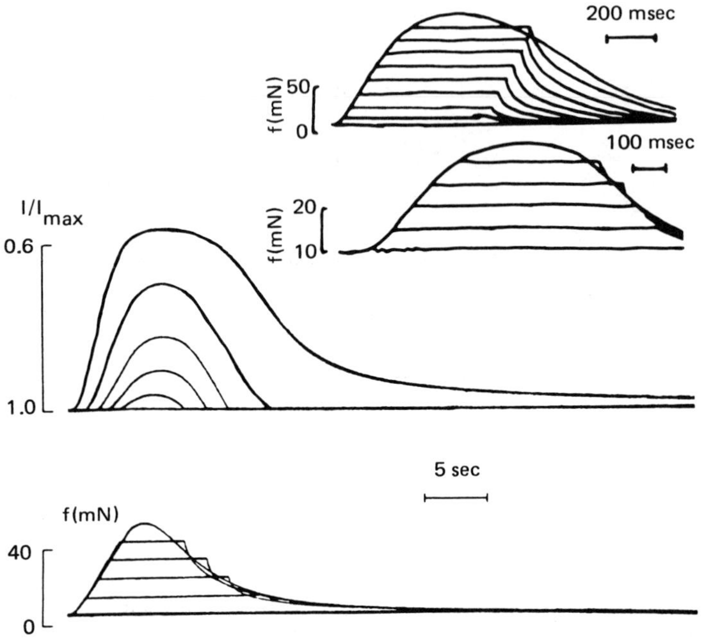

Figure 28 Curves of length (as a fraction of l_{max}) and force as functions of time during conventional afterloaded isotonic contractions taken from a single experiment. The inset shows similar force-time curves reported by Brutsaert et al. for cat heart papillary (upper) and frog ventricular (lower) muscles (from Stephens and Brutsaert, 1982).

in airway smooth muscle could contribute to the bronchoconstriction of asthma. We have studied the relaxation process in control strips of canine trachealis but have not yet studied ovalbumen-sensitized muscle.

Brutsaert et al. (1978) have shown that in cat heart papillary muscle relaxation is of the so-called load dependent type. Jewell and Wilkie (1960) have shown that frog skeletal muscle behaves similarly.

The upper set of force tracings in the inset in Figure 28 shows force twitch curves for the papillary muscle. The uppermost curve in this series represents isometric contraction and the ones below this are afterloaded isotonic contractions for different loads. The relaxation pathways for each of the latter differs and all are more rapid than that for the isometric. The load dependence of the relaxation is evident. This behavior has been ascribed to rapid resequestration of calcium by the relatively rich sarcoplasmic reticulum. Relaxation therefore sets in rapidly and is subsequently determined by the load.

The lower set of force traces in the inset is from frog ventricular muscle, which is characterized by a very slow rate of contraction and a paucity of sarcoplasmic reticulum. The relaxation pathways for the afterloaded contractions are quite different and all follow the isometric relaxation pathway. This type of relaxation has been termed inactivation-dependent relaxation by Brutsaert et al. (1978). Since the calcium resequestration mechanism is poor, the muscle remains activated for much longer and therefore relaxation depends not on the load but on the completion of the resequestration process and therefore of muscle inactivation. It is interesting that Brutsaert also noted that if he treated the cat heart papillary muscle with Brij-58, a detergent, and thus removed its sarcoplasmic reticulum, relaxation changed from load-dependent to inactivation-dependent.

Two plots in the main part of Figure 28 are taken from canine tracheal smooth muscle. The lower of these depicts force-time records that demonstrate that relaxation in this muscle is also of the inactivation-dependent type.

Alterations in Mechanical Properties of Tracheal Smooth Muscle from a Canine Model of Allergic Bronchoconstriction

While a fair amount of research has been carried out on the pharmacology (Suzuki et al., 1976; Russell, 1980) and electrophysiology (Souhrada and Souhrada, 1981) of sensitized airway smooth muscle, relatively little has been directed at elucidating the changes in mechanical properties. Dr. Kepron of our Immunology Department has developed an excellent canine model of allergic bronchoconstriction (Kepron et al., 1977). Using tracheal muscle strips, we have demonstrated that a well-defined Schultz-Dale response develops on challenge with specific antigen. At least in vitro, the response appears to be mediated by histamine since it can be completely blocked with an H_1 antagonist We have noted similar responses with 3 mm wide bronchi. Furthermore, Schultz-Dale responses were also elicited from the pulmonary vein (Kong and Stephens, 1981) and the hepatic vein, terminal ileum, and ureter (unpublished observations). This suggests that, in the model, sensitization is widespread. The shock organ or organs for the allergic or anaphylactic response would be determined by the portal of entry of the antigen into the subject. The pulmonary vein and the trachealis demonstrated increased sensitivity (leftward shift of dose-response curve) and reactivity (upward shift) to histamine. The pulmonary artery, which did not demonstrate a Schultz-Dale response, nevertheless showed abnormal responsiveness to histamine.

With respect to the sensitized trachealis we have found (Antonissen et al., 1979) that its maximum capacity to shorten (ΔL_{max}) is greater than that of the littermate control muscle; this is the in vitro counterpart of the increased bronchoconstriction of "asthma." The reasons for this behavior were speculated upon in the section on length-tension properties of smooth muscle.

In addition we found that while the maximum isometric force (P_o) developed by the sensitized muscle was unchanged, the maximum velocity of unloaded shortening (V_o) was increased. This suggests that the properties of the actomyosin ATPase are altered. These are discussed in the following section.

IV. Molecular Physiology of Airway Smooth Muscle Contraction

Very little work has been done in this area especially with regard to changes that may have developed because of sensitization. We are currently interested in establishing biochemical techniques that will enable us to understand molecular mechanisms of contraction of airway smooth muscle. Our studies to date have dealt with some aspects of energy production (oxidative phosphorylation), energy utilization (actomyosin ATPase) activity, and biochemical regulation of muscle contraction (myosin light chain phosphorylation).

A. Oxidative Phosphorylation

Pantesco et al. (1962) have reported that the extent to which different smooth muscles rely on glycolysis as an energy source varies considerably. It seemed useful to determine the role of oxidative phosphorylation in airway smooth muscle.

We isolated mitochondria from canine trachealis using a modified Chance and Hagihara (1963) procedure. The average mitochondrial protein yield was 0.43 ± 0.05 (SE) mg/g wet weight of muscle. Oxidative phosphorylation was determined polarographically with a Clarke-type electrode.

Ultrastructurally the mitochondria resembled those of skeletal muscle. They possessed a double membrane with cristae, the latter were present in smaller number than in striated muscle mitochondria. Under resting nonphosphorylating conditions the mitochondria, when suitably fixed and stained, showed the typical "orthodox" configuration described by Hackenbrock (1966). Under maximally phosphorylating conditions they presented the typical condensed configuration.

The oxidative phosphorylation parameters for smooth muscle mitochondria are very similar to those for skeletal muscle mitochondria and are given in Table 1. The substrate used for the above experiments was 5 mM pyruvate and 1 mM L-malate (P/M). The P:0 ratio, a measure of efficiency of phosphorylation, was within the low normal units for hamster skeletal muscle mitochondria. The respiratory control ratio (RCR), which is a more sensitive index for assessing the tightness of coupling of phosphorylation to respiration, was also within normal limits for hamster skeletal muscle mitochondria. Using NADH oxidase and cytochrome oxidase as markers, we measured mitochondrial protein content per gram wet weight of muscle. Knowing the phosphorylation rate (see Table 1) we

Table 1 Oxidative Phosphorylation Parameters in Smooth Muscle Mitochondria

Exp no.	O_2 uptake rate (moles O_2/min/g mitochondrial protein)	RCR	ADP/O (moles ADP added/ atoms O_2 used)	P Rate (moles ADP phosphorylated/min g mitochondrial protein)
1	118	4.6	1.9	441
2	85	3.5	2.2	376
3	95	4.2	2.2	409
4		4.9	2.4	
5		5.5	2.2	
6		5.1	2.0	
7		4.4	2.3	
8		3.6	2.4	
9	79	5.7	2.4	373
10	68	2.6	2.2	298
11	98	5.8	2.3	457
12	78	4.5	2.2	335
13	99	4.5	2.3	455
14		4.5	2.3	
Mean ± SE	94 ± 5	4.5 ± 0.2	2.30 ± 0.03	393 ± 21

From Stephens and Wrogemann, 1970.

were able to compute the phosphorylation capacity of the muscle. This of course is the phosphorylation rate per gram of muscle and is an important parameter in understanding smooth muscle bioenergetics. The capacity value of 1.40 mol of ADP phosphorylation per minute per gram wet weight of muscle was only about 10% of the value for skeletal muscle, and proved that the anaerobic glycolytic pathway provides comparatively more energy for smooth muscle contraction than for skeletal.

B. Anaerobic Glycolysis

Our studies of anaerobic glycolysis of high-energy phosphate levels are limited (Kroeger and Stephens, 1971). Lundholm (1956) has made fairly extensive studies of glycolysis in bovine tracheal smooth muscle. It appears that the pathways for carbohydrate metabolism are very similar to those for striated muscle. The presence of the pentose shunt has not been determined in airway smooth muscle;

however it has been shown to be present in aortic smooth muscle (Mandel and Kempf, 1963). For this [1-^{14}C] glucose was used.

The prominence of glycosis and of the lactate pathway raises questions as to the status of the Pasteur effect in smooth muscle. Only a weak Pasteur effect was found in bovine tracheal smooth muscle by the Lundholms (1960).

C. Contractile and Regulatory Proteins

While considerable work has been done in this area in a variety of smooth muscles, very little has been carried out in airway smooth muscle. Perhaps only three or four groups (De Lanerolle and Stull, 1980; Bose and Stephens, 1977) have paid attention to airway smooth muscle. Our interest in this area was engendered by wanting to determine the biochemical processes controlling the mechanical properties of the canine trachealis.

For smooth muscle in general the velocity of its unloaded shortening is probably controlled by its actomyosin ATPase activity. This activity is almost 100 times less than that of the frog sartorius. Not unexpectedly, the ATPase activity is also 100 times less.

We were led into a study of myofibrillar actomyosin ATPase activity in sensitized canine tracheal and pulmonary vascular smooth muscle because we had found that the maximum velocity of unloaded shortening of the muscles was considerably greater than that of the control muscles.

Tracheal and pulmonary arterial myofibrillar washed pellets were prepared by modification of a method developed by Sobieszek and Bremel (1975). Triton X-100 was used to eliminate contaminating ATPases of membranous origin. These pellets were subjected to ATPase activity measurement. The solution for the assay contained 0.1 mM $CaCl_2$, 1 mM $MgCl_2$, 1 mM cystine; 60 mM KCl, 1 mM MgATP, and 40 mM imidazole buffer to pH 6.9 at 25°C. The myofibrillar concentration was 14-16 mg/ml. Assay solutions (without MgATP) were preincubated at 25°C for 15 min and the reaction begun by adding MgATP and mixing gently. The reaction was stopped after 20 sec by adding 10% (to a final concentration) of trichloroacetic acid. The precipitate protein was pelleted by centrifugation. Inorganic phosphate in the supernatant fraction was measured by the method of Taussky and Shorr (1953). Enzyme activity was expressed as a function of unit myosin content, the latter being determined by quantitative sodium dodecyl sulfate (SDS) gel electrophoresis using bovine serum albumen as a standard. Protein concentrations were determined by the Bio-Rad protein assay.

The myofibrillar ATPase activities of sensitized tracheal and pulmonary arterial smooth muscle were 499 nmoles Pi/mg myosin per min ± 11.5 (SE); n = 7; and 359 nmoles Pi/mg myosin per min ± 12.6 (SE); n = 7, respectively. Those for the control tracheal and arterial muscles were 345 nmoles Pi/mg myosin per min ± 5.6 (SE), n = 7, and 272 nmoles Pi/mg myosin per min ± 5.6

(SE). The differences between the sensitized and control muscles were significantly different.

These studies indicated that the increased velocity of shortening of the smooth muscle could be accounted for by increased ATPase activity. These results bear a striking resemblance to those for the thyrotoxic heart muscle. Our proposal for the future is to follow the same tack laid down by heart muscle investigators. We plan therefore to determine whether tracheal smooth muscle myosin isozymes exist, and if so, to determine what their relative ATPase rates are, and finally to find out if they change from a slow isozyme pattern in control trachealis to a more rapid one in the sensitized muscle. No studies of this kind have been undertaken for airway smooth muscle. With respect to the smooth muscle field in general, the position is extremely confused, some groups reporting the existence of isozymes (Paganni et al., 1985) and others denying it (Murphy, personal communication).

The ultimate goal for us, in the area of asthma research, is to carry out all these studies in human central and peripheral airway smooth muscle. If similar results are found, then the process of gene expression will need to be studied. All of these projects will require technologic development.

D. Myosin Light Chain Phosphorylation

Following the era of cyclic AMP and cyclic GMP research, perhaps the most exciting development in smooth muscle research has been in the area of phosphorylation of contractile and regulatory proteins. This has extended to areas beyond muscle itself and therefore assumed major importance. It is now recognized that a host of nonmuscular contractile systems, such as spermatozoa, mucosal cilia, platelets, slime molds, exocytosis at presynaptic nerve terminals, and migrating cancer cells, to name a few, all utilize a regulatory system much like that of the smooth muscle.

There are two major differences between skeletal and smooth muscle: (1) the latter possesses no troponin system; tropomyosin however is present; (2) purified skeletal muscle actin and myosin, when mixed, display abrupt quasimaximal ATPase activity. Magnesium ions inhibit this activity while calcium also inhibits it to a lesser extent. Hence the effect of calcium, by producing reduced inhibition, manifests what appears as a stimulatory effect. The steplike ATPase activity is regulated by a tropomyosin-troponin-calcium-like system that converts the response into a graded one displaying calcium sensitivity. Myosin light chain phosphorylation has been demonstrated in skeletal muscle but its role has not yet been defined. Considerable controversy exists in the field. The current consensus is that it does not affect mechanical function.

In smooth muscle the role of myosin light chain (20,000 dalton) phosphorylation is fairly clear, although here some controversy exists also. Ebashi (1984) has reported that an actin-linked nonphosphorylatable protein, which

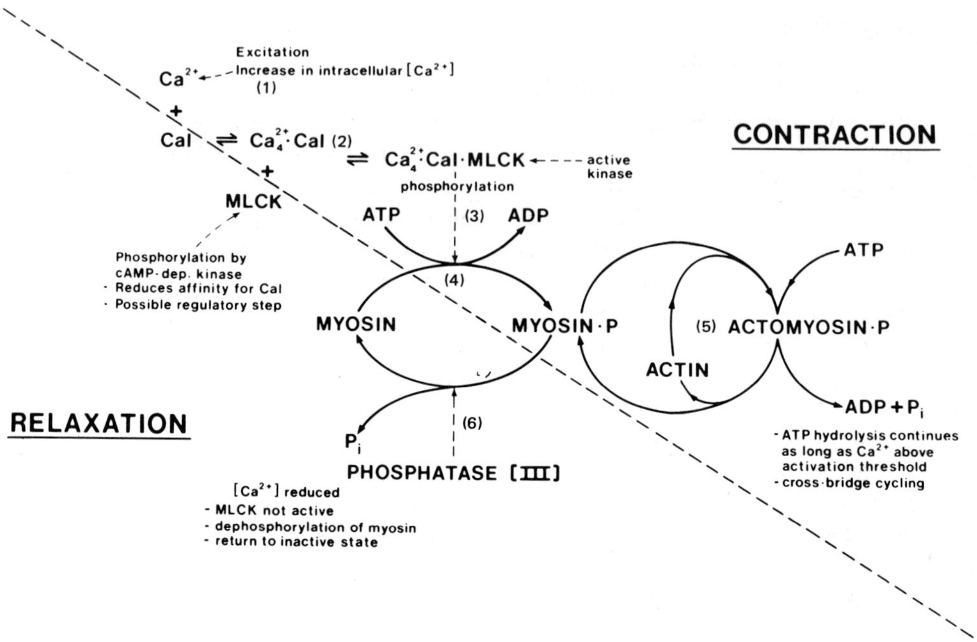

Figure 29 Outline of phosphorylation theory of regulation in smooth muscle. The dashed line indicates the protein species thought to exist and the events thought to occur in contracting and relaxing muscle. Numbers in brackets (1-6) indicate the sequence of events thought to occur following excitation of the muscle and proceeding through a contraction-relaxation cycle. Cal, Calmodulin; myosin-P, phosphorylated myosin; MLCK, myosin light chain kinase (from Hartshorne and Persechini, 1984).

he calls leiotonin, is responsible for smooth muscle regulation. Marston et al. (1980) reported that in mammalian vascular and avian gizzard smooth muscle a dual system of regulation exists in which both myosin phosphorylation and a thin, filament-linked control system were involved. The protein in the actin filament was found to be a specific, basic protein (Marston et al., 1980) which underwent phosphorylation. Currently the status of these two theories of regulation is uncertain.

The major theory in the field is that regulation is brought about by a calcium-sensitive phosphorylation of the 20,000 dalton myosin light chain.

Figure 29 is a schematic diagram published by Hartshorne and Persechini (1984), which provides an excellent overview. However Hartshorne himself offers a caveat to the effect that his group has found that under some conditions myosin phosphorylation is not sufficient for complete activation of ATPase activity (Persechini and Hartshorne, 1981) and that other components in addition to tropomyosin are involved. Whether the in vitro activity of these activators is artifactual has not been settled. With depolarization of the smooth muscle membrane by neurotransmitters or by binding of agonists to membrane receptors, intracellular calcium concentration rises from about 10^{-7} to 10^{-5} M. The ionic calcium binds to calmodulin, which possesses a very high affinity for it. Calmodulin contains four binding sites for calcium. Another protein, myosin light chain kinase, is also present in the cell but in the resting state is not associated with calmodulin. Once the Ca^{2+}-calmodulin complex is formed it develops a high affinity for myosin light chain kinase to which it binds. This activates the kinase, which phosphorylates the 20,000 dalton light chain. This phosphorylation results in the actin activation of myosin Mg-ATPase, development of cross-bridge cycling, and thus either force or shortening generation by the muscle.

Once the stimulus is turned off no more calcium enters the myoplasm and the activated, ATP-dependent calcium pumps either resequester calcium inside the sarcoplasmic reticulum or extrude it across the sarcolemma. Since the calcium level falls, myosin light chain phosphorylation does not occur any more. However this per se does not result in relaxation. A specific myosin light chain phosphatase is activated which dephosphorylates the light chain and this results in smooth muscle relaxation. Pato and Adelstein (1980) have described different smooth muscle phosphatases: SMP-I, SMP-II, and SMP-III. Recently Pato et al. (1984) have isolated another phosphatase, SMP-IV.

Adelstein and Eisenberg (1980) have also described cAMP-dependent phosphorylation of myosin light chain kinase, which results in impaired binding of Ca^{2+}-calmodulin to the kinases. This results in reduced light chain phosphorylation and reduced contraction. When calmodulin binds to myosin light chain kinase, only 1 mole of phosphate is incorporated with no effect on kinase activity. When phosphorylation occurs in the absence of bound calmodulin, 2 moles of phosphate are incorporated and the activity of the enzyme is reduced. The doubly phosphorylated kinase has an affinity for calmodulin almost 20 times lower than that of the unphosphorylated enzyme. The role of cellular cAMP in controlling mechanical activity can be best understood by assuming that the balance between myosin light chain kinase and myosin light chain phosphatase activities determines the extent of myosin light chain phosphorylation, and that not every molecule of myosin kinase is bound by calmodulin. Under these conditions a rise in concentration of cAMP would result in a decrease in myosin light chain kinase activity. Were cAMP levels to rise when the muscle was relaxed and the myosin light chain unphosphorylated, then kinase phosphorylation would prevent contraction, but if the rise occurred during the course of a contraction then kinase phosphorylation would lead to relaxation.

Using the above as a background and our findings that myofibrillar actomyosin MgATPase activity was increased in sensitized tracheal smooth muscle, we compared myosin light chain phosphorylation in control and sensitized muscles. Another reason for studying phosphorylation was that there is a close association between the extent of phosphorylation of myosin light chain and actomyosin ATPase activity. Whether the relationship is linear (Sobieszek and Small, 1977) or nonlinear (Persechini and Hartshorne, 1981) has not yet been settled.

We have (Stephens et al., 1985) used two-dimensional gel analysis to measure the stoichiometry of myosin light chain phosphorylation in control canine tracheal smooth muscle and have commenced studies of ovalbumen-sensitized muscles. Studies to determine the relation between myosin light chain phosphorylation and isometric force development are discussed here. Among the questions we addressed was: Does phosphorylation regulate contraction? The crucial measurement is to determine whether phosphorylation precedes muscle contraction. We have obtained evidence (using zero load clamp shortening) showing (Stephens et al., 1985) that mechanical activation commences within 600 msec ± 72 (SE) of supramaximal electrical stimulus onset. Phosphorylation should therefore precede this. As far as we are aware such data have never been published.

We developed a system by which the very thin (0.5 mm wide, weighing 2 mg) strip of trachealis could be frozen within 100 msec. We were thus able to carry out biomedical studies at 400 msec after stimulus onset and at 4 sec, which is midway during the development phase and at the peak of the contraction (30 sec), at which time a force plateau has emerged and after which the stimulus is switched off. The muscle relaxes back to normal at 90 sec. The muscle was superfused and essentially was suspended in room air, which facilitated rapid freezing. Under these conditions the contraction is almost three times slower compared to that in bathing medium. The tension trace was simultaneously obtained.

The two-dimensional gel electrophoresis technique developed by O'Farrell (1975) was used to separate the 20,000 dalton myosin light chain from the other proteins. The first dimension was isoelectric focusing (IEF; pH 4 0-6.5) in a tube gel, and the second was 12% SDS-polyacrylamide slab gel. The gels were stained with 0.25% Coomassie blue R250.

To demonstrate phosphorylation of the light chain we employed radioactive phosphorus for radioautography. Figure 30 shows the slab gel. The lower panel picture is the same as in the upper except that autoradiography was carried out. Appropriate standardizations were employed to determine the stoichiometry of phosphorylation. Figure 31 shows that light chain phosphorylation jumps from basal to maximal levels at 400 msec, which is well before the 600 msec mark for onset of mechanical activation. Thereafter the level of phosphorylation is unchanged throughout the contraction. When relaxation is complete

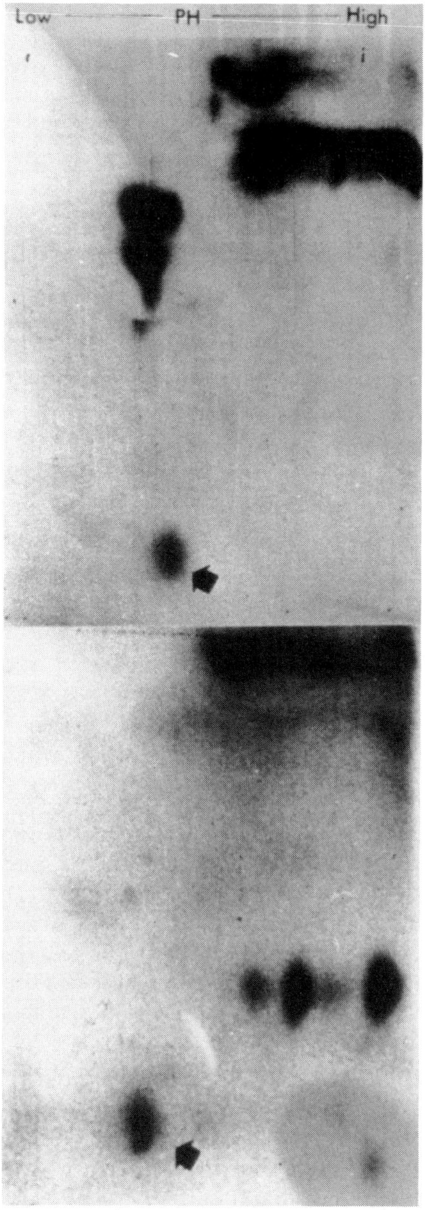

Figure 30 Two-dimensional gel electrophoresis. The upper panel shows the gel staining profile and the lower panel shows the autoradiographic profile. Arrows indicate the positions of the 20,000 dalton myosin light chain (from Stephens et al., 1986).

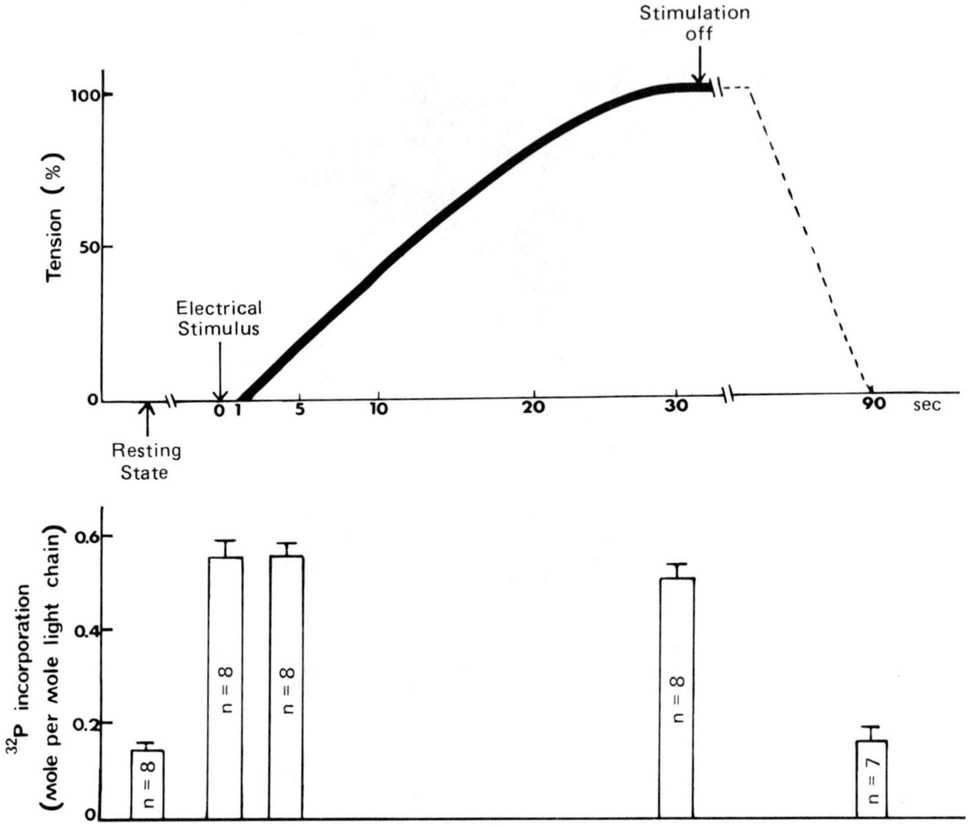

Figure 31 The upper panel shows the time course of tension development, when the muscle was stimulated in midair. The muscle samples were frozen at 0.4 sec, 4 sec, and 30 sec (plateau of maximal tension) after the electrical stimulation. The frozen sample of the relaxing muscle was obtained at 60 sec after the electrical stimulation had been turned off. The resting muscle without any stimulation was also frozen. The lower panel shows the phosphorylation level of myosin light chain of the corresponding frozen muscle. SE bars are shown.

(90 sec) phosphorylation also returns to basal level. Since there is no significant difference in phosphorylation between the 400 msec, 4 sec, and 30 sec marks while the tension has increased from 0 to 0.10 P_0 to P_0 we conclude that phosphorylation is not dependent on the numbers of cross-bridges. From this we conclude that while phosphorylation may be responsible for tension development in early contraction, the development of latch bridges in the late phase is not

phosphorylation dependent as reported by Dillon et al. (1981) for hog carotid arterial smooth muscle. While De Lanerolle and Stull (1980) find results similar to those of Dillon et al., others (Hacherk et al., 1985; Siegman et al., 1977) have reported results similar to ours.

F. The Role of Caldesmon

A number of smooth muscle calmodulin-binding proteins have been isolated by Ngai and Walsh (1985) from chicken gizzard using calmodulin-sepharose affinity chromatography. Among these was caldesmon, which exists in very large intracellular concentrations 11.1 μM (compared to 4.6 μM for myosin light chain kinase). Caldesmon could be phosphorylated by a Ca^{2+}, calmodulin-dependent caldesmon kinase and dephosphorylated by a phosphatase. It appeared to inhibit myosin light-chain kinase activity by competing for calmodulin. It could therefore play an important role in muscle relaxation. It may be exerting its effect by mechanisms other than simple competition and may well turn out to be an important factor in the regulation of smooth muscle contraction. Its status needs to be evaluated in airway smooth muscle, both control and sensitized.

G. The Role of Inositol Triphosphate and Protein Kinase-C Activation in Smooth Muscle Contraction

This represents perhaps one of the most important developments in cell biology over the last 2 or 3 years. Its role in smooth muscle contraction also appears to be important. Its manifestation in the muscle system is only one of those found to operate in a large variety of cells where excitation-contraction or excitation-secretion is involved. The model described by Rasmussen and Barrett (1984) is one in which the flow of information from cell surface to cell interior in the calcium messenger system proceeds by two operationally distinct branches. The first is a calmodulin (CaM) branch that is activated by a transient rise in cytosolic calcium concentration and responsible for the initial phase of the cell response. The second is a protein C-kinase-system that is stimulated by rises in calcium concentration and in diacylglycerol content of the plasma membrane and responsible for the sustained phase of cell response. This dual response is common in smooth muscle where the mechanical response to a variety of agonists is an initial phasic transient, followed rapidly by a more prolonged tonic one.

A review of the pathways in phosphoinositide biochemistry relevant to cell activation now follows. The phosphoinositides play a central role in cellular signal relaying for a variety of neurotransmitters, hormones, and growth factors. Binding of neurotransmitter, for example, to its receptor activates phosphatidyl -4.5-biphosphate (PlP_2) phosphodiesterase (Irvine et al., 1984). This hydrolyzes PlP_2 to diacylglycerol (DG), which activates protein kinase C (Rando and Young, 1984), and inositol triphosphate (IP_3) which releases calcium ions from intracellular stores (Berridge and Irvine, 1984). The DG is converted to phosphatidic acid (PA) by DG-kinase and then to cytidine diphosphate -1,2-diacylglycerol (CDP-DG) by CTD phosphatidate cytidyltransferase. CDP-DG and inositol are combined by CDP-DG inositol phosphatidyl transferase to produce phosphatidyl inositol (PI) (Paulus and Kennedy, 1960). PI is phosphorylated at the 4-position of its inositol group by PI kinase to produce phosphatidyl-phosphate (PIP) (Jergil and Sundler, 1983). Phosphorylation of PIP at the 5-position of its inositol group by PIP kinase leads to formation of PIP_2. Resynthesis of PIP_2 also involves the conversion of IP_3 to inositol by stepwise removal of the three phosphate groups. The first enzyme involved in this progression (inositol-1-phosphatase) is markedly inhibited by lithium (Berridge and Irvine, 1984) a drug extensively used to treat psychiatric disorders.

Studies have also shown that the products of ras and src oncogenes can act as lipid kinases and phosphorylate Pl, PIP, and DG. Sirhan et al. (1981) have also reported that phosphatic acid acts as an endogenous calcium ionophore in cells.

An important research tool in this area has been the recognition that ionophore A23187 will increase cytoplasmic cellular concentrations of calcium without activating the C-kinase branch, and the phorbol ester TPA (tetradecanolyl phorbol acetate) will activate the protein kinase-C branch without causing a rise in intracellular calcium concentrations.

Rasmussen reports that angiotensin II and norepinephrine are vascular smooth muscle agonists. The mechanical response shows an initial phase response followed by tonic. Rasmussen's unpublished results indicate that TPA induces a slowly progressive, Ca^{2+}-dependent increase in the active tension developed by vascular smooth muscle and that either A23187 or brief electrical trains of impulses augment this response. Furthermore the TPA-induced contraction is reversed by forskolin, an adenylate cyclase activator. So the second Ca^{2+}-dependent mechanism by which the tonic phase of smooth muscle contraction is maintained appears to be the C-kinase pathway of the Ca^{2+} messenger system.

Analysis suggests that the phasic response most likely is subserved by normally cycling smooth muscle cross-bridges and the tonic by latch bridges. If this turns out to be true (and this can be easily substantiated by measuring muscle shortening velocities under zero load clamps), then TPA and A23187 will provide us with an easy way to separate functionally the two types of crossbridges for independent study.

Acknowledgment

This work was supported by an operating grant from the Medical Research Council of Canada.

Dr. Kong was the recipient of a Canadian Heart Foundation studentship.

References

Abe, Y., and Tomita, T. (1968). Cable properties of smooth muscle. *J. Physiol. (Lond.) 196*: 87-100.

Adelstein, R. S., and Eisenberg, E. (1980). Regulation and kinetics of the actin-myosin-ATP interaction. *Annu. Rev. Biochem. 49*: 921-956.

Akasaka, K., Konno, K., Ono, Y., Mue, S., Abe, C., Kumagai, M., and Tse, T. (1975). A new electrode for electromyographic study of bronchial smooth muscle. *Tohoku J. Exp. Med. 117*: 49-54.

Antonissen, L. A., Mitchell, R. W., Kroeger, E. A., Kepron, W., Tse, K. S., and Stephens, N. L. (1979). Mechanical alterations of airway smooth muscle in a canine asthmatic model. *J. Appl. Physiol. 46*: 681-687.

Bagby, R. M. (1983). Organization of contractile/cytoskeletal elements. In *Biochemistry of Smooth Muscle,* Vol. 1. Edited by N. L. Stephens, Boca Raton, Florida, CRC Press, pp. 1-84.

Bai, T. R., Macklem, P. T., and Martin, J. A. (1984). The effects of partial or complete vagosympathetic section on induced bronchoconstriction in the cat. *Am. Rev. Respir. Dis. 129*: A 293.

Barsotti, R., Ikebe, M., and Hartshorne, D. (1985). Effects of Ca^{2+} and Mg^{2+} on myosin and shortening velocity of gizzard smooth muscle. *Biophys. J. 47* (no. 2 part 2): 2999.

Bergen, J. M., and Kroeger, E. A. (1980). Isometric tension responses to non-epinephrine in canine tracheal smooth muscle. *Fed. Proc. 39*: 1175A.

Berridge, M. J., and Irvine, R. F. (1984). Inositol triphosphate a novel second messenger in cellular signal transduction. *Nature 312*: 315-321.

Bose, R., and Stephens, N. L. (1977). Mechanism of action of hypoxia in smooth muscle: Role of contractile proteins. In *The Biochemistry of Smooth Muscle.* Edited by N. L. Stephens. Baltimore, University Park Press, pp. 499-512.

Bruns, R. R., and Palade, G. (1968). Studies on blood capillaries. II. Transport of ferritin molecules across the wall of mouse capillaries. *J. Cell. Biol. 37*: 277-299.

Brutsaert, D. L., de Clerck, N. M., Goethals, M. A., and Housmans, P. R. (1978). Relaxation of ventricular cardiac muscle. *J. Physiol. 283*: 469-480.

Burnstock, G. (1970) Structure of smooth muscle and its innervation. In *Smooth Muscle.* Edited by E. Bulbring, A. Brading, A. N. Jones, and T. Tomita. London, Edward Arnold, pp. 1-69.

Burnstock, G. (1975). Ultrastructure of autonomic nerves and neuroeffector junctions: analysis of drug action. In *Methods in Pharmacol.* Vol. 3,

Smooth Muscle. Edited by E. E. Daniel and D. M. Paton. New York, Plenum Press, pp. 133-137.

Cameron, A. R., and Kirkpatrick, C. T. (1976). The distribution of autonomic nerves within the smooth muscle layer of the bovine trachea. *J. Physiol. (Lond.) 259*: 48.

Chamley, J., Groschel-Stewart, U., Campbell, G. R., and Burnstock, G. R. (1977). Distinction between smooth muscle, fibroblasts and endothelial cells in culture by the use of fluorescinated antibodies against smooth muscle action. *Cell. Tissue Res. 177*: 445.

Chance, B., and Hagihara, B. (1963). Direct spectroscopic measurements of interaction of compounds of the respiratory chain with ATP, ADP, phosphate and uncoupling agents. *Proc. Intern. Congr. Biochem, 5th, Moscow, 1961 5*: 3-37.

Chand, N., and Eyre, P. (1978). Spasmolytic action of histamine in airway smooth muscle of horse. *Agents Action 9*: 191-198.

Chatterjee, M., and Murphy, R. (1983). Calcium-dependent stress maintenance without myosin phosphorylation in skinned smooth muscle. *Science 221*: 464-466.

Cooke, P. (1976). A filamentous cytoskeleton in vertebrate smooth muscle fibres. *J. Cell. Biol. 68*: 539-556.

Cooke, P., and Fay, F. (1972). Correlation between fibre length, ultrastructure and the length-tension relationship of mammalian smooth muscle. *J. Cell. Biol. 52*: 105-116.

De Lanerolle, P., and Stull, J. T. (1980). Myosin phosphorylation during contraction and relaxation of tracheal smooth muscle. *J. Biol. Chem. 255*: 9993-10000.

Dey, R. D., and Said, S. I. (1981). Localization of substance P-like immunofluorescence in nerves within dog airways and pulmonary vessels. *Fed. Proc. 40*: 595.

Dey, R. D., Shannon, W. A., and Said, S. I. (1981). Localization of VIP immunoreactive nerves in airways and pulmonary vessels of dogs, cats, and human subjects. *Fed. Proc. 40*: 595.

Dillon, P. F., Aksoy, M. O., Driska, S. P., and Murphy, R. A. (1981). Myosin phosphorylation and the crossbridge cycle in arterial smooth muscle. *Science 211*: 494-497.

Douglas, J. S., Dennis, M. O., Ridway, P., Bouhuys, A. (1973). Airway constriction in guinea pigs: Interaction of histamine and autonomic drugs. *J. Pharmacol. Exp. Ther. 184*: 169-70.

Ebashi, S. (1984). Actin-linked mechanism: Leiotonin system. In *Smooth Muscle Contraction.* Edited by N. L. Stephens. New York, Marcel Dekker, pp. 317-327.

Eyre, P. (1973). Histamine H_2-receptors in the sheep bronchus and cat trachea: the actions of burimamide. *Br. J. Pharmacol. 48*; 321.

Fay, F. S. (1976). Structural and functional features of isolated smooth muscle cells. In *Cell Motility: Molecules and Organization.* Edited by S. Hatano, H. Ishikawa, and H. Sato. Tokyo, University of Tokyo Press, p. 185.

Fay, F. S., Fogarty, K., and Fujiwara, K. (1983). The organization of the contractile apparatus in single isolated smooth muscle cells. In *Smooth Muscle Contraction.* Edited by N. L. Stephens. Boca Raton, Florida, CRC Press, pp. 1-84.

Fleisch, J. H., Shaethe, S. M., and Johnson, W. D. (1980). Drug-induced effects on the longitudinal smooth muscle of rat bronchus. *Proc. Soc. Exp. Biol. Med. 164*: 196-198.

Furchgott, O. H., and Zawadski, J. V. (1980). The obligatory role of endothelial cells in the relaxation of arterial smooth muscle by acetylcholine. *Nature 288*: 373-376.

Gabella, G. (1984). Structural apparatus for force transmission in smooth muscles. *Physiol. Rev. 64(2)*: 455-477.

Gabella, G., and Blundell, D. (1978). Effect of stretch and contraction on caveolae of smooth muscle cells. *Cell Tissue Res. 190*: 255-271.

Gabella, G., and Blundell, D. (1979). Nexuses between the smooth muscle cells of the guinea pig ileum. *J. Cell. Biol. 82*: 239-247.

Gaskin, F., and Shelanski, M. L. (1976). Microtubules and intermediate filaments. *Essays Biochem. 12*: 115-146.

Goldman, R., and Knipe, D. (1973). Functions of cytoplasmic fibres in nonmuscle cell motility. *Cold Spring Harbor Symp. Quant. Biol. 37*: 523-534.

Groschel-Stewart, U., Chamley, J. H., McConnell, J. D., and Buenstock, G. (1975). Comparison of the reaction of cultured smooth and cardiac muscle cells and fibroblasts to specific antibodies to myosin, *Histochemistry 43*: 215.

Hacherk, J., Hathaway, D. R., and De Paoli-Roach, A. A. (1985). The effects of an exogenous phosphatase on isometric force maintenance and myosin phosphorylation of glycerinated uterine smooth muscle. *Biophys. J. 42* (2, part 2): 1869.

Hackenbrock, C. R. (1966). Ultrastructural basis for metabolically linked mechanical activity in mitochondria I. Reversible ultrastructural changes with change in metabolic steady state in isolated liver mitochondria. *J. Cell. Biol. 30*: 269-297.

Hartshorne, D. J., and Persechini, A. (1984). Regulatory mechanisms in smooth muscle: the role of myosin phosphorylation. In *Smooth Muscle Contraction.* Edited by N. L. Stephens, New York, Marcel Dekker, pp. 271-282.

Hill, A. V. (1938). The heat of shortening and the dynamic constants of muscle. *Proc. R. Soc. London* [B] *126*: 136-195.

Henderson, R. M., Duchon, G., and Daniel, E. E. (1971). Cell contacts in duodenal smooth muscle layers. *Am. J. Physiol. 221*: 564-574.

Huxley, H. E. (1977). Summary of discussion on "Structural Aspects." In *Excitation-Contraction Coupling in Smooth Muscle.* Edited by R.Castells, T. Goodfriend, and J. C. Ruegg. Elsevier/N. Holland Biomedical Press, New York.

Huxley, A. F., and Simmons, R. M. (1971). Proposed mechanism of force generation in striated muscle. *Nature 233*: 533-538.

Irvine, R. F., Letcher, A. J., Lander, D. J., and Downes, C. P. (1984). Inositol triphosphates in carbachol-stimulated rat parotid glands. *Biochem. J. 223*: 237-243.

Ishikawa, H., Bischoff, R., and Holtzer, H. (1968). Mitosis and intermediate sized filaments in developing skeletal muscle. *J. Cell. Biol. 38*: 538-555.

Jennings, M. A., Marchesi, V. T., and Florey, H. (1962). The transport of particles across the walls of small blood vessels. *Proc. R. Soc* [B] *156*: 14-19.

Jergil, B., and Sundler, R. (1983). Phosphorylation of phosphatidylinositol in rat liver Golgi. *J. Biol. Chem. 258*(13): 7968-7973.

Jewell, B. R., and Wilkie, D. R. (1958). An analysis of the mechanical components in frog's striated muscle. *J. Physiol. (London) 143*: 575-540.

Jewell, B. R., and Wilkie, D. R. (1960). The mechanical properties of relaxing muscle. *J. Physiol. (London) 152*: 30-47.

Johnson, R., Hammer, M., Shendan, S. D., and Revel, J. P. (1974). Gap junction formation between reaggreated hepatoma cells. *Proc. Natl. Acad. Sci. USA 71*: 4536-4540.

Kannan, M. S., and Daniel, E. E. (1978). Formation of gap junctions by treatment in vitro with potassium conductance blockers. *J. Cell. Biol. 78*: 338-348.

Kannan, M. S., and Daniel, E. E. (1980). Structural and functional study of control of canine tracheal smooth muscle. *Am. J. Physiol. 238*: C27-C33.

Kepron, W., James, J. M., Kirk, B., Sehon, A. H., and Tse, K. S. (1977). A canine model for reaginic hypersensitivity and allergic bronchoconstriction. *J. Allergy Clin. Immunol. 59*: 64-69.

Kirkpatrick, C. H. (1975). Excitation and contraction in bovine tracheal smooth muscle. *J. Physiol. (London) 244*: 263-281.

Kong, K. S., and Stephens, N. L. (1981). Pharmacological studies of sensitized canine pulmonary blood vessels. *J. Pharmacol. Exp. Ther. 219*: 551.

Krahl, V. (1964). Anatomy of the mammalian lung. In *Handbook of Physiology,* Sec. 3, Respiration, Vol. 1. Edited by W. O. Fenn and H. Rahn. Washington, DC, Am. Physiol. Soc., pp. 213-284.

Kroeger, E. A., and Stephens, N. L. (1971). Effect of hypoxia on energy and metabolism in airway smooth muscle. *Am. J. Physiol. 220*(5): 1199-1204.

Kroeger, E. A., and Stephens, N. L. (1975). Effect of tetraethylammonium on tonic airway smooth muscle: Initiation of phasic electrical activity. *Am. J. Physiol. 228*: 633-663.

Kromer, U., and Stephens, N. L. (1983). Airway smooth muscle mechanics: reduced activation and relaxation. *J. Appl. Physiol. 54*(2): 345-348.

Lazarides, E., and Hubbard, B. (1976). Immunological characterization of the subunit of the 100A filaments from smooth muscle cells. *Proc. Natl. Acad. Sci. USA 73*: 4344-4348.

Lowenstein, W. R., and Rose, B. (1978). Calcium in (junctional) intercellular communication and a thought on its behaviour in intracellular communication. *Ann. N.Y. Acad. Sci. 307*: 285-307.

Lowy, J., Poulsen, F. R., and Vibert, P. J. (1970). Myosin filaments in vertebrate smooth muscle. *Nature 225*: 1053-1054.

Lullich, K. M., Mitchell, H. W., and Sparrow, M. P. (1976). The cat lung strip as an in vitro preparation of peripheral airways. *Br. J. Pharmacol. 58*: 71-79.

Lundberg, J. M., Saria, A. (1983). Capsaicin-induced desensitization of airway mucosa to cigarette smoke, mechanical and chemical irritants. *Nature 152*: 183.

Lundholm, E. (1956). Effect of adrenaline, nor-adrenaline isopropyl-noradrenaline and ephedrine on tone and lactic acid formation in bovine tracheal muscle. *Acta Physiol. Scand. 37*: 1-4.

Lundholm, L., and Mohme-Lundholm, E. (1960). The carbohydrate metabolism and tone of smooth muscle. *Acta Pharmacol. Toxicol. 16*: 374-388.

Mandel, P., and Kempf, E. (1963). The pentose phosphate pathway in the degradation of glucose by aortic tissue. *J. Atheroscler. Res. 3*: 233-236.

Marston, R. B., Trevett, R. M., and Walters, M. (1980). Calcium ion-regulated thin filaments from vascular smooth muscle. *Biochem. J. 185*: 355-365.

Merrillees, N. C. R., Burnstock, G., and Holman, M. E. (1963). Correlation of fine structure and physiology of the innervation of smooth muscle in the guinea pig vas deferens. *J. Cell. Biol. 19*: 529-550.

Miller, M. D., and Marshall, J. M. (1975). Uterine response to nerve stimulation: relation to hormonal status and catecholamines. *Am. J. Physiol. 209*: 859-865.

Mitchell, R. W., and Stephens, N. L. (1983). Maximum shortening velocity of smooth muscle: zero load clamp vs. afterloaded method. *J. Appl. Physiol. 55*(5): 1630-1633.

Ngai, P. K., and Walsh, M. P. (1985). Smooth muscle calmodulin binding proteins. *Biophys. J. 47* (no. 2, Part 2): 187a.

O'Farrell, P. H. (1975). High resolution two-dimensional electrophoresis of protein. *J. Biol. Chem. 250*: 4007-4021.

Paganni, E. D., Faris, R., Shemin, R., Julian, F. J. (1985). Evidence for smooth muscle myosin isozymes. *Biophys. J. 47*: (no. 2, part 2): 301a.

Palade, G. E. (1960). Transport of quenita across the endothelium of blood capillaries. *Anat. Rec. 136*: 254.

Pantesco, V., Kempf, E., Mendel, P., and Fontaine, R. (1962). Studies metabolique comparés des parois arterielles et veineuse chez les bovides. Leurs variation au cours du vieillissement. *Pathol. Biol. Sem. Hop. 10*: 1301-1306.

Pato, M. D., and Adelstein, R. S. (1980). Dephosphorylation of the 20,000 dalton light chain of myosin by two different phosphatases from smooth muscle. *J. Biol. Chem. 255*: 6535-6538.

Pato, M. D., Sellers, J. R., Conti, M. A., and Adelstein, R. S. (1984). Reversible phosphorylation of smooth muscle myosin and myosin kinase. In *Smooth Muscle Contraction.* Edited by N. L. Stephens. New York. Marcel Dekker, pp. 329-345.

Paul, R. J., and Peterson, J. W. (1975). Relation between length, isometric force and O_2 consumption rate in vascular smooth muscle. *Am. J. Physiol. 228*: 915-922.

Paulus, H., and Kennedy, E. P. (1960). The enzymatic synthesis of inositol monophosphatide. *J. Biol. Chem. 235*: 1301-1311.

Persecchini, A., and Hartshorne, D. J. (1981). Phosphorylation of smooth muscle myosin: evidence for cooperativity between the myosin heads. *Science 213*: 1383.

Rando, R. R., and Young, N. (1984). The stereospecific activation of protein kinase C. *J. Biochem. Biophys. Res. Commun. 122*: 818-823.

Rasmussen, H., and Barrett, P. O. (1984). Calcium messenger system: An integrated view. *Physiol. Rev. 64*(3): 938-984.

Rice, R. V., McManus, G. M., Devine, C. E., and Somlyo, A. D. (1971). A regular organization of thick filaments in mammalian smooth muscle. *Nature New Biol. 231*: 242-243.

Richardson, J. B., and Beland, J. (1976). Nonadrenergic inhibitory nervous system in human airway. *J. Appl. Physiol. 41*: 764-771.

Russell, J. A. (1978a). Innervation of beta-adrenergic receptors in airway smooth muscle of dog. *Fed. Proc. 37*: 81A.

Russell, J. A. (1978b). Responses of isolated canine airways to electric stimulation and acetylcholine. *J. Appl. Physiol. 45*(5): 690-698.

Russell, J. A. (1980). Nonadrenergic inhibitory innervation of canine airways. *J. Appl. Physiol. 48*(1): 16-22.

Shibata, S., Kurahashi, K., and Kuchii, M. (1973). A possible etiology of contractility impairment of vascular smooth muscle from spontaneously hypertensive rats. *J. Pharmacol. Exp. Ther. 185*: 406-417.

Shoenberg, C. F., and Haseltone, J. (1974). Filaments and ribbons in vertebrate smooth muscle. *Nature 249*: 152-154.

Siegman, M., Butler, J., Mooers, S., and Davies, R. (1977). Mechanical and energetic correlates of isometric relaxation. In *Excitation-Contraction Coupling in Smooth Muscle.* Edited by R. Casteels, T. Godfraind, and J. G. Ruegg. New York, Elsevier/North Holland, pp. 449-453.

Siegman, M. J., Davidheiser, S., Butler, T. M., and Moeers, S. U. (1985). What is the length-tension relation in smooth muscle? *Fed. Proc. 44*(3): 456A.

Sirhan, C., Anderson, P., Goodman, E., Dunham, P., and Weissman, G. (1981). Phosphatide and oxidized fatty acids are calcium ionophores. *J. Biol. Chem. 256*: 2736-2741.

Small, J. V. (1977). Studies on smooth muscle cells: the contractile apparatus. *J. Cell. Sci. 24*: 327-349.

Small, J. V., and Celis, J. (1978). Direct visualization of the 10 nm (100A) filament network in whole and enucleated cultured cells. *J. Cell. Sci. 31*: 393-409.

Sobieszek, A., and Bremel, R. D. (1975). Preparation and properties of vertebrate smooth muscle myofibrils and actomyosin. *Eur. J. Biochem. 15*: 49-60.

Sobieszek, A., and Small, J. (1976). Myosin-linked calcium regulation in vertebrate smooth muscle. *J. Mol. Biol. 102*: 75-92.

Sobieszek, A., and Small, J. V. (1977). Regulation of the actin-myosin interaction in vertebrate smooth muscle. Activation via a myosin light-chain kinase and the effect of tropomyosin. *J. Mol. Biol. 112*: 559-576.

Somlyo, A. P., and Somlyo, A. V. (1975). Ultrastructure of smooth muscle. In *Methods in Pharmacology.* Edited by E. E. Daniel and D. M. Paton. New York, Plenum Press, pp. 3-45.

Somlyo, A. P., Devine, C. E., and Somlyo, A. V. (1972). Sarcoplasmic reticulum mitochondria and filament organization in vascular smooth muscle. In *Vascular Smooth Muscle. A Symposium.* Edited by E. Betz. Heidelberg, Springer-Verlag, pp. 119-121.

Somlyo, A. P., Devine, C. E., Somlyo, A. V., and Rice, R. V. (1973). Filament organization in vertebrate smooth muscle. *Phil. Trans. R. Soc. Lond.* [B] *265*: 223-229.

Somlyo, A. V., Bond, M., Berner, P. F., Ashton, F. T., Holtzer, H., Somlyo, A. P., and Butler, T. M. (1984). The contractile apparatus of smooth muscle: An update. In *Smooth Muscle Contraction.* Edited by N. L. Stephens. New York, Marcel Dekker, pp. 1-20.

Souhrada, M., and Souhrada, J. F. (1981). Reassessment of electrophysiological and contractile characteristics of sensitized airway smooth muscle. *Respir. Physiol. 46*: 17-27.

Stephens, N. L., and Wrogemann (1970). Oxidative phosphorylation in smooth muscle. *Am. J. Physiol. 219*: 1796-1801.

Stephens, N. L. (1975). Physical properties of contractile systems. In *Methods in Pharmacology. Vol. 3. Smooth Muscle.* Edited by E. E. Daniel and D. M. Paton. New York, Plenum Press, pp. 265-296.

Stephens, N. L., and Brutsaert, D. (1982). Maximum force potential of tetanized mammalian smooth muscle. *Am. J. Physiol. 242*: C283-C287.

Stephens, N. L., Meyers, J. L., and Cherniack, R. M. (1968). Oxygen carbon dioxide, H^+ ion, and bronchial length-tension relationships. *J. Appl. Physiol. 25*(4): 376-383.

Stephens, N. L., and Kroeger, E. A. (1980). Ultrastructure, Biophysics and Biochemistry of Airway Smooth Muscle. In *Physiology and Pharmacology of the Airways.* Edited by J. A. Nadel. New York, Marcel Dekker, pp. 31-121.

Stephens, N. L., Kroeger, E. A., and Mehta, J. A. (1969). Force-velocity characteristics of respiratory airway smooth muscle. *J. Appl. Physiol. 26*: 685-692.

Stephens, N. L., and Skoog, C. M. (1974). Tracheal smooth muscle and rate of oxygen uptake. *Am. J. Physiol. 226(6)*: 1462-1467.

Stephens, N. L., Cardinal, R., and Simmons, B. (1977). Mechanical properties of tracheal smooth muscle: effects of temperature. *Am. J. Physiol. 2*(2): C92-C98.

Stephens, N. L., Morgan, G., Packer, C. S., and Kong, S. K. (1985). Smooth muscle contractility: effects of hypoxia. *Chest 88S*: 223S-229S.

Stephens, N. L. (1985). Airway smooth muscle: Physiology, bronchomotor tone, pharmacology, and relation to asthma. In *Bronchial Asthma. Mechanisms and Therapeutics.* Second edition. Edited by E. B. Weiss, M. S. Segal, and M. Stein. Little Brown & Co., Boston, 96-110.

Stephens, N. L., Parker, C. F., and Mitchell, R. W. (1986). Mechanical properties of airway smooth muscle. *Bull. Europ. Physiopath. Respir. 22*, Suppl. 7: 178-190.

Sugi, H., and Daimon, T. (1977). Translocation of intracellularly stored calcium during the contraction-relaxation cycle in guinea pig taenia coli. *Nature 269*: 436-438.

Suzuki, H., Monita, K., and Kuriyama, H. (1976). Innervation and properties of the smooth muscle of the dog trachea. *Jpn. J. Physiol. 26*: 303-320.

Szentivanyi, A. (1968). The B-adrenergic theory of the atopic abnormality in bronchial asthma. *J. Allergy 42*: 203.

Taussky, H. H., and Shorr, E. (1953). A microcolorimetric method for the determination of inorganic phosphorus. *J. Biol. Chem. 202*: 675-685.

Taylor, S. R. (1976). Decreased activation in skeletal muscle fibres at short lengths. In *The Physiological Basis of Starling's Law of the Heart.* Edited by R. Porter and D. W. Fitzsimmons. London, Elsevier/Excerpta, pp. 93-116.

Uddman, R., Alumets, J., Densert, O., Hakason, R., and Sundler, F. (1978). Occurrence and distribution of VIP nerves in the nasal mucosa and tracheobronchial wall. *Acta Otolaryngol. 86*(5-6): 443-448.

Uehara, Y., and Burnstock, G. (1972). Postsynaptic specialization of smooth muscle at close neuromuscular junctions in the guinea pig sphincter pupillae. *J. Cell. Biol. 53*: 849-853.

Verbeke, N., Morel, N., and Godfraind, T. (1977). Microsomal and mitochondrial calcium pumps in smooth muscle. In *Excitation-Contraction Coupling in Smooth Muscle.* Edited by R. Casteels T. Godfraind, and J. C. Ruegg. North Holland, pp. 219-224.

Vermeire, P., and Vanhoutte, P. (1979). Inhibitory effects of catecholamines in isolated canine bronchial smooth muscle. *J. Appl. Physiol. 46*: 787-791.

Vibert, P. J., Haselgrove, J. C., and Poulsen, F. R. (1972). Structural changes in actin-containing filaments of muscle. *Nature New Biol. 236*: 182-183.

Van Hayuk, H. *The Human Lung.* Hafner, New York, 1960.

Wharton, J., Polak, J. M., Bloom, S. R., Will, J. A., Brown, M. R., and Pearse, A.G. (1979). Substance P-like immunoreactive nerves in mammalian lung. *Invest. Cell. Pathol. 2*: 3-10.

Yamauchi, A., and Burnstock, G. (1969). Post-natal development of smooth muscle cells in the mouse vas deferens. A fine structural study. *J. Anat. 104*: 1-5.

Yeatman, L. A., Jr., Parmley, W. W., and Sonnenblick, E. H. (1969). Effects of temperature on series elasticity and contractile element motion in heart muscle. *Am. J. Physiol. 217*: 1030-1034.

2

Airway Receptors

PETER J. BARNES

Cardiothoracic Institute
Brompton Hospital
London, England

Airway tone is influenced by many hormones, neurotransmitters, drugs, and mediators. These agents produce their effects by binding to specific recognition sites or receptors on the external surface of the various target cells in the airway. It is therefore possible to view bronchoconstriction and bronchodilatation in terms of receptor activation or blockade. There have recently been considerable advances in our understanding of receptor function and many new selective drugs that interact with receptors have been developed. A great impetus to research into basic mechanisms of receptor function has been provided by the technique of radioligand binding, in which a radiolabeled agonist or antagonist permits direct study and isolation of receptors. As most of the bronchodilators in current use produce their effects by interacting with various airway receptors, a knowledge of receptor function is fundamental to understanding their mechanism of action in depth.

Much emphasis has been placed on contraction of airway smooth muscle as the cause of bronchoconstriction in asthma, and it is likely that the immediate effects of bronchodilators can be explained by smooth muscle relaxation. However, airway narrowing in asthma is also due to edema of the bronchial wall (due to microvascular leakiness and inflammatory cell infiltration), and to luminal plugging by viscous mucus secretions, and these pathologic events may be produced by mediators released from inflammatory cells, including mast cells and eosinophils. In discussing airway receptors, it is therefore important to consider not only the receptors on airway smooth muscle, but also receptors on other target cells, such as submucosal glands, airway epithelium, mast cells, and other inflammatory cells.

Airway tone is regulated by the autonomic nervous system, via the release of neurotransmitters that activate specific autonomic receptors. The role of autonomic receptors and their possible abnormalities in asthma is discussed in the first part of this chapter. Bronchoconstriction in asthma is probably explained by the combined effects of several inflammatory mediators that cause airway obstruction by stimulating specific receptors. These receptors are discussed in the second part of the chapter.

I. Receptor Pharmacology

A. Molecular Pharmacology

Receptors are proteins located on the external surface of cells, which specifically combine with their agonist. Recently several receptors have been isolated and most have proved to be glycoproteins, which consist of several subunits linked by disulfide bridges. Receptors appear to float in the phospholipid bilayer of the cell membrane. When a specific agonist binds to the receptor there is a change in the physical properties of the receptor that may lead to an increase in its mobility in the cell membrane; this then activates a series of intracellular events resulting in the final response. With some receptors, such as muscarinic cholinergic receptors or α-adrenoceptors there may be an increase in calcium ion influx into the cell. Other types of receptor such as β-adrenoceptors or vasoactive intestinal polypeptide receptors activate the enzyme adenylate cyclase, which converts ATP to cyclic AMP, triggering the production of protein kinases that bring about the characteristic cellular response. The linking of receptors to adenylate cyclase involves a coupling protein regulated by guanine nucleotides (nucleotide regulatory protein; N). Two related forms of N are now recognized; one stimulates adenylate cyclase (N_s) and the other inhibits this enzyme (N_i) (Fig. 1). Although some receptors are located on the cell surface membrane, some receptors are intracellular. Thus steroids bind to specific cytoplasmic receptors, which then translocate the molecule to the nucleus.

B. Receptors and Disease

It is now recognized that receptors are not static but have a rapid turnover, and that receptors may change in various disease states, and as the result of treat-

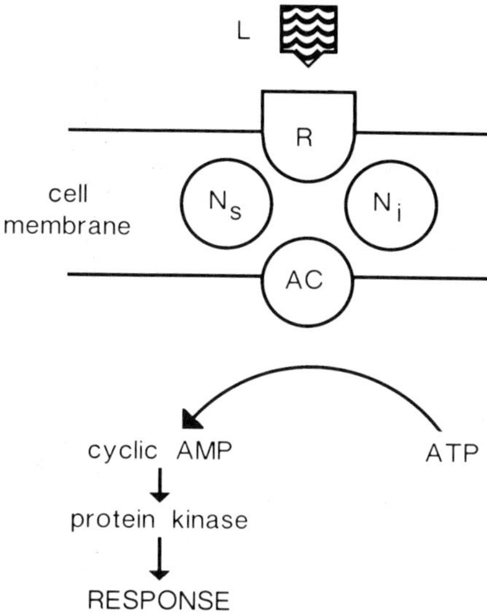

Figure 1 Receptor activation involving adenylate cyclase. A ligand (L) binds to its specific receptor (R) located on the outside of the cell surface membrane. If the ligand is an agonist, it leads to activation or inhibition of adenylate cyclase (AC). This activation involves a coupling protein, guanine nucleotide regulatory protein (N_s). ATP is then converted to cyclic AMP which leads to the response via specific protein kinases. Some agonists inhibit adenylate cyclase via the intermediary of an inhibitory coupling protein (N_i).

ment (Pollett and Levey, 1980). Since receptors determine tissue responsiveness, it may be possible to explain the abnormal responsiveness in some conditions by an abnormality in specific receptors. The most convincing example of this is seen with myasthenia gravis, in which a blocking antibody to nicotinic cholinergic receptors is found, which accounts for the defect in neuromuscular transmission in skeletal muscle. In asthma a similar mechanism has been proposed, with autoantibodies to β-receptors, to explain the apparent defects in β-adrenergic function in asthma (Venter et al., 1980).

C. Receptor Subtypes

Each homrone, neurotransmitter, and mediator has a specific receptor to which it binds with high specificity and affinity. Several endogenous agonists have more than one type of receptor. Thus two types of receptor for acetylcholine can be recognized pharmacologically; the nicotinic cholinergic receptor (in

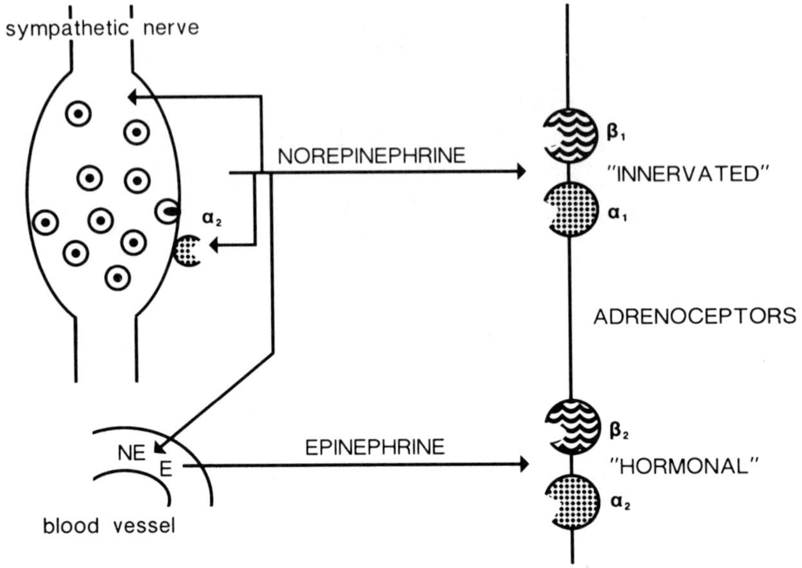

Figure 2 Regulation of adrenoceptor subtypes. Norepinephrine released from sympathetic nerves activates β_1 and α_1-adrenoceptors, which are therefore "innervated." Circulating epinephrine however activates β_2- and probably α_2-receptors, which are therefore "hormonal."

ganglia) is blocked by hexamethonium, whereas the muscarinic cholinergic receptor (in airway smooth muscle) is blocked by atropine. Molecular pharmacology techniques have indeed shown that two quite distinct receptor proteins exist.

Catecholamines may have different effects in different tissues and Ahlquist in 1948 first recognized that this could be best explained not by two different catecholamines, but by assuming the presence of two different receptors. Thus in some tissues the rank order of potency norepinephrine = epinephrine > isoproterenol was found, whereas in others the rank order isoproterenol > epinephrine > norepinephrine was found; these receptors were designated α- and β-adrenergic receptors, respectively. The existence of separate receptors for the same hormone allows the hormone to have different effects, depending on the preponderance of each receptor in the tissue. Thus norepinephrine contracts pulmonary vessels because α-receptors predominate, but causes relaxation of airways because β-receptors outnumber α-receptors.

With the development of specific blockers it became possible to differentiate further subtypes of each receptor. Thus β-receptors were differentiated into β_1-receptors, which mediate cardiac stimulation and lipolysis, and β_2-receptors, mediating relaxation of smooth muscle in bronchi, vessels, and uterus (Lands et al., 1967). The existence of these subtypes was subsequently confirmed by radioligand binding studies, and there are probably two distinct molecular structures (Stiles et al., 1984). Similarly, with the development of selective blocking drugs α-adrenoceptors have now been subclassified into α_1- and α_2-subtypes, muscarinic receptors into M_1- and M_2-receptors, and histamine receptors into H_1- and H_2-receptors. Although the biological significance of these receptor subtypes is not always clear, they usually subserve different physiological functions. As an example β_1- and α_1-receptors are probably regulated by the neurotransmitter norepinephrine, whereas β_2- and α_2-receptors may be regulated by the circulating catecholamine epinephrine (Ariëns and Simonis, 1983) (Fig. 2).

II. Autonomic Receptors

A. Autonomic Control of Airways

Autonomic innervation of the airways is complex (Nadel and Barnes, 1984). In addition to classic cholinergic pathways that cause bronchoconstriction and adrenergic mechanisms which are usually bronchodilator, there is a more recently recognized component of autonomic control that is neither cholinergic nor adrenergic (Barnes, 1984c). These nervous pathways influence airway tone by activating specific receptors (Fig. 3, Table 1). In the case of cholinergic pathways, acetylcholine released from postganglionic nerve endings stimulates muscarinic cholinergic receptors on target cells. Adrenergic mechanisms include sympathetic nerves, which release norepinephrine, and circulating epinephrine secreted from the adrenal medulla. These catecholamines activate α- or β-adrenoceptors on target cells. The neurotransmitter of the nonadrenergic noncholinergic (NANC) nervous system is not certain, but the most likely candidate for the inhibitory nervous system is vasoactive intestinal polypeptide (VIP), whereas that of noncholinergic excitatory nerves is probably substance P or a related peptide. These neuropeptides interact with specific receptors on target cells.

The different components of the autonomic nervous system interact with each other in a complex way, both by affecting release of neurotransmitter (via presynaptic receptors), at ganglia in the airways, and by interaction at postsynaptic receptors. Thus airway tone may be determined by a complex interplay between different components of the autonomic nervous system.

B. Autonomic Abnormalities in Asthma

Because asthma is characterized by exaggerated bronchoconstrictor responses to a wide variety of apparently unrelated stimuli, this has suggested that there

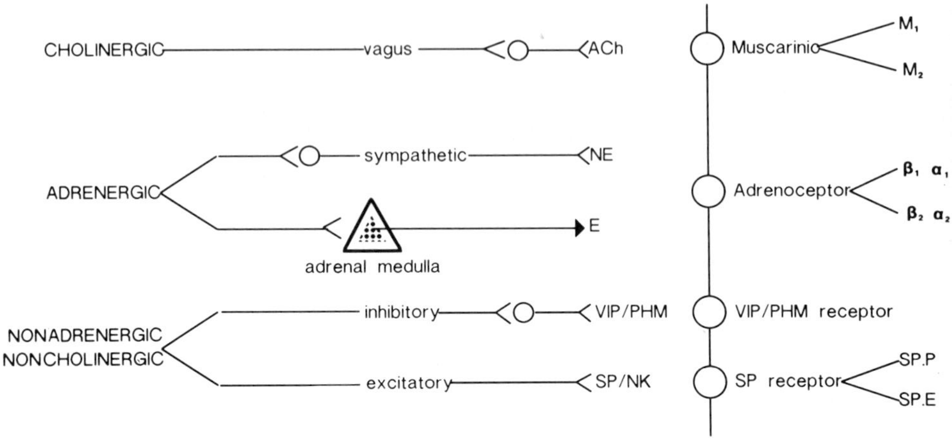

Figure 3 Autonomic innervation and receptors in airways. Cholinergic nerves release acetylcholine (ACh), sympathetic nerves norepinephrine (NE), and the adrenal medulla epinephrine (E). The nonadrenergic inhibitory nerves probably release vasoactive intestinal peptide (VIP) and peptide histidine methionine (PHM). Noncholinergic excitatory nerves may release substance P (SP) or neurokinins (NK), acting on the two types of SP receptor.

may be an abnormality in either airway smooth muscle or its control. Recent studies of airway smooth muscle from nonasthmatic patients show no correlation between in vivo and in vitro reactivity to histamine (Armour et al., 1984), suggesting that bronchial hyperreactivity at least in COPD cannot be explained by an abnormality of airway smooth muscle, and suggest that the defect is more likely to be in autonomic control. This might be due to an exaggeration of excitatory mechanisms (cholinergic, α-adrenergic, or noncholinergic excitatory) or a deficiency in inhibitory mechanisms (β-adrenergic or nonadrenergic inhibitory) (Nadel and Barnes, 1984) (Fig. 4). Many studies have now examined the possibility that autonomic receptor function may be normal in asthma (Kaliner et al., 1982).

C. β-Adrenergic Receptors

Control

Sympathetic innervation of human airways is very scanty in contrast to the rich parasympathetic nerve supply. Histochemical studies have shown that adrenergic fibers supply submucosal glands, bronchial vessels, and airway ganglia, but there is little or no direct innervation of airway smooth muscle (Richardson,

Table 1 Autonomic Receptors of Airways

	β-Adrenergic	α-Adrenergic	Muscarinic	VIP	Substance P
Smooth muscle–large	relax+++	contract+	contract+++	relax+++	contract+
–small	relax+++	contract+	contract+	relax+	contract+
Submucosal gland	↑ secretion+	↑ secretion+	↑ secretion++	↑ secretion++	↑ secretion++
Airway epithelium	↑ secretion+	↑ secretion+	↑ secretion++	↑ secretion++	↑ secretion+
Clara cell	↑ secretion+	?	?	?	?
Mast cell	↓ secretion+++	↑ secretion ?	↑ secretion ?	↓ secretion ?	↑ secretion
Bronchial microvascular	↓ leak+	?	?	?	↑ leak++

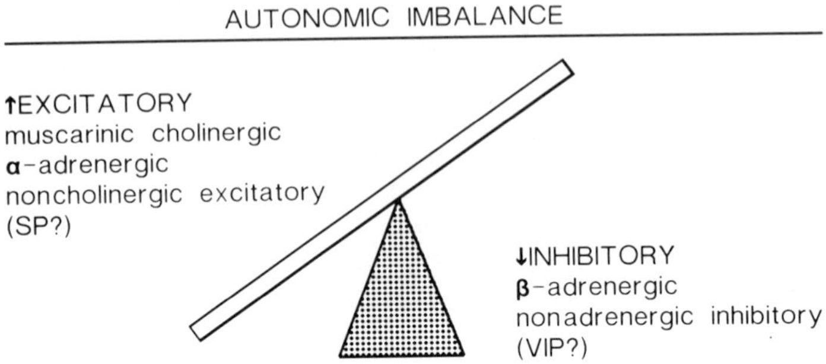

Figure 4 Autonomic receptor imbalance in asthma. Increased excitatory effects and/or lack of inhibitory effects tips the balance in favor of bronchoconstriction.

1979). This anatomical evidence is supported by functional studies in which nerves are activated by electrical field stimulation; in human airways in vitro there is a cholinergic contractile response and an inhibitory response that is not affected by adrenergic blockers (Richardson and Beland, 1976; Davis et al., 1982).

In normal subjects β-antagonists have no effect on airway function, indicating the tonic adrenergic influence, but in asthmatics they cause bronchoconstriction, suggesting that adrenergic mechanisms are important in counteracting bronchospasm. In the absence of functional sympathetic innervation, this suggests that circulating catecholamines exert this tonic influence. While norepinephrine has no significant effects within its physiological range, epinephrine has potent effects on airway and metabolic function. Surprisingly epinephrine concentrations are not elevated in asthmatic subjects, even during acute exacerbations, and the expected rise in epinephrine on exercise does not occur in asthmatics, suggesting that there may be a defect in epinephrine secretion in asthma (Barnes, 1983).

Localization and Function

Radioligand binding studies have demonstrated a high density of β-receptors in lung of many species, including humans (Rugg et al., 1979; Barnes et al., 1980c). More recent autoradiographic techniques have revealed that β-receptors are found on many different cell types within lung (Barnes et al., 1982a; Carstairs et al., 1984). β-Receptors are found in airway smooth muscle from all airways, as expected, since β-agonists are potent relaxants of bronchial smooth muscle, bronchioles, and peripheral lung strips (Goldie et al., 1982; Zaagsma et al., 1983).

β-Agonists also stimulate secretion of mucus in several species, including humans (Nadel et al., 1979; Phipps et al., 1982), resulting in a more viscous secretion by selective stimulation of mucous rather than serous cells in submucosal glands. Autoradiographic studies confirm a high density of β-receptors in airway glands (Barnes and Basbaum, 1983), with greater labeling of mucous cells. In addition, β-agonists stimulate ion transport across human airway epithelium in vitro (Knowles et al., 1984) and a high density of β-receptors is seen on airway epithelial cells. Thus β-agonists may increase mucus and water secretion into airways, which should result in increased mucociliary clearance, thereby reversing the deficit in clearance found in asthma (Pavia et al., 1980). Clara cells, which secrete a lipid into the airway and are present in human bronchiolar epithelium, are also stimulated by β-agonists (Massaro et al., 1981). Their function is not certain, but this secretion may function as an antiglue, preventing closure of small airways.

β-Agonists inhibit antigen-induced release of mast cell mediators from human lung fragments and isolated lung mast cells in vitro (Peters et al., 1982), suggesting the presence of inhibitory β-receptors on human mast cells. Whether this contributes to the bronchodilator effect of β-agonists in asthma is not certain, however. In vivo the infusion of epinephrine in asthmatic subjects lowers plasma histamine concentrations (Barnes et al., 1980b), and a β-agonist prevents the rise in plasma histamine after an antigen challenge (Holgate et al., 1984).

Histamine-induced microvascular leakiness in airways of guinea pigs is reduced by prior treatment with β-agonists, suggesting that β-receptors also regulate bronchial microvascular permeability (Persson et al., 1982). β-Agonists also modulate cholinergic neurotransmission in animals, either at the level of cholinergic ganglia or at postsynaptic nerve terminals (Skoogh, 1983).

β-Agonists therefore have several beneficial actions on airway obstruction. In addition to relaxing airway smooth muscle they also reduce release of mediators from mast cells, reduce cholinergic tone, and possibly reduce mucosal edema and increase clearance of airway mucus (Barnes, 1984a).

Subtypes

Although originally β-receptors of airway smooth muscle were classified as β_2-receptors (Lands et al., 1967), later studies showed that in several species relaxation of tracheal smooth muscle was intermediate between a β_1- and β_2-mediated response. This suggested the presence of β_1 in addition to β_2-receptors. Using direct receptor binding techniques and selective β-antagonists, the coexistence of β_1 and β_2 receptors was confirmed in animal and human lung (Rugg et al., 1979; Engel, 1981). In dog tracheal smooth muscle, while β_2 receptors predominate, 20% of receptors are of the β_1-subtype (Barnes et al., 1983b). Functional studies of the same tissue in vitro show that relaxation to exogenous β-agonists is mediated by β_2-receptors, but relaxation to sympathetic nerve stimulation is mediated by β_1-receptors. These findings are consistent with hypothesis that β_1-receptors are regulated by sympathetic nerves ("neuronal β-receptors), whereas β_2-receptors are regulated by circulating epinephrine ("hormonal β-receptors") (Ariëns and Simonis, 1983) (Fig. 2).

Further support for this data is provided by studies of airway β-receptor function in other species. Thus in guinea pig trachea, which has a sparse sympathetic innervation, mixed β_1- and β_2-responses are found, and binding studies show that approximately 15% of β-receptors are of the β_1-subtype (Carswell and Nahorski, 1983). In cat trachea, which has a dense sympathetic nerve supply, relaxation to β-agonists is mediated predominantly by β_1-receptors, whereas in lung strips containing bronchioles devoid of sympathetic nerves, responses are mediated by β_2-receptors (Lulich et al., 1976). In human airway smooth muscle, with its absence of significant sympathetic innervation, no β_1-receptor mediated effects would be expected. This has been confirmed in functional studies in vitro, in which relaxation of central and peripheral airways is mediated by β_2-receptors (Goldie et al., 1982; Zaagsma et al., 1983). Similarly prenalterol, a β_1-selective agonist, in vivo has no bronchodilator effect in asthmatic subjects, despite significant cardiac effects (Löfdahl and Svedmyr, 1982). Recent autoradiographic studies of human lung have confirmed that the β-receptors of human airway smooth muscle from bronchi to terminal bronchioles are entirely of the β_2-subtype (Carstairs et al., 1985).

Submucosal glands, which receive a sparse sympathetic nerve supply have a small population (10%) of β_1-receptors as expected, and functional studies show that mucus secretion is mediated by β_1 and β_2-receptors (Phipps et al., 1982). Epithelial β-receptors, which are not adrenergically innervated, are entirely of the β_2-subtype. It is remarkable that autoradiographic studies have shown that $>90\%$ of all β-receptors in lung are localized to alveolar walls (Barnes et al., 1982a; Carstairs et al., 1984). Surfactant secretion by type 2 pneumocytes is stimulated by β-agonists, but these cells make up only 7% of the alveolar wall; this must mean that β-receptors are located on capillary endothelial cells and/or type 1 pneumocytes. Approximately one-third of these alveolar receptors are of the β_1-subtype, which goes against the notion that β_1-receptors are always "innervated." The functional significance of these alveolar β-receptors is not yet established.

Function in Asthma

Because β-agonists reverse the bronchospasm in asthmatic airways it was logical to suggest that there might be a defect in β-receptor function underlying asthma (Szentivanyi, 1968). There is unlikely to be a fundamental defect in β-receptor function in asthma, however, since blockade of β-receptors does not produce asthma or bronchial hyperreactivity in normal individuals. There is still debate about whether there may be an impairment in β-receptor function in asthma secondary to the disease (reviewed in Barnes et al., 1984). A defect in β-receptors would not only apply to airway smooth muscle (tipping the balance in favor of cholinergic and possibly α-adrenergic constriction) but may also increase mediator release and increase bronchial wall edema.

Early studies showed that cardiovascular, metabolic, and leukocyte responses to β-agonists were impaired in asthmatic patients when compared with normal controls and that there was a decreased number of β-receptors on circulating leukocytes. These changes could be explained by tachyphylaxis as a result of prior adrenergic therapy. Studies of β-receptor function in untreated asthmatics are conflicting. Some studies show no significant differences compared with normal subjects, whereas others show impaired cardiovascular or metabolic responses to β-agonists, although the magnitude of these changes is very small. It has been suggested that the cause of this impairment of β-receptor function might be autoantibodies to β_2-receptors (Venter et al., 1980) but this seems unlikely since these antibodies have been detected in only a small proportion of asthmatic patients and also occur in normal subjects. After antigen challenge, asthmatics show a reduction in leukocyte β-receptor numbers and responses, suggesting that any defect in β-receptors might be secondary to the disease (Meurs et al., 1982).

Studies of cardiovascular, metabolic, and leukocyte β-receptors may not reflect an abnormality of airway β-receptors. It has been difficult to determine whether airway β-receptor function is impaired in asthma however. No significant difference in bronchodilator dose-responses to inhaled β-agonist was found in mild asthmatics (Harvey and Tattersfield, 1979), but more severe asthmatics appeared less sensitive to β-agonists (Barnes and Pride, 1983). This could be explained by functional antagonism due to greater initial bronchoconstriction, rather than a defect in β-receptor, function per se. Some of the difficulties encountered in vivo may be overcome by studying β-receptors in isolated airways, but asthmatic tissue is only rarely available. In three asthmatics who died during an attack, an apparent reduction in isoproterenol responsiveness was found (Paterson et al., 1982), although in another study no impairment in β-receptor responses could be measured (Svedmyr et al., 1976).

Because airway β-receptor function has been difficult to study in asthma, various animal models have been used, although none closely mimics human disease. In the Basenji greyhound, a crossbreed with bronchial hyperreactivity, impaired leukocyte β-receptor function has been found (Peters et al., 1981). In a guinea pig model of asthma, while a 20% reduction in pulmonary β-receptor density was found, there was no change in β-agonist-induced adenylate cyclase activation, suggesting no significant functional defect (Barnes et al., 1980a).

Whether β-receptor function is impaired in asthma is not yet determined, but such a defect is probably of little clinical significance, since asthmatics bronchodilate so readily to β-agonists. The apparent failure of asthmatics to respond to β-agonists during acute exacerbations is more likely to be explained by luminal mucus plugging. In one such patient who died, the airways were subsequently found to respond normally to β-agonists in vitro (Svedmyr et al., 1976).

Tolerance

There is considerable controversy over the occurrence and importance of β-receptor tolerance or tachyphylaxis (Jenne, 1982). Tachyphylaxis circulatory and metabolic responses to β-agonists is readily produced in asthmatic and normal subjects. Tachyphylaxis has been demonstrated in vivo in canine airways (Stephan et al., 1980), accompanied by a reduction both in β-receptor density ("down-regulation") and a fall in the proportion of receptors in a high-affinity state (Brown et al., 1986). In human airways the concentration of β-agonist required to produce desensitization is high and the degree of tachyphylaxis variable (Davis and Conolly, 1980). In vivo β-agonist tolerance has been demonstrated in normal subjects in some studies (Holgate et al., 1977) but not in others (Higgs et al., 1982). In asthmatic subjects there is no convincing evidence for tolerance to β-agonists when they are given over prolonged periods of times in conventional dosages. The reasons why the airways are spared from the development of tolerance is not known, but may be related to the presence of "spare receptors."

Steroids and β-Receptor Function

Corticosteroids modify β-receptor function, but it is unlikely that this contributes significantly to their therapeutic effect in asthma. In vitro steroids potentiate the effects of β-agonists on bronchial smooth muscle and prevent the development of tachyphylaxis (Mackenzie, 1982). In vivo steroids reverse tolerance to inhaled β-agonists in dogs (Stephan et al., 1980) and in normal humans (Holgate et al., 1977).

The mechanism by which steroids affect β-receptor expression has been investigated by radioligand binding. Steroids increase the density of β-receptors in rat lung (Mano et al., 1979), and this may involve the synthesis of new β-receptor protein (Fraser and Venter, 1980). Steroids increase the proportion of β-receptors in the high-affinity binding state in human leukocytes (Davis et al., 1982), and reverse the fall in β-receptors after exposure to β-agonists in leukocytes of normal and asthmatic subjects (Hui et al., 1982). Steroids could play a beneficial role in asthma by preventing or reversing β-receptor desensitization. Clinically significant desensitization has not clearly been demonstrated in asthmatics with conventional doses of β-agonists, but whether it might occur with the higher doses given by nebulizer is not known. If so, steroids might prevent this potential problem.

D. α-Adrenoceptors

Localization and Function

α-Receptors that mediate contraction of airway smooth muscle have been demonstrated in many species, including humans (Kneussl and Richardson, 1978), although it may only be possible to demonstrate their presence under certain conditions. Human peripheral lung strips contract with α-agonists, although it is likely that contractile elements other than airway smooth muscle are responsible (Black et al., 1981). Autoradiographic studies confirm a very low density of α_1-receptors in smooth muscle of large airways, but have revealed surprisingly high density in small airways (Barnes et al., 1983a).

α-Agonists stimulate mucus secretion and α_1-receptors have been demonstrated autoradiographically on serous cells of submucosal glands (Barnes and Basbaum, 1983). α-Agonists also facilitate mediator release from human lung fragments (Kaliner et al., 1972), although others have failed to confirm this finding.

Subtypes

As with β-receptors, two subtypes of α-receptor have now been recognized with the development of selective α-agonists (Hoffman and Lefkowitz, 1980). The classic α-receptor-mediating contractile effect is known as an α_1-receptor and selectively blocked by prazosin, whereas presynaptic α-receptors mediating negative feedback of norepinephrine release and selectively blocked by yohimbine are termed α_2-receptors. More recently α_2-receptors have also been found postsynaptically. It was suggested that α_1-receptors were regulated physiologically by norepinephrine and α_2-receptors by epinephrine (Fig. 2), but there is now little evidence to support this. There have been few studies on α-receptor subtypes in airways; in dog tracheal smooth muscle the contractile response to both sympathetic nerve stimulation and to exogenous α-agonists is mediated almost entirely by α_2-receptors, and the majority of α-receptors measured by radioligand binding in the same tissue are of this subtype (Barnes et al., 1983d).

Function in Asthma

There is some evidence that α-adrenergic responses may be increased in asthma and may therefore contribute to bronchial hyperreactivity. The α-agonist methoxamine causes bronchoconstriction in asthmatic but not in normal subjects (Snashall et al., 1978), even in the absence of β-blockade (Black et al., 1982).

This suggests that α-adrenergic responses are increased in the airways of asthmatics, and there is even evidence for α-adrenergic hyperresponsiveness in pupillary and vascular responses in asthmatics (Henderson et al., 1979).

No α-adrenergic response can be demonstrated in normal canine or human airway smooth muscle in vitro, even after β-blockade, but a marked α-adrenergic contractile response is seen with diseased human airways or pretreatment of normal canine airways with histamine or serotonin (Kneussl and Richardson, 1978; Barnes et al., 1983c), suggesting an activation of α-adrenergic responses by mediators or disease. This is not an artifact of the in vitro situation, since similar activation of α-adrenergic responses can also be demonstrated in dogs in vivo Brown et al., 1983). This suggests that inflammatory mediators may "turn on" α-adrenergic mechanisms in asthma. The mechanism for this activation does not involve any change in airway α-receptor density or affinity, and is likely to be a postreceptor mechanism, possibly involving voltage-dependent calcium channels (Barnes et al., 1983c). In the guinea pig model of asthma there is an increase in lung α_1-receptors (Barnes et al., 1980a), but no increased α-adrenergic responsiveness has been found in airway smooth muscle (Turner et al., 1983).

If exaggerated α-responses were an important factor in bronchial hyperreactivity, then α-blockers should be beneficial in asthma. α-Antagonists, such as phentolamine and thymoxamine, have been shown to inhibit bronchoconstriction induced by histamine, allergen, and exercise, but such drugs lack specificity and their protective effects may be explained by other pharmacologic actions such as antihistamine activity (Barnes, 1984b). The specific α_1-blocker prazosin given by inhalation has no bronchodilator effect in asthmatics, who readily bronchodilate with a β-agonist, suggesting that α-hyperresponsiveness does not contribute to resting bronchomotor tone in asthma (Barnes et al., 1981a). Similarly, prazosin has no effect on histamine-induced bronchoconstriction, but has a weak protective effect against exercise-induced bronchospasm (Barnes et al., 1981b), suggesting that under some circumstances α-receptor activation may contribute to bronchoconstriction, but it is unlikely to be of major significance. The effects of specific α_2-blockers on airway function have not yet been reported.

E. Cholinergic Receptors

Localization and Function

In normal human airways there is a small amount of resting tone due to vagal motor activity with release of acetylcholine in the vicinity of airway smooth muscle. This suggests that cholinergic mechanisms might be exaggerated in asthma. Acetylcholine causes contraction of airway smooth muscle by activating muscarinic receptors, which are blocked by atropine. The mechanisms by which occupation of muscarinic receptors causes contraction of smooth muscle is not certain, but evidence is now accumulating that the breakdown of phosphatidylinositol in the cell membrane is involved in triggering the release of intracellular calcium ions (Baron et al., 1984). The receptors involved in cholinergic neurotransmission through airway ganglia are nicotinic and blocked by hexamethonium. Ganglion blockers should therefore produce bronchodilatation by blocking tonic vagal ganglionic neurotransmission, but in practice these drugs are not useful since they affect ganglia in other systems such as the cardiovascular system, leading to profound hypotension.

Direct receptor binding studies have demonstrated a high density of muscarinic receptors in smooth muscle of large airways (Murlas et al., 1982), and this has been confirmed autoradiographically (Barnes et al., 1983). The density of muscarinic receptors decreases as airways become smaller, so that terminal bronchioles are almost devoid of muscarinic receptors (Barnes et al., 1983). This is consistent with physiological studies in dogs using tantalum bronchography, showing that vagal stimulation has a marked effect on large airways but little effect on bronchioles (Nadel et al., 1971). In humans anticholinergic drugs have more effect on large than on small airways, as measured by helium-oxygen flow-volume curves, whereas β-agonists relax all airways (McFadden et al., 1977).

Vagus nerve stimulation and cholinergic agonists are potent at causing mucus secretion in animals and humans (Nadel et al., 1979; Baker et al., 1985) and submucosal glands have a high density of muscarinic receptors. Cholinergic agonists are also reported to stimulate histamine secretion from human lung fragments (Kaliner et al., 1972), suggesting that there may be muscarinic receptors on human lung mast cells.

Muscarinic Receptor Subtypes

There is now evidence from binding and functional studies that muscarinic receptors may be subclassified into at least two types, based on the development of selective blocking drugs such as pirenzipine (Hammer et al., 1980). In the gut M_1-receptors, which are selectively blocked by pirenzipine, are localized to nerve terminals and ganglia, whereas M_2-receptors are localized to smooth muscle. The functional significance of muscarinic receptor subtypes in airways has not yet been determined.

F. Nonadrenergic Noncholinergic Receptors

The demonstration that there is a third component of the autonomic nervous system in airways is of considerable interest, particularly since it may function abnormally in airway disease (Richardson, 1981; Barnes, 1984c). A nonadrenergic inhibitory nervous pathway has been found in airways of several species, and in human airways it is the only inhibitory nervous mechanism (Richardson and Beland, 1976; Davis et al., 1982). In guinea pigs a noncholinergic excitatory pathway has also been described (Anderson and Gundström, 1983).

Nonadrenergic Inhibitory Receptors

The neurotransmitter of nonadrenergic inhibitory nerves is not yet certain, but VIP is the most likely candidate (Said, 1982). VIP-immunoreactive nerves are found in human airways (Dey et al., 1981) and VIP is a potent relaxant of isolated human bronchi, mimicking the effect of nonadrenergic nerve stimulation (Palmer et al., 1985). In guinea pig and bovine trachea VIP is released on nonadrenergic nerve stimulation (Matsuzaki et al., 1980; Cameron et al., 1983). A closely related peptide, peptide histidine isoleucine (PHI) and in humans peptide histidine methionine (PHM) coexists with VIP in airway curves (Lundberg et al., 1984), and is equipotent with VIP in causing relaxation of human airways (Palmer et al., 1985). Both VIP and PHM activate specific receptors, which have been identified in homogenized lung by direct binding techniques (Robberech et al., 1981). Activation of these peptide receptors stimulates adenylate cyclase to increase intracellular cyclic AMP (Frandsen et al., 1978).

VIP also stimulates mucus secretion and fluid transport across airway epithelium (Peatfield et al., 1983; Nathanson et al., 1983). Immunocytochemical studies have demonstrated that VIP increases the cyclic AMP content in submucosal glands, airway epithelium, and airway smooth muscle, indicating the presence of VIP receptors on these cells (Lazarus et al., 1985).

VIP and PHM appear to coexist with acetylcholine in airway vagal nerves, and these peptides may therefore interact functionally with cholinergic mechanisms. In salivary glands VIP increases the affinity of muscarinic receptors (Lundberg et al., 1982), but in airway smooth muscle VIP is a functional antagonist of acetylcholine and has no effect on muscarinic receptors.

Noncholinergic Excitatory Receptors

Electrical stimulation of the vagus causes bronchoconstriction in guinea pigs that is not entirely blocked by atropine (Anderson and Gundström, 1983) but is blocked by a substance P antagonist (Lundberg et al., 1983). Substance P is localized to afferent nerves in the airway and may be released by antidromic conduction. Substance P causes contraction of airway smooth muscle, increased mucus secretion, mucosal edema, and may increase mediator release from mast cells. Its actions are produced by stimulation of specific substance P receptors. Using a series of related peptides (tachykinins) isolated from nonmammalian species, it has been possible to differentiate at least two types of substance P receptor. For SP.P receptors substance P is more potent than the peptides physalaemin and eledoisin, whereas for SP.E receptors eledoisin is more potent than substance P. In airway smooth muscle the receptors appear to be SP.E subtype (Karlsson et al., 1984), whereas the receptor-mediating mast cell mediator release in skin is probably of the SP.P subtype (Foreman et al., 1983). Recently endogenous tachykinins, which are active at SP.E receptors (neurokinin A and B), have been isolated from mammalian tissues (Kangawa et al., 1983), and more potently contract airway smooth muscle than substance P.

III. Mediator Receptors

Several inflammatory mediators have now been implicated in asthma, although certain evidence of their contribution to asthmatic bronchoconstriction is often lacking. These mediators have several actions on the airways that contribute to bronchial obstruction, including contraction of airway smooth muscle, mucus hypersecretion, chemotaxis of inflammatory cells, which themselves then release further mediators (Table 2). The cellular origin of the various mediators is uncertain. Mast cells, macrophages, eosinophils, and neutrophils are all probably involved. Mediators produce their effects by activating specific receptors on target cells in the airway and there is increasing information about the characteristics of these receptors and their antagonism. Because many mediators are involved in asthma it seems unlikely that antagonism of a single mediator receptor will produce significant clinical benefit. Furthermore there is likely to be complex interaction between the different mediators. Preliminary evidence suggests that some mediators, such as prostaglandin D_2, potentiate the effects of other mediators such as histamine and methacholine (Fuller et al., 1985).

A. Histamine Receptors

Histamine produces its effects by activation of two types of receptor, termed H_1 and H_2 receptors. Inhaled histamine causes bronchoconstriction in vivo and contraction of large and small human airways in vitro by activating H_1-receptors, which are antagonized by the classic antihistamines such as chlorpheniramine (White and Eiser, 1983; Persson and Ekman, 1976). Studies with radiolabeled H_1-antagonists have demonstrated a high density of H_1-receptors in guinea pig lung, but these receptors have not yet been localized (Carswell and Nahorski, 1982). In human airways there is little evidence for H_2-receptor-mediated bronchodilatation, as has been reported in other species (White and Eiser, 1983; Braude et al., 1984). Histamine increases airway mucosal edema by an H_1-mediated contraction of bronchial vein endothelial cells, thus increasing microvascular permeability (Persson et al., 1982). Histamine also increases bronchial mucus production in human airways by an H_2-mediated effect (Shelhammer et al., 1980), and increases lung epithelial permeability (and therefore perhaps airway mucosal permeability) via H_2-receptors (Braude et al., 1984). Antihistamines have been disappointing in asthma, and even in high doses given by inhalation have little protective effect against various bronchial challenges, presumably because other mediators are involved.

B. Leukotriene Receptors

There is now good evidence that leukotriene B_4 and the sulfidopeptide leukotrienes C_4, D_4, and E_4 (which comprise slow-reacting substance of anaphylaxis) are involved in asthmatic bronchoconstriction (Lewis and Austen, 1984). There

Table 2 Mediator Receptors in Airways

Mediator	Receptor	SM Muscle	Mucus secretion	Permeability	Chemotaxis
Histamine	H_1	++	-	++	+
	H_2	-	+	+	-
Leukotrienes	LTB_4	-	-	-	+++
	LTC_4				
	LTD_4	+++	+++	+++	-
Prostaglandins	PGF_2a				
	PGD_2	++	++	+	+
	PGE_2				
	Thromboxane	++	?	?	?
	PGI_2	-	-	-	-
Adenosine	A_1	+ (2°?)	?	+	+
	A_2	-	?	-	-
Platelet-activating factor	PAF	++ (2°)	?	+++ (2°)	++
Bradykinin	Bradykinin	++ (2°)	?	++	?

is increasing evidence that they produce their effects by activating specific and probably distinct receptors. LTB_4 has potent chemotactic activity, particularly for neutrophils and, using $[^3H]LTB_4$-specific binding sites, have been identified on human neutrophils (Goldman and Goetzl, 1982). Functional studies with LTC_4 and LTD_4 indicate that there are probably discrete receptors for each leukotriene and the leukotriene antagonist FPL 55712 appears to inhibit the LTD_4 receptor selectively. This is confirmed by binding studies that show specific, stereoselective and distinct binding sites for $[^3H]LTC_4$ and $[^3H]LTD_4$ in guinea pig lung membranes (Bruns et al., 1983) and autoradiographic studies have indicated that the receptors are differentially distributed (Barnes et al., 1985). The sulfopeptide leukotrienes are potent bronchoconstrictors in human airways in vivo and in vitro, with an order of potency $LTD_4 > LTC_4 > LTE_4$ (Lewis and Austen 1984). They are also potent stimulants of mucus secretion in human airways in vitro (Marom et al., 1981) and produce microvascular leakiness and marked bronchial edema in guinea pigs.

C. Prostaglandin Receptors

Several prostaglandins have effects on airways, although their role in asthma is uncertain since inhibition of cyclo-oxygenase (by drugs such as aspirin and indomethacin), which blocks their synthesis, usually has no effect on asthma. However, a few individuals (estimated at 5% of all asthmatics) develop bronchoconstriction, suggesting that prostaglandins may be beneficial in these individuals. Prostaglandin receptors have not been well characterized since no specific blockers are available. Specific prostacyclin receptors have been identified in guinea pig lung by radioligand binding, although they are probably localized to vascular rather than to airway tissues (MacDermot et al., 1981). Prostaglandin D_2 (the major prostaglandin produced by human lung mast cells) and $PGF_2\alpha$ are both potent bronchoconstrictors of human airways, whereas PGE_2 is a bronchodilator. These prostaglandins presumably produce their effects by activating specific receptors on airway smooth muscle. Thromboxane A_2, which is also a cyclo-oxygenase product, is also a potent bronchoconstrictor that activates specific receptors, for which selective antagonists have recently been developed. Prostaglandins have a variety of other actions on the respiratory tract including mucus secretion (Marom et al., 1981), bronchial edema formation, and chemotaxis.

D. Adenosine Receptors

Adenosine is produced under conditions of hypoxia and its concentration increases in plasma after antigen challenge (Mann et al., 1983). At least two specific adenosine receptors have been recognized, with the development of a series of adenosine analogs (Londos et al., 1980). A_1-receptors are usually excitatory and associated with a fall in intracellular cyclic AMP, whereas A_2-receptors are inhibitory and associated with a rise in cyclic AMP. Adenosine given by inhalation causes bronchoconstriction in asthmatic subjects (Cushley et al., 1983), but has little effect on isolated human airways in vitro (Finney et al., 1985), suggesting that its bronchoconstrictor action is indirect, possibly involving a reflex mechanism. Adenosine may potentiate mast cell mediator release, probably via an A_2-receptor. Theophylline is a specific antagonist of both A_1 and A_2-receptors at concentrations within its therapeutic range, but there is compelling evidence against this as its mechanism of bronchodilatation (Persson, 1986).

E. Other Mediator Receptors

Platelet-activating factor (PAF) is a potent bronchoconstrictor in animals, producing its effects by causing release of factors (predominantly thromboxane) from platelets and probably also from other cells such as neutrophils. Specific receptors for PAF have been identified in human neutrophils (Valone and Goetzl, 1983) and specific antagonists have been developed.

Bradykinin is generated in inflammatory processes by the action of an enzyme, kallikrein, on a plasma kininogen. Bradykinin has potent bronchoconstrictor effects and may activate specific bradykinin receptors, which have been identified in other tissues by radioligand binding (Odya et al., 1980). Bradykinin is also potent at causing bronchial edema.

IV. Conclusions

Airway caliber is determined by a balance between many constrictor and dilator agents, which bring about their effects on the various target cells of the airway by activating specific cell surface receptors. Bronchodilator drugs can be viewed in terms of their interaction with these receptors, either stimulating dilator receptors (e.g., β-agonists), or inhibiting constrictor receptors (e.g., muscarinic antagonists). Airway receptors can be classified into receptors mediating the effects of the autonomic nervous control of the airways (autonomic receptors) and receptors mediating the effects of the various mediators that may be generated in asthma. Recently, there has been a great increase in our understanding of the properties of these receptors. This not only throws light on the mechanism of action of existing bronchodilators, but may also lead to the development of novel classes of bronchodilator drug in the future.

References

Ahlquist, R. P. (1948). A study of the adrenotropic receptors. *Am. J. Physiol. 153*: 586-600.

Anderson, R. G. G., and Grundström, N. (1983). The excitatory non-cholinergic, non-adrenergic nervous system of the guinea-pig airways. *Eur. J. Respir. Dis. 64 (Suppl. 131)*: 141-157.

Ariëns, E. J., and Simonis, A. M. (1983). Physiological and pharmacological aspects of adrenergic receptor classification. *Biochem. Pharmacol. 32*: 1539-1545.

Armour, C. L., Lazar, N. M., Schellenberg, R. R., Taylor, S. M., Chan, N., Hogg, J. C., and Pare, P. D. (1984). A comparison of in vivo and in vitro human airway reactivity to histamine. *Am. Rev. Respir. Dis. 129*: 907-910.

Avner, C. P., and Jenne, J. W. (1981). Desensitization of isolated human bronchial smooth muscle to beta-receptor agonists. *J. Allergy Clin. Immunol. 68*: 51-57.

Baker, B., Peatfield, A. C., and Richardson, P. S. (1985). The nervous control of mucus secretion from human bronchus. *J. Physiol. 365*: 297-305.

Barnes, P. J. (1983). Endogenous plasma adrenaline in asthma. *Eur. J. Respir. Dis. 64*: 559-563.

Barnes, P. J. (1984a). Beta-adrenoceptors in lung tissue. In *Beta Adrenoceptors in Asthma.* Edited by J. Morley. London, Academic Press, pp. 67-90.

Barnes, P. J. (1984b). Adrenergic receptors of normal and asthmatic airways. *Eur. J. Respir. Dis. 65* (suppl. 135) 72-79.

Barnes, P. J. (1984c). The third nervous system in the lung: physiology and clinical perspectives. *Thorax 39*: 561-567.

Barnes, P. J., and Basbaum, C. B. (1983). Mapping of adrenergic receptors in mammalian trachea using an autoradiographic method. *Exp. Lung Res. 5*: 183-192.

Barnes, P. J., and Pride, N. B. (1983). Dose-response curves to inhaled beta-adrenergic agonists in normal and asthmatic subjects. *Br. J. Clin. Pharmacol. 15*: 677-682.

Barnes, P. J., Dollery, C. T., and MacDermot, J. (1980a). Increased pulmonary alpha-adrenergic receptors in experimental asthma. *Nature 285*: 569-571.

Barnes, P. J., Fitzgerald, G., Brown, M., and Dollery, C. (1980b). Nocturnal asthma and changes in circulating epinephrine, histamine and cortisol. *N. Engl. J. Med. 303*: 263-267.

Barnes, P. J., Karliner, J. S., and Dollery, C. T. (1980c). Human lung adrenoceptors studied by radioligand binding. *Clin. Sci. 58*: 457-461.

Barnes, P. J., Ind, P. W., and Dollery, C. T. (1981a). Inhaled prazosin in asthma. *Thorax 36*: 378-381.

Barnes, P. J., Basbaum, C. B., Nadel, J. A., and Roberts, J. M. (1982a). Localization of beta-adrenoceptors in mammalian lung by light microscopic autoradiography. *Nature 299*: 444-447.

Barnes, P. J., Nadel, J. A., Roberts, J. M., and Basbaum, C. B. (1982b). Muscarinic receptors in lung and trachea: autoradiographic localization using [^{3}H] quinuclidinyl benzilate. *Eur. J. Pharmacol. 86*: 103-106.

Barnes, P. J., Basbaum, C. B., and Nadel, J. A. (1983a). Autoradiographic localization of autonomic receptors in airway smooth muscle: marked differences between large and small airways. *Am. Rev. Respir. Dis. 127*: 758-762.

Barnes, P. J., Nadel, J. A., Skoogh, B-E., and Roberts, J. M. (1983b). Characterization of beta adrenoceptor subtypes in canine airway smooth muscle by radioligand binding and physiological responses. *J. Pharmacol. Exp. Ther. 225*: 456-461.

Barnes, P. J., Skoogh, B-E., Brown, J. R., and Nadel, J. A. (1983c). Activation of alpha-adrenergic responses in tracheal smooth muscle: a post-receptor mechanism. *J. Appl. Physiol. 54*: 1469-1476.

Barnes, P. J., Skoogh, B-E., Nadel, J. A., and Roberts, J. M. (1983d). Postsynaptic alpha$_2$-adrenoceptors predominant over alpha$_1$-adrenoceptors in canine tracheal smooth muscle and mediate neuronal and hormonal alpha-adrenergic contraction. *Mol. Pharmacol. 23*: 570-575.

Barnes, P. J., Ind., P. W., and Dollery, C. T. (1984). Beta-adrenoceptors in asthma and their response to agonists. In *Asthma: Physiology, Immunopharmacology and Treatment.* Edited by A. B. Kay, K. F. Austen, and L. M. Lichtenstein. London, Academic Press, pp. 339-358.

Barnes, P. J., Carstairs, J. R., Norman, P., and Abram, T. S. (1985). Autoradiographic localization of leukotriene receptors in guinea pig lung and trachea. *Am. Rev. Respir. Dis. 131*: A29.

Baron, C. B., Cunningham, M., Strauss, J. F., and Coburn, R. F. (1984). Pharmacomechanical coupling in smooth muscle may involve phosphatidylinositol metabolism. *Proc. Natl. Acad. Sci. USA 82*: 6899-6903.

Black, J., Turner, A., and Shaw, J. (1981). Alpha-adrenoceptors in human peripheral lung. *Eur. J. Pharmacol. 72*: 83-86.

Black, J. L., Salome, C. M., Yan, K., and Shaw, J. (1982). Comparison between airways response to an alpha-adrenoceptor agonist and histamine in asthmatic and non-asthmatic subjects. *Br. J. Clin. Pharmacol. 14*: 464-465.

Braude, S., Royston, D., Coe, C., and Barnes, P. J. (1984). Histamine increases lung permeability by an H$_2$-receptor mechanism. *Lancet 2*: 372-374.

Brown, J. K., Shields, R., Jones, C., and Gold, W. M. (1983). Augmentation of alpha-adrenergic responsiveness in tracheitis muscle of living dogs. *J. Appl. Physiol. 54*: 1558-1566.

Brown, J. K., Jones, C. A., Walters, E. H., Barnes, P. J., Nadel, J. A., and Roberts, J. M. (1986). Isoproterenol down regulates beta-adrenergic receptors in airway smooth muscle. *Am. Rev. Respir. Dis.* (in press).

Bruns, R. T., Thomsen, W. J., and Pugsley, T. A. (1983). Binding of leukotrienes C_4 and D_4 to membranes from guinea pig lung: Regulation by ions and guanine nucleotides. *Life Sci. 33*: 645-653.

Cameron, A. R., Johnston, C. F., Kirkpatrick, C. T., and Kirkpatrick, M. C. A. (1983). The quest for the inhibitory neurotransmitter in bovine tracheal smooth muscle. *Q. J. Exp. Physiol. 68*: 413-426.

Carstairs, J. R., Nimmo, A. J., and Barnes, P. J. (1984). Autoradiographic localisation of beta-adrenoceptors in human lung. *Eur. J. Pharmacol. 103*: 189-190.

Carstairs, J. R., Nimmo, A. J., and Barnes, P. J. (1985). Autoradiographic visualization of beta-adrenoceptor subtypes in human lung. *Am. Rev. Respir. Dis. 132*: 541-547.

Carswell, H., and Nahorski, S. R. (1982). Distribution and characteristics of histamine H_1-receptors in guinea-pig airways identified by [^{3}H] mepyramine. *Eur. J. Pharmacol. 81*: 301-307.

Carswell, H., and Nahorski, S. R. (1983). Beta-adrenoceptor heterogeneity in guinea-pig airways: comparison of functional and receptor labelling studies. *Br. J. Pharmacol. 79*: 965-971.

Cushley, M. J., Tattersfield, A. E., and Holgate, S. T. (1983). Inhaled adrenosine and guanosine on airway resistance in normal and asthmatic subjects. *Br. J. Clin. Pharmacol. 15*: 161-165.

Davis, C., and Connolly, M. E. (1980). Tachyphylaxis to beta-adrenoceptor agonists in human bronchial smooth muscle: Studies in vitro. *Br. J. Clin. Pharmacol. 10*: 417-423.

Davis, A. O., and Lefkowitz, R. J. (1983). In vitro desensitization of beta-adrenergic receptors in human neutorphils. Attenuation by corticosteroids. *J. Clin. Invest. 71*: 565-571.

Davis, C., Kannan, M. S., Jones, T. R., and Daniel, E. E. (1982). Control of human airway smooth muscles: in vitro studies. *J. Appl. Physiol. 53*: 1080-1087.

Dey, R. D., Shannon, W. A., and Said, S. I. (1981). Localization of VIP-immunoreactive nerves in airways and pulmonary vessels of dogs, cats and human subjects. *Cell Tissue Res. 220*: 231-238.

Engel, G. (1981). Subclasses of beta-adrenoceptors—a quantitative estimation of $beta_1$- and $beta_2$-adrenoceptors in guinea pig and human lung. *Postgrad. Med. J. 57* (suppl. 1): 77-83.

Finney, M. J. B., Karlsson, J-A., and Persson, C. G. A. (1985). Effects of bronchoconstrictors and bronchodilators on a novel human small airway preparation. *Br. J. Pharmacol. 85*: 29-36.

Foreman, J. C., Jordan, C. C., Oehme, P., and Renner, H. (1983). Structure-activity relationships for some substance P-related peptides that cause wheal and flair reactions in human skin. *J. Physiol. 335*: 449-465.

Frandsen, E. K., Krishna, G. A., and Said, S. I. (1978). Vasoactive intestinal polypeptide promotes cyclic adenosine 3′, 5′ mono-phosphate accumulation in guinea pig trachea. *Br. J. Pharmacol. 62*: 367-369.

Fraser, C. M., and Venter, J. C. (1980). The synthesis of beta-adrenergic receptors in cultured human lung cells: induction by glucocorticoids. *Biochem. Biophys. Res. Commun. 94*: 390-397.

Fuller, R. W., Dixon, C. M. S., Dollery, C. T., and Barnes, P. J. (1985). Prostaglandin D_2 potentiates airway responses to histamine and methacholine. *Am. Rev. Respir. Dis. 133*: 252-254.

Goldie, R. G., Paterson, J. W., and Wale, J. L. (1982). A comparative study of beta-adrenoceptors in human and porcine lung parenchyma strip. *Br. J. Pharmacol. 76*: 523-526.

Goldman, D. W., and Goetzl, E. J. (1982). Specific binding of leukotriene B_4 to receptors on human polymorphonuclear leukocytes. *J. Immunol. 129*: 1600-1604.

Hammer, R., Berrie, C. P., Birdsall, N. J. M., Burgen, A. S. V., and Hulme, E. C. (1980). Pirenzipine distinguishes between different subclasses of muscarinic receptors. *Nature 283*: 90-92.

Harvey, J. E., and Tattersfield, A. E. (1979). Beta-adrenergic responsiveness in asthmatic and atopic non-asthmatic subjects. *Thorax 34*: 416-417.

Henderson, W. R., Shelhamer, J. H., and Reingold, D. B. (1979). Alpha-adrenergic hyperresponsiveness in asthma. *N. Engl. J. Med. 300*: 642-647.

Higgs, C. M. B., Richardson, R. B., and Laszlo, G. (1982). The effect of regular inhaled salbutamol on the airway responsiveness of normal subjects. *Clin. Sci. 63*: 513-517.

Hoffman, B. B., and Lefkowitz, R. J. (1980). Alpha-adrenergic receptor subtypes. *N. Engl. J. Med. 302*: 1390-1396.

Holgate, S. T., Baldwin, C. J., and Tattersfield, A. E. (1977). Beta-adrenergic agonist resistance in normal human airways. *Lancet 2*: 375-377.

Holgate, S. T., Church, M. K., Cushley, M. J., Robinson, C., Mann, J. S., and Howarth, P. H. (1984). Pharmacological modulation of airway calibre and mediator release in human models of bronchial asthma. In *Asthma III.* Edited by A. B. Kay, K. F. Austen, and L. M. Lichtenstein. London, Academic Press, pp. 391-413.

Hui, K. P., Conolly, M. E., and Tashkin, D. P. (1982). Reversal of human lymphocyte beta-adrenoceptor desensitization by glucocorticoids. *Clin. Pharmacol. Ther. 32*: 566-571.

Jenne, J. W. (1982). Whither beta-adrenergic tachyphylaxis? *J. Allergy Clin. Immunol. 70*: 413-416.

Kaliner, M., Orange, R. P., Austen, K. F. (1972). Immunological release of histamine and slow secreting substance of anaphylaxis from human lung. IV. Enhancement by cholinergic and alpha-adrenergic stimulation. *J. Exp. Med. 136*: 556-567.

Kaliner, M., Shelhamer, J., Davis, P. B., Smith, L. J., and Venter, J. C. (1982). Autonomic nervous system abnormalities and allergy. *Ann. Intern. Med. 96*: 349-357.

Kangawa, K., Minamino, N., Fukuda, A., and Hisayuki, M. (1983). Neuromedin K: a novel mammalian tachykinin identified in porcine spinal cord. *Biochem. Biophys. Res. Comm., 114*: 533-540.

Karlsson, J-A., Finney, M. J. B., Persson, C. G. A., and Post, C. (1984). Substance P antagonists and the role of tachykinins in non-cholinergic bronchoconstriction. *Life Sci. 35*: 2681-2691.

Kneussl, M. P., and Richardson, J. B. (1978). Alpha-adrenergic receptors in human and canine tracheal and bronchial smooth muscle. *J. Appl. Physiol. 45*: 307-311.

Knowles, M., Murray, G., Shallal, J., Askin, F., Ranga, V., Gatzy, J., and Boucher, P. (1984). Bioelectric properties and ion flow across excised human bronchi. *J. Appl. Physiol. 56*: 868-877.

Lands, A. M., Arnold, A., McAuliff, J. P., Luduena, F. P., and Brown, T. G. (1967). Differentiation of receptor systems activated by sympathomimetic amines. *Nature 214*: 597-598.

Lazarus, S. C., Basbaum, C. B., Barnes, P. J., and Gold, W. M. (1986). Mapping of VIP receptors by use of an immunocytochemical probe for the intracellular mediator cyclic AMP. *Am. J. Physiol.* (in press).

Lewis, R. A., and Austen, K. F. (1984). The biologically active leukotrienes. *J. Clin. Invest. 73*: 889-897.

Löfdahl, C-G., and Svedmyr, N. (1982). Effects of prenalterol in asthmatic patients. *Eur. J. Clin. Pharmacol. 23*: 297-303.

Londos, C., Cooper, D. M. F., and Wolff, J. (1980). Subclassification of external adenosine receptors. *Proc. Natl. Acad. Sci. USA 77*: 2551-2554.

Lulich, V. M., Mitchell, H. W., and Sparrow, M. P. (1976). The cat lung strip as an in vitro preparation of peripheral airways: A comparison of beta-adrenoceptor agonists, autocoids and anaphylactic challenge of the lung strip and trachea. *Br. J. Pharmacol. 58*: 71-79.

Lundberg, J. M., Hedlund, B., and Bartfai, T. (1982). Vasoactive intestinal polypeptide enhances muscarinic ligand binding in cat submandibular salivary gland. *Nature 295*: 147-149.

Lundberg, J. M., Martling, C-R., and Saria, A. (1983). Substance P and capsaicin-induced contraction of human bronchi. *Acta Physiol. Scand. 119*: 49-53.

Lundberg, J. M., Fahrenkrug, J., Hökfelt, T., Matling, C-R., Larsson, O., Tatemoto, K., and Anggard, A. (1984). Coexistence of peptide H_1 (PHI) and VIP in nerves regulating blood flow and bronchial smooth muscle tone in various mammals including man. *Peptides 5*: 593-606.

MacDermot, J., Barnes, P. J., Wadell, K., Dollery, C. T., and Blair, I. A. (1981). Prostaglandin binding to guinea pig pulmonary receptors. *Eur. J. Pharmacol. 68*: 127-130.

McFadden, E. R., Ingram, R. H., Haynes, R. L., and Wellman, J. J. (1977). Predominant site of flow limitation and mechanisms of post exertional asthma. *J. Appl. Physiol. 42*: 76-752.

Mackenzie, C. W. (1982). Dexamethasone inhibits isoproterenol desensitization of bovine tracheal strips. *Fed. Proc. 42*: 1048.

Mann, J. S., Renwick, A. G., and Holgate, S. T. (1983). Antigen bronchial provocation causes an increase in plasma adenosine levels in asthma. *Clin. Sci. 65*: 22P.

Mano, K., Akbarzadeh, A., and Townley, R. G. (1979). Effect of hydrocortisone on beta-adrenergic receptors in lung membranes. *Life Sci. 26*: 1925-1930.

Marom, Z., Shelhamer, J. H., and Kaliner, M. (1981). The effects of arachadonic acid, monohydroxyeicosatetranoic acid and prostaglandins on the release of mucous glycoproteins from human airways in vitro. *J. Clin. Invest. 67*: 1695-1703.

Massaro, G. O., Fischman, C. M., Chiang, M. J., Amado, C., and Massaro, D. (1981). Regulation of secretion in Clara cells. Studies using the isolated perfused lung. *J. Clin. Invest. 67*: 345-351.

Matsuzaki, Y., Hamasaki, Y., and Said, S. I. (1980). Vasoactive intestinal peptide: A possible transmitter of non-adrenergic relaxation of guinea pig airways. *Science 210*: 1252-1253.

Meurs, H., Koëter, G. H., De Vries, K., and Kauffman, H. F. (1982). The beta-adrenergic system and allergic bronchial asthma: changes in lymphocytes beta-adrenergic receptor number and adenylate cyclase activity after an allergen-induced attack. *J. Allergy Clin. Immunol. 70*: 272-280.

Murlas, C., Nadel, J. A., and Roberts, J. M. (1982). The muscarinic receptors of airway smooth muscle: their characterization in vitro. *J. Appl. Physiol. 52*: 1084-1091.

Nadel, J. A., and Barnes, P. J. (1984). Autonomic regulation of the airways. *Annu. Rev. Med. 35*: 451-467.

Nadel, J. A., Cabezas, G. A., and Austin, J. H. M. (1971). In vivo roentgenographic examination of parasympathetic innervation of small airways: use of powdered tantalum and a fine focal spot X-ray tube. *Invest. Radiol. 6*: 9-17.

Nadel, J. A., Davis, B., and Phipps, R. J. (1979). Control of mucus secretion and ion transport in airways. *Annu. Rev. Physiol. 41*: 369-381.

Nathanson, I., Widdicombe, J. H., and Barnes, P. J. (1983). Effect of vasoactive intestinal peptide across dog tracheal epithelium. *J. Appl. Physiol. 55*: 1844-1848.

Odya, C. E., Goodfriend, T. L., and Pena, C. (1980). Bradykinin receptor-like binding studied with iodinated analogues. *Biochem. Pharmacol. 29*: 175-183.

Orange, R. P., Kaliner, M. A., Laraia, P. J., and Austen, K. F. (1971). Immunological release of histamine and slow secreting substance of anaphylaxis from human lung. II. Influence of cellular levels of cyclic AMP. *Fed. Proc. 30*: 1725-1729.

Palmer, J. B., Cuss, F. M., and Barnes, P. J. (1986). Vasoactive intestinal peptide, peptide histidine methionine, and nor-adrenergic inhibitory nerves in human airways. *J. Appl. Physiol.* (in press).

Paterson, J. W., Lulich, K. M., and Goldie, R. G. (1982). The role of beta-adrenoceptors in bronchial hyperreactivity. In *Bronchial Hyperreactivity*. Edited by J. Morley. London, Academic Press, pp. 19-38.

Pavia, D., Bateman, J. R. M., and Clarke, S. W. (1980). Deposition and clearance of inhaled particles. *Clin. Respir. Physiol. 16*: 335-366.

Peatfield, A. C., Barnes, P. J., Bratcher, C., Nadel, J. A., and Davis, B. (1983). Vasoactive intestinal peptide stimulates tracheal submucosal gland secretion in ferret. *Am. Rev. Respir. Dis. 128*: 89-93.

Persson, C. G. A. (1986). The pharmacology of antiasthmatic xanthines and the role of adenosine. In *Asthma Reviews*. Edited by J. Morley. London, Academic Press (in press).

Persson, C. G. A., and Ekman, M. (1976). Contractile effects of histamine in large and small respiratory airways. *Agents Actions 6*: 389-393.

Persson, C. G. A., Ejefält, I., Grega, G. J., and Svensjo, E. (1982). The role of beta-receptor agonists in the inhibition of pulmonary edema. *N.Y. Acad. Sci. 384*: 544-556.

Peters, J. E., Chan, S. C., Hanifin, J. M., and Hirshman, C. A. (1981). The Basenji-Greyhound dog model of asthma: defective leukocyte nucleotide response. *Clin. Sci. 29*: 171A.

Peters, S. P., Schulman, E. S., Schleimer, R. P., MacGlashan, D. W., Newball, H. H., and Lichtenstein, L. M. (1982). Dispersed human lung mast cells. Pharmacologica aspects and comparison with human lung tissue fragments. *Am. Rev. Respir. Dis. 126*: 1034-1039.

Phipps, R. J., Williams, I. P., Richardson, P. S., Pell, J., Pack, R. J., and Wright, N. (1982). Sympathetic drugs stimulate the output of secretory glycoprotein from human bronchi in vitro. *Clin. Sci. 63*: 23-28.

Pollett, R. J., and Levey, G. S. (1980). Principles of membrane receptor physiology and their application to clinical medicine. *Am. Intern. Med. 92*: 663-680.

Richardson, J. B. (1979). Nerve supply to the lungs. *Am. Rev. Respir. Dis. 119*: 785-802.

Richardson, J. B. (1981). Non-adrenergic inhibitory innervation of the lung. *Lung 159*: 315-322.

Richardson, J., and Beland, J. (1976). Non-adrenergic inhibitory nervous system in human airways. *J. Appl. Physiol. 41*: 764-771.

Robberech, P., Chatelain, P., De Neef, P., Camus, J-C., Waelbroeck, M., and Christophe, J. (1981). Presence of vasoactive intestinal peptide receptors coupled to adenylate cyclase in rat lung membranes. *Biochem. Biophys. Acta 678*: 76-82.

Roberts, J. A., Raeburn, D., Rodger, I. W., and Thomson, N. C. (1984). Comparison of in vivo airway responsiveness and in vitro sensitivity to methacholine in man. *Thorax 39*: 837-843.

Rugg, E. L., Barnett, D. B., and Nahorski, S. R. (1979). Coexistence of $beta_1$- and $beta_2$-adrenoceptors in mammalian lung: Evidence from direct binding studies. *Mol. Pharmacol. 14*: 996-1005.

Said, S. I. (1982). Vasoactive peptides in the lung, with special reference to vasoactive intestinal peptide. *Exp. Lung. Res. 3*: 343-348.

Shelhamer, J., Marom, Z., and Kaliner, M. (1980). Immunologic and neuropharmacologic stimulation of glycoprotein release from human airways in vitro. *J. Clin. Invest. 66*: 1400-14.

Skoogh, B-E. (1983). Transmission through airway ganglia. *Eur. J. Respir. Dis. 64 (suppl. 131)*: 159-170.

Snashall, P. D., Boother, F. A., and Sterling, G. A. (1978). The effect of alpha-adrenoceptor stimulation on the airways of normal and asthmatic man. *Clin. Sci. Mol. Med. 54*: 283-289.

Stephan, W. C., Chick, T. W., Avner, B. P., and Jenne, J. W. (1980). Tachyphylaxis to inhaled isoproterenol and the effect of methyl prednisolone in dogs. *J. Allergy Clin. Immunol. 65*: 105-109.

Stiles, G. L., Caron, M., and Lefkowitz, R. J. (1984). Beta-adrenergic receptors. *Pharmacol. Rev. 64*: 661-743.

Svedmyr, N. A., Larsson, A. L., and Thiringer, G. K. (1976). Development of "resistance" in beta-adrenergic receptors of asthmatic patients. *Chest 69*: 479-483.

Szentivanyi, A. (1968). The beta adrenergic theory of the atopic abnormality in bronchial asthma. *J. Allergy 42*: 203-232.

Turner, A. J., Seale, J. P., and Shaw, J. (1983). Antigen sensitization does not alter response of guinea-pig lung strips to noradrenaline. *Eur. J. Pharmacol. 87*: 141-144.

Valone, F. H., and Goetzl, E. J. (1983). Specific binding by human polymorphonuclear leukocytes of the immunological mediator 1-0-hexadecyl/octadecyl 2-acetyl-glycero-3 phosphorylcholine. *Immunology 48*: 141-149.

Venter, J. C., Fraser, C. M., and Harrison, L. C. (1980). Autoantibodies to beta$_2$-adrenergic receptors: A possible cause of adrenergic hyporesponsiveness in allergic rhinitis and asthma. *Science 207*: 1361-1363.
White, J., and Eiser, N. M. (1983). The role of histamine and its receptors in the pathogenesis of asthma. *Br. J. Dis. Chest. 77*: 215-226.
Zaagsma, J., van der Heijden, P. J. C. M., van der Schaar, M. W. G., and Bank, C. M. C. (1983). Comparison of functional beta-adrenoceptor heterogeneity in central and peripheral airway smooth muscle of guinea pig and man. *J. Receptor. Res. 3*: 89-106.

3

Receptor-Mediated Regulation of Tension in Smooth Muscle Cells

J. FREDERICK KRALL

Veterans Administration Medical Center
Sepulveda, California

I. Introduction

Although our understanding is very far from complete, few mechanisms of cellular regulation are understood in extent or detail as well as the cyclic AMP-mediated pathways. In this instance, understanding has been the beneficiary of a control process that is both fundamental and evolutionarily conservative. As a consequence, wide-ranging interest in cyclic AMP in a variety of tissues and species has led to an appreciation that its mechanisms of action are ubiquitous in general and specific only in detail. Burgeoning knowledge of cyclic AMP naturally stimulates interest in cyclic GMP, but to date it remains the more obscure of the cyclic nucleotides with respect to function.

Smooth muscle has received its fair share of attention with respect to cyclic nucleotide metabolism because of its widespread distribution and obvious clinical importance in the respiratory, cardiovascular, gastrointestinal, and urogenital systems. There are marked similarities in the properties and sensitivity of smooth muscle from any of these organs, so advances in understanding the role of cyclic AMP in one of them provide potential insight into the regulation of all of them. To an extent the same is probably also true of regulation by cyclic GMP, but the greater immediate interest may be differences recently discovered between the regulation of cyclic GMP production in vascular smooth muscle compared to that from other sources.

In the same sense, advances in cyclic nucleotide biochemistry in general are useful in our understanding of their role in smooth muscle, specifically since many aspects of regulation are similar or the same in most vertebrate cells. Of course this is true only so long as it is possible to distinguish where differences in detail diverge from fundamental similarities and properties. Although these points are monotonously indistinct in biology and medicine and further obscured by real species differences, important insight into the regulation of smooth muscle tone in the lung benefits from a broader understanding of cyclic nucleotide biochemistry where this is appropriate.

II. Regulation by Protein Phosphorylation

Despite the occasionally poor correlation between tension and cyclic AMP levels observed in smooth muscle strips, most investigators conclude that cyclic AMP has profound effects on the smooth muscle contraction-relaxation cycle in general and regulation by β-adrenergic catecholamines specifically (Hardman, 1981; Krall et al., 1983). The disparity sometimes observed between an agonist's physiological potency (relaxation) and its potency in stimulating smooth muscle cyclic AMP production is accounted for by the likelihood that immeasurably small increases in cyclic AMP production have large physiological consequences. The cyclic-nucleotide-dependent protein kinases are key enzymes in this powerful amplification network and exert their diverse effects by stimulating the covalent modification of enzymatic or structural proteins. These modifications are catalyzed by the transfer of the terminal (gamma) phosphate from ATP to a specific protein substrate by protein kinase. Intracellular phosphatases have the capacity subsequently to remove the phosphate, so the function of the modified protein is altered depending upon whether it exists in its phospho- or dephospho- state.

Protein kinase activation is precipitated by cyclic nucleotide binding by the phosphorylating enzyme and dissociation of the bound cyclic nucleotide leads to protein kinase inactivation. The kinetics of inactivation are different for the different cyclic nucleotides by virtue of the structure of the cyclic-nucleotide-specific protein kinases. Thus, cGMP binds to and dissociates from a single peptide chain that contains both the protein kinase catalytic site and the cGMP binding site. The kinetics of inactivation are therefore appropriately simple. Cyclic-AMP-dependent protein kinase has a more complex subunit structure, however, so the kinetics are expectedly more complex. The cAMP binding site and the catalytic site are on different subunits, and the activation process is characterized by dissociation of the cAMP-regulatory subunit complex from the catalytic subunit with concomitant activation. Inactivation therefore requires not only dissociation of cAMP from the regulatory subunit but the subsequent reassociation of the free and activated catalytic subunit with the unoccupied regulatory subunit. The kinetics of inactivation are further complicated by the fact that some but not all regulatory subunits are in turn protein kinase substrates and the rate at which they reassociate with the catalytic subunit depends on whether they are in a phospho- or dephospho- state. These properties of the two kinds of cyclic nucleotide-dependent protein kinase are summarized below, where R and C are, respectively, the regulatory and catalytic subunits of cyclic AMP-dependent protein kinase while PK represents the simpler structure of cyclic GMP-dependent protein kinase:

$$\text{cGMP} + \text{PK} \rightleftharpoons \text{cGMP}\cdot\text{PK (active)} \qquad (1)$$

$$\text{cAMP} + \text{R}\cdot\text{C} \rightleftharpoons \text{cAMP}\cdot\text{R} + \text{C (active)} \qquad (2)$$

Thus, the determination of the magnitude of change in the number of occupied protein kinase regulatory subunits and the extent of increase in the protein kinase activity ratio (enzyme activity in the absence of cyclic AMP/activity in the presence of cyclic AMP) in broken cell preparations or the extent of cyclic AMP-dependent protein kinase substrate phosphorylation (by autoradiographic analysis of radiophosphate-labelled peptides separated electrophoretically) in intact cells are more reliable methods of measuring the effects of low agonist doses than quantification of cyclic nucleotide levels.

Several important smooth muscle cell phosphoproteins are specific substrates for smooth muscle cyclic-AMP-dependent protein kinases and these figure prominently in the regulation of tension. Among the best characterized of the smooth muscle phosphoproteins are myosin light chain kinase (MK) and its substrate, the 20,000 dalton myosin light chain (Adelstein et al., 1981). In its dephospho- state MK phosphorylates the myosin light chain, which favors actomyosin formation and therefore contraction. Active MK is actually a complex between MK and calmodulin that forms in the presence but not in the absence of Ca^{+2}. Phosphorylation of MK by cyclic AMP-dependent (or other) protein kinase produces a form of the enzyme that cannot bind calmodulin at the concentration of free Ca^{2+} present in the resting cell. This favors dephosphorylation of the myosin light chain by intrinsic phosphatase activity and therefore relaxation. The regulation of the phosphorylation of the myosin light chain by Ca^{+2}:calmodulin-dependent MK is summarized in Figure 1.

This protein-kinase-mediated mechanism of force development has been shown to be correct in principle in several kinds of smooth muscle. There is good agreement, for instance, between the isoproterenol-dependent decrease in tension and cyclic AMP-dependent protein kinase activation in smooth muscle

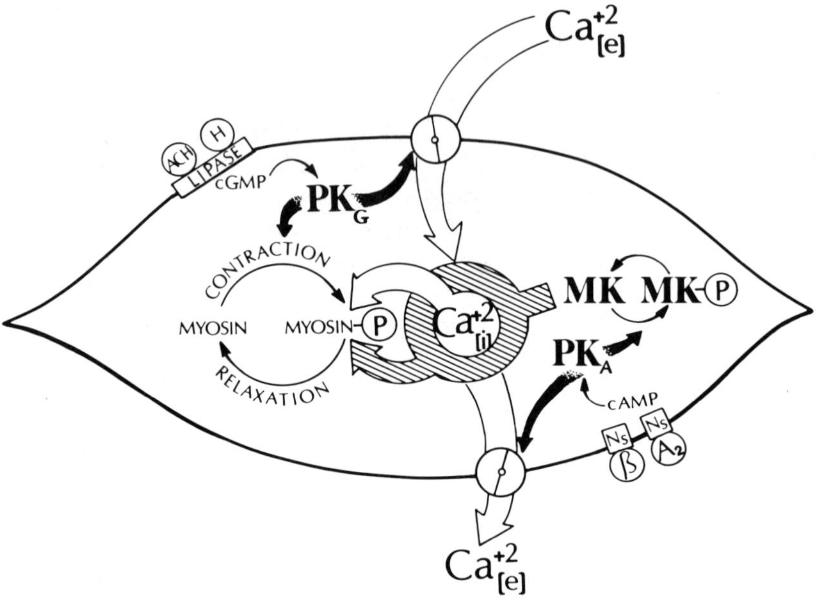

Figure 1 The regulation of smooth muscle tension by protein kinase and Ca^{2+}. The production of cyclic AMP and cyclic GMP by smooth muscle cells is probably stimulated in numerous ways but only the better characterized are shown here: N_S-dependent coupling of the β-adrenergic (β) and adenosine (A_2) receptors with adenylate cyclase and the phospholipase-mediated coupling of the cholinergic (ACh) and histamine (H) receptors with guanylate cyclase. Activation of cyclic-AMP-dependent protein kinase (PK_A) regulates the activity of a number of phosphoprotein substrates directly, and some oı these change the distribution of Ca^{2+} between the intracellular ($Ca^{2+}{}_{[i]}$) and extracellular ($Ca^{2+}{}_{[e]}$) compartments. PK_A regulates the state of phosphorylation of the myosin light chain in an indirect manner, through the phosphorylation of myosin light chain kinase (MK) converting it from the Ca^{2+} (and calmodulin–) sensitive active form which phosphorylates myosin (⇧) to the inactive form. Cyclic-AMP-dependent phosphorylation of MK therefore favors dephosphorylation of the myosin light chain by intrinsic phosphatase activity and subsequently relaxation.

In contrast to PK_A, cyclic-GMP-dependent protein kinase (PK_G) seems to lack an indirect mechanism of action and acts directly on Ca^{2+} distribution and perhaps on the actomyosin complex. Both cyclic nucleotides may affect a second Ca^{2+}-dependent process that functions independently of MK (⇧) and accounts for the Ca^{2+} sensitivity of dephosphomyosin.

from the frog stomach and bovine coronary artery (Scheid et al., 1979; Silver et al., 1982). Forskolin, a potent stimulator of cyclic AMP production in both intact and broken cell smooth muscle preparations, partially relaxes methacholine-treated tracheal muscle strips, decreases myosin light chain phosphate content, and increases the phosphorylation of MK as determined by specific immunoprecipitation (DeLanerolle et al., 1984). In confirmation of its importance, the addition of the purified catalytic subunit of cyclic AMP-dependent protein kinase decreases tension developed in the presence of elevated Ca^{2+} in skinned smooth muscle fibers from chicken gizzard, teleost aorta, pulmonary and carotid artery, and from guinea pig trachealis (Kerrick and Hoar, 1981; Ruegg and Paul, 1982; Sparrow et al., 1984).

Measurement of tension developed as a function of myosin light chain phosphorylation during the course of Ca^{2+} contracture has been simulateously determined by freeze-clamping followed by electrophoretic analysis of the ratio of dephosphorylated/phosphorylated myosin light chain by isoelectric focusing in the first dimension and acrylamide gel electrophoresis in the presence of sodium dodecyl sulfate (SDS) in the second dimension (Driska et al., 1981; Chatterjee and Murphy, 1983; Gerthoffer and Murphy, 1983; Aksoy et al., 1983). These studies show that there is a good correlation between Ca^{2+}-dependent tension development and myosin light chain phosphorylation. Force is subsequently maintained even if the extracellular Ca^{2+} concentration is reduced, however, conditions under which partial or even complete myosin dephosphorylation occurs. In agreement with this apparent dependence of tension development but not maintenance on myosin light chain phosphorylation, relaxation of skinned tracheal smooth muscle fibers induced by the addition of purified cyclic AMP-dependent protein kinase catalytic subunit proceeds much more slowly than relaxation induced by Ca^{2+} withdrawal (Sparrow et al., 1984). The Ca^{2+}-sensitive mechanism of tension regulation that functions independently of MK is summarized in a simplified fashion in Figure 1.

Two possibilities have been proposed for the mechanism by which the dephosphorylated myosin light chain can still impart Ca^{2+} sensitivity to the actomyosin complex: (1), phosphorylation of the myosin light chain greatly increases myosin Ca^{2+} sensitivity in a manner that is reversed slowly relative to the rate of dephosphorylation, or (2), two varieties of Ca^{2+}-sensitive cross-bridges are formed in smooth muscle and only one of these is sensitive to the effects of phosphorylation by MK. These possibilities, although still unresolved, focus renewed attention on the importance of the regulation of intracellular Ca^{2+} levels in smooth muscle cell function. Like MK and myosin light chain phosphorylation, Ca^{2+} transport in the smooth muscle cell is probably also regulated by protein kinase-mediated phosphorylation. These Ca^{2+}-regulating phosphorylations may therefore be of principal importance in the regulation of the contraction-relaxation cycle of the smooth muscle cell and are summarized in Figure 1.

Mitochondria, sarcoplasmic reticulum, and the smooth muscle cell plasma membrane (sarcolemma) have all been proposed to function as intracellular Ca^{2+} storage sites in smooth muscle from which Ca^{2+} can be recruited or released for activation of contraction. The properties of these compartments in smooth muscle from a variety of sources have been recently reviewed by Daniel et al. (1983). Cyclic AMP stimulates the ATP-dependent Ca^{2+} transport activity of smooth muscle microsomes from uterus, intestine, and aorta (Andersson and Nilsson, 1972; Baudouin-Legros and Meyer, 1973; Krall et al., 1976; Nishikori and Maeno, 1979), as well as in purified sarcolemmal fractions from aorta (Brockbank and England, 1980). Stimulation of Ca^{2+} transport activity by cyclic AMP is associated with increased phosphorylation of a specific and similar membrane protein in both uterine microsomes and arterial sarcolemma (Nishikori and Maeno, 1979; Brockbank and England, 1980). Addition of exogenous protein kinase stimulates the Ca^{2+} uptake activity of arterial sarcolemma, and different membrane proteins are phosphorylated by cyclic AMP- compared to cyclic GMP-dependent protein kinase (Brockbank and England, 1980; Suematsu et al., 1984b).

The $^{45}Ca^{2+}$-uptake activity of the sarcolemma from porcine aorta is stimulated by calmodulin and by the addition of purified cyclic AMP- and cyclic-GMP-dependent protein kinase. Moreover, while stimulation by cyclic AMP-dependent protein kinase is associated with the phosphorylation of 22,000 and 28,000 dalton proteins, stimulation by cyclic GMP-dependent protein kinase is associated with the phosphorylation of a different (35,000 dalton) membrane protein. Like cyclic AMP-dependent protein kinase, calmodulin stimulates the phosphorylation of the 22,000 protein in aortic smooth muscle. In trachea, however, calmodulin and cyclic GMP increase the phosphorylation of 130,000 and 80,000 dalton proteins to a much greater extent than either increases the phosphorylation of a 22,000 dalton protein (Hogaboom et al., 1982). Both the Ca^{2+} pump and Ca^{2+}, Mg^{2+}-ATPase are calmodulin-sensitive in microsomal preparations from aorta and trachea, so the 22,000 dalton protein could be a cyclic AMP-sensitive part of that pump that can be independently regulated by a Ca^{2+}/calmodulin complex in aortic smooth muscle (Morel et al., 1981; Hogaboom and Fedan, 1981). In tracheal smooth muscle, on the other hand, cyclic GMP and calmodulin might regulate the same pump through the phosphorylation of different, higher-molecular-weight subunits. Although speculative, differences like these at the level of the cyclic nucleotide-dependent protein kinases and their intrinsic cell substrates could explain why cyclic GMP is associated with relaxation in aorta but contraction in trachea.

Despite the better characterized role of cyclic AMP-dependent protein kinase in the regulation of contraction and relaxation, smooth muscle in general and tracheal smooth muscle and lung specifically are particularly rich in cyclic-GMP-dependent protein kinase (Nakazawa and Sano, 1975; Lincoln et al., 1976;

Torphy et al., 1982). In addition, smooth muscle from ductus deferens, small intestine, aorta, and uterus have the same or markedly similar integral membrane proteins that are phosphorylated in a cyclic·GMP-dependent manner under conditions that stimulate contraction as well as cyclic GMP production (Casnellie and Greengard, 1974; Ives et al., 1980; Casnellie et al., 1980). The marked similarity between the action of potent vasodilators such as acetylcholine, nitroprusside, and isosorbide and their potency in elevating vascular cyclic GMP levels has accentuated the putative role of cyclic GMP in vascular smooth muscle relaxation (Katsuki and Murad, 1977; Lincoln, 1983; Galvas and DiSalvo, 1983). Acetylcholine, nitroprusside, and 8-bromocyclic GMP induce phosphorylation of the same proteins in intact rat aorta and, in addition, reduce myosin light chain phosphorylation (Rapoport and Murad, 1983b; Rapoport et al., 1983).

The action of acetylcholine but not nitroprusside or 8-bromo cyclic GMP is diminished by removal of the vascular endothelium, which implies that interaction between these two tissues plays an important role in cyclic GMP-dependent protein kinase activation in the smooth muscle layers (Rapoport and Murad, 1983a, b).

III. Regulation of Cyclic Nucleotide Production

A. Cyclic AMP

Mammalian adenylate cyclase is composed of several subunits including a catalytic subunit (C), the hormone receptor (R), and a guanine nucleotide-binding complex (N) that couples the other subunits (Kaslow et al., 1979; Strittmatter and Neer, 1980; Ross, 1982). N is complex and present in two forms in membranes, stimulatory (N_s) and inhibitory (N_i), which have opposite effects on C (Sternweiss et al., 1981; Katada and Ui, 1982; Hildebrandt et al., 1983; Bokoch et al., 1984). Best characterized of the cell surface receptors that regulate adenylate cyclase activity are those for β-adrenergic catecholamines.

B. Regulation by β-Adrenergic Receptors

In general there is a positive correlation between β-adrenergic receptor concentration and target cell sensitivity. β-Adrenergic receptors in respiratory tissues are principally of the β_2 subtype as classified by physiological responsiveness (Boe and Simonsson, 1980; Davis et al., 1980) and by specific binding of both radioagonists and radioantagonists to isolated cell membranes (Minneman et al., 1979; Heidenreich et al., 1980; U'Prichard et al., 1978; Witkin and Harden, 1981). About 85% of the β-adrenergic receptors in rat lung are of the β_2 and 15% of the β_1 variety by unlabeled agonist competition of specific radioantagonist binding (Minneman et al., 1979), and β_2 selectivity appears constant throughout the trachea and bronchial tree (Niewoehner et al., 1979; Davis et al., 1980). β-Adrenergic receptors have been purified from rat, canine, and guinea pig lung and consist in each case of a single peptide (Cerione et al., 1983a; Homcy et al., 1983). The simple single chain structure of the purified lung receptor has been verified by its reconstitution into artificial membranes where it confers catecholamine sensitivity to adenylate cyclase (Cerione et al., 1983b).

In detergent solutions of the purified subunits, dissociable interactions play an indispensable role in the activation and inactivation precipitated by guanine and nucleotide binding. The slow and rate-limiting step in the coupling of inhibitory as well as stimulatory receptors in these solubilized and purified systems is the dissociation of the subunits of N_s or N_i and the subsequent effect they have on the catalytic (C) subunit (see Gilman, 1984, for review). The extent to which this complex mechanisms of regulation involving dissociable subunit interactions and diffusion in detergent extracts reflects regulation in intact cells is so far uncertain. The inhibitory or stimulatory nature of receptors regulating cyclic-AMP-mediated pathways probably depends on whether they are coupled with C through N_i or N_s, however. The adenosine receptor is an example of a receptor that is coupled both ways in some tissues, although probably not in smooth muscle.

C. Regulation by Adenosine Receptors and Methylxanthine Action

Separate and distinct receptors account for the inhibitory effect adenosine has on cyclic AMP production in adipocytes, cardiac muscle, and brain and its stimulatory effect in platelets, adrenal cells, lung, and smooth muscle (Fain and Malbon, 1979; Wolff et al., 1981). The two kinds of adenosine receptor (A_1 and A_2) are readily distinguished by the relative potencies of adenosine compared to the analogs 5′-N-ethylcarboxamide adenosine (NECA), and N_6-phenylisopropyladenosine (PIA): A_2, NECA>adenosine>PIA; A_1, PIA>adenosine> NECA (Wolff et al., 1981). The action of both kinds of adenosine receptors are guanine nucleotide requiring.

There is little evidence of A_1 receptors in smooth muscle where adenosine has, in general, relaxing effects shown to be mediated by A_2 receptor-dependent cyclic AMP production in both vascular and tracheal muscle (Brown and Collis, 1982; Anand-Srivastava et al., 1982; Collis and Brown, 1983). In guinea pig trachea, however, adenosine caused relaxation of pilocarpine-induced contraction but contraction suggestive of an A_1 receptor in the absence of drug-induced contraction (Fredholm et al., 1979). Adenosine, added in the absence of pilocarpine, antagonized the relaxing effects of theophylline in these preparations but whether theophylline in turn antagonized adenosine-induced contraction, an important characteristic of A_1-receptor function, was not determined. The predominant relaxing effect adenosine has on smooth muscle in general can be attributed, therefore, to adenosine-dependent cyclic AMP production mediated by A_2-receptors.

Besides the adenylate cyclase-coupled adenosine receptors, a second site of adenosine action is closely coupled with the adenylate cyclase catalytic subunit (C) in a nonguanine-nucleotide-dependent manner, the so-called P site (Wolff et al., 1981). The P site exerts an inhibitory effect on C in broken cell adanylate cyclase preparations, but it has been difficult to assign it a physiological role in intact cells. The disparity between the adenylate cyclase-inhibiting potency of a variety of adenosine analogs and their potency in relaxing intestinal smooth muscle might be best explained by action at the P site, however (McKenzie et al., 1977). Adenosine action at the different sites can be distinguished by ribose modification, which destroys receptor but not P site activity, and by the fact that methylxanthines are potent antagonists of receptor- but not P site-mediated action (Wolff et al., 1981). This is a ubiquitous property of the methylxanthines which vary in potency: methyl-isobutylxanthine>theophylline>caffeine. As expected from the A_2 properties of their receptors, methylxanthines block adenosine-induced relaxation in intestinal, vascular, and tracheal smooth muscle (McKenzie et al., 1977; Jones et al., 1980; Collis and Brown, 1983).

Adenosine antagonism is not the sole mechanism of action of the methylxanthines, however, as reflected by the complex effects theophylline has on intestinal smooth muscle where it potentiates the relaxing effects of isoproterenol and concomitantly antagonizes those of adenosine (McKenzie et al., 1977). Moreover, chemical modification produces methylxanthine analogs that have lost their adenosine antagonizing properties but retained their bronchodilating properties (Persson et al., 1982; Karlsson et al., 1982). Although it is difficult to ascribe the relaxing effects of the methylxanthines to their antagonism of smooth muscle adenosine-dependent cyclic AMP production which also mediates relaxation, they remain much more potent A_2-adenosine receptor antagonists than they are phosphodiesterase inhibitors (Wolff et al., 1981).

As phosphodiesterase inhibitors, methylxanthines stimulate the accumulation of both cyclic AMP and cyclic GMP in tracheal smooth muscle (Katsuki and Murad, 1977; Lohmann et al., 1977). There is a correlation between the physiological potency of methylxanthines and their capacity to inhibit crude or partially purified bronchial and tracheal phosphodiesterase activity from guinea pig and dog (Triner et al., 1977; Fredholm et al., 1979; Polson et al., 1979; 1982), but not between physiological potency and capacity to induce cyclic nucleotide accumulation in intact smooth muscle (Lohmann et al., 1977; Kolbeck et al., 1979). Nevertheless, theophylline pretreatment increases the sensitivity of the isolated trachea to the relaxing effects of isoproterenol which are known to be cyclic AMP-mediated. There is a perfect correlation between isoproterenol and theophylline sensitivity in five different tracheal and bronchiole preparations from three different species (Niewoehner et al., 1979). It is also significant that theophylline concentrations too low to cause detectable increases in cyclic nucleotide concentration stimulate $^{45}Ca^{2+}$-uptake and sequestration in guinea pig and canine tracheal muscle strips since both of these activities may be cyclic AMP or cyclic GMP mediated (Kolbeck et al., 1979).

These effects on tracheal $^{45}Ca^{2+}$ flux seem specific since theophylline as well as caffeine stimulates $^{45}Ca^{2+}$ efflux in aortic smooth muscle but inhibits it in ileal, vas deferens, and bladder smooth muscle (Deth and Casteels, 1977; Deth and Lynch, 1981; Huddart et al., 1983). Methyl-isobutylxanthine, caffeine, theophylline, and RO-20-1724 all increase aortic smooth muscle cyclic AMP levels while over a limited concentration range only caffeine and theophylline also stimulate $^{45}Ca^{2+}$ efflux (Deth and Lynch, 1981). It is uncertain therefore, whether this particular effect of theophylline and caffeine on aortic smooth muscle is mediated by cyclic AMP, although a role for cyclic GMP has not been ruled out. The latter is an important consideration in view of the role cyclic GMP may play in vascular smooth muscle relaxation.

Although the capacity of the methylxanthines to relax smooth muscle is better explained by their properties as phosphodiesterase inhibitors than by their ability specifically to inhibit adenosine-dependent cyclic AMP production under experimental conditions, it remains uncertain that the drugs reach the levels required in situ to explain their therapeutic value by a similar mechanism (Hendeles and Weinberger, 1983). One indication that they do is the report that theophylline has a desensitizing effect on lymphocyte β-adrenergic receptors when administered to human subjects by itself and also potentiates the desensitizing effects of metaproterenol (Scarpace et al., 1982). Even though methylxanthine effects can be largely explained by their cyclic nucleotide-elevating properties, they also have properties unrelated to either adenosine antagonism or phosphodiesterease inhibition. Among these are effects on protein kinase activation, membrane phospholipase activity, and protein methylation (Miech et al., 1979; Hong, 1983; MacFarlane, 1984).

D. Regulation by Ca^{2+}

In addition to cyclic AMP production regulated by receptors for hormones and neurotransmitters, at least some kinds of smooth muscle have adenylate cyclase activity that is Ca^{2+}-sensitive. Smooth muscle cells cultured from the rat uterus have adenylate cyclase activity simulated by micromolar concentrations of Ca^{2+} while bovine aortic activity is stimulated by Ca^{2+} concentrations below 1 μmol but inhibited by higher concentrations (Fortier et al., 1983; Piascik et al., 1983). The Ca^{2+} sensitivity of the vascular enzyme is calmodulin dependent, but neither the vascular nor the uterine form requires guanine nucleotide. The absence of a guanine nucleotide requirement is a property distinctly different from hormone regulation of adenylate cyclase in these same cells and demonstrates that Ca^{2+}-sensitive cyclic AMP production is independent of receptor function.

The role of Ca^{2+}-sensitive cyclic AMP synthesis in smooth muscle is unknown, but it may serve as an independent mechanism for regulating intracellular Ca^{2+} levels in the uterine smooth muscle cells (Fortier et al., 1983).

E. Cyclic GMP Production

Compared with cyclic AMP, little is understood about the regulation of cyclic GMP production. Smooth muscle guanylate cyclase exists in both soluble (cytosolic) and particulate forms (Leiber and Harbon, 1979; Katsuki et al., 1977), and lung is a particularly rich source of the soluble form of the enzyme (Garbers, 1979). While hydroxylamine stimulates both soluble and particulate guanylate cyclase in tracheal smooth muscle, nitroprusside stimulates only the soluble form of the enzyme (Katsuki et al., 1977). Although the significance of this curious property remains obscure, it suggests that special and unique mechanisms for the regulation of cyclic GMP production may exist in some types of smooth muscle.

Guanylate cyclase activation by nitric oxide free radicals accounts for the relaxing effects nitrovasodilators have on most varieties of smooth muscle (Bohme et al., 1984). While these nitrovasodilators activate guanylate cyclase in broken cell preparations, activation as well as relaxation induced by hormones and neurotransmitters requires intact cells and extracellular Ca^{2+}. In these instances, both the elevation of intracellular cyclic GMP and relaxation induced in vascular smooth muscle are suppressed by inhibitors of phospholipase and lipoxygenase. Investigators have been appropriately cautious in interpreting these inhibitor studies, but the results suggest that oxidation of membrane phospholipid fatty acyl chains produces oxygen radicals and peroxides that activate guanylate cyclase in some smooth muscle cells (Rapoport and Murad, 1983a).

Removal of the endothelium, shown to be required for acetylcholine-induced vasodilation (Furchgott and Zawadski, 1980), abolishes or reduces agonist-dependent cyclic GMP accumulation in rat, rabbit, and cow aortic strips (Rapoport and Murad, 1983b; Rapoport et al., 1982; Holzmann, 1982). It is possible, therefore, that the vascular endothelium is the origin of the membrane fatty acids oxidized to stimulate cyclic GMP production by vascular smooth muscle cells, as recently proposed by Rapoport and Murad. Similar interaction between smooth muscle and its associated epithelium does not seem to occur in myometrium, vas deferens, or taenia coli where nitroprusside and hydroxylamine elevate cyclic GMP levels without an effect on tension (Diamond and Chu, 1983; Diamond, 1983). Thus, the important role assigned the endothelium in acetylcholine-induced smooth muscle relaxation and guanylate cyclase activation (discussed below) is either unique to the vasculature or characterizes an epithelial requirement of smooth muscle cyclic GMP production in some but not all organs.

IV. Regulation of Sensitivity

A. Desensitization

Exposure of target tissues to β-adrenergic catecholamines results in progressive refractoriness to stimulation that persists even if the agonists are removed by extensive washing. This refractoriness characterizes the desensitized state and accounts for the onset of tachyphylaxis in most tissues including lung and human bronchial smooth muscle (Holgate et al., 1977; Stephan et al., 1980; Conolly, 1980). Desensitization is complex biochemically, and to a limited extent might be rapidly reversible and an intrinsic property of the formation of the agonist-receptor complex rather than the result of protracted stimulation. Since antagonists are tightly bound by the receptor without these concomitant decreases, desensitizing effects are another criterion that distinguishes agonists from antagonists.

In intact cells, desensitization is associated with increasing cell refractoriness to stimulation by the desensitizing agonist and has been characterized as a two-stage process involving (1) a rapid decrease in the affinity of the receptor for the agonist and concomitant uncoupling from adenylate cyclase, and; (2) eventual diminution of receptors from the cell surface (Toews et al., 1983; Waldo et al., 1983). Since guanine nucleotides also cause a decrease in the affinity of β-adrenergic receptors for agonists but not antagonists, desensitization may encompass the GTP-binding coupling factor N_s. Because of possible effects at the level of receptor coupling, changes in β-adrenergic receptor affinity for agonists or the distribution of multiple affinity states ("high" and "low") for agonists detectable by competition of radioantagonist binding are frequently interpreted as effects on the coupling process in lung and in other tissues (Scarpace and Abrass, 1982b; Davies and Lefkowitz, 1984; Feldman et al., 1984). The significance of these differences may actually be more obscure.

When the affinity of β-adrenergic receptors for unlabeled agonists is determined by competition of specific radioantagonist binding by isolated cell membranes under initial velocity (>10% radioantagonist binding) rather than equilibrium-binding conditions, there is good agreement between the lower IC_{50} of agonist binding and the activation association constant (K_a) for agonist-dependent cyclic AMP production (Toews et al., 1983; Hoyer et al., 1984). The affinity of the receptors for agonists is also in better agreement with that observed in living cells using these initial velocity conditions (Toews et al., 1983).

The significance of the difference in the properties of the receptor using initial velocity compared to equilibrium-binding methods may be that protracted exposure to agonists (but not to antagonists) under equilibrium conditions produces a desensitized state of the receptor even in isolated membranes. The difference in observed agonist affinity using the two binding methods obscures, at any rate, the significance of the relative distribution of multiple or altered affinity states of β-adrenergic receptors sometimes observed as a consequence of desensitizing intact cells.

More direct approaches reveal that while desensitization always effects the receptor, it is only sometimes associated with decreased guanine nucleotide sensitivity of adenylate cyclase (Green et al., 1981; Iyengar et al., 1981; Kirchick et al., 1983; Krall et al., 1984). Consequently, desensitization probably begins at the receptor and only occasionally or subsequently envelopes other adenylate cyclase subunits. The initial receptor phase of desensitization is associated with almost immediate membrane alterations and perhaps eventual endocytosis or internalization to account for the disappearance of receptors from the cell surface (Waldo et al., 1983; Stadel et al., 1983a). Some or all of these stages of receptor desensitization may be accompanied by or actually regulated by protein kinase-mediated phosphorylation of the receptor (Stadel et al., 1983b).

In some but perhaps not all cells, protracted elevation of intracellular cyclic AMP levels by exposure to exogenously added cyclic AMP analogs or to agents that stimulate cyclic AMP production by non-receptor-mediated mechanisms causes desensitization to β-adrenergic catecholamines (Nickols and Brooker, 1979; Moylan et al., 1982). Cyclic AMP-mediated desensitization may be another important mechanism of action of the methylxanthines, for instance. Exposing guinea pig trachealis to theophylline or to dibutyryl cyclic AMP and dibutyryl cyclic GMP induces tachyphylaxis to isoproterenol (Douglas et al., 1977). This cyclic-nucleotide-mediated desensitization does not reduce the sensitivity of the muscle strips to the subsequent relaxing effects of reexposure to dibutyryl-cyclic AMP, which suggests that desensitization does not include the protein kinase-mediated pathway distal to cyclic AMP production. Moreover, uterine smooth muscle strips exposed to theophylline or isobutylmethylxanthine in vitro rapidly lose sensitivity to series E prostaglandins as well as to isoproterenol (Tougui et al., 1980). Since receptors for these different agonists might regulate cyclic AMP production through the same population of N_s or C in this tissue (Tougui et al., 1980; Krall et al., 1984), cyclic AMP-mediated desensitization might also extend to these subunits in some types of smooth muscle.

In experiments performed in vivo, there is a decrease in both isoproterenol-dependent cyclic AMP production and β-adrenergic receptor concentration of peripheral lymphocytes isolated from human subjects given adrenergic catecholamines (Conolly and Greenacre, 1976; Galant et al., 1978; Scarpace et al., 1982). Few differences are detected using these methods between asthmatic and normal subjects with respect to the desensitizing effects of adrenergic therapy. In one study, however, normal subjects receiving metaproterenol alone or metaproterenol with theophylline had fewer lymphocyte β-adrenergic receptors, but when asthmatic subjects received the same treatment, only about half responded with lowered lymphocyte receptor concentration (Scarpace et al., 1982).

When normal subjects received theophylline alone for 1 week in this study, lymphocyte β-adrenergic receptor concentration was also lowered, although not to the extent observed with metaproterenol administered by itself or with theophylline. These results suggest that nonreceptor- as well as receptor-mediated desensitization may be a consequence of methylxanthine therapy in some cases. Cyclic AMP-mediated desensitization may also explain some of the effects glucocorticoids have on the properties of the β_2-adrenergic receptor-regulated adenylate cyclase system of the human lymphocyte and, perhaps, lung as well (discussed below). Resensitization and sometimes supersensitization follow withdrawal of agonist and in some tissues, including those of the respiratory system, resensitization is facilitated by glucocorticoids. This may be because corticosteroids have direct effects on the adenylate cyclase system of some cells as well as anti-inflammatory effects.

B. Glucocorticoids

Glucocorticoids increase the density of β-adrenergic receptors in rat lung membranes, although the effects of adrenalectomy remain equivocal (Mano et al., 1979; Scarpace and Abrass, 1982a). The steroids also increase receptor density in fetal rabbit lung and in cultured lung cells (Fraser and Venter, 1980; Cheng et al., 1980). Although hydrocortisone and methylprednisolone reverse or block airway tachyphylaxis to catecholamines (Conolly and Greenacre, 1976; Holgate et al., 1977; Stephen et al., 1980), few studies to date provide insight into the biochemistry of reversal in respiratory tissue.

In one study metaproterenol administered to rats decreased lung β-adrenergic receptor concentration and isoproterenol-dependent cyclic AMP production in a manner that was inhibited by concomitant methylprednisolone administration (Scarpace and Abrass, 1982b), much as the corticosteroid blocks airway tachyphylaxis (Stephan et al., 1980). Lung receptor loss occurs over 3-5 days in the rat. During that period β-adrenergic receptor number can be completely restored but isoproterenol-dependent cyclic AMP production only partially restored by methylprednisolone administration. Thus, despite replenishment, some receptors remained in an uncoupled state incapable of activating the catalytic subunit of adenylate cyclase. Experiments in human tissues more accessible than lung suggest that glucocorticoids exert similar effects on the β-adrenergic catecholamine-sensitive adenylate cyclase system in the management of asthma.

As in lung and bronchus, cyclic AMP production in peripheral lymphocytes is regulated by β_2-adrenergic receptors (Davis et al., 1980). Moreover, changes in the properties of these leukocyte receptors seem to mirror changes in the catecholamine sensitivity of the respiratory system. Thus, cyclic AMP levels are reduced in tracheal muscle from asthmatic dogs (Rinard et al., 1979), and lymphocytes from asthmatic humans have similarly reduced responsiveness to isoproterenol with respect to cyclic AMP production, which can be reversed by glucocorticoid exposure (Conolly and Greenacre, 1976; Lee et al., 1977; Logsdon et al., 1972). Hydrocortisone inhibits isproterenol-induced receptor loss and desensitization of human neutrophils if the two hormones are administered simultaneously in vivo (Davies and Lefkowitz, 1983). A single dose of methylprednisolone restores the receptor density of lymphocytes from asthmatic as well as normal human subjects desensitized in vivo with terbutaline (Hui et al., 1982). Even high concentrations of hydrocortisone fail to inhibit isoproterenol-dependent desensitization carried out in vitro, however, suggesting that the mechanism of steroid action is complex (Marone et al., 1980).

Although glucocorticoids have profound effects on β-adrenergic catecholamine sensitivity in general, the mechanism through which regulation is achieved remains unknown. Glucocorticoids increase the rate of de novo β-adrenergic receptor synthesis in lung cells in vitro at a rate somewhat similar to the time it takes glucocorticoids to reverse airway tachyphylaxis in vitro and in vivo (Holgate et al., 1977; Conolly, 1980).

Glucocorticoid-dependent replacement of receptors in desensitized rat lung (in vivo) appears to take much longer, however (Scarpace and Abrass, 1982b). A much more acute mechanism of glucocorticoid regulation might better explain, therefore, corticosteroid-dependent resensitization. In fact, a variety of glucocorticoids both stimulate basal and potentiate isoprotrenol- and PGE_1-dependent cyclic AMP production in human lymphocytes (Lee and Reed, 1977; Marone et al., 1980). There are marked differences between corticosteroid potency in vivo and ability to stimulate lymphocyte cyclic AMP production, so the mechanism of steroid action seems to be independent of the conventional glucocorticoid receptor (Lee and Reed, 1977). Glucocorticoids do not elevate lymphocyte cyclic AMP levels by phosphodiesterase inhibition like the methylxanthines, and the effects are not only too rapid to involve de novo protein synthesis but are not affected by inhibitors of RNA or protein synthesis (Lee and Reed, 1977). Direct effects of the glucocorticoids on the plasma membrane cannot be ruled out, but hydrocortisone does not affect the rate or extent of lymphocyte desensitization when this is carried out in vitro using high concentrations of isoproterenol (Marone et al., 1980). In contrast, quite different results were obtained when isoproterenol-induced tachyphylaxis was reversed within a few hours in human bronchial smooth muscle also treated with glucocorticoid in vitro (Conolly, 1980).

Paradoxically, these acute glucocorticoid effects on lymphocyte adenylate cyclase better explain some possible desensitizing effects the steroids seem to have rather than do their airway resensitizing properties. Exposing cells to hydrocortisone alone in vitro results in persistent elevation of intracellular cyclic AMP so long as the steroid remains. A similar elevation in lymphocyte cyclic AMP in vivo may mediate the cortisone-induced decrease in β-adrenergic receptors that occurs 4 hr after oral administration (Marone et al., 1980; Davies and Lefkowitz, 1980). Desensitization is transient under these conditions, however, and receptor concentration returns and slightly exceeds normal values after 24 hr, despite additional cortisone administration.

Clearly, a single mechanism of action fails to explain all of the effects glucocorticoids have on β-adrenergic catecholamine sensitivity. The ability of corticosteroids to block, reverse, or actually promote β-adrenergic receptor desensitization appears enigmatic, but may only represent real differences between the mechanism of regulation in lung and leukocyte or its properties in vivo and in vitro. Much higher concentrations of agonist can be achieved in vitro than in vivo, for instance, and these differences can markedly alter the properties of lymphocyte desensitization (Krall et al., 1980). It seems that some actions of the glucocorticoids can be attributed largely to the stimulatory effect they have on leukocyte cyclic AMP production since this might be expected to produce cyclic AMP- but not receptor-mediated desensitization. How recovery might be achieved and the extent to which a similar mechanism functions in lung remains to be determined.

C. Senescence

Sensitivity of tracheal smooth muscle to the relaxing effects of β-adrenergic catecholamines decreases with age in some species (Melville et al., 1979). In the rat sensitivity of lung adenylate cyclase to stimulation by guanine nucleotide, sodium fluoride, forskolin, and by isoproterenol decreases with age relative to basal activity (Scarpace and Abrass, 1983). These age-related decreases occur without concomitant changes in β-adrenergic receptor density, which suggests that many of the receptors are uncoupled.

Basal as well as isoproterenol-dependent cyclic AMP production also decreases in an age-related fashion in bovine trachealis (Andersson et al., 1978). Although age affects cyclic AMP production under conditions of basal or spontaneous tone, it does not affect the degree to which isoproterenol relaxes histamine-induced contraction. This apparent disparity might be explained by an effect of tension on hormone-sensitivity. Indeed, both cyclic AMP production and the degree of relaxation induced by isoproterenol differ depending on whether determinations are made on spontaneously contracting muscle strips or strips contracted with carbachol or histamine. The method of contracture does not affect theophylline- or papaverine-induced relaxation, however (Andersson et al., 1978).

Similar effects occur in guinea pig trachea, where isoproterenol and theophylline relax to the same extent both spontaneous contraction and that induced by low concentrations of carbachol, although isoproterenol is much more potent (Karlsson and Persson, 1981). As the concentration of carbachol is increased, however, isoproterenol sensitivity decreases more than theophylline sensitivity until relative potency has fallen from 15,000 to 1,500 and the maximal isoproterenol response is only a fraction of that achieved with theophylline. Like carbachol-dependent cyclic GMP production, its effects on isoproterenol sensitivity also require extracellular Ca^{2+} in the guinea pig trachea (Wong and Buckner, 1978). Somewhat paradoxically, the cholinergic agonist seems to have no effect on $^{45}Ca^{2+}$ uptake by tracheal smooth muscle rings despite this Ca^{2+} dependency (Kolbeck and Speir, 1984). Carbachol might be expected to facilitate or potentiate theophylline-dependent cyclic GMP accumulation during the course of β-adrenergic receptor desensitization under these conditions to explain, in part, the complex relationship between tension regulation by the cholinergic and adrenergic receptors. Events are probably not so straightforward, however, since carbachol is reported to decrease tracheal cyclic GMP in the guinea pig in sharp contrast to its effects on cyclic GMP levels in bovine trachea (Kolbeck and Speir, 1984).

Since these effects on β-adrenergic catecholamine sensitivity do not seem to extend to the relaxing effects of phosphodiesterase inhibitors, aging seems to affect a step proximal to the activation of cyclic-AMP-dependent protein kinase, possibly at the level at which the receptor is coupled with the adenylate cyclase catalytic subunit. For the same reason, altered catecholamine sensitivity seems to reflect interaction between the β-adrenergic receptor and the cholinergic and histamine receptors rather than the effect of tension on sensitivity per se. As expected of this kind of interaction, methacholine antagonizes isoproterenol-dependent cyclic AMP production and protein kinase activation in dog trachea (Torphy et al., 1983). Both carbachol and histamine promote the synthesis of cyclic GMP as well as contraction in bovine trachealis (Katsuki and Murad, 1977) which suggests that interactions may be mediated in a cyclic GMP-dependent manner.

D. Acetylcholine

Besides stimulating cyclic GMP production and the turnover of membrane phosphatidylinositol (described below), cholinergic agonists are inhibitors of smooth muscle cyclic AMP synthesis (Lee et al., 1972; Triner et al., 1972; Lohman et al., 1977). These inhibitory effects are mediated by the muscarinic cholinergic receptor, which has been partially purified from ileum smooth muscle (Venter, 1983). The mechanism of inhibition is most likely complex. In some cells it requires the activation of the inhibitory form of the N regulatory protein (N_i) which suppresses agonist-dependent (but not basal) adenylate cyclase (Gilman, 1984; Hughes et al., 1984). Inhibition also occurs through an entirely different mechanism that is not antagonized by the bacterial toxin that inhibits N_i activity (Hughes et al., 1984). The nature of this alternative mechanism remains obscure, but phosphodiesterase activation has been ruled out. It may, on the other hand, be related to the role of other N (not N_s or N_i) regulatory proteins in membrane phospholipid metabolism.

Muscarinic receptor-dependent stimulation of membrane phosphatidylinositol turnover is mediated by an N regulatory protein as well, but one with properties that are different from either N_s or N_i (Masters et al., 1985). The N regulatory proteins seem to constitute, therefore, a structurally homologous but functionally heterogeneous class of guanine nucleotide-binding membrane proteins (Roof et al., 1986; Mumby et al., 1986). Although acetylcholine is a potent inhibitor of smooth muscle cell cyclic AMP production, tracheal smooth muscle seems to have less N_i than other tissues when levels are quantified using polyclonal antibodies against the purified regulatory proteins (Mumby et al., 1986).

Instead, a larger though structurally homologous protein which is absent from brain, adrenal medulla, heart, or retinal rod outer segment is present in adrenal cortex and tracheal smooth muscle. The function of this protein, which is not necessarily an N regulatory protein despite its homology, is not known. Although speculative, these properties are consistent with a cholinergic inhibitory pathway in smooth muscle that is not mediated by N_i.

Another membrane phospholipid, phosphatic acid, has been shown to inhibit cyclic AMP synthesis in a manner that resembles cholinergic inhibition (Clark et al., 1980). As described more fully below, acetylcholine stimulates phosphatidic acid production through the diacylglycerol pathway. Moreover, phosphatidic acid causes contration in at least some kinds of smooth muscle (Salmon and Honeyman, 1980). Like some of the inhibitory effects of the muscarinic receptor, however, phosphatidic acid inhibition of cyclic AMP synthesis seems to be mediated by N_i in fibroblasts (Proll et al., 1985). Phosphatidic acid inhibition of cyclic AMP production could serve as an alternative or amplifying mechanism of the component of cholinergic inhibition mediated by N_i. The importance of this secondary inhibitory pathway might then differ with the capacity of the target cell to form phosphatidic acid from diacylglycerol.

Clearly, the interaction between the muscarinic cholinergic receptor and cyclic AMP-dependent smooth muscle relaxation is complex. It may have elements that encompass several kinds of N regulatory proteins, the degradation and synthesis of several membrane phospholipids, Ca^{2+} mobilization, and, in some instances, cyclic GMP synthesis as well. It is possible, however, that the complex mechanism of cholinergic receptor function is only the best understood of a ubiquitous mechanism through which receptors that regulate contraction interact with those that induce relaxation.

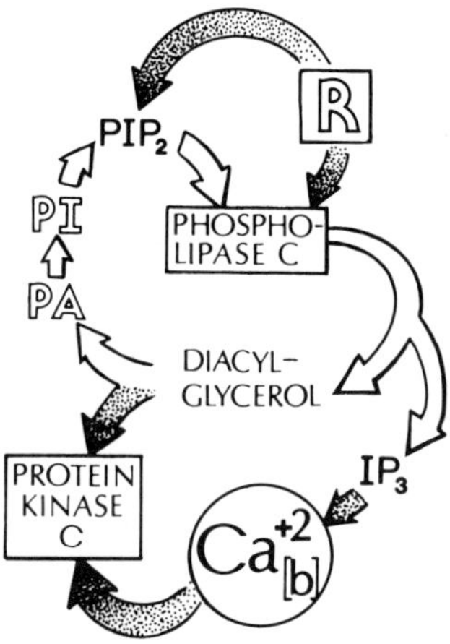

Figure 2 Regulation of intracellular calcium by membrane phosphatidylinositol breakdown. A small amount of phosphatidylinositol (PI) is converted to phosphatidylinositol 4,5-biphosphate (PIP_2) by membrane phosphorylating pathways. A hormone or neurotransmitter receptor (R) regulates the concentration of the intracellular PIP_2 breakdown products myoinositol 1,4,5-triphosphate (IP_3) and diacylglycerol, either by activating a membrane lipase (phospholipase C) or by increasing the size of the PIP_2 pool. IP_3 is short-lived, but has the capacity to release calcium by a poorly understood mechanism from intracellular storage sites ($Ca^{2+}{}_{[b]}$), probably the cisternae of the sarcoplasmic reticulum. Diacylglycerol activates a specific calcium-dependent and cyclic-nucleotide-*independent* protein kinase (protein kinase C) by increasing its sensitivity to cytoplasmic levels of the Ca^{2+}/calmodulin complex. Protein kinase C has a variety of specific phosphoprotein substrates, but the only one with a well-characterized function is the myosin light chain. Membrane PI is resynthesized from diacylglycerol by way of phosphatidic acid (PA). The rate-limiting stimulatory pathways are shown by (↑).

V. Cyclic-Nucleotide-Independent Mechanisms

The regulatory mechanisms described above are all related to the control of cyclic nucleotide-sensitive pathways in the smooth muscle cell. Despite the importance of the cyclic nucleotides in the regulation of tension, there are smooth muscle cell receptors that regulate contraction and relaxation without demonstrable effects on cyclic nucleotide production; how might these function? Noncyclic nucleotide-dependent mechanisms that regulate intracellular calcium are beginning to be characterized in a variety of cell types and may be of special importance in the regulation of tension in the smooth muscle cell.

Smooth muscle contraction induced by several different neurotransmitters has been known for some time to be associated with the degradation of the membrane lipid phosphatidylinositol (PI) (Jafferji and Michell, 1976; Salmon and Honeyman, 1979 and 1980). A small amount of PI in the plasma membrane is doubly phosphorylated by kinases or esterases and the resultant PIP_2 may be the actual form of the phospholipid regulated by the receptors for a variety of hormones and neurotransmitters in many mammalian cell types including smooth muscle (Suematsu et al., 1984a; Exton, 1985).

In vascular smooth muscle, as in nonmuscular tissue, receptors for α-adrenergic catecholamines, serotonin, and acetylcholine stimulate the hydrolysis of PIP_2 by phospholipase C. As shown in Figure 2, there are two principal products of PIP_2 hydrolysis: diacylglycerol and the inositol polyphosphate IP_3. IP_3 is short-lived and rapidly dephosphorylated or further phosphorylated. During its brief life span, however, it probably triggers the release of calcium from intracellular storage sites much as IP_3 release stored calcium when added to cells first permeabilized to the exogenously added IP_3 by destruction of integrity of the plasma membrane (Suematsu et al., 1984a; Exton, 1985). In the absence of an intact plasma membrane, the calcium released is undoubtedly from intracellular storage sites, principally the endoplasmic reticulum. This has been verified in several cell types by IP_3 addition to suspensions of endoplasmic reticulum-enriched vesicles preloaded with calcium.

Diacylglycerol, the other hydrolytic product of PIP_2, is a potent intracellular signal in its own right and activates calcium-dependent protein kinase C by increasing its calcium sensitivity. The more calcium-sensitive form of protein kinase C is then able to function at resting cell calcium levels and phosphorylates a number of specific phosphoproteins including the myosin light chain, which is also an MK (myosin light chain kinase, Fig. 1) substrate in smooth muscle. Protein kinase C phosphorylation probably decreases in turn the rate of phosphorylation of the myosin light chain by MK and also decreases actin-dependent ATPase activity (Nishikawa et al., 1984). Although both of these decreases would favor relaxation in the intact muscle cell, receptor-mediated PI breakdown, which should lead to an increase in diacylglycerol production and concomitant activation of protein kinase C, is generally associated with smooth muscle cell contraction. Clearly, these complex phospholipid pathways are not yet well enough understood to provide an unambiguous picture of how they contribute to the regulation of smooth muscle function.

Like IP_3, diacylglycerol is also short-lived and is rapidly rephosphorylated to form phosphatidic acid, which accounts for the appreciable increase in the level of phosphatidic acid (PA) that accompanies the breakdown of phosphatidylinositol in several varieties of smooth muscle (Salmon and Honeyman, 1979, 1980; Putney et al., 1980). PA is a precursor of membrane PI, and its phosphorylation to form PI completes the PI turnover cycle even though resynthesis may not take place in the plasma membrane.

VI. Conclusions

Most neurotransmitters and hormones regulate smooth muscle tension by binding to ligand-specific receptors on the cell surface. Many of these agonist-receptor complexes modulate the production of cyclic nucleotides with diverse intracellular consequences. Even steroid hormones that generally function at the level of the cell nucleus may affect changes in tension only indirectly by the effect they have on the synthesis of smooth muscle receptors or the proteins that couple them with cyclic nucleotide production.

A number of different pathways are probably regulated by cyclic-nucleotide-dependent phosphorylation in the control of smooth muscle tension but only the phosphorylation of the myosin light chain by MK and Ca^{2+} transport activity have been characterized in depth. Although the two pathways are regulated in a seemingly independent fashion by cyclic AMP and cyclic GMP in vitro, they must be integrated at the molecular level to account for the complex patterns of contraction and relaxation that occur in situ. Regulation of cyclic nucleotide production and destruction, activity of protein kinase or (protein) substrate accessibility, and interaction with epithelium are all levels at which integration might be achieved.

It is becoming equally clear, however, that the same agonist may have different mechanisms of action in different cells. Thus, the endothelial cell cholinergic receptor indirectly mediates cyclic GMP production by smooth muscle cells in the aorta and other vessels but stimulates phosphatidylinositol breakdown in nonvascular smooth muscle. The two forms of the α-adrenergic catecholamine receptor are another example in which the α_2 receptor inhibits agonist-dependent cyclic AMP production while the α_1 receptor stimulates the breakdown of membrane PI and mobilizes intracellular calcium in the smooth muscle cell (Fain and Garcia-Sainz, 1980; Brown et al., 1984).

In the final analysis, the relative importance of these different and complex mechanisms to normal physiological function, their differences in health and disease, and whether they may be therapeutically manipulated to restore normal function are the anticipated consequences of further research into the basic mechanisms of smooth muscle cell regulation.

Acknowledgment

This work was supported by funds from the Veterans Administration and by NIH Grant No. HD-9285.

References

Adelstein, R. S., Pato, M. D., and Conti, M. A. (1981). The role of phosphorylation in regulating contractile proteins. In *Advances in Cyclic Nucleotide Research,* Vol. 14. Edited by J. Dumont, P. Greengard, and G. A. Robison. New York, Raven Press, pp. 361-373.

Aksoy, M. O., Mras, S., Kamm, K. E., and Murphy, R. A. (1983). Ca^{+2}, cAMP, and changes in myosin phosphorylation during contraction of smooth muscle. *Am. J. Physiol. 245*: C255-C270.

Anand-Srivastava, M. B., Franks, D. J., Cantin, M., and Genest, J. (1982). Presence of "Ra" and "P"-site receptors for adenosine coupled to adenylate cyclase in cultured vascular smooth muscle cells. *Biochem. Biophys. Res. Commun. 108*: 213-219.

Andersson, R., and Nilsson, K. (1972). Cyclic AMP and calcium in relaxation in intestinal smooth muscle. *Nature 238*: 119-120.

Andersson, R. G., Kovesi, G., and Ericsson, E. (1978). Beta-adrenoceptor stimulation and cyclic AMP levels in bovine tracheal muscle of old and young animals. *Acta Pharmacol. Toxicol. 43*: 323-327.

Baudouin-Legros, M., and Meyer, P. (1973). Effects of angiotensin, catecholamines, and cAMP on calcium storage in aortic microsomes. *Br. J. Pharmacol. 47*: 377-385.

Boe, J., and Simonsson, B. G. (1980). Adrenergic receptors and sympathetic agents in isolated human pulmonary arteries. *Eur. J. Respir. Dis. 61*: 195-202.

Bohme, E., Grossmann, G., Herz, J., Musch, A., Spies, C., and Schultz, G. (1984). Regulation of cyclic GMP formation by soluble guanylate cyclase: Stimulation by NO-containing compounds. In *Advances in Cyclic Nucleotide and Protein Phosphorylation Research,* Vol. 17. Edited by P. Greengard, G. A. Robison, R. Paoletti, and S. Nicosia. New York, Raven Press, pp. 259-266.

Bokoch, G. M., Katada, T., Northup, J. K., Ui, M., and Gilman, A. G. (1984). Purification and properties of the inhibitory guanine nucleotide-binding regulatory components of adenylate cyclase. *J. Biol. Chem. 259*: 3560-3567.

Brockbank, K. J., and England, P. J. (1980). A rapid method for the preparation of sarcolemma vesicles from rat aorta and the stimulation of Ca-uptake into the vesicles by cAMP-dependent protein kinase. *FEBS Lett 122*: 67-71.

Brown, C. M., and Collis, M. G. (1982). Evidence for an A_2/Ra adenosine receptor in the guinea pig trachea. *Br. J. Pharmacol. 76*: 381-388.

Brown, R. D., Berger, K. D., and Taylor, P. (1984). $Alpha_1$-adrenergic receptor activation mobilizes cellular Ca^{2+} in a muscle cell line. *J. Biol. Chem. 259*: 7554-7562.

Casnellie, J. E., and Greengard, P. (1974). Guanosine 3′:5′-monophosphate-dependent phosphorylation of endogenous substrate proteins in membranes of mammalian smooth muscle. *Proc. Natl. Acad. Sci. USA 71*: 1891-1895.

Casnellie, J. E., Ives, H. E., Jamieson, J. D., and Greengard, P. (1980). Cyclic

GMP-dependent phosphorylation in intact medial tissue and isolated cells from vascular smooth muscle. *J. Biol. Chem. 255*: 3770-3776.

Cerione, R. A., Strulovici, B., Benovic, J. L., Lefkowitz, R. J., and Caron, M. G. (1983a). Pure beta-adrenergic receptor: The single polypeptide confers catecholamine responsiveness to adenylate cyclase. *Nature 306*: 562-566.

Cerione, R. A., Strulovici, B., Benovic, J. L., Strader, C. D., Caron, M. G., and Lefkowitz, R. J. (1983b). Reconstitution of beta-adrenergic receptors in lipid vesicles: Affinity chromatography-purified receptors confer catecholamine responsiveness on a heterologous adenylate cyclase system. *Proc. Natl. Acad. Sci. USA 80*: 4899-4903.

Chatterjee, M., and Murphy, R. A. (1983). Calcium-dependent stress maintenance without myosin phosphorylation in skinned smooth muscle. *Science 221*: 464-466.

Cheng, J. B., Goldfien, A., Ballard, P. L., and Roberts, J. M. (1980). Glucocorticoids increase pulmonary beta-adrenergic receptors in fetal rabbit. *Endocrinology 86*: 154-159.

Clark, R., Salmon, D., and Honeyman, T. (1980). Phosphatidic acid inhibition of PGE-stimulated cAMP accumulation in WI-38 fibroblast: similarities with carbachol inhibition. *J. Cyc. Nuc. Res. 6*:37-49.

Collis, M. G., and Brown, C. M. (1983). Adenosine relaxes the aorta by interacting with an A_2 receptor and an intracellular site. *Eur. J. Pharmacol. 96*: 61-69.

Conolly, M. E. (1980). Cyclic nucleotides, beta receptors, and bronchial asthma. In *Advances in Cyclic Nucleotide Research,* Vol. 12. Edited by P. Hamet and H. Sands. New York, Raven Press, pp. 151-159.

Conolly, M. E., and Greenacre, J. K. (1976). The lymphocyte beta-adrenoreceptor in normal subjects and patients with bronchial asthma. The effect of different forms of treatment on receptor function. *J. Clin. Invest. 58*: 1307-1316.

Daniel, E. E., Grover, A. K., and Kwan, C. Y. (1983). Calcium. In *Biochemistry of Smooth Muscle,* Vol. III. Edited by N. L. Stephens. Boca Raton, CRC Press, pp. 2-88.

Davies, A. O., and Lefkowitz, R. J. (1980). Corticosteroid-induced differential receptors in circulating human polymorphonuclear leukocytes and mononuclear leukocytes. *J. Clin. Endocrinol. Metab. 51*: 599-605.

Davies, A. O., and Lefkowitz, R. J. (1983). In vitro desensitization of beta adrenergic receptors in human neutrophils. Attenuation by corticosteroids. *J. Clin. Invest. 71*: 565-571.

Davies, A. O., and Lefkowitz, R. J. (1984). Regulation of beta-adrenergic receptors by steroid hormones. *Annu. Rev. Physiol. 46*: 119-130.

Davis, C., Conolly, M. E., and Greenacre, J. K. (1980). Beta-adrenoceptors in human lung, bronchus, and lymphocytes. *Br. J. Clin. Pharmacol. 10*: 425-432.

DeLanerolle, P., Nishikawa, M., Yost, D. A., and Adelstein, R. S. (1984). Increased phosphorylation of myosin light chain kinase after an increase in cyclic AMP in intact smooth muscle. *Science 223*: 1415-1417.

Deth, R. C., and Lynch, C. J. (1981). Mobilization of a common source of smooth muscle Ca^{+2} by norepinephrine and methylxanthines. *Am. J. Physiol. 240*: C239-C247.

Deth, R., and Casteels, R. (1977). A study of releasable Ca fractions in smooth muscle cells of the rabbit aorta. *J. Gen. Physiol. 69*: 401-416.

Diamond, J. (1983). Lack of correlation between cyclic GMP elevation and relaxation of nonvascular smooth muscle by nitroglycerine, nitroprusside, hydroxylamine, and sodium azide. *J. Pharmacol. Exp. Ther. 225*: 422-426.

Diamond, J., and Chu, E. B. (1983). Possible role for cyclic GMP in endothelium-dependent relaxation of rabbit aorta by acetylcholine. Comparison with nitroglycerine. *Res. Commun. Chem. Pathol. Pharmacol. 41*: 369-381.

Douglas, J. S., Lewis, A. J., Ridgway, P., Brink, C., and Bouhuys, A. (1977). Tachyphylaxis to beta-adrenoceptor agonists in guinea pig airway smooth muscle in vivo and in vitro. *Eur. J. Pharmacol. 42*: 195-205.

Driska, S. P., Aksoy, M. O., and Murphy, R. A. (1981). Myosin light chain phosphorylation associated with contraction in arterial smooth muscle. *Am. J. Physiol. 240*: C222-C233.

Exton, J. (1985). Role of calcium and phosphoinositides in the actions of certain hormones and neurotransmitters. *J. Clin. Invest. 75*: 1753-1757.

Fain, J. N., and Garcia-Sainz, J. A. (1980). Role of phosphatidylinositol turnover in $alpha_1$ and of adenylate cyclase inhibition in $alpha_2$ effects of catecholamines. *Life Sci. 26*: 1183-1194.

Fain, J. N., and Malbon, C. C. (1979). Regulation of adenylate cyclase by adenosine. *Mol. Cell. Biochem. 25*: 143-169.

Feldman, R. D., Limbird, L. E., Nadeau, J., FitzGerald, G. A., Robertson, D., and Wood, J. J. (1983). Dynamic regulation of leukocyte beta adrenergic receptor-agonist interactions by physiological changes in circulating catecholamines. *J. Clin. Invest. 72*: 164-170.

Fortier, M., Chase, D., Korenman, S. G., and Krall, J. F. (1983). Beta-adrenergic catecholamine-dependent properties of rat myometrium primary cultures. *Am. J. Physiol. 245*: C84-C90.

Fraser, C. M., and Venter, J. C. (1980). The synthesis of beta-adrenergic receptors in cultured human lung cells: induction by glucocorticoids. *Biochem. Biophys. Res. Commun. 94*: 390-397.

Fredholm, B. B., Brodin, K., and Strandberg, K. (1979). On the mechanism of relaxation of tracheal muscle by theophylline and other cyclic nucleotide phosphodiesterease inhibitors. *Acta Pharmacol. Toxicol. 45*: 336-344.

Furchgott, R. F., and Zawadski, J. V. (1980). The obligatory role of endothelial cells in the relaxation of arterial smooth muscle by acetylcholine. *Nature 288*: 373-376.

Galant, S. P., Duriseti, L., Underwood, S., Insel, P. A. (1978). Decreased beta-adrenergic receptors on polymorphonuclear leukocytes after adrenergic therapy. *N. Engl. J. Med. 299*: 933-936.

Galvas, P. E., and DiSalvo, J. (1983). Concentration and time-dependent relationships between isosorbide dinitrate-induced relaxation and formation of cyclic GMP in coronary arterial smooth muscle. *J. Pharmacol. Exp. Ther. 224*; 373-378.

Garbers, D. L. (1979). Purification of soluble guanylate cyclase from rat lung. *J. Biol. Chem. 254*: 240-243.

Gerthoffer, W. T., and Murphy, R. A. (1983). Ca^{2+}, myosin phosphorylation, and relaxation of arterial smooth muscle. *Am. J. Physiol. 245*: C271-C277.

Gilman, A. G. (1984). Guanine nucleotide-binding regulatory proteins and dual control of adenylate cyclase. *J. Clin. Invest. 73*: 1-4.

Green, D. A., Friedman, J., Clark, R. B. (1981). Epinephrine desensitization of adenylate cyclase from cyc^- and S49 cultured lymphoma cells. *J. Cyclic Nucleotide Res. 7*: 161-172.

Hardman, J. G. (1981). Cyclic nucleotides and smooth muscle contraction: some conceptual and experimental considerations. In *Smooth Muscle: An Assessment of Current Knowledge*. Edited by E. Bulbring, A. F. Brading, A. W. Jones, and T. Tomita. Austin, University of Texas Press, pp. 249-262.

Heidenreich, K. A., Weiland, G. A., and Molinoff, P. B. (1980). Characterization of radiolabeled agonist binding to beta-adrenergic receptors in mammalian tissues. *J. Cyclic Nucleotide Res. 6*: 217-230.

Hendeles, L., and Weinberger, M. (1983). Theophylline. A "state of the art" review. *Pharmacotherapy 3*: 2-44.

Hildebrandt, J. D., Sekura, R. D., Codina, J., Iyengar, R., Manclark, C. R., and Birnbaumer, L. (1983). Stimulation of adenylyl cyclases mediated by distinct regulatory proteins. *Nature 302*: 706-709.

Hogaboom, G. K., and Fedan, J. S. (1981). Calmodulin stimulation of calcium uptake and (Ca^{2+}-Mg^{2+})-ATPase activities in microsomes from canine tracheal smooth muscle. *Biochem. Biophys. Res. Commun. 99*: 737-744.

Hogaboom, G. K., Emler, C. A., Butcher, F. R., and Fedan, J. S. (1982). Concerted phosphorylation of endogenous tracheal smooth muscle membrane proteins by Ca^{+2}-modulin, cyclic GMP- and cyclic AMP-dependent protein kinases. *FEBS Lett. 139*: 309-312.

Holgate, S. T., Baldwin, C. J., and Tattersfield, A. E. (1977). Beta-adrenergic agonist resistance in normal human airways. *Lancet 2*: 375-377.

Holzmann, S. (1982). Endothelium-induced relaxation by acetylcholine associated with larger rises in cyclic GMP in coronary arterial strips. *J. Cyclic Nucleotide Res.* *8*: 409-419.

Homey, C. J., Rockson, S. G., Countaway, J., and Egan, D. A. (1983). Purification and characterization of the mammalian β_2-adrenergic receptor. *Biochemistry 22*: 660-668.

Hong, S. L. (1983). Inhibition of prostacyclin synthesis in endothelial cells by methylisobutylxanthine is not mediated through elevated cAMP level. *Biochim. Biophys. Acta 754*: 258-263.

Hoyer, D., Reynolds, E. E., and Molinoff, P. (1984). Agonist-induced changes in the properties of beta-adrenergic receptors on intact S49 lymphoma cells. Time-dependent changes in the affinity of the receptors for agonists. *Mol. Pharmacol. 25*: 209-218.

Huddart, H., Bayton, E., and Shanklin, J. (1983). Influence of some common methylxanthines on contractile responses and calcium mobilization of ileal, vas deferens and bladder smooth muscle. *J. Exp. Biol. 107*: 73-93.

Hughes, A., Martin, M., and Harden, T. (1984). Pertussis toxin differentiates between two mechanisms of attenuation of cyclic AMP accumulation by muscarinic cholinergic receptors. *Proc. Natl. Acad. Sci. USA. 81*:5680-5684.

Hui, K. K., Conolly, M. E., and Tashkin, D. (1982). Reversal of human lymphocyte beta-adrenoceptor desensitization by glucocorticoids. *Clin. Pharmacol. Ther. 32*: 566-571.

Ives, H. E., Casnellie, J. E., Greengard, P., and Jamieson, J. D. (1980). Subcellular localization of cyclic GMP-dependent protein kinase and its substrates in vascular smooth muscle. *J. Biol. Chem. 255*: 3777-3785.

Iyengar, R., Bhat, M. K., Riser, M. E., and Birnbaumer, L. (1981). Receptor-specific desensitization of the S49 lymphoma cell adenylyl cyclase. Unaltered behavior of the regulatory component. *J. Biol. Chem. 256*: 4810-4815.

Jafferji, S., and Michell, R. (1976). Muscarinic cholinergic stimulation of phosphatidylinosotiol turnover in the longitudinal smooth muscle of guinea-pig ileum. *Biochem. J. 154*: 653-657.

Jones, T. R., Lefcoe, N. M., and Hamilton, J. T. (1980). Pharmacological study of adenosine and related compounds on isolated guinea pig trachea: Evidence for more than one type of purine receptor. *Can. J. Physiol. Pharmacol. 58*: 1356-1365.

Karlsson, J.-A., and Persson, C. G. A. (1981). Influence of tracheal contraction on relaxant effects in vitro of theophylline and isoproterenol. *Br. J. Pharmacol. 74*: 73-79.

Karlsson, J.-A., Kjellin, G., and Persson, C. (1982). Effects on tracheal smooth muscle of adenosine and methylxanthines, and their interaction. *J. Pharmacol. 34*: 788-793.

Kaslow, H. R., Farfel, Z., Johnson, G. L., and Bourne, H. R. (1979). Adenylate cyclase assembled in vitro: cholera toxin substrates determine different patterns of regulation by isoproterenol and guanosine 5′-triphosphate. *Mol. Pharmacol. 15*: 472-483.

Katada, T., and Ui, M. (1982). ADP ribosylation of the specific membrane protein of C6 cells by islet-activating protein associated with modification of adenylate cyclase activity. *J. Biol. Chem. 257*: 7210-7216.

Katsuki, S., and Murad, F. (1977). Regulation of adenosine cyclic 3′:5′-monophosphate and guanosine cyclic 3′:5′ cyclic monophosphate levels and contractility in bovine tracheal smooth muscle. *Mol. Pharmacol. 13*: 330-341.

Katsuki, S., Arnold, W., Mittal, C., and Murad, F. (1977). Stimulation of guanylate cyclase by sodium nitroprusside, nitroglycerine and nitric oxide in various tissue preparations and comparison to the effects of sodium azide and hydroxylamine. *J. Cyclic Nucleotide Res. 3*: 23-35.

Kerrick, W. G. L., and Hoar, P. E. (1981). Inhibition of smooth muscle tension by cyclic AMP-dependent protein kinase. *Nature 292*: 253-255.

Kirchick, H. J., Iyengar, R., and Birnbaumer, L. (1983). Human chorionic gonadotropin-induced heterologous desensitization of adenylyl cyclase from highly luteinized rat ovaries: Attenuation of regulatory N component activity. *Endocrinology 113*: 1638-1646.

Kolbeck, R. C., and Speir, W. A. (1984). Temporal relationship of cyclic nucleotide levels and calcium exchange to histamine-induced tension development. *Proc. Soc. Exp. Biol. Med. 177*: 126-131.

Kolbeck, R. C., Speir, W. A., Carrier, G. O., and Bransome, E. D. (1979). Apparent irrelevance of cyclic nucleotides to the relaxation of tracheal smooth muscle induced by theophylline. *Lung 156*: 73-183.

Krall, J. F., Swensen, J. L., and Korenman, S. G. (1976). Hormonal control of uterine contraction. Characterization of cyclic AMP-dependent membrane properties in the myometrium. *Biochim. Biophys. Acta 448*: 578-588.

Krall, J. F., Connelly, M., and Tuck, M. L. (1980). Acute regulation of beta-adrenergic catecholamine sensitivity in human lymphocytes. *J. Pharmacol. Exp. Ther. 214*: 554-560.

Krall, J. F., Fortier, M., and Korenman, S. G. (1983). Smooth muscle cyclic nucleotide biochemistry. In *Biochemistry of Smooth Muscle*, Vol. III. Edited by N. L. Stephens. Boca Raton, CRC Press, pp. 89-128.

Krall, J. F., Barrett, J. D., Jamgotchian, N., and Korenman, S. G. (1984). Interaction of series E prostaglandins and beta-adrenergic catecholamines in the regulation of uterine smooth muscle motility and adenylate cyclase. *J. Endocrinol. 102*: 329-336.

Lee, T.-P., Kuo, J., and Greengard, P. (1972). Role of muscarinic cholinergic receptors in regulation of guanosine 3′:5′-cyclic monophosphate content in mammalian brain, heart muscle, and intestinal smooth muscle. *Proc. Nat. Acad. Sci. USA. 69*:3287-3291.

Lee, T.-P., and Reed, C. E. (1977). Effects of steroids on the regulation of the levels of cyclic AMP in human lymphocytes. *Biochem. Biophys. Res. Commun. 78*: 998-1004.

Lee, T.P., Busse, W. W., and Reed, C. E. (1977). Effect of beta adrenergic agonist, prostaglandins, and cortisol on lymphocyte levels of cyclic adenosine monophosphate and glycogen. *Allergy Clin. Immunol. 59*: 408-413.

Leiber, D., and Harbon, S. (1979). Modulation of rat myometrial guanylate cyclase activities by sodium nitroprusside and unsaturated fatty acids. *Biochem. Biophys. Res. Commun. 89*: 598-606.

Lincoln, T. M. (1983). Effects of nitroprusside and 8-bromo-cyclic GMP on the contractile activity of the rat aorta. *J. Pharmacol. Exp. Ther. 224*: 100-107.

Lincoln, T. M., Hall, C. L., Park, C. R., and Corbin, J. D. (1976). Guanosine 3′:5′-cyclic monophosphate binding proteins in rat tissues. *Proc. Natl. Acad. Sci. USA 73*: 2559-2563.

Logsdon, P. J., Middleton, E., Jr., and Coffey, R. G. (1972). Stimulation of leukocyte adenyl cyclase by hydrocortisone and isoproterenol in asthmatic and nonasthmatic subjects. *J. Allergy Clin. Immunol. 50*: 45-56.

Lohmann, S. M., Miech, R. P., and Butcher, F. R. (1977). Effects of isoproterenol, theophylline and carbachol on cyclic nucleotide levels and relaxation of bovine tracheal smooth muscle. *Biochim. Biophys. Acta 499*: 238-250.

MacFarlane, D. E. (1984). Inhibitors of cyclic nucleotide phosphodiesterases inhibit protein carboxyl methylation in intact blood platelets. *J. Biol. Chem. 259*: 1357-1362.

Mano, K., Akbarzadeh, A., and Townley, R. G. (1979). Effect of hydrocortisone on beta-adrenergic receptors in lung membranes. *Life Sci. 25*: 1925-1930.

Marone, G., Lichtenstein, L. M., and Plaut, M. (1980). Hydrocortisone and human lymphocytes: increases in cyclic adenosine 3′:5′-monophosphate and potentiation of adenylate cyclase-activating agents. *J. Pharmacol. Exp. Ther. 215*: 469-478.

Masters, S., Martin, M., Harden, T., and brown, J. (1985). Pertussis toxin does not inhibit muscarinic-receptor-mediated phosphoinositide hydrolysis or calcium mobilization. *Biochem. J. 227*:933-937.

McKenzie, S. G., Frew, R., and Bar, H.-P. (1977). Effects of adenosine and related compounds on adenylate cyclase and cyclic AMP levels in smooth muscle. *Eur. J. Pharmacol. 41*: 193-203.

Melville, G. N., Irvani, J., Vassell, M., and Minnis, J. (1979). Airway response to adrenergic agonists and antagonists in 3-day- to 2-year-old rats. *Respiration 38*: 74-80.

Miech, R. P., Niedzwicki, J. G., and Smith, T. R. (1979). Effect of theophylline on the binding of cAMP to soluble protein from tracheal smooth muscle *Biochem. Pharmacol. 28*: 3687-3688.

Minneman, K. P., Hegstrand, L. R., and Molinoff, P. B. (1979). Simultaneous determination of β_1-x and β_2-x adrenergic receptors in tissues containing both receptor subtypes. *Mol. Pharmacol. 16*: 34-36.

Morel, N., Wibo, M., and Goddfraind, T. (1981). A calmodulin-stimulated Ca^{+2} pump in rat aorta plasma membranes. *Biochim. Biophys. Acta 644*: 82-88.

Moylan, R. D., Barovsky, K., and Brooker, G. (1982). N^6,O^2-Dibutyryl cyclic AMP and cholera toxin-induced beta-adrenergic receptor loss in cultured cells. *J. Biol. Chem. 257*: 4947-4950.

Mumby, S., Kahn, R., Manning, D., and Gilman, A. (1986). Antisera of designed specificity for subunits of guanine nucleotide-binding regulatory proteins. *Proc. Natl. Acad. Sci. USA. 83*:265-269.

Nakazawa, K., and Sano, M. (1975). Partial purification and properties of guanosine 3′:5′-monophosphate-dependent protein kinase from lung. *J. Biol. Chem. 250*: 7415-7419.

Nickols, G. A., and Brooker, G. (1979). Induction of refractoriness to isoproterenol by prior treatment of C6-2B rat astrocytoma cells with cholera toxin. *J. Cyclic Nucleotide Res. 5*: 435-447.

Niewoehner, D. E., Campe, H., Duane, S., McGowan, T., and Montgomery, M. R. (1979). Mechanisms of airway smooth muscle response to isoproterenol and theophylline. *J. Appl. Physiol. 47*: 330-336.

Nishikawa, M., Sellars, J., Adelstein, R., and Hidaka, H. (1984). Protein kinase C modulates *in vitro* phosphorylation of the smooth muscle heavy meromyson by myosin light chain kinase. *J. Biol. Chem. 259*: 8808-814.

Nishikori, K., and Maeno, H. (1979). Close relationship between adenosine 3′:5′-monophosphate dependent endogenous phosphorylation of a specific protein and stimulation of Ca uptake in rat uterine microsomes. *J. Biol. Chem. 254*: 6099-6105.

Persson, C., Karlsson, J.-A., and Erjefalt, I. (1982). Differentiation between bronchodilation and universal adenosine antagonism among xanthine derivatives. *Life Sci. 30*: 2181-2189.

Piascik, M. T., Babich, M., and Rush, M. E. (1983). Calmodulin stimulation and calcium regulation of smooth muscle adenylate cyclase activity. *J. Biol. Chem. 258*: 10913-10918.

Polson, J. B., Krzanowski, J. J., Anderson, W. H., Fitzpatrick, D. F., Hwang, D. P. C., and Szentivanyi, A. (1979). Analysis of the relationship between pharmacological inhibition of cyclic nucleotide phosphodiesterase and relaxation of canine tracheal smooth muscle. *Biochem. Pharmacol. 28*: 1391-1395.

Polson, J. B., Krzanowski, J. J., and Szentivanyi, A. (1982). Inhibition of a high affinity cyclic AMP phosphodiesterase and relaxation of canine tracheal smooth muscle. *Biochem. Pharmacol. 31*: 3403-3406.

Proll, M., Clark, R., and Butcher, R. (1985). Phosphatidate and monooleylphosphatidate inhibition of fibroblast adenylate cyclase is mediated by the inhibitory coupling protein, N_i. *Mol. Pharmacol. 28*:331-337.

Putney, J. W. Jr., Weiss, S. J., Van De Walle, C. M., and Haddas, R. A. (1980). Is phosphatidic acid a calcium ionophore under neurohumoral control? *Nature 284*:343-347.

Rapoport, R. M., and Murad, F. (1983a). Endothelium-dependent and nitrovasodilator-induced relaxation of vascular smooth muscle role of cyclic GMP. *J. Cyclic Nucleotide Protein Phosphate Res. 9*: 281-296.

Rapoport, R. M., and Murad, F. (1983b). Agonist-induced endothelium-dependent relaxation in rat thoracic aorta may be mediated through GMP. *Circ. Res. 52*: 352-357.

Rapoport, R. M., Draznin, M. B., and Murad, F. (1982). Sodium nitroprusside-induced protein phosphorylation in intact rat aorta is mimicked by 8-bromo-cyclic GMP. *Proc. Natl. Acad. Sci. USA 79*: 6470-6474.

Rapoport, R. M., Draznin, M. B., and Murad, F. (1983). Endothelium-dependent relaxation in rat aorta may be mediated through cyclic GMP-dependent protein phosphorylation. *Nature 306*: 174-176.

Rinard, G. A., Rubinfeld, A. R., Brunton, L. L., and Mayer, S. E. (1979). Depressed cyclic AMP levels in airway smooth muscle from asthmatic dogs. *Proc. Natl. Acad. Sci. USA 76*: 1472-1476.

Roof, D., Applebury, M., and Sternweis, P. (1985). Relationships within the family of GTP-binding proteins isolated from bovine central nervous system. *J. Biol. Chem. 260*:16242-16249.

Ross, E. (1982). Physical separation of the catalytic and regulatory proteins of hepatic adenylate cyclase. *J. Biol. Chem. 257*: 10751-10758.

Ruegg, J. C., and Paul, R. J. (1982). Vascular smooth muscle: calmodulin and cyclic AMP-dependent protein kinase alter calcium sensitivity in porcine carotid skinned fibers. *Circ. Res. 50*: 394-399.

Salmon, D. M., and Honeyman, T. W. (1979). Increased phosphatidase accumulation during single contractions of isolated-smooth muscle cells. *Biochem. Soc. Trans. 7*: 986-988.

Salmon, D. M., and Honeyman, T. W. (1980). Proposed mechanisms of cholinergic action in smooth muscle. *Nature 284*: 344-345.

Scarpace, P. J., and Abrass, I. B. (1982a). Glucocorticoid regulation of lung beta-adrenergic receptors. *Drug. Dev. Res. 2*: 91-94.

Scarpace, P. J., and Abrass, I. B. (1982b). Desensitization of adenylate cyclase and down regulation of beta-adrenergic receptors after *in vivo* administration of beta-agonist. *J. Pharmacol. Exp. Ther. 223*: 327-331.

Scarpace, P. J., and Abrass, I. B. (1983). Decreased beta-adrenergic agonist affinity and adenylate cyclase activity in senescent rat lung. *J. Gerontol. 38*: 143-147.

Scarpace, P. J., Littner, M. R., Tashkin, D. P., and Abrass, I. B. (1982). Lymphocyte beta-adrenergic refractoriness induced by theophylline or metaproterenol in healthy and asthmatic subjects. *Life Sci. 31*: 1567-1573.

Scheid, C. R., Honeyman, T. W., and Fay, F. B. (1979). Mechanism of beta-adrenergic relaxation of smooth muscle. *Nature 277*: 32-36.

Silver, P. J., Schmidt-Silver, C., and DiSalvo, J. (1982). Beta-adrenergic relaxation and cAMP kinase activation in coronary arterial smooth muscle. *Am. J. Physiol. 242*: H177-H184.

Sparrow, M. P., Pfitzer, G., Gagelman, M., and Ruegg, J. C. (1984). Effect of calmodulin, Ca^{+2}, and cAMP protein kinase on skinned tracheal smooth muscle. *Am. J. Physiol. 246*: C308-C314.

Stadel, J. M., Strulovici, B., Nambi, P., Lavin, T. H., Briggs, M. M., Caron, M. G., and Lefkowitz, R. J. (1983a). Desensitization of the beta-adrenergic receptor of frog erthyrocytes. Recovery and characterization of the down-regulated receptors in sequestered vesicles. *J. Biol. Chem. 258*: 3032-3038.

Stadel, J. M., Nambi, P., Shorr, R. G. L., Sawyer, D. F., Caron, M. G., and Lefkowitz, R. J. (1983b). Catecholamine-induced desensitization of turkey erythrocyte adenylate cyclase is associated with phosphorylation of the beta-adrenergic receptor. *Proc. Natl. Acad. Sci. USA 80*: 3173-3177.

Stephan, W. C.. Chick, T. W., Avner, B. P., and Jenne, J. W. (1980). Tachyphylaxis to inhaled isoproterenol and the effect of methylprednisolone in dogs. *J. Allergy Clin. Immunol. 65*: 105-109.

Sternweiss, P. C., Northrup, J. K., Smigel, M. D., and Gilman, A. G. (1981). The regulatory component of adenylate cyclase. Purification and properties. *J. Biol. Chem. 256*: 11517-11526.

Strittmatter, S., and Neer, E. J. (1980). Properties of the separated catalytic and regulatory units of brain adenylate cyclase. *Proc. Natl. Acad. Sci. USA 77*: 6344-6348.

Suematsu, E., Hirata, M., Hasimoto, T., and Kuriyama, H. (1984a). Inositol 1,4,5-triphosphate releases Ca^{2+} from intracellular store sites in skinned single cells of porcine coronary artery. *Biochem. Biophys. Res. Commun. 120*: 481-485.

Suematsu, E., Hirata, M., and Kuriyama, H. (1984b). Effects of cAMP- and cGMP-dependent protein kinases, and calmodulin on Ca^{+2} uptake by highly purified sarcolemmal vesicles of vascular smooth muscle. *Biochim. Biophys. Acta 773*: 83-90.

Toews, m. L., Harden, T. K., and Perkins, J. P. (1983). High-affinity binding of agonists to beta-adrenergic receptors on intact cells. *Proc. Natl. Acad. Sci. USA 80*: 3553-3557.

Torphy, T. J., Freese, W. B., Rinard, G. A., Brunton, L. L., and Mayer, S. E. (1982). Cyclic nucleotide-dependent protein kinases in airway smooth muscle. *J. Biol. Chem. 257*: 11609-11616.

Torphy, T. J., Rinard, G. A., Rietow, M. G., and Mayer, S. E. (1983). Functional antagonism in canine tracheal smooth muscle: Inhibition by methacholine of the mechanical and biochemical responses to isoproterenol. *J. Pharmacol. Exp. Ther. 227*: 694-700.

Tougui, Z., Do Khac, L., and Harbon, S. (1980). Modulation of cyclic AMP content of the rat myometrium:desensitization to isoproterenol, PGE_2, and prostacyclin. *Mol. Cell. Endocrinol. 20*: 17-34.

Triner, L., Vulliemoz, Y., Verosky, M., and Nahas, G. (1972). Acetylcholine and the cyclic AMP system in smooth muscle. *Biochem. Biophys. Res. Comm. 46*:1866-1873.

Triner, L., Vulliemoz, Y., and Verosky, M. (1977). Cyclic 3′:5′-adenosine monophosphate and bronchial tone. *Eur. J. Pharmacol. 41*: 37-46.

U'Prichard, D. C., Bylund, D. B., and Snyder, S. H. (1978). (±)-[^{3}H] Epinephrine and (-)-[^{3}H] dihydroalprenolol binding to β_1- and β_2-noradrenergic receptors in brain, heart, and lung membranes. *J. Biol. Chem. 253*: 5090-5102.

Venter, J. (1983). Muscarinic cholinergic receptor structure. Receptor size, membrane size, membrane orientation, and absence of major phylogenetic structural diversity. *J. Biol. Chem. 258*:4842-4848.

Waldo, G. I., Northrup, J. K., Perkins, J. P., and Harden, T. K. (1983). Characterization of an altered membrane form of the beta-adrenergic receptor produced during agonist-induced desensitization. *J. Biol. Chem. 258*: 13900-13908.

Witkin, K. M., and Harden, T. K. (1981). A sensitive equilibrium binding assay for soluble beta-adrenergic receptors. *J. Cyclic Nucleotide Res. 7*: 235-246.

Wolff, J., Londos, C., and Cooper, D. M. F. (1981). Adenosine receptors and the regulation of adenylate cyclase. In *Advances in Cyclic Nucleotide Research,* Vol. 14. Edited by J. Dumont, P. Greengard, and G. A. Robison. New York, Raven Press, pp. 199-214.

Wong, S. K., and Buckner, C. K. (1978). Studies on β-adrenorecetors mediating changes in mechanical events and adenosine 3′,5′-monophosphate levels. Guinea pig trachea. *Eur. J. Pharmacol. 47*: 273-280.

4

In Vitro Responses to Bronchodilator Drugs

CARL G. A. PERSSON

University Hospital and
AB Draco
Lund, Sweden

JAN-ANDERS KARLSSON

AB Draco
Lund, Sweden

I. Introduction

Bronchodilator drugs characteristically improve breathing in patients with asthma and other lung diseases involving reversible airways obstruction. Due to its rapid onset, the induced reduction of airway resistance would be best explained by a bronchial smooth muscle relaxatory effect. It cannot be excluded, however, that other lung actions of the bronchodilator drugs may contribute to the therapeutic response, particularly during prolonged treatment. A microvascular antipermeability effect of xanthines and β-receptor agonists may reduce airway edema (Persson 1986). These drugs have also been shown to produce a number of effects on the epithelial lining, one of which is to increase the mucociliary transport rate (Pavia et al., 1983; Wanner, 1977). Stationary and blood-borne inflammatory cells may be important drug targets and xanthines and β-receptor agonists have the capacity of inhibiting the release of mediators from such cells (Lichtenstein and Margolis, 1968; Kaliner and Austen 1974; Bussolino and Benveniste, 1980). The present overview does not discuss anti-inflammatory effects but is based on the assumption that the airway smooth muscle responsiveness is a major link between the pathophysiology of asthma and the action of bronchodilator drugs.

Although many imaginative and useful in vivo methods have been devised (Hahn and Nadel, 1979), isolated tissue preparations offer better possibilities for studying actions of drugs on the airway smooth muscle. The emphasis of the present chapter is on pragmatic observations of relaxatory effectiveness, tolerance development, age-dependent effects, interactions with proposed mediators of asthma, and novel findings related to structure activity. Whether or not the actual observations fit proposed mechanisms of action of bronchodilators will be noted.

II. Relevance of In Vitro Findings

Asthma is a disease unique to humans and one may question whether studies employing animal bronchi in vitro (a major focus of this chapter) can generate relevant data. ". . . Any sort of translation from an experimental model to real asthma will be fraught with disaster" (Turner-Warwick, 1984). While it must be recognized that adequate animal models of asthma are lacking, this does not mean that all aspects of the disease have to be examined in the asthmatic subject. Perhaps studies of pathophysiological rather than pharmacologic mechanisms have given experimental models a bad reputation. The work designed to determine individual roles of putative mediators of asthma will clearly have serious flaws. In the disease, a large number of known and unknown mediators would be released, produced, and interact with each other in many intricate ways, which would be hard to mimic experimentally. A further complication is the existence of many qualitative and quantitative differences in mediator actions between different-sized airways, between species, and between in vitro and in vivo conditions. Moreover, for no single mediator do we know its concentration in vivo at relevant sites, such as in the biophase adjacent to the bronchial smooth muscle receptors.

It is suggested that the prospects for relevant in vitro experiments may be better with bronchodilators than with many aspects of asthma pathophysiology. The development of improved bronchodilator compounds has certainly been guided by data obtained in isolated airway smooth muscle preparations. With established bronchodilator drugs there is usually no problem identifying the compound (including active metabolites) and we know much about the plasma and tissue drug levels that are clinically relevant. Furthermore, there may be a good correlation between the relaxatory effects of bronchodilators in vitro and in vivo in animals and humans (including asthmatic subjects). All in vitro data must nevertheless be interpreted with great caution, and different techniques need to be used to improve relevancy. If a study deals with novel types of compounds or some other conceptually new aspect of bronchodilator action, it is particularly desirable that experiments on human bronchi be included.

Bronchi from asthmatic subjects are rarely available for in vitro experiments. However, the hitherto reported findings do suggest that the smooth muscle responsiveness in vitro is not different between airway preparations from normal and asthmatic individuals (Paterson et al., 1984; Vincenc et al., 1983; Roberts et al., 1984, 1985; Dahlen et al., 1983).

The in vitro pharmacology of bronchodilator drugs may provide significant insights into asthma and show ways of finding new and improved therapeutic agents. This is said with many reservations, however. For example, we have to recognize that the prototype drugs of the bronchodilator principles in use today were discovered not in rational pharmacologic in vitro work but through shrewd, prescient observations in asthmatic subjects (Salter, 1859; Gandevia, 1975; Persson, 1985a).

III. Isolated Airway Preparations

A. Trachea and Bronchi

In 1840, Williams used isolated lungs to demonstrate convincingly the contractile mechanism of the bronchi. In 1912 Trendelenburg devised a simple and useful large airway preparation in the form of an opened ring mounted for the recording of isotonic circular smooth muscle activity. He could use it with the cartilage present or, as he preferred, with the cartilage carefully dissected away. With this technique he showed that xanthines (caffeine) relax airway smooth muscle and confirmed the bronchodilator property of adrenaline (cf. Kahn, 1907; Januschke and Pollak, 1911) and atropine (cf. Roy and Brown, 1885; Einthoven, 1892). Many tracheobronchial chain and spiral preparation techniques have been devised through the years (Castillo and De Beer, 1947; Rosa and McDowall, 1951; Akcasu, 1952; Patterson, 1958; Foster, 1960; Constantine, 1965), some of which may seem unnecessarily complicated. The modern counterparts to the Trendelenburg methods can be represented by the single, open or closed, airway rings (Persson and Ekman, 1976; Hooker et al., 1977; Karlsson and Persson, 1981) and the isolated trachealis muscle (Kirkpatrick, 1975; Stephens and Kroeger, 1980). For convenience, isometric tension changes are now the most frequently recorded variable. It is noteworthy that the early workers who had to resort to isotonic recording techniques (the preparation was connected to the short arm of a lever, the long arm of which was arranged to write on a slowly moving kymograph to record changes in muscular length) were studying directly how the smooth muscle activity would change the caliber or the airway lumen. For pharmacologic evaluations, there is probably a quite acceptable correlation between isometric and isotonic evaluations of contractile and relaxatory activities (see Stephens and Van Niekerk, 1977). However, this aspect has not been examined in detail and systematically with mediators and bronchodilators. Advice on preparations of tissue and organ baths for in vitro experiments can be found in the literature (e.g., Perry, 1968). Many aspects of bronchodilator actions in vitro concern drug-receptor interactions. Theoretical and practical considerations for in vitro studies of drug distribution to the receptor, and the subsequent events leading to the functional effect, have been well discussed by Ruffolo (1982) and Kenakin (1984).

B. Small Airways

Tracheal and bronchial preparations are the most frequently employed tissues in vitro but they do not a priori exhibit the same responsiveness as small airways. This is particularly important to recognize since the small airways (diameter < 2 mm) may be a major location of obstruction (Hogg et al., 1968; Despas et al., 1972). Small airways narrowing and expansion can be examined in vitro in bronchial perfusion experiments (Sollmann and Von Oettingen, 1928; Thornton, 1932; Tainter et al., 1934) and by microscopic observations (Sollmann and Gilbert, 1937; Young and Gilbert, 1941; Iravani and Schuller, 1971). The perfusion experiments have been rather crude, involving scarring of lung surface to provide a fluid outlet. The technique is nevertheless sufficient to demonstrate bronchodilator effects of sympathomimetics and xanthines (Tainter et al., 1934; Luduena, 1942). A further development with perfused dissected small airways seems desirable, in which the involved tissues are better defined and quantitation of drug actions is possible. Likewise, the technique devised by Sollman and Gilbert (1937), using microscopic observation of thin sections of fresh lungs in vitro, could be further developed and used. For example, it might be a method of studying the pharmacology of small airways closure.

Tubal segments of dissected small airways are suitable preparations for quantitative recording of isometric tension changes. They can readily be dissected from lungs of different species (Persson and Ekman, 1976; Hooker et al., 1977; Finney et al., 1985). From human lungs, terminal bronchioles 0.5–1 mm in diameter have thus been mounted on two thin prongs of steel, one of which is fixed and the other finely adjustable (Finney et al.,1 985; Fig. 1). With such preparations, small airways responsiveness, in terms of graded contractile and relaxatory actions of drugs, can repeatedly be examined in vitro.

C. Lung Parenchymal Strips

Simultaneous with the description of dissected small airways preparations, the lung parenchymal strip preparation, cut from the surface of lung lobes, was developed as an in vitro preparation for the study of drug effects on peripheral airways (Kapanci et al., 1974; Lulich et al., 1976; Drazen and Schneider, 1978; Kleinstiver and Eyre, 1980; Ghelani et al., 1980; Chand et al., 1979). As such it has now been used in numerous studies. Among its merits are ease

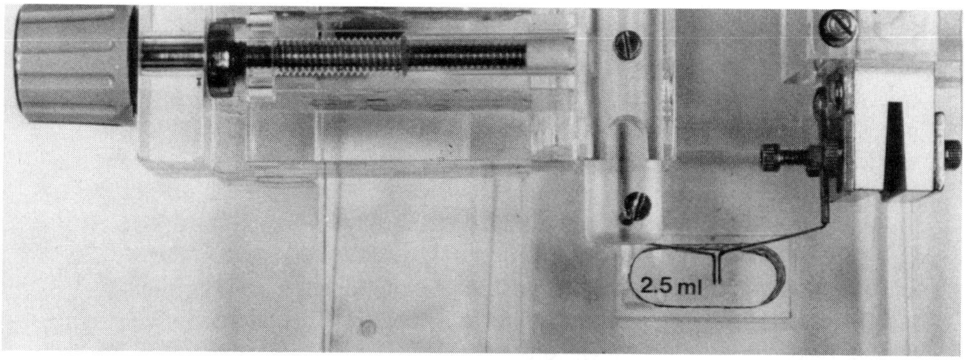

Figure 1(a) A small (2.5 ml) organ bath for studying small airways contractility. Two tissue prongs in the bath are connected to a force-displacement transducer (to the right) and to an adjustable sled (to the left), respectively. The bath is circulated by heating water and contains an outlet for gassing the buffer.

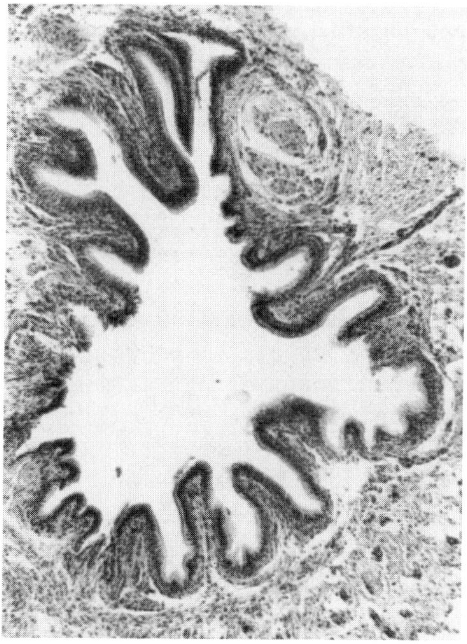

Figure 1(b) Photomicrograph of a cross-section of a human bronchiolar preparation used in the set-up illustrated in (a). The bronchiole has a maximum luminal diameter of about 0.6 mm (0.8 μm thick preparation, stained with hematoxylin and eosin).

of preparation, which may explain its popularity. Its drawbacks must include the fact that it does not reflect small airways responsiveness. About 5% or less of the tissue volume is airway smooth muscle and a number of other cell types with contractile activity, including a variable proportion of vascular smooth muscle, are also present (Bertram et al., 1983; Finney et al., 1984). It is, therefore, unfortunate that the wealth of data generated on lung strips is uncritically accepted as relevant for small airways. However, it cannot be discounted that results obtained with lung strips may have some significance. Due to the variability of the composition of these preparations each investigator must show the particular relevance that should be lent to his or her lung parenchymal strip findings. In the discussions of bronchodilator actions on small airways below, data obtained on lung strips have not been included.

D. Perfused Lungs

The airway's responsiveness can be studied under close to in situ conditions in experiments with the whole lung in vitro. From the simple observations of bronchoconstriction and bronchodilation in isolated lungs (Williams, 1840), techniques have now been developed in which lung resistance and compliance are recorded in excised lungs that are ventilated in an artificial thoracic chamber by an alternating negative pressure. The pulmonary vessels are perfused with an oxygenized, osmotically balanced buffer producing viable lungs and maintaining the significant metabolizing capacity of the pulmonary vascular bed (Fig. 2). Different modifications of the technique have been described (Delaunois, 1964; Niemeier and Bingham, 1972; Ryrfeldt and Nilsson, 1978; Smith and Bend, 1981; Kröll et al., 1986) and various aspects of lung viability discussed (Fisher et al., 1980; Mehendale et al., 1981; Longmore, 1982; Kröll et al., 1986). It is difficult to perfuse the tracheobronchial arteries in vitro. However, the nutritional microcirculation of the large airways can obviously be well supplied through perfusion of only the pulmonary artery (unpublished observations by Kroll, Karlsson, and Persson). This observation suggests an increased usefulness of the isolated perfused lung preparation, because the richly developed bronchial subepithelial microcirculation may play important roles in the pathophysiology and pharmacology of asthma (e.g., Persson, 1986).

In isolated lungs, bronchodilator effects can be examined after airway or pulmonary intravascular application of drugs. The preparation has found considerable use for determining mediators and various factors that appear in the perfusate leaving the lung (after provocation and drug treatments). By proper handling, the rat or guinea pig perfused lung preparation will usually work without significant problems of edema formation or air trapping. Many aspects of the effects of bronchodilator drugs remain to be studied in this type of preparation.

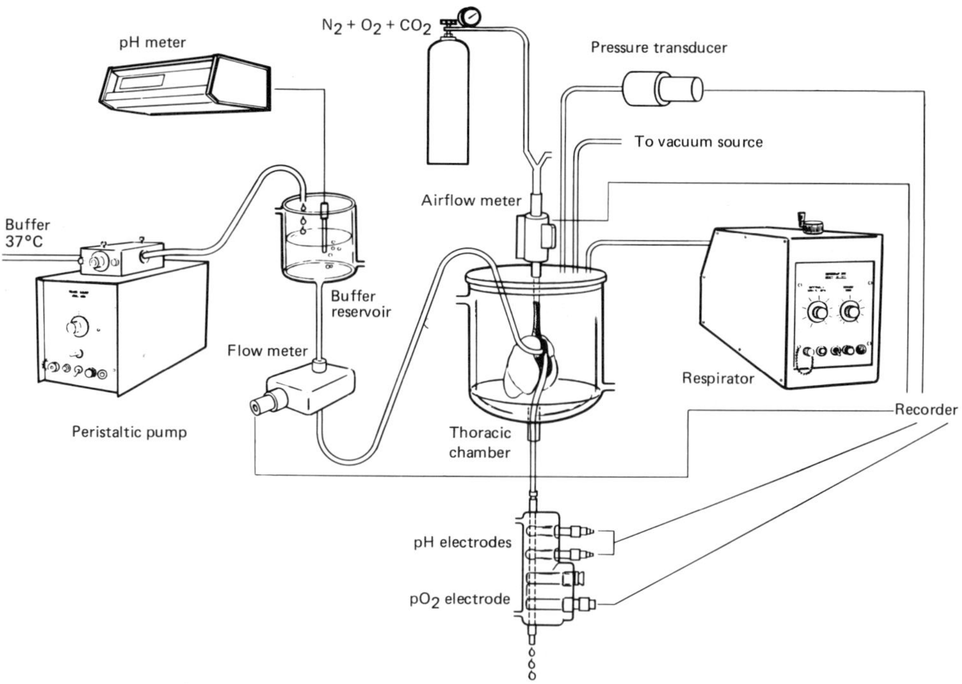

Figure 2 Experimental set-up for studying effects in isolated perfused lungs. Lungs excised from anesthetized guinea pigs are mounted in a water-vapor-saturated artificial thoracic chamber. Ventilation is carried out using a variable negative pressure (0- –10 cmH_2O) from a respirator and a vacuum source. The lung is breathing a gas mixture of 1/3 carbogen (95% O_2, 5% CO_2), and 2/3 N_2 gas. The pressure inside the thoracic chamber, the tracheal air flow, and the tidal volume are recorded on a Grass polygraph. On-line computer calculations of lung resistance and dynamic compliance are used. The pulmonary circulation is perfused with Krebs bicarbonate buffer (1% glucose, 4.5% albumin) at a pH of 7.4-7.5. The buffer level in the reservoir is kept constant by means of a peristaltic pump. The perfusion flow, the PO_2, and the pH of the buffer effluent are also recorded. Drugs can be administered intravascularly or intratracheally (figure kindly supplied by Kröll and Franziska).

E. Other Preparations

In the excised lung described above, proper contribution to airways responsiveness of many different lung cells is allowed. Other composite preparations are those in which autonomic nerves of the tracheal tube have been codissected and used in vitro for selective stimulation (Bouhuys, 1974; Blackman and McCaig, 1983; Waldeck and Widmark, 1986). Preparations obtained from different organs have also been mounted in the same bath in studies of selectivity of drug actions on airways vs. the heart (Persson and Johnson, 1970). In principle, in vitro arrangements of airway smooth muscle preparations allow inclusion, one by one, of select in vivo factors or combinations of these. For example, a stepwise increase in complexity, by adding different types of inflammatory cells to simple tracheobronchial preparations, carry interesting potentials for elucidating control of airway responsiveness and actions of bronchodilator drugs.

Another recent development is to reduce the complexity already present in the simple tracheobronchial preparations. There is now some focus on the role of epithelial lining (which may be seriously deranged in asthma) in airway smooth muscle and responsiveness. In deepithelialized isolated airways, little changes may be recorded (Thompson et al., 1986; unpublished observations by Lunddlad, Karlson, and Persson) on contraction may be increased and relaxation decreased (Flavahan et al., 1985; Barnes et al., 19856). Bronchodilator drugs may also be examined in airway smooth muscle cells ridded of their membrane (Sparrow et al., 1984).

F. Induced Tone

Isolated airway smooth muscle variably gains tone spontaneously in vitro. Preparations of human large and small airways and particularly of guinea pig trachea may develop considerable intrinsic isometric tone. When stabilized, the tension may be entertained for hours, allowing repeated evaluations of bronchodilator effects. The tone is largely nonnervous in origin. It may be produced by generation of contractile products of arachidonate metabolism (Farmer et al., 1974; Orehek et al., 1975), but it has not been fully explained. The tone in vitro may not correspond to the tone maintained in vivo, where there is a pronounced cholinergic component (Boushey et al., 1980; Nadel, 1980). Additional contractions, or contractions in preparations such as the rat trachea, that lack intrinsic tone, can readily be produced by a variety of contractile mediators and analogues. If sustained contractions are obtained, which is usually the case, it is convenient to evaluate concentration-response relationships by adding bronchodilators to the organ bath in cumulatively increasing concentrations

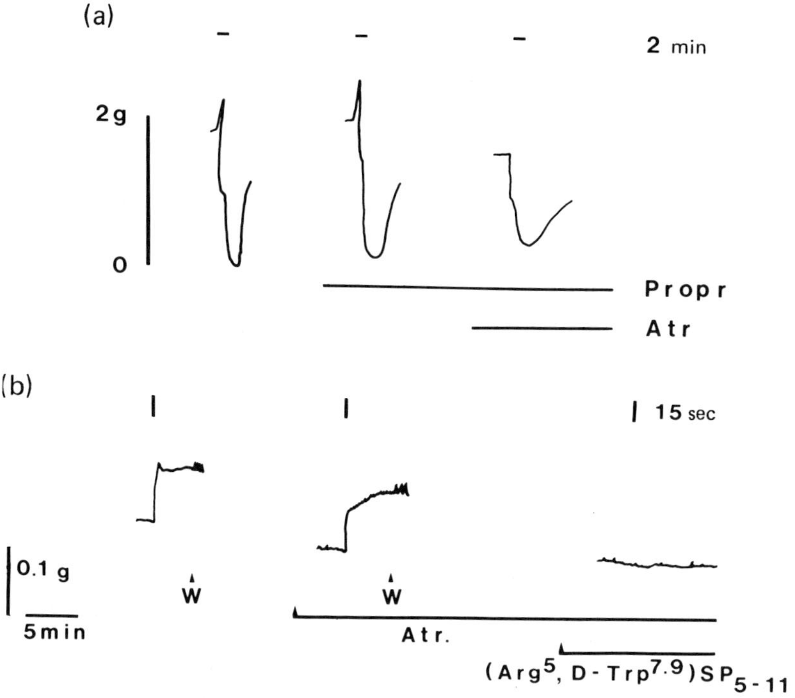

Figure 3 Tracings from electrical-field-stimulated (trains of pulses at supramaximal voltage) guinea pig isolated tracheal (a: 20 Hz, 0.5 msec pulse duration) and bronchial (b: 15 Hz, 0.3 msec) preparations having a spontaneous tone. Periods of stimulation are indicated above tracings. In the trachea, the biphasic response is almost unaffected by propranolol (Propr, 0.1 μM) whereas the contractile component is blocked by atropine (Atr, 1 μM). All tension changes including the inhibitory response are abolished by tetrodotoxin (3 μM). The bronchial contraction is reduced by atropine (1 μM) and the remaining contractile response is inhibited by a tachykinin antagonist (0.1 mM).

(van Rossum, 1963). Addition of bronchodilators prior to a bronchoconstrictor will entail the difficulty of a varying baseline (in intrinsic tone preparations).

It is noteworthy that some compounds will be variably bronchoconstrictors and bronchodilators, depending on how much tone is present. Thus in low-tone guinea pig tracheas, prostaglandin E_2 (and analogues), ATP, adenosine, and bradykinin produce significant contractions; in high-tone preparations they are monophasic relaxatory agents (Kamikawa and Shimo, 1976; Karlsson et al.,

1982; Lundblad et al., 1985). The specific ways of inducing tone in vitro may be used to categorize different types of bronchodilator compounds.

G. Neurogenic Tone

By electrical field stimulation of isolated airway preparations, four different types of innervation that affect smooth muscle tone may be discernible (Fig. 3). The cholinergic innervation releases acetylcholine that will produce constriction via activation of smooth muscle muscarinic receptors. This effect is antagonized by antimuscarinic drugs, which have long been used as bronchodilators (Gandevia, 1975). Especially in guinea pig bronchi (this is not established in other species), there is an additional contractile and inflammatory innervation, possibly releasing tachykinin peptides (Lundberg et al., 1983; Karlsson and Persson, 1983; Karlsson et al., 1984, Saria et al., 1985; Persson et al., 1985a). The sympathetic innervation of airway smooth muscle is usually sparse or lacking (Richardson, 1979) but some relaxation may be attributed to this system in vitro, at least in animal airways (Ito and Tajima, 1981; Taylor et al., 1984). In vivo adrenergic inhibition would be produced by circulating epinephrine, released by adrenal activation (Barnes, 1983) and acting on bronchial β_2 adrenoceptors. Finally, there is a potent nonadrenergic, noncholinergic inhibitory innervation of the airways of many species including humans (Macklin, 1929; Richardson, 1979). (The vagus of the salamander may contain only bronchodilator fibers; see Macklin, 1929.) This system has been much studied in vitro and there is currently a debate over the identity of the neurotransmitter(s) involved (Matsuzaki et al., 1980; Ito and Takeda, 1982; Cameron et al., 1983; Karlsson and Persson, 1984). No bronchodilator drugs have so far been developed that activate or mimic this system. Putative neurotransmitter peptides and purines have already been examined and found to be of little or no value as bronchodilators in asthmatic subjects (Cushley et al., 1983; Bundgaard et al., 1983; Barnes et al., 1984).

IV. Drugs

A. Anticholinergic Drugs

Theoretically, many types of drugs may exert anticholinergic bronchodilator effects. Inhibition of vagal tone may thus be produced at the central nervous system level, at the level of ganglionic transmission, at the prejunctional level modulating release of acetylcholine, and at the postjunctional muscarinic receptor sites. In vitro the three latter drug target levels can be studied readily (Skoogh, 1986). Hexamethonium blocks ganglionic transmission and is also effective clinically (Boushey, 1984), but has no role in asthma therapy. Adrenoceptors may be located on cholinergic nerves and have inhibitory functions.

Skoogh (1986) has shown that β_2-receptor stimulation inhibits transmission through parasympathetic ganglia in ferret trachea. In intestinal tissue stimulation of prejunctional α-receptors inhibits release of acetylcholine (Paton and Vizi, 1969). The latter possibility seems to be transferable to airways tissue, (Grandstrom and Andersson, 1985; Martin and Collier, 1985).

Atropine and its quarternary derivatives effectively inhibit vagal bronchoconstriction in asthma. Atropine-like drugs have a considerable degree of specificity as pharmacologic antagonists of muscarinic actions of acetylcholine. However, at concentrations in vitro slightly greater than those required for antimuscarinic effects atropine has been reported to inhibit thromboxane A_2-formation (Bertie et al., 1980). Still larger concentrations will nonspecifically inhibit effects of a number of contractile mediators (Weiner, 1980; Folco et al., 1982) other than acetylcholine and its analogues (carbachol, bethanechol, methacholine, etc.)

Structure-activity studies of atropine alkaloids in asthma have been limited. A degree of lung specificity is obtained by inhalation of quarternary derivatives that have little ability to pass lipid membranes. On the pharmacodynamic side, attempts have been made to separate antimuscarinic effects on smooth muscle from those on secretory cells (Engelhardt and Klupp, 1975; Madison et al., 1985). Acetylcholine is known to increase watery secretions in airway epithelium and increase mucociliary transport rate in vitro and in vivo (see Gross and Skorodin, 1984). Inhibition of this effect by antimuscarinics can be considered a drawback of these compounds.

The need for new drugs in this area may be limited by the fact that antimuscarinics, probably because they antagonize just one of many mediators of asthma, generally are less effective bronchodilator drugs than are xanthines and sympathomimetics (Paterson et al., 1979).

B. Tachykinin Antagonists

The undecapeptide substance P has been suggested to be the neurotransmitter of the bronchoconstrictory noncholinergic innervation of guinea pig bronchi (Lundberg and Saria, 1982; Lundberg et al., 1983; Karlsson and Persson, 1983). Synthetic analogues of substance P containing D-amino acids in select positions have been shown to possess substance-P-antagonistic properties (Rosell and Folkers, 1982; Leander et al., 1983; Regoli et al., 1984) (Fig. 4). Further studies in guinea pig bronchi in vitro have shown that such antagonists inhibit contractions caused by other tachykinins or by stimulation of noncholinergic nerves more efficiently than those produced by exogenously added substance P (Karlsson et al., 1984). The substance P antagonists should perhaps rather be called tachykinin antagonists and it obviously remains to be established which member(s) of the tachykinin family may be involved in noncholinergic bronchocon-

Arg-Pro-Lys-Pro-Gln-Gln-Phe-Phe-Gly-Leu-Met-NH_2	Substance P
Pyr-Ala-Asp-Pro-Asn-Lys-Phe-Tyr-Gly-Leu-Met-NH_2	Physalaemin
Pyr-Pro-Ser-Lys-Asp-Ala-Phe-Ile-Gly-Leu-Met-NH_2	Eledoisin
His-Lys-Thr-Asp-Ser-Phe-Val-Gly-Leu-Met-NH_2	Neurokinin A
Arg-pro*-Lys-Pro-Gln-Gln-trp-Phe-trp-Leu-Met-NH_2	Tachykinin antagonist
Arg-Gln-trp-Phe-trp-Leu-Met-NH_2	Tachykinin antagonist

* small letters indicate D-amino acid

Figure 4 Amino acid sequences of tachykinins and of two tachykinin antagonists.

striction of guinea pig bronchi (Karlsson et al., 1984; Karlsson and Persson, 1985a).

Structure-activity studies with tachykinin antagonists must tackle problems of potency and specificity. The analogues variably have the ability to contract airway smooth muscle themselves (Karlsson and Persson, 1985a), to release histamine (Foreman et al., 1983; Hakanson et al., 1983), and to produce local anesthetic effects (Karlsson and Persson, 1983; Karlsson et al., 1984; Post et al., 1985). It would be useful to have a potent and specific analogue that can be studied in humans to evaluate the role, if any, of noncholinergic tachykinergic nerves in asthmatic subjects.

C. Mediator Antagonists

Since the number of bronchoconstrictory agents proposed to be mediators of asthma is large and growing it is becoming less probable that pharmacologic antagonism of a single mediator could produce an acceptable clinical bronchodilator response. The fact that atropine, which presumably counteracts only acetylcholine, is effective in some patients does not increase the likelihood that specific antagonism of another single mediator could also result in significant antiasthmatic effects. Nevertheless, we might wish that for each putative mediator a specific pharmacologic antagonist will be found. If in vitro studies can establish a high degree of specificity, such antagonist compounds will be important tools for defining individual roles of bronchoconstrictory mediators in asthma.

Histamine H_1-receptor antagonists relax histamine-induced bronchoconstriction whereas histamine analogues, which specifically stimulate H_2-receptors, may themselves be bronchodilators in vitro (Chand et al., 1980; Chand and Eyre, 1980; Tomioka and Yamada, 1982). Bronchodilation via H_2-receptor stimulation may not be seen in humans, however (Eiser and White, 1985). The histamine-induced bronchoconstriction is dependent on species as well as on size of the airway. Isolated airway preparations of cat and rhesus monkey are barely responsive, except for dissected small airways that will contract readily to histamine as will large and small airways from animals and humans (Persson and Ekman, 1976; Chand et al., 1980). There is presently some renewed interest in the effect of H_1-receptor antagonists. Some such compounds may have lung actions in addition to those explainable by histamine antagonism (Arnoux et al., 1985).

Leukotriene C_4 and D_4 are potent bronchoconstrictors in vitro in large (Dahlén et al., 1980; Hanna et al., 1981) and small human airways (Karlsson and Persson, 1985b). As with other mediators, asthmatic subjects may exhibit exaggerated responses (in vivo) to these agents compared with healthy volunteers (see Leitch and Drazen, 1984; Barnes et al., 1985c; Piper and Costello, 1985). One leukotriene antagonist, FPL 55712, is available (Augstein et al., 1973). It is effective in vitro, with some degree of specificity, to antagonize bronchoconstriction induced by LTC_4 and LTD_4 in bronchial preparations from many species (Chand, 1979) but may be poorly effective in vivo (Holroyde et al., 1981). Many experimental drugs proposed specifically to inhibit endogenous leukotriene production have recently become available. However, little is known about their effect in asthma.

Two recently proposed mediators of asthma, adenosine and PAF-acether, will not readily contract ordinary tracheobronchial preparations. However, they consistently produce marked bronchoconstriction in isolated perfused lungs from guinea pigs (Kröll et al., 1985; Hamasaki et al., 1984; Lefort et al., 1984). The latter in vitro preparation may thus be suitable for studying bronchodilation caused by pharmacologic antagonism of these two mediators.

Many mediators do not exert bronchoconstrictory effects in vitro solely by pharmacomechanical coupling in the smooth muscle cells. There may be indirect constrictory effects via release of agents such as thromboxane A_2 (e.g., by bradykinin and leukotrienes) or indirect attenuating effects via release of relaxatory cyclo-oxygenase products (e.g., by histamine; Orehek et al., 1975; Adcock and Garland, 1980; Mitchell, 1982). Many types of cells, including inflammatory cells, epithelium, and endothelium, can be an important source for modulatory agents. Although the indirect actions may be receptor-operated mechanisms, this aspect of mediator actions will complicate studies of pharmacologic antagonism.

D. Calcium Antagonists

Vascular, gastrointestinal, and uterine smooth muscle usually has a spontaneous contractile activity in vitro (Bortoff, 1972; Persson, 1973). It is largely a nonner-

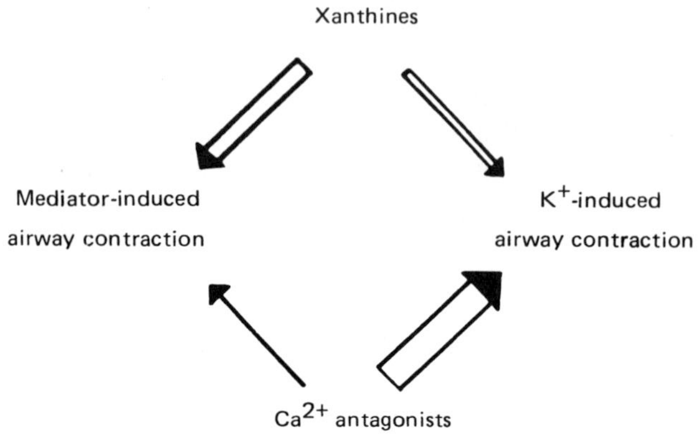

Figure 5 Xanthines and Ca^{2+} antagonists preferentially relax mediator- and potassium depolarization-induced airways contractions, respectively.

vous myogenic activity and it is readily inhibited by a group of relaxant drugs called calcium antagonists (Fleckenstein et al., 1971; Forman et al., 1979). These drugs are thought to act by inhibiting a voltage-dependent inward calcium current (e.g., Andersson and Högestätt, 1984) and, hence, they are also effective relaxants of contractions induced by depolarizing solutions of potassium. Calcium antagonist drugs have attracted a great deal of interest lately as novel bronchodilator drugs with great theoretical promise (Middleton, 1984). Although some reports show a protective effect against exercise-induced bronchoconstriction (Barnes et al., 1981; Cerrina et al., 1981; Patel, 1981) these drugs apparently have a limited effect in asthma (see Russi and Ahmed, 1984). Also in vitro calcium antagonists are poor relaxants of mediator-induced compared with depolarization-induced bronchoconstriction (Cerrina et al., 1983, Duncan and Douglas, 1984; Ahmed et al., 1985; Nielsen-Kudsk et al., 1986). It is not typical for tracheobronchial preparations to exhibit rhythmic spontaneous mechanical activity, but when they do, this activity may be inhibited by calcium antagonists (unpublished observations by Karlsson, Persson, and Waldeck). Xanthines and sympathomimetic bronchodilators may not be particularly effective relaxants of spontaneous phasic activity nor of potassium-induced airway contraction (Spilker and Minatoya, 1975; Cerrina et al., 1983; Nielsen-Kudsk et al., 1986). Thus, calcium antagonists preferentially relax depolarization-induced contractions whereas the clinically effective bronchodilator drugs preferentially relax airways contracted by proposed mediators of asthma (which apparently do not operate via voltage-dependent calcium channels) (Fig. 5).

V. Xanthines and β-Receptor Agonists

The usefulness of these types of drugs in asthma was probably discovered by Dr. Henry Hyde Salter. In 1859 he described in detail the curative influence of coffee and mental excitements in asthmatic subjects (see Persson, 1985a). Caffeine, the active ingredient contained in coffee, was much later on shown to be a bronchodilator in vitro (Trendelenburg, 1912). Since 1922 (Hirsch) theophylline, which is very similar to caffeine in its actions, has been repeatedly characterized clinically as an effective antiasthma drug. Further development with novel types of xanthines has occurred.

About 40 years after Salter's note of an instantaneous "cure" by mental excitements (1859), Solis-Cohen (1900) found that intake of adrenal extract was effective in patients with asthma. Solis-Cohen used the adrenal extract because of its recently discovered vasoconstrictor property. (His patients suffered from asthma caused by "vasomotor ataxia of the relaxing variety.") A few years later Kahn (1907) showed that epinephrine relaxed dog tracheal tone. Later developments include the introduction of isoprenaline. This potent β-receptor agonist was characterized by Konzett in 1941, 7 years before Ahlquist (1948), by employing isoprenaline, could announce his concept of α- and β-receptors. Two specific $\beta\text{-}_2$ receptor agonists, terbutaline and salbutamol, were described in 1966 (patent applications) just before Lands et al. (1967) suggested that β-receptors could be subdivided into β_1- and β_2-receptors (Fig. 6).

Xanthines and β-receptor agonists have been shown to exert many lung actions experimentally, but this discussion is confined to their bronchorelaxatory effects.

A. New Aspects of β-Receptor Agonists

A number of reviews cover the vast developments in studies of ligand binding to β-receptors and subcellular events following receptor activation (Minneman et al., 1979; Lefkowitz et al., 1982; Wikberg, 1982). Many detailed aspects of how β-receptor-mediated responses should be studied have also evolved in recent years (Furchgott, 1972; Ruffolo, 1982; O'Donnell and Wanstall, 1979). Quite specific β_2-adrenoceptor agonist molecules, such as procaterol (Yabuuchi, 1977), have been synthetized. However, the novel compounds do not seem to offer advantages over terbutaline and salbutamol. The structure-activity relationships of many β-receptor agonists including these two drugs have been reported (Bergman et al., 1969; Brittain et al., 1976).

Autoradiographic techniques combined with ligand binding studies have provided an insight into density and distribution of β-receptors in the lung (Barnes et al., 1982; Barnes et al., 1985a). For β-adrenoceptor antagonists, results of binding experiments may correlate with functional in vitro and in vivo

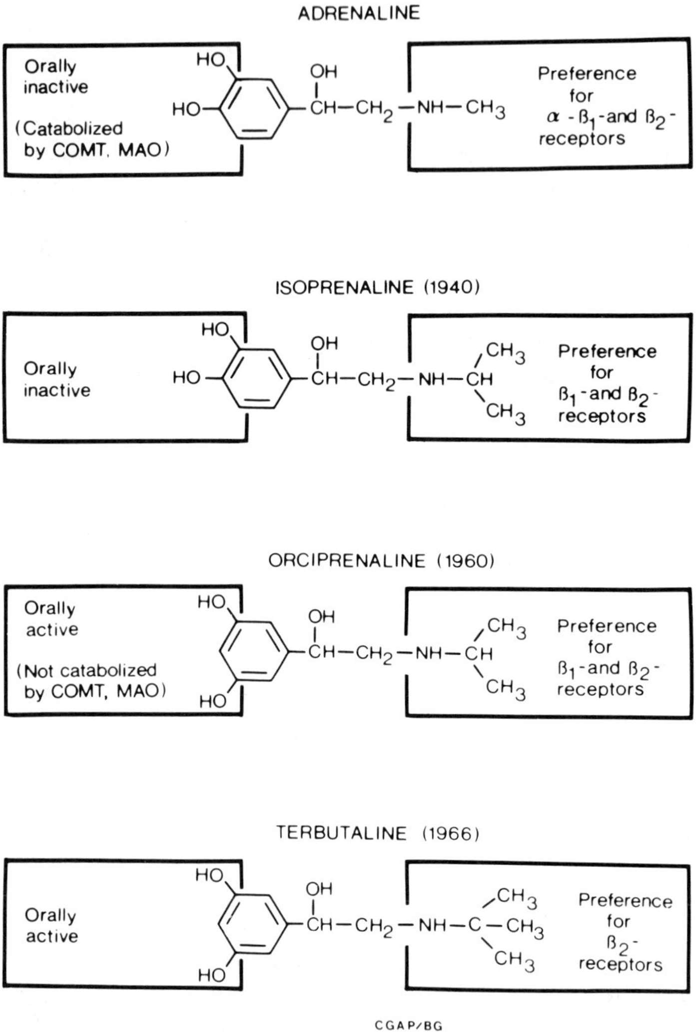

Figure 6 These compounds illustrate how slight changes in the chemical structure of the sympathomimetic prototype drug epinephrine have stepwise generated potent bronchodilator drugs with increased specificity in action and increased metabolic stability. A number of alternative chemical structures with selective sympathomimetic bronchodilation comparable to that of terbutaline are now available. COMT, Catechol-O-methyltransferase; MAO, Monoamino-oxidase.

data (Kenakin, 1984). This may not be so with β-adrenoceptor agonists. It is noteworthy that β_2-receptor specificity of bronchodilator drugs, as determined by ligand receptor binding, has been found to be different from that determined by functional studies (Minneman et al., 1979; Bieth et al., 1980; Hedberg and Mattsson, 1981). Had binding studies been dominating at the time when terbutaline and salbutamol were being developed, it is unlikely that these compounds would have been given priority for further evaluations in humans.

Choice of species is also critical for studies with bronchoselective β-receptor agonists. Functional in vitro experiments have revealed a marked variation in the distribution of β_1 and β_2-receptors in airway smooth muscle. In trachea from cats and ferrets β_1-receptors dominate (Lulich et al., 1976; Skoogh et al., 1985). In guinea pigs there is a preponderance of β_2 over β_1-receptors (O'Donnell and Wanstall, 1979; Johansson and Waldeck, 1981) and the human airways seem to harbor only β_2-receptors (Davies et al., 1980; Goldie et al., 1984; Barnes et al., 1985a).

The relaxatory characteristics of a β_2-adrenoceptor agonist include potency and maximum effect. The most commonly used parameter to describe a "dose"-response relationship is potency, which usually is expressed as an EC_{50} value (concentration necessary to produce 50% of its maximum response; $-\log EC_{50} = pD_2$). The maximum obtainable relaxation with a β_2-receptor stimulant (intrinsic activity) can be expressed as a fraction of the tissue response induced by a full agonist, the intrinsic activity of which equals 1. However, with β_2-adrenoceptor agonists one has to consider the concept of spare receptors, which means that not all receptors must be occupied by a full agonist for induction of a maximum response (Furchgott, 1955; Stephenson, 1956; Nickerson, 1956). Thus, for a full agonist, efficacy (ability to activate the receptor subsequent to binding) will be high, whereas a partial agonist will have a low efficacy and a competitive antagonist almost none (see Ruffolo, 1982; Kenakin, 1984). Receptor occupancy can be examined in functional studies employing agonists and irreversible antagonists, or by use of ligand binding techniques. Half-maximal receptor occupancy is expressed as a K_d-value ($-\log K_d = pK_d$).

Structure-activity studies in vitro that well characterize both desired bronchodilator effects and undesired cardiac stimulant, and tremor-inducing effects (Persson and Johnson, 1970; Olsson et al., 1979; Andersson et al., 1982) suggest that few additions can be made to the characteristics illustrated by terbutaline. It was discovered that in some newly synthetized phenylethylamines, β_2-receptor agonist and α_1-receptor antagonist properties were combined in the same molecule (Olsson et al., 1981). However, as with many other attempts of combining different classes of drugs in one molecule (Nicolaus, 1983) this combination of β-receptor agonist and α-receptor antagonist properties did not seem successful (Löfdahl and Svedmyr, 1984).

Other aspects of the β_2-receptor agonist compounds in which in vitro evaluations are less essential, are now being worked on to improve further their therapeutic characteristics. An increased duration of action after both oral and aerosol administration may be achieved by novel compounds which are active as such, or by prodrugs in which the active compound is produced in vivo at a suitable rate (Svensson, 1985).

B. New Aspects of Xanthines

Structure Activity

Misunderstandings concerning the relationship between structure and activity of xanthines have flourished in pharmacomedical textbook literature. Some are serious mistakes, which have led people to calculate how much theophylline is contained in clinically used xanthine derivatives (Bussey, 1981; Magnusson et al., 1985) which are different molecules from theophylline (cf. Persson, 1982a). (This is just as impossible as calculating how much epinephrine is contained in isoprenaline.) However, the structure-activity relationships with xanthines form a fascinating field. Knowledge is accumulating as to which positions, and what kind of substitutions at these, determine the bronchodilator potency and how this property may covary with other effects. It is further clear that many actions generally thought to be inherent in the xanthines will vary with very slight changes in chemical structure.

Armitage et al. (1961) published an extensive in vitro study of structure-activity relationships for tracheal relaxant effects of xanthines (thioxanthines) but could not confirm their findings in vivo. In particular the high potency that they expected was not present in vivo (Armitage and Wooldridge, 1960). This apparent inconsistency may be explained by the fact that xanthines may exhibit biphasic relaxant responses. The incomplete relaxatory effect produced by very low concentrations of some derivatives in isolated guinea pig tracheas (also used by Armitage et al., 1961) has not been observed in vivo (Persson, 1985b). However, if the potency determination is based on the full concentration response line obtained in the isolated trachea there is usually a good correlation with in vivo bronchodilator potency (Persson, 1985b). Xanthine derivatives exhibit a wide range of airway relaxatory potencies and compounds that consistently are 20-30 times more potent than theophylline can readily be produced (Persson, 1985c). Figure 7 is an attempt at a condensed summary of the structure-activity of xanthines with an emphasis on bronchorelaxatory properties. It is based on in vitro and in vivo data obtained with some 300 derivatives (Persson and Kjellin, 1981; Persson et al., 1982; Karlsson et al., 1982; and unpublished observations by Persson, Kjellin, Ekman, Erjefält, and Gustafsson). The structure-activity relationships in vitro may also be powerful instruments to evaluate proposed cellular mechanisms of action of the xanthines.

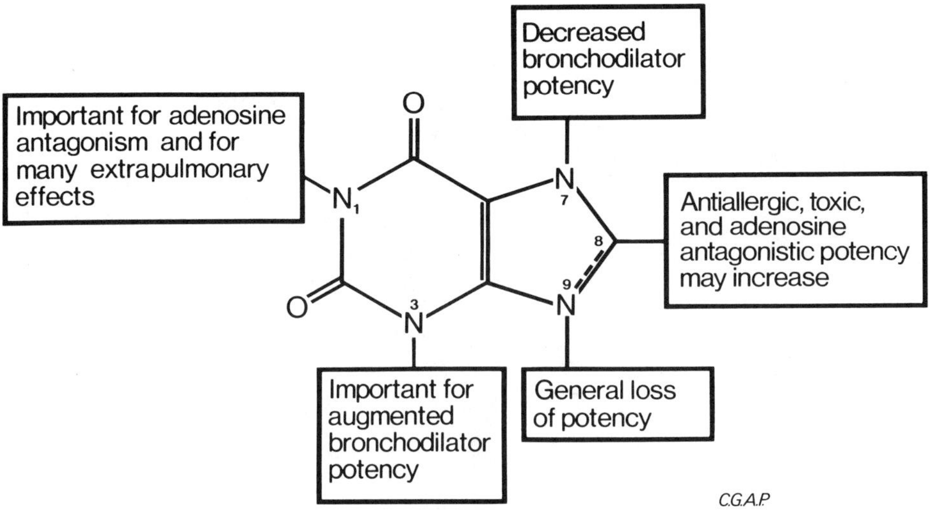

Figure 7 Some important features of alkyl substitution at various positions of the xanthine molecule. (When the 9-nitrogen is substituted, the 8-9 double bond is moved to the 7-8 position.)

Phosphodiesterase Inhibition

There is generally a good correlation between the rank order of tracheal relaxant potency and that of inhibition of the cyclic AMP catabolizing phosphodiesterase enzyme in lung homogenates (Triner et al., 1977; Polson et al., 1978; Bergstrand, 1980; Persson, 1985b). However, this has become a weak support for a mechanism against which many arguments have accumulated. It is now agreed that at therapeutic levels theophylline is only a poor inhibitor of phosphodiesterase enzymes (Lohman et al., 1977; Kolbeck et al., 1979; Bergstrand, 1980). Theophylline relaxes airways in vitro apparently without changes in cyclic nucleotide levels (Lohmann et al., 1977; Kolbeck et al., 1979). It is also timely to analyze and conclude from the available facts that several types of potent phosphodiesterase inhibitory compounds have been found since the mechanism was first proposed (Sutherland et al., 1968) but none has shown an acceptable clinical effect in asthma (see Persson, 1982a). Following the discovery that potent relaxatory nitroderivatives were inhibitors of cyclic GMP phosphodiesterase, there has been a growing interest in whether this nucleotide causes smooth muscle to relax (Itoh et al., 1985; Murad, 1985; Polson et al., 1985). Effects of xanthines may contribute to this discussion. Select xanthine derivatives have been shown to exert potent (> 200 times that of theophylline) and specific inhibition of cyclic GMP phosphodiesterase (purified from human

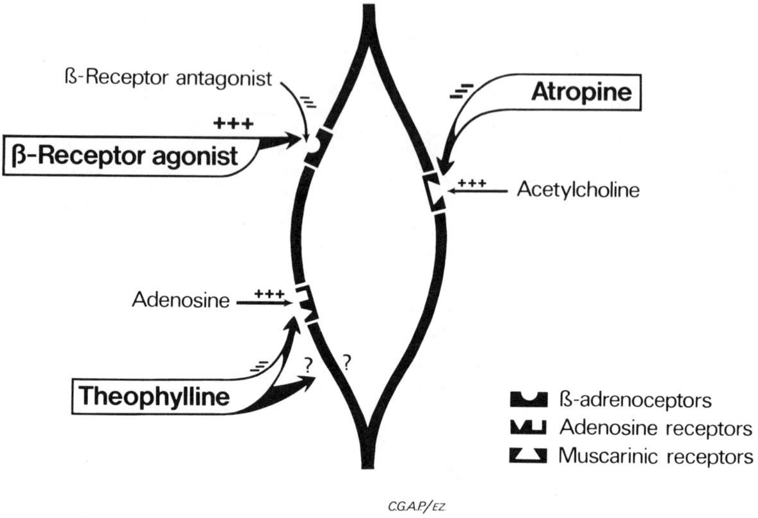

Figure 8 Interactions between bronchodilators and different types of cell surface receptors. Whereas stimulation of β-adrenoceptors and blockade of muscarinic receptors are essential bronchodilator mechanisms, adenosine receptor antagonism apparently is not (see text).

lung tissue (Bergstrand, 1980). However, structure-activity relationships illustrate clearly that this property is not at all paralleled by in vitro and in vivo bronchodilator potency (unpublished observations by Bergstrand, Kjellin, and Persson; see Persson, 1985b). Furthermore, a well-known cyclic GMP phosphodiesterase inhibitory and smooth muscle relaxatory drug, nitroglycerine, has been found to produce little but side effects in asthmatic subjects (Miller and Shultz, 1979). At the present state of knowledge it seems unlikely that inhibition of either cyclic AMP or cyclic GMP phosphodiesterase is a significant mechanism behind xanthine-induced bronchodilation.

Adenosine Receptor Antagonism

It has been established that theophylline, within concentrations comprising the therapeutic levels, is an effective adenosine receptor antagonist (Fig. 8) (Rall, 1980). The purine nucleoside adenosine is formed by intracellular and ectoenzyme pathways, and inactivated by catabolism and uptake into cells (Baer and Drummond, 1979). Biochemical and cell biology research has shown that adenosine activates two types of membranal receptors, A_1 (or R_i) and A_2- (or R_a), frequently differentiated by their inhibitory and stimulatory interaction, respectively, with the adenylate cyclase system (Van Calker et al., 1978; Londos et al., 1980). Adenosine exerts pharmacologic effects in most tissues, but the role of cyclic AMP in the functional responses remains to be established. It has been suggested that adenosine has many important physiological actions (Oswald et al., 1980; Phillips et al., 1979; Johannesson et al., 1985).

Some characteristics of adenosine may be compatible with a role as a mediator of asthma. It may increase allergen-induced release of mediators (Marquardt et al., 1978). As in other organs the lung tissue level of adenosine is increased by stresses such as hypoxia (Mentzer et al., 1975) and allergen provocation (see Holgate et al., 1985). The intriguing observation has been made that atopic as well as nonatopic asthmatic subjects, but not normal subjects, respond with a marked bronchoconstriction to inhaled adenosine (Cushley et al., 1983). Inferentially, adenosine antagonism would be an attractive explanation of anti-asthma effects of xanthines as has also been suggested (Marquardt et al., 1978; Fredholm, 1980; Welton and Simko, 1980; Snyder, 1981; Cushley et al., 1983). Considering the clinical effectiveness of xanthines, this possibility, if true, would make adenosine the most significant single agent among the numerous proposed mediators of asthma. A number of observations discussed below suggest, however, that any role of adenosine in asthma is hardly supported by the pharmacology of xanthines.

Besides its asthma-like actions adenosine has been shown to produce anti-inflammatory and bronchorelaxatory effects in various in vitro systems (Farmer and Farrar, 1976; Marone et al., 1979; Karlsson et al., 1982; Cronstein et al., 1984). This is not surprising because adenosine has dual complex actions in several systems. Theophylline antagonizes, with some specificity, both bronchoconstrictor and bronchodilator effects (Karlsson et al., 1982; Pauwels et al., 1985; Holgate et al., 1985; Kröll et al., 1985), in line with the view that adenosine blocking xanthines are general antagonists that do not differentiate between adenosine cell surface receptor types (Londos et al., 1980). Conversely, those xanthines that are weak antagonists may not appreciably interfere with any pharmacologic or physiological action of adenosine (Persson et al., 1985).

As is clear from structure-activity relationships, the airway relaxatory potencies of xanthine derivatives are completely unrelated to their ability to antagonize adenosine (Persson and Kjellin, 1981; Persson et al., 1981; Karlsson et al., 1982) (Fig. 9). The lung actions of one xanthine derivative, enprofylline (3-propylxanthine), that is practically without antagonism of different functional effects of adenosine, have been studied extensively in vitro and in vivo in animals and humans. Enprofylline is more potent than theophylline as a bronchodilator and this concerns also findings in patients treated for up to a fortnight (Persson and Kjellin, 1981; Lunell et al., 1982; Laursen et al., 1985; Persson, 1985a,b). Enprofylline has potent anti-inflammatory and antiallergic actions in animals (Persson et al., 1985b; Andersson et al., 1985) and obviously in asthmatics too (Pauwels et al., 1985), indicating that many potentially impor-

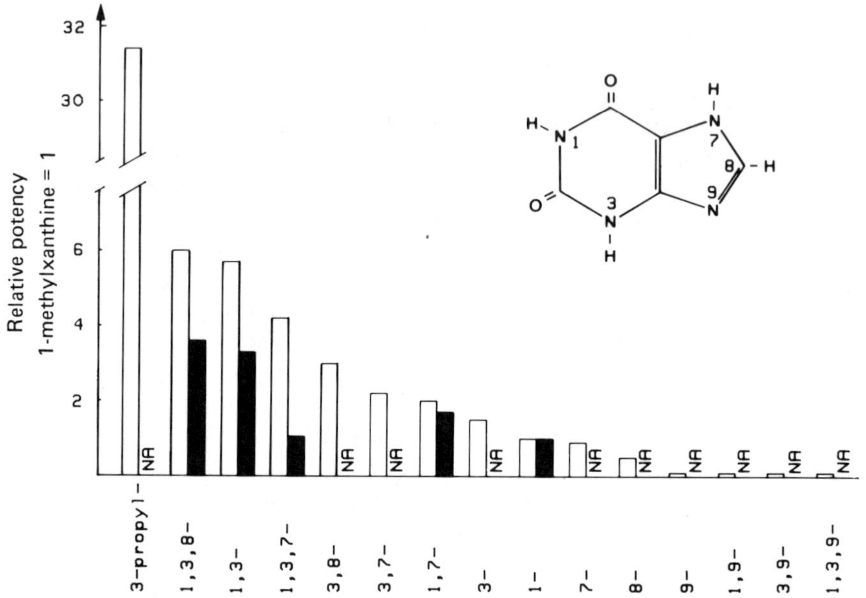

Figure 9 Effects on the isolated guinea pig trachea of 3-propylxanthine (enprofylline) and different methylxanthines. The positions for methylsubstitution of the xanthine molecule are indicated (see insert). The open bars illustrate tracheal relaxatory potencies based on EC_{50} values of the xanthines (n=4) compared with that of 1-methylxanthine (EC_{50}, mean ± SEM-1.8±0.07 mM, n-4; potency =1). At EC_{50}, SEM is less than 15% for all compounds. The filled bars illustrate adenosine antagonism. Schild plots (data not shown) calculated from three concentrations of each active compound (n-4–10 at each concentration) had slopes that did not differ from 1, the theoretical value for competitive antagonism. Relative potencies were obtained by comparing the pA_2 values with that of 1-methylxanthine (pA_2=4.40; potency = 1). NA = compounds not active as adenosine antagonists (data from Persson et al., 1982; Karlsson et al., 1982; and unpublished findings).

tant antiasthma lung actions of xanthines would have to be explained by mechanisms unrelated to adenosine. This does not preclude a role for adenosine, but it would not be a major factor in asthma.

On the other hand adenosine may well have significant physiological roles in extrapulmonary tissues. This is in fact both supported and suggested by enprofylline data obtained in comparisons with theophylline in animals and humans (Persson, 1982a; Anderson and Persson, 1985). A number of theophylline-like stimulant actions (CNS stimulant behavioral effects, diuresis, gastric

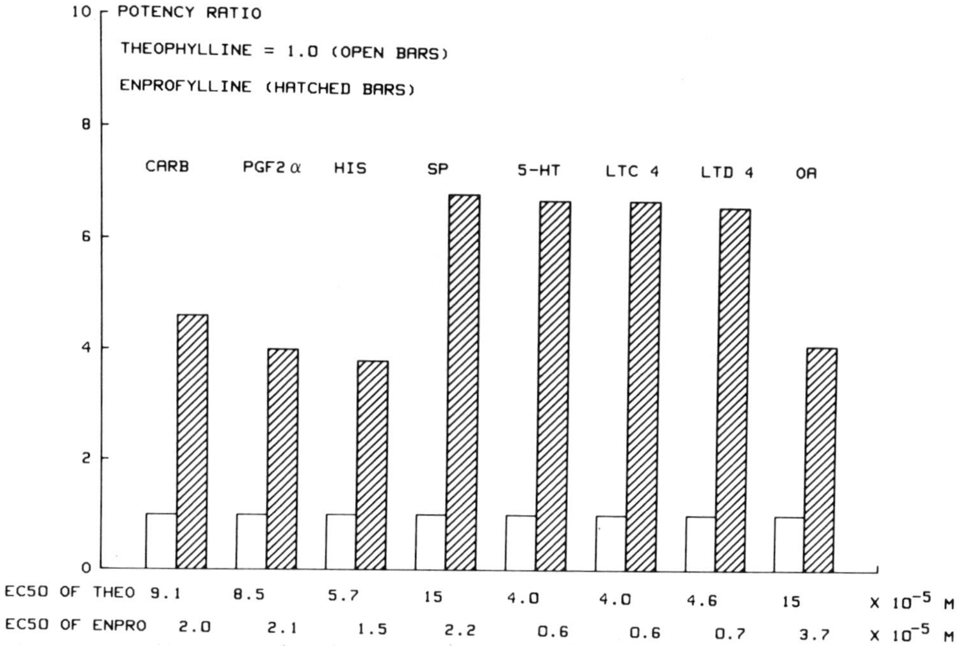

Figure 10 Potency ratios and EC_{50} values to theophylline (Theo) and enprofylline (Enpro) obtained in guinea pig isolated tracheal preparations contracted by various mediators. Cumulative relaxatory concentration-response relationship to theophylline and enprofylline were obtained in tracheas that had been contracted to about 1.4 g by carbachol (Carb, 6×10^{-8} M), prostaglandin $F_2\alpha$ ($PGF_2\alpha$, 1.8×10^{-6} M), histamine (His, 1×10^{-6})M, substance P (SP, 3.7×10^{-6} M), 5-hydroxytryptamine (5-HT, 2×10^{-7} M), leukotriene C_4 (LTC_4, 1×10^{-8} M), leukotriene D_4 (LTD_4, 10^{-8} M), and ovalbumin (OA, 0.1 μg/ml to tracheas from sensitized animals). The potency ratio was calculated as EC_{50} value to theo/EC_{50} to enpro. Each EC_{50} value is the mean results obtained in at least four animals; SEM was always less than 27%. The potency ratio between Theo and Enpro was consistently about 1:5, irrespective of which mediator had contracted the trachea. Both xanthines were somewhat more potent for relaxing leukotriene- and serotonin-induced contractions.

secretion, release of free fatty acids) may well reflect adenosine antagonism because they are not produced by enprofylline.

C. Functional Antagonism

The action of atropine and the discovery of adenosine-receptor antagonistic properties of theophylline suggest the possibility that bronchodilator drugs may not be equally effective in the presence of different proposed bronchoconstrictory mediators of asthma. Also, as stated above there may be some smooth muscle contractions that are not readily relaxed by xanthines and β-receptor agonists. It was, therefore, of interest to study more systematically the interaction between bronchodilators and different mediators. In in vitro experiments employing guinea pig tracheal preparations the relaxatory effects of terbutaline, enprofylline, and theophylline were examined on contractions induced by LTD_4, LTC_4, carbachol, substance P, $PGF_2\alpha$, 5-HT, or histamine. Throughout these experiments the three bronchodilators produced potent relaxation without interacting specifically (see below) with any one particular mediator (Fig. 10). They simply produced an effect opposite to that induced by the mediator, that is, they were functional antagonists (van den Brink, 1973; Offermeier and Van den Brink, 1974). This does not mean that xanthines and β-receptor agonists have a relaxatory potency completely independent of which type of mediator has induced the contraction. The example of potassium-induced contractions that may be poorly relaxed by these agents has already been given. It was also found that both enprofylline and theophylline had slightly increased potencies in the presence of 5HT, LTC_4, or LTD_4 compared with other mediators (Fig. 10). The finding of a somewhat variable interaction is compatible with the view that different subcellular pathways are coupled to the activation of cell surface mediator-receptors and that relaxatory drugs may differ depending on whether or not they interfere with some step in the same pathway postreceptor as the mediator (cf Baron et al., 1984; Berridge and Irvine, 1984). Normal mediator inhibitory concentrations of the two xanthines were needed to relax allergen-induced tracheal constriction in vitro, and it did not matter if the xanthines were given on top of an established contraction (Fig. 10) or prior to the addition of allergen (to guinea pig trachea and lung strips; unpublished observations by Hillery, Persson, and Andersson). This observation is in contrast to findings in vivo in sensitized guinea pigs (Andersson, 1982; Andersson et al., 1985), in which exceedingly low doses of theophylline and enprofylline inhibit allergen-induced bronchoconstriction. The relevance of allergen-induced bronchoconstriction in vitro may thus be questioned. It is possible that in vivo in guinea pigs the xanthines inhibit the allergen-induced activation of some cell type not present in vitro by critically involved in the in vivo bronchoconstriction. Further studies with addition of immunocompetent inflammatory cells to the in vitro preparations may solve this problem.

D. Relaxatory Effectiveness

Under many in vitro conditions the maximal relaxatory effects of xanthines and β-receptor agonists do not differ. However, in particular in human isolated

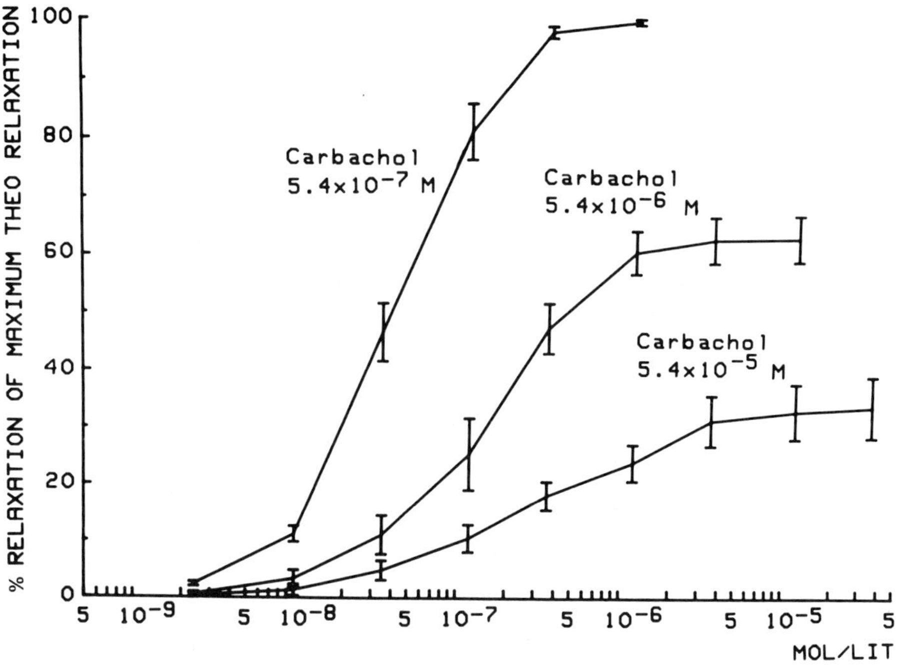

Figure 11 Cumulative concentration-response curves for isoprenaline-induced relaxation of guinea pig isolated trachea. On the ordinate scale, relaxation is expressed as a percentage of the maximum theophylline (THEO) effect. The effect of isoprenaline was evaluated on trachea contracted by different concentrations of carbachol.

airways xanthines may produce larger relaxations than β-receptor agonists. Such a difference can also consistently be induced by increasing the severity of constriction in guinea pig tracheas. The relaxatory activity of the potent β-receptor agonist isoprenaline was thus compared with that of theophylline in guinea pig isolated tracheal ring preparations contracted by carbachol (Karlsson and Persson, 1981). It was found that the more contracted the trachea the less potent and effective was isoprenaline (Fig. 11). The effect of theophylline was also reduced but not as much as that of isoprenaline. Similar observations have been made in isolated contracted bronchi obtained from humans (unpublished observations) and in vivo in dogs (Jenne et al., 1985). The ability to induce large relaxations is shared by other xanthines, notably enprofylline. Isoprenaline is a potent stimulant of the production of cyclic AMP and could be expected to show the relaxatory capacity of this second messenger (provided that cyclic

AMP is causally involved in smooth muscle relaxation, which is debatable) (Cauvin et al., 1984). The greater relaxatory effectiveness of xanthines is, therefore, difficult to reconcile with the belief that these drugs act via the inhibition of cyclic AMP degradation (Sutherland et al., 1968).

In human isolated small and large airways (apparently normal airways dissected from surgical specimens obtained at lung carcinoma operations on nonasthmatic patients) the xanthines have been shown to be consistent relaxatory agents also in preparations that are nonresponsive or almost nonresponsive to β-receptor agonists (Finney et al., 1983, 1985; Guillot et al., 1984). There is as yet no explanation of this "spontaneous" insensitivity to β-receptor stimulation observed in vitro. Whether the cause is to be found in disease processes such as bronchitis has been speculated (Guillot et al., 1984). However, there apparently was no consistent pattern in the history of the patients delivering the nonresponsive bronchi. It seems important that this β-receptor agonist resistance can be explained. Are the in vitro conditions somehow irrelevant for the test of β-receptor-mediated effects on human bronchi, or should we question the view that β-receptor agonists are general bronchorelaxants in humans?

E. Development of Tolerance

Prolonged exposure of airway smooth muscle (or other tissues) to high concentrations of a drug may induce tolerance, that is, a decreased responsiveness to subsequent exposure to the drug or to drugs acting via a common mechanism. This phenomenon can be acutely induced in vitro by treating animal and human airway preparations with large concentrations of β-receptor agonists (Lin et al., 1977; Davis and Conolly, 1980; Avner and Jenne, 1981). The desensitization is present in isolated tracheobronchial preparations obtained from animals subjected to prolonged treatment with high doses of β-receptor agonist drugs (Avner and Noland, 1978). Moderate doses of β-receptor agonists are also effective (Holmberg et al., 1981; Paynter et al., 1985). Holmberg and co-workers (1981) showed that tolerance to β-receptor stimulation developed much more readily in skeletal muscle than in airways. This difference is evident in asthmatic subjects who rapidly become tolerant to the tremor-inducing ability of β-receptor agonists (Svedmyr, 1984). However, bronchodilation by these drugs may not be attenuated during prolonged treatment (Jenne, 1979, 1981; Svedmyr and Simonsson, 1981).

Avner and Noland (1978) observed that the response to theophylline was unchanged in preparations made tolerant to β-receptor stimulation. Moreover, they found no difference between relaxatory effects of theophylline in tracheas obtained from placebo-treated and theophylline-treated (5-day period) rats. Treatment with large oral doses of enprofylline has been extended up to 6 months, which is a considerable part of the life span of these animals. Still, the

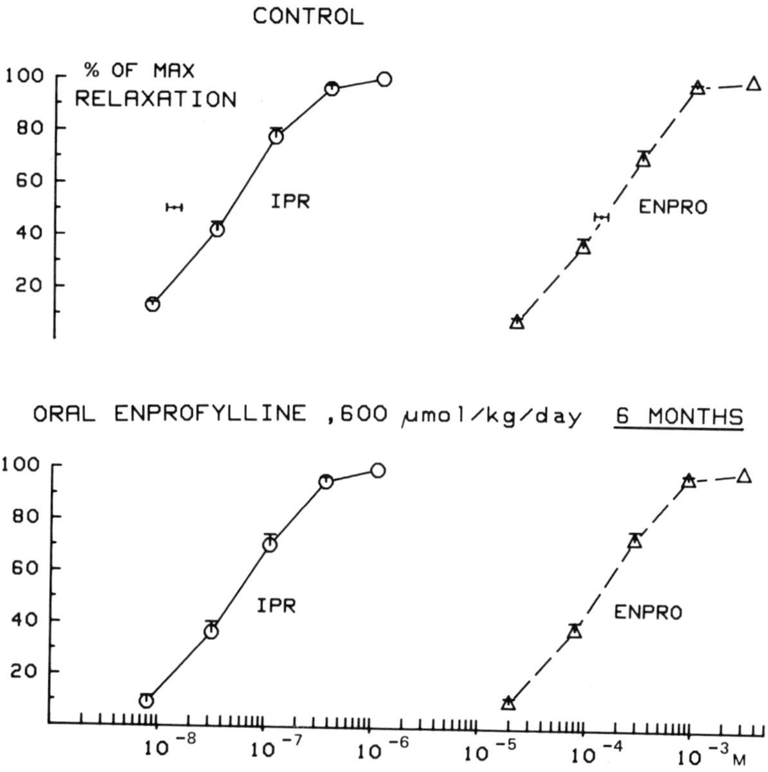

Figure 12 A large oral dose of enprofylline (ENPRO) given daily to rats for 6 months did not change the responsiveness of the tracheal smooth muscle to this xanthine or to isoprenaline (IPR). Results in tracheas obtained from the active dose groups are shown below and above are data from placebo-treated control animals. Above are also indicated mean tracheal relaxatory EC_{50} values of isoprenaline (⊢○⊣) and enprofylline (-△-) obtained in young rats, 1.5 months old. (These values should be compared to the tracheal concentration response lines from 7.5 months old rats.) Only isoprenaline showed a decreased potency with age.

isolated tracheas from enprofylline- and placebo-treated rats did not differ in their sensitivity and degree of response to enprofylline (Fig. 12). Also, the exposure to this drug had not reduced the effect of isoprenaline (Karlsson and Persson, 1982) (Fig. 11). It must be noted that human airways in vitro, which must have been exposed in vivo to caffeine for many years (through the intake of beverages), showed a consistent responsiveness to the relaxatory xanthines (but not to β-receptor agonists) (Finney et al., 1983, 1985; Guillot et al., 1984).

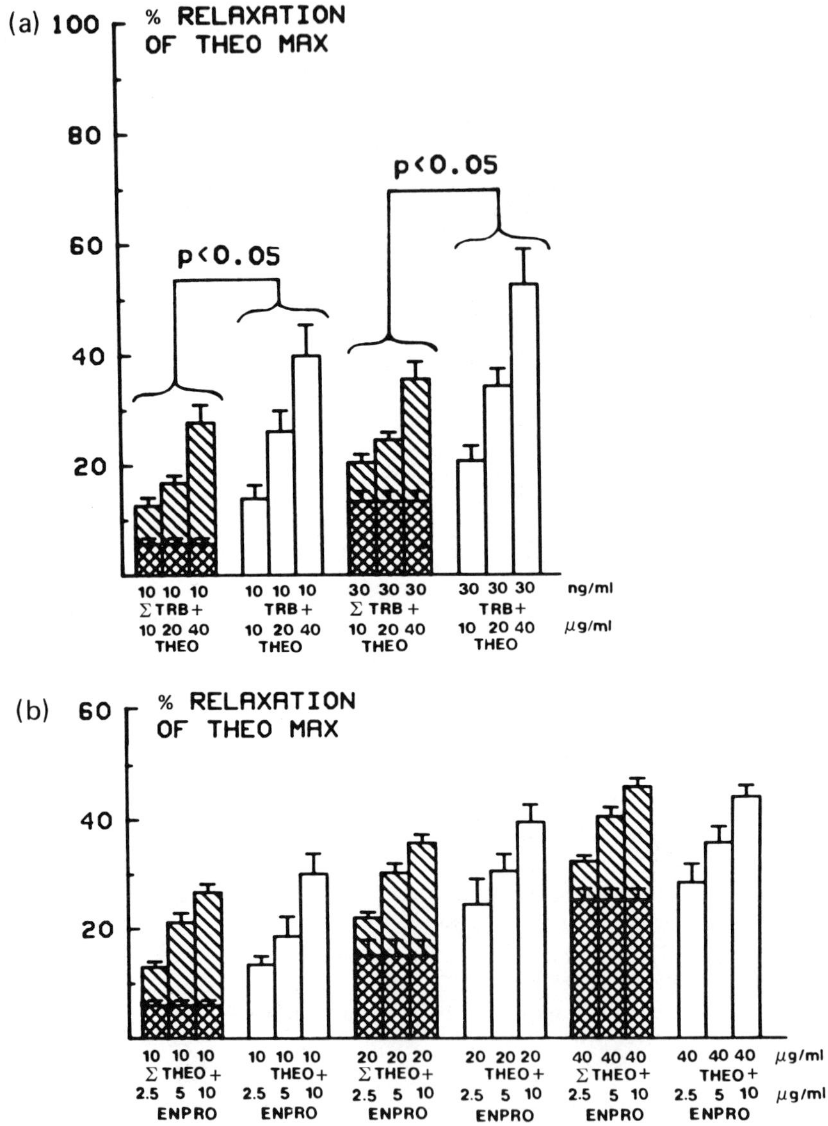
(a)
% RELAXATION OF THEO MAX
100
80
60
40
20
p<0.05
p<0.05
10 10 10 ΣTRB+ 10 20 40 THEO
10 10 10 TRB+ 10 20 40 THEO
30 30 30 ΣTRB+ 10 20 40 THEO
30 30 30 TRB+ 10 20 40 THEO
ng/ml
μg/ml
(b)
% RELAXATION OF THEO MAX
60
40
20
10 10 10 ΣTHEO+ 2.5 5 10 ENPRO
10 10 10 THEO+ 2.5 5 10 ENPRO
20 20 20 ΣTHEO+ 2.5 5 10 ENPRO
20 20 20 THEO+ 2.5 5 10 ENPRO
40 40 40 ΣTHEO+ 2.5 5 10 ENPRO
40 40 40 THEO+ 2.5 5 10 ENPRO
μg/ml
μg/ml

Figure 13

It is generally considered that tolerance to the bronchodilator effect of theophylline does not occur during long-term treatment of asthma (Paterson et al., 1979; Jenne, 1979; Svedmyr, 1984).

A major factor that, in experimental settings, seems to determine the degree of tolerance development to β-receptor stimulation is the concentration of the drug. Based on findings with human airways in vitro (Davis and Conolly, 1980; Avner and Jenne, 1981) a risk for tolerance should be largest when huge doses of β-receptor agonists are being inhaled directly onto the airways. Nevertheless, such a treatment of acute severe asthmatic conditions is frequently effective and is now gaining popularity in many countries.

F. Age-Dependent Effects

In rats and guinea-pigs it has been demonstrated that effects of β-receptor stimulation may decrease significantly with age (Ericsson and Lundholm, 1975; Brink et al., 1980). Accordingly, it has been shown that isolated tracheal preparations from 7-month-old rats are 5-10 times less sensitive to isoprenaline than tracheas from young (1.5 months) animals (Karlsson and Persson, 1982). (It has also been reported that tracheas obtained from newborn [2-3 weeks old] guinea pigs had a reduced sensitivity to isoprenaline [Bretz et al., 1984]). Age dependency has not been systematically examined in humans. That little age dependency may occur in humans is maintained by Svedmyr (1984), who had studied human airways in vitro obtained from adults with a wide range in age. Moreover, a fetal tracheal preparation (20th week of gestation) has been found to respond well to terbutaline (Persson, 1982b).

Figure 13 (a) The open bars show the recorded relaxatory effects (in percent of a maximal effect of theophylline) of combinations of theophylline (THEO) and terbutaline (TRB). For comparison, algebraic sums (hatched bars) of the effects of these agents given singly are illustrated. Significant supraadditive interactions occurred between theophylline and terbutaline (enprofylline showed the same or larger supraadditive responses with terbutaline) (data are from Persson and Gustafsson, 1985). (b) The open bars show the recorded relaxatory effects (in percent of a maximal effect of theophylline) of combinations of enprofylline (ENPRO) and theophylline (THEO) and the hatched bars illustrate the algebraic sums of effects of the two xanthines given singly. No difference between observed and calculated values was found. It is evident that for each combination the recorded additive effect was larger than that obtained with one of the drugs at the employed concentration. (2.5; 5; 10 μg/ml of enprofylline correspond to 12.9; 25.7; 51.5 μM. 10; 20; 40 μg/ml of theophylline correspond to 50,0; 100.9; 201.8 μM) (data from Persson and Gustafsson, 1985).

Xanthines do not seem to exhibit age-dependent effects: An unchanged responsiveness to enprofylline but a significantly reduced responsiveness to isoprenaline was observed in tracheas obtained from old compared with young rats (Karlsson and Persson, 1982) (Fig. 12).

G. Interactions Between Xanthines and β-Receptor Agonists

Bronchodilator drugs are frequently combined in asthma therapy. In particular, there is a concomitant use of xanthines and β_2-receptor stimulants. Through their proposed mechanisms of action of increasing cyclic AMP levels by inhibiting breakdown and stimulating production, respectively, xanthines and β-receptor agonists have been postulated to cooperate positively to produce much more than additive bronchodilation (Sutherland et al., 1968). A large number of clinical and experimental studies have now been performed in a search for synergistic effects of this combination of drugs, but generally only additive bronchodilator effects have been demonstrated (Marlin et al., 1978; Wolfe et al., 1978; Svedmyr and Svedmyr, 1980; Handslip et al., 1981; Billing et al., 1982). Because of the complexity involved in these in vivo studies (including variable responses between patients, and potential antiasthma effects of the drugs other than bronchorelaxation) it may be preferable to evaluate the quantitative aspects of interaction between xanthines and β-receptor agonists in vitro at the level of bronchial smooth muscle. So far, quantitative evaluation of this interaction has been done in a few studies of airway smooth muscle obtained from animals. The reported findings are conflicting and difficult to interpret. They suggested that less than additive (Hanna and Roth, 1979), additive (Hanna and Roth, 1979; Jeppson et al., 1982), or more than additive airway smooth relaxant effects (Bertelli et al., 1973; Philajamäki, et al., 1972) will result from combinations of sympathomimetics and xanthines.

In an in vitro study using moderately contracted guinea pig tracheal preparations, interactions were examined between theophylline and enprofylline and between terbutaline and either of the two xanthines (Persson and Gustafsson, 1985). There was a strict additive interaction when enprofylline was combined with theophylline, which is to be expected with two agents that have the same mechanism of action (Fig. 13). With terbutaline, both enprofylline and theophylline cooperated consistently in a slightly more than additive fashion (Fig. 13). This interaction is compatible with different cellular mechanisms of action of xanthines and β-receptor agonists but does not reveal those mechanisms.

Presently the recommendations for a combined drug regimen in asthma are based largely on the fact that xanthines and β_2-receptor agonists do not have the same side effects. It cannot be excluded, however, that the two types of bronchodilator drugs may also produce more than additive bronchorelaxatory effects when given together.

VI. Conclusion

Although many interesting types of bronchodilator compounds have been developed, modern research has not produced any novel pharmacologic principle with improved properties than the three traditional remedies (xanthines, sympathomimetics, and antimuscarinics). However, novel sympathomimetics with an increased lung selectivity have been developed; similar xanthines may also be synthesized soon. These advancements have been based to a large extent on structure-activity data obtained in vitro.

Our views on asthma are very much formed by the accepted opinion as to how those drugs operate to affect asthmatic symptoms. It is noteworthy, therefore, that xanthines and β_2-receptor agonists exert a number of potentially important "antiasthma" actions in addition to effecting bronchial smooth muscle relaxation. Many aspects of target cells as well as cellular mechanisms of action for these drugs remain to be investigated in detail. Further in vitro experiments will no doubt provide important and specific information on these points.

Acknowledgment

We thank Ingegerd Källén and Ulla Larsson for their expert secretarial help.

References

Adcock, J. J., and Garland, L. G. (1980). A possible role for lipoxygenase products as regulators of airway smooth muscle reactivity. *Br. J. Pharmacol. 69*: 167-169.

Adelroth, E., Morris, M., Hargreave, F. E., and O'Byrne, P. M. (1985). Airway responsiveness to leukotrienes C_4 and D_4: relationship to airway responsiveness to methacholine. *Am. Rev. Respir. Dis. 131*: A4.

Ahlquist, R. P. (1948). A study of the adrenotropic receptors. *Am. J. Physiol. 153*: 586-600.

Ahmed, F., Foster, R. W., and Small, R. C. (1985). Some effects of nifedipine in guinea-pig isolated trachealis. *Br. J. Pharmacol. 84*: 861-869.

Akcasu, A. (1952). The actions of drugs on the isolated trachea. *J. Pharm. Pharmacol. 84*: 861-869.

Andersson, K.-E., and Högestätt, E. D. (1984). On the mechanism of action of calcium antagonists. *Acta Med. Scand.* (suppl.) *681*: 11-24.

Andersson, K.-E., and Persson, C. G. A. (1985). The clinical pharmacology of enprofylline and theophylline. In *Antiasthma Xanthines and Adenosine.* Edited by K.-E. Andersson, and C. G. A. Persson, Excerpta Medica, Amsterdam.

Andersson, P. (1982). Studies on antigen-induced bronchial anaphylaxis in actively sensitized guinea-pigs. Differentiation of two models with respect to immunological parameters and drug effects. Thesis, University of Lund, Sweden.

Andersson, P., Olsson, O. A. T., and Waldeck, B. (1982). Some problems encountered in the evaluation of new bronchodilating β-adrenoceptor agonists. *Acta Pharmacol. Toxicol. 51*: 358-364.

Andersson, P., Brange, C., Sonmark, B., Stahre, G., Erjefält, I., Wieslander, E., and Persson, C. G. A. (1985). Anti-anaphylactic and anti-inflammatory effects of xanthines in the lung. In *Antiasthma Xanthines and Adenosine.* Edited by K.-E. Andersson and C. G. A. Persson. Excerpta Medica, Amsterdam.

Armitage, A. K. J., and Wooldridge, K. R. H. (1960). 1,3-Dialkyl-6-thioxanthines: A new series of bronchodilators and coronary vasodilators. *Nature 188*: 1107-1108.

Armitage, A. K., Boswood, J., and Large, B. J. (1961). Structure activity relationships in a series of 6-thioxanthines with bronchodilator and coronary dilator properties. *Br. J. Pharmacol. 17*: 196-207.

Arnoux, B., Denjean, A., Page, C. P., Morley, J., and Benveniste, J. (1985). Pulmonary effects of platelet activating factor in primate are inhibited by ketotifen. *Am. Rev. Respir. Dis. 131*: A2.

Augstein, J., Farmer, J. B., Lee, T. B., Sheard, P., and Tattersall, M. L. (1973). Selective inhibitor of slow reacting substance of anaphylaxis. *Nature New Biol. 245*: 215-217.

Avner, B. P., and Jenne, J. W. (1981). Desensitization of isolated human bronchial smooth muscle to beta-receptor agonists. *J. Allergy Clin. Immunol. 68*: 51-57.

Avner, B. P., and Noland, B. (1978). In vivo desensitization to beta receptor mediated bronchodilator drugs in the rat: Decreased beta receptor affinity. *J. Pharmacol. Exp. Ther. 207*: 23-33.

Baer, H. P., and Drummond, G. I. Eds. (1979). *Physiology and Regulatory Functions of Adenosine and Adenine Nucleotides.* New York, Raven Press.

Barnes, P. J. (1983). Endogenous plasma adrenaline in asthma. *Eur. J. Respir. Dis. 64*: 559-563.

Barnes, P. J., Wilson, N. M., and Brown, M. J. (1981). A calcium antagonist, nifedipine, modifies exercise-induced asthma. *Thorax 36*: 726-730.

Barnes, P. J., Basbaum, C. B., Nadel, J. A., and Roberts, J. M. (1982). Localization of β-adrenoceptors in mammalian lung by light microscopic autoradiography. *Nature 299*: 444-447.

Barnes, P. J., Bloom, S. R., and Dixon, C. M. S. (1984). VIP and asthma. *Lancet 1*: 112.

Barnes, P. J., Carstairs, J. A., and Nimmo, A. J. (1985a). Visualization of beta-adrenoceptor subtypes in human lung. *Am. Rev. Respir. Dis. 131*: A387.

Barnes, P. J., Cuss, F. M., and Palmer, J. B. (1985b). The effect of airway epithelium on smooth muscle contractility in bovine trachea. *Br. J. Pharmacol. 86*: 685-691.

Barnes, N. C., Piper, P. J., and Costello, J. F. (1985c). Hyper-responsiveness of asthmatics to inhaled leukotriene D_4. *Am. Rev. Respir. Dis. 131*: A24.

Baron, C. B., Cunningham, M., Strauss, J. F., and Coburn, R. F. (1984). Pharmacomechanical coupling in smooth muscle may involve phosphatidylinositol metabolism. *Proc. Natl. Acad. Sci. 81*: 6899-6903.

Bergman, J., Persson, H., and Wetterlin, K. (1969). Two new groups of selective stimulants of adrenergic β-receptors. *Experientia 25*: 899-901.

Bergstrand, H. (1980). Phosphodiesterase inhibition and theophylline. *Eur. J. Respir. Dis. 61* (suppl. 109): 37-44.

Berridge, M. J., and Irvine, R. F. (1984). Inositol triphosphate, a novel second messenger in cellular signal transduction. *Nature 312*: 315-321.

Bertelli, A., Bianchi, C., and Beani, L. (1973). Interaction between β-adrenergic stimulant and phosphodiesterase inhibiting drugs on the bronchial muscle. *Experientia 29*: 300-302.

Bertie, F., Folco, G. C., Giachetti, A., Malandrino, S., Omini, C., and Vigiano, T. (1980). Atropine inhibits thromboxane A_2 generation in isolated guinea-pig lungs. *Br. J. Pharmacol. 68*: 467-472.

Bertram, J. F., Goldie, R. G., Papadimitriou, J. M., and Paterson, J. W. (1983). Correlations between pharmacological responses and structure of human lung parenchyma strips. *Br. J. Pharmacol. 80*: 107-114.

Bieth, N., Rouot, B., Schwartz, J., and Velly, J. (1980). Comparison of pharmacological and binding assays for ten β-adrenoceptor blocking agents and two β-adrenoceptor agonists. *Br. J. Pharmac. 68*: 563-569.

Billing, B., Dahlquist, R., Garle, M., Hornblad, Y., and Ripe, E. (1982). Separate and combined use of terbutaline and theophylline in asthmatics—effects related to plasma levels. *Eur. J. Respir. Dis. 63*: 399-406.

Blackman, J. G., and McCaig, D. J. (1983). Studies on an isolated innervated preparation of guinea-pig trachea. *Br. J. Pharmacol. 80*: 703-710.

Bortoff, A. (1972). Digestion: Motility. *Am. Rev. Physiol. 34*: 261-290.

Bouhuys, A. (1974). Bronchial asthma. In *Breathing, Physiology, Environment and Lung Disease.* Edited by A. Bouhuys. New York & London, Grune & Stratton, pp. 441-489.

Boushey, H. A. (1984). The role of the parasympathetic system in the regulation of bronchial smooth muscle. *Eur. J. Respir. Dis. 65* (suppl. 135): 80-90.

Boushey, H. A., Holtzman, M. J., Sheller, J. R., and Nadel, J. A. (1980). Bronchial hyperreactivity. *Am. Rev. Respir. Dis. 121*: 389-413.

Bretz, U., Martin, U., and Ney, U. M. (1984). Drug effects on β-adrenoceptor function in experimental animals. In *Beta-adrenoceptors in Asthma.* Edited by J. Morley, London, Academic Press, pp. 227-238.

Brink, van den F. G. (1973). The model of functional interaction. II. Experimental verification of a new model: The antagonism of β-adrenoceptor stimulants and other agonists. *Eur. J. Pharmacol. 22*: 279-286.

Brink, C., Duncan, P. G., Midzenski, M., and Douglas, J. S. (1980). Response and sensitivity of female guinea-pig respiratory tissues to agonists during ontogenesis. *J. Pharmacol. Exp. Ther. 215*: 426-433.

Brittain, R. T., Dean, C. M., and Jack, D. (1976). Sympathomimetic bronchodilator drugs. *Pharmacol. Ther.* (B) *2*: 423-462.

Bundgaard, A., Enehjelm, S. D., and Aggestrup, S. (1983). Pretreatment of exercise-induced asthma with inhaled vasoactive intestinal peptide (VIP). *Eur. J. Respir. Dis. 64* (suppl. 128): 427-429.

Bussey, H. (1981). Theophylline toxicity after dyphylline therapy. *Am. Rev. Respir. Dis. 124*: 504.

Bussolino, F., and Benveniste, J. (1980). Pharmacologic modulation of platelet activating factor (PAF) release from rabbit leukocytes. *Immunology 49*: 367-376.

Calker, van D., Muller, M., and Hamprecht, B. (1978). Adenosine inhibits the accumulation of cyclic AMP in cultured brain cells. *Nature 276*: 839-841.

Cameron, A. R., Johnston, C. F., Kirkpatrick, C. T., and Kirkpatrick, M. C. A. (1983). The quest for the inhibitory neurotransmitter in bovine tracheal smooth muscle. *Q. J. Exp. Physiol. 68*: 413-426.

Castillo, J. C., and DeBeer, E. J. (1947). The tracheal chain. I. A preparation for the study of antispasmodics with particular reference to bronchodilator drugs. *J. Pharmacol. Exp. Ther. 90*: 104-109.

Cauvin, C., Meisheri, K., Mueller, E., Saida, K., and van Breeman, C. (1984). Beta-adrenergic relaxation of smooth muscle and second messengers. In *Beta-Adrenoceptors in Asthma.* Edited by J. Morley. London. Academic Press, pp. 25-40.

Cerrina, J., Denjean, A., Alexandre, G., Lockhart, A., and Duroux, P. (1981). Inhibition of exercise-induced asthma by a calcium antagonist, nifedipine. *Am. Rev. Respir. Dis. 123*: 156-160.

Cerrina, J., Advenier, C., Renier, A., Floch, A., and Duroux, P. (1983). Effects of diltiazem and other Ca^{2+} antagonists on guinea-pig tracheal muscle. *Eur. J. Pharmacol. 94*: 241-249.

Chand, N. (1979). FPL 55712–an antagonist of slow reacting substance of anaphylaxis (SRS-A): A review. *Agents Actions 9*: 133-140.

Chand, N., and Eyre, P. (1980). Further studies of dog tracheobronchial smooth muscle. *Res. Commun. Chem. Pathol. Pharmacol. 28*: 245-254.

Chand, N., Deroth, L., and Eyre, P. (1979). Pharmacology of Schultz-Dale reaction in canine lung strip in vitro: Possible model for allergic asthma. *Br. J. Pharmacol. 66*: 511-516.

Chand, N., Dhawan, B. N., Srimal, R. C., Rahmani, N. H., Shukla, R. K., and Altura, B. M. (1980). Reactivity of trachea, bronchi, and lung strips to histamine and carbachol in rhesus monkeys. *J. Appl. Physiol. 49*: 729-734.

Constantine, J. W. (1965). The spirally cut tracheal strip preparation. *J. Pharm. Pharmacol. 17*: 384-385.

Cronstein, B. N., Kramer, S. B., Weissman, G., and Hinsellhorn, R. (1983). Adenosine: A physiological modulator of superoxide anion generation by human neutrophils. *J. Exp. Med. 158*: 1160-1177.

Cushley, M. J., Tattersfield, A. E., and Holgate, S. T. (1983). Inhaled adenosine and guanosine on airway resistance in normal and asthmatic subjects. *Br. J. Clin. Pharmacol. 15*: 161-165.

Dahlén, S.-E., Hedqvist, P., Hammarström, S., and Samuelsson, B. (1980). Leukotrienes are potent constrictors of human bronchi. *Nature 288*: 484-486.

Dahlén, S.-E., Hansson, G., Hedqvist, P., Bjorck, T., Granstrom, E., and Dahlén, B. (1983). Allergen challenge of lung tissue from asthmatics elicits bronchial contraction that correlates with the release of leukotrienes C_4, D_4, and E_4. *Proc. Natl. Acad. Sci. USA 80*: 1712-1716.

Davis, C., and Conolly, M. E. (1980). Tachyphylaxis to β-adrenoceptor agonists in human bronchial smooth muscle: Studies in vitro. *Br. J. Clin. Pharmacol. 10*: 417-423.

Davis, C., Conolly, M. E., and Greenacre, J. K. (1980). β-adrenoceptors in human lung, bronchus and lymphocytes. *Br. J. Clin. Pharmacol. 10*: 425-432.

Delaunois, A. L. (1964). A new isolated lung apparatus. *Arch. Int. Pharmacodyn. 148*: 597-606.

Despas, P. J., Leroux, M., and Macklem, P. T. (1972). Site of airway obstruction in asthma as determined by measuring maximal expiratory flow breathing air and a helium-oxygen mixture. *J. Clin. Invest. 51*: 3235-3243.

Drazen, J. M., and Schneider, M. W. (1978). Comparative responses of tracheal spirals and parenchymal strips to histamine and carbachol in vitro. *J. Clin. Invest. 61*: 1441-1447.

Duncan, P. G., and Douglas, J. S. (1984). Sensitivity and responsiveness of tracheal and bronchial tissues from young and old guinea pigs: Effect of calcium antagonists. *J. Pharmacol. Exp. Ther. 228*: 612-619.

Einthoven, W. (1892). Ueber die Wirkung der Bronchial-muskeln, nach einer neuen Method untersucht, und ueber Asthma nervosum. *Pflüger's Arch li*: 367-445.

Eiser, N. M., and White, J. (1985). The effects of histamine H_1- and H_2-receptor agonists on large and small airways in normal and asthmatic subjects. *Am. Rev. Respir. Dis. 131*: A285.

Engelhardt, A., and Klupp, H. (1975). The pharmacology and toxicology of a new tropane alkaloid derivative. *Postgrad. Med. J. 51*: suppl 7, 82-84.

Ericsson, E., and Lundholm, L. (1975). Adrenergic β-receptor activity and cyclic AMP metabolism in vascular smooth muscle; variations with age. *Mechanisms Ageing Dev. 4*: 1-6.

Farmer, J. B., and Farrar, D. G. (1976). Pharmacological studies with adenine, adenosine and some phosphorylated derivatives on guinea-pig tracheal muscle. *J. Pharm. Pharmacol. 28*: 748-752.

Farmer, J. B., Farrar, D. G., and Wilson, J. (1974). Antagonism of tone and prostaglandin-mediated responses in a tracheal preparation by indomethacin and SC-19220. *Br. J. Pharmacol. 52*: 559-565.

Finney, M. J. B., Karlsson, J.-A., and Persson, C. G. A. (1983). An alternative human small airway preparation. *Br. J. Pharmacol. 80*: 709P.

Finney, M. J. B., Berend, N., and Black, J. L. (1984). Cholinergic responses in the human lung parenchymal strip: A structure-function correlation. *Eur. J. Respir. Dis. 65*: 447-455.

Finney, M. J. B., Karlsson, J.-A., and Persson, C. G. A. (1985). Effects of bronchoconstrictors and bronchodilators on a novel human small airway preparation. *Br. J. Pharmacol. 85*: 29-36.

Fisher, A. B., Dodia, C., and Linask, J. (1980). Perfusate composition and edema formation in isolated rat lungs. *Exp. Lung Res. 1*: 13-21.

Flavahan, N. A., Aarhus, L. L., Rimele, T. J., and Vanhoutte, P. M. (1985). Respiratory epithelium inhibits bronchial smooth muscle tone. *J. Appl. Physiol. 58*(3): 834-838.

Fleckenstein, A., Grun, G., Tritthart, H., and Byon, K. (1971). Uterus-Relaxation durch hochaktive Ca^{2+}-antagonistische Hemmstoffe der electromechanischen Koppelung wie Isoptin (Verapamil, Iproveratril), Substanz D600 und Segontin (Prenylamin) (Versuchen am isolierten Uterus virginellen Ratten). *Klin. Wochenschr. 49*: 32-41.

Folco, G., Omini, C., Rossoni, G., Vigano, T., and Berti, F. (1982). Anticholinergic agents prevent guinea-pig airway constriction induced by histamine, bradykinin and leukotriene C_4: Relationship to circulating TXA_2. *Eur. J. Pharmacol. 78*: 159-165.

Foreman, J. C., Jordan, C. C., Oehme, P., and Renner, H. (1983). Structure-activity relationships for some substance P-related peptides that cause wheal and flare reactions in human skin. *J. Physiol. 335*: 449-465.

Forman, A., Andersson, K.-E., Persson, C. G. A., and Ulmsten, U. (1979). Relaxant effects of nifedipine on isolated, human myometrium. *Acta Pharmacol. Toxicol. 45*: 81-86.

Foster, R. W. (1960). The paired tracheal chain preparation. *J. Pharm. Pharmacol. 12*: 189-191.

Fredholm, B. B. (1980). Theophylline actions on adenosine receptors. *Eur. J. Respir. Dis. 61* (suppl. 109): 29-36.

Furchgott, R. F. (1955). The pharmacology of vascular smooth muscle. *Pharmacol. Rev.* 7: 183-265.

Furchgott, R. F. (1972). The classification of adrenoceptors (adrenergic receptors). An evaluation from the standpoint of receptor theory. In *Handbook of Experimental Pharmacology, Catecholamines,* vol. 33. Edited by H. Blaschko and E. Muscholl. New York, Springer-Verlag, pp. 283-335.

Gandevia, B. (1975). Historical view of the use of parasympatholytic agents in the treatment of respiratory disorders. *Postgrad. Med. J. 51* (suppl 7): 13-20.

Ghelani, A. M., Holroyde, M. C., and Sheard, P. (1980). Response of human isolated bronchial and lung parenchymal strips to SRS-A and other mediators of asthmatic bronchospasm. *Br. J. Pharmacol. 71*: 107-112.

Goldie, R. G., Paterson, J. W., Spina, D., and Wale, J. L. (1984). Classification of β-adrenoceptors in human isolated bronchus. *Br. J. Pharmacol. 81*: 611-615.

Gross, N. J. and Skorodin, M. S. (1984). Anticholinergic, antimuscarinic bronchodilators. *Am. Rev. Respir. Dis. 129*: 856-870.

Grundstöm, N., and Andersson, R. G. G. (1985). Inhibition of the cholinergic neurotransmission in human airways via prejunctional alpha-2-adrenoceptors. *Acta Physiol. Scand. 125*: 513-517.

Guillot, C., Fornaris, M., Badier, M., and Orehek, J. (1984). Spontaneous and provoked resistance to isoproterenol in isolated human bronchi. *J. Allergy Clin. Immunol. 74*: 713-718.

Hahn, H. L., and Nadel, J. A. (1979). Methods of study of airway smooth muscle and its physiology. *Pharmacol. Ther.* 7: 253-295.

Hakanson, R., Leander, S., Andersson, R. G. G., and Hörig, J. (1983). Substance P antagonists release histamine from peritoneal mast cells. *Acta Physiol. Scand. 117*: 319-320.

Hamasaki, Y., Mojarad, M., Saga, T., Tai, H-H., and Said, S. I. (1984). Platelet-activating factor raises airway and vascular pressures and induces edema in lungs perfused with platelet-free solution. *Am. Rev. Respir. Dis. 129*: 742-748.

Handslip, P. D., Dart, A. M., and Davies, B. H. (1981). Intravenous salbutamol and aminophylline in asthma: A search for synergy. *Thorax 36*: 741-744.

Hanna, C. J., and Roth, S. H. (1979). Combination bronchodilators: Antagonism of airway smooth muscle contractions in vitro. *Agents Actions 9*: 18-23.

Hanna, C. J., Bach, M. K., Paré, P. D., and Schellenberg, R. R. (1981). Slow reacting substances (leukotrienes) contract human airway and pulmonary vascular smooth muscle in vitro. *Nature 290*: 343-344.

Harihara, M., Angevine, L. S., and Ohmiya, Y. (1981). The isolated perfused lung: A critical evaluation. *Toxicology 21*: 1-36.

Hedberg, A., and Mattsson, H. (1981). Beta-adrenoceptor interaction of full and partial agonists in the cat heart and soleus muscle. *J. Pharmacol. Exp. Ther. 219*: 798-808.

Hirsch, S. (1922). Klinischer und Experimenteller Beitrag zur Krampflösenden Wirkung der Purinderivate. *Klin. Wochenschr. 1*: 615-618.

Hogg, J. C., Macklem, P. T., and Thurlbeck, W. M (1968). Site and nature of airway obstruction in chronic obstructive lung disease. *N. Engl. J. Med. 278*: 1355-1360.

Holgate, S., Cushley, M. J., Church, M. K., Hughes, P., and Mann, J. S. (1985). Adenosine–a potential mediator of bronchial asthma and its antagonism by methylxanthines. In *Antiasthma Xanthines and Adenosine.* Edited by K-E. Andersson and C. G. A. Persson. Amsterdam, Excerpta Medica.

Holmberg, E., Jeppsson, A.-B., and Waldeck, B. (1981). Selective development of tolerance to β-adrenoceptor agonists in skeletal muscle as compared with airway smooth muscle from the guinea-pig. *Clin. Exp. Pharmacol. Physiol. 8*: 49-56.

Holroyde, M. C., Altounyan, R. E. C., Cole, M., Dixon, M., and Elliott, E. V. (1981). Bronchoconstriction produced in man by leukotrienes C and D. *Lancet 2*: 17-18.

Hooker, C. S., Calkins, P. J., and Fleisch, J. H. (1977). On the measurement of vascular and respiratory smooth muscle responses in vitro. *Blood Vessels 14*: 1-11.

Iravani, J., and Schuller, K. G. (1971). In-vitro-Untersuchungen der Bronchomotorik der Ratte. *Pneumologie 144*: 253-265.

Ito, Y., and Tajima, K. (1981). Actions of indomethacin and prostaglandins on neuro-effector transmission in the dog trachea. *J. Physiol. 319*: 379-392.

Ito, Y., and Takeda, K. (1982). Non-adrenergic inhibitory nerves and putative transmitters in the smooth muscle of the cat trachea. *J. Physiol. 330*: 497-511.

Itoh, T., Kanamura, Y., Kuriyama, H., and Sasaguri, T. (1985). Nitroglycerine- and isoprenaline-induced vasodilation: Assessment from the actions of cyclic nucleotides. *Br. J. Pharmacol. 84*: 393-406.

Januschke, H., and Pollak, L. (1911). Zur Pharmakologie der Bronchialmuskulatur. *Arch. Exp. Pathol. Pharmacol. 66*: 205-220.

Jenne, J. W. (1979). Beta adrenergic agents–how much is enough? *J. Allergy Clin. Immunol. 63*: 74-76.

Jenne, J. W. (1981). A critique of dosing strategies for beta-2-adrenergic agents and theophylline. *Lung 159*: 295-314.

Jenne, J. W., Shaughnessy, T. K., Manfredi, C. J., and Druz, W. S. (1985). Bronchodilation by isoproterenol depends on both dose and nature of the constricting stimulus in the dog. *Am. Rev. Respir. Dis. 131*: A280.

Jeppsson, A. B., Johansson, U., and Waldeck, B. (1982). Dissociation between the effects of some xanthine derivatives on the tracheal smooth muscle and on skeletal muscle. *Acta Pharmacol. Toxicol. 51*: 115-121.

Johannesson, N., Andersson, K.-E., Joelsson, B., and Persson, C. G. A. (1985). Relaxation of lower esophageal sphincter and stimulation of gastric secretion and diuresis by antiasthmatic xanthines. Role of adenosine antagonism. *Am. Rev. Respir. Dis. 131*: 26-31.

Johansson, U., and Waldeck, B. (1981). β_1-Adrenoceptors mediating relaxation of the guinea-pig trachea: experiments with prenalterol, a β_1-selective adrenoceptor agonist. *J. Pharm. Pharmacol. 33*: 353-356.

Kahn, R. H. (1907). Zur Physiologie der Trachea. *Arch. Anat. Physiol.* 398-418.

Kaliner, M., and Austen, K. F. (1974). Cyclic nucleotides and modulation of effector systems of inflammation. *Biochem. Pharmacol. 23*: 763-771.

Kamikawa, Y., and Shimo, Y. (1976). Pharmacological differences of non-adrenergic inhibitory response and of ATP-induced relaxation in guinea-pig tracheal strip-chains. *J. Pharm. Pharmacol. 28*: 854-855.

Kapanci, Y., Assimacopoulos, A., Irle, C., Zwahlen, A., and Gabbiani, G. (1974). Contractile interstitial cells in pulmonary alveolar septa: A possible regulator of ventilation/perfusion ratio. *J. Cell Biol. 60*: 375-392.

Karlsson, J.-A., and Persson, C. G. A. (1981). Influence of tracheal contraction on relaxant effects in vitro of theophylline and isoprenaline. *Br. J. Pharmacol. 74*: 73-79.

Karlsson, J.-A., and Persson, C. G. A. (1982). Unchanged responsiveness to bronchodilators in tracheas obtained from rats treated with enprofylline for six months. *Br. J. Pharmacol. 77*: 396P.

Karlsson, J.-A., and Persson, C. G. A. (1983). Evidence against vasoactive intestinal polypeptide (VIP) as a dilator and in favour of substance P as a constrictor in airway neurogenic responses. *Br. J. Pharmacol. 79*: 634-636.

Karlsson, J.-A., and Persson, C. G. A. (1984). Neither vasoactive intestinal peptide (VIP) nor purine derivatives may mediate non-adrenergic tracheal inhibiton. *Acta Physiol. Scand. 122*: 589-598.

Karlsson, J.-A., and Persson, C. G. A. (1985a). Effects of different substance P analogues on tachykinin-induced contractions of airway smooth muscle. In *Tachykinin Antagonists.* Edited by R. Hakanson and F. Sundler. Amsterdam, Elsevier.

Karlsson, J.-A., and Persson, C. G. A. (1985b). Effects of LTC_4 and tachykinins in dissected human small airways. *Am. Rev. Respir. Dis. 131*: A286.

Karlsson, J.-A., Kjellin, G., and Persson, C. G. A. (1982). Effects on tracheal smooth muscle on relaxant effects in vitro of theophylline and isoprenaline. *Br. J. Pharmacol. 74*: 73-79.

Karlsson, J.-A., Finney, M. J. B., Persson, C. G. A., and Post, C. (1984). Substance P antagonists and the role of tachykinins in non-cholinergic bronchoconstriction. *Life Sci. 35*: 2681-2691.

Kenakin, T. P. (1984). The classification of drugs and drug receptors in isolated tissues. *Pharmacol. Rev. 36*: 165-222.

Kirkpatrick, C. T. (1975). Excitation and contraction in bovine tracheal smooth muscle. *J. Physiol. 244*: 263-281.

Kleinstiver, P. W., and Eyre, P. (1980). The lung parenchyma strip preparation of the cat and dog. Responses to anaphylactic mediators and sympathetic bronchodilators. *Res. Commun. Chem. Pathol. Pharmacol. 27*: 451-467.

Kolbeck, R. C., Speir, W. A. Jr., Carrier, G. O., and Bransome, E. D. Jr. (1979). Apparent irrelevance of cyclic nucleotides to the relaxation of tracheal smooth muscle induced by theophylline. *Lung 156*: 173-183.

Konzett, H. (1941) Neue broncholytische, hochwirksame Körper der Adrenalinreihe. *Arch. Exp. Pathol. Pharmacol. 197*: 27-32.

Kröll, F., Karlsson, J.-A., Persson, C. G. A., and Ryrfeldt, A. (1985). Interactions between xanthines, mepyramine, and adenosine in the guinea-pig lung. In *Antiasthma Xanthines and Adenosine.* Edited by K.-E. Andersson and C. G. A. Persson. Amsterdam, Excerpta Medica, pp. 193-196.

Kröll, F., Karlsson, J.-A., Persson, C. G. A., and Ryrfeldt, A. (1986). The isolated perfused lung used for spirometric evaluation. *Acta Physiol. Scand.* (in press).

Lands, A. M., Arnold, A., McAuliff, J. P., Luduena, F. P., and Brown, T. G. Jr. (1967). Differentiation of receptor systems activated by sympathomimetic amines. *Nature 214*: 597-598.

Laursen, L. C., Eriksson, G., and Weeke, B. (1985). Comparison of two weeks treatment with enprofylline and theophylline twice daily in asthmatic patients. In *Antiasthma Xanthines and Adenosine.* Edited by K.-E. Andersson and C. G. A. Persson. Amsterdam, Excerpta Medica.

Leander, S., Hakanson, R., Hörig, J., and Folkers, K. (1983). Screening of substance P antagonists. In *Substance P.* Edited by P. Skrabanek and D. Powell. Dublin, Boole Press, pp. 12-13.

Lefkowitz, R. J., Caron, M. G., Michel, T., and Stadel, J. M. (1982). Mechanisms of hormone receptor-effector coupling: The β-adrenergic receptor and adenylate cyclase. *Fed. Proc. 41*: 2664-2670.

Lefort, J., Rotilio, D., and Vargaftig, B. B. (1984). The platelet-independent release of thromboxane A_2 by Paf-acether from guinea-pig lungs involves mechanisms distinct from those for leukotrienes. *Br. J. Pharmacol. 82*: 565-575.

Leitch, A. G., and Drazen, J. M. (1984). Pulmonary mechanical responses to leukotriene administration in vivo. In *Asthma, Physiology, Immunopharmacology and Treatment.* Edited by A. B. Kay, K. F. Austen, and L. M. Lichtenstein. Orlando, Academic Press, pp. 85-99.

Lichtenstein, L. M., and Margolis, S. (1968). Histamine release in vitro: Inhibition by catecholamines and methylxanthines. *Science 161*: 902-903.

Lin, C-S., Hurwitz, L., Jenne, J., and Avner, B. P. (1977). Mechanism of isoproterenol-induced desensitization of tracheal smooth muscle. *J. Pharmacol. Exp. Ther. 202*: 12-22.

Lohmann, S. M., Miech, R. P., and Butcher, F. R. (1977). Effects of isoproterenol, theophylline and carbachol on cyclic nucleotide levels and relaxation of bovine tracheal smooth muscle. *Biochim. Biophys. Acta 499*: 238-250.

Londos, C., Cooper, D. M. F., and Wolff, J. (1980). Subclasses of external adenosine receptors. *Proc. Natl. Acad. Sci. 77*: 2551-2554.

Longmore, W. J. (1982). The isolated perfused lung as a model for studies of lung metabolism. In *Lung Development: Biological and Clinical Perspectives,* Vol. 1. Edited by P. Farrell. pp. 101-110.

Luduena, F. P. (1942). Bronchial antispasmodic actions of theophylline derivatives, including effects of continued administration. *J. Pharmacol. Exp. Ther. 75*: 316-327.

Lulich, K. M., Mitchell, H. W., and Sparrow, M. P. (1976). The cat lung strip as an in vitro preparation of peripheral airways: A comparison of β-adrenoceptor agonists, autacoids and anaphylactic challenge in the lung strip and trachea. *Br. J. Pharmacol. 58*: 71-79.

Lundberg, J. M., and Saria, A. (1982). Bronchial smooth muscle contraction induced by stimulation of capsaicin-sensitive sensory neurons. *Acta Physiol. Scand. 116*: 473-476.

Lundberg, J. M., Saria, A., Brodin, E., Rosell, S., and Folkers, K. (1983). A substance P antagonist inhibits vagally induced increase in vascular permeability and bronchial smooth muscle contraction in the guinea pig. *Proc. Natl. Acad. Sci. USA 80*: 1120-1124.

Lundblad, K. A. L., Karlsson, J.-A., and Persson, C. G. A. (1985). On the actions of ATP on tracheal tissue. *Acta Physiol. Scand. 124* (suppl. 542): 331.

Lunell, E., Svedmyr, N., Andersson, K.-E., and Persson, C. G. A. (1982). Effects of enprofylline, a xanthine lacking adenosine receptor antagonism, in patients with chronic obstructive lung disease. *Eur. J. Clin, Pharmacol. 22*: 395-402.

Löfdahl, C.-G., and Svedmyr, N. (1984). A new β_2-adrenoceptor agonist—D2343—with long duration. *Allergy 39*: 485-489.

Macklin, C. C. (1929). The musculature of the bronchi and lungs. *Physiol. Rev. 9*: 1-60.

Madison, J. M., Jones, C. A., Tom-Moy, M., and Brown, J. K. (1985). Characterization of muscarinic cholinergic receptor subtypes in bovine airway smooth muscle and epithelium. *Am. Rev. Respir. Dis. 131*: A281.

Magnusson, H., Litt, M., Reuss, G., Jörres, R., and Hartmann, V. (1985). Efficacy of methylxanthines in bronchial asthma: bronchodilation versus protection. *Am. Rev. Respir. Dis. 131*: A49.

Marlin, G. E., Jartnett, B. J. S., Berend, N., and Hacker, N. B. (1978). Assessment of combined oral theophylline and inhaled β-adrenoceptor agonist bronchodilator therapy. *Br. J. Clin. Pharmacol. 5*: 45-50.

Marone, G., Findlay, S. R., and Lichtenstein, L. M. (1979). Adenosine receptor on human basophils: Modulation of histamine release. *J. Immunol. 123*: 1473-1477.

Marquardt, D. L., Parker, C. W., and Sullivan, T. J. (1978). Potentiation of mast cell mediator release by adenosine. *J. Immunol. 120*: 871-878.

Martin, J. G., and Collier, B. (1985). Norepinephrine does not modulate peripheral cholinergic neurotransmission in isolated canine trachealis. *Am. Rev. Respir. Dis. 131*: A282.

Matsuzaki, Y., Hamasaki, Y., and Said, S. I. (1980). Vasoactive intestinal peptide: A possible transmitter of nonadrenergic relaxation of guinea-pig airways. *Science 210*: 1252-1253.

Mentzer, Jr. R. M., Rubio, R., and Berne, R. M. (1975). Release of adenosine by hypoxic canine lung tissue and its possible role in pulmonary circulation. *Am. J. Physiol. 229*: 1625-1631.

Middleton, E. Jr. (1984). Airway smooth muscle, asthma, and calcium ions. *J. Allergy Clin. Immunol. 73*: 643-650.

Miller, W. C., and Shultz, T. F. (1979). Failure of nitroglycerin as a bronchodilator. *Am. Rev. Respir. Dis. 120*: 471.

Minneman, K. P., Hedberg, A., and Molinoff, P. B. (1979). Comparison of beta adrenergic receptor subtypes in mammalian tissues. *J. Pharmacol. Exp. Ther. 211*: 502-508.

Mitchell, H. W. (1982). The effect of contraction and Ca^{2+} removal on the indomethacin-induced increase in tracheal smooth muscle reactivity. *Arch. Int. Pharmacodyn. 260*: 54-62.

Murad, F. (1985). Effects of phosphodiesterase inhibitors and a role of cyclic nucleotides in smooth muscle relaxation. In *Antiasthma Xanthines and Adenosine.* Edited by K.-E. Andersson and C. G. A. Persson. Amsterdam, Excerpta Medica.

Nadel, J. A. (1980). Autonomic regulation of airway smooth muscle. In *Physiology and Pharmacology of the Airways.* Edited by J. A. Nadel. New York, Marcel Dekker, pp. 217-257.

Nickerson, M. (1956). Receptor occupancy and tissue response. *Nature (Lond) 178*: 697-698.

Nicolaus, B. J. R. (1983). Symbiotic approach to drug design. In *Decision Making in Drug Research.* Edited by F. Gross. New York, Raven Press, pp. 173-186.

Nielsen-Kudsk, J. E., Karlsson, J.-A., and Persson, C. G. A. (1986). Relaxatory effects of xanthines, a β_2-receptor agonist and Ca^{2+}-antagonists in guinea-pig tracheal preparations contracted by potassium or carbachol. *Eur. J. Pharmacol.,* in press.

Niemeier, R. W., and Bingham, E. (1972). An isolated perfused lung preparation for metabolic studies. *Life Sci. 11*: 807-820.

O'Donnell, S. R., and Wanstall, J. C. (1979). The importance of choice of agonist in studies designed to predict $\beta_2:\beta_1$ adrenoceptor selectivity of antagonists from pA_2 values on guinea-pig trachea and atria. *Naunyn-Schmiedebergs Arch. Pharmacol. 308*: 183-190.

Offermeier, J., and Brink, van den F. G. (1974). The antagonism between cholinomimetic agonists and β-adrenoceptor stimulants, the differentiation between functional and metaffinoid antagonism. *Eur. J. Pharmacol. 27*: 206-213.

Olsson, O. A. T., Swanberg, E., Svedinger, I., and Waldeck, B. (1979). Effects of β-adrenoceptor agonists on airway smooth muscle and on slow-contracting skeletal muscle: In vitro and in vivo results compared. *Acta Pharmacol. Toxicol. 44*: 272-276.

Olsson, O. A. T., Ahlquist, B., and Gustafsson, B. (1981). A new β_2-adrenoceptor agonist with α_1-adrenoceptor blocking properties. *Acta Pharmacol. Toxicol. 48*: 340-348.

Orehek, J., Douglas, J. S., and Bouhuys, A. (1975). Contractile responses of the guinea-pig trachea in vitro: Modification by prostaglandin synthesis-inhibiting drugs. *J. Pharmacol. Exp. Ther. 194*: 554-564.

Osswald, H., Nabarovski, G., and Hermes, H. (1980). Adenosine as a possible mediator of metabolic control of glomerular filtration rate. *Int. J. Biochem. 12*: 263-267.

Patel, K. R. (1981). The effect of calcium antagonist, nifedipine in exercise-induced asthma. *Clin. Allergy 11*: 429-432.

Paterson, J. W., Wooolcock, A. J., and Shenfield, G. M. (1979). Bronchodilator drugs. *Am. Rev. Respir. Dis. 120*: 1149-1188.

Paterson, J. W., Goldie, R. G., Spina, D., Lulich, K. M., and Henry, P. J. (1984). Responsiveness of human isolated asthmatic bronchi to relaxant and spasmogenic agonists. *Clin. Exp. Pharmacol. Physiol.* suppl. *8*: 123.

Paton, W. D. M., and Vizi, E. S. (1969). The inhibitory action of noradrenaline and adrenaline on acetylcholine output by guinea-pig ileum longitudinal muscle strip. *Br. J. Pharmacol. 35*: 10-28.

Patterson, R. (1958). The tracheal strip: Observations on the response of tracheal muscle. *J. Allergy 29*: 165-172.

Pauwels, R., and Van Der Stracten, M. (1985). Experimental asthma and xanthines. In *Antiasthma Xanthines and Adenosine.* Edited by K.-E. Andersson and C. G. A. Persson. Amsterdam, Excerpta Medica.

Pauwels, R., Van Renterghen, D., Van Der Straeten, M., Johannesson, N., and Persson, C. G. A. (1985). The effect of theophylline and enprofylline on allergen induced bronchoconstriction. *J. Allergy Clin. Immunol. 76*: 583-590.

Pavia, D., Sutton, P. P., Lopez-Vidriero, M. T., Agnew, J. E., and Clarke, S. W. (1983). Drug effects on mucociliary function. *Eur. J. Respir. Dis. 64* (Suppl 128): 304-317.

Paynter, D. E., Hiller, F. C., Coronett, L. E., Norris, J. S., and Popovich, K. J. (1985). Beta-adrenergic desensitization in airway smooth muscle. *Am. Rev. Respir. Dis. 131*: A363.

Perry, W. L. M., Ed. (1968). *Pharmacological Experiments on Isolated Preparations.* Edinburgh and London, E & S Livingstone.

Persson, C. G. A. (1973). Adrenergic, cholecystokinetic and morphine-induced effects on extra-hepatic biliary motility. *Acta Physiol. Scand. 87*: suppl. 383.

Persson, C. G. A. (1982a). The profile of action of enprofylline, or why adenosine antagonism seems less desirable with xanthine antiasthmatics. In *Pharmacology of Asthma.* Edited by J. Morley and K. D. Rainsford. Basel, Birkhäuser Verlag, pp. 115-129.

Persson, C. G. A. (1982b). Some β-adrenoceptor functions of therapeutic interest. *Acta Obstet. Gynecol. Scand* suppl. *108*: 7-12.

Persson, C. G. A. (1985a). On the medical history of xanthines and other remedies for asthma. A tribute to H. H. Salter. *Thorax 40*: 881-886.

Persson, C. G. A. (1985b). Experimental lung actions of xanthines. In *Antiasthma Xanthines and Adenosine.* Edited by K.-E. Andersson and C. G. A. Persson. Amsterdam, Excerpta Medica.

Persson, C. G. A. (1985c). Subdivision of xanthines. In *Antiasthma Xanthines and Adenosine.* Edited by K.-E. Andersson and C. G. A. Persson. Amsterdam, Excerpta Medica.

Persson, C. G. A., and Ekman, M. (1976). Contractile effects of histamine in large and small respiratory airways. *Agents Actions 6/4*: 389-393.

Persson, C. G. A. (1986). Leakage of macromolecules from the tracheobronchial microcirculation. *Am. Rev. Respir. Dis.,* in press.

Persson, C. G. A., and Gustafsson, B. (1985). Tracheal relaxation of combinations between xanthines and between a β_2-receptor agonist and xanthines. *Lung 164*: 33-40.

Persson, C. G. A., and Kjellin, G. (1981). Enprofylline, a principally new antiasthmatic xanthine. *Acta Pharmacol. Toxicol. 49*: 313-316.

Persson, C. G. A., Erjefält, I., and Karlsson, J.-A. (1981). Adenosine antagonism, a less desirable characteristic of xanthine asthma drugs? *Acta Pharmacol. Toxicol. 49*: 317-320.

Persson, C. G. A., Karlsson, J.-A., and Erjefält, I. (1982). Differentiation between bronchodilation and universal adenosine antagonism among xanthine derivatives. *Life Sci. 30*: 2182-2189.

Persson, C. G. A., Erjefält, I., and Andersson, P. (1986). Leakage of macromolecules from guinea-pig tracheobronchial microcirculation. Effects of allergen, leukotrienes, tachykinins, and antiasthma drugs. *Acta Physiol. Scand. 127*: 95-106.

Persson, C. G. A., Erjefält, I., and Karlsson, J.-A. (1985b). Effects of tachykinin and tachykinin-antagonists on the tracheobronchial microcirculation. In *Tachykinin-antagonists.* Edited by R. Hakanson and F. Sundler. Amsterdam, Elsevier.

Persson, C. G. A., Gustafsson, B., and Kjellin, G. (1985b). Tracheal relaxation and adenosine antagonism by 1- and/or 3-alkylxanthines. In *Antiasthma Xanthines and Adenosine.* Edited by K.-E. Andersson and C. G. A. Persson. Amsterdam, Excerpta Medica.

Persson, H., and Johnson, B. (1970). Adrenergic receptors in the guinea-pig trachea and lung. *Acta Pharmacol. (Kbh) 28*: 49-56.

Philajamäki, K., Kanto, J., and Iisalo, E. (1972). Human and animal studies on the interactions between glyphylline and isoprenaline. *J. Asthma Res. 9*: 255-261.

Phillis, J. W., Edstrom, J. P., Kostopoulos, G. K., and Kirkpatrick, J. R. (1979). Effects of adenosine and adenine nucleotides on synaptic transmission in the cerebral cortex. *Can. J. Physiol. Pharmacol. 57*: 1289-1312.

Polson, J. B., Krzanowski, J. J., Fitzpatrick, D. F., and Szentivanyi, A. (1978). Studies on the inhibition of phosphodiesterase-catalyzed cyclic AMP and cyclic GMP breakdown and relaxation of canine tracheal smooth muscle. *Biochem. Pharmacol. 27*: 254-256.

Polson, J. B., Krzanowski, J. J., and Szentivanyi, A. (1985). Correlation between inhibition of a cyclic GMP phosphodiesterase and relaxation of canine tracheal smooth muscle. *Biochem. Pharmacol. 34*: 1875-1879.

Post, C., Butterworth, J. F., Strichartz, G. R., Karlsson, J.-A., and Persson, C. G. A. (1985). Tachykinin antagonists have potent local anaesthetic actions. *Eur. J. Pharmacol. 117*: 347-354.

Rall, T. W. (1980). Central nervous stimulants. The xanthines. In *The Pharmacological Basis of Therapeutics.* Edited by A. Goodman Gilman, L. S. Goodman, and A. Gilman. New York, Macmillan, pp. 592-607.

Regoli, D., Escher, E., Drapeau, G., D'Orleans-Juste, P., and Mizrahi, J. (1984). Receptors for substance P. III. Classification by competitive antagonists. *Eur. J. Pharmacol. 97*: 179-189.

Richardson, J. B. (1979). Nerve supply to the lungs. *Am. Rev. Respir. Dis. 119*: 785-801.

Roberts, J., Raeburn, D., Rodger, I. W., and Thomson, N. C. (1984). Comparison of in vivo airway responsiveness and in vitro smooth muscle sensitivity to methacholine in man. *Thorax 39*: 837-843.

Roberts, J. A., Rodger, I. W., and Thomson, N. C. (1985). Airway responsiveness to histamine in man: Effect of atropine on in vivo and in vitro comparison. *Thorax 40*: 261-267.

Rosa, L. M., and McDowall, R. J. S. (1951). The action of the local hormones on the isolated human bronchus. *Acta Allergol. IV*: 293-304.

Rosell, S., and Folkers, K. (1982). Substance P-antagonists: a new type of pharmacological tool. *Trends Pharmacol. Sci. 3*: 211-212.

Rossum, J. M. van (1963). Cumulative dose-response curves. II. Technique for the making of dose-response curves in isolated organs and the evaluation of drug parameters. *Arch. Int. Pharmacodyn. 143*: 299-330.

Roy, S. C., and Brown, G. (1885). On bronchial contraction. *J. Physiol. 6*: 21-25.

Ruffolo, R. R. (1982). Important concepts of receptor theory. *J. Autonom. Pharmacol. 2*: 277-295.

Russi, E. W., and Ahmed, R. (1984). Calcium and calcium antagonists in airway disease. A review. *Chest 86*: 475-482.

Ryrfeldt, A., and Nilsson, E. (1978). Uptake and biotransformation of ibuterol and terbutaline in isolated perfused rat and guinea pig lungs. *Biochem. Pharmacol. 27*: 301-305.

Salter, H. (1859). On some points in the treatment and clinical history of asthma. *Edinburgh Med. J. 4*: 1109-1115.

Saria, A., Theodorsson-Norheim, E., Gamse, R., and Lundberg, J. M. (1985). Release of substance P- and substance K-like immunoreactivities from the isolated perfused guinea-pig lung. *Eur. J. Pharmacol. 106*: 207-208.

Skoogh, B.-E., (1986). Parasympathetic ganglia in the airways. *Bull. Physiopathol. Respir. 20*(Suppl 7): 143-147.

Skoogh, B.-E., Löfdahl, L.-G., and Svedmyr, N. (1985). Beta-adrenoceptors in ferret tracheal smooth muscle subtyped as beta-1. *Am. Rev. Respir. Dis. 131*: A284.

Smith, B. R., and Bend, J. R. (1981). Lung perfusion techniques for xenobiotic metabolism and toxicity studies. *Methods Enzymol. 77*: 105-120.

Snyder, S. H. (1981). Adenosine receptors and the actions of methylxanthines. *Trends Neurosci. 4*: 242-244.

Solis-Cohen, S. (1900). The use of adrenal substance in the treatment of asthma. *JAMA 34*: 1164-1166.

Sollmann, T., and Gilbert, A. J. (1937). Microscopic observations of bronchiolar reactions. *J. Pharmacol. Exp. Ther. 61*: 272-285.

Sollmann, T., and Oettingen, von W. F. (1928). Bronchial perfusion of isolated lung as a method for studying pharmacologic reactions of bronchiolar muscle. *Proc. Soc. Exp. Biol. Med. 25*: 692-695.

Sparrow, M. P., Pfitzer, G., Gagelmann, M., and Ruegg, J. C. (1984). Effect of calmodulin, Ca^{2+} and cAMP protein kinase on skinned tracheal smooth muscle. *Am. J. Physiol. 246*: C308-C314.

Spilker, B., and Minatoya, H. (1975). The role of bronchoconstrictors in evaluating smooth muscle relaxant activity. *Arch. Int. Pharmacodyn. 217*: 201-217.

Stephens, N. L., and Kroeger, E. A. (1980). Ultrastructure, biophysics, and biochemistry of airway smooth muscle. In *Physiology and Pharmacology of the Airways.* Edited by J. A. Nadel. New York, Marcel Dekker, pp. 31-121.

Stephens, N. L., and Van Niekerk, W. (1977). Isometric and isotonic contractions in airway smooth muscle. *Can. J. Physiol. Pharmacol. 55*: 833-838.

Stephenson, R. P. (1956). A modification of receptor theory. *Br. J. Pharmacol. 11*: 379-393.

Sutherland, E. W., Robison, G. A., and Butcher, R. W. (1968). Some aspects of the biological role of adenosine 3′,5′-monophosphate (cyclic AMP). *Circulation 37*: 279-306.

Svedmyr, N. (1984). Is beta-adrenoceptor sensitivity a limiting factor in asthma therapy? In *Beta-Adrenoceptors in Asthma.* Edited by J. Morley. London, Academic Press, pp. 181-199.

Svedmyr, N., and Simonsson, B. G. (1981). Drugs in the treatment of asthma (review). In *Respiratory Pharmacology* (International Encyclopedia of Pharmacology and Therapeutics, section 104). Edited by J. Widdicombe. Oxford, Pergamon Press, pp. 657-701.

Svedmyr, N., and Svedmyr, K. (1980). In vitro and in vivo effects of theophylline and β_2-adrenoceptor stimulants in combination. *Eur. J. Respir. Dis.* (suppl 61): 83-91.

Svensson, L. A. (1985). Sympathomimetic bronchodilators: increased selectivity with lung specific prodrugs. *Pharmaceutical Res.* 156-162.

Tainter, M. L., Pedden, J. R., and James, M. (1934). Comparative actions of sympathomimetic compounds: bronchodilator actions in perfused guinea pig lungs. *J. Pharmacol. Exp. Ther. 51*: 371-386.

Taylor, S. M., Paré, P. D., and Schellenberg, R. R. (1984). Cholinergic and nonadrenergic mechanisms in human and guinea pig airways. *J. Appl. Physiol. 56*: 958-965.

Thompson, D. C., Wells, J. L., Altiere, R. J., and Diamond, L. (1986). The effect of epithelium removal on nonadrenergic, noncholinergic (NANC) inhibitory responses in the isolated central airways of the cat and guinea pig. *Am. Rev. Respir. Dis. 133*: A172.

Thornton, J. W. (1932). Reactions of isolated bronchi. *Q. J. Exp. Physiol. 21*: 305-314.

Tomioka, K., and Yamada, T. (1982). Effects of histamine H_2-receptor agonists and antagonists on isolated guinea-pig airway muscles. *Arch. Int. Pharmacodyn. 255*: 16-26.

Trendelenburg, P. (1912). Physiologische und pharmakologische Untersuchungen an der isolierten Bronchialmuskulatur. *N. S. Arch. Exp. Pathol. Pharmakol. 69*: 79-107.

Triner, L., Vulliemoz, Y., and Verosky, M. (1977). Cyclic 3′5′-adenosine monophosphate and bronchial tone. *Eur. J. Pharmacol. 41*: 37-46.

Turner-Warwick, M. (1984). Summing up. In *Asthma, Physiology, Immunopharmacology and Treatment.* Edited by A. B. Kay, K. F. Austen, and L. M. Lichtenstein. Orlando, Academic Press, pp. 417-425.

Vincenc, K., Black, J., Yan, K., Armour, C. L., Donelly, P. D., and Woolcock, A. J. (1983). Comparison of in vivo and in vitro responses to histamine in human airways. *Am. Rev. Respir. Dis. 128*: 875-879.

Wanner, A. (1977). Clinical aspects of mucociliary transport. *Am. Rev. Respir. Dis. 116*: 73-125.

Weiner, N. (1980). Atropine, scopolamine and related antimuscarinic drugs. In *The Pharmacological Basis of Therapeutics.* Edited by A. Goodman Gilman, L. S. Goodman, and A. Gilman. New York, Macmillan, pp. 120-137.

Welton, A. F., and Simko, B. A. (1980). Regulatory role of adenosine in antigen-induced histamine release from the lung tissue of actively sensitized guinea pigs. *Biochem. Pharmacol. 29*: 1085-1092.

Widmark, E., and Waldeck, B. (1986). Physiological and pharmacological characterization of an in vitro vagus nerve-trachea preparation from guine-pig. *J. Auton. Pharmacol.*, in press.

Wikberg, J. E. S. (1982). Adrenergic receptors: Classification, ligand binding and molecular properties. *Acta Med. Scand.* suppl. 665: 19-36.

Williams, C. J. B. (1840). Report of experiments on the physiology of the lungs and air-tubes. British Association for the Advancement of Science. Report of the Annual Meeting, Glasgow, pp. 411-420.

Wolfe, J. D., Tashkin, D. P., Calvarese, B., and Simmons, M. (1978). Bronchodilator effects of terbutaline and aminophylline alone and in combination in asthmatic patients. *N. Engl. J. Med. 298*: 363-367.

Yabuuchi, Y. (1977). The β-adrenoceptor stimulant properties of OPC-2009 on guinea-pig isolated tracheal, right atrial and left atrial preparations. *Br. J. Pharmacol. 61*: 513-521.

Young, R. H., and Gilbert, R. P. (1941). The use of theophylline with ethylenediamine (aminophyllin) for the control of bronchial spasm. A pharmacologic study. *J. Allergy 12*: 235-241.

5

Physiology and Pharmacodynamics of Beta-Adrenergic Agonists

NILS SVEDMYR and CLAES-GORAN LÖFDAHL

Sahlgrenska University Hospital
Gothenburg, Sweden

I. Introduction

Ephedrine is our oldest adrenoceptor stimulant. It has been used by the Chinese for some 5000 years and, in Greece, it was extracted from the ephedra plant 2000 years ago (Chen and Schmidt, 1930). The indications for this drug have been extensive and, apart from the treatment of venereal diseases, it enjoyed a good reputation for treating respiratory disorders.

In 1910, Barger and Dale described the activity of several adrenaline-like amines that stimulated the sympathetic nervous system; they introduced the term "sympathomimetic" to describe them.

Isoprenaline was introduced by Konzett in 1940 as a very effective bronchodilator given by aerosol. Isoprenaline came to be of great importance for subsequent research and still serves as both a therapeutic agent and a reference substance in drug trials. Ahlquist later (1948) postulated the presence of two distinct types of adrenergic receptors, the α and β receptors. In 1967, Lands and co-workers made it clear that the β-receptors could be separated into two distinct groups, a β_1-type in the heart, adipose tissue, and small intestine, and a β_2-type in the bronchiolus, vascular bed, uterus, and diaphragm. Since β_2-receptor activation was found to be necessary for bronchodilation, the search for selective β_2-stimulants intensified, eventually leading to the development of highly selective β_2-stimulating drugs.

During the last 15 years, the treatment of asthma has changed considerably. Epinephrine and isoprenaline have been replaced by selective β_2-stimulants, disodium cromoglycate has been introduced, and inhaled glucocorticosteroids have replaced oral steroids to a large extent. Theophylline therapy has improved due to better monitoring of the plasma levels, evaluation of its pharmacokinetics, and introduction of slow-release preparations.

The first β_2-adrenoceptor-stimulating drug with certain selectivity was metaproterenol, introduced for clinical use in Europe in 1961 under the name orciprenaline. The three selective β_2-stimulants most used today,—fenoterol, albuterol (salbutamol in Europe), and terbutaline—were in fact discovered before Lands and co-workers subdivided the β-receptors into β_1 and β_2. Albuterol and terbutaline were registered in Europe about 1970 and fenoterol a few years later.

When evaluating the advantages and disadvantages of the different drugs, we unfortunately have to rely upon our knowledge of their pharmacodynamics and clinical effects which, in turn, are based on acute and rather short-term studies. No long-term studies are available.

II. Physiology of β-Stimulation

A. β_1- and β_2-Receptors

Receptor-binding studies have demonstrated that both β_1- and β_2-adrenoceptors are present in *lung* tissues from animals and humans. The ratio of β_1- to β_2-receptors in peripheral tissue from human lung is about 1:3 (Engel, 1981). However, since there are about 60 different cell populations in the lung, this does not necessarily mean that these receptors are present in the bronchial smooth muscle (see Chapter 2).

Several animal species have been found to have β_1-adrenoceptor-mediated relaxation of bronchial muscle, as in the guinea pig, where approximately 25% of the relaxation is mediated via β_1-adrenoceptors (Zaagsma et al., 1984; Johansson and Waldeck, 1981). In the cat and ferret, however, trachea relaxation is mediated *mainly* via β_1-adrenoceptors (Lulich et al., 1976; Skoogh et al., 1985), both species having a dense adrenergic innervation in the bronchial smooth muscle.

In human bronchial muscle, relaxation is mediated only by β_2-receptors as shown in vitro (Zaagsma et al., 1984) and in asthmatic patients using both selective β_1-agonists and antagonists (Löfdahl and Svedmyr, 1982; Löfdahl et al., 1983). To date, no one has been able to demonstrate sympathetic innervation of human bronchial muscle, despite its existence in several other species. This illustrates the importance of confirming animal results with studies in human asthmatics.

So far all studies show a correlation between sympathetic innervation and β_1-receptors in the tissues. This supports the concept that β_1-receptors are receptors for sympathetic stimulation by released norepinephrine and that β_2-receptors are mainly receptors for endogenous epinephrine stimulation (Ariens and Simonis, 1976).

The β-receptors of *skeletal muscle* are important in asthma treatment since β-receptor-induced tremor is the dose-limiting side effect of treatment with modern β_2-agonists (Larsson and Svedmyr, 1977a; Larsson, 1977). It has been shown in several studies that the skeletal muscle has β_2-receptors in the slow-contracting fibers mediating tremor (Larsson and Svedmyr, 1977a,c; Bowman, 1981; Perucca et al., 1981; Arnold and McDevitt, 1983a), and in the fast-contracting fibers sometimes mediating local cramps (K. Svedmyr, 1981).

In vitro animal models for studying muscle provided some evidence for an increased efficiency in bronchial muscle relaxation compared to the skeletal muscle effects, indicating that β_2-receptors in the organs are different (Andersson et al., 1982). However, clinical dose-response studies could not confirm any difference in potency of the new drugs on β_2-receptors in bronchi and skeletal muscle compared to terbutaline or salbutamol (Löfdahl et al., 1982, 1984). Consequently, there is still no evidence that the β_2-receptors in skeletal muscle are different from those in the bronchial muscle.

β-Receptors in the *heart* have been shown to be heterogeneous in several species: both β_1- and β_2-receptors mediated increased heart rate (Carlsson et al., 1972, 1977; Hedberg et al., 1980). Chronotropy was mediated about 20% by β_2-receptors while inotropy was almost solely β_1-adrenoceptor-mediated (Carlsson et al., 1977). Thus, there is a possibility that β_2-agonist-induced tachycardia is mediated directly by β_2-adrenoceptors in the heart and more recent studies support a small direct β_2 effect (Arnold and McDevitt, 1983b; Brown et al., 1983). Nevertheless, the most important reason for tachycardia during β_2-agonist treatment is a reflex tachycardia due to β_2-receptor-mediated vasodilation (Robinson et al., 1966; Arnold and McDevitt, 1983b).

B. Therapeutic Effects of β_2-Adrenoceptor Stimulation

The following effects of β_2-adrenoceptor stimulation have been proposed to be of therapeutic importance in asthma:

1. Bronchial smooth muscle relaxation
2. Increase in mucociliary transport
3. Inhibition of release of mediators
4. Suppression of permeability edema
5. Decrease in pulmonary hypertension and increase in right ventricular ejection fraction

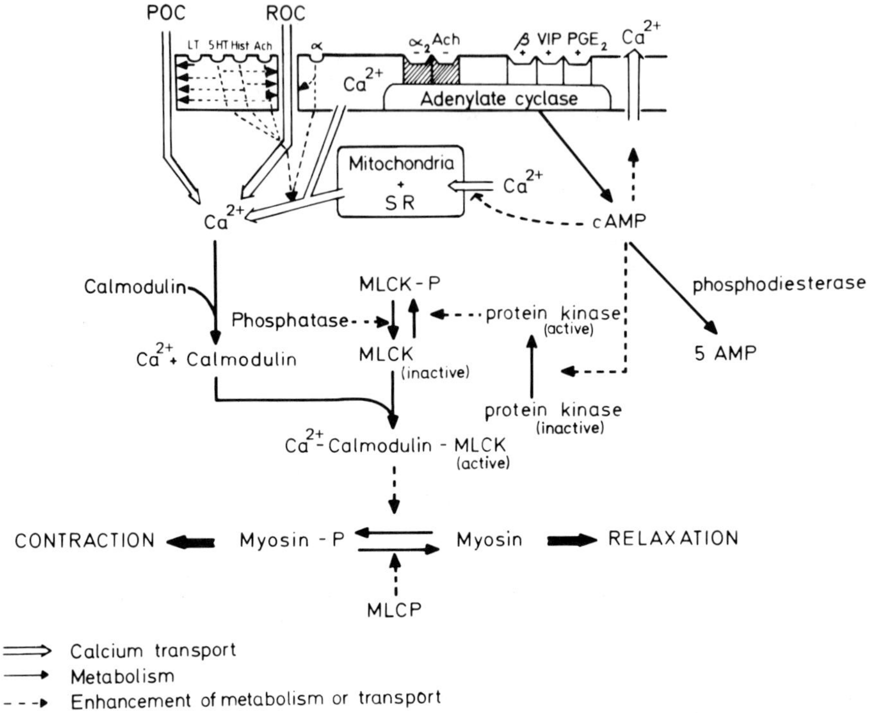

Figure 1 Schematic representation of the biochemistry of the smooth muscle cell and the intracellular events leading to contraction and relaxation. To the left are the factors contributing to contraction and to the right the factors contributing to relaxation. The membrane is shown in the upper part of the figure.

Contraction of the airway smooth muscle occurs when free calcium increases due to stimulation by several agonists: leukotrienes (LT), 5-hydroxytryptamine (5-HT), histamine (Hist), acetylcholine (ACh), and α-adrenoceptor agonists (α). The contraction is dependent upon phosphorylated myosin bound to actin and ATP. The phosphorylation of myosin is catalyzed by myosin light chain kinase (MLCK) activated by calcium and calmodulin. Dephosphorylation of myosin-phosphate is catalyzed by myosin light chain phosphatase (MLCP), and causes relaxation. One possibility for decreasing the amount of active MLCK is to stimulate protein kinases, which phosphorylates MLCK and thereby makes it less prone to react with calcium and calmodulin. The protein kinases are dependent on the level of cAMP, which is increased by stimulation of, for example, β-adrenoceptors on the cellular membrane via activation of adenylate cyclase. An increased level of cAMP also increases the internalization of calcium into the sarcoplasmic reticulum and the mitochondria. Furthermore, cAMP increases the

6. Improved contractility of fatigued diaphragmatic muscle
7. Inhibition of transmission through airway parasympathetic ganglia

The first six of these effects are shared by theophylline and β_2-stimulants. The most important in the treatment of asthma is bronchial smooth muscle relaxation, but the other effects may also contribute to the antiasthmatic effect, especially when the drugs are given regularly and prophylactically. Unfortunately, it is difficult to evaluate the clinical significance of the other effects.

Bronchial Smooth Muscle Relaxation

Figure 1 gives an overview of the intracellular events after β_2-adrenoceptor stimulation leading to contraction of the smooth muscle.

Potency

Figure 2 shows one of our earlier experiments on isolated human bronchial muscle contracted by a moderate dose of carbachol. The different β-adrenoceptor stimulants and theophylline derivatives all had the same maximum relaxant effect, the relative potency being proportional to the potencies found clinically. Thus, the β_2-agonists are about 1,000 times more potent than theophylline.

When the concentration of carbachol was increased to a maximum of 5.4×10^{-5} M, the potency difference between relaxation induced by isoprenaline and by theophylline was gradually reduced (Karlsson and Persson, 1981) (see Chapter 4). O'Donnell and Wanstall (1978) have also shown that the relative bronchodilating potency of fenoterol compared to albuterol increases in bronchial muscle contracted with high doses of carbachol. The concentration of theophylline used in these studies, however, was far above the therapeutic range as was the concentration of carbachol. Therefore the significance of these differences is difficult to assess. In fact, they may have no significance,

---

Figure 1 (continued) extrusion of calcium by the calcium extrusion pump and the Na-Ca exchange. An increased level of cAMP thus decreases the internal level of free calcium and stimulates protein kinases, both of which contribute to relaxation. Other agonists than β-adrenoceptor agonists, such as VIP and prostaglandin E_2, also activate adenylate cyclase. This activation occurs via a stimulating guanine-nucleotide-binding protein, whereas an inhibition of adenylate cyclase occurs by cholinergic and α_2-receptor stimulation via inhibitory guanine nucleotide binding protein (Birnbaumer et al., 1984).

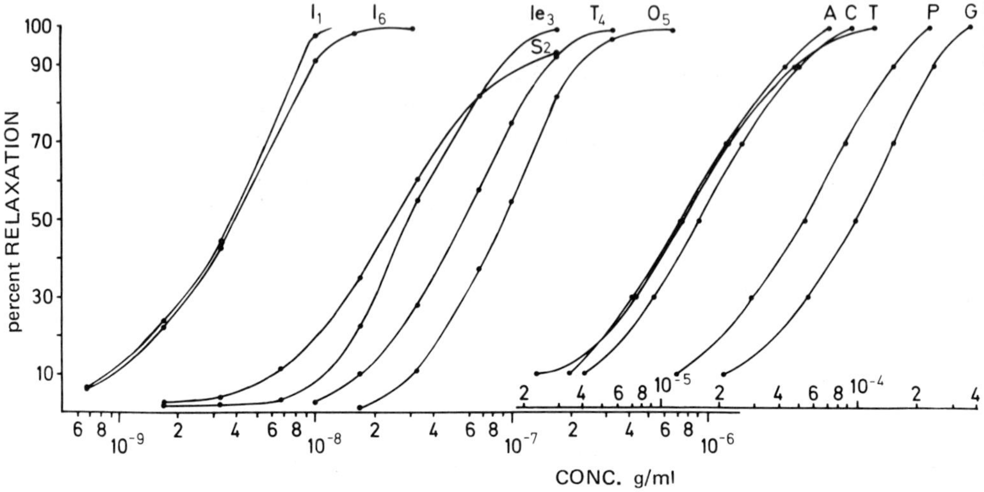

Figure 2 Dose-response curves for different β-adrenoceptor stimulants and theophylline preparations on carbachol-contracted human bronchial muscles in vitro. Means from 13 experiments. I_1, isoprenaline given as first drug; I_6, isoprenaline given as sixth drug; S_2, salbutamol; Ie_3, isoetharine; T_4, terbutaline; O_5, orciprenaline; A, aminophylline; C, choline theophylline; T, theophylline-sodium-glycinate; P, proxyphylline; G, glyphylline or dyphylline (modified with permission from Svedmyr, 1977).

since clinical studies have not shown a better antiasthmatic effect with theophylline or fenoterol compared to the other β_2-adrenoceptor stimulants.

Experiments with isolated airway preparations from animals and humans (Karlsson and Persson, 1984) show that both theophylline and β_2-stimulants relax smooth muscle in large and small airways, irrespective of whether they have been contracted by different asthma mediators such as carbacholine, histamine, 5-hydroxytryptamine, prostaglandin $F_{2}\alpha$, LTC_4, LTD_4, or substance P (see Chapter 4, Fig. 10, pp. 151-152).

Thus, terbutaline and theophylline are effective *functional* antagonists of a large variety of potential asthma mediators at the level of the smooth muscle, probably accounting for their excellent therapeutic effect. Their effects are superior to those of anticholinergics which only block acetylcholine and, consequently, only the reflex-mediated bronchoconstriction. The β_2-agonists and xanthines are also more effective than cromoglycate.

Selectivity

There have been difficulties in evaluating selectivity in vitro and in transferring the results to the clinical situation.

Table 1 Relative Potencies of Intravenous β-Stimulants in the Anesthetized Guinea Pig

β-Stimulant	50% Decrease in in intratracheal pressure	50% Decrease in skeletal muscle tension during submaximal tetanus	25% Increase in heart rate
Isoprenaline	1	1	1
Fenoterol	4.3	3.2	83
Orciprenaline	56	63	226
Salbutamol	5.2	5.2	245
Terbutaline	15	18.5	266

From Brittain et al., 1981.

One difficulty is that drugs can be full or partial agonists. In vitro dose-response studies in isolated guinea-pig *heart* muscle show metaproterenol and fenoterol to be full β_1-adrenoceptor agonists but with lower potency than isoproterenol (Table 1). Albuterol and terbutaline are partial agonists: maximal heart stimulation is not achieved, even at very high concentrations. The selectivity for the different drugs therefore varies, depending on the level of heart stimulation at which selectivity comparisons are performed. At very high in vitro concentrations, the β_2-selectivity of fenoterol ought to be lower because it is a full β_1-agonist. Partial agonists cannot even reach that high level of stimulation. Whether this is of any clinical importance can only be evaluated in dose-response comparisons in asthma patients, using objective recording of the bronchodilating and heart stimulating effects. Figure 3 shows the results of such a study comparing cumulatively increasing doses of oral fenoterol and albuterol. The doses of albuterol were 2, 6, and 18 mg, given at 2-hr intervals; the corresponding bronchodilating doses of fenoterol were 2.5, 5, and 15 mg. It is evident from the figure that, even after relative overdoses, no difference in β_2-selectivity can be detected between these drugs. From a clinical point of view, this indicates that there is no difference in their therapeutic efficacy or selectivity. Furthermore, this shows that in vitro results cannot always be transferred to the clinical situation. Approximately the same clinical β_2-selectivity has been established for albuterol, fenoterol, and terbutaline (Svedmyr, 1985).

Increase in Mucociliary Transport

Both β_2-stimulants and theophylline have been proven to increase mucociliary transport in asthmatics, an effect which may contribute to their therapeutic

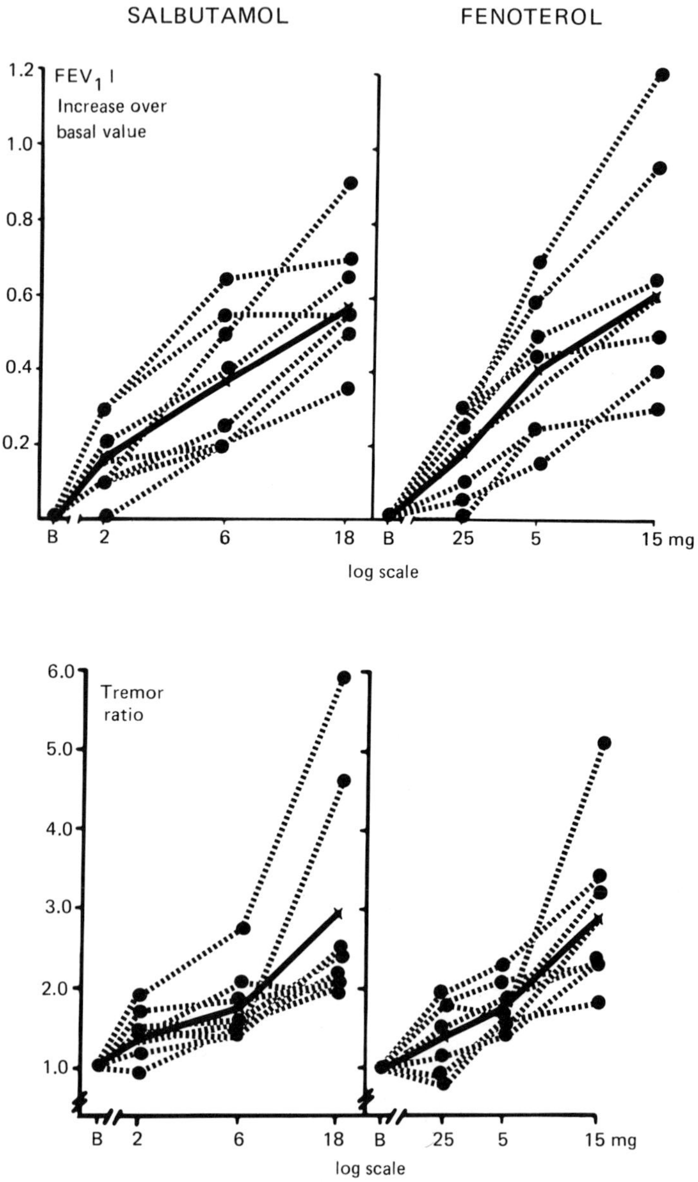

Figure 3 Effects of increasing dosages of fenoterol and albuterol (salbutamol) on FEV_1, tremor ratio, and heart rate. The heavy line is the mean value from eight asthmatic patients; the dotted line shows individual values (modified with permission from Larsson and Svedmyr, 1977b).

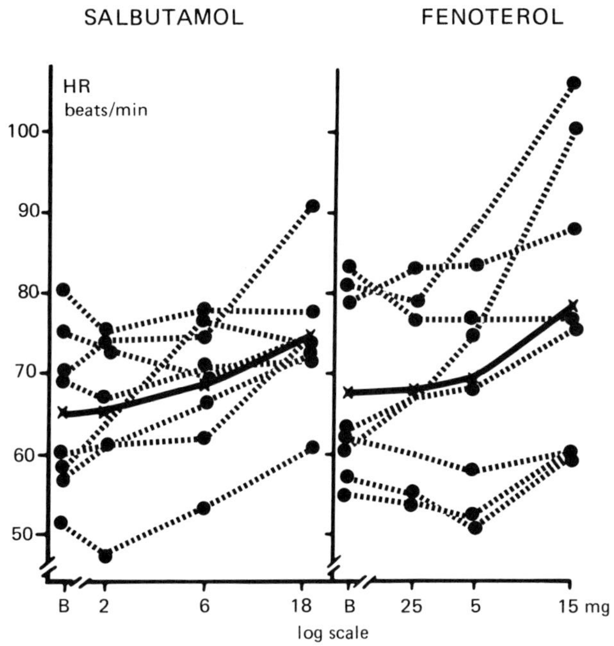

Figure 3 (continued)

efficacy (Mossberg et al., 1976; Matthys and Köhler, 1980). Matthys and co-workers (1984) have also shown that β_2-stimulants and theophylline only have an additive effect on this parameter. The clinical importance of this effect has been questioned by Sutton et al. (1981). β_2-Stimulants have also been shown to increase the chloride ion and water secretion into the bronchial lumen (Al-Bazzaz and Cheng, 1979; Borson et al., 1980). This may be one mechanism behind the increase in mucociliary transport.

Inhibition of Anaphylactic Release of Mediators

Histamine release from human lung mast cells is inhibited to a larger extent by β_2-agonists than by cromoglycate (Holgate and Church, 1984). Martin and co-workers showed in 1980 that both terbutaline and theophylline given orally to asthmatics protect against antigen provocation and at the same time partly inhibit the release of histamine and neutrophil chemotactic factors (NCF) Borum and Mygind (1980) found that a nasal aerosol application of fenoterol protected against nasal antigen challenge. These studies show that the effects on human basophils and mast cells may be of clinical relevance but other clinical studies (Hegardt, 1981) throw doubts on the relative importance of inhibition of mast cell histamine release.

Suppression of Permeability Edema

The vasoconstrictor action of α-adrenoceptor-stimulating sympathomimetics is the important mechanism behind their well-known decongestant action in the nasal airways. However, Svensjö et al. (1977) showed that isoprenaline and terbutaline effectively prevented the mediator-induced extravasation of macromolecules in spite of an increased local blood flow. β-Adrenoceptor stimulants have clearly been shown to have a venular antipermeability effect in many different microvascular beds, such as skin, skeletal muscle, trachea, lung, and mesentery (Persson and Svensjö, 1983). The experimental evidence suggests that these drugs have direct effects on the microvascular membrane, presumably the venular endothelial cells, inhibiting macromolecular permeability. This inhibition is blocked by β-blockers. The antipermeability effect is exerted against various types of mediators. Thus, irrespective of whether the mediator is an amine, peptide, or a lipid metabolite, β-adrenoceptor stimulation is an effective way of preventing the increased venular permeability.

All experiments to date have used concentrations of β_2-receptor stimulants larger than those obtained in plasma after systemic administration of these drugs. By inhaled administration, the antipermeability action of these drugs may have increased importance due to higher concentrations in the target tissue. Thus, the effect of inhalation therapy with β-receptor agonists may be partly due to an effect on bronchial venules, where asthma mediators apparently increase macromolecular permeability. The therapeutic value of this antipermeability effect, however, remains to be proven.

Decrease in Pulmonary Hypertension and Increase in Right Ventricular Ejection Fraction

Normal systemic doses of both theophylline and β_2-stimulants reduce the pulmonary artery pressure and increase the right ventricular ejection fraction in patients with hypoxia (Parker et al., 1967; Amory et al., 1974; Teule and Majid, 1980; Jones et al., 1982; MacKnee et al., 1983; Winter et al., 1984a,b). These effects can hardly be important in the normal treatment of asthma, but they might be important in patients with COPD in whom pulmonary hypertension and right ventricular failure carry a poor prognosis (Wetzenblum et al., 1981). These vascular effects cause a further unevenness of ventilation perfusion resulting in a temporary fall in oxygen tension.

Improved Contractility of Fatigued Diaphragmatic Muscle

Theophylline improves the contractility of fatigued diaphragmatic muscle (Aubier et al., 1981). The same effect has also been shown with β_2-stimulants in animal studies, in which these drugs seem to have an additive effect (Howell and Roussos, 1984). This effect is probably without clinical relevance in usual asthma treatment, with a comparatively low PCO_2. It might be of importance, however, when the asthmatic is no longer able to maintain ventilation the PCO_2 begins to increase, and a respirator may be needed. This effect may also be of clinical importance in patients with chronic obstructive pulmonary disease COPD.

Inhibition of Transmission Through Airway Parasympathetic Ganglia

β_2-Agonists block the parasympathetic ganglion transmission in the vagal nerve of ferret trachea (Skoogh and Svedmyr, 1984). The effect starts after some delay compared to the effect on the bronchial muscle. It is impossible to evaluate the clinical importance of this effect at the moment, but these studies indicate the possibility that part of the β-agonist effect is mediated via yet another airway target cell than the bronchial muscle.

C. Side Effects

Skeletal muscle tremor is a dose-limiting factor when β_2-agonists are given systemically, as in maintenance therapy (Formgren, 1975). Side effects are minor after *inhalation* of normal doses of all selective β_2-adrenoceptor stimulants, if they occur at all. Tachycardia, palpitation, a slight increase in blood glucose and free fatty acids, hypokalemia, and a certain degree of nervousness sometimes occur, especially when systemic treatment is begun. Inhaled β_2-stimulants cause a temporary fall of PO_2 in acute severe asthma but this can be prevented by oxygen treatment (Svedmyr and Simonsson, 1981).

Tremor

There is no evidence to date that β_2-receptors in skeletal muscle and bronchial muscle are different (Löfdahl et al., 1982, 1984). The effect elicited by β-adrenoceptor agonists on skeletal muscle is dependent on the fiber type involved. In slow-contracting muscles the tension and degree of fusion in subtetanic contractions are decreased, whereas fast-contracting muscles respond with an increase in these parameters (Bowman, 1981). The depression of slow-contracting muscles is thought to be responsible for the muscle tremor observed. Although there is a considerable individual variation in tremor response, the most regular responders may shake so much that fine movements are impossible (Thiringer and Svedmyr, 1975). There is a close relationship between the initial individual tremor response to β_2-stimulants and the basal tremor (Jenne et al., 1982). Moreover, the perception of tremor seems to be related to the relative increase over the basal tremor produced by the drug. However, prolonged treatment with β_2-stimulants makes the skeletal muscle tolerant, whereas the sensitivity of the airway smooth muscle remains essentially unchanged. This

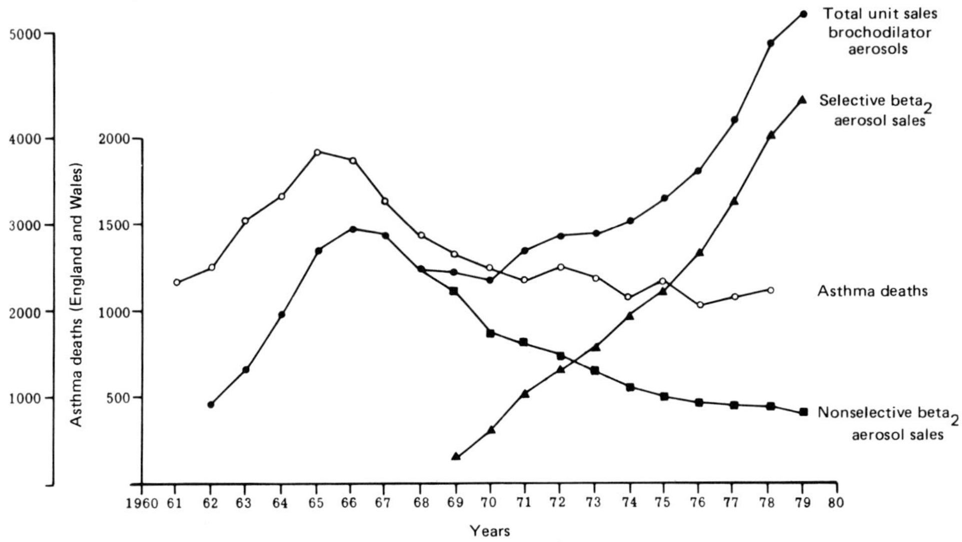

Figure 4 Relation between unit aerosol sales and asthma deaths, 1961-1979, in United Kingdom. There has been no increase in asthma deaths since the introduction of selective β_2-adrenoceptor stimulants in 1969 (reprinted with kind permission from Clark, 1982a).

has been observed clinically in humans (Larsson et al., 1977) and experimentally in guinea pigs (Holmberg et al., 1981). Thus, these drugs should be introduced in a reduced dosage until skeletal muscle tolerance develops. Despite this, some individuals cannot tolerate even reduced systemic dosages.

Cardiovascular Effects

The heart stimulation is mainly reflexogenic through β_2-mediated peripheral vasodilation. Thus both tremor and tachycardia are, in principle, β_2-mediated effects and both are dose-dependent.

At equipotent bronchodilating doses, β_2-adrenoceptor-stimulating drugs given systemically induce more tachycardia than theophylline (K. Svedmyr, 1981). The tachycardia induced by β_2-agonists however, is mainly a reflex effect of peripheral vasodilation and is a specific β_2 action.

Cardiac arrhythmia was not seen in a case of self-poisoning by albuterol (K. Svedmyr, 1981).

Cardiac side effects may occur with theophylline at a lower plasma concentration when combined with systemically administered β_2-stimulants than when given alone. A recent study from New Zealand (Wilson and Sutherland,

1981) reported an apparent increase in the sudden death rate among young asthmatics, when the combination of theophylline and β_2-agonists became more prevalent. Laursen et al. (1985) found an increased rate of arrhythmias in asthma patients when they were treated with a combination of theophylline and β_2-stimulants by oral route. This was seen only when the agents were combined at high dosages. At low dosages, or with single drugs high dosages, no arrhythmias were seen. The combination of oral β_2-stimulants and theophylline provides additive bronchodilating effects and fewer side effects than single drugs dosed to give equal bronchodilation (K. Svedmyr, 1981).

In the late 1960s, a connection was suspected between the sale of β-stimulant aerosol inhalers and an increased mortality in asthma in Great Britain and several other countries (Speizer et al., 1968a,b; Fraizer et al., 1971). Figure 4 shows that this increased asthma mortality dropped when isoprenaline prescriptions were decreased and has remained unchanged despite a more than doubling of prescriptions for selective β_2-bronchodilator aerosols (Clark, 1982a).

In animal studies, heart muscle necrosis has been observed after very high doses of isoprenaline. This does not seem to be relevant to asthma treatment with selective β_2-adrenoceptor stimulants (Rona et al., 1959; Balazs, 1972; Balazs and Herman, 1976).

III. Routes of Administration

A. Systemic Administration

Complete dose-response curves in patients with asthma show that nonselective and selective β_2-stimulants attain the same maximal bronchodilating effect when given intravenously (Fig. 5) just as in the previously discussed in vitro studies. The bronchodilator and cardiac stimulant effects of isoprenaline run parallel, suggesting that β_1- and β_2-receptors are equally stimulated. However, with a very high dose of isoprenaline giving maximal bronchodilation, the heart rate continues to increase until it is nearly double at the highest dose (a cumulative total dose of 190 μg racemic isoprenaline given during 2.5 hr). This should limit the use of intravenous isoprenaline (non-β-selective) in asthma. In the same patients the selective β_2-stimulant albuterol (salbutamol) gave the same maximal bronchodilation but was initially not associated with any pulse increase (sign of selective β_2 effect). The pulse did not begin to increase until almost half of the maximal bronchial relaxation had been achieved and it increased thereafter with increasing albuterol dose (total cumulative dose 600 μg racemic salbutamol). Yet, even with selective β_2-stimulants given parenterally or orally, it is not possible to achieve maximal bronchodilation in moderately obstructed patients without a simultaneous increase in pulse rate, owing to peripheral vasodilation with an ensuing chronotropic reflex.

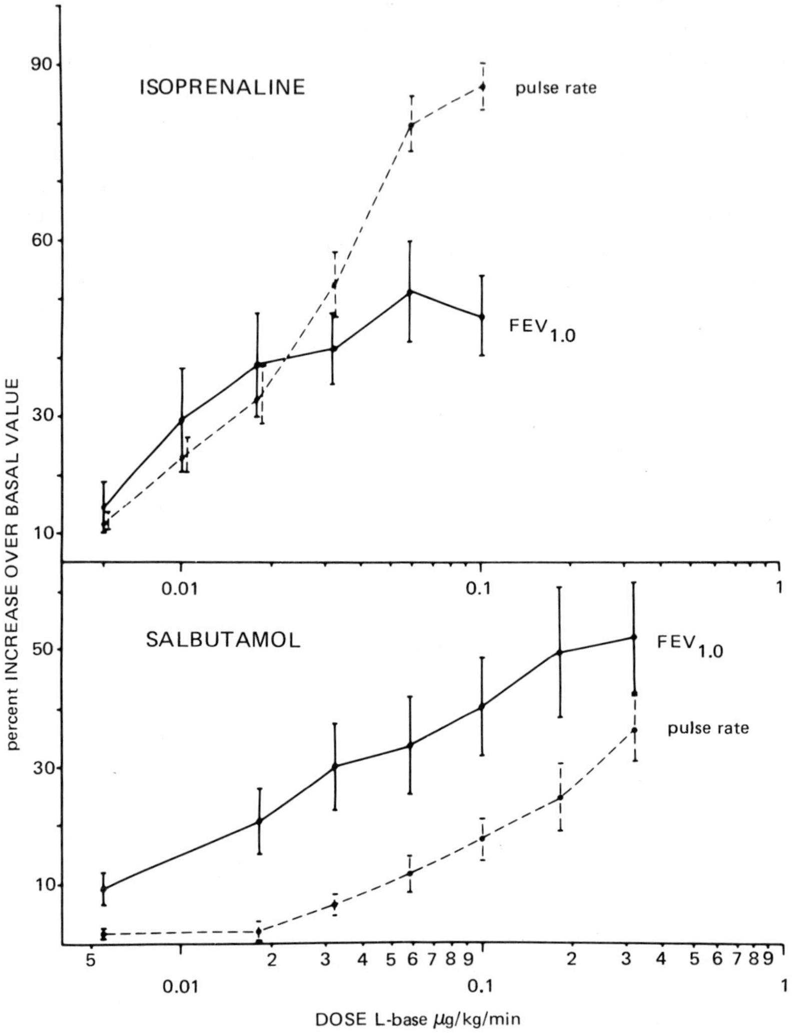

Figure 5 Mean dose-response curves ± SEM for isoprenaline and salbutamol (albuterol) for 10 patients with asthma. Each dose was infused during 6 min with 30-min intervals (modified with permission from Svedmyr and Thiringer, 1971).

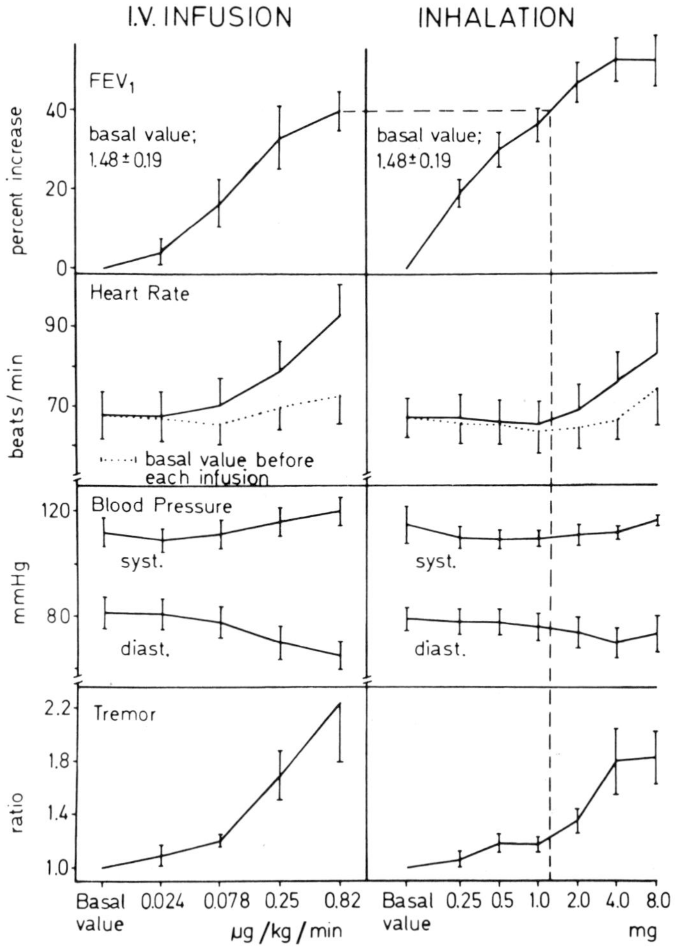

Figure 6 Effects of increasing dosages of terbutaline by intravenous infusion (during 6 min) and by dose aerosol on FEV_1, heart rate, blood pressure, and skeletal muscle tremor in asthmatics (dotted line-heart rate just before the next dose). Mean ± SEM from 10 patients (modified with permission from Thiringer and Svedmyr, 1975).

B. Inhalation

Isoprenaline has been used as a metered dose inhaler for about 40 years. Despite its lack of β_2-selectivity, one or two inhalations can be given without any tachycardia.

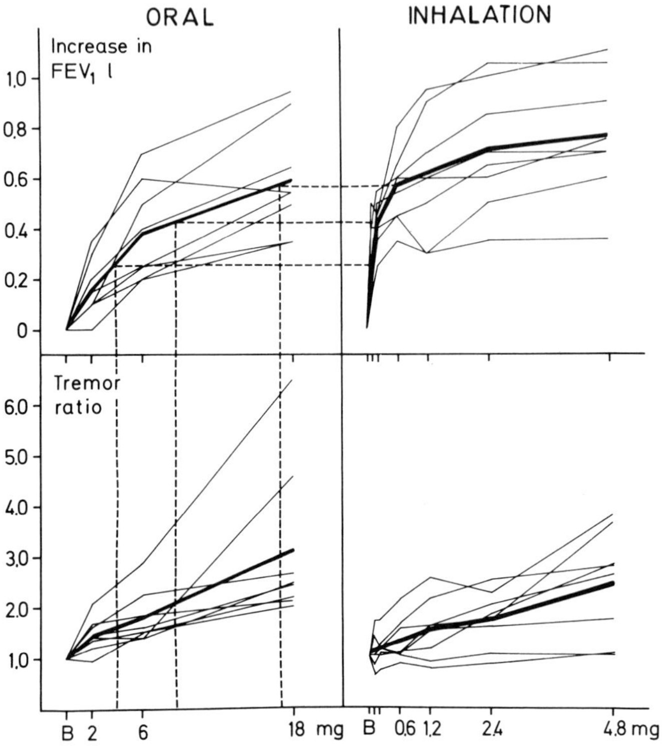

Figure 7 Effects on 1-sec forced expired volume (FEV_1) and tremor ratio of increasing inhaled and oral doses of salbutamol. Arrows point to FEV_1 values caused by oral and inhaled doses giving the same effect on FEV_1. These identical FEV_1 values are connected by the broken line (reprinted with permission from Larsson and Svedmyr, 1977c).

The administration of a drug by inhalation has many advantages since the drug is delivered directly to the affected area. Rapid onset of action and high efficacy can be obtained from a low dose and the incidence of unwanted side effects can thereby be reduced. Maximal β_2-selective stimulation in the lung can be achieved with one of the new β_2-selective agonists given by the inhaled route.

Figure 6 shows a comparison of the bronchodilating effect and the side effects of terbutaline given intravenously and by a metered dose inhaler (MDI) (Thiringer and Svedmyr, 1976). Intravenous doses exceeding the recommended therapeutic levels did not produce maximal relaxation of the bronchial muscle in patients with endogenous asthma, but they did increase the heart rate by 25 beats/min and more than doubled the skeletal muscle tremor. When terbutaline

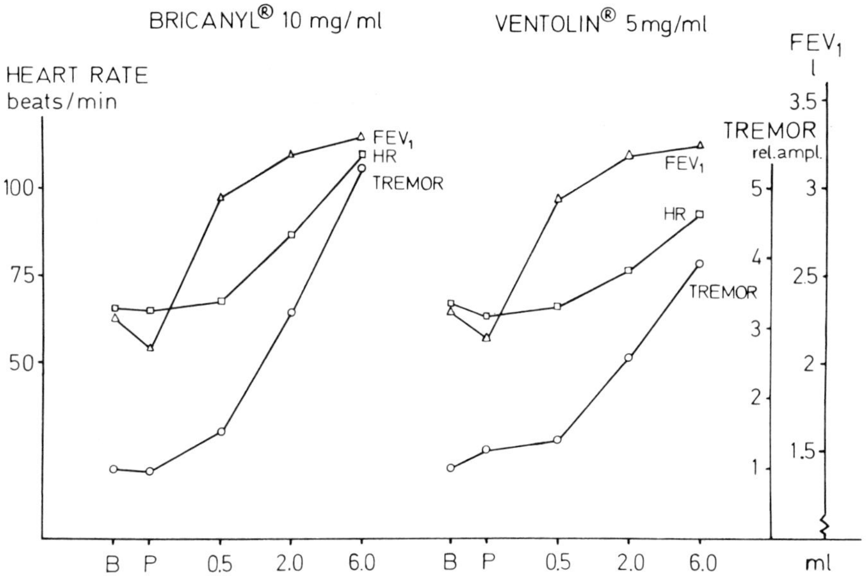

Figure 8 Effects of Bricanyl® (terbutaline) and Ventoline® (salbutamol) inhaled by IPPB on FEV_1, heart rate, and skeletal muscle tremor in asthmatics. Each dose was inhaled during 15 min, with 60-min intervals between the start of each inhalation. Means from nine patients in a double-blind crossover study (modified with permission from Bennis and Svedmyr, 1977).

was given by inhalation, the same degree of bronchial relaxation was obtained without any effect on heart rate, blood pressure, or tremor, indicating a local effect and increased therapeutic range.

Figure 7 shows the result of a controlled crossover study comparing inhaled and oral albuterol (Larsson and Svedmyr, 1977c). Oral doses giving the same bronchodilating effect as the three lowest inhaled doses have been intrapolated. Significantly less tremor was produced by inhaled doses than by calculated oral doses, giving the same effect on FEV_1. Inhalations from a metered aerosol are therefore superior to tablets in producing an increase in FEV_1 without side effects. However, there is a considerable variation of the bronchodilating effect of inhaled salbutamol. One patient had a maximal bronchodilating effect after one inhalation. Up to 93 inhalations during 2.5 hr did not produce more bronchodilation in this patient. Most of the patients, however, had an increasing bronchodilatory effect, with about 80% of the mean maximal effect attained after 6 inhalations. In the clinic, therefore, it is also important to individualize an inhaled drug and give as high a dose as is tolerated or as can be regarded to be safe from the point of view of drug tolerance. In the presently used doses, clinically important tolerance has not been shown.

The margin of safety of acutely inhaled β_2-stimulants given alone is very large and very high doses can be inhaled by continuous wet nebulization as shown in Figure 8. Here 5, 20, and 60 mg of terbutaline and 2.5, 10, and 30 mg of salbutamol were inhaled with IPPB with 60 min intervals between the doses in a crossover study (Bennis and Svedmyr, 1977). These results contrast strongly with the effect of a nonselective β-stimulant such as isoprenaline (Svedmyr et al., 1972) and, with other similar studies, favoring inhalation as the route of choice (Clark, 1982b). However, it is extremely important that the inhalation technique be correct (see Chaps. 15 and 17).

β_2-Stimulant aerosols are normally prescribed in a dose of one or two inhalations every 4-6 hr. In Sweden, up to six inhalations are given in severe cases. When patients are taking two inhalations, the package insert states that the inhalations should be taken with a 3 min interval. The rationale for the 3 min interval is to allow time for the first to open up the obstructed airways, so that the second can better penetrate into the lung periphery. However, the two doses are often taken in rapid succession. In two studies, 33% and 45% of the patients (Epstein et al., 1979; Arvaston et al., 1976) took their inhalations less than 30 sec apart. Only 5 of 33 patients waited for 3 min before the second inhalation.

Several reports compare the relative merits of doses given at one time and doses given as sequential inhalations. With metaproterenol, rimiterol, and isoprenaline, it was found that divided doses separated by 10, 15, and 20 min produced a greater overall effect than the same dose given at one time (Riley et al., 1979; Heimer et al., 1980; Shim and Williams, 1980). Terbutaline sulfate 500 μg delivered as either one, two, or four inhalations, however, did not show any difference in effect (Dulfano et al., 1977). The main difference between these investigations is the time factor. In the first three studies there is at least a 10 min interval between the doses, while in the last interval is only 30 sec. The explanation may be that the distribution of the inhaled drug is improved when the doses are separated by at least 10 min. For practical reasons this is a difficult mode of administration.

Even if this technique is used, the maximal effect will usually not be achieved after 5-10 inhalations taken in rapid succession from a pressurized aerosol (Svedmyr, 1981). Britton and Tattersfield (1984) have shown that sequential administration of inhaled β_2-stimulants given with a 20 min interval had a better bronchodilating effect than when the same dose was given in one administration. However, the same effect can more easily be achieved, with a low oral bronchodilating dose given 1-2 hr before the inhalations or given regularly by continuous oral treatment (K. Svedmyr, 1981).

The duration of bronchodilator activity is to some degree related to the inhaled dose (Ruffin et al., 1978). Higher doses of inhaled bronchodilators at

Table 2 Comparison of β_2-Stimulants and Theophylline in Maintenance Treatment of Asthma

	β_2-Stimulants	Theophylline
Antiasthmatic effect (systemic)	+	+
Antiasthmatic effect (inhalation)	++	-
Duration of action	Too short	Long (in slow-release form)
Therapeutic margin	Very wide	Narrow
Development of tolerance	Perhaps, but probably without clinical importance	No

+ Moderate effect; ++ pronounced effect; – no effect.

bedtime may be more effective than standard doses in the prophylaxis of nocturnal bronchoconstriction and related symptoms, but the duration of the presently available β_2-stimulants is too short to last the whole night, even when given in high doses.

IV. Combinations of β_2-Receptor Stimulants and Other Drugs

A. β_2-Stimulants and Theophylline

Table 2 compares β-receptor stimulants and theophylline in the maintenance treatment of asthma. When given by the systemic route they seem to have the same antiasthmatic effect. However, only β_2-stimulants, can be given by inhalation and their acute antiasthmatic effect is much better. Consequently, in many countries inhaled β_2-stimulants are considered the drugs of choice, both for treating acute asthma attacks and for maintenance therapy. However, the duration of action of inhaled β_2-stimulants, even the longest acting preparations, is too short. Optimal 24-hr stabilization of the airways is unlikely and they will probably suffice only in mild asthma. Therefore, in more severe cases, they must be combined with oral long-acting bronchodilators or steroids.

Oral β_2-stimulants have a wide margin of safety but, when combined with an individualized inhaled dose, often induce troublesome tremor. Therefore, in most cases slow-release theophylline is preferred and a moderate and safe theophylline dose can be used in preference to "high dose theophylline." Fear of developing tolerance to β_2-stimulants is exaggerated in some countries, as is the fear of theophylline toxicity in others. Both of these risks are dose-dependent, and therefore it is advantageous to combine oral β_2-stimulants and theophylline in moderate doses for the maintenance treatment of asthma. Their antiasthmatic effects are additive, while their side effects differ, as shown by several acute and long-term studies (Wolfe et al., 1978; K. Svedmyr, 1981; Marlin et al., 1978; von Dorow, 1979; Galant et al., 1979; Leopold and Handslip, 1979; Roddick et al., 1979; Blumenthal, 1980; Clark and Boyd, 1980; Groggins et al., 1980; Lönnerholm et al., 1981). The disadvantage of this combined therapy is that the patient must take two drugs instead of one.

One would expect theophylline given together with a β-agonist to have at least an additive effect, and, at best, true potentiation. Even an additive bronchodilating effect combined with less side effects would be a clinical advantage. Unfortunately, the earlier studies with β-agonists and theophylline were carried out with ephedrine, a somewhat less potent β-agonist than those currently used. Ephedrine also gives more side effects, especially central nervous system (CNS) stimulation, which is also a side effect of theophylline. Consequently, a combination of these two drugs is not ideal.

It has sometimes been claimed that different drugs act synergistically with β-receptor agonists. However, the evaluation of interactions is very difficult and conclusions about synergism are often misleading. Studies have been performed in which it is impossible to judge whether there is a synergistic action (Berenbaum, 1981).

The therapeutic value of the newer β_2-agonist and theophylline in combination has still not been thoroughly evaluated in long-term studies. In 1977, it was shown by K. Svedmyr that systemically administered bronchodilators (both theophylline and terbutaline) increase the efficacy of inhaled terbutaline in patients with endogenous (intrinsic) asthma (K. Svedmyr, 1981). As shown in Figure 9, oral theophylline and terbutaline with the same bronchodilating effect increased the efficacy of inhaled terbutaline to the same degree. This indicates that systemic bronchodilation enhances the effect of inhaled bronchodilation, probably by producing a better distribution of the inhaled drug in these asthmatics who often have expectoration problems. However, the study did not show any pharmacologic potentiation between theophylline and terbutaline, indicating that the combination of theophylline and terbutaline has only an additive effect. This finding is consistent with the view that phosphodiesterase inhibition does not explain the bronchodilating effects of xanthines.

In severe asthma, bronchoconstriction is only partly responsible for the airway obstruction. There is also mucosal thickening, edema in the bronchial wall, and mucus plugging. The bronchoconstriction may respond to inhaled bronchodilators but the airway obstruction may prevent the access of inhaled

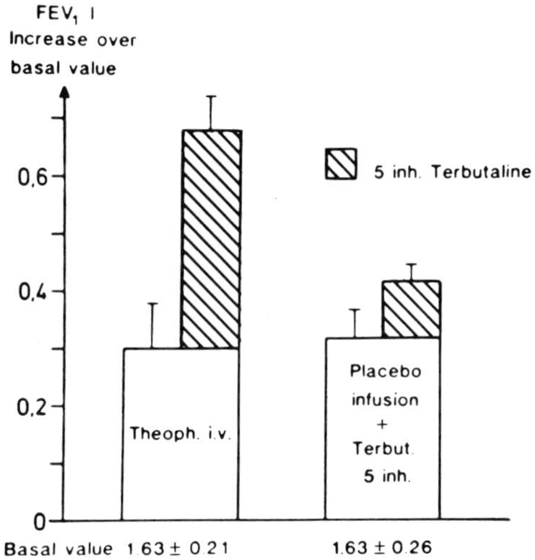

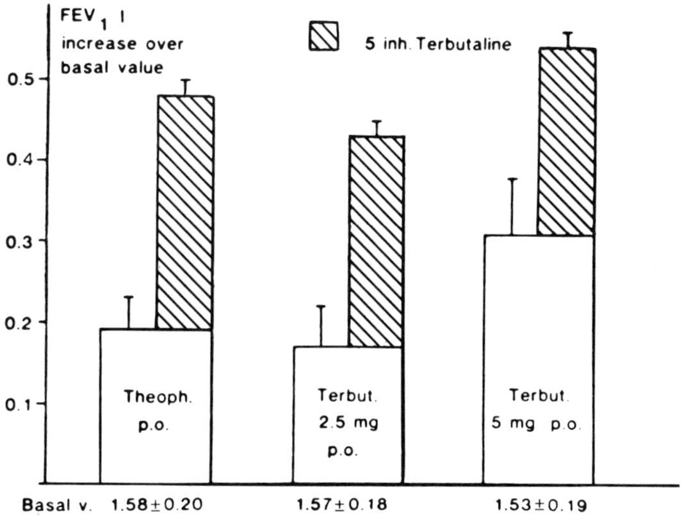

Figure 9 Effect on FEV_1 of five metered aerosol doses of terbutaline after pretreatment with equipotent doses of aminophylline intravenously or terbutaline by inhalation (upper panel) and after oral theophylline (280 mg anhydrous) or oral terbutaline (2.5 mg and 5 mg) (lower panel). Increase in FEV_1 over basal values in six and eight patients, respectively (reprinted with permission from K. Svedmyr, 1981).

drugs to all parts of the lung. If these patients are only given inhaled β_2-stimulants from a metered dose aerosol as maintenance treatment, the FEV_1 increases to a lesser degree than when the combination of inhaled and oral bronchodilators is used. The enhancement produced by the combined treatment may be important only as the patient deteriorates and may be difficult to demonstrate in those patients with mild to moderate asthma without expectoration problems or airway closure.

In a long-term study, an increased peak expiratory flow rate was noted when theophylline was added to terbutaline aerosol (Smith et al., 1980). This effect was particularly pronounced in the early morning, when the asthma symptoms normally are also more pronounced.

B. β_2-Stimulants and Ipratropium Bromide

The addition of ipratropium bromide to conventional doses of a β_2-agonist usually produces slightly greater bronchodilation than either drug alone. Increasing the dosage of β_2-agonists, however, gives better bronchodilation than this combination and may also block the parasympathetic pathway via ganglionic blockade.

C. β_2-Stimulants and Steroids

Corticosteroids have been shown to have a permissive effect on β-agonist stimulation in vitro (Svemyr and Simonsson, 1981). It has been shown also that there is an up-regulation of β-receptors with corticosteroid treatment (Hui et al., 1982), Corticosteroids have been shown to restore the airway responsiveness to β_2-agonists in resistant asthmatic patients (Ellul-Micaleff and Fenech, 1975). This could be due either to an anti-inflammatory effect on pronounced mucosal edema or to a direct effect on β-receptor function. However, studies in patients with stable asthma have only shown an additive effect between corticosteroids and β_2-agonists and not the synergistic effect one would expect, if corticosteroids indeed increased receptor responsiveness (Harrison and MacKay, 1980; Dahl and Johansson, 1982). Thus, the clinical relevance of the up-regulation of β-receptor numbers is not clear.

D. β_2-Stimulants and Calcium Channel Blockers

Calcium channel blockers have very small effects on resting bronchial tone in vivo, in spite of a good bronchorelaxing effect in vitro (Löfdahl and Barnes, 1986). However, in vitro studies have shown that there is a synergistic effect with β-agonists on inhibition of phasic contraction by field stimulation in ferret tracheal rings (Löfdahl et al., 1984). A clinical study also showed a synergistic action with terbutaline on bronchodilation in asthmatic patients (K. Svedmyr et al., 1984). The mechanism for this synergistic action could be one of many. Decreased release of bronchoconstricting mediators has been discussed as an explanation for the synergism. Other possibilities include influences on the neural regulation of airway tone or an intracellular interaction in the airway smooth muscle, as both intracellular free calcium and cAMP act on active myosin light chain kinase to control activation (see Fig. 1).

V. Development of Tolerance to β_2-Adrenoceptor Stimulants

Reports in the late 1960s from Great Britain (Speizer et al., 1968a,b) strongly indicated a connection between the sale of β-adrenergic stimulants in spray form and an increased mortality from asthma. This soon focused attention on the development of tolerance to these drugs (Conolly et al., 1971).

Continued exposure to a hormonal agonist often leads to a blunted response to that agonist. This process has been termed desensitization, tolerance, tachyphylaxis, or refractoriness, and it is a well-known pharmacologic phenomenon. It normally functions as a physiological feedback mechanism to modulate the effect of the continuous presence of high concentrations of the hormone. It is probable that the mechanism exists to protect the cell against excessive levels of a stimulating ligand (see Chaps. 3, 7).

It is quite clear that the administration of β_2-adrenoceptor stimulants can result in tolerance in animal studies (in vitro and in vivo) and in nonbronchial β_2-adrenoceptor responses in humans (tremor, heart rate, lymphocyte and leukocyte cAMP levels and also down-regulation of the β-receptor number; for further details see Chaps. 3, 7). Development of tachyphylaxis to the bronchodilating effect of β_2-agonists in healthy individuals has also been shown, but there was no tachyphylaxis in asthmatic patients under the same test conditions (Holgate et al., 1977; Harvey et al., 1981; van den Berg et al., 1982; Tashkin et al., 1982). About 40 controlled studies on β-agonists given both by the oral and the inhaled route in normal dosages suggest that asthmatics do not develop clinically important tachyphylaxis to conventional dosages of β_2-agonists (Jenne 1982; Tattersfield, 1982; Svedmyr, 1984). Fear of developing tolerance to the antiasthmatic effect of β_2-adrenoceptor stimulants has led to the increased use of theophylline in many countries.

Any study on the development of tolerance to the bronchodilating effect of β-agonists during treatment with these drugs encounters several difficulties. Asthmatics, even rather large groups of asthmatics, show spontaneous fluctuations in basal values for ventilation probably caused by factors such as climatic variations, air pollution, and respiratory tract infections. Such variations can mask the development of tolerance or falsely indicate tolerance. Patients in a tolerance study, therefore, must be evaluated for a long time. A period of one year would be necessary, unless a parallel control group with no treatment is used (Svedmyr, 1984).

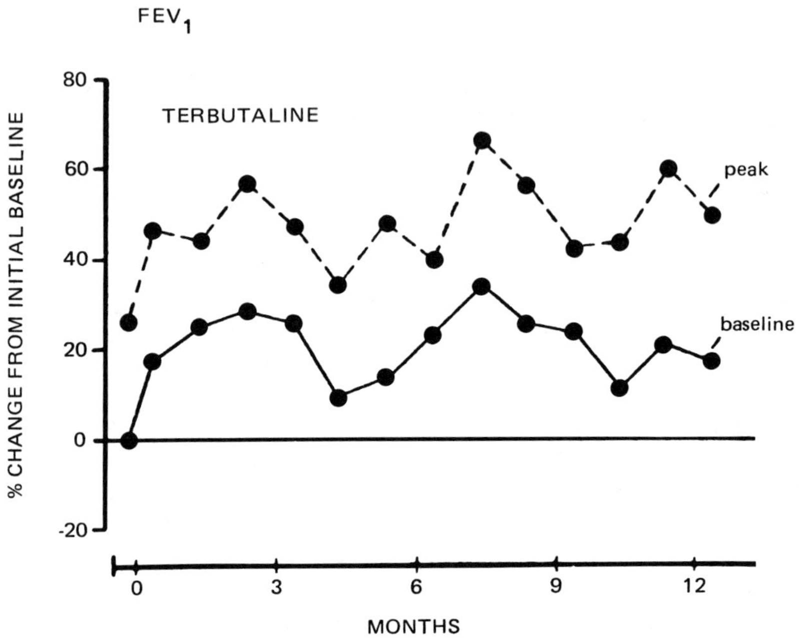

Figure 10 Effects of oral terbutaline on baseline and peak FEV_1 values during a 12-month tolerance study (reprinted with permission from Wilson, 1976).

According to a review by Nelson (1982), patients entering a tolerance study must not have been treated with β_2-agonists for at least 2 weeks in order to exclude adrenergic subsensitivity before starting the study. He states that failure to exclude all adrenergic medication, oral and inhaled, for at least 2 weeks prior to initiating drug tolerance studies has resulted in failure to detect the development of slight subsensitivity during many drug trials. A parallel control group or an observation period of at least 1 year is probably much more important.

The study by Wilson and co-workers (1976) (Fig. 10) has been heavily criticized because it lacks a washout period. This might have masked a slight subsensitivity at the start, mostly of academic interest, since the bronchodilating effect was maintained throughout the year without a decrease in basal FEV_1. On the contrary, however, there was a tendency towards an increase in basal FEV_1. But if, for instance, a tolerance study was started at month 7 and the patients were evaluated for 2 months (9 in the figure), the results would falsely indicate the development of tolerance.

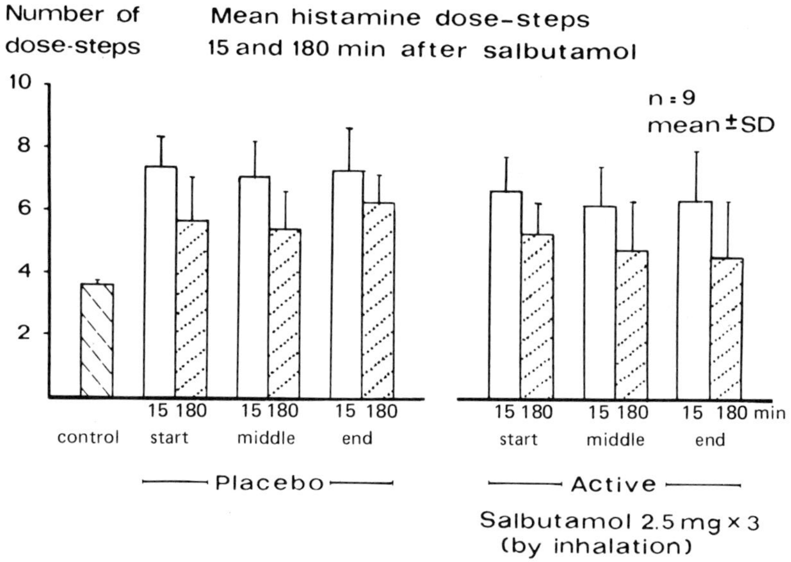

Figure 11 Effects of regular treatment with continuous nebulized salbutamol in high doses at home (2.5 mg t.i.d.) on the acute protective effect of salbutamol on histamine provocation tests. The control value is the number of histamine-steps inducing a decrease in FEV_1 of 25% before the start of the study. It is followed by two provocations before the home placebo or salbutamol treatment period, 15 min and 3 hr after an individualized acute preventive salbutamol treatment. The next two columns show corresponding recordings made after 1.5 week of home treatment and the following two columns after 3 weeks of treatment. There are no statistically significant differences between placebo treatment and active treatment in this randomized, double-blind, crossover study in 9 hyperactive asthmatics without previous β_2-stimulant therapy.

Most studies postulating tolerance development are short-term studies without a control group. These results could therefore also be due to a temporary, spontaneously occurring change in the status of the patients. Therefore, it is difficult to draw conclusions from such studies.

The most sensitive measure of β_2-agonists inducing tolerance seems to be a decreasing duration of action (Jenne, 1981). The development of tolerance is also dose-dependent and, if the doses administered are high enough, a clinically important tolerance at the β_2-receptor level in the lung wall might occur.

In a recent study, the development of tolerance was investigated during regular treatment at home with continuous nebulized albuterol in high doses (2.5 mg t.i.d.) in a double-blind, crossover study (Lowhagen et al., 1985). The patients included 9 hyperreactive asthmatics who were asymptomatic except for rare attacks and were only occasionally on therapy. These patients reacted to treatment much like healthy people, in whom it is easy to demonstrate development of tolerance in the bronchi after inhalation of β_2-agonists (Holgate et al., 1977). Figure 11 shows the results of the study and the number of histamine dose-steps that caused a 25% reduction of base-line FEV_1 (PC 25). The conclusion we draw from this study is that development of tolerance in the bronchial β_2-adrenoceptors is not a general phenomenon of clinical importance in this group of patients during treatment with high dosages of inhaled salbutamol.

In a study of emergency treatment of asthma, 2.5 mg isoprenaline inhaled three times every 20 min gave as great an antiasthmatic effect when combined with a placebo infusion as when administered with an acute loading dose of aminophylline, producing a mean theophylline concentration of 21 mg/liter (Fanta et al., 1982). There was no significant difference in the mean bronchodilating effect, in the number of patients who could leave the emergency ward after 1 hr, or in the number of patients who required admission after 4 hr. Thus the β_2-receptors in the lung were still mediating a very good acute antiasthmatic effect. However, all the patients were on maintenance treatment with theophylline and had a mean theophylline blood concentration of 7 mg/liter at admission. We have previously shown in several acute studies (K. Svedmyr, 1981) that this theophylline concentration increases the effect of inhaled β_2-agonists. The study by Fanta et al. (1982) therefore does not exclude an important role for intravenous theophylline in the treatment of acute severe asthma. It should be noted, however, that modern selective β_2-stimulants can be given in considerably more potent antiasthmatic dosages than the isoprenaline dosage given in that study. It is becoming more and more usual to start treatment of acute severe asthma with a nebulized β_2-stimulant in high dosages at admission and to give theophylline intravenously after 1 hr only if the patient has not improved.

In asthmatics there is an obvious difference between β_2-receptors in the lung and other β_2-receptors when it comes to development of tolerance. A clear development of tolerance in the β_2-receptors in the skeletal muscle but not in the bronchial muscle of asthmatics was shown during a 1-year tolerance study (Larsson et al., 1977). This shows that tolerance development must be studied in the pertinent organ and that conclusions cannot be drawn from other organs or from healthy individuals.

One explanation for this difference in the development of tolerance may be a large number of "spare receptors," or a more efficient signal transmission, in the lungs of asthmatics. In such cases, stimulation of a small part of the total β_2-receptor population would give a maximal bronchodilating effect. Another possibility is that the β_2-receptors in the lung are not down-regulated in the same way in asthmatics as in healthy individuals.

There is no convincing evidence today that tolerance of clinical importance occurs in asthmatics receiving normal dosages of β_2-receptor stimulants. On the contrary, these agents are very potent when inhaled and it is easy for the patient to rely on this normally very effective treatment. However, in a severe prolonged asthma attack, other factors than muscular spasm may dominate, such as mucosal edema and mucus plugging. Therefore, the patient must be instructed to contact the doctor or the hospital immediately if the aerosol must be taken more often than every third hour. Other treatments are needed then, such as corticosteroids, antibiotics.

VI. Concluding Remarks

Our new antiasthmatic drugs have undoubtedly increased the quality of life for asthmatics. Unfortunately, there are no good long-term studies to elucidate which of these drugs is the most beneficial for long-term treatment. Studies of that kind could perhaps explain why the number of acute asthma deaths has not decreased during the last 15 years. There is a great need for well-performed, prospective, long-term studies in asthmatics. Both the effect on lung function and the overall asthma symptoms need to be measured in large groups of patients. Such studies are very difficult to perform and very expensive. Today no such studies are available for the β_2-agonists, theophylline, or any of the other antiasthmatic drugs.

References

Ahlquist, R. P. (1948). A study of the adrenotropic receptors. *Am. J. Physiol. 153*: 586-600.

Al-Bazzaz, F. J., and Cheng, E. (1979). Effect of catecholamines on ion transport in dog tracheal epithelium. *J. Appl. Physiol. 47*: 397.

Amory, D. W., Burnham, S. C., and Cheney, F. W. J. (1974). Comparison of the cardio-pulmonary effects of subcutaneously administered epinephrine and terbutaline in patients with reversible airway obstruction. *Chest 67*: 279.

Anderson, P., Olsson, O. A. T., and Waldeck, B. (1982). Some problems encountered in the evaluation of new bronchodilating β-adrenoceptor agonists. *Acta Pharmacol. Toxicol. 51*: 358-364.

Ariens, E. J., and Simonis, A. M. (1976). Receptors and receptor mechanisms. In *Beta-Adrenoceptor Blocking Agents. The Pharmacological Basis of Clinical Use.* Edited by P. R. Saxena and R. P. Forsyth. Amsterdam, North Holland Publishing Co., pp. 3-27.

Arnold, J. M. O., and McDevitt, D. G. (1983a). An assessment of physiological finger tremor as an indicator of β-adrenoceptor function. *Br. J. Clin. Pharmacol. 16*: 167-174.

Arnold, J. M. O., and McDevitt, D. G. (1983b). Heart rate and blood pressure responses to intravenous boluses of isoprenaline in the presence of propranolol, practolol and atropine. *Br. J. Clin. Pharmacol. 16*: 175-184.

Aubier, M., DeTroier, A., and Sampson, M. (1981). Aminophylline improves diaphragmatic contractility. *N. Engl. J. Med. 305*: 249.

Balazs, T. (1972). Cardiotoxicity of isoproterenol in experimental animals: Influence of stress, obesity, and repeated dosage. In *Recent Advances in Studies of Cardiac Structure and Metabolism.* Edited by E. Bajuzs and G. Rona. Baltimore, University Park Press, pp. 770-778.

Balazs, T., and Herman, H. E. (1976). Toxic cardiomyopathies. *Ann. Clin. Lab. Sci. 6*: 467-474.

Barger, G., and Dale, H. H. (1910). Chemical structure and sympathomimetic action of amines. *J. Physiol. Lond. 41*: 19-59.

Bennis, J., and Svedmyr, N. (1977). A controlled comparison of salbutamol and terbutaline inhaled by IPPV in asthmatic patients: A dose-response study. *Scand. J. Respir. Dis.* suppl. *10*: 113-117.

Berenbaum, M. (1981). Criteria for analysing interactions between biologically active agents. *Adv. Cancer Res. 35*: 269-335.

van den Berg, M. D., Leferink, J. G., Fokkens, J. K., Kreuknict, J., Maes, R. A. A., and Bruynzeel, P. L. B. (1982). Clinical implications of drug-induced desensitization of the β-receptor after continuous oral use of terbutaline. *J. Allergy Clin. Immunol. 69*: 410-417.

Birnbaumer, L., Codina, J., Mattera, R., Rojas, R. J., Hildebrandt, J. D., Rosenthal, W., and Sunyer, T. (1984). Structural and regulatory properties of nucleotide binding regulatory N proteins of adenylate cyclase and their effects on hormone receptors. In *IUPHAR 9th International Congress of Pharmacology, London 1984.* Edited by W. Paton, J. Mitchell, and P. Turner. London, Macmillan Press, pp. 279-286.

Blumenthal, I. (1980). A comparative trial of slow-release aminophylline, salbutamol and a half dose combination in the prevention of childhood asthma. *J. Inte. Med. Res. 8*: 400-403.

Borson, D. B., Chinn, R. A., Davies, B., and Nadel, J. A. (1980). Adrenergic and cholinergic nerves mediate fluid secretion from tracheal glands of ferrets. *J. Appl. Physiol. 49*: 1027-1031.

Borum, P., and Mygind, N. (1980). Inhibition of the immediate allergic reaction of the nose by β_2-adrenostimulant fenoterol. *J. Allergy Clin. Immunol. 66*: 25.

Bowman, W. C. (1981). Effects of adrenergic activators and inhibitors on the skeletal muscle. In *Handbook of Experimental Pharmacology,* vol. 54/II. Edited by L. Szekeres. Berlin, Springer Verlag, pp. 47-128.

Brittain, R. T., Dean, C. M., and Jack, D. (1981). Sympathomimetic bronchodilating drugs. In *Respiratory Pharmacology.* Edited by J. Widdicombe. Oxford, Pergamon Press, pp. 613-652.

Britton, J., and Tattersfield, N. A. (1984). Comparison of cumulative and non-cumulative techniques to measure dose-response curves for β-agonists in patients with asthma. *Thorax 39*: 597-599.

Brown, J. E., McLeod, A. A., and Shand, S. G. (1983). Evidence for cardiac β_2-adrenoceptors in man. *Clin. Pharmacol. Ther. 33*: 424-428.

Carlsson, E., Ablad, B., Brändström, A., and Carlsson, B. (1972). Differentiated blockade of the chronotropic effects of various adrenergic stimuli in the cat heart. *Life Sci. 11*: 953-958.

Carlsson, E., Dahlöf, C. E., Hedberg, A., Persson, H., and Tangstrand, B. (1977). Differentiation of cardiac chronotropic and inotropic effects of β-adrenoceptor agonists. *Naunyn Schmiedebergs Arch. Pharmacol. 300*: 101-105.

Chen, K. K., and Schmidt, C. F. (1930). Ephedrine and related substances. *Medicine 9*: 1-117.

Clark, C. J., and Boyd, G. (1980). Combination of aminophylline (Phyllocontin continuous tablets) and salbutamol in the management of chronic obstructive airways disease. *Br. J. Clin. Pharmacol. 9*: 359-364.

Clark, T. J. H. (1982a). The inhaled route as the route of choice in airway disease therapy. In *New Concepts in the Topical Treatment of Asthma and Related Disorders.* Greenwich, Conn., Cliggott Publ. Co., p. 15.

Clark, T. J. H. (1982b). Choice of drug treatment in asthma. *Pharmacol. Ther. 17*: 221-228.

Conolly, M. E., Davies, D. S., Dollery, C. T., and George, C. F. (1971). Resistance to β-adrenoceptor stimulants (a possible explanation for the rise in asthma deaths). *Br. J. Pharmacol. 43*: 389-402.

Dahl, R., and Johansson, S. A. (1982). Effect on lung function of budesonide by inhalation, terbutaline s.c. and placebo given simultaneously or as single treatment. *Eur. J. Respir. Dis.* suppl. *122*: 132.

Dorow, P. von (1979). Langzeituntersuchung mit einem neuen β_2-Sympathikomimetikum (Hexoprenalin) und einer Kombination (orales Theophyllin-Ethylendiaminpräparat mit Retardwirkung + Hexprenalin). *Arzneim. Forsch./Drug Res. 29*: 145-147.

Dulfano, M. J., Glass, P., and McPhillips, J. J. A. (1977). A comparison of the bronchodilator effects of the same amounts of terbutaline aerosol given as a single or in divided doses. *Ann. Allergy 39*: 266-271.

Ellul-Micaleff, R., and Fenech, F. F. (1975). Effect on intravenous prednisolone in asthmatics with diminished adrenergic responsiveness. *Lancet 2*: 1269-1271.

Engel, G. (1981). Subclasses of β-adrenoceptors—a quantitative estimation of β_1- and β_2-adrenoceptors in guinea pig and human lung. *Postgrad. Med. J. 57* (suppl. 1): 77-83.

Epstein, S. W., Manning, C. P. R., Ashley, M. J., and Corey, P. N. (1979). Survey of the clinical use of pressurized aerosol inhalers. *Can. Med. Assoc. J. 20*: 813-816.

Fanta, C. H., Rossing, T. H., and McFadden, E. R. Jr. (1982). Emergency room treatment of asthma. *Am. J. Med. 72*: 416.

Formgren, H. (1975). The therapeutic value of oral long-term treatment with terbutaline (Bricanyl®) in asthma. *Scand. J. Respir. Dis. 56*: 321-328.

Fraizer, P. M., Speizer, F. E., Waters, S. D. M., Doll, R., and Mann, N. M. (1971). The circumstances preceding death from asthma in young people in 1968-1969. *Br. J. Dis. Chest 65*: 71-84.

Galant, S. P., Groncy, C. E., Duriseti, S., and Strick, L. (1979). The effect of metaproterenol in chronic asthmatic children receiving therapeutic doses of theophylline. *J. Allergy Clin. Immunol. 61*: 2:73-79.

Groggins, R. C., Lenney, W., Milner, A. D., and Stokes, G. M. (1980). Efficacy of oral administered salbutamol and theophylline in preschool children with asthma. *Arch. Dis. Child. 55*: 204-206.

Harrison, R. N., and MacKay, A. D. (1980). Hydrocortisone and bronchial β-adrenergic responsiveness. *Thorax 35*: 238.

Harvey, J. E., Baldwin, C. J., Wood, P. J., Alberti, K. G., and Tattersfield, A. E. (1981). Airway and metabolic responsiveness to intravenous salbutamol in asthma: Effect of regular inhaled salbutamol. *Clin. Sci. 60*: 579-585.

Hedberg, A., Minneman, K. D., and Molinoff, P. B. (1980). Differential distribution of beta-1 and beta-2 adrenergic receptors in cat and guinea pig heart. *J. Pharmacol. Exp. Ther. 213*: 503-508.

Hegardt, B. (1981). Evaluation of the anti-allergic property of the β-adrenoceptor agonist KWD 2131 in asthmatics. Thesis. *Eur. J. Respir. Dis. 62* (suppl. 115): 1-54.

Heimer, D., Shim, C., and Williams, M. H. Jr. (1980). The effect of sequential inhalations of metaproterenol aerosol in asthma. *J. Allergy Clin. Immunol. 66*: 75.

Holgate, S. T., Baldwin, C. J., and Tattersfield, A. E. (1977). β-Adrenergic agonist resistance in normal human airways. *Lancet 2*: 375.

Holgate, S. T., and Church, M. K. (1984). Mediator release from human lung mast cells. *Respiration 46* (suppl. 1): 22.

Holmberg, E., Jeppsson, A. B., and Waldeck, B. (1981). Selective development of tolerance to β-adrenoceptor agonists in skeletal muscle as compared with airway smooth muscle from the guinea-pig. *Clin. Exp. Pharmacol. Physiol. 8*: 49-56.

Howell, S., and Roussos, C. (1984). Isoproterenol and aminophylline improve contractility of fatigued canine diaphragmae. *Am. Rev. Respir. Dis. 129*: 118.

Hui, K. K. P., Conolly, M. E., and Tashkin, D. P. (1982). Methylprednisolone reverses the β-agonist-induced decrease in β-receptor number in human lymphocytes. *Clin. Pharmacol. Ther. 32*: 566.

Jenne, J. W. (1981). Reviews. A critic of dosing strategies for β_2-adrenergic agents and theophylline. *Lung 159*: 295-314.

Jenne, J. W., Ridley, D. J., Marcucci, R. A., Druz, W. S., and Rook, J. C. (1982). Objective and subjective tremor responses to oral β_2-agents on first exposure. A comparison of metaproterenol and terbutaline. *Am. Rev. Respir. Dis. 126*: 4:607-610.

Jenne, J. W. (1982). Whither beta-adrenergic tachyphylaxis? *J. Allergy Clin. Immunol. 70*: 413-416.

Johansson, U., and Waldeck, B. (1981). β_1-Adrenoceptors mediating relaxation of the guinea-pig trachea: experiments with prenalterol, a β_1-selective adrenoceptor agonist. *J. Pharm. Pharmacol. 33*: 353-356.

Jones, R. M., Stockley, R. A., and Bishop, J. M. (1982). Early effects of intravenous terbutaline and cardiac pulmonary function in chronic obstructive bronchitis and pulmonary hypertension. *Thorax 37*: 746-750.

Karlsson, J. A., and Persson, C. G. A. (1981). Influence of tracheal contraction on relaxant effects in vitro of theophylline and isoprenaline. *Br. J. Pharmacol. 74*: 73-79.

Karlsson, J. A., and Persson, C. G. A. (1984). Asthma mediators functional antagonized by theophylline, enprofylline and terbutaline. Thesis, University of Lund, p. 83.

Konzett, H. (1940). Neue broncholytisch hochwirksame Körper der Adrenalinreibe. *Arch. Exp. Pathol. Pharmakol. 197*: 27-40.

Lands, A. M., Arnold, A., McAuliff, J. P., Luduena, F. P., and Brown, T. G. (1967). Differentiation of receptor systems activated by sympathomimetic amines. *Nature 214*: 597-598.

Larsson, S. (1977). Long-term treatment with β_2-adrenostimulants in asthma. Side effects, selectivity, tolerance and routes of administration. *Acta Med. Scand.* suppl. *608*.

Larsson, S., and Svedmyr, N. (1977a). Tremor caused by sympathomimetics is mediated by β_2-adrenoceptors. *Scand. J. Respir. Dis. 58*: 5-10.

Larsson, S., and Svedmyr, N. (1977b). Cumulative dose-response curves for comparisons of oral bronchodilating drugs. A study of salbutamol and fenoterol. *Ann. Allergy 39*: 5:362-366.

Larsson, S., and Svedmyr, N. (1977c). Bronchodilating effect and side effects of β_2-adrenoceptor stimulants by different modes of administration (tablets, metered aerosol and combinations thereof). A study with salbutamol and asthmatics. *Am. Rev. Respir. Dis. 116*: 861-869.

Larsson, S., Svedmyr, N., and Thiringer, G. (1977). Lack of bronchial β-adrenoceptor resistance in asthmatics during long term treatment with terbutaline. *J. Allergy Clin. Immunol. 59*: 93-100.

Laursen, L. C., Taudorf, E., Gnospelius, Y., Gymose, E., and Weeke, B. (1985).

Long-term oral therapy of asthma with terbutaline and theophylline, alone and combined. *Eur. J. Respir. Dis. 66*: 82-90.

Leopold, D., and Handslip, P. (1979). Additive interaction of aminophylline and salbutamol in asthma: An in vivo study using dose-response curves. *J. Int. Med. Res. 7* (suppl. 1): 52.

Löfdahl, C. G., and Barnes, P. J. (1986). Calcium, calcium channel blockade, and airways function. *Acta Pharmacol. Toxicol. 58* (Suppl 2): 98-111.

Löfdahl, C. G., Bengtsson, B., Svedmyr, K., and Svedmyr, N. (1982). Two new β_2-adrenoceptor agonists, D 2343 and QH 25, studied in asthmatic patients. *Allergy 37*: 351-357.

Löfdahl, C. G., Marlin, G. E., and Svedmyr, N. (1983). Pafenolol, a highly selective β_1-adrenoceptor antagonist studied in asthmatic patients. Interaction with terbutaline. *Clin. Pharmacol. Ther. 33*: 1-9.

Löfdahl, C. G., Svedmyr, K., Svedmyr, N., Andersson, P., Bengtsson, B., Olsson, O. A. T., and Waldeck, B. (1984). Comparison of β_2-adrenoceptor stimulation in bronchial and skeletal muscle in experimental and clinical studies. *Eur. J. Respir. Dis.* (suppl. 135): 124-127.

Löfdahl, C. G., and Svedmyr, N. (1982). Effects of prenalterol in asthmatic patients. *Eur. J. Clin. Pharmacol. 22*: 535-539.

Löwhagen, O., Larsson, S., Lindholm, N., and Svedmyr, N. (1985). Does continuous domiciliary treatment with high doses of nebulized β_2-stimulants give tolerance development. *Am. Rev. Respir. Dis.*, in press.

Lulich, K. M., Mitchell, H. W., and Sparrow, M. P. (1976). The cat lung strip as an in vitro preparation of peripheral airways: A comparison of β-adrenoceptor agonists, autacoids and anaphylactic challenge of the lung strip and trachea. *Br. J. Pharmacol. 58*: 71-79.

MacKnee, W. J., Wathen, C. G., Hannan, W. J., Flenley, D. C., and Muir, A. L. (1983). Effects of pirbuterol and sodium nitroprusside on pulmonary hemodynamics in hypoxic cor pulmonale. *Br. Med. J. 287*: 1169.

Marlin, G. E., Hartnett, B. J. S., Berend, W., and Hacket, N. B. (1978). Assessment of combinred oral theophylline and inhaled β-adrenoceptor agonist bronchodilator therapy. *Br. J. Clin. Pharmacol. 5*: 45-50.

Martin, G. L., Atkins, P. C., Dynsky, E. H., and Zweiman, B. (1980). Effects of theophylline, terbutaline and prednisolone on antigen-induced bronchospasm and mediator release. *J. Allergy Clin. Immunol. 66*: 204.

Matthys, H., and Köhler, D. (1980). Effect of theophylline on mucociliary clearance in man. *Eur. J. Respir. Dis. 61* (suppl. 109): 98.

Matthys, H., Köhler, D., and Daikeler, G. (1984). Additive actions of bronchodilators on mucous transport. *Respiration 46* (suppl. 1): 34.

Mossberg, B., Strandberg, K., Philipson, K., and Camner, P. (1976). Tracheobronchial clearance in bronchial asthma response to β-adrenoceptor stimulation. *Scand. J. Respir. Dis. 57*: 119.

Nelson, H. S. (1982). β-Adrenergic agonists. *Chest* suppl.: 33-38.

O'Donnell, S. R., and Wanstall, J. C. (1978). Evidence that the efficacy (intrinsic activity) of fenoterol is higher than that of salbutamol on β-adrenoceptors in guinea pig trachea. *Eur. J. Pharmacol. 37*: 333-340.

Parker, J. O., Ashekian, P. B., Di Georgi, S., and West, R. O. (1967). Hemodynamic effects of aminophylline in chronic obstructive pulmonary disease. *Circulation 35*: 365.

Persson, C. G. A., and Svensjö, E. (1983). Airway hyperreactivity and microvascular permeability to large molecules. *Eur. J. Respir. Dis. 64*: (suppl. 131): 183.

Perucca, E., Pickles, H., and Richens, A. (1981). Effect of atenolol, metoprolol and propranolol on isoproterenol induced tremor and tachycardia in normal subjects. *Clin. Pharmacol. Ther. 29*: 425-433.

Riley, D. J., Liu, R., and Edelman, N. H. (1979). Enhanced responses to aerosolized bronchodilator therapy in asthma using respiratory manoeuvres. *Chest 76*: 501-507.

Robinson, B. F., Epstein, S. E., Beiser, G. D., and Braunwald, E. (1966). Control of heart rate by the autonomic nervous system. *Circ. Res. 19*: 400-411.

Roddick, L. G., South, R. T., and Mellis, C. M. (1979). Value of combining an oral sympathomimetic agent with oral theophylline in asthmatic children. *Med. J. Ausr. 2*: 118:153-154.

Rona, G., Chappel, C. I., Balazs, T., and Gaudri, R. (1959). An infarct-like myocardial lesion and other toxic manifestations produced by isoproterenol in the rat. *Arch. Pathol. 67*: 443-455.

Ruffin, R. E., Obminski, G., and Newhouse, M. G. (1978). Aerosol salbutamol administration by IPPB: Lowest effective dose. *Thorax 33*: 689-693.

Shim, C., and Williams, M. H. Jr. (1980). Bronchial response to oral versus aerosol metaproterenol in asthma. *Ann. Intern. Med. 93*: 428-431.

Skoogh, B. E., Löfdahl, C. G., and Svedmyr, N. (1985). β-Adrenoceptors in ferret tracheal smooth muscle subtyped as β_1. *Am. Rev. Respir. Dis. 131*: A284.

Skoogh, B. E., and Svedmyr, N. (1984). β_2-Adrenoceptor stimulation inhibits ganglionic transmission in ferret trachea. *Am. Rev. Respir. Dis. 129*, suppl. A232.

Smith, J. A., Weber, R. W., and Nelson, H. S. (1980). Theophylline and aerosolized terbutaline in the treatment of bronchial asthma. Double-blind comparison of optimal doses. *Chest 78*: 816.

Speizer, F. E., Doll, R., and Heaf, P. (1968a). Observations on recent increase in mortality from asthma. *Br. Med. J. I*: 335-339.

Speizer, F. E., Doll, R., Heaf, P., and Strang, L. B. (1968b). Investigation in the use of drugs preceding death from asthma. *Br. Med. J. I*: 339-343.

Sutton, P. P., Pavia, D., Bateman, J. R. M., and Clarke, S. W. (1981). The effect of oral aminophylline on lung mucociliary clearance in man. *Chest 80*: 889.

Svedmyr, K. (1981). β_2-Adrenoceptor stimulants and theophylline in asthma therapy. Thesis. *Eur. J. Respir. Dis. 62* (suppl. 116): 1-48.

Svedmyr, K., Löfdahl, C. G., and Svedmyr, N. (1984). Nifedipine–a calcium channel blocker–in asthmatic patients. *Allergy 39*: 17-22.

Svedmyr, N. (1984). Is beta-adrenoceptor sensitivity a limiting factor in asthma therapy? In *Perspectives in Asthma. II. Beta-Adrenoceptors in Asthma.* Edited by J. Morley. London, Academic Press, pp. 181-199.

Svedmyr, N. (1985). Fenoterol: A β_2-adrenerigc agonist for use in asthma. Pharmacology, pharmacokinetics, clinical efficacy and adverse effects. *Pharmacotherapy 5*: 109-125.

Svedmyr, N., Malmberg, R., and Thiringer, G. (1972). The effect of a new adrenergic β_2-receptor-stimulating agent (rimiterol, R 798) in patients with chronic obstructive lung disease. *Scand. J. Respir. Dis. 53*: 302-313.

Svedmyr, N., and Simonsson, B. G. (1981). Drugs in the treatment of asthma. In *Respiratory Pharmacology*. Edited by J. Widdicombe. Oxford, Pergamon Press, p. 657.

Svedmyr, N., and Thiringer, G. (1971). The effects of salbutamol and isoprenaline on β-receptors in patients with C.O.P.D. *Postgrad. Med. J. 47* (suppl.): 44-46.

Svensjö, E., Persson, C. G. A., and Rutili, G. (1977). Inhibition of bradykinin-induced macromolecular leakage from postcapillary venules by a β_2-adrenoceptor stimulant, terbutaline. *Acta Physiol. Scand. 101*: 504.

Tashkin, D. P., Conolly, M. E., Deutch, R. I., Ka Kit, H. I., Littner, M., Scarpace, P., and Abrass, I. (1982). Subsensitization of β-adrenoceptors in airways and lymphocytes of healthy and asthmatic subjects. *Am. Rev. Respir. Dis. 125*: 185-193.

Tattersfield, A. E. (1982). Bronchodilator drugs. *Pharmacol. Ther. 17*: 299-313.

Teule, G. J. J., and Majid, P. A. (1980). Hemodynamic effects of terbutaline in chronic obstructive airway disease. *Thorax 35*: 536-542.

Thiringer, G., and Svedmyr, N. (1975). Evaluation of skeletal muscle tremor due to bronchodilator agents. *Scand. J. Respir. Dis. 65*: 93-102.

Thiringer, G., and Svedmyr, N. (1976). Comparison of infused and inhaled terbutaline in patients with asthma. *Scand. J. Respir. Dis. 57*: 17-24.

Weitzenblum, E., Hirth, C., Dulolone, A., and Mirhom, R. (1981). Prognostic value of pulmonary artery pressure in chronic obstructive pulmonary disease. *Thorax 36*: 752.

Wilson, A. F., Novey, H. S., Cloninger, P., Davies, J., and White, D. (1976). Cardiopulmonary effects of longterm bronchodilator administration. *J. Allergy 58*: 204-212.

Wilson, J. D., and Sutherland, D. C. (1981). Has the change to β-agonists combined with oral theophylline increased cases of fatal asthma? *Lancet 1*: 12-35.

Winter, R. J. D., Langford, J. A., George, R. J. D., and Rudd, R. M. (1984a). The effects of theophylline and salbutamol on right and left ventricular function in chronic bronchitis and emphysema. *Br. J. Dis. Chest. 78*: 358.

Winter, R. J. D., Langford, J. A., and Rudd, R. M. (1984b). Effects of oral and inhaled salbutamol and oral pirbuterol on right and left ventricular function in chronic bronchitis. *Br. Med. J. 288*: 824.

Wolfe, J. D., Tashkin, D. P., Calvarese, B., and Simmons, M. (1978). Bronchodilator effects of terbutaline and aminophylline alone and in combination in asthmatic patients. *N. Engl. J. Med. 298*(7): 363-3667.

Zaagsma, J., van der Hejden, P. J. C. M., van der Schaar, M. W. G., and Bank, C. M. C. (1984). Differentiation of functional adrenoceptors in human and guinea pig. *Eur. J. Respir. Dis. 65* (suppl. 135): 16-33.

6

Pharmacokinetics of Beta-Adrenergic Compounds

JOHN W. JENNE

Loyola-Stritch School of Medicine
Maywood, and
Edward Hines, Jr. Veterans
Administration Hospital
Hines, Illinois

RICHARD C. AHRENS

University of Iowa
Iowa City, Iowa

I. Introduction

Why pharmacokinetics? Pharmacokinetics is the study of behavior of drug products in the body over time and is essential in optimizing treatment. Clinicians should be asking "Why is the oral dosage of terbutaline so much greater than the parenteral dose? How rapidly should my patient respond to this dosage by mouth, and how long will the effect last? How does it compare to the inhaled dosage? Is there a greater effect after multiple dosing? Should I be giving all my patients the same dosage, and if not, are the differences due to variability in response or variability in drug levels? Are toxic effects likely to occur at the usual dosages if my patient has liver, kidney, or heart disease?"

These questions fall in the realm of pharmacokinetics. Their answers require the development of a sufficiently sensitive assay for the drug. Unfortunately, technological limitations delayed these assays for $beta_2$-adrenergic compounds since plasma levels of the unchanged drug are only a few ng/ml. Once a suitable assay is obtained, pharmacokinetic information rapidly follows, aided by the use of established pharmacokinetic models. Yet obtaining the data is still rather painstaking, since patients must be studied under single- and multiple-dose conditions and in various disease states before an adequate groundwork is laid for clinical use.

In the following discussions, we will outline general pharmacokinetic principles underlying systemic administration of these drugs using existing data recently obtained for terbutaline and albuterol with new methods employing mass spectrometry, and will apply these principles to their clinical use. Much of the pharmacokinetic information is owed to a discussion by Benet (1984). We will then shift to the pharmacokinetics of the inhaled route, with special emphasis on the implications for protection against bronchoprovocation as well as bronchodilation.

II. Systemic Route

A. Absorption, Metabolism, and Excretion

The fate of any drug and its ability to produce the desired effect is determined by the extent of its absorption, and the degree to which it resists inactivation and excretion by various routes. There is a common pattern for oral beta-adrenergic drugs in their extensive "first-pass" metabolism by gut and liver sulfatases on their way to the systemic circulation. Moreover, absorption may be incomplete.

For example, following intravenous (IV) injection of terbutaline sulfate in normals, about three-quarters of the recovered urinary products consist of unchanged drug, and about two-thirds of the clearance is by the kidney. Following oral absorption, however, only about 25% of the drug remains unchanged and the remainder is largely present as the sulfate conjugate (Davies et al., 1974). A small fraction has also been identified as the glucuronide (Hornblad et al., 1976). Thus, about 70% of the drug is inactivated by presystemic conjugation and it is believed that more of this occurs in the gut mucosa than the liver. There is no evidence for oxidation by monoamine oxidase or for methylation by O-methyltransferase, and less than 1% is excreted in the bile (Tegner et al., 1984).

An additional loss of activity occurs through incomplete oral absorption, absorption ranging from 30 to 61% in five fasting subjects. This gives a net mean bioavailability of only about 15% into the circulation (Davies, 1984a). Bioavailability falls to about 10% (7–26%) under nonfasting conditions (Davies et al., 1974; Leferink et al., 1982). The combination of first-pass effects and incomplete absorption thus accounts for the discrepancy between parental and oral dose of this drug. Furthermore, the individual variability in both metabolism and absorption will result in large variations in blood levels between individuals taking the same dosage, but the absorption differences predominate (Davies, 1984b).

The situation differs slightly for albuterol. While the first-pass effect is similar to terbutaline, absorption by mouth is more complete, over 90% in one

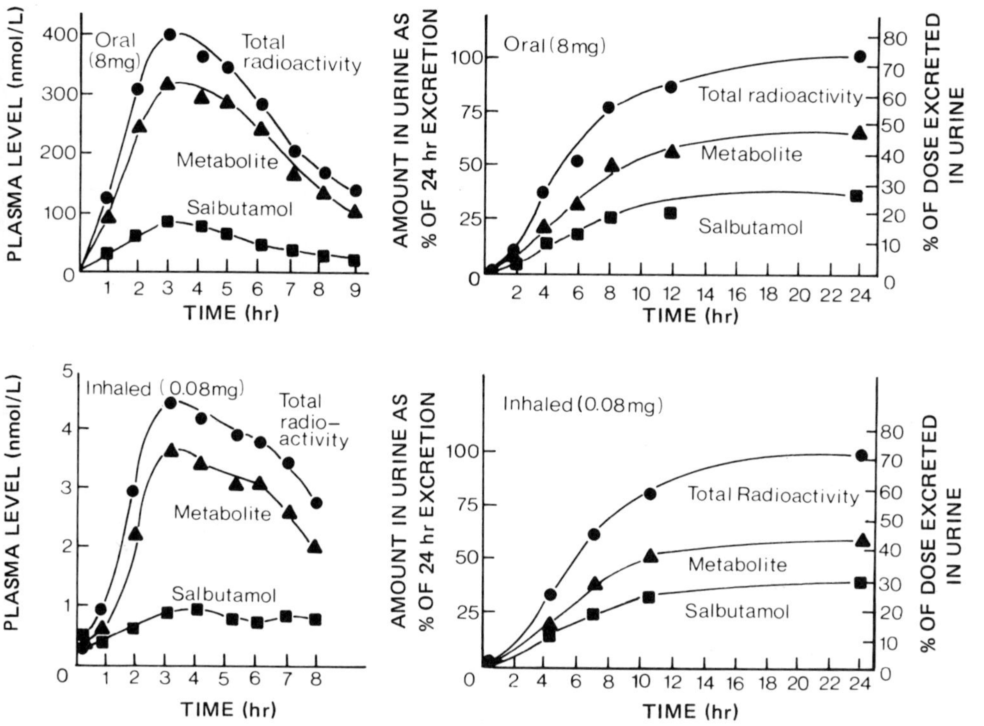

Figure 1 Plasma and urine levels of unchanged salbutamol (albuterol), its major metabolite, and total radioactivity in plasma and urine after 9.0 mg [^{3}H] salbutamol by mouth and 0.08 mg by positive pressure aerosol. The peak bronchodilator effect of the aerosol was a little more than half that of the oral drug. The experiment clearly proves that the response to inhaled drug is due to local deposition, although the paper chromatographic methodology at the time was not as precise as current methods (reproduced from Walker et al., 1972, with permission).

study (Martin et al., 1971), with overall bioavailability of nearly 30% in three subjects (Walker et al., 1972). About 60% is conjugated when given by mouth, or by aerosol (mostly swallowed) (Fig. 1), but this figure drops to a mean value of 27% when given IV (Evans et al., 1973). Again the conjugated form in humans is a sulfate ester at the 4-OH position, identified after prolonged hydrolysis with sulfatase (Lin et al., 1977), but the conjugation differs qualitatively between species (Fig. 2).

The same conjugation behavior exists for other beta agonists. Those with the 3,4 O-H catechol nucleus, such as isoproterenol, are especially vulnerable to

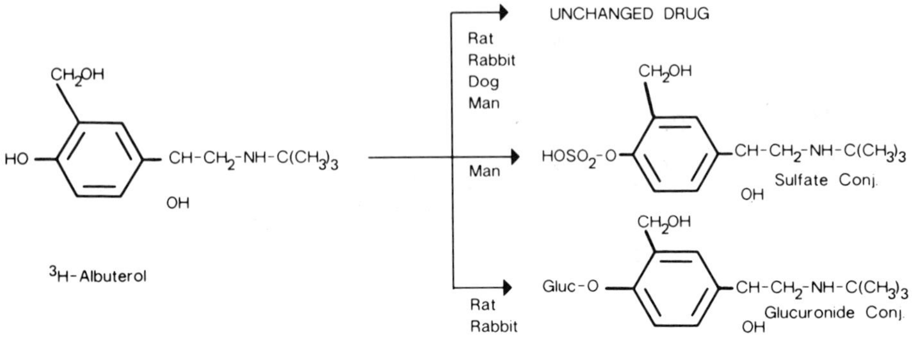

URINARY METABOLITES OF ^3H-ALBUTEROL

	Rat	Rabbit	Dog	Man
Unchanged Drug	+++	+	++++	+++
Sulfate Conjugate	--	--	--	+++
Glucuronide Conjugate	+++	++++	--	--

Figure 2 Conjugation pathways of [^{3}H]albuterol in various animal species. Data summarized from Martin et al., 1971; Evans et al., 1973; Lin et al., 1977 (drawing courtesy of Schering Corporation).

conjugation by the oral route, but also undergo O-methylation by catechol-O-methyltransferase in the tissues leading to very low levels, unless given in large doses. Oxidation of the side chain by monoamine oxidases (MAO) is resisted by substitution of the amino group. It does not occur with terbutaline, and isoproterenol < epinephrine < tyramine (Tegner et al., 1984). The catecholamines epinephrine and norepinephrine are cleared rapidly from extracellular fluid by uptake into the sympathetic postganglionic neurones (uptake$_1$) where they are stored or broken down by MAO. This is a high-affinity, low-capacity system that does not take up isoproterenol. All three catecholamines are also inactivated by the low-affinity, high-capacity extraneuronal (uptake$_2$) catechol-O-methyltransferase system in other tissues, however (Cryer, 1980).

B. Clearance

Clearance (Cl) is a measure of drug elimination from the body by all routes expressed as ml/min or ml/kg per min of some drug-containing fluid, usually plasma. It can be subdivided by organ or pathway. Plasma clearance is expressed as the product of a rate constant, K_{el}, times the volume, V_d, of the apparent space in the body available to the drug, assuming a uniform concentration. Thus,

$$Cl = V_d \times K_{el} \tag{1}$$

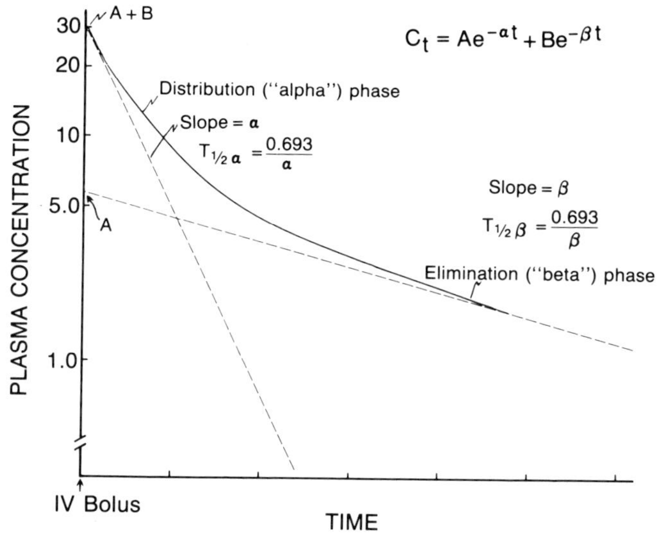

Figure 3 Plasma decay curve after intravenous bolus of a drug, showing basis of constants that constitute the overall elimination equation, $C_t = Ae^{-\alpha t} + Be^{-\beta t}$. See text for further details.

where K_{el} is the sum of all the separate disposition rate constants removing drug from that compartment. $K_{el} = k_{metabol} + k_{renal} + k_{others}$.

For terbutaline, the renal rate constant is about twice all others combined. For the clinician, clearance is the most important index for determining a dosing regimen once the drug has reached the systemic circulation. Thus, for a desired serum level at steady state, C_{ss}, the dosing rate, can be approximated from the clearance

$$\text{Dosing rate} = Cl \times C_{ss} \qquad (2)$$

if one assumes complete bioavailability. Likewise, clearance can be calculated from the dosing rate, given C_{ss}. Since steady-state levels require a dosing period of at least four half-lives, and since levels vary over the dosing interval, the formula has limited clinical usefulness from a single random level. On a multiple dose or continuous IV or subcutaneous schedule, the formula can still be utilized providing sufficient points are measured during a dosing interval to calculate the mean C_{ss}.

C. Intravenous Bolus Determination of Kinetic Parameters Clearance Half-Life and Distribution Volume

Following IV injection of a drug, its decline is very rapid at first as it distributes into the tissue compartment ("alpha" or "distribution" phase) (Fig. 3). A slower decay then emerges during which plasma drug levels are in rough equilibrium with the tissues ("beta" or "elimination" phase). The rate of decline can be characterized by its half-life, T-1/2, and an elimination rate constant K_{el} or K_d as follows:

$$T\text{-}1/2 = \frac{0.693}{K_{el}} \quad (3)$$

Substituting for K_{el} from (Eq. 3), we get

$$T\text{-}1/2 = \frac{0.693}{Cl} \times V_d \quad (4)$$

T-1/2 not only depends on CL but also on V_d. For a given clearance, the larger the V_d, the longer the T-1/2. C_p at any time during the beta phase is

$$C_{p_t} = C_{p_o} e^{-K_{el}t} \quad (5)$$

Multiple Compartments

The V_d can be broken down into smaller compartments beginning with the central compartment, in close approximation with plasma levels, and those hypothetical compartments that seek to equilibrate with the central compartment. The equilibration process may be discerned by analysis of the disposition curve after IV injection if the compartment is large enough. Most drugs, including theophylline, have been adequately described by only a two-compartment model, consisting of a central compartment and a peripheral compartment whose decay constants are alpha and beta, each being hybrids of rate constants of drug between the compartments and intercept terms. The equation for declining drug concentration in a two-compartment model is

$$C_p = Ae^{-\alpha t} + Be^{-\beta t} \quad (6)$$

These constants and the various associated kinetic parameters can be calculated from a nonlin program (Metzler et al., 1974).

As many as three compartments can be discerned from the decay curve in some cases, and then

$$C_p = A_1 e^{-k_1 t} + A_2 e^{-k_2 t} + A_3 e^{-k_3 t} \quad (7)$$

The constants, k_1, k_2, and k_3 are calculated by curve-fitting procedures. Each of these components represents a distribution volume that dominates the curve at that particular point. The last constant, k_3, the contribution from the slowest equilibrating compartment, may not become a significant portion of the curve until its levels have reached steady state from previous doses. The total area under the curve, AUC, can be calculated as

$$AUC = A_1/k_1 + A_2/k_2 + A_3/k_3 \quad (8)$$

and the contribution of any individual to the AUC as (Wagner, 1976)

$$AUC_n = A_n/k_n \quad (9)$$

This multiple-compartment approach is strikingly successful in describing the kinetics of terbutaline. Although the mean overall half-life after subcutaneous injection has been assumed to be slightly less than 4 hr (Van den Berg et al., 1982), attention to the terminal portion of the decay curve using tritiated drug or urine measurements reveals a much longer component, in the neighborhood of 16 hr. With the terminal half-life accurately obtained from urine measurements, the entire terbutaline elimination curve can be well described as a composite of three half-lives that dominate the elimination curve from 0-2 hr, 3-12 hr, and 12 hr to infinity as illustrated in Figure 4. The decay curve in this subject was found to conform to the equation

$$C_p \; 5.3\,e^{-3.61t} + 3.8e^{-0.68t} + 0.46e^{-0.053t}$$

Using (Eqs. 8 and 9), the contributions of the three components to the AUC are in the proportion

$$\frac{5.3}{3.6} + \frac{3.8}{0.68} + \frac{0.46}{0.053} \quad \text{or } 9.3\% + 35.5\% + 55.2\%$$

the terminal component contributing 55.2%.

Effector Tissue Compartments

The effect of a drug on a given organ does not necessarily correspond precisely to plasma levels, either with respect to timing or extent. The timing of the effect may be delayed, depending on the rate of equilibration of plasma levels with the effector compartment. An extreme case, although commonly encountered, is the difference in half-life of equilibration of the effect of lidocaine compared to digoxin. The half-life for lidocaine effect has been calculated to be under 2 min, while that for digoxin is about 200 min. Lidocaine effectiveness thus closely parallels plasma levels while digoxin effectiveness is delayed for several hours (Benet, 1984; Holford and Sheiner, 1981).

The effectiveness of drug or a toxic effect may correspond more closely to the amount in the body (Benet, 1984). Distinction between these alternatives requires calculation of the area under the moment curve, or AUMC, also known as

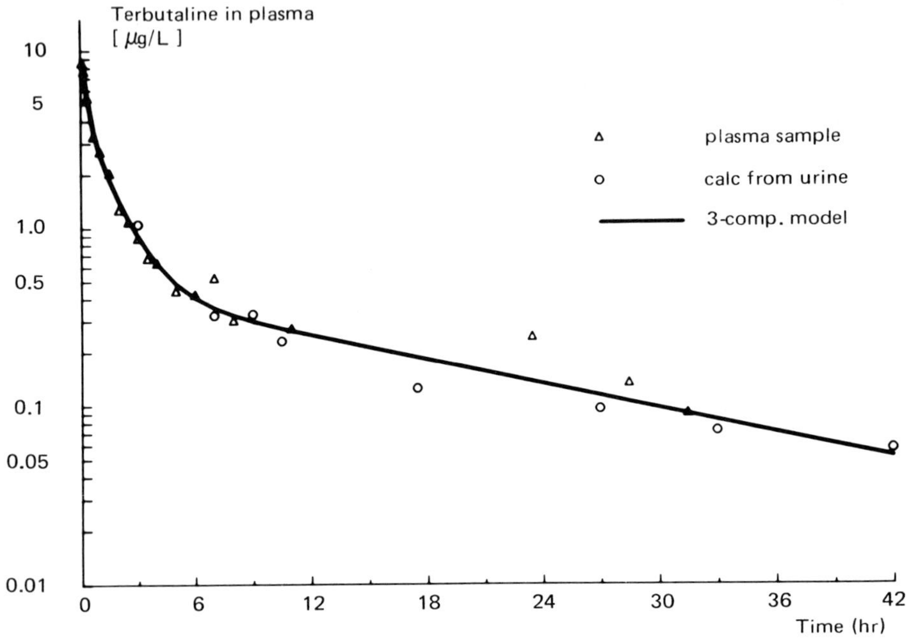

Figure 4 Measured and derived plasma concentrations of terbutaline following IV injection in a single subject receiving 210 μg terbutaline sulfate. The simulated curve, based on a three-compartment model, has the constant $C_p(t) = 5.3\ e^{-3.61t} + 3.8\ e^{-0.68t} + 0.46\ e^{-0.053t}$ (reproduced from Fagerstrom, 1983, with permission).

the first moment of the plasma-time curve, $C_p \times$ time vs. time, and V_{ss}; the volume at steady-state. Thus

$$A_{ss} = C_{ss} \times V_{ss} \tag{10}$$

where A_{ss} is the amount in the body at steady state, and V_{ss} the steady-state volume (Benet and Galeazzi, 1979).

$$V_{ss} = \frac{(\text{Dose}_{IV})\ (\text{AUMC})}{(\text{AUC})^2} \tag{11}$$

in this calculation, AUMC is derived as

$$\text{AUMC} = A_1/k_1{}^2 + A_2/k_2{}^2 + A_3/k_3{}^2. \tag{12}$$

For example, the relative plasma AUC for gentamicin at steady state and the amount in the body, A_{ss}, at steady state differ considerably when calculated by the two methods, because of the differing contribution of the terminal component of half-life. When an IV dose of 90 mg gentamicin is given, the plasma decay curve is represented by two components $C_p = 5.38\ e^{-0.195t} + 0.060\ e^{-0.013t}$ consisting of a predominant half-life of 3.56 hr and a terminal half-life of 53.3 hr (Schentag et al., 1979). The terminal component contributes only 14% of the AUC when calculated by (Eq. 9), using the ratios of the coefficients and exponents, AUC = 27.6 (86%) + 4.6 (14%), and this also applies to its contribution to the plasma curve at steady state. On the other hand, when the amount in the body is calculated by the AUMC method, the major portion of the A_{ss} is contributed by the terminal component. Thus, the A_{ss} with the terminal component included is 2.9 times the A_{ss} when it is excluded (Benet, 1984).

It remains to be seen what the significance of the amount of terbutaline in the body calculated by this method is to its action. In any case, this large body reservoir will exert a stabilizing effect on drug levels, and prolong the action when drug is deliberately or inadvertently discontinued.

Model-Independent Parameters and Mean Residence Time

The plasma decay data may also be analyzed in a model-independent manner, often considered to be the most relevant way of looking at a compound's pharmacokinetics (Benet, 1984). This approach avoids the necessity of dealing with multiple compartment calculations. The AUC and the AUMC extrapolated to infinity are calculated directly by curve-fitting techniques or by the trapezoidal method, using urine values if necessary to extrapolate plasma levels not directly measurable. This approach allows calculation of the mean residence time (MRT) or mean transit time, that is, the time the average molecule remains in the body, and includes calculation of Vd_{ss}, the distribution volume at steady state, and the corresponding clearance.

Thus, after IV infusion $\mathrm{MRT} = \dfrac{\mathrm{AUMC}(\infty);}{\mathrm{AUC}\ (\infty)}$ $\mathrm{Cl} = \dfrac{\mathrm{Dose}}{\mathrm{AUC}\ (\infty)}$; and $V_{ss} = \mathrm{Cl} \cdot \mathrm{MRT} = \mathrm{Dose} \times \dfrac{\mathrm{AUMC}(\infty)}{\mathrm{AUC}^2\ (\infty)}$ or (Eq. 11) which must be corrected for loss during the infusion.

In six adult male subjects, plasma and urine terbutaline levels were sampled out to 48 hr after intravenous injection and the plasma levels calculated from urine levels. Mean body clearance, Cl, was 213 ml/min (range, 165-270), mean residence time (MRT) 7.5 hr (range, 7.3-11.7), and mean V_{ss} 96L (range, 83-140) (Fagerstrom, 1984). An even longer MRT value, 9.0 hr, was calculated from urine decay curves extrapolated to infinity and this is considered the most accurate value.

D. Oral Dosing

Single Oral Dose

Following an oral dose, plasma concentrations in a two-compartment open model with first-order absorption kinetics are described by the equation

$$C_p = A_1 e^{-\alpha t'} + A_2 e^{-\beta t'} - A_3 e^{-k_a t'} \tag{13}$$

when α is the disposition rate constant of the distribution (alpha) phase, β is the disposition rate constant in the elimination phase, k_a the absorption rate constant, and A_1, A_2, and A_3 are coefficients of the rate constants, α, β, and k_a, respectively. In addition, t' represents the absorption time corrected for lag time ($t' = t - t$ lag), the time at which absorption begins (Powell et al., 1985).

Following an oral dose of 5.0 mg terbutaline (expressed as the sulfate salt), mean peak plasma levels were 6.6 ng/ml in fasting men (Bengtsson and Fagerstrom, 1982), but only 3.3 ng/ml if nonfasting (Leferink et al., 1982) (Van den Berg et al., 1980) (Table 1; Fig. 5). An oral dose of 4 mg albuterol (expressed as the base) produced peak plasma levels of about 12–14 ng/ml in 12 fasting men (Powell, 1985) but these values appeared to the authors to be population-related, since more commonly the level was 7-9 ng/ml (Powell, personal communication). Another laboratory reported mean peak levels of about 8.0 ng/ml in nine fasting men (Maconochie and Fowler, 1983), and levels of 8-10 ng/ml are found by another laboratory (Glaxo, personal communication, 1981).

From the terbutaline data cited, the fasting state appears to be important when comparing drug levels and physiological responses, but no data are currently available on fasting vs. nonfasting levels for albuterol. The plasma levels of albuterol in the fasting state are similar to or slightly higher than those of terbutaline.

In the nonfasting state, the bronchodilator responses to albuterol and terbutaline are similar (Fig. 6) (Wolfe et al., 1985). This is puzzling since the potency of albuterol in vitro and by inhalation on a mg/mg basis exceeds that of terbutaline by a factor of at least two (Svedmyr and Thiringer, 1971). Some clues to this mystery come from recent quantitative tremor comparisons between the two drugs. When these same doses were compared in 20 fasting men with chronic obstructive pulmonary disease, albuterol initially produced only one-third the mean tremor response to terbutaline (Jenne et al., 1985) and this has been confirmed (Levy et al., 1986). An earlier comparison of 8 mg albuterol and 10 mg terbutaline in six subjects also showed a smaller tremor response to albuterol (Watson and Richens, 1974). In our studies, plasma responses of cyclic AMP, pulse elevation, and the drop in diastolic pressure were also less in proportion to the tremor response, while the increase in FEV_1 was more nearly the same between the two drugs.

Table 1 Summary of Terbutaline Pharmacokinetics and Dosing Characteristics[a]

	Pharmacokinetics	Dosing characteristics		
		Dosage form	Tmax	Cmax (ng/ml)
Bioavailability	15% (fasting)	*Single dose*		
	10% (nonfasting)	5 mg orally		
Protein binding	14-25%	fasting (11 men)	2.5 hr (1.5-4.0)	6.6 (4.1-11.2)
		fasting (3 men)		7.9 (5.4-10.0)
V_{ss}	1.37 (0.87-1.85) liters/kg	nonfasting (8 men)	3.0 hr (1-4.0)	3.3 (2.3-5.5)
		nonfasting (3 men)		4.6 (4.3-5.1)
	1.61 (1.23-2.03) liters/kg (corrected to 9.0 MRT)	0.5 mg SC	22 min (16-30)	7.4 (5.8-11.1)
Total body clearance	3.02 (2.60-3.90) ml/min/kg	0.25 mg IV		10 ng/ml
Renal clearance	1.99 ± 0.43 ml/min/kg	*Steady state*		
T-1/2 (3-12 hr IV)	4.7 hr	5 mg every 8 hr orally		
T-1/2 (terminal)	17 (11.5-23.0) hr	nonfasting (4 men)		3.3 (1.9-3.6)
T-1/2 steady state	17, 20 hr	nonfasting (4 women)		6.5 (4.7-10.5)
MRT	9.0 hr			

[a]All values are found in the text with references.

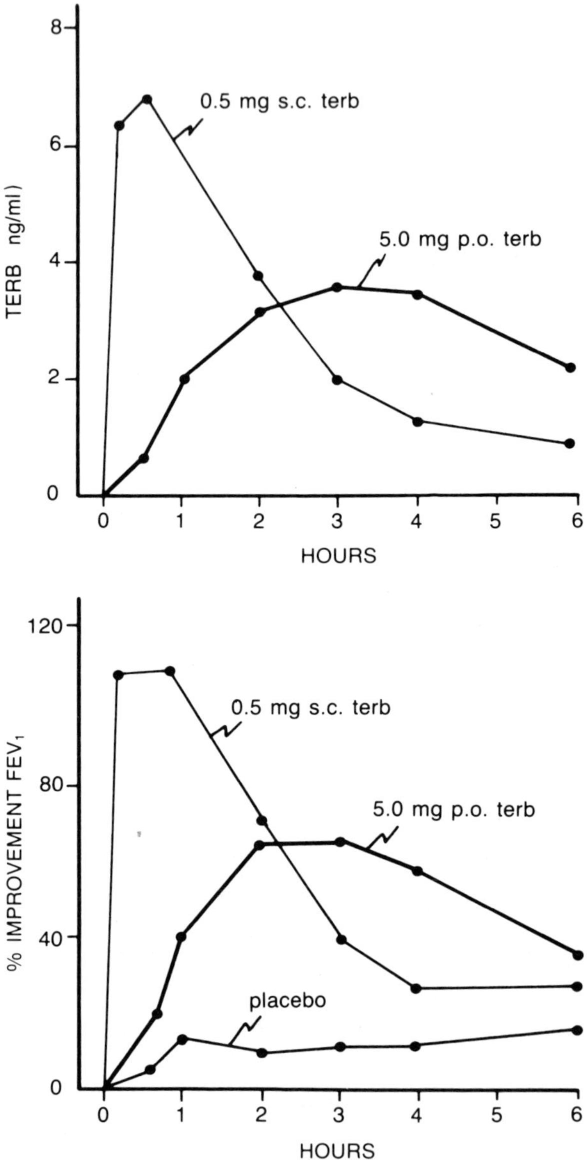

Figure 5 Comparison of plasma levels and % improvement in forced expired volume in 1 sec to 5.0 mg oral terbutaline and 0.5 terbutaline subcutaneously over time. The oral dose was given nonfasting. Values are the means in eight asthmatic subjects. Note the close correspondence between FEV_1 response and drug levels (reproduced from Van den Berg et al., 1984, with permission).

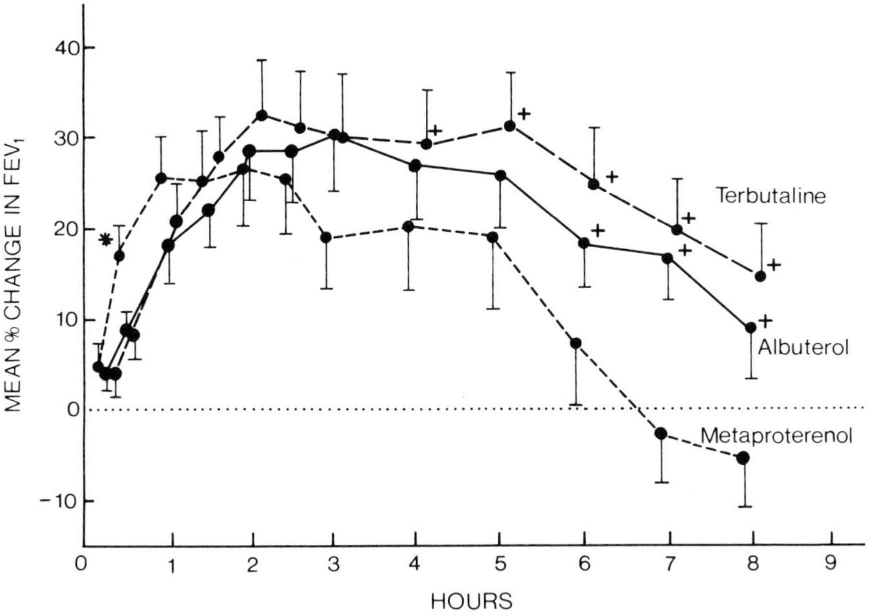

Figure 6 Mean percent improvement (SEM) in forced expired volume in 1 sec (FEV_1) with time following oral (nonfasting) administration of albuterol 4 mg, metaproterenol sulfate 20 mg, and terbutaline sulfate 5 mg. Plus signs indicate significant differences from metaproterenol (P = 0.05) (reproduced from Wolfe et al., 1985).

These discrepancies could be explained by assuming a smaller rate or extent of distribution of albuterol from the central compartment to the effector compartments. The delay is not present by the inhaled route. In time, the concentration of the two drugs in the effector compartments becomes more comparable although albuterol may still not be as well distributed. Continued administration of both drugs three times daily for 3 weeks produced roughly equal baseline tremor elevations 16 hr after the last dose, but yet the tremor response to a single further dose of albuterol was less, although not statistically so (Jenne et al., 1986). This same rising basal tremor on terbutaline three times daily with lesser response to each single dose had been previously noted (Van den Berg, 1982). Further comparisons between the two drugs are needed at steady state.

Differences in receptor specificity might also explain the discrepancy between tremor and FEV_1 responses to the two drugs. This seems unlikely, since, to date, no convincing evidence has emerged that the $beta_2$ receptor specificity of skeletal and bronchial smooth muscle differs (Andersson et al., 1982; Olsson et al., 1979).

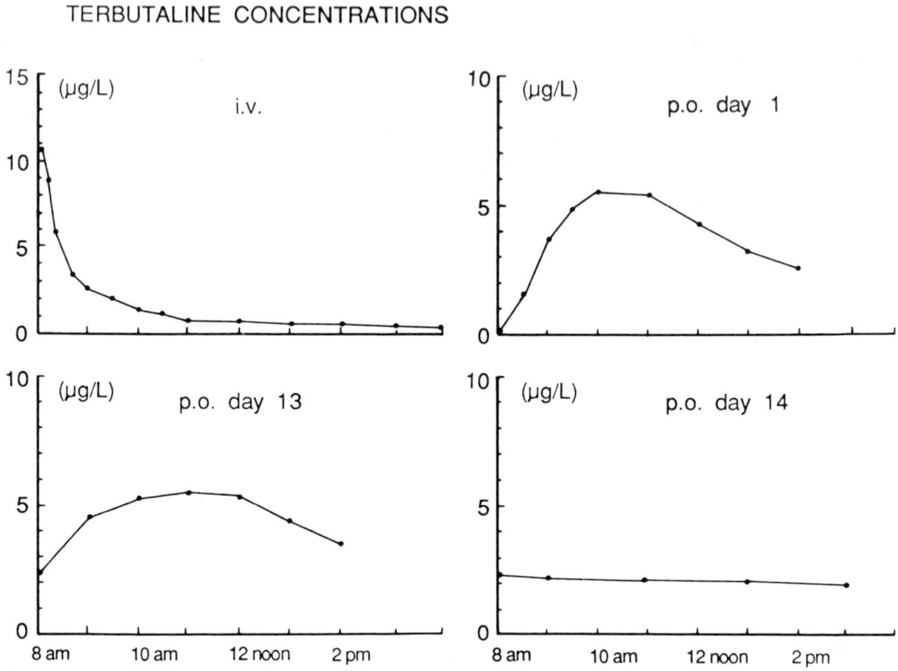

Figure 7 Plasma terbutaline concentrations after intravenous infusion of 250 μg terbutaline sulfate over 5 min (upper left), and after oral dosing of 5 mg three times daily for 13 days, the last dose taken at 8 P.M. on day 13. Note slow decay on day 14. Values represent means of 11 subjects (adapted with permission from Bengtsson and Fagerstrom, 1982).

Multiple Oral Dosing and Accumulation to Steady State

When a drug is dosed repeatedly, the ratio of the AUC for a single dosing interval at steady state to the AUC over the same interval with the initial dose, R_c, is a measure of drug accumulation and can be described by the formula

$$R_c = \frac{1}{1 - e^{\beta T}} \tag{14}$$

where T is the dosing interval and β the elimination rate constant (Wagner, 1976).

When terbutaline was administered at 5.0 mg for 13 days to 11 fasting male adult subjects, mean plasma levels peaked at about 5 ng/ml, no higher than after the first dose, but the troughs remain elevated between peaks. Levels 12 hr

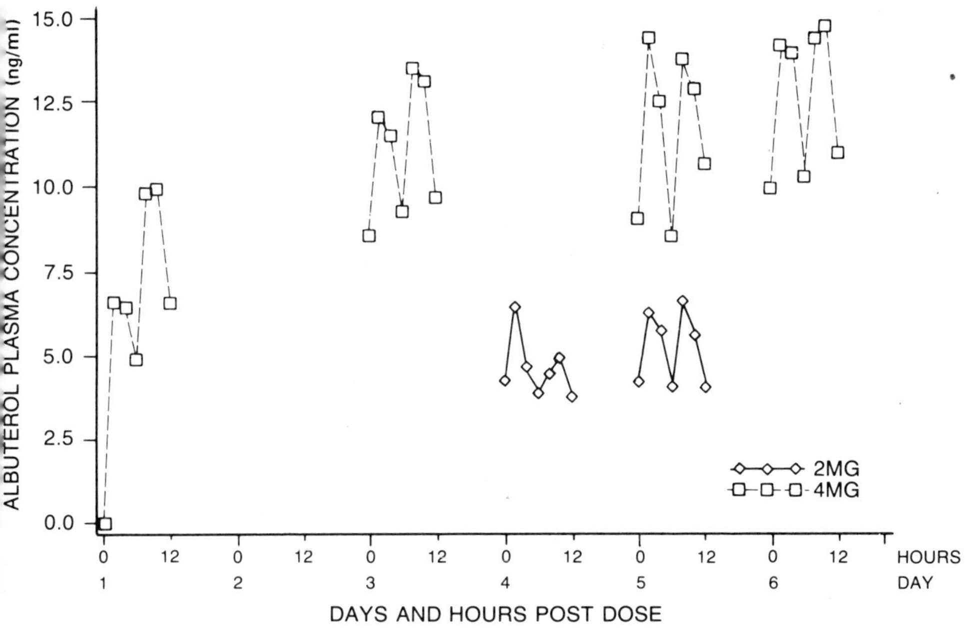

Figure 8 Mean plasma concentration–time curves of albuterol following multiple oral administration of 2- and 4-mg tablets showing cumulative kinetics. Note that the increase in plasma level is greater on the first dose than increases after subsequent doses of the 4-mg tablet (figure courtesy of Schering, Inc.).

after the last dose were still 2.3 ng/ml and declined thereafter with a half-life of 20 hr (Bengtsson and Fagerstrom, 1982) (Fig. 7). When 2.5 mg was administered similarly three times daily to eight adult subjects, plasma levels 6 hr after the last dose averaged 1.0 ng/ml and terminal T-1/2s ranged from 11.5 to 23.0 hr with a mean of 17.0 hr (Nyberg and Kennedy, 1984). These long terminal half-lives indicate the slow unloading of drug from a large slowly equilibrating compartment, and have been calculated to be responsible for 40-50% of the AUC (Nyberg, 1984). They explain the observation that adult asthmatics on a three times daily schedule of terbutaline show a prolonged elevation of cyclic AMP in their urine following drug discontinuation (Morris et al., 1983), paralleling the slow loss of terbutaline from a large body reservoir, consistent with the large V_{ss} of 96 liter.

Although less information is available for albuterol, the circumstances are likely to be the same for this drug. When either 2.0 mg or 4.0 mg albuterol is administered orally on a four times daily schedule to adults, there is a rising plasma level that plateaus by 3 days at levels proportional to the dose (Powell

M, personal communication) (Fig. 8). Even when adjusted to a three times daily schedule, the accumulation would occur. A mean half-life from steady state has been measured as 6.5 hr by these authors.

With either terbutaline or albuterol, the peak-trough differences at steady state are less than with the initial dose. Trough levels are maintained by the "buffering" action of the reservoir compartment, which begins to unload between each dose.

As shown in Table 1, summarizing plasma levels reached with single and multiple doses of terbutaline, the nonfasting state markedly reduces peak levels. Gender also appears to play a significant role, levels on multiple dosing being twice as high in females in these small study groups. Added to these variables is the variability existing in the pharmacodynamic response to a given level. The variability in FEV_1 response has been studied over a range of terbutaline levels (Billings et al., 1984) and the variability for tremor shown in the large individual differences in both basal tremor and tremor response to terbutaline in 24 fasting COPD patients (Jenne et al., 1982). In this case, basal tremor and the response to 5.0 mg terbutaline were correlated, suggesting that the largest component of variability resided in the skeletal muscle $beta_2$ receptors.

Individuality of Steady-State Levels

It has now been shown that individual terbutaline levels vary considerably on the same dose. Terbutaline given three times daily to nine children and increased weekly (40-80-120-160 μg/kg) produced a fourfold range of plasma levels between individuals when levels were obtained before and 2 hr after the 2 P.M. dose on the seventh day each week (Lonnerholm, 1984). Most individuals maintained their rank order each week as the dosage was increased, indicating a surprising constancy of individual absorption metabolic and excretory behavior (Fig. 9). There was a linear relationship between dosage and plasma levels, with progressively increasing pulse, tremor, and PEFR as the dosage was increased. Side effects became intolerable for some children at the larger dosage.

E. Parenteral Routes

Subcutaneous Injection

Published levels after injection are only available for terbutaline; a dosage of 0.5 mg was used. Peak levels of 7.4 ng/ml in one study were reached an average of 22 min later, with a subsequent half-life of 3.6 hr; levels fell to about 2 ng/ml at 3 hr (Leferink et al., 1982). Similar peak levels of 7.2-7.6 ng/ml were recorded in another series, with a maximum reached between 15 and 30 min (Van den Berg et al., 1984). These levels are shown in Figure 5, compared to levels after 5.0 mg terbutaline sulfate by mouth. The bronchodilator response

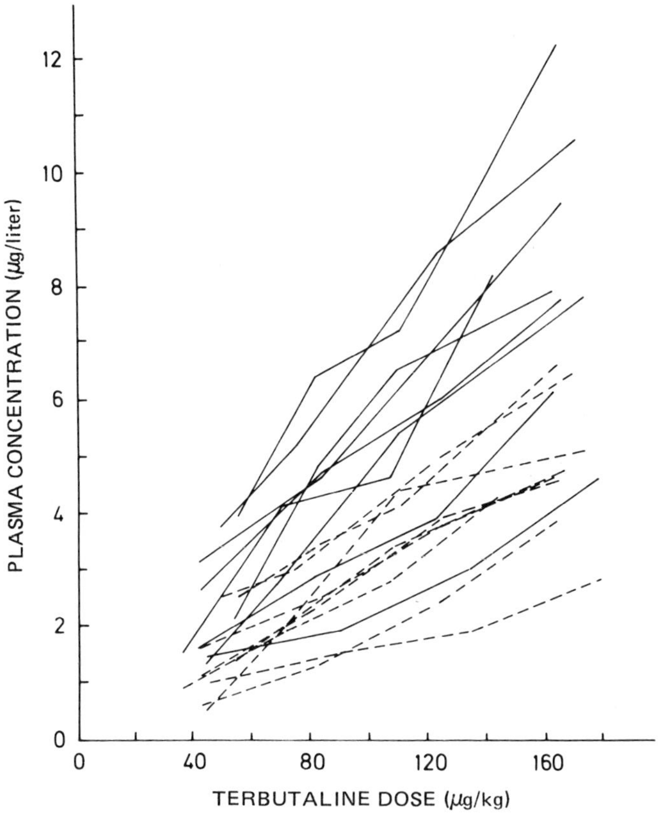

Figure 9 Terbutaline plasma concentrations before (dashed lines) and 2 hr after intake (solid lines) on day 7 of a 7-day three times daily schedule at increasing dosages ranging from approximately 40 μg/kg to 160 μg/kg (reproduced from Lonnerholm et al., 1984, with permission).

closely parallels plasma levels. It is important to note that over half the peak level is reached by 5 min after subcutaneous injections.

Although 0.5 mg provides slightly greater bronchodilation than 0.25 mg (Dulfano and Glass, 1976) (Fig. 10), most authors have concluded, based on results in stable asthmatics, that the optimal dosage is 0.25 mg (Sackner et al., 1974, 1975; Pierce et al., 1981), with larger dosages producing more side effects (Buck and Bangaard, 1984). However, if the response to 0.25 mg is not satisfactory, an additional dose at 20 min may be used, as recommended by the manufacturer, since some additional bronchodilation will clearly occur, and in more severe bronchospasm, a larger dosage may be needed. The duration of action of the 0.25 mg dose is 3-4 hr (Freedman, 1971).

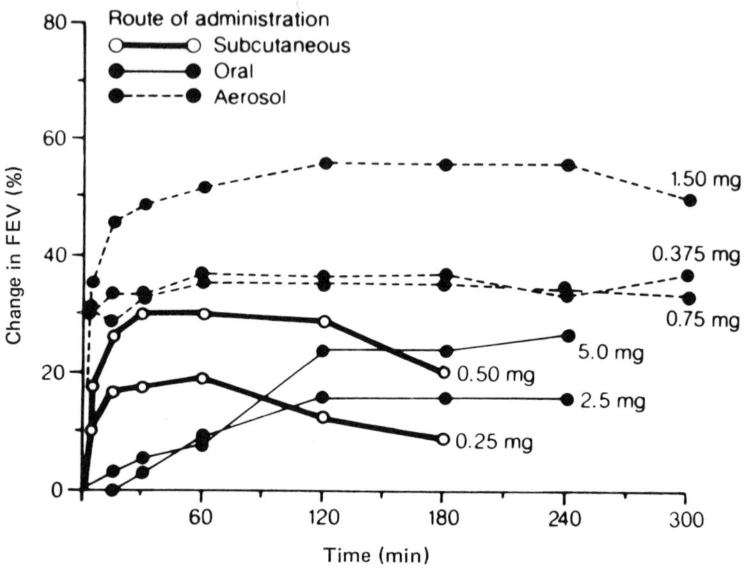

Figure 10 Changes in FEV_1 following these different routes of administration of terbutaline. There were 15 patients in the subcutaneous study, 26 in the oral study, and 15 in the inhaled study. Since the patients were not crossed over between groups, the comparison is only approximate (reprinted from Dulfano and Glass, 1976, with permission).

Compared to terbutaline, an equal dosage of epinephrine produces a less intense bronchodilation of shorter duration (Schwartz et al., 1976) and a smaller rise in pulse and cardiac output (Sackner et al., 1975).

Intravenous Administration

Beta$_2$ Agonists

The principal use of intravenous beta$_2$ agonists is in suppression of premature labor (tocolysis). Pharmacokinetic data are available on the continuous infusion of terbutaline. At a dosage of 10 μg/min in the gravid woman, plasma levels of 5-16 ng/ml are reached at 30-60 min infusion and are still rising. Thus, *the infusion rate must be cut back,* for example, to 2.5 μg/min to maintain these levels (Berg et al., 1984). Higher levels may be necessary to relax the uterus, but are frequently associated with uncomfortable side effects.

A single IV infusion of terbutaline of 0.25 mg over 5 min also produces peak levels of about 10 ng/ml, but levels decline precipitously as shown in Figure 7. Infusions of albuterol have been advocated in the treatment of severe acute asthma as an alternative to the inhaled route (Bloomfield et al., 1979; Williams and Seaton, 1977). A dose of 10 μg/min for 60

Table 2 Changes in Plasma Concentrations of Epinephrine During a 60-Min Infusion of 1-Epinephrine at a Mean Rate of 0.083 μg/kg/min

Time (min)	Plasma epinephrine (nmol/liter)
-6.0	0.29 ± 0.06
1.8	0.63 ± 0.23
3.75	2.86 ± 1.74
7.5	3.50 ± 0.57
10.0	3.54 ± 0.61
15.0	3.65 ± 0.57
20.0	4.36 ± 0.60
30.0	4.51 ± 0.65
45.0	4.32 ± 0.0
55.0	4.38 ± 0.95
60.0	4.35 ± 1.07

Values are mean ± SEM
Reproduced with permission from Fitzgerald et al., 1980.

min, used in one study, produced no further rise in pulse (Williams et al., 1975) while a dose of 20 μg/min for 45 min in another study produced excessive side effects and tachycardia (Lawford et al., 1978). Thus, the lower dosage, 10 μg/min for 60 min, is probably better suited for therapy, although, like terbutaline, the dosage must be cut back after the loading period to avoid a continued rise into toxic levels (see Appendix for current schedules).

Catecholamines

The rapidity of disposition of IV catecholamines is impressive. A half-life of 75 sec was described for epinephrine and isoproterenol (Brown et al., 1983) while a slightly longer initial half-life of about 3 min followed by a longer half-life of 9-12 min was described for epinephrine (Fitzgerald et al., 1980) and mean clearance of 9.41 (range 4.86-14.61) liters/min. In any case with these kinetics, physiological responses to IV infusions begin almost immediately, maximizing at about 20 min. They abruptly decline on terminating infusion, but require 30-60 min to level off (Brown et al., 1983; Fitzgerald et al., 1980).

Table 2 illustrates the early plateau reached during epinephrine infusion at 0.0893 ± 0.06 μg/kg/min, full equilibrium being reached at about 20 min at plasma epinephrine levels of 4.4 nm/liter or about 0.800 ng/ml and near equilibrium by 7.5 min. Lower infusion rates gave proportionately lower equilibrium levels. This dosage produced an increase of 10 beats/min in heart rate.

There are very few data correlating bronchodilator effects with plasma levels of epinephrine. In a recent study 0.06 μg/kg min were infused for 15 min (Sands et al., 1985), producing plasma levels of 0.690 ± 0.290 ng/ml in normals and 0.52 ± 0.02 ng/ml in asthmatics, from basal levels of 1/10th to 1/20th of this. There was complete reversal of methacholine-induced bronchospasm at this dose. Some idea can be gained from this study of the levels following a subcutaneous dose of epinephrine. The usual dosage of 0.3 mg in the adult is likely to produce somewhat higher levels than the approximately 0.06-ng total dose over 15 min in this study, but measurements are not available.

From the epinephrine kinetics, we can assume similar kinetic behavior for infused isoproterenol. Bronchodilating effect and pulse elevations will reach near-equilibrium by 10 min and remain constantly influenced by the infusion rate.

F. Summary of Systemic Terbutaline Pharmacokinetics and Clinical Relevance

Table 1 summarizes the pharmacokinetic data and plasma levels obtained by various routes and circumstances for terbutaline, the compound for which we have the most information.

The renal clearance of terbutaline approximates the creatinine clearance, and accounts for about 2/3 of total body clearance (Fagerstrom, 1984), being slightly lower in older subjects (Hornblad et al., 1976). Plasma protein binding is low. Terbutaline has been shown to accumulate to twice the plasma value in erythrocytes, and the V_{ss} for terbutaline is considerably in excess of body water, indicating accumulation in tissues and contributing to its prolonged T-1/2 at steady state. Studies in various disease states have not yet been done, but obviously, the dose should be reduced in renal insufficiency. Some of the clinically useful inferences from this pharmacokinetic background are discussed below.

1. In the acute asthmatic attack, subcutaneous terbutaline provides therapeutic levels in minutes, and is the obvious mode of choice for the first stages of treatment if systemic beta-agonists are used. Following the initial dose, subsequent doses should be given at fairly frequent intervals (e.g., 0.25 mg every 4 hr) consistent with the approximate half-life in the early, unequilibrated stages.
2. With continued dosing of either terbutaline or salbutamol, a "floor" of drugs develops that maintains troughs at about 50% of the peak levels and continues levels for some time following discontinuation of drug. Patients beginning maintenance dosing will require several doses before this floor is fully established, with steady state reached by 72 hr.

3. There is a spread of plasma levels between individuals, shown with terbutaline, which reflects individual differences in their handling of this drug, and probably others in this class. Existence of these differences speaks against rigid adherence to dosing guidelines, and suggest that, within limits, dosages should be tailored to the response.
4. In contrast to infused catecholamines, intravenous infusions of terbutaline or albuterol do not rapidly equilibrate. Once loading is achieved to the desired level, the infusion rate must be markedly reduced to prevent further elevations into toxic levels.

III. Inhaled Route

A. Background

Aerosols generated by compressed-air-driven jet nebulizers, ultrasonic nebulizers, and freon-propelled metered dose inhalers are commonly used to deliver beta$_2$-agonist sympathomimetics to the respiratory tract. This route of administration has the potential of maximizing the beneficial antiasthmatic effects of these agents and minimizing their adverse systemic effects by concentrating drug in the lung. Consequently, inhaled beta$_2$-agonists have seen increasing use, often in preference to systemically administered drugs, for a number of clinically important purposes in the treatment of asthma (Ahrens and Smith, 1984). These include the initial treatment of acute symptoms of asthma in both hospitalized (Williams and Seaton, 1977; Lawford et al., 1978) and ambulatory patients (Larsson and Svedmyr, 1977), intermittent administration for the prevention of bronchospasm triggered by predictable specific inciting factors such as vigorous exercise (Anderson et al., 1976; Francis et al., 1980), and routinely scheduled treatment for prophylactic maintenance therapy in chronic asthma (Larsson and Svedmyr, 1977; Woolcock, 1977). As is true for systemically administered beta$_2$-agonists, optimal dosing strategies for inhaled beta$_2$-agonist use in each of these clinical settings should be based at least in part upon knowledge of behavior of these agents in the body. Therefore, this section reviews what is known about the mechanisms by which inhaled beta$_2$-agonists arrive at and are subsequently eliminated from the vicinity of beta$_2$-agonist receptors in the lung and rates at which these processes occur.

All currently used inhaled beta$_2$-agonists have structures that are modifications of the basic phenylethanolamine structure of the naturally occurring sympathomimetics. In terms of their behavior in the body, inhaled sympathomimetics may be classified into three groups: (1) agents administered as active catecholamines (e.g., epinephrine, isoproterenol, isoetharine); (2) agents administered as active, noncatecholamines (e.g., metaproterenol, albuterol, terbutaline, fenoterol); (3) agents administered as inactive prodrugs that must be metabolized to active form (bitolterol is the only currently available drug fitting this description).

B. Absorption and Disposition

For inhaled $beta_2$-agonists to exert their antiasthmatic effects, they must first reach the location of the receptors responsible for producing these effects. These receptors appear to be located in the lung and not in the upper respiratory tract (Ruffin et al., 1978). Furthermore, it appears that inhaled $beta_2$ agonists reach these receptors by a direct entry into the lungs via airways rather than by way of the systemic circulation after absorption from the oral mucosa or GI tract (Ruffin et al., 1978; Newman et al., 1981; Davies, 1984b). It has been widely assumed that the receptors responsible for inhaled $beta_2$-agonist therapeutic effect are located diffusely throughout the conducting airways on the surface of airway smooth muscle cells. However, receptors located on neural structures (Richardson, 1977), mast cells (Assem and Schild, 1969; Lichtenstein and Margolis, 1968; Howarth et al., 1985) or other respiratory structures may also be of importance.

Adequate knowledge of and control over the quantity of administered $beta_2$-agonist actually deposited in the airways, and the pattern of deposition in the lungs, is critical to the successful clinical use of these agents. Influential factors include the quantity of drug retained in the device used to generate and deliver the aerosol (Dennis, 1977), the quantity of drug lost into the room because of a lack of synchronization of aerosol delivery with inspiration (Clay et al., 1983), the quantities of drug deposited in the oropharynx (Newman et al., 1981), degree of airway obstruction present in the lung (Dolovich et al., 1976), and the quantity of drug entering the lower respiratory tract that fails to be deposited and is exhaled (American Conference, 1978). These often-neglected aspects of clinical aerosol therapy are covered extensively elsewhere in this book.

Once the inhaled $beta_2$-agonist has reached the airways, it must be transported across epithelial surfaces to the actual receptor site on airway smooth muscle, tissue mass cell, or other respiratory structure before a clinical effect can occur. Unfortunately, little is known about the mechanism or kinetics of this process. For the drug bitolterol, one additional step is also necessary. Unlike all other $beta_2$-agonists currently in use, this drug is administered as an inactive, di-p-toluate ester which must be hydrolyzed to the active catecholamine, colterol, by tissue esterases. This process appears to occur over several hours (Orgel et al., 1985).

The length of time over which therapeutic effects of $beta_2$-agonists other than bitolterol persist will depend upon the length of time that sufficient concentrations of drug remain at the receptor site. This in turn will depend not only on the quantity of active drug delivered to this site but also on the rate at which drug is removed. Elimination of active drug from the receptor site appears to occur by three mechanisms. First, epinephrine, synthetic catecholamines such as isoetharine, isoproterenol, and the active form of bitolterol, colterol (but not the parent prodrug itself) are subject to active uptake into various types of cells in the lung. This is known as type II uptake to differentiate it from norepinephrine uptake into postganglionic sympathetic nerve terminals (type I uptake) (Gryglewski and Vane, 1970). Noncatecholamine agents such as metaproterenol, fenoterol, terbutaline, and albuterol are not subject to rapid removal from the sight of action by type II uptake. Second, catecholamines are also subject to inactivation by enzymatic metabolism in the lung. Catechol-orthomethyl-transferase, present in lung tissue (Axelrod and Cohn, 1971), rapidly inactivates all catecholamines. The enzyme MAO inactivates epinephrine but not isoproterenol (Blackwell et al., 1974) or colterol (Shargel et al., 1976). Noncatecholamine agents currently in clinical use are unaffected by either of these enzymes (Davies et al., 1974; Lin et al., 1977). Resistance to type II uptake and enzymatic degradation appears to explain the significantly longer persistence of clinical effect seen for noncatecholamine agents as compared to the catecholamines. Third, all $beta_2$ agonists are removed from the lungs by absorption into the systemic circulation (Blackwell et al., 1974; Shenfield et al., 1976). This appears to be the only means by which the noncatecholamines studied to date are removed from their site of action. This process may not occur at the same rate for different $beta_2$-agonists since rate of absorption from the lung appears to vary directly with a drug's lipid solubility and inversely with its molecular weight (Enna and Schanker, 1972). This could, in part, account for the apparent differences in duration of action of the noncatecholamines albuterol, fenoterol, and terbutaline suggested by some studies (Huhti and Poukkula, 1978; Freedman, 1971).

Unchanged albuterol and terbutaline have been shown to appear in the plasma promptly after deposition directly in the airways (Shenfield et al., 1976; Davies, 1984). However, this may in large part reflect rapid absorption from the alveoli rather than the true rate of absorption from the vicinity of the beta receptor in the airways. The catecholamines isoproterenol, isoetharine, and rimiterol appear in the plasma more slowly after direct administration to the airways and are largely metabolized before being absorbed from the lung (Shenfield et al., 1976; Blackwell et al., 1974; Williams et al., 1974). This delayed appearance in the plasma after intratracheal administration may result from a small portion of the drug being immediately absorbed, with the rest of the drug being taken up by the lung by type II uptake, metabolized, and then more slowly released (Shenfield et al., 1976). When clinically used dosages of albuterol and terbutaline are administered by metered dose inhaler, plasma concentrations of active drug are in the range of 1-5 nM. These levels are approximately 10 times lower than occur after the same drugs are administered in recommended dosages orally (Walker et al., 1972; Davies, 1984b).

The major portion of both catecholamines and noncatecholamine beta$_2$-agonists absorbed into the circulation after metered dose aerosol administration arrives there after initially being deposited in the oropharynx, swallowed, and absorbed from the gastrointestinal tract (Walker et al., 1972; Davies, 1984b; Blackwell et al., 1974). Beta$_2$-agonist absorbed unchanged from the lung into the circulatory system is subject to the same kind of metabolism and excretion as it would if it had been initially administered parenterally. Similarly, a beta$_2$-agonist that fails to reach the lung and is deposited in the oropharynx (Newman et al., 1981) behaves as an orally administered drug (Walker et al., 1972).

C. In Vivo Measurements of Antiasthmatic Effects: Pharmacokinetic Implications

When drugs are administered systemically, the concentration present in the plasma often has a known relationship to the pharmacologic effects achieved. The kinetics of plasma concentrations can therefore be used to determine optimal dosages and dosing frequencies. However, when drugs are administered topically, such as aerosol to the lung, the desired therapeutic effects depend on local tissue drug concentrations, which may bear no direct relationship to plasma drug concentrations. Since beta$_2$ agonist concentrations in the lung cannot, of course, be routinely measured in clinical patients and are difficult to measure even in experimental animals, nearly all the information we have concerning the rates at which pharmacokinetic processes occur after aerosol beta$_2$-agonist administration has come from examining the pharmacodynamics of these agents (i.e., the observed effects of these drugs on the lungs). Changes in drug concentrations in the lung must be inferred from these pharmacodynamic observations.

Onset of Action

Numerous studies of beta$_2$-agonist-induced bronchodilation (Ahrens and Smith, 1984; Svedmyr, 1985) have shown that the catecholamines isoetharine and isoproterenol exert their maximal level of effect within 5 min after aerosol administration. In contrast, the noncatecholamines such as albuterol, fenoterol, and terbutaline produce about 80% of their effects within 5 min, but require 15-60 min to reach maximal effect. As an explanation for this, Jack (1971) speculated that catecholamines crossed the airway epithelium and arrived at the smooth muscle beta$_2$-receptor more rapidly than the noncatecholamine agents. In support of this concept, he noted two additional observations, which suggest that catecholamines are capable of crossing epithelial barriers more quickly. First, catecholamines also appear in vitro to relax isolated guinea pig airway smooth muscle more rapidly than noncatecholamines. Second, if sufficient quantities of isoproterenol are placed on the buccal mucosa, significant bronchodilation and tachycardia promptly ensue. This does not appear to be the case for noncatecholamines. Jack went on to postulate that an active transport system for catecholamines similar to that associated with type II uptake was involved.

No apparent differences in the time required for onset of effect of the different noncatecholamine bronchodilators have been demonstrated. Like the noncatecholamine bronchodilators, bitolterol also requires 15-60 min (Cockcroft et al., 1981). This probably reflects the rate not only at which it is transported from the bronchial lumen to the receptor site, but also at which it is hydrolyzed to its active form, the catecholamine colterol.

Choosing an agent with a more rapid onset of effects may be important for a few specific clinical situations. For example, when assessing bronchodilator responsiveness during pulmonary function testing, it may be desirable to be able to perform postbronchodilator spirometry after just 5 min, rather than after 15-60 min. However, for most therapeutic settings, speed of onset of effect will not have a significant influence on the choice of a specific $beta_2$-agonist.

Measurement of Intensity and Duration of Action

Probably of greatest interest to the clinician are studies of the intensity and duration of effectiveness of inhaled $beta_2$-agonists. This type of study is currently the only practical way in which the length of time that clinically relevant concentrations of $beta_2$-agonist remain in the vicinity of the $beta_2$-receptor can be estimated. These studies determine the average length of time required for $beta_2$-agonist effects on the airway to become undetectable or fall below some arbitrary level deemed by the investigator to be the least that is clinically relevant. Often, one or two selected dosages of each drug are compared, usually the dosage(s) recommended by the manufacturer.

Intelligent choice of a specific $beta_2$-agent, dosage, and dosing interval for clinical treatment must be based at least in part upon information provided by these studies. This is especially true when around-the-clock efficacy is needed such as for the treatment of a prolonged exacerbation of symptoms of asthma, or for preventive, maintenance therapy of chronic asthma. The dosing strategy used in these two situations should be designed so that each successive dose is administered before the effects of the prior dose have become insufficient to control symptoms.

The mean duration of effect of a given inhaled $beta_2$-agonist is a function of three independent factors, each of which is under the control of the clinician by his or her choice of the specific drug and dosage to be administered. First, the rate at which the effects of the drug diminish with time influences the overall duration of action (Fig. 11, panel A). This probably reflects the rate at which the drug is eliminated from the vicinity of the $beta_2$-receptors that mediate airway relaxation. Second, the higher the dosage of a specific $beta_2$-agonist

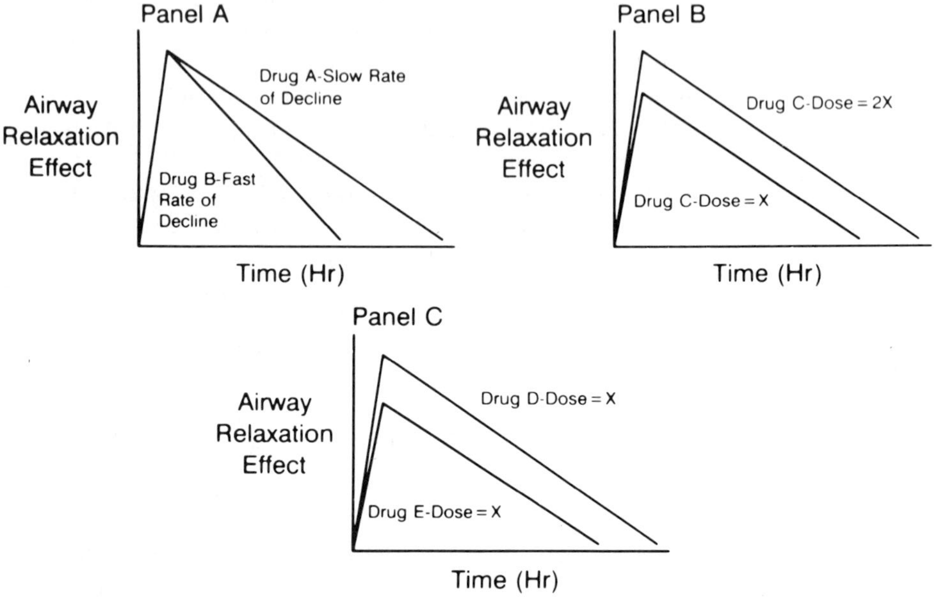

Figure 11 Hypothetical examples of factors affecting duration of action of inhaled $beta_2$-agonists. Panel A: Rate at which effects diminish with time. If two drugs are given in dosages that produce identical initial effects, the drug with the lower rate of decline will have effects detectable for longer. Panel B: Dosage. For any given $beta_2$-agonist, the higher the dosage administered, the longer the effects will be detectable. Panel C: Relative potency. If two drugs are given in identical dosages and have identical rates of decline in effect, the more potent drug will have effects detectable longer. These hypothetical curves assume a linear relationship between effect and log of $beta_2$-agonist in the vicinity of the $beta_2$-receptor and a first-order decline of this concentration with time.

administered, the longer the overall duration of action for that drug will be (Fig. 11, panel B). Third, the relative potency of a drug on a milligram for milligram (or, in the case of metered dose inhalers, puff for puff) basis also plays an important role. If, for example, two drugs with equal rates of decline in effect are given in equal, milligram for milligram (or puff for puff) doses, the more potent drug will tend to produce a greater initial effect, and therefore will have a longer duration of action (Fig. 11, Panel C). These later two factors are similar in that they both influence the magnitude of the initial effects of the inhaled $beta_2$ agonist administered.

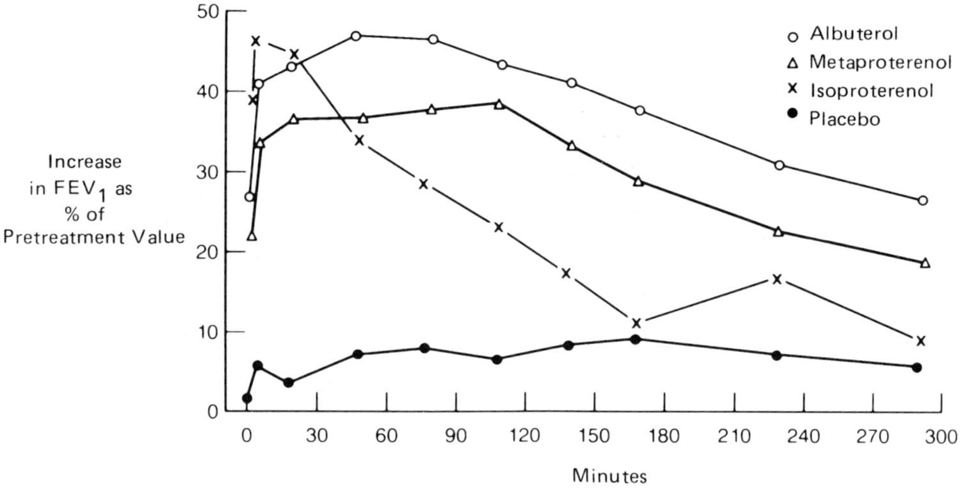

Figure 12 Percentage increase in FEV_1 after metered dose aerosol inhalation of albuterol (200 μg -O), metaproterenol sulfate (1500 μg - △), isoproterenol sulfate (1000 μg - X), and placebo (●). Effects of metaproterenol and albuterol were sustained for greater than 3 hr, but effects of isoproterenol were not significantly different from placebo after 2 hr (from Choo-Kang et al., 1969).

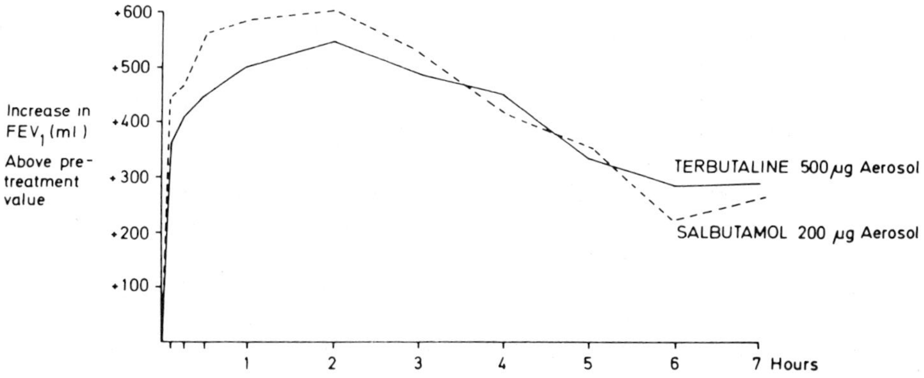

Figure 13 Percent increase in FEV_1 after metered dose aerosol inhalation of albuterol (salbutamol) and terbutaline. Effects of the two drugs were not significantly different at any point (from Choo-Kang et al., 1973).

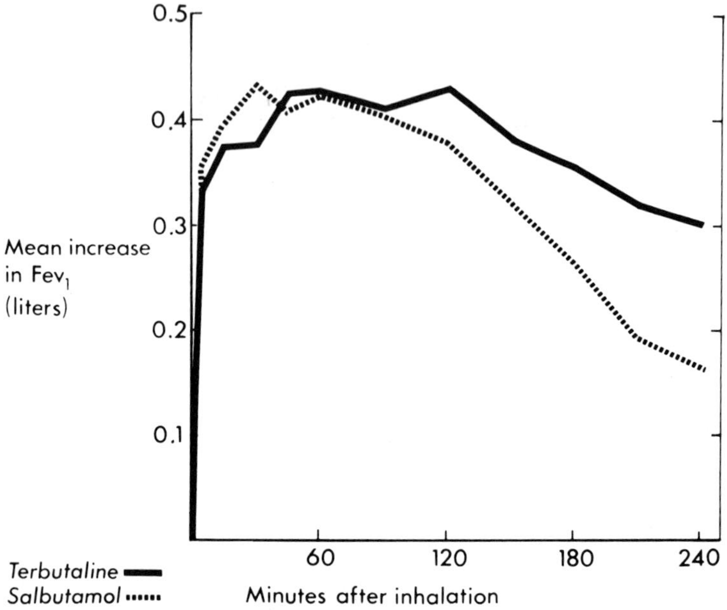

Figure 14 Increase in FEV_1 (liters) after metered dose aerosol inhalation of albuterol (salbutamol, 100 μg) and terbutaline (250 μg). Effects of the two drugs were significantly different only at 180 min and thereafter (from Freedman, 1972).

Use of Bronchodilation to Determine Duration of Action

Studies of drug-induced bronchodilatation have been most commonly employed to provide information about the intensity and duration of action of inhaled $beta_2$-agonists. This clinical experimental model has provided very useful information, but it also has significant limitations.

Studies of bronchodilatation have clearly shown that the effects of catecholamine agents diminish much more rapidly than do those of the noncatecholamine agents (Fig. 12), or bitolterol (Choo-Kang et al., 1969; Kass and Mingo, 1980). This results in an overall duration of action of only 1-1.5 hr for clinically recommended dosage of inhaled catecholamines. This of course might be expected since, as noted previously, catecholamines are subject to removal from the vicinity of the receptor by both type II uptake and enzymatic degradation. The noncatecholamine agents are not. The rapid rate at which the clinical effects of catecholamine $beta_2$-agonists diminish with time and the resultant short overall duration of action has made them obsolete as therapeutic agents for any clinical situation in which more than transient airway relaxation is required.

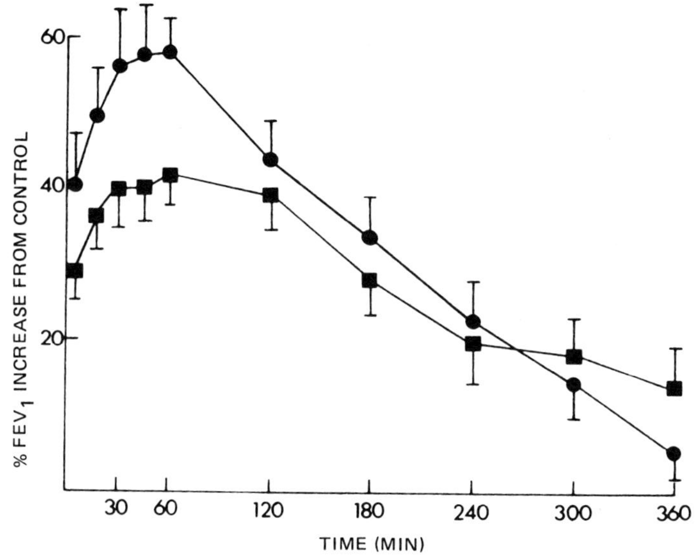

Figure 15 Percentage increase in FEV_1 after metered dose aerosol inhalation of albuterol (200 μg – ●) and terbutaline (500 μg – ■). Effect of the two drugs was significantly different for only the first 60 min (from Hartnett and Marlin, 1977).

The limitations of studies of bronchodilation become apparent when comparisons among various longer-acting noncatecholamine agents are examined. Results of these studies are often conflicting and usually do not allow the reader to discern clearly whether differences in apparent duration of action of the inhaled $beta_2$-agonists being compared are related to differences in magnitude of their initial effects, differences in the rates at which the effects of the drugs decline with time, or both. For example, several published studies have compared equal numbers of metered dose inhaler puffs of terbutaline (250 μg/puff) and albuterol (100 μg/puff). Depending upon the study cited, it is possible to reach entirely different conclusions concerning these drugs. It may be concluded that, puff for puff, terbutaline has virtually the same initial effect, rate of decline of effect, and duration of action as albuterol (Choo-Kang et al., 1973) (Fig. 13), has the same initial effect, but a slower rate of decline of effect, and therefore, a longer duration of action than albuterol (Freedman et al., 1972) (Fig. 14), or has a lesser initial potency, a slower rate of decline, and consequently, a similar duration of action to albuterol (Harnett and Marlin, 1977) (Fig. 15).

The reasons for these inconsistent and conflicting results are not completely clear. A possible explanation is that intersubject and intrasubject variabil-

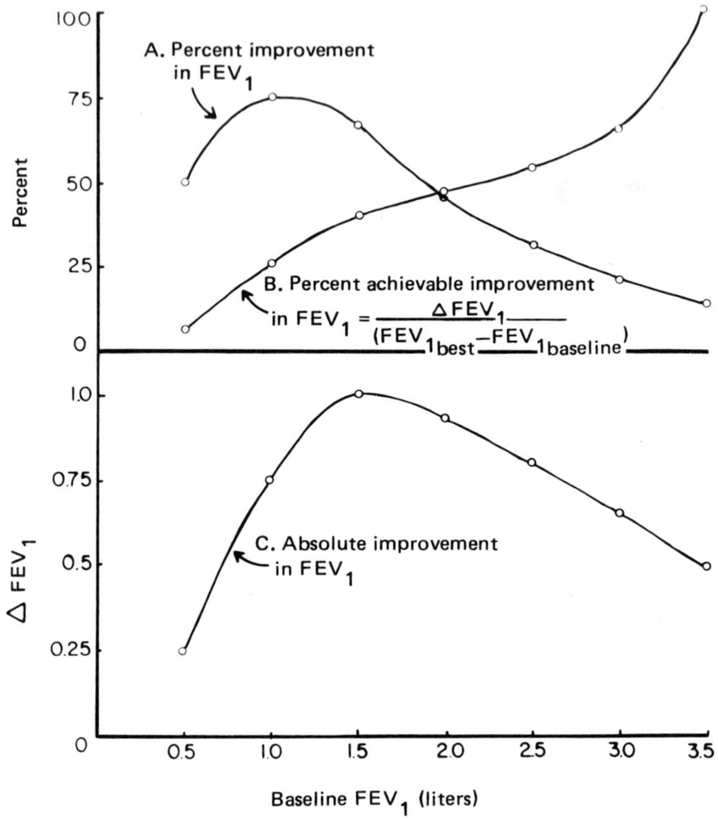

Figure 16 Three ways of representing the bronchodilator responses in a hypothetical patient studied on seven different occasions at seven different baseline values (FEV_1 ranging from 0.5 to 3.5) with seven different arbitrary responses (from Jenne and Tashkin, 1983).

ity in "baseline" pulmonary function status, and potential for bronchodilator response, can significantly influence the study outcome (Weber et al., 1979; Jenne and Tashkin, 1983) (Fig. 16). Subjects with small amounts of initial bronchospasm cannot be expected to show more than small amounts of bronchodilator response on inhaled $beta_2$-agonist. Maximal response may occur in these subjects after relatively low dosages of the inhaled agent (Williams and Kane, 1975). Once this maximal response is achieved, even relatively large changes in $beta_2$-agonist dose and potential airway relaxant effect will not be reflected by changes in bronchodilator effect. This may obscure comparisons of both the magnitude of initial effects and rates at which effects diminish with time. Furthermore, when results are expressed as "percent bronchodilation" (as they most commonly are), low initial pulmonary function values tend to magnify bronchodilator responses because this initially small value becomes the denominator in calculations of percent response to beta$_2$-agonist. Conversely, apparent bronchodilator responses will be minimized in subjects with near to normal initial pulmonary function values. Attempts have been made to remedy these problems. Reporting absolute increase in FEV_1, FEF_{25-75}, or other indicator of airway obstruction appears to be an improvement, since there is no denominator to magnify or minimize the responses in individuals with high or low initial pulmonary function values. Reporting "percent achievable bronchodilation" is probably the most logical method, but even this may have limitations. Neither of these methods of expressing bronchodilatation can overcome the fact that individuals with small amounts of initial bronchospasm are capable of demonstrating only small amounts of bronchodilatation, no matter how potent the bronchodilator administered.

A second limitation of studies of beta$_2$-agonist bronchodilatation relates to the clinical relevance of these studies. Numerous reports have shown that the bronchodilatation induced by oral and inhaled beta$_2$-agonists does not correlate well with, and, in fact, overestimates, ability of these agents to inhibit exercise-induced bronchospasm (Eggleston and Beasley, 1981; Anderson et al., 1976; Del Bono et al., 1979; Konig et al., 1981; Eggleston and McMahan, 1978) and to inhibit bronchospasm induced by pharmacologic agents (Salome et al., 1983). Sly et al. (1968) demonstrated that while inhaled metaproterenol completely inhibited exercise-induced bronchospasm immediately after it was administered, it provided virtually no protection between 3 and 4 hr later despite the persistence of significant bronchodilation. Similarly, Ahrens et al. (1984) demonstrated that measureable effects of recommended dosages of inhaled metaproterenol on airway responsiveness to methacholine persist for only 2-3 hr, while bronchodilatation remained near maximal after 4 hr (Fig. 17). These studies suggest that bronchodilatation overestimates the length of time that clinically important quantities of beta$_2$-agonist remain in the vicinity of the beta$_2$-receptor.

A possible explanation for this discrepancy between bronchodilator effects and effects on airway responsiveness to exercise, methacholine, and histamine relates to the fact that studies of bronchodilatation are performed with very specific subject populations (clinically stable, chronic asthmatics) who are experiencing a very specific and carefully controlled clinical situation. They are sitting quietly in a pulmonary function lab, repeatedly blowing into a pulmonary function machine. The physiological stimulus to develop bronchospasm is clearly less intense than that present in the same individuals after exercise or inhalation of histamine or methacholine, since these forms of bronchial provocation produce additional degrees of bronchospasm. The quantity of beta$_2$-agonist activity necessary to counteract the more intense bronchospasm occurring after bronchial

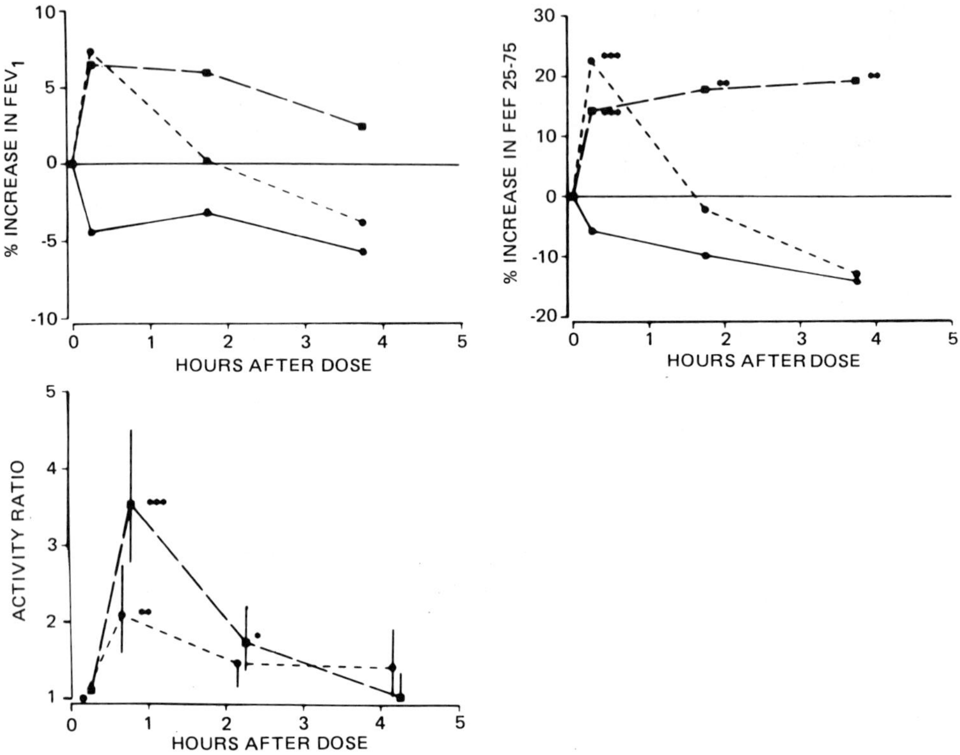

Figure 17 The effects of aerosol metaproterenol (1,300 μg – ■), isoetharine (305 μg - - -), and placebo (——) on FEV_1 (top left), FEF_{25-75} (top right panel), and nonspecific airway responsiveness as reflected by the activity ratio (bottom panel). Activity ratio is PD_{20} FEV_1 after drug divided by PD_{20} FEV_1 after drug. The effect of metaproterenol on nonspecific airway responsiveness diminishes much more rapidly than its bronchodilator effect. Brackets indicate standard error of the mean. Tests of significance are against zero for percent increase in FEV_1 and $FEF_{25\text{-}75}$, and against 1 for activity ratio (* = $P < 0.05$, ** = $P < 0.01$, *** = $P < 0.001$) (from Ahrens et al., 1984).

provocation may simply be greater, and a direct function of the intensity of that bronchospasm. This type of relationship, known pharmacologically as "functional antagonism" (Van den Brink, 1973), has been confirmed in in vitro and in vivo canine and guinea pig airway smooth muscle (O'Donnell and Wanstall, 1978; Torphy et al., 1983) and confirmed in vivo (Jenne et al., 1985). If this kind of relationship exists for inhaled $beta_2$-agonists in humans, the clinical consequences will be that the intensity and duration of effectiveness of these

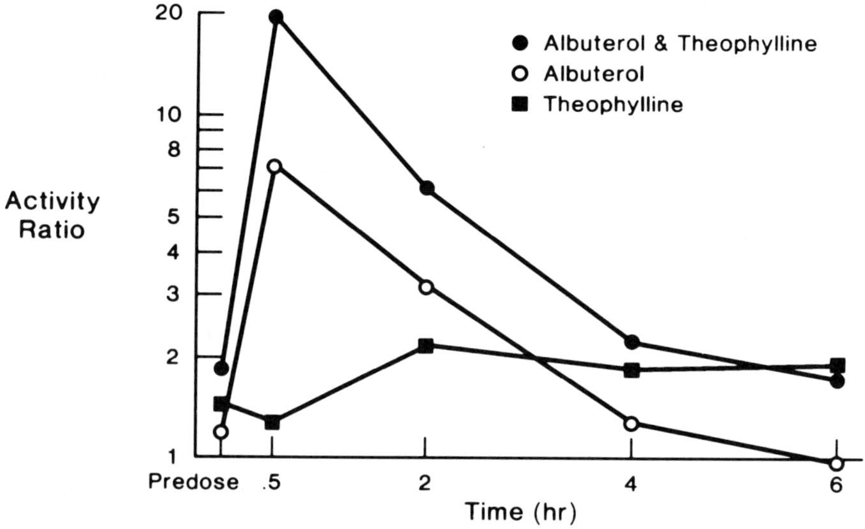

Figure 18 Effect of inhaled albuterol (180 μg, four times daily), slow-release theophylline (peak serum concentration, 10-20 μg/ml), and the combination on airway responsiveness over 6 hr after the morning doses of each drug (activity ratio defined as in Fig. 17) (from Joad et al., 1986).

agents in reversing bronchospasm in asthmatic subjects in the laboratory will consistently overestimate the ability of these agents to prevent or reverse bronchospasm in any clinical situations where more intense bronchospasm is present (e.g., after exposure to exercise, cold air, allergic antigen, etc.).

Use of Bronchial Provocation to Quantitate Duration of Action

An alternative to studies of bronchodilation is to measure the ability of inhaled $beta_2$-agonists to inhibit bronchospasm induced by various types of bronchial provocation. With appropriate study design, this approach may more accurately reflect the clinical efficacy of these agents. In simple forms, experimental models using bronchospasm induced by exercise and pharmacologic agents have been used for many years to quantitate the initial antiasthmatic effects of inhaled $beta_2$-agonists (Herschfus et al., 1951). More recently, these types of bronchial provocation have been employed to document not only the initial intensity of various antiasthmatic drugs, but also to quantitate the duration of effectiveness of various inhaled agents (Massey et al., 1986). Exercise, however, has an important technical limitation that appears to have prevented it from being extensively employed. Exercise challenges cannot be performed at intervals of less than about 3 hr without the development of significant refractoriness to exercise-induced bronchospasm even in the absence of any therapeutic agent (Stearns et al., 1981; Ben-Dov et al., 1982). On the other hand, nonspecific airway responsiveness can be measured with histamine at intervals of 1 hr or less without evidence of the development of tolerance to histamine-induced bronchospasm (Ruffin et al., 1981). The use of bronchial provocation with histamine to measure changes in inhaled $beta_2$-agonist effectiveness in the lung also has other advantages. Measurement of nonspecific airway responsiveness with histamine or methacholine is highly reproducible (Juniper et al., 1978). $Beta_2$-agonist effects on airway responsiveness appear to diminish in an appropriately linear fashion over time (Ahrens et al., 1986). In contrast, decreases in $beta_2$-agonist bronchodilator effects are nonlinear. As a result, airway responses can reflect broad changes in inhaled $beta_2$-agonist activity under conditions where bronchodilatation has "plateaued" near maximal achievable levels (Ahrens et al., 1984). Information obtained appears to be at least as clinically relevant as that obtained from studies of bronchodilatation since airway responsiveness itself correlates with exercise-induced bronchospasm (Anderton et al., 1979), cold air-induced bronchospasm (O'Byrne et al., 1982), asthmatic medication requirements (Juniper et al., 1981; Cockcroft et al., 1977), and the severity of asthma symptoms (Makino, 1966).

Furthermore, when the inhaled $beta_2$-agonist albuterol is administered on a regularly scheduled basis, the pattern of drug-induced changes in airway responsiveness closely correlates with the frequency of asthmatic symptoms experienced by the patients. Joad and co-workers (1987) recently demonstrated that the effects of albuterol on nonspecific airway responsiveness as measured with histamine go from being highly significant to being undetectable in only a little more than 4 hr (Fig. 18). Asthma symptom control relative to the length of time since the last albuterol dose was administered was also documented in this study using patient symptom diaries. This showed symptoms of asthma increasing rapidly between 4 and 5 hr after albuterol administration (Fig. 19). As a consequence, administered four times daily albuterol was significantly less effective in controlling symptoms of asthma in this study than was sustained-release theophylline or their combination in spite of the much greater initial effects of albuterol on airway responsiveness. Thus, the effects of albuterol appeared to "wear off" too quickly to provide optimal, around-the-clock protection against asthma symptoms with four times daily dosing. The close temporal correlation between the disappearance of the effects on nonspecific airway responsiveness and the increase in symptoms of asthma suggest that nonspecific airway responsiveness will be a useful tool for designing inhaled $beta_2$-agonist dosing strategies that provide better around-the-clock effectiveness than does four times daily dosing with recommended doses of albuterol.

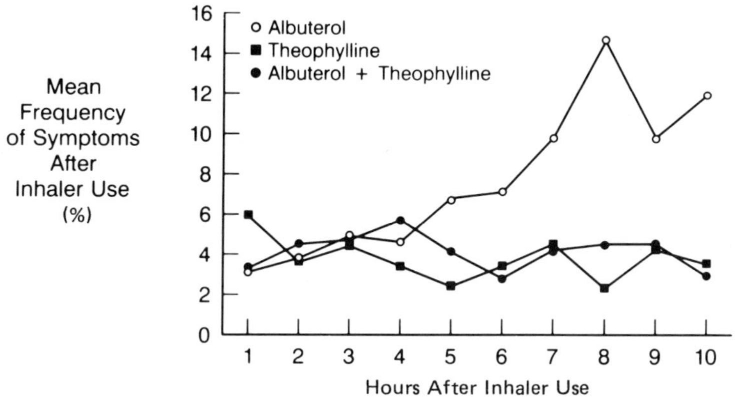

Figure 19 Relationship of time after metered aerosol inhalation of albuterol or placebo to mean frequency of symptoms. Regimens: Albuterol, active albuterol inhaler plus placebo theophylline capsules; theophylline, placebo inhaler plus active theophylline; combination, active albuterol plus active theophylline. Mean symptom frequency correlated significantly with hour after inhaler for albuterol alone ($p < 0.001$) but not the other regimens ($p > 0.05$) (Joad et al., 1987).

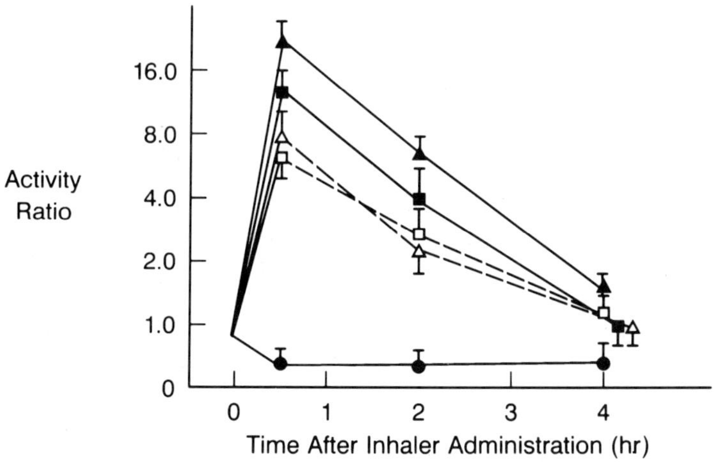

Figure 20 Effect of metaproterenol (4 puffs –■, 2 puffs – □), albuterol (2 puffs – ▲, 1 puff – △), and placebo (●) on airway responsiveness. Activity ratio defined as in Figure 17. Brackets indicate standard error of the mean (Ahrens et al., 1985).

Table 3 Comparison of Selected Metered-Dose Aerosol Beta$_2$-Receptor Agonists[a]

Drug and recommended dosage[b]	Relative aerosol potency[c]	Mean rate of decline in effect	Projected T 1/2 of conc. at beta$_2$ receptor site	Duration of effect on airway responsiveness of recommended dose (hr)
Albuterol (180 μg/2 puffs)	1	0.77 ± 0.07[d] log units/hr	1.43 ± 0.46[d] hr	4-5
Metaproterenol (1300 μg/2 puffs)	0.37 (0.22-0.53)	0.72 ± 0.11 log units/hr	1.01 ± 0.48 hr	3-4
Terbutaline (400 μg/2 puffs)	0.43 (0.22-0.59)	0.37 ∓ 0.04 log units/hr	2.3 hr	4-5
Bitolterol (1050 μg/3 puffs)	not estimated	0.57 ± 0.05 log units/hr	not estimated	4-5
Fenoterol (400 μg/2 puffs)	1.88 (1.01-4.23)[e]	not estimated	not estimated	5-6

[a]Based on studies of effects on airway responsiveness.
[b]Based on products available in the United States (fenoterol excepted).
[c]Equivalent number of puffs of albuterol required to produce initial effects equal to 1 puff of the drug being tested. Ninety-five percent confidence levels are in parentheses.
[d]Standard error of the mean.
[e]Based on a study of bronchodilatation.

Considerations for Improving Inhaled $Beta_2$-Agonist Therapy

One possible way to increase the duration of effectiveness of inhaled albuterol would be to increase the dosage above that currently recommended by the maufacturer. However, this approach may be limited by undesirable extrapulmonary effects. A second alternative may be to choose a $beta_2$-agent with effects that diminish much more slowly than did those of albuterol in the above study. Regularly scheduled administration of such a $beta_2$-agonist might be more effective in controlling chronic asthma symptoms.

With these possibilities in mind, several studies have recently used effects on nonspecific airway responsiveness to histamine to evaluate the relative potencies and rates of decline in effect (Table 3) of some of the longer-acting inhaled $beta_2$-agonists available in metered dose inhaler form (metaproterenol, albuterol, terbutaline, bitolterol, and fenoterol). It is interesting to note that two puffs of metaproterenol appear to have a shorter overall duration of action than two puffs of albuterol (Fig. 20) simply because this dosage of metaproterenol produces a less intense initial effect than does the albuterol (Ahrens et al., 1986). The effects of both drugs appear to diminish at similar rates. Two puffs of terbutaline, on the other hand, appear to be less potent than two puffs of albuterol, but have effects that wear off more slowly than those of albuterol (Harris et al., 1986a). These two differences between terbutaline and albuterol counterbalance one another and, as a result, the overall duration of action of recommended doses is similar. This suggests that if terbutaline were given in a dosage equipotent with two puffs of albuterol, it would have a significantly longer duration of action. However, this needs to be confirmed experimentally. A comparison between two puffs of albuterol and three puffs of bitolterol suggests that in these recommended dosages the drugs have similar initial potencies, but that bitolterol has a slower rate of decline in effect and therefore a slightly longer overall duration of action (Harris et al., 1986b). This is compatible with a study of the duration of bronchodilator effects of these agents (Orgel et al., 1985). Salome et al. (1983) reported a duration of effectiveness on airway responsiveness for recommended dosages of fenoterol (400 μg) that was 5-6 hr (1-2 hr longer than that seen in other studies for albuterol, bitolterol, or terbutaline in other studies). However, since this study did not directly compare fenoterol with any other drug, comparisons of relative potency and rate of decline in effect are not possible from these data. Shenfield and Paterson (1973) used bronchodilatation to compare the relative potency of recommended doses (two puffs) of albuterol and fenoterol. Application of standard statistical methods for calculation of relative potency (Finney, 1978) to data presented in their paper suggest that, puff for puff, fenoterol is significantly more potent than albuterol. This may account for the longer apparent duration of action of fenoterol noted above.

Another useful way to compare inhaled $beta_2$-agonists may be to estimate their half-lives of disappearance from the vicinity of the $beta_2$ receptor in the lung. Using the data summarized in Table 3, we have calculated this half-life for albuterol, metaproterenol, and terbutaline. This was accomplished by first estimating how much a two-fold change in $beta_2$-agonist concentration in the lung altered airway responsiveness. This was done by examining differences in the initial effects on airway responsiveness produced by doses of the same inhaled $beta_2$ agonists that differed by a factor of 2 (e.g., one vs. two puffs). The time required for the effects of the larger dose (e.g., two puffs) to diminish until it was equal to the *initial* effects of the two-fold smaller dose was then taken as the half-life of disappearance from the vicinity of the $beta_2$ receptor. This was approximately 1.4 hr for albuterol, 1.0 hr for metaproterenol, and 2.3 hr for terbutaline. If these estimates are correct, they indicate that each doubling of the dosage of metaproterenol or albuterol will result in an increased duration of action of approximately 1 hr, and each doubling of the terbutaline dosage will result in an increase of over 2 hr. This again suggests that terbutaline could be a much more effective drug for around-the-clock asthma prophylaxis than albuterol if it was used in a dosage with initial effects similar to two puffs of albuterol.

D. Summary of Inhaled Pharmacokinetics and Clinical Relevance

Based on their behavior in the body, available inhaled $beta_2$-agonists can be classified into three groups: drugs administered as active catecholamines (e.g., isoproterenol and isoetharine), drugs administered as active noncatecholamines (e.g., albuterol, fenoterol, metaproterenol, and terbutaline), and bitolterol, which is administered as an inactive prodrug and must be metabolized to active form. Catecholamine agents are obsolete because of their rapid elimination from the lung and consequent short duration of action. The noncatecholamine agents and bitolterol appear to remain in the vicinity of the receptor in clinically important concentrations for longer periods of time. The potent initial effects and relatively long duration of action of recommended doses of these drugs make them excellent agents for the management of acute exacerbations of asthma symptoms. Studies of the duration of bronchodilator effects of the noncatecholamines suggest that they would also be suitable for regularly scheduled, prophylactic maintenance therapy of asthma. However, bronchodilatation studies may overestimate the duration of effectiveness of these agents in preventing symptoms provoked by exercise and various environmental stimuli. The magnitude and persistence of effect of these agents in preventing airway obstruction triggered by various types of bronchial provocation may more accurately predict their efficacy for prophylactic therapy. Studies of this type suggest that currently recommended dosing schedules for inhaled beta$_2$-agonists leave patients unprotected at the end of longer dosing intervals and thus do not provide around-the-clock effectiveness. Studies using bronchial provocation may be useful in designing improved inhaled beta$_2$-agonist dosing strategies for regularly scheduled maintenance therapy for asthma.

Acknowledgments

The authors are grateful to Dr. Mark Powell of Schering, Inc. for information and manuscript review regarding albuterol.

References

Ahrens, R. C., Bonham, A. C., Maxwell, G. A. et al. (1984). A method for comparing the peak intensity and duration of action of aerosolized bronchodilators using bronchoprovocation with methacholine. *Am. Rev. Respir. Dis. 129*: 903-906.

Ahrens, R. C., Harris, J. B., Milavetz, G., Annis, L., Ries, R. (1986). Use of bronchial provocation with histamine to compare the pharmacodynamics of inhaled albuterol and metaproterenol in asthmatic patients. *J. Allergy Clin. Immunol.* (in press).

Ahrens, R. C., and Smith, G. D. (1984). Albuterol: An adrenergic agent for use in the treatment of asthma; pharmacology, pharmacokinetics and clinical use. *Pharmacotherapy 4*: 105-121.

American Conference of Governmental Industrial Hygienists (1978). Air Sampling Instruments. Cincinnati, OH, Edition 5: F9-F10.

Anderson, S. D., Seale, J. P., Rozea, P., et al. (1976). Inhaled and oral salbutamol in exercise-induced asthma. *Am. Rev. Respir. Dis. 114*: 493-500.

Andersson, P., Olsson, O. A. T., and Waldeck, B. (1982). Some problems encountered in the evaluation of new bronchodilating beta-adrenoceptor agonists. *Acta Pharmacol. Toxicol. 51*: 358-364.

Anderton, R. C., Cuff, M. T., and Frith, P. A. et al. (1979). Bronchial responsiveness to inhaled histamine and exercise. *J. Allergy Clin. Immunol. 63*: 315-320.

Assem, E. S. K., and Schild, H. O. (1969). Inhibition by sympathomimetic amines of histamine release induced by antigen in passively sensitized human lung. *Nature 224*: 1028-1029.

Axelrod, J., and Cohn, C. K. (1971). Methyltransferase enzymes in red blood cells. *J. Pharmacol. Exp. Ther. 176*: 650-654.

Ben-Dov, I., Bar-Yishay, E., and Godfrey, S. (1982). Refractory period following exercise-induced asthma unexplained by respiratory heat loss. *Am. Rev. Respir. Dis. 125*: 530-534.

Benet, L. Z. (1984). Pharmacokinetic parameters: Which are necessary to define a drug substance? *Eur. J. Respir. Dis. 65* (Suppl) 134: 45-61.

Benet, L. Z., and Galeazzi, R. L. (1979). Noncompartment determination of the steady-state volume of distribution. *J. Pharm. Sci. 68*: 1071-1074.

Bengtsson, B., and Fagerstrom, P.-O. (1982). Extrapulmonary effects of terbutaline during prolonged administration. *Clin. Pharmacol. Ther. 31*: 726-732.

Berg, G., Lindberg, C., and Ryden, G. (1984). Terbutaline in the treatment of preterm labor. *Eur. J. Respir. Dis. 65*, Suppl. 134: 219-230.

Billing, B., Dahlquist, R., Garle, M., Hornblad, I., and Ripe, E. (1984). Simultaneous treatment with terbutaline and theophylline. *Eur. J. Respir. Dis. 65* (Suppl) 134: 211-218.

Blackwell, E. W., Briant, R. H., Conolly, M. E., et al. (1974). Metabolism of Isoprenaline after aerosol and direct intra-bronchial administration in man and dog. *Br. J. Pharmacol. 50*: 587-591.

Bloomfield, P., Carmichael, J., Petrie, G. R., Jewell, N. P., and Crompton, G. K. (1979). Comparison of salbutamol given intravenously and by positive pressure breathing in life-threatening asthma. *Br. Med. J. 1*: 848-850.

Brown, M. J., Brown, D. C., and Murphy, M. B. (1983). Hypokelemia from $beta_2$-receptor stimulation by circulating epinephrine. *N. Engl. J. Med. 309*: 1414-1419.

Buck, J., and Bundegaard, A. (1984). Cardiovascular effects of intramuscular or inhaled terbutaline in asthmatics. *Acta Pharmacol. Toxicol. 54*: 183-188.

Choo-Kang, Y. F. J., Simpson, W. T., and Grant, I. W. B. (1969). Controlled comparison of the bronchodilator effects of three beta-adrenergig stimulant drugs administered by inhalation to patients with asthma. *Br. Med. J. 2*: 287-289.

Choo-Kang, Y. F. J., MacDonald, H. L., and Horne, N. W. (1973). A comparison of salbutamol and terbutaline aerosols in bronchial asthma. *Practitioner 211*: 802-803.

Clay, M. M., Pavia, D., Newman, S. P., et al. (1983). Assessment of jet nebulizers for lung aerosol therapy. *Lancet 2*: 592-594.

Clutter, W. E., Bier, D. M., Shah, S. D., and Cryer, P. E. (1980). Epinephrine plasma metabolic clearance rates and physiological thresholds for metabolic and hemodynamic actions in man. *J. Clin. Invest. 66*: 94-101.

Cockroft, D. W., Killian, D. N., Mellon, J. J. A., et al. (1977). Bronchial reactivity to inhaled histamine: A method and clinical survey. *Clin. Allergy 7*: 235-243.

Cockroft, D. W., Berschied, B. A., Dosman, J A., et al. (1981). Comparison of bitolterol mesylate and metaproterenol sulfate. *Cur. Ther. Res. 30*: 817-824.

Cryer, P. E. (1980). Physiology and pathophysiology of the human sympathoadrenal neuroendocrine system. *N. Engl. J. Med. 303*: 436-444.

Davies, D. S., George, C. F., Blackwell, E., Conolly, M. E., and Dollery, C. T. (1974). Metabolism of terbutaline in man and dog. *Br. J. Clin. Pharmacol. 1*: 129-136.

Davies, D. S. (1984a). Pharmacokinetics of terbutaline after oral absorption. *Eur. J. Resp. Dis. 65, Suppl. 134*: 111-117.

Davies, D. S. (1984b). The fate of inhaled terbutaline. *Eur. J. Respir. Dis. 65* Suppl. 134: 141-147.

Del Bono, N., Quartieri, F., and Vibelli, C. (1979). Aerosolized clenbuterol (NAB 365) and salbutamol in exercise-induced asthma. *Curr. Med. Res. Opin. 6*(4): 237-243.

Dennis, R. R. (ed.) (1977). Handbook of Aerosols. Washington, D.C., Energy Research and Developmental Administration, Publication # TID-26608.

Dolovich, M. B., Sanchis, J., Rossman, C., et al. (1976). Aerosol penetrance: A sensitive index of peripheral airways obstruction. *J. Appl. Physiol. 40*: 468-471.

Dulfano, M. J., and Glass, P. (1976). The bronchodilator effects of terbutaline: Route of administration and patterns of response. *Ann. Allergy 37*: 357-366.

Eggleston, P. A., and Beasley, P. P. (1981). Bronchodilation and inhibition of exercise induced bronchospasm. *Clin. Pharmacol. Ther. 29*: 505-510.

Eggleston, P. A., and McMahan, S. A. (1978). The effects of fenoterol, ephedrine, and placebo on exercise induced asthma. *Chest 73*: 1006-1008.

Enna, S. J., and Schanker, L. S. (1972). Absorption of drugs from the rat lung. *Am. J. Physiol. 223*: 1227-1231.

Evans, M. E., Walker, S. R., Brittain, R. T., and Paterson, J. W. (1973). The metabolism of salbutamol in man. *Xenobiotica 3*: 113-120.

Fagerstrom, P.-O. (1984). Pharmacokinetics of terbutaline after parenteral administration. *Eur. J. Respir. Dis. 54* Suppl 134: 101-110.

Finney, D. J. (1978). *Statistical Method in Biological Assay,* ed. 3. London, Charles Griffin and Company, pp. 112-115.

Fitzgerald, G. A., Barnes, P., Hamilton, C. A., and Dollery, C. T. (1980). Circulating adrenaline and blood pressure: The metabolic effects and kinetics of infused adrenalin in man. *Eur. J. Clin. Invest. 10*: 401-406.

Francis, P. W. J., Krastins, I. R. B., and Levison, H. (1980). Oral and inhaled salbutamol in exercise-induced bronchospasm. *Pediatrics 66*: 103-108.

Freedman, B. J. (1971). Trial of new bronchodilator, terbutaline in asthma. *Br. Med. J. 1*: 633-636.

Freedman, B. J. (1972). Trial of a terbutaline aerosol in the treatment of asthma and comparison of its effects with those of salbutamol aerosol. *Br. J. Dis. Chest 66*: 222-229.

Gryglewski, R., and Vane, J. R. (1970). The inactivation of noradrenaline and isoprenaline in dogs. *Br. J. Pharmacol. 39*: 573-584.

Harris, J. B., Ahrens, R. C., Annis, L., et al. (1986a). Comparison of the intervals and duration of effect of albuterol and bitolterol using bronchial provocation with histamine. *Ann. Allergy 56*(6): 250.

Harris, J. B., Ahrens, R. C., Milavetz, G., et al. (1986b). Relative potencies and rates of decline in effect of inhaled albuterol (A) and terbutaline (T). *J. Allergy Clin. Immunol. 77*, No. 1, part 2, 147.

Hartnett, B. J. S., and Marlin, G. E. (1977). Comparison of terbutaline and salbutamol aerosols. *Aust. N.Z. J. Med. 7*(1): 13-15.

Herschfus, J. A., Bresnick, E., Levison, L., et al. (1951). A new sympathomimetic amine ("neosuprel") in the treatment of bronchial asthma. *Ann. Allergy 9*: 769-773.

Hornblad, Y., Ripe, E., Magnusson, P. O., and Tegner, K. (1976). The metabolism and clinical activity of terbutaline and its prodrug ibuterol. *Eur. J. Clin. Pharmacol. 10*: 9-18.

Holford, N. H. G., and Sheiner, L. B. (1981). Understanding the dose-effect relationship: Clinical application of pharmacokinetic-pharmacodynamic models. *Clin. Pharm. 6*: 420-453.

Howarth, P. H., Durham, S. R., Lee, T. H., et al. (1985). Influence of albuterol, cromolyn sodium and ipratorium bromide on the airway and circulating mediator response to allergen bronchial provocation in asthma. *Am. Rev. Respir. Dis. 132*: 986-992.

Huhti, E., and Poukkula, A. (1978). Clinical comparison of fenoterol and albuterol administered by inhalation. A double-blind study. *Chest 73*: 348-351.

Jack, D. (1971). An introduction to salbutamol and other modern beta-adrenoreceptor stimulants. *Postgrad. Med. J. 47* (Suppl): 8-11.

Jenne, J. W., and Tashkin, D. P. (1983). Bronchodilators as a bronchial challenge: A critical assessment. In *Provocation Challenge Procedures: Bronchial, Oral Nasal and Exercise.* Edited by S. L. Spector. Boca Raton, Florida, CRC Press, pp. 19-74.

Jenne, J. W., Ridley, D. J., Marcucci, R. A., Druz, W. S., and Rook, J. C. (1982). Objective and subjective tremor responses to oral $beta_2$ adrenergic agents on first exposure. A comparison of metaproterenol and terbutaline. *Am. Rev. Respir. Dis. 126*: 607-610.

Jenne, J. W., Shaughnessy, T. K., Manfredi, C. J., and Druz, W. S. (1985). Bronchodilation by isoproterenol depends on both dose and nature of the constricting stimulus in the dog. *Am. Rev. Respir. Dis. 131*, No. 4, part 2, A280 (abstract).

Jenne, J. W., Valcarenghi, G., Druz, W. S., Starkey, P. W., Yu, C., and Shaughnessy, T. (1986). Comparison of tremor responses to oral albuterol. *Am. Rev. Respir. Dis. 134*: 708-713.

Joad, S., Ahrens, R. C., Lindgren, S., and Weinberger, M. M. (1987). Relative efficacy of maintenance therapy with theophylline, inhaled albuterol, and the combination for chronic asthma. *J. Allergy Clin. Immunol.* (in press).

Juniper, E. F., Frith, P. A., Dunnett, C., et al. (1978). Reproducibility and comparison of responses to inhaled histamine and methacholine. *Thorax 33*: 705-710.

Juniper, E. F., Frith, P. A., and Hargreave, F. E. (1981). Airway responsiveness to histamine and methacholine: Relationship of minimum treatment to control symptoms of asthma. *Thorax 36*: 575-579.

Kass, I., and Mingo, T. S. (1980). Bitolterol mesylate aerosol. A new long acting bronchodilator with reduced chronotropic effects. *Chest 78*: 283-287.

Konig, P., Eggleston, P., and Serby, C. (1981). Oral and inhaled metaproterenol in exercise induced asthma. *J. Allergy Clin. Immunol. 67* (Suppl): 110.

Larsson, S., and Svedmyr, N. (1977). Bronchodilating effect and side effects of $beta_2$-adrenoceptor stimulants by different modes of administration (tablets, metered-dose aerosol, and combination thereof). *Am. Rev. Respir. Dis. 116*: 861-869.

Lawford, P., Jones, B. J. M., and Milledge, J. S. (1978). Comparison of intravenous and nebulized salbutamol in initial treatment of severe asthma. *Br. Med. J. 1*: 84.

Leferink, J. G., Van den Berg, W., Wagemaker-Engels, J., Kruekneit, J., and Maes, R. A. A. (1982). Pharmacokinetics of terbutaline, a $beta_2$-sympathomimetic in healthy volunteers and asthmatic patients. *Arzneim Forsch. 32*: 159-164.

Leitch, A. G., Clancy, L. J., Costello, J. F., and Flenley, O. C. (1976). Effect of intravenous infusion of salbutamol on ventilatory response, heart rate and plasma potassium in normal men. *Br. Med. J. 1*: 365-367.

Levy, S., Mallett, S., and Levine, S. (1986). Comparison of the effects of two $beta_2$ (β_2) agonists with respect to bronchodilator and skeletal muscle tremor responses. *Am. Rev. Respir. Dis. 133*, No. 4, part 2: A63.

Liechtenstein, L. M., and Margolis, S. (1968). Histamine release *in vitro*: Inhibition by catecholamines and methylxanthines. *Science 161*: 902-903.

Lin, C., Li, Y., McGlothlen, J., and Symchowikz, S. (1977). Isolation and identification of the major metabolite of albuterol in human urine. *Drug Metab. Dispos. 5*: 234-238.

Lonnerholm, G., Foucard, T., and Lindstrom, B. (1984). Dose, plasma concentration and effect of oral terbutaline in long-term treatment of childhood asthma. *J. Allergy Clin. Immunol. 73*: 508.

Maconochie, M. L., and Fowler, P. (1983). Plasma concentrations of salbutamol after an oral slow release preparation. *Curr. Med. Res. Opin. 8*: 634-640.

Makino, S. (1966). Clinical significance of bronchial sensitivity to acetylcholine and histamine. *J. Allergy 38*: 127-142.

Martin, L. E., Hobson, J. C., Page, J. A., and Harrison, C. (1971). Metabolic studies of salbutamol ^{3}H: A new bronchodilator in rat, rabbit, dog and man. *Eur. J. Pharmacol. 14*: 183-199.

Massey, K. L., Hendeles, L., Harman, E., et al. (1986). The effect of increasing doses of inhaled gallopamil on airway reactivity to methacholine in intermittent asthmatics. *Am. Rev. Respir. Dis.* (abstract) *133(4)*: A57.

Metzler, C. m., Lefering, G. L., and McEwen, A. J. (1974). A package of computer programs for pharmacokinetic modeling. *Biometrics 30*: 562.

Morris, H. G., Sherman, N. A., Silvers, W. S., Mills, D., and Shepperdson, F. T. (1983). Timed effects of an oral adrenergic bronchodilator on pulmonary function and measurement of plasma and leukocyte cyclic AMP. Divergence in duration of drug action and development of tolerance. *J. Allergy Clin. Immunol. 71*: 266-276.

Newman, S. P., Pavia, D., and Clarke, S. W. (1981). How should pressurized aerosols be inhaled? *Eur. J. Respir. Dis. 62*: 3-21.

Nyberg, L. (1984). Pharmacokinetic parameters of terbutaline in healthy men. An overview. *Eur. J. Respir. Dis. 65* (Suppl) 134: 149-160.

Nyberg, L., and Kennedy, B.-M. (1984). Pharmacokinetics of terbutaline given in slow-release tablets. *Eur. J. Respir. Dis. 65* (Suppl) 132: 119-139.

O'Byrne, P. M., Ryan, G., Morris, M., et al. (1982). Asthma induced by cold air and its relationship to nonspecific bronchial responsiveness to methacholine. *Am. Rev. Respir. Dis. 125*: 281-289.

O'Donnell, S. R., and Wanstall, J. C. (1978). Evidence that the efficacy (intrinsic activity) of fenoterol is higher than that of salbutamol in beta-adrenoceptors in guinea-pig trachea. *Eur. J. Pharmacol. 47*: 333-340.

Olsson, O. A. T., Swanberg, E., Svedinger, I., and Waldeck, B. (1979). Effect of beta-adrenoceptor agonists on airway smooth muscle and on slow-contracting skeletal muscle: In vitro and in vivo results compared. *Acta Pharmacol. Toxicol (Copnh) 44*: 272-276.

Orgel, H. A., Kemp, J. P., Tinkelman, D. G., et al. (1985). Bitolterol and albuterol metered-dose aerosols: Comparison of two long-acting beta$_2$-adrenergic bronchodilators for treatment of asthma. *J. Allergy Clin. Immunol. 75*: 55-62.

Pierce, R. J., Payne, C. R., Williams, S. J., Denison, and Clark, T. J. H. (1981). Comparison of intravenous and inhaled terbutaline in the treatment of asthma. *Chest 79*: 506-511.

Richardson, J. B. (1977). The neural control of human tracheobronchial smooth muscle. In *Asthma: Physiology, Immunopharmacology, and Treatment.* Edited by L. M. Lichtenstein and K. F. Austen. Academic Press, New York.

Ruffin, R. E., Montgomery, J. M., and Newhouse, M. (1978). Site of beta-adrenergic receptors in the respiratory tract. *Chest 74*: 256-260.

Ruffin, R. E., Alpers, M. B., Crockett, A. J., et al. (1981). Repeated histamine inhalation tests in asthmatic patients. *J. Allergy Clin. Immunol. 67*: 285-289.

Sackner, M. A., Greeneitch, N., Silva, G., Wanner, A. (1974). Bronchodilator effects of terbutaline and epinephrine in obstructive lung disease. *Clin. Pharmacol. Ther. 16*: 499-506.

Sackner, M. A., Dougherty, R., Watson, H., and Wanner, A. (1975). Hemodynamic effects of epinephrine and terbutaline in normal man. *Chest 68*: 616-624.

Salome, C. M., Schoeffel, R. E., Yan, K., et al. (1983). Fenoterol on the severity of bronchial hyperreactivity in patients with asthma. *Thorax 38*: 854-858.

Sando, M. F., Douglas, F. L., Green, J., Banner, A. S., and Leff, A. R. (1985). Homeostatic regulation of bronchodilator tone by sympathetic activation during bronchoconstriction in normal and asthmatic humans. *Am. Rev. Respir. Dis. 132*: 993-998.

Schentag, J. J., Jusko, W. J., Vance, J. W., Cumbo, T. J., Abrutyn, E., DeLattre, M., and Gerbracht, L. M. (1979). Gentamycin disposition and tissue accumulation in multiple dosing. *J. Pharmacokinet. Biopharm. 5*: 559-577.

Schwartz, H. J., Trautlein, J. J., and Goldstein, A. R. (1976). Acute effects of terbutaline and epinephrine in asthma. *J. Allergy Clin. Immunol. 58*: 516-522.

Shargel, L., Dorrbecker, S. A., and Levitt, M. (1976). Physiological disposition and metabolism of N-t-butylarterenol and its Di-p-toluate ester (bitolterol) in the rat. *Drug. Metab. Dispos. 4*(1): 65-71.

Shenfield, G. M., Evans, M. E., and Paterson, J. W. (1976). Absorption of drugs by the lung. *Br. J. Clin. Pharmacol. 3*: 583-589.

Shenfield, G. M., and Paterson, J. W. (1973). Clinical assessment of bronchodilator drugs delivered by aerosol. *Thorax 28*: 124-128.

Sly, M., Heimlich, E. M., Ginsburg, J., et al. (1968). Exercise-induced bronchospasm: Evaluation of metaproterenol. *Ann. Allergy 26*: 253-258.

Stearns, D. R., McFadden, E. R., Breslin, F. J., et al. (1981). Reanalysis of the refractory period in exertional asthma. *J. Appl. Physiol. 50*: 503-508.

Svedmyr, N. (1985). Fenoterol: A $beta_2$-adrenergic agonist for use in asthma. Pharmacology, pharmacokinetics, clinical efficacy, and adverse effects. *Pharmacotherapy 5*: 109-125.

Svedmyr, N., and Thiringer, G. (1971). The effects of salbutamol and isoproterenol on beta-2 receptors in patients with chronic obstructive lung disease. *Postgrad. Med. 44* (Suppl): 44-46.

Tegner, K., Nilsson, H. T., Persson, C. G. A., Persson, K., and Ryrfeldt, A. (1984). Elimination pathways of terbutaline. *Eur. J. Respir. Dis. 65*: Suppl 124: 93-100.

Torphy, T. J., Rinard, G. A., Rietow, M. G., et al. (1983). Functional antagonism in canine tracheal smooth muscle: Inhibition by methacholine of mechanical and biochemical responses to isproterenol. *J. Pharmacol. Exp. Ther. 227*: 694-699.

Van den Berg, W. (1982). Clinical implications of drug-induced desensitization of the beta receptor after continuous oral use of terbutaline. *J. Allergy Clin. Immunol. 69*: 410.

Van den Berg, W., Leferink, J. G., Maes, R. A. A., Kerukneit, J., and Bruynzeel, P. L. B. (1980). Correlation between terbutaline serum levels, cAMP plasma levels and FEV_1 in normals and asthmatics after subcutaneous administration. *Ann. Allergy 44*: 235-239.

Van den Berg, W., Leferink, J. G., Maes, R. A. A., Fokkens, J. K., Krueukniet, J., and Bruynzeel, P. L. B. (1984). The effects of oral and subcutaneous administration of terbutaline in asthmatic patients. *Eur. J. Respir. Dis. 65* (Suppl) 134: 181-193.

Van Den Brink, F. G. (1973). The model of functional interaction. 1. Development and first check of a new model of functional synergism·and antagonism. *Eur. J. Pharmacol. 22*: 270-278.

Wagner, J. G. (1976). Linear pharmacokinetic equations during direct calculation of needed pharmacokinetic parameters from the coefficients and exponents of polyexponential equations which have been fitted to data. *J. Pharmacokin. Biopharm. 4*: 443-467.

Walker, S. R., Evans, M. E., Richards, A. J., and Paterson, J. W. (1972). The clinical pharmacology of oral and inhaled salbutamol. *Clin. Pharmacol. Ther. 13*: 861-867.

Watson, E. M., and Richens, A. (1974). The effect of salbutamol and terbutaline on physiological tremor, bronchial tone and heart rate. *Br. J. Clin. Pharmacol. 1*: 223-227.

Weber, R. W., Petty, W. E., and Nelson, H. S. (1979). Aerosolized terbutaline in asthmatics: Comparison of dosage, strength, schedule, and method of administration. *J. Allergy Clin. Immunol. 63*: 116-121.

Williams, M., and Kane, C. (1975). Dose response of patients with asthma to inhaled isoproterenol. *Am. Rev. Respir. Dis. 11*: 321-324.

Williams, S., and Seaton, A. (1977). Intravenous or inhaled salbutamol in severe acute asthma? *Thorax 32*: 555-558.

Williams, F. M., Briant, R. H., Dollery, C. T., et al. (1974). The influence of route of administration on urinary metabolites of isoetharine. *Xenobiotica 4*: 345-353.

William, S. J., Parrish, R. W., and Seaton, A. (1975). Comparison of intravenous aminophylline and salbutamol in severe asthma. *Br. Med. J. 4*: 685.

Wolfe, J. D., Yamate, M., Bieder, A. A., and Chu, T. J. (1985). Comparison of the acute cardiopulmonary effects of oral albuterol, metaproterenol and terbutaline in asthmatics. *JAMA 253*: 2068-2072.

Woolcock, A. J. (1977). Inhaled drugs in the prevention of asthma. *Am. Rev. Respir. Dis. 115*: 191-194.

7

Beta-Adrenergic Tachyphylaxis (Desensitization) and Functional Antagonism

MATTHEW E. CONOLLY, KA KIT HUI, and STEVEN E. BORST

UCLA School of Medicine
Los Angeles, California

JOHN. W. JENNE

Loyola-Stritch School of Medicine, Maywood, and Edward Hines, Jr. Veterans Administration Hospital
Hines, Illinois

I. Tachyphylaxis

If music be the food of love, play on
Give me excess of it, that surfeiting,
the appetite may sicken and so die

Twelfth Night
Act I, Scene I

The immortal bard reminds us that there is nothing new under the sun, and that the concept of a waning response to oft-repeated stimuli is long established.

A. Historical Highlights

The work of Sir Henry Dale and others in the early years of this century led to the recognition of the existence of cell surface receptors specific to given agonists. With this recognition, it has become possible to envisage mechanisms whereby agonist-induced desensitization (and denervation supersensitivity too, for that matter) might occur. Within the last decade, the development of highly radioactive ligands that also exhibit high pharmacologic specificity has enormously aided investigations in these areas. Several receptors including those for acetylcholine, insulin, and angiotensin have been studied using these techniques, as well as beta-adrenergic receptors (adrenoceptors), which form the focus of this chapter.

Beta-adrenoceptors and bronchial asthma have been linked in the minds of clinicians ever since 1909, when Matthews in England (1900) and Ephraim in Germany (1910) first applied epinephrine to the respiratory tract in an attempt to treat asthma. Over the ensuing two to three decades, an increasing trickle of reports on this form of therapy appeared. It received a major boost in the 1940s when Konsett synthesized isoproterenol, the first adrenergic agonist without significant alpha-adrenergic activity. In a sense, this paved the way for Alqvist's (1948) classic studies which, for the first time, clearly identified the alpha- and beta-adrenoceptor subtypes. Lands and his co-workers (1967) built on this when, almost twenty years later, they showed that beta-receptors could be further subdivided into $beta_1$ and $beta_2$ subcategories.

Therapeutics marched in step with these developments, as physicians first substituted the predominantly beta agonist isoproterenol for epinephrine, and then later salbutamol, terbutaline, fenoterol, and others, all of which exhibit a degree of selectivity for the $beta_2$-receptor.

Another advance in the use of beta-agonists in asthma has been the development of small pressurized aerosols that deliver precisely metered doses of the bronchodilator, which is suspended, in microfine crystalline form, in the freon propellant. These unobtrusive devices were introduced in 1960. By virtue of their own convenience they won quick acceptance by physicians and patients alike, and thus the almost totally unregulated use of adrenergic bronchodilators soared, more so in some countries than others.

With hindsight, it is possible to perceive an increasingly frequent incidence of sudden asthmatic deaths associated with the use of adrenergic bronchodilators, beginning before World War II. It began with a report by Graeser (1939) of two patients who died of asthma after inhaling excessive amounts of a 1% epinephrine spray. An autopsy performed on one of them revealed extensive mucus plugging of the smaller bronchi. Benson and Perlman (1948) reviewed a series of 2236 asthmatic patients under their care. Epinephrine aerosols had been used by 648 patients, of whom 48 (7.4%) had died of asthma, whereas out of 1588 patients who had not used the spray, only 22 (1.4%) had so died. The inherent severity of asthma in the two groups was not recorded. It was, however, noted that in many of the patients using epinephrine, its efficacy declined with prolonged use, necessitating the consumption of larger and larger doses. In a report of isoproterenol inhalation therapy, Lowell et al. (1949) reported the sudden and unexpected deaths of two patients who had taken progressively increasing dosages of the aerosol. Keighley (1966) reported three patients whose obstructive airways disease was made worse by the inhalation of isoproterenol, and van Metre (1968) gave an account of nine patients dying of asthma who has used aerosols of isoproterenol to excess. Twelve other patients were described in whom a similar picture resolved only when the isoproterenol was withdrawn. Adverse effects were further described by Reisman (1970) in chronic "overusers." The sulfite in these bronchodilator solutions may have been a factor (Koepke et al., 1983).

This issue was brought into sharp and stark focus when Speizer and his colleagues (1968a,b) published two papers showing that from the time that the small pressurized aerosols had become available, the asthma death rate for England and Wales had risen sharply among patients aged 5-34 years. The increase was greatest among those between 10 and 14 years old, in whom the mortality rate increase was 830%. During this period 1961-1966, there were in England and Wales, 3,500 more asthmatic deaths among 5-34 year olds than would have been predicted on the basis of the mortality rate for this age range over the preceding decade. The factors responsible for this are complex and may never be fully understood. Autopsies were performed on many of these patients because their deaths were considered sudden and unexpected. It was found that almost all had changes typical of an asthmatic death, with mucus plugging of the small airways and hyperinflated lungs, and 77% were found to have received little or no steroids. It was also noted that 83% had used pressurized aerosols, most of which contained isoproterenol. Several patients were found dead, with empty aerosol cannisters beside them, and it seems clear that there had been widespread misuse of these devices with inadequate medical supervision.

This sequence of events has helped to focus considerable attention on the question of beta-adrenoceptor function, and there has been a considerable debate of the chicken-and-egg variety on whether there is an inherent defect in beta-adrenoceptor function that actually causes patients to be asthmatic, or whether asthmatics have inherently normal beta-receptors that become abnormal as a result of the disease or the drugs used to treat it. The concept of an inherent defect of the beta-receptor drew support from clinical observations of blunted physiological and metabolic responses to adrenergic agonists in asthmatics (Cookson and Reed, 1963; Lockey et al., 1967; Inoue, 1967). These data were augmented by the experimental studies of Szentivanyi (1968). He observed an apparent reduction in beta receptor responses in guinea pigs when they had been sensitized with *B. pertussis* vaccine, and Szentivanyi has most vigorously argued that the primary defect in the asthmatic lies in the beta-receptor (Krzenowski and Szentivanyi, 1983). This concept gained support from studies showing depressed beta adrenoceptor function in leukocytes of asthmatics during acute exacerbations (Parker and Smith, 1973). The alternative hypothesis, first explored by Conolly and Greenacre (1976), was that the reduced beta-adrenergic responses seen in asthmatics is not a primary feature, but is a result of prolonged exposure to beta-adrenergic bronchodilators. Studying lymphocyte beta-receptor function, they found marked depression of the cyclic AMP response to isoproterenol in asthmatics using adrenergic drugs, but not in asthmatics of comparable severity who were treated exclusively with nonadrenergic medications such as cromolyn or beclomethasone (Fig. 1). Asthmatics weaned off adrenergic drugs

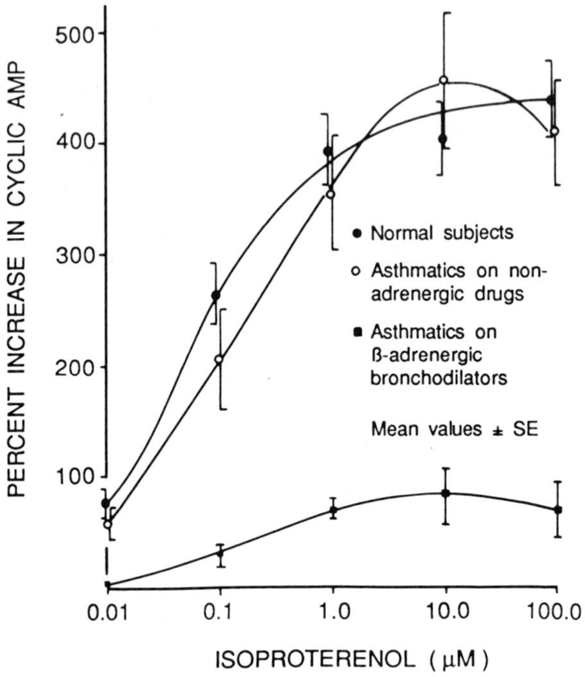

Figure 1 Percentage increase in cyclic AMP in lymphocytes after a 15-min incubation at 37°C with isoproterenol. Lymphocytes were taken from normal subjects (O-----O); asthmatic patients receiving only nonadrenergic drugs (O-----O); asthmatic patients taking excessive dosages of β-adrenergic bronchodilators (——) (reproduced with permission from Conolly and Greenacre, 1976).

reverted to a normal pattern of response, while previously normal (nonasthmatic) obstetric patients developed a marked attentuation of the lymphocyte cyclic AMP response after a 48 hr infusion of a beta-agonist, given to prevent the onset of premature labor. Other early workers expanded on this theme (Morris et al., 1977; Svedmyr et al., 1976; Jenne et al., 1977a; Nelson et al., 1977; Plummer, 1978; Galant et al., 1978.

B. Prospective Studies in Humans

From this beginning, numerous groups have studied the development of tachyphylaxis as a clinical phenomenon, and the mechanisms whereby such tachyphylaxis might develop have been extensively investigated. Studies performed in vitro utilizing a variety of animal tissues, cultured cells, human leukocytes, and human bronchial smooth muscle uniformly show that the response to beta-agonists is lessened with prolonged exposure to these compounds, even though the mechanism involved may not be the same in each case (see below).

In contrast to the uniformity of the in vitro studies, clinical studies have produced disturbingly conflicting results, in that not every study of asthmatics has been able to produce evidence of bronchial tolerance to adrenergic bronchodilators. The reason for this discrepancy is far from clear, although in early studies preceding beta-adrenergic drugs were not scrupulously withdrawn. It may be related to factors other than the actual process of tachyphylaxis, such as the route of administration, effectiveness of drug delivery, the sensitivity of the tests used to demonstrate the onset of desensitization, and finally, of course, the population being studied. In treating a disease with the complexity of asthma, it should be remembered that reversible airways obstruction, which all asthmatics exhibit, may be due to a variety of causes, so that susceptibility to drug-induced changes, and the impact they have, may differ greatly. Thus, Jenne et al. (1977a), Nelson et al. (1977), Miller (1978), Chervinsky (1978), Van Arsdel et al. (1978), Plummer (1978), Weber and co-workers (1982), and Repsher et al. (1984) all showed the development of a degree of tolerance to bronchodilators after their prolonged use, while, in contrast, Taylor and Heimlick (1965), Wilson et al. (1976), Larsson and colleagues (1976), Sims and co-workers (1978), and Peel and Gibson (1980) all failed to demonstrate the development of any tolerance.

The complexities, precautions, and distinctions made in conducting these studies have been analyzed (Larsson, 1979; Jenne, 1982) and are discussed below.

1. Many earlier studies neglected to withdraw patients from their usual sympathomimetic therapy for a sufficient period (2 weeks) before commencing the study, thus diluting the effect of the new beta-agonist exposure.

2. A concurrent placebo group has usually been absent. Thus, seasonal factors could contaminate the data (Chap. 5). A concurrent placebo group with a crossover design was employed by Löwhagen et al. (1985) in one negative study. A partial solution is to follow the test period with a period off the drug to ensure that original sensitivity returns (Jenne et al., 1977a; Weber et al., 1982).

3. Rising or falling baseline pulmonary function during the study precludes valid use of "percent increase" or "change" in bronchodilator response. Yet this approach is still in use. Only if baseline functions remain unchanged is such use warranted. To compensate for changing baseline function, the bronchodilator responses should be expressed as absolute peak values at that time (Jenne et al., 1977), or "percent achievable response" (Tashkin et al., 1982; Conolly et al., 1982).

4. Peak responses may be less sensitive than the duration of response of the area under the response curve (AUC). Therefore, the total response over time

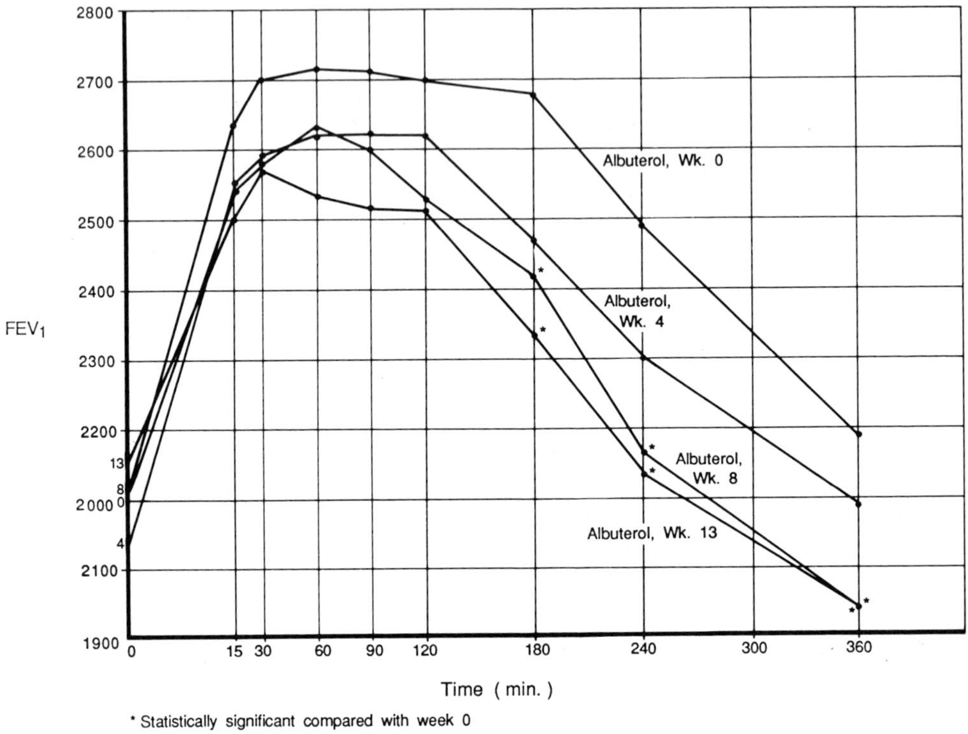

Figure 2 Absolute values of mean FEV_1 after inhalation of albuterol aerosol at study weeks, 0.4, 8, and 13. There is no significant difference in peak bronchodilation, but there is a significant difference in duration of bronchodilation between week 0 and weeks 8 and 13 (reproduced with permission from Repsher et al., 1984).

should be documented. An example of this distinction is one in which 58 asthmatics using albuterol by inhaler showed significant tachyphylaxis by the AUC or duration criteria, but an insignificant response by the peak improvement, although all studies were done in absolute terms (Repsher et al., 1984) (Fig. 2). These authors could not document tachyphylaxis to isoproterenol in an identical study design, a finding that also raises the question of differing beta-agonists.

5. Concurrent drug therapy must remain constant. Corticosteroids may reduce any development of tachyphylaxis as suggested by the data of Weber and colleagues (1982), Holgate et al. (1977), and Ellul-Micallef and Fenech (1975).

6. The pulmonary function tests selected to measure response may miss a positive response if they measure different things. For example, asthmatics

inhaling terbutaline developed tachyphylaxis when analyzed by measurements of specific airway conductance, which measures large airway effects, but did not develop tachyphylaxis when analyzed by measurements of flow which reflected small airway function. The difference was attributed to the greater deposition of beta-agonist particles in the large airways. Systemic delivery of drug (5.0 mg terbutaline orally three times daily) did not produce tachyphylaxis as measured by either test (Tashkin et al., 1982).

7. Tests of improvement in spirometry or specific airway conductance may reflect different airway responses than tests of improvement in airway reactivity. In the first case, relaxation of airway tone is involved. In the second, a sudden increase in tone is being resisted by the bronchodilator. Examples of the second variety include studies by Peel and Gibson (1980), Löwhagen et al. (1985), and Tashkin et al. (1982) using histamine or methacholine provocation. All were negative for tachyphylaxis. The nature of the provoking stimulus may also make a difference. Antigenic challenge represents a mixture of signals, some of which may be altered by the beta-agonist. In one of these studies, there was a suggestion of tachyphylaxis to protection from antigen challenge, but none to methacholine (Tashkin et al., 1982).

8. Population differences may be a factor. The most striking example of this to date is the ease with which tachyphylaxis can be induced in normals, and the difficulty of producing it in asthmatics (Harvey and Tattersfield, 1979, 1982; Tashkin et al., 1982).

9. Results may vary with the duration of exposure. Tachyphylaxis may continue to develop beyond the 4-week period (Repsher et al., 1984; Plummer, 1978).

10. Individual differences in susceptibility are hidden in the analysis of the whole group, and may also lead to either a false-positive or -negative result if the study group is too small.

11. Developing tachyphylaxis may not only show up in single bronchodilator responses but also be reflected in a deterioration of baseline function (Weber et al., 1982).

The central questions still to be asked, even if tachyphylaxis is shown, is whether the degree of tachyphylaxis is clinically important. Most positive studies would suggest that it is not. The therapeutic response still occurs, although the dosage may have to be increased slightly. What has not been answered is (1) whether more intense beta agonist stimulation will cause more significant tachyphylaxis (although both Larsson et al., 1976; and Löwhagen, 1985, used relatively large dosages) and (2) whether some few individuals are particularly at risk of severe tachyphylaxis. Only further studies with preselected individuals can answer this question.

Continuing in this vein, it is interesting to compare the inconsistencies in results of Lichterfield and Lollgen (1974) with those of Paterson et al. (1971). The first group gave repeated infusions of isoproterenol to 12 asthmatics, and failed to demonstrate any tachyphylaxis. No ill effects were reported. The second group gave a dose ranging infusion of isoproterenol to 15 asthmatics, at the end of which four developed severe rebound bronchoconstriction, were relatively refractory or resistant to further adrenergic bronchodilators, two responding only to aminophylline and corticosteroid. There is now even inconsistency in the development of desensitization reported by Harvey and Tattersfield (1979) and by Tashkin et al. (1982) in normal subjects but not in similarly treated asthmatics. The latter group has shown such desensitization to develop in other similar asthmatics after prolonged bronchodilator therapy (Conolly et al., unpublished observations).

C. Studies in Intact Animals and Excised Airways

In Vivo

In vivo production of airway smooth muscle subsensitivity by systemic administration of beta-agonists in the guinea pig using histamine provocation has been accomplished by a number of investigators (Conolly et al., 1971; Bouhuys et al., 1972; Benoy et al., 1975; Watanabe et al., 1976; Spilker and Tyll, 1976; Anderson and Lees, 1976; Douglas et al., 1977; Elfellah and Turnbull, 1978; Williams et al., 1983; Ward and Tomlinson, 1976), in the rat using methacholine provocation (Avner and Noland, 1978), and in the dog following large dosages of inhaled isoproterenol using methacholine provocation (Cho et al., 1968; Stephan et al., 1980). Interference with the natural ability of the adrenergic nervous system to protect the guinea pig against histamine was shown with repeated injection of isoproterenol, terbutaline, or salbutamol (Conolly et al., 1971). The degree of subsensitivity production by isoproterenol or terbutaline in the rat was shown to be dosage- and time-related, and to wear off progressively over 96 hr following discontinuation of these drugs (Avner and Noland, 1978).

Subsensitivity Production In Vitro in Airway Smooth Muscle

Extending the work of Fleisch and Titus (1972), Lin et al. studied rat tracheal rings under isometric conditions at a constant baseline tension, contracted with carbachol, and then caused to relax with successively increasing concentrations of isoproterenol to produce a cumulative dose-response curve (Lin et al., 1977). After exposure to 5×10^{-6} M isoproterenol for 30 min, these tissues showed a considerable loss of responsiveness to isoproterenol. The affinity for isoproterenol was reduced 180-fold by the method of Furchgott using propranolol. The rings were now also cross-resistant to terbutaline, isoetharine, and epinephrine. They still responded normally to theophylline, D600, sodium nitrate, and hydralazine with relaxation. Preincubation of the tissues with 5×10^{-5} M methylprednisolone did *not* protect against desensitization.

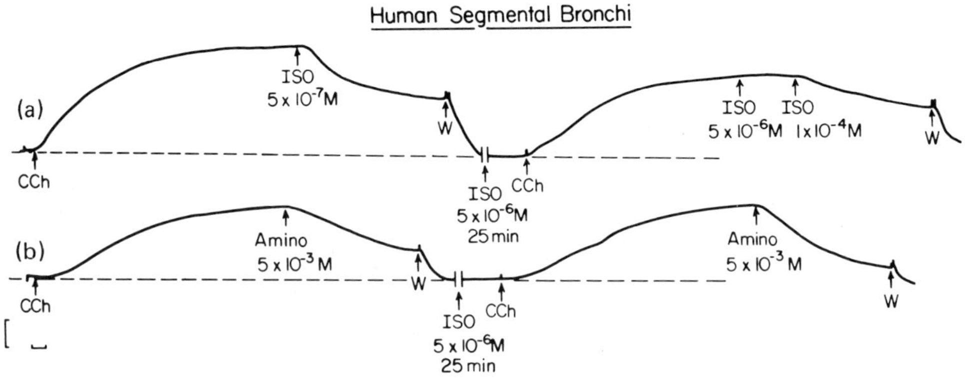

Figure 3 Responsiveness of isolated human bronchi to ISO (a) and AMINO (b) before and after pretreatment with ISO (5×10^{-6} M, 25 min). Dashed line, basal tension (1 g). The vertical and horizontal markers (lower left) represent 1 g tension and 1 min, respectively (reproduced with permission from Avner and Jenne, 1981).

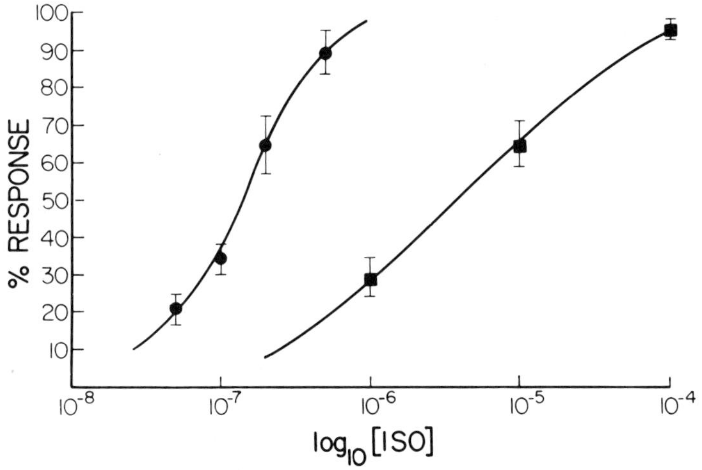

Figure 4 Log_{10} concentration vs. response relationships for ISO in control (o) and desensitized (1×10^{-6} M, 25 min) human bronchial preparations. The means are plotted with the brackets denoting the SEM (reproduced with permission from Avner and Jenne, 1981).

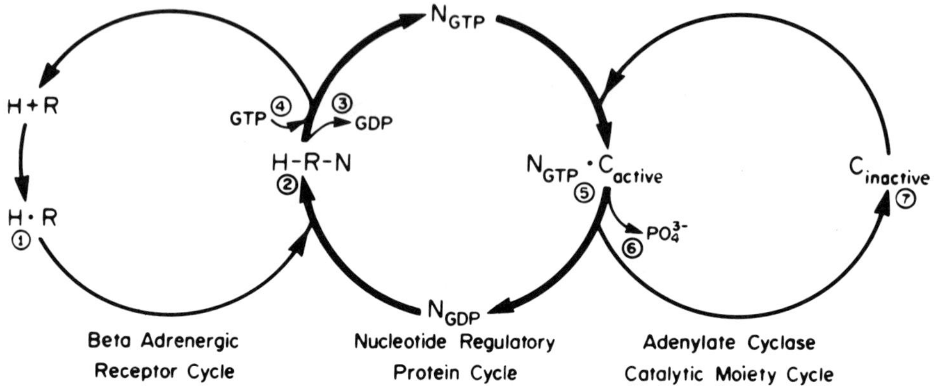

Figure 5 Working model incorporating present concepts for adenylate cyclase activity by hormone agonists and guanine nucleotides. See text for explanation (reproduced with permission from Lefkowitz, 1982).

Using the same approach, the production of subsensitivity in vitro is also possible with bronchi from humans, dog, rat, and rabbit (Avner and Jenne, 1977a,b, 1981). Human bronchi exposed to isoproterenol or to terbutaline in concentrations of 10^{-6} M and 10^{-4} M, respectively, underwent desensitization and a similar loss of affinity, as shown in Figure 3.

After 10^{-6} M isoproterenol for 25 min, there was again a sizable shift in the dose-response curve to the right (Fig. 4) with a reduction in slope. There was also cross-resistance between isoproterenol and terbutaline. Unfortunately, the desensitized tissues were not exposed to corticosteroid to determine whether they would revert towards their normal state.

However, such an experiment was performed by Davis and Conolly (1980) with human bronchi. Those investigators also produced subsensitivity with isoproterenol using a concentration of 4×10^{-4} M for 60 min. The tissues also showed cross-resistance to albuterol. In the presence of only 10^{-9} M isoproterenol, persistence of subsensitivity was prolonged. When drug was removed, 60% of the original sensitivity returned over a period of 3 hr. Its return was complete at 3 hr in the presence of 1.5×10^{-4} M hydrocortisone. Thus, corticosteroid moderately hastened recovery. At a sensitizing concentration of 10^{-6} M isoporterenol, there was considerable interindividual *variation in susceptibility* to desensitization, which may have important clinical implications.

In this connection, it should also be mentioned that in canine tracheal smooth muscle, hydrocortisone has been shown to increase sensitivity to isoproterenol and the production of cyclic AMP by the tissues (Rinard et al., 1983).

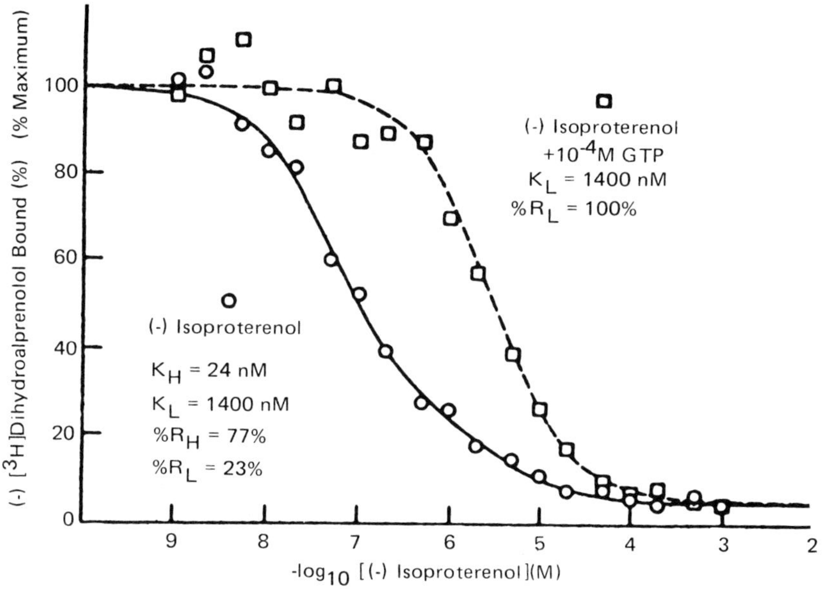

Figure 6 Computer-modeled curves for inhibition of (–) [^{3}H] dihydroapreno-lol binding ([^{3}H] DHA) to frog erythrocyte membranes by (–) isoproterenol in presence and absence of GTP. K_H, the high-affinity dissociation constant; K_L, the low affinity dissociation constant; % R_H, the % receptors in the high-affinity state; %R_L, the % receptors in the low-affinity state. The addition of GTP corresponding to (4) in Figure 5 causes the high-affinity complex H-R-N (2) to dissociate to low-affinity complex (3) and to N_{GTP}, which then activates adenylate cyclase (5) (reproduced with permission from Kent et al., 1980).

D. Mechanisms of Tachyphylaxis

Normal Beta-Receptor Physiology

The relationship between the receptor and adenylate cyclase is thought to be constantly changing as agonist or hormone (H) interacts with the receptor (Fig. 5). The agonist and the receptor first form a complex (H-R) by reversible binding, which then interacts with a nucleotide-binding protein (N) (or G/F in the Harden nomenclature, 1983) causing the release of GDP bound to it. This new complex (H-R-N), which represents the high affinity form of the receptor for agonist, then binds GTP. The H-R-N-GTP complex next dissociates to give H-R (the low-affinity form of the receptor from which the agonist can dissociate), while N-GTP interacts with the catalytic subunit of adenylate cyclase (C), to give N-GTP-C, the active form of the enzyme. Cyclase activity is increased until

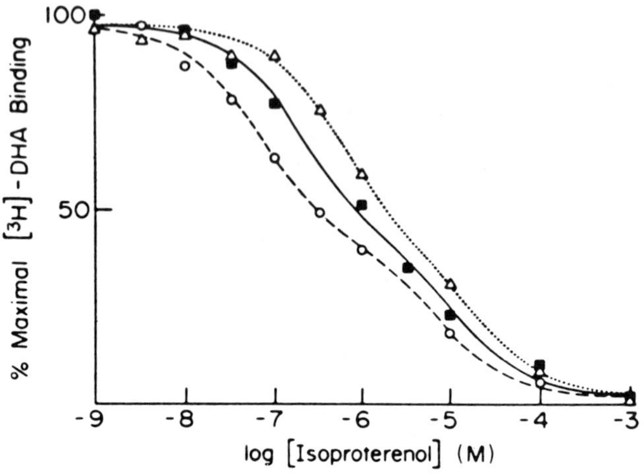

Figure 7 Composite curve for the competition of isoproterenol for [^{3}H] DHA bound expressed as the percentage of maximal [^{3}H] DHA bound in the abscissa represents the concentration of isoproterenol competing for [^{3}H] DNA bound expressed as the percentage of maximal [^{3}H] DNA bound in the absence of isoproterenol. These are composite means of several experiments. The medium contained 80% plasma. Hydrocortisone was added to give a free concentration of about 20 μg/dl (0.5 μM), which simulates its concentration during severe stress of major steroid therapy. Isoproterenol addition at μM shifted the curve to the right with an eightfold increase in EC_{50}, a greater increase in K_H than K_L, and a reduced K_L/K_H ratio. Hydrocortisone partly prevents these changes (reprinted with permission from Davies and Lefkowitz, 1983).

GTPase degrades the GTP moiety, and N-GDP then dissociates from the cyclase, thus allowing it to revert to its basal state.

Figure 6 shows the composite curves constructed from the mean binding values for the radioligand antagonist [^{3}H] DHA (dihydroxyprenolol) in the presence of competing isoproterenol concentrations. While beta-agonists variably bind to either the low- or high-affinity form of the receptor (R or RN), antagonists show equal affinity for either form. Adding GTP shifts all receptors into the low-affinity state with dissociation of agonist.

Computer-assisted modeling methods (Kent et al., 1980) were used to derive the binding constants of isoproterenol for the low- and high-affinity states of the receptor, K_L and K_H, and the proportions of receptor present in each form can be derived, as well as the EC_{50}, the value of isoproterenol giving half-maximum velocity of adenylate cyclase activity. The ratio of K_L/K_H has been found to correlate with a drug's intrinsic affinity (higher ratio and smaller

Table 1 Binding Parameters Derived from Beta-Adrenergic Receptors Exposed to Control Hydrocortisone, Isoproterenol plus Hydrocortisone, or Isoproterenol Treatment

	Control medium	Hydrocortisone	Isoproterenol plus hydrocortisone	Isoproterenol
EC_{50} (nM)	340 ± 75	360 ± 61	930 ± 340	2600 ± 400
K_H (nM)	9.4 ± 2.1	10 ± 3.5	26 ± 11	260 ± 43
K_L (nM)	1,100 ± 300	1,800 ± 270	1,500 ± 570	9,900 ± 2,600
K_L/K_H	120 ± 3.7	180 ± 5.0	57 ± 4.2	39 ± 1.9

See Davies and Lefkowitz, 1983, for details.

EC_{50}). Administration of corticosteroids at high therapeutic levels prior to cell collection, or their presence in an equivalent concentration during incubation, promotes the formation of the high-affinity form of the receptor-agonist (HRN), increases K_L/K_H, and the ability to generate cyclic AMP. On the other hand, preincubation with isoproterenol causes a shift of the curve to the right, reduces K_L/K_H, increases EC_{50}, and reduces generated cyclic AMP.

The binding curve for neutrophils from human subjects in the control state, preincubated with isoproterenol to produce desensitization, and the ameliorating effects of hydrocortisone incubation on the system are shown in Figure 7, along with the derived binding constants in Table 1 (Davies and Lefkowitz, 1984). While pretreatment with isoproterenol alone increased the EC_{50} eightfold with a proportional reduction in cyclic AMP production and reduced K_L/K_H, only a threefold increase in EC_{50} occurred in the presence of hydrocortisone, reflected in partial restoration of activity. Similar changes have been shown in the neutrophils of patients on oral terbutaline therapy (Samuelson and Davies, 1984).

Receptor Modification

Numerous laboratories have demonstrated a diminished cyclic AMP response to beta agonists and/or a reduction in the number of cell surface receptors by taking normal cells and exposing them in vitro to a beta-agonist (Mickey et al., 1975; Greenacre et al., 1978; Chuang and Costa, 1979), or by exposing an intact individual to a beta-agonist and examining the appropriate cells before and after this maneuver (Greenacre et al., 1978; Galant et al., 1978; Scarpace et al., 1982). Studies of this nature have utilized avian and amphibian erythrocytes, mammalian leukocytes, and cultured tumor cells.

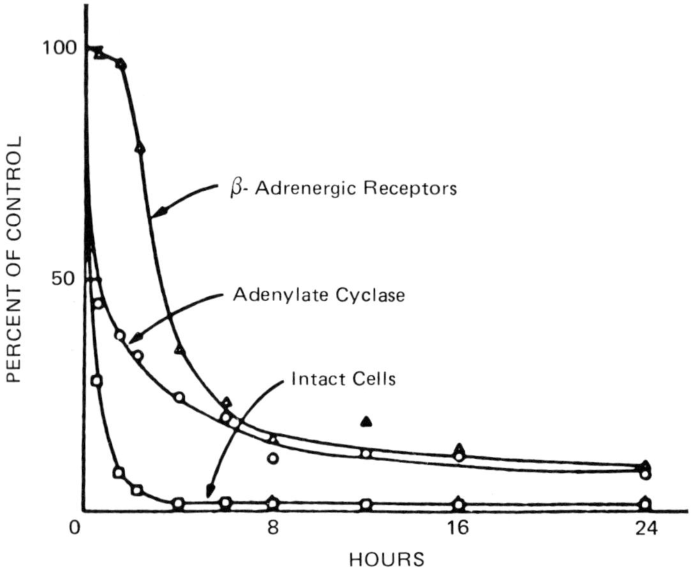

Figure 8 Time course of decrease in beta receptor density, isoproterenol-stimulated adenylate cyclase activity, and isoproterenol-stimulated cAMP accumulation during incubation of 1321N1 astrocytoma cells with 1 μM isoproterenol. At the indicated times cells were withdrawn, washed, and reincubated with 10 μM isoproterenol for determination of adenylate cyclase activity with formation of cAMP in membrane preparations (——O——) and intact cells (——□——). The binding of ^{125}I-HYP (——△——) is also shown representing receptor number. All values are given as percent of control cells. The slide illustrates the more rapid loss of adenylate cyclase function than receptor number, contrasting "uncoupling" with "internalization," respectively, as two distinct processes (reprinted with permission from Su et al., 1980).

Uncoupling Followed by Internalization (Down-Regulation)

As discussed by Lefkowitz and associates (1984), desensitization in a number of systems (astrocytoma cells, frog erythrocytes, lymphocytes) is a two-step process. The first, most immediate, reaction, occurring within minutes of exposure to isoproterenol, is an uncoupling of the receptor, which occurs at low concentrations of drug, is not associated with a reduction in receptor number, and is rapidly reversed as soon as the drug is removed. The second process occurs with more prolonged exposure or exposure more briefly to a higher concentration of drug. It is not readily reversible, and is associated with a loss of receptors (down-regulation). It apparently is due to internalization of the receptors into vesicles, removing them from the cell surface and therefore reducing the number of receptors available for binding studies. Once internalized, receptors remain intact for a while, as shown by ingenious fusion experiments (Strulovici et al., 1983), but will slowly recycle back to the cell membrane if agonist is removed. If agonist is not removed, they are destroyed by lysosomal proteases, and must be resynthesized.

The difference between these processes is nicely exemplified in 1321N1 astrocytoma cells incubated in the presence of 1 μM isoproterenol (Su et al., 1980) (Fig. 8).

The ability to generate cyclic AMP is lost most rapidly with the intact cells, but still occurs rapidly with cell membranes as determined from radioligand binding with ^{125}IHYP. This loss of receptor number is a slower process. When overall desensitization is nearly complete, the receptor loss is incomplete, usually amounting to 50-80% after 24 hr or more. The uncoupling component is rapidly reversible after removal of isoproterenol from the system, but total recovery is limited by the still-reduced number of normal receptors.

The exact signal either for initial uncoupling or for the loss of receptor number remains to be elucidated, and it may not be the same for all cells. In human astrocytoma cells, isoproterenol-induced reduction in cell number occurs in cells deficient in the catalytic subunit of adenylate cyclase, but not in cells lacking a functional regulatory protein (Su et al., 1980). Such results suggest that receptor occupancy and formation of the high-affinity hormone-receptor-regulatory protein complex (HRN) is required for receptor internalization, but that cyclic AMP formation is not. Accompanying receptor phosphorylation, independent of cyclic AMP, has been shown to occur in some systems (Lefkowitz and Caron, 1985).

The spontaneous reversal of uncoupling, once isoproterenol is removed from the system, has implications for tissue removed from the host. Subsequent testing of the tissue may underestimate the uncoupling that existed in situ. Loss of receptor number, on the other hand, would still be present since return of receptor number is very slow: longer than 2 weeks in some patients (Tashkin et al., 1982).

Uncoupling with Covalent Modification of the Receptor

In the turkey erythrocyte, a different sequence takes place upon exposure to the same 1 μM concentration or isoproterenol. Using $^{32}P_i$ incorporation, it has been shown that the beta-adrenergic receptor is phosphorylated, and that, coincidental with desensitization, the amount of phosphate incorporated into the receptor increases two- to threefold (Stadel et al., 1983a). In this system, in contrast to the two-step system described above, the rate of phosphorylation is closely correlated in time with the rate of desensitization, and requires 2-6 hr

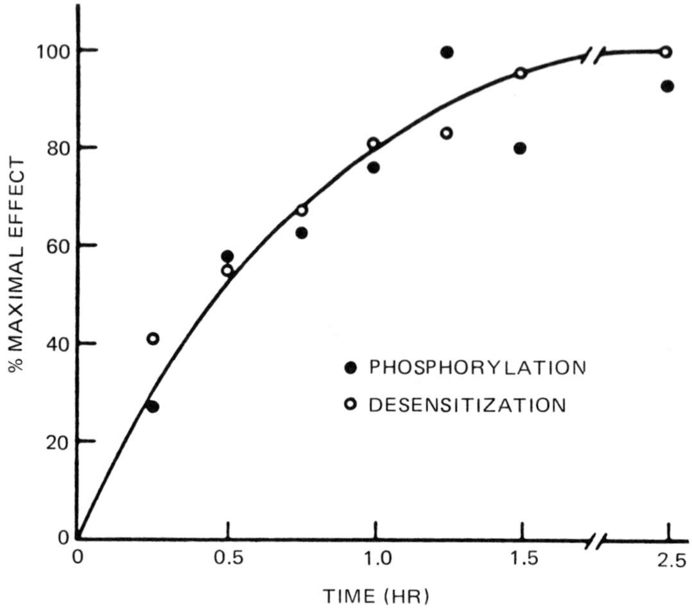

Figure 9 Time course for isoproterenol-induced beta-adrenergic receptor phosphorylation and adenylate cyclase desensitization in turkey erythrocytes. This figure shows an alternative form of desensitization to the internalization seen with frog erythrocytes, namely, phosphorylation of the receptor. Turkey erythrocytes were preincubated with ^{32}Pi. Isoproterenol 1 μM was then added and the cells incubated for various times. ^{32}Pi uptake into the receptors (——●——) paralleled desensitization as measured by cAMP formation (——O——) expressed as the % of maximum desensitization (about 51%). Resensitization (not shown) occurs on a similar time scale when isoproterenol is removed (reproduced with permission from Sibley et al., 1984).

to become complete (Fig. 9). Cyclic AMP is required in part for this process, possibly through a cyclic AMP-dependent protein kinase (Sibley et al., 1984), but other kinases are also involved (Nambi et al., 1985).

Recently it has been shown that mammalian lung beta-adrenergic receptor can be similarly phosphorylated with some reduction in activity (Benovic et al., 1985). Using a reconstituted system containing purified mouse lung receptor, it has been shown that phosphorylation slightly reduces its ability to stimulate adenylate cyclase and that combination with beta-agonist appears to induce conformational changes that facilitate its phosphorylation and dephosphorylation. The reader is referred to a current review for more details of this rapidly evolving field (Lefkowitz and Caron, 1985).

Table 2 Patterns of Desensitization for Adenylate Cyclase Systems

	Heterologous	Homologous
Agonist-specific	No	Yes
F-GppNHp activity	Decreased	Unchanged
Time course	Slow	Fast
cAMP mediation	Yes	No
Receptor sequestration	No	Yes
Receptor phosphorylation	Yes	Yes

See Lefkowitz and Caron, 1985, for details.

Homologous and Heterologous Desensitization

Desensitization of adenylate cyclase systems can be broadly categorized into *homologous,* specific for a particular class of agonists such as beta adrenergic drugs or prostaglandin E_1, and *heterologous,* stimulated by all classes of agonists using that adenylate cyclase system. Thus, the latter effects could arise from either impairment of the guanine regulatory protein or adenylate cyclase or enhancement of phosphodiesterase activity, all resulting in a net reduction in ability to generate cyclic AMP (Harden, 1983). The principal receptor modifications and other general features of these two categories are summarized in Table 2, as listed by Lefkowitz and Caron (1985).

Cell Studies in Humans

In humans, the lymphocytes have been used extensively as a substitute for smooth muscle cells. In a very good parallel to the astrocytoma cell work, intact lymphocytes incubated in the presence of 1 μM isoproterenol show a progressive loss of cyclic AMP response when removed from the incubation system at various times, washed thoroughly, and restimulated (Krall et al., 1980). There is rapid fall in total activity within minutes, and a slower and less complete fall in receptor number. One cannot safely produce this isoproterenol concentration in humans. In fact, the upper limit is about 0.01-0.1 nM, or 1/10,000-1/100,000th as much. When lymphocytes are exposed to 0.01 nM isoproterenol in vitro, there is still a rapid loss of overall activity while the receptor number remains constant. When human subjects are infused with isoproterenol to approximate this low level (1.8 ± 0.3 μg/min), enough to raise the pulse rate by 20%, their lymphocytes also lose overall activity although there is no loss of receptor number over a few hours. Evidently, transferring cells out of their in vivo milieu still allows demonstration of uncoupling, despite the concerns mentioned above. In summary, short-term incubation at low drug levels, or exposure

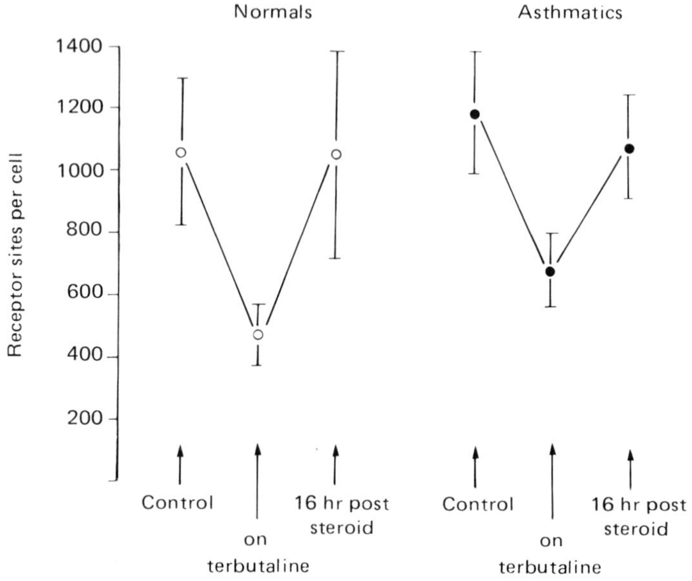

Figure 10 [^{3}H] DHA binding sites in four normal subjects and four asthmatic subjects before terbutaline, at the end of 3-5 weeks on 5 mg three times daily, and 16 hr after 2 mg/kg IV methylprednisolone. Bars show the SEM (reproduced from Hui et al., 1982).

for short periods in vivo produces only uncoupling while higher concentrations in vitro produce loss of receptors.

What happens to lymphocytes upon exposure for long periods at in vivo concentrations? Over time, there is a definite loss of receptor number, even at these low drug levels. In asthmatics after 3-5 weeks on oral terbutaline maintenance, there was approximately a 40% loss of receptor number (Hui et al., 1982). When analyzed by Scatchard binding of the radioligand ^{3}H DHA (dihydroalprenolol), there was no change in affinity. Most interesting is the fact that an injection of 2 mg/kg methylprednisolone restored the receptor number when tested 16 hr later (see below) (Fig. 10). These authors did not study cyclic AMP generation. In another study, the same authors found that while the lymphocyte receptor number was initially equal in both normals and asthmatics and decreased during terbutaline therapy, cyclic AMP production ability decreased significantly only in the normals while lower to begin with in the asthmatics and did not fall further after prolonged exposure to terbutaline (Tashkin et al., 1982).

The question arises whether lymphocytes are suitable models of bronchial smooth muscle when one is studying subsensitivity, and to what extent. It may be quite useful to study changes in receptor number. For example, Aarons and Molinoff (1982) compared the change in receptor number of rat lymphocytes, lung, and heart and found parallel increases in receptor number in each tissue while the animals were receiving propranolol. We are not aware of studies of bronchial smooth muscle per se. However, rat myometrial smooth muscle has been studied in this fashion by Levin et al. (1980). Only 10 min after an injection of 100 mg/kg isoproterenol (admittedly, an enormous dose) there was a considerable loss of receptor number which paralleled the loss of receptors when muscle cells were incubated with 10 μM isoproterenol. Scatchard analysis of [^{3}H]DHA binding showed no loss of affinity. The receptor number was rapidly restored by adding guanyl nucleotide, indicating that a conformational change in receptor caused the apparent loss of receptor number.

The Allergic Host

A degree of uncoupling may already exist in the lymphocytes of asthmatics at the outset, as suggested by Tashkin et al. (1982). Other authors have also reported an innate decrease in ability to generate cyclic AMP in asthmatic lymphocytes and deficient beta-adrenergic responses of other tissues (for review, see Krzenowski and Szentivanyi, 1983). It has been shown that bronchial smooth muscle of those dogs sensitive to *Ascaris* antigen with asthmatic reactions is also impaired in its ability to generate cyclic AMP (Rinard et al., 1979).

Some inroads are being made into possible reasons for depression of beta-adrenergic function in the asthmatic other than the effects of drug-induced tachyphylaxis. Peripheral lymphocytes in asthmatics studied at 0 and 24 hr following inhaled antigen challenge underwent a 20% reduction in beta-receptor number and a 40% mean drop in adenylate cyclase response to isoproterenol, GppNHp, and NaF, but no change in K_d for [^{3}H]DHA) (Meurs et al., 1982). This work suggests that substances released during the allergic response react adversely on the beta-adrenergic system.

One such substance may be the phospholipid platelet-activating factor (PAF;PAF-acethar). An exciting series of studies has shown that this substance released from a variety of inflammatory cells during the allergic response not only activates platelets to release platelet factor 4 but also acts directly on capillaries and bronchioles to produce edema, muscle spasm, and inflammation (Page et al., 1985). It also causes airway hyperreactivity when injected repeatedly into rabbits and guinea pigs (Page et al., 1985a,b). It has now been shown to produce desensitization of beta-adrenergic responses in lymphocytes (Morley, personal communication) with the implications that it may contribute in this way to the severity of an asthmatic attack. If this proves to be the case, the potential for drug-induced tachyphylaxis would be augmented by the allergic response, with possible diastrous consequences.

Augmentation of characteristic alpha-adrenergic responses and diminution of beta-adrenergic responses has been reported in allergic asthmatics off drug therapy using infused isoproterenol and phenylephrine to produce cardiovascular responses (Conolly et al., unpublished work) and earlier with infused isoproterenol and topical phenylephrine to the pupil (Shelhamer, 1980). Asthmatics on only minimal beta-adrenergic therapy by inhalation had greater depression of several metabolic beta-adrenergic responses than chronic bronchitics on similar therapy (Jenne et al., 1977b). These observations suggest that the alpha- and beta-receptors regulating production of mediators by lung mast cells could be similarly involved by both tachyphylaxis and inherent abnormalities, resulting in augmented mediator release (Orange et al., 1971).

Finally, autoantibodies specific for beta-adrenergic receptors in calf lung membranes have been found in the plasma IgG fraction of 3 of 19 normal nonatopic subjects, 1 of 9 normal atopic subjects, 4 of 17 subjects with mild allergic asthma, and 1 of 7 subjects with cystic fibrosis (Fraser et al., 1981), but their significance is uncertain. The group with antibodies differed from the others in showing the abnormal autonomic responses characterized by alpha-adrenergic and cholinergic hypersensitivity and beta-adrenergic hyposensitivity, as previously reported by this group in allergic subjects (Shelhamer, 1980). While suggesting that these autoantibodies may play a role in the development of autonomic abnormalities, the lack of correlation with the clinical manifestations of allergic disease would seem to relegate them to a minor role at best in the pathogenesis of asthma.

Mediator Release

Thus far, we have considered only tachyphylaxis of beta-adrenergic control of airway tone, showing that it is relatively resistant to developing tachyphylaxis from ordinary beta-adrenergic drug therapy. Another site of potential tachyphylaxis is in the modulation of mediator release from the lung during such challenges as antigen inhalation or exercise. As pointed out by Bruynzeel (1984), there is some evidence that these processes are more susceptible to developing tachyphylaxis. Thus, while there was no decline in the ability of subcutaneous terbutaline to protect against methacholine challenge after prolonged oral terbutaline therapy, there was a 10-15-fold reduction in its ability to protect against antigen-induced bronchospasm in two of three asthmatics, and a fourfold reduction in the other (Tashkin et al., 1982). Oral prednisone taken 16 hr before challenge restored sensitivity (Fig. 11) in the one patient in whom this was tried. Similarly, following daily therapy with oral salbutamol, there was a fall in protection by inhaled salbutamol against exercise-induced asthma (Gibson et al., 1978), but no fall in histamine reactivity (Peel and Gibson, 1980).

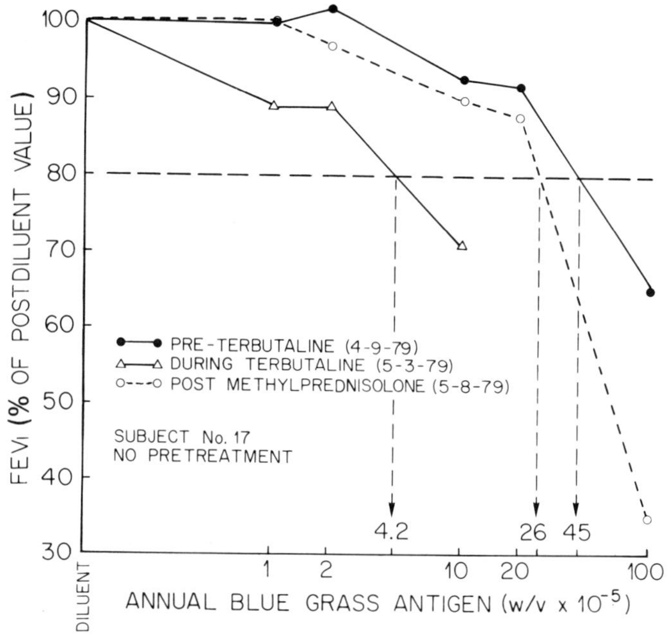

Figure 11 Percentage changes in FEV_1 in subject 17 after inhalation of serial cumulative doses of annual blue grass antigen (wt/vol) during the preterbutaline control period, during the period of daily terbutaline therapy, and 16 hr after a single dose of methylprednisolone (2 mg/kg) administered intravenously at the end of the terbutaline period (see text). Provocative concentrations of antigen (wt/vol) required to decrease FEV_1 by 20% from the diluent control are determined by graphic interpolation and are indicated by numbers on the abscissa opposite arrows ($\times 10^{-5}$). Reproduced with permission from Tashkin et al., 1982.

Beta-adrenergic control of mediator release could be exerted both at the level of tissue inflammatory cells and the capillaries through which mediators pass in the inflamed area. It is quite remarkable that 200 μg of inhaled salbutamol completely suppresses the appearance of histamine and neutrophil chemotactic factor into the blood following antigen challenge (Howarth et al., 1985), and it is also somewhat surprising that some beta-adrenergic tachyphylaxis of circulating granulocyte lysosomal release is seen after continuous inhaled salbutamol therapy (Busse et al., 1979). This area of tachyphylaxis research deserves further study, since it is important in the acute asthmatic attack.

E. Prevention and Reversal of Beta-Adrenergic Tachyphylaxis

To the extent that beta-adrenergic subsensitivity plays a role in the aggravation of the asthmatic state, on or off beta-adrenergic therapy, its prevention or reversal will prevent worsening of the disease. Two common drugs used in treating asthma, glucocorticosteroid and ketotifen, have among their properties the ability to reverse at least some aspects of beta-adrenergic tachyphylaxis. In addition, certain drugs not used for therapy, namely antimalarials, and, in some systems, indomethacin, have been shown experimentally to counter tachyphylaxis.

Glucocorticoids

Despite multiple effects of steroids on the inflammatory and allergic processes, some of glucocorticoids antiasthmatic effect may be secondary to an interaction with the beta-adrenergic system (Schleimer, 1985) in two possible ways: (1) enhancement of several beta-adrenergic-mediated physiological processes (Davies and Lefkowitz, 1984), and (2) restoration of responsiveness to a beta-agonist, as shown in asthmatics on beta agonist therapy who have become unresponsive (Ellul-Micallef and Fenech, 1975) and in normal subjects made unresponsive by large dosages (Holgate et al., 1977). Similar findings have been demonstrated in dogs (Stephen et al., 1980) as well as in human bronchial muscle, in which steroids hastened recovery from tachyphylaxis induced in vitro (Davis and Conolly, 1980).

At the biochemical level, several laboratories have shown a reversal of the diminished cyclic AMP response of asthmatics to beta-agonists by exposure to glucocorticoids either in vivo or in vitro (Conolly, 1980). In lymphocytes, hydrocortisone not only increases cyclic AMP production by itself but also potentiates other adenylate-cyclase stimulating agonists including the beta-adrenergic drugs (Marone et al., 1980). In the canine bronchus, hydrocortisone potentiates cyclic AMP production with a dose-response curve shift that almost superimposes its potentiation of isoproterenol relaxation, but does not potentiate relaxation by prostaglandin E_2 (Rinard et al., 1983). These authors questioned the hypothesis (Geddes et al., 1974) that the potentiating action is due to inhibition of isoproterenol removal by $uptake_2$ mechanisms, because they found that potentiation occurred even at saturating isoproterenol concentrations.

At the receptor level, glucocorticoids have been found to increase beta-adrenergic receptor density in numerous tissues and cell types including human lung tissues and leukocytes (Davies and Lefkowitz, 1984). Prednisone has been found to increase beta-receptor density in leukocytes from asthmatics (Sano et al., 1980). In another study, a single large dose of intravenous methylprednisolone (2 mg/kg) reversed terbutaline down-regulation of beta-receptors in human lymphocytes obtained from asthmatics and volunteers treated with maintenance doses of terbutaline (Fig. 10) and to normalize impaired cardiovascular responses to isoproterenol and phenylephrine (Hui et al., 1982), while a smaller oral dose of prednisone, 20 mg four times daily, has no similar protective effect (Hui et al., unpublished observations). Female rats treated for 1-5 days with metaproterenol developed progressive loss of β receptors in their excised lungs, and an uncoupling of receptors into the low-affinity state for isoproterenol as well as a reduction in ability to generate cyclic AMP (Scarpace and Abrass, 1982). Concomitant methylprednisolone prior to sacrifice restored receptor density, but failed fully to normalize cyclic AMP production or improve receptor affinity.

However, hydrocortisone has been shown to regulate beta-adrenoceptor function in other cell systems by facilitating the formation of the high-affinity coupled state as previously mentioned, and shown in Figure 7 (Davies and Lefkowitz, 1981). In desensitized neutrophils, obtained from volunteers treated with terbutaline, hydrocortisone reversed prior agonist-induced uncoupling as the K_L/K_H ratio shifted back towards control values (Davies and Lefkowitz, 1983; Samuelson and Davies, 1984). In this system, hydrocortisone had no effect in restoring the reduced beta-receptor density.

How glucocorticoids achieve these effects on desensitized tissues, and whether different dosages or preparations have different effects on the various aspects of tachyphylaxis uncoupling, reduction in receptor density, and adenylate cyclase activity remain to be determined. A theory currently attracting attention is based on the ability of corticosteroids to produce macrocortin or lipomodulin, a protein inhibitor of phospholipase A_2 (Blackwell et al., 1980). There is a good correlation between the ability of certain compounds such as quinacrine and tetracaine to inhibit phospholipase A_2 and their ability to block isoproterenol-induced desensitization in tissues of some species, while compounds enhancing activity of this enzyme induce desensitization (Mallorga et al., 1980; Torda et al., 1981). Corticosteroids may operate through the same mechanism by blocking some phospholipase-A_2-mediated reaction.

Ketotifen

Ketotifen, a drug used in other parts of the world for the prophylaxis of asthma and currently under study in the United States, has interesting properties, including inhibition of the release of myotonic mediators, calcium antagonistic properties, and the reversal and prevention of diminished beta-adrenergic sensitivity in some systems (Craps and Ney, 1984). As measured by inhibition of the passive cutaneous anaphylaxis, the acute isoproterenol protective effect in the rat decreased 600-fold after a subcutaneous infusion of isoproterenol by minipump for 7-10 days. This tachyphylaxis has been found to be completely reversed by a single oral dose (1 mg/kg) of ketotifen that has no antitachyphylaxis activity per se. Pretreatment with ketotifen also prevented tachyphylaxis (Bretz et al., 1983). The cellular and biochemical basis for the antitachyphylaxis action of ketotifen remains to be shown. It is uncertain whether this pharmacologic property is of therapeutic value, particularly at the dosages used in humans. Ketotifen did not reverse isoproterenol tachyphylaxis produced in guinea pig trachea in vitro (Bretz et al., 1983).

Indomethacin

In guinea pigs with airways made tachyphylactic to isoproterenol by 7 days of isoproterenol injections, indomethacin added to the incubation media restored the original sensitivity (Douglas et al., 1977). Added indomethacin also prevented the production of tachyphylaxis in vitro by either isoproterenol or theophylline (an exception to the belief that theophylline does not produce tachyphylaxis to itself).

There is also interest in the ability of arachidonic acid and its metabolites to modulate relaxation of smooth muscle to beta agonists (Adcock and Garland, 1980; Mitchell, 1982; Omini et al., 1981). For example, isoproterenol relaxation of bovine coronary artery appears to be inhibited by arachidonic acid and lipoxygenase products, but stimulated by cyclooxygenase products, although the mechanisms are uncertain (Rubanyi and Paul, 1985).

Calcium Channel Blockers

The fall in agonist affinity upon incubation of lymphocytes with isoproterenol can be reduced by a number of compounds that affect calcium transport, such as nifedipine and verapamil. However, loss of receptors from the cell surface is not prevented, nor is the reduction in adenylate cyclase activity (Borst et al., 1985).

II. Functional Antagonism

The term functional antagonism was used by Van den Brink (1973) to describe the inverse relationship between the protective effect of isoproterenol and the degrees of constriction produced by methacholine or histamine in guinea pig trachea (Van den Brink, 1973). As such, the phenomenon is of potential importance in governing the response to a bronchodilator and therefore can be considered in the same chapter as tachyphylaxis. Indeed, if the dosage of a cholinergic constrictant is sufficient, there is no response in vitro to a beta agonist (Torphy et al., 1983). Early further work on this subject was done by Jones and co-workers (1974) and Buckner and Saini (1975) in guinea pig trachea. More recently, functional antagonism to methacholine has been studied in detail in the guinea pig trachea (Karlsson and Persson, 1981), canine trachealis (Torphy et al., 1983, 1985), to acetylcholine, histamine, and serotonin in canine trachealis (Russell, 1984), and to carbacholine and histamine in human bronchial muscle strips (Raffestin et al., 1985). The Russell studies bring out qualitative

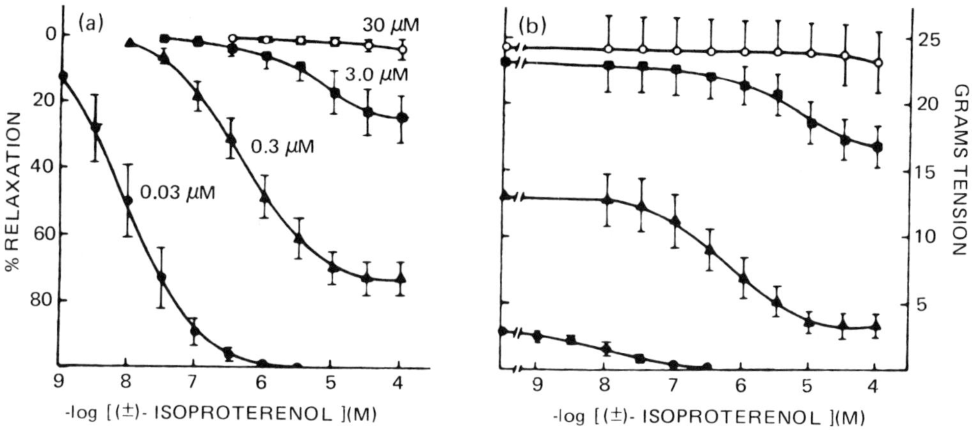

Figure 12 Cumulative concentration-response curves to (–) isoproterenol in canine trachealis strips contracted with various concentrations of methacholine indicated by figures to the right of each curve. Data are expressed both as percentage of relaxation compared to the resting state (A) and absolute tension (B) using four strips from each of six dogs with means and SEM. Note that there is approximately a two-log increase in EC_{50} with only a 10-fold increase in methacholine, from 0.03 to 0.3 μM. Also note that virtually no relaxation takes place at 30 μM methacholine at any isoproterenol concentration (reproduced with permission from Torphy et al., 1983).

differences in the functional antagonism to isoproterenol with the three antagonists mentioned, with the loss of protection with increased dose being greatest with acetylcholine, and only slight with serotonin.

A. Dependence on Type and Dosage of Constrictant

Methacholine

Figure 12, using canine trachealis, shows that as the dosage of methacholine increases from 0.03 to 3.0 μM, the EC_{50} for isoproterenol increases almost 500-fold (Torphy et al., 1983). An in vivo human counterpart is the demonstration that salbutamol effectiveness decreases (in terms of the dosage required to produce maximum bronchodilation) as the degree of bronchospasm in the asthmatic increases (Barnes and Pride, 1983). The dosage of salbutamol required in normal persons is less than in asthmatics. Likewise, in an in vivo canine model using pulses of bronchospasm produced by inhaled methacholine or histamine, the protective effect of infused isoproterenol was reduced approximately 50% by a fourfold increase in dosage of either methacholine or histamine, as stated in the preliminary report (Jenne et al., 1985) (Table 3).

Table 3 Effect of a Fourfold Increase in Methacholine or Histamine Aerosol Concentration (Low R_L, High R_L) on Protection by Infused Isoproterenol in the Intact Dog

	Methacholine (6)		Histamine (4)	
	Low R_L	High R_L	Low R_L	High R_L
Mean % Increase R_L	79.0	262.9	82.4	216.3
Mean % Protection	60.1	21.1	60.5	31.8
	(P = 0.002)		(P = 0.06)	

Data from Jenne et al., 1985.

Further observations have borne this out (Jenne et al., submitted for publication).

The biochemical basis for the isoproterenol methacholine antagonism has been explored in a series of elegant papers (Torphy et al., 1983, 1985) and found to center on the effect of these two competing influences (isoproterenol and methacholine) on the concentrations of cyclic AMP and cyclic-AMP-dependent protein kinase activity in the muscle. The depressant effect of a cholinergic antagonist on these compounds can confuse the picture in smooth muscle when investigations of cyclic nucleotide changes with relaxants are made (Lohman et al., 1977), since cAMP levels are distorted or do not rise. A recent investigation used bullfrog hemilung with its natural intrinsic tone to avoid such an artifact (Taylor and Downes, 1982).

The mechanism whereby cholinergic agents depress cyclic AMP and cyclic-AMP-dependent kinase is thought to be due either to depression of adenylate cyclase or to an increase in activity of phosphodiesterase (Torphy, 1985). Muscle contraction is associated with a rise in Ca^{2+}, and it is known that calcium activation of calmodulin can activate the high K_m phosphodiesterase activity by several times (Wolff and Brostrom, 1979; Meeker and Harden, 1982) in a manner analogous to the activation of myosin light-chain kinase by Ca^{2+}.

Serotonin

Serotonin relaxes human bronchial smooth muscle (Raffestin, 1985), but constricts canine trachealis (Russell, 1984). Relaxation by isoproterenol against serotonin is not as seriously impaired by a dosage increase as smooth muscle contracted with acetylcholine (Russell, 1984). Thus, when intravenous (IV) serotonin infusion was varied to adjust R_L in the canine model, there was little loss of protective effect with a large increase in R_L (Jenne et al., 1985). Once bronchospasm had been initiated and stabilized at a low level over baseline, only a small increase in serotonin dosage was needed to increase R_L by 340%, and there was only a slight reduction in the effectiveness of infused isoproterenol from what had been required at the low elevation in R_L. This is in sharp contrast with the reduction in protective effect of infused isoproterenol against the fourfold increases in inhaled dosage of methacholine or histamine (Table 3) and suggests that the dosage of antagonist, rather than the resistance produced by it, is the crucial factor in functional antagonism. However, in addition to the difference in type and route of constricting agent in these contrasting results, there was also a difference in the nature of the response. With the nebulized constrictants, isoproterenol was protecting against a rapidly increased muscle constriction. With the infused constrictant, isoproterenol was relaxing sustained bronchospasm.

Leukotriene D

Leukotriene D_4 is another constrictant that deviates from the methacholine picture of functional antagonism. With guinea pig trachealis, although LTD_4 and methacholine had nearly parallel dose-response curves, the decrease in effectiveness produced by a 10-fold increase in methacholine was much greater than by an equal increase in LTD_4 (Torphy, 1984). In other words, there was less functional antagonism, whether related to dosage or the increase in resistance.

Phorbal Esters

Phorbal myristate acetate (PMA) causes contraction of a guinea pig parenchymal strip, containing a mixture of respiratory and vascular smooth muscle, but predominantly the former. Compared to its relaxing effect against histamine contraction, isoproterenol is relatively ineffective (Dale and Obianine, 1985). Phorbal esters are thought to activate protein kinase C directly in the polyphosphoinositol pathway of calcium activation, as demonstrated in guinea pig ileal and canine tracheal smooth muscle (Baron et al., 1984). This is of particular interest because the involvement of the polyphosphoinositol pathway is probable in respiratory smooth muscle contraction but not fully explored. Activation of this pathway allows actin-myosin contraction at much lower Ca^{2+} levels, and may be pertinent in the tonic phase.

B. Implications for the Treatment of Asthma by Beta-Adrenergic Drugs

Obviously, the continuing research into these various constrictants and their antagonism by isoproterenol and other relaxants is of considerable importance to the various asthmatic states and their treatment. Particularly interesting is work on the leukotrienes, since these are thought to constitute a large proportion of the stimulus to bronchospasm in the antigenic response of the airways (Dahlen et al., 1983). This research may also explain the effectiveness of anticholinergics over beta-agonists in conditions such as chronic bronchitis in which vagal tone is apparently enhanced.

One of the most fascinating questions is whether the acute bronchospastic impulses ("reactive airways") respond differently to beta-agonists than the chronically increased tone of the stable asthmatic. Here, the question of the formation and lysis of latched state cross-bridges may enter, discussed by Stephens and by Krall in earlier chapters.

Awareness that respiratory smooth muscle enters a tonic contraction by passing through the rapid cycling cross-bridge phase to a slowly cycling latched bridge phase, with different energetics and calcium relationships (Askoy et al., 1983; Gerthoffer and Murphy, 1983) introduces the possibility that the action of bronchodilators may differ depending upon the phase of contraction. As discussed by Ahrens in the chapter on pharmacokinetics of beta-adrenergic agonists, prevention of bronchoconstriction may not be the equivalent of bronchodilation from a state of bronchospasm. Likewise, in the in vivo canine studies cited (Jenne et al., 1985) the dose-response relation of infused isoproterenol in preventing a pulse of methacholine or histamine induced bronchospasm may differ from the dose-response relation in relaxing serotonin-induced spasm because the latter case is a sustained contraction, presumably a latched state. While the former may have a developing element of latched state physiology, one is principally preventing a developing contraction. Could differing dose-response curves account for the more rapid decline of protective effect after aerosolized beta-agonist than the decline in FEV_1, as shown by Ahrens et al. (1984) and discussed in Chapter 6.

Finally, all the evidence for functional antagonism against various bronchoconstrictant is a strong argument for adjusting the dosage of a beta-agonist according to the severity of the asthmatic attack. However, here we may be running the danger of producing tachyphylaxis. From what we have learned about the amelioration of tachyphylaxis with glucocorticosteroids, the answer to this problem may be in our hands. Severe attacks require increased beta-agonist therapy along with corticosteroids.

References

Aarons, R. D., and Molinoff, P. B. (1982). Changes in the density of beta adrenergic receptors in rat lymphocytes, heart and lung after chronic treatment with propranolol. *J. Pharmacol. Exp. Ther. 221*: 439-443.

Adcock, T. T., and Garland, L. G. (1980). A possible role for lipoxygenase products as regulators of airway smooth muscle reactivity. *Br. J. Pharmacol. 69*: 167-169.

Ahrens, R. C., Bonham, A. C., Maxwell, G. A., and Weinberger, M. M. (1984). A method for comparing the peak intensity and duration of action of aerosolized bronchodilators using bronchoprovocation with methacholine. *Am. Rev. Respir. Dis. 129*: 903-906.

Ahlqvist, R. P. (1948). A study of adrenotropic receptors. *Am. J. Physiol. 153*: 586-600.

Anderson, A. A., and Lees, G. M. (1976). Investigation of occurrence of tolerance to bronchodilator drugs in chronically pretreated guinea pigs. *Br. J. Pharmacol. 56*: 331-338.

Askoy, M. O., Mros, S., Kamm, K. E., and Murphy, R. A. (1983). Ca^{++}, cAMP and changes in myosin phosphorylation during contraction of smooth muscle. *Am. J. Physiol. 245*: C255-C270.

Avner, B. P., and Jenne, J. W. (1977a). Comparison of in vitro isoproterenol-induced desensitization in human, dog, rat and rabbit respiratory smooth muscle. (abstract) *Am. Rev. Respir. Dis. 114*: Suppl. 45.

Avner, B. P., and Jenne, J. W. (1977b). Desensitization of human bronchial smooth muscle to beta receptor agonists. *Proc. West. Pharmacol. Soc. 20*: 25-31.

Avner, B. P., and Jenne, J. W. (1981). Desensitization of isolated human bronchial smooth muscle to β-receptor agonists. *J. Allergy Clin. Immunol. 68*: 51-57.

Avner, B. P., and Noland, B. (1978). In vivo desensitization to beta receptor mediated bronchodilator drugs in the rat: Decreased beta receptor affinity. *J. Pharmacol. Exp. Ther. 207*: 23-33.

Barnes, P. J., and Pride, N. B. (1983). Dose-response curves to inhaled B-adrenoceptor agonists in normal and asthmatic subjects. *Br. J. Clin. Pharmacol. 15*: 677-682.

Baron, C. B., Cunningham, M., Strauss, J., and Coburn, R. F. (1984). Pharmacomechanical coupling in smooth muscle may involve phosphatidylinositol metabolism. *Proc. Natl. Acad. Sci. USA 81*: 6899-6903.

Benovic, J. L., Pike, L. J., Cerione, R. A., Staniszewski, C., Yashimasa, T., Codina, J., Caron, M. C., and Lefkowitz, R. J. (1985). Phosphorylation of the mammalian beta-adrenergic receptor by cyclic AMP-dependent protein kinase. *J. Biol. Chem. 260*: 7094-7101.

Benson, R. L., and Perlman, F. (1948). Clinical effects of epinephrine by inhalation. *J. Allergy 19*: 129-140.

Benoy, C. J., El-Fellah, M. S., Schneider, R., and Wade, O. L. (1975). Tolerance to sympathomimetic bronchodilators in guinea pig isolated lung following chronic administration in vivo. *Br. J. Pharmacol. 55*: 547-554.

Blackwell, G. J., Carnuccio, R., DiRosa, M., Flower, R. J., Parente, L., and Persico, P. (1980). Macrocortin: A polypeptide causing the antiphospholipase activity of corticoid. *Nature 287*: 147-149.

Borst, S. E., Hui, K. K., and Conolly, M. E. (1985). Verapamil inhibits agonist induced desensitization of human lymphocyte beta-adrenergic receptors. *Fed. Proc. 44*(5): 1640 (abstract).

Bouhuys, A., Douglas, J. W., and Lewis, A. J. (1972). Hypersensitivity to adrenoceptor agents in the guinea pig in vitro and in vivo. *Br. J. Pharmacol. 42*: 195-105.

Bretz, U., Martin, W., and Mazzoni, L. (1983) β-adrenergic tachyphylaxis in the rat and its reversal and prevention by ketotifen. *Eur. J. Pharmacol. 86*: 321, 1983.

Bruynzeel, P. L. (1984). Changes in the beta-adrenergic system due to beta adrenergic therapy: Clinical consequences. *Eur. J. Respir. Dis.* (Suppl 135): 62-71.

Buckner, C. K., and Saini, R. K. (1975). On the use of functional antagonism to estimate dissociation constants for beta adrenergic receptor agonists in isolated guinea pig trachea. *J. Pharmacol. Exp. Ther. 194*: 565-574.

Busse, W. W., Bush, R. K., and Cooper, W. (1979). Granulocyte responses in vitro to isoproterenol histamine and prostaglandin E_1 during treatment with beta-adrenergic aerosols in asthma. *Am. Rev. Respir. Dis. 120*: 377.

Chervinsky, P. (1978). A comparative evaluation of fenoterol and terbutaline in the treatment of asthma. *Ann. Allergy 40*: 189-194.

Cho, Y. W., Aviado, D. M., and Lish, P. M. (1968). Efficacy of a new bronchodilator, soterenol, on experimental locked-lung syndrome in dogs. *J. Allergy 42*: 36-48.

Chuang, D. (1981). Inhibitors of transglutaminase prevent agonist-mediated internalization of beta adrenergic receptors. *J. Biol. Chem. 256*(16): 8291-8293.

Chuang, D., and Costa, E. (1979). Evidence for internalization of the recognition site of beta-adrenergic receptors during receptor subsensitivity induced by (-) isoproterenol. *Proc. Natl. Acad. Sci. 76*: 3024-3028.

Clayberger, C. A., Goodman, D. B., and Rasmussen, H. (1981). Regulation of cyclic AMP metabolism in the rat erythrocyte during chronic beta adrenergic stimulation: evidence for calmodulin mediated alteration of membrane-bound phosphodiesterase activity. *J. Membrane Biol. 58*: 191-201.

Conolly, M. E. (1980). Cyclic nucleotides, β receptors and bronchial asthma. *Adv. Cyclic Nucl. Res. 12*: 151-159.

Conolly, M. E., and Greenacre, J. K. (1976). The lymphocyte beta-adrenoceptor in normal subjects and patients with bronchial asthma. *J. Clin. Invest. 58*: 1307-1316.

Conolly, M. E., Davies, D. S., Dollery, C. T., and George, C. F. (1971). Resistance to beta-adrenoceptor stimulants (a possible explanation for the rise in asthma deaths). *Br. J. Pharmacol. 43*: 389.

Conolly, M. E., Tashkin, D. P., Hui, K. K. P., Littner, M. R., and Wolfe, R. N. (1982). Selective subsensitization of beta-adrenergic receptors in central airways of asthmatics and normal subjects during long-term therapy with inhaled salbutamol. *J. Allergy Clin. Immunol. 20*: 423.

Cookson, D. H., and Reed, C. E. (1963). A comparison of the effect of isoproterenol in the normal and asthmatic subject. *Am. Rev. Respir. Dis. 88*: 636-643.

Craps, L. P., and Ney, U. M. (1984). Ketotifen. Current views on its mechanism of action and their therapeutic implications. *Respiration 45*: 411-421.

Dahlen, S. E., Hansson, G., Hedqvist, P., Bjorck, T., Granstrom, E., and Dahlen, B. (1983). Allergen challenge of lung tissue from asthmatics elicits bronchial contraction that correlates with the release of leukotrienes C_4, D_4, and E_4. *Proc. Natl. Acad. Sci. 80*: 1712-

Dale, M. M., and Obianine, L. (1985). Phorbol myristate acetate causes in guinea pig parenchymal strip, a maintained bronchospasm which is relatively resistant to isoproterenol. *FEBS Letters 190*: 6-10.

Davies, A. O., and Lefkowitz, R. J. (1981). Agonist-promoted high affinity state of the β-adrenergic receptor in human neutrophils: Modulation by corticosteroids. *J. Clin. Endocrinol. Metab. 53*: 703-708.

Davies, A. O., and Lefkowitz, R. J. (1983). In vitro desensitization of β-adrenergic receptors in human neutrophils: Attentuation by corticosteroids. *J. Clin. Invest. 71*: 565-571.

Davies, A. O., and Lefkowitz, R. J. (1984). Regulation of beta adrenergic receptors by steroid hormones. *Annu. Rev. Physiol. 46*: 119-130.

Davis, C., and Conolly, M. E. (1980) Tachyphylaxis to β-adrenoceptor agonists in human bronchial smooth muscle: Studies in vitro. *Br. J. Clin. Pharmacol. 10*: 417-423.

Douglas, J. S., Lewis, A. J., Ridgeway, P., Brink, C., and Bouhuys, A. (1977). Tachyphylaxis to beta-adrenoceptor agonists in guinea pig airway smooth muscle in vitro and in vivo. *Eur. J. Pharmacol. 42*: 195-205.

Elfellah, M. S., and Turnbull, M. J. (1978). Effect of pretreatment with bronchodilator drugs on in vitro responsiveness of guinea pig lung adenylate cyclase. *Eur. J. Pharmacol. 51*: 211-217.

Ellul-Micallef, R., and Fenech, F. F. (1975). Effect of intravenous prednisolone in asthmatics with diminished adrenergic responsiveness *Lancet 2*: 1269-1271.

Ephraim, A. (1910). Uber endobronchiale therapié Berliner. *Klin. Wochenchr. 47*: 1317-1320.

Falliers, C. J. (1981). Acute effects of albuterol aerosol in reversible obstructive airway disease. *Ann. Allergy 47*: 387.

Fleisch, J. H., and Titus, E. (1972). The prevention of isoproterenol desensitization and isoproterenol reversal. *J. Pharmacol. Exp. Ther. 181*: 425-433.

Forder, J., Scriabine, A., and Rasmussen, H. (1985). Plasma membrane calcium flux protein kinase C activation and smooth muscle contraction. 235: 267-273.

Fraser, C. M., Venter, J. C., and Kaliner, M. (1981). Autonomic abnormalities and autoantibodies to β-adrenergic receptors. *N. Engl. J. Med. 305*: 1165-1170.

Galant, S. P., Duriseta, S., Underwood, S., and Insel, P. A. (1978). Decreased beta-adrenergic receptors on polymorphonuclear leukocytes after adrenergic therapy. *N. Engl. J. Med. 229*: 933-936.

Geddes, B., Jones, T. R., Dvorsky, R. J., and Lefcoe, N. M. (1974). Interaction of glucocorticoids and bronchodilators on isolated guinea pig tracheal and human bronchial smooth muscle. *Am. Rev. Respir. Dis. 110*: 420-427.

Gerthoffer, W. T., and Murphy, R. A. (1983). Myosin phosphorylation and regulation of cross-bridge cycle in tracheal smooth muscle. *Am. J. Physiol. 244*: (Cell Physiol 13): C182-187.

Graesser, J. N. (1939). Inhalation therapy of bronchial asthma. *JAMA 112*: 1223-1226.

Greenacre, J. K., Schofield, P., and Conolly, M. E. (1978). Desensitization of the beta-adrenoceptor of lymphocytes from normal subjects and asthmatic patients in vitro. *Br. J. Clin. Pharmacol. 5*: 199-206.

Harden, T. K. (1983). Agonist-induced desensitization of the B-adrenergic receptor-linked adenylate cyclase. *Pharmacol. Rev. 35*: 5-33.

Harvey, J. E., and Tattersfield, A. E. (1979). Beta-adrenergic responsiveness in asthmatics and atopic non-asthmatics. *Thorax 34*: 416.

Harvey, J. E., and Tattersfield, A. E. (1982). Airway response to salbutamol. Effect of regular salbutamol inhalations in normal, atopic and asthmatic subjects. *Thorax 37*: 280.

Holgate, A. T., Baldwin, C. J., and Tattersfield, A. C. (1977). Beta adrenergic resistance in normal human airways. *Lancet 2*: 375-377.

Hui, K. K. P., Conolly, M. E., and Tashkin, D. P. (1982). Reversal of human lymphocyte β-adrenoceptor desensitization by glucocorticoids. *Clin. Pharmacol. Ther. 32*: 566-571.

Inoue, S. (1967). Effect of epinephrine on blood glucose, pulmonary function and heart rate in children with asthma of varying severity. *J. Allergy 40*: 337-348.

Jenne, J. W. (1982). Whither beta-adrenergic tachyphylaxis? *J. Allergy Clin. Immunol. 70*: 413-416.

Jenne, J. W., Chick, T. W., Strickland, R. D., and Wall, F. J. (1977a). Subsensitivity of beta responses during therapy with a long acting beta-2 preparation. *J. Allergy Clin. Immunol. 59*: 383.

Jenne, J. W., Chick, T. W., Strickland, R. D., and Wall, F. J. (1977b). A comparison of beta-adrenergic function in asthma and chronic bronchitis. *J. Allergy Clin. Immunol. 60*: 346-356.

Jenne, J. W., Manfredi, C., and Druz, W. S. (1985). A canine model of chronic bronchial beta adrenergic subsensitivity and the effect of methyl prednisolone. *J. Allergy Clin. Immunol. 73*: No. 1, part 2, 129 (abstract).

Jones, T. R., Hamilton, J. T., and Lefcoe, N. M. (1974). Variations in the relative potencies of bronchodilators in the presence and absence of carbachol-induced tone. *Can. J. Physiol. Pharmacol. 52*: 358-361.

Karlsson, A.-J., and Persson, C. G. A. (1981). Influences of tracheal contraction on relaxant effects in vitro of theophylline and isoproterenol. *Br. J. Pharmacol. 74*: 73-79.

Keighley, J. F. (1966). Iatrogenic asthma associated with adrenergic aerosols. *Ann. Intern. Med. 65*: 985.

Kent, R. S., DeLean, A., and Lefkowitz, R. J. (1980). A quantitative analysis of beta-adrenergic receptor interactions: Resolution of the high and low affinity states of the receptor by computer modelling of ligand binding data. *Mol. Pharmacol. 17*: 14-23.

Krall, J. F., Conolly, M., and Tuck, M. L. (1980). Acute regulation of beta-adrenergic receptor catecholamine sensitivity. *J. Pharmacol. Exp. Ther. 214*: 554-560.

Krzenowski, J. J., and Szentivanyi, A. (1983). Reflections on some aspects of current research in asthma. *J. Allergy Clin. Immunol. 72*: 433-442.

Lands, A. M., Luduena, F. P., and Buzzo, H. J. (1967). Differentiation of receptors responsive to isoproterenol. *Life Sci. 6*: 2241-2249.

Larsson, S. (1979). Aspects of bronchial $beta_2$-receptor tolerance. *Scand. J. Respir. Dis. 103* (Suppl): 84.

Larsson, S., Svedmyr, N., and Thiringer, G. (1976). Lack of bronchial beta-adrenoceptor resistance in asthmatics during long term treatment with terbutaline. *J. Allergy Clin. Immunol. 59*: 93-100.

Lefkowitz, R. J. (1982). Clinical physiology of adrenergic receptor regulation. *Am. J. Physiol 243*: E43-47.

Lefkowitz, R. J., and Caron, M. C. (1985). Adrenergic receptors: Molecular mechanism of clinically relevant regulation. *Clin. Res.* 395-406.

Lefkowitz, R. J., Caron, M. G., and Stiles, G. L. (1984). Mechanisms of membrane receptor regulation. *N. Engl. J. Med. 310*: 1570-1579.

Levin, L. C., Korenman, S. G., and Kroll, J. F. (1980). Agonist-dependent desensitization of symmetrical β-adrenergic catecholamine-sensitive adenylate cyclase. *Biol. Reprod. 22*: 493-499.

Lichterfield, A., and Lollgen, H. (1974). Investigation into isoprenaline resistance in patients with obstructive lung disease. *Eur. J. Clin. Pharmacol. 7*: 347-351.

Lin, C. S., Hurwitz, L., Jenne, J. W., and Avner, B. P. (1977). Mechanism of isoproterenol-induced desensitization of tracheal smooth muscle. *J. Pharmacol. Exp. Ther. 203*: 12-22.

Lockey, S. D., Jr., Glennon, J. A., and Reed, C. E. (1967). Comparison of some metabolic responses in normal and asthmatic subjects to epinephrine and glucagon. *J. Allergy 40*: 349-354.

Lohman, S. M., Miech, R. P., and Butcher, F. R. (1977). Effects of isoproterenol, theophylline and carbachol on cyclic nucleotide levels and relaxation of bovine tracheal smooth muscle. *Biochem. Biophys. Acta 499*: 238-250.

Lowell, F. C., Curry, J. J., and Schiller, I. W. (1949). A clinical and experimental study of isuprel in spontaneous and induced asthma. *N. Engl. J. Med. 240*: 45-51.

Lowhagen, O., Larsson, S., Lindholm, N., and Svedmyr, N. (1985). Does continuous domiciliary treatment with high doses of beta stimulants give tolerance development? *Am. Rev. Respir. Dis.* (Submitted for publication).

Mallorga, P., Tallman, J. F., Henneberry, R. C., Hirata, F., Strittmatter, W. T., and Axelrod, J. (1980). Mepacrin blocks beta-adrenergic agonist induced desensitization in astrocytoma cells. *Proc. Natl. Acad. Sci. USA 77*: 1341-1345.

Marone, G., Lichtenstein, L. M., and Plaut, M. (1980). Hydrocortisone and human lymphocytes: Increases in cyclic adenosine 3′5′-monophosphate and potentiation of adenylate cyclase-activating agents. *J. Pharmacol. Exp. Ther. 215*: 469-478.

Meeker, R. B., and Harden, T. K. (1982). Muscarinic cholinergic receptor mediated activation of phosphodiesterase. *Mol. Pharmacol. 22*: 310-319.

Mickey, J. V., Caron, M. G., and Lefkowitz, R. J. (1975). Subsensitivity of adenylate cyclase and decreased beta-adrenergic receptor binding after chronic exposure to (–) isoproterenol in vitro. *J. Biol. Chem. 250*: 5727-5729.

Miller, W. C. (1978). Long-term $beta_2$ bronchodilator therapy and the question of tolerance. *Chest 73* (suppl)1000-1001.

Minetoya, H., and Spilker, B. A. (1975). Lack of cardiac or bronchodilator tachyphylaxis to isoprenaline in the dog. *Br. J. Pharmacol. 53*: 333-340.

Mitchell, N. W. (1982). The effect of inhibition of arachidonic acid metabolism on drug-induced contractions in isolated tracheal smooth muscle of the pig. *Br. J. Pharmacol. 755*: 129-136.

Muers, H., Koeter, G. H., deVries, K., and Kauffman, H. F. (1982). The beta-adrenergic system and allergic bronchial asthma: Changes in lymphocyte beta-adrenergic receptor number after an allergen induced asthmatic attack. *J. Allergy Clin. Immunol. 70*: 272-280.

Nelson, H. S., Black, J. W., Branch, L. B., et al. (1975). Subsensitivity to epinephrine following administration of epinephrine and ephedrine to normals. *J. Allergy Clin. Immunol. 55*: 299-309.

Nelson, A. S., Rain, D., Jr., Doner, H. C., and Posey, W. C. (1977). Subsensitivity to bronchodilator action of albuterol produced by chronic administration. *Am. Rev. Respir. Dis. 116*: 871.

Omini, C., Folco, G., Sautebin, L., Nava, G., Madelli, V., and Berti, F. (1981). Beta adrenoceptor activation induces prostaglandin E_2 generation in guinea-pig trachea. *Eur. J. Pharmacol. 72*: 227-231.

Orange, R. P., Austin, W. G., and Austin, K. F. (1971). Immunological release of histamine and slow reactive substance of anaphylaxis from human lung. 1. Modulation by agents influencing cellular levels of cyclic 3′5′ adenosine monophosphate. *J. Exp. Med.* (Suppl) *134*: 136.

Page, C. P., Mazzoni, L., and Sanjar, S. (1985a). Induction of non-specific hyper-reactivity by platelet activating factor (PAF) and its inhibition by anti-asthmatic drugs. *Am. Rev. Respir. Dis. 131* (part 2): A44.

Page, C. P., Paul, W., Basron, G. S., and Morley, J. (1985b). Platelet activating in asthma. In *Bronchial Asthma. Mechanisms and Therapeutics,* 2nd Ed. Edited by E. B. Weiss, M. S. Segal, and M. Stein. Boston, Little, Brown, pp. 266-269.

Parker, C. W., and Smith, J. W. (1973). Alterations in cyclic adenosine monophosphate metabolism in human bronchial asthma. 1. Leukocyte responsiveness to B-adrenergic agents. *J. Clin. Invest. 52*: 48-59.

Paterson, J. W., Conolly, M. E., Davies, D. S., and Dollery, C. T. (1968). Isoprenaline resistance and the use of pressurized aerosols in asthma. *Lancet 2*: 21-38.

Paterson, J. W., Courteney, R. J., Evans, R. S., and Prime, F. J. (1971). Selectivity of bronchodilator action on salbutamol in asthmatic patients. *Br. J. Dis. Chest 65*: 21-38.

Peel, E. T., and Gibson, G. J. (1980). Effects of long-term salbutamol inhalation therapy on the provocation of asthma by histamine. *Am. Rev. Respir. Dis. 121*: 973-983.

Perkins, J. P., Harden, T. K., and Harper, J. F. (1984). Acute and chronic modulation of the responsiveness of receptor associated adenylate cyclase. In *Handbook of Experimental Pharmacology.* Edited by J. Nathanson and J. Kebabian. New York, Springer-Verlag, pp. 185-223.

Plummer, A. L. (1978). Development of drug tolerance to beta$_2$ adrenergic agents in asthmatic patients. *Chest 73* (suppl): 749-757.

Raffestin, B., Cerrina, J., Boullet, C., Labat, C., Benveniste, J., and Brink, C. (1985). Response and sensitizing of isolated human pulmonary muscle preparation to pharmacological agents. *J. Pharmacol. Exp. Ther. 233*: 186-194

Reisman, R. E. (1970). Asthma induced by adrenergic aerosols. *J. Allergy 46*: 169-177.

Repsher, L. H., Anderson, J. A., Bush, R. K., Falliers, C. J., Kass, F., Kemp, J. P., Reed, C., Siegel, S., and Webb, D. (1984). Assessment of tachyphylaxis following prolonged therapy of asthma with inhaled albuterol. *Chest 85*: 34-38.

Rinard, G. A., Rubinfeld, A. R., Brunton, L. L., and Mayer, S. E. (1979). Depressed cyclic AMP levels in airway smooth muscle from asthmatic dogs. *Proc. Natl. Acad. Sci. 76*: 1472-1476.

Rinard, G. A., Jensen, A., and Puckett, A. M. (1983). Hydrocortisone and isoproterenol effects on trachealis cAMP and relaxtation. *J. Appl. Physiol. 55*(5): 1609-1613.

Rubanyi, G. M., and Paul, R. J. (1985). Modulation of beta adrenergic responsiveness by arachidonic acid metabolites in isolated bovine coronary arteries. *J. Pharmacol. Exp. Ther. 234*: 555-560.

Russell, J. A. (1984). Differential inhibitory effect of isoproterenol on contractions of canine airways. *J. Appl. Physiol. 57*: 801-807.

Samuelson, W. M., and Davies, A. O. (1984). Hydrocortisone-induced reversal of beta-adrenergic receptor uncoupling. *Am. Rev. Respir. Dis. 130*: 1023-1026.

Sano, Y., Ford, L., Begley, M., et al. (1980). Effect of in vivo anti-asthmatic drugs on human leukocyte b-adrenergic receptors. *Clin. Res. 28*: 431A.

Scarpace, P. J., and Abrass, I. B. (1982). Desensitization of adenylate cyclase and down-regulation of beta adrenergic receptors in vivo by administration of beta agonists. *J. Pharmacol. Exp. Ther. 223*: 327-331.

Scarpace, P. J., Littner, M. J., Tashkin, D. P., and Abrass, I. B. (1982). Lymphocyte beta-adrenergic refractoriness induced by theophylline or metaproterenol in healthy and asthmatic subjects. *J. Allergy Clin. Immunol. 57*: 88-89.

Schleimer, R. P. (1985). The mechanisms of antiinflammatory steroid action in allergic diseases. *Annu. Rev. Pharmacol. Toxicol. 25*: 381-412.

Shelhamer, J. M. (1980). Abnormal adrenergic responsiveness in allergic subjects: Analysis of isoproterenol-induced cardiovascular and plasma cyclic adenosine monophosphate responses. *J. Allergy Clin. Immunol. 66*: 52.

Sibley, D. R., Peters, J. R., Nambi, P., Caron, M. G., and Lefkowitz, R. J. (1984). Desensitization of turkey erythrocyte adenylate cyclase. B-adrenergic receptor phosphorylation is correlated with attenuation of adenylate cyclase activity. *J. Biol. Chem. 259*: 9742-9749.

Sims, J. A., doPico, G. A., and Reed, C. E. (1978). Bronchodilating effect of oral theophylline-ephedrine combination. *J. Allergy Clin. Immunol. 62*: 15-21.

Speizer, F., Doll, E. R., and Heaf, P. (1968a). Observations on the recent increase in mortality from asthma. *Br. Med. J. 1*: 335-339.

Speizer, F., Doll, E. R., Heaf, P., and Strang, L. B. (1968b). Investigation into the use of drugs proceeding death from asthma. *Br. Med. J. 1*: 339-343.

Spilker, B., and Tyll, J. (1976). On the question of tachyphylaxis to isoproterenol in guinea pigs. *Eur. J. Pharmacol. 36*: 283-288.

Stadel, J. M., Nambi, P., Shorr, R. G. L., Sawyer, D. F., Caron, M. G., and Lefkowitz, R. J. (1983a). Catecholamine induced desensitization of turkey erythrocyte adenylate cyclase is associated with phosphorylation of the β-adrenergic receptor. *Proc. Natl. Acad. Sci. USA 80*: 3173-3177.

Stadel, J. M., Strulovici, B., Nambi, P., Lavin, T. N., Briggs, M. M., Caron, M. G., and Lefkowitz, R. J. (1983b). Desensitization of the beta-adrenergic receptor of frog erythrocytes. Recovery and characterization of the down-regulated receptors in sequestered vesicles. *J. Biol. Chem. 258*: 3032.

Stephan, W. C., Chick, T. W., Avner, B. P., and Jenne, J. W. (1980). Tachyphylaxis to inhaled isoproterenol and the effect of methyl prednisolone in dogs. *J. Allergy Clin. Immunol. 65*: 105.

Strulovici, B., Stadel, J. M., and Lefkowitz, R. J. (1983). Functional integrity of desensitized β-adrenergic receptors internalized receptors reconstitute catecholamine stimulated adenylate cyclase activity. *J. Biol. Chem. 258*: 6410-6414.

Su, Y. F., Harden, T. K., and Perkins, J. P. (1980). Catecholamine-specific desensitization of adenylate cyclase: Evidence for a multistep process. *J. Biol. Chem. 255*: (15): 7410-7419.

Svedmyr, N. L. V., Larsson, S. A., and Thiringer, G. K. (1976). Development of "resistance" in beta drenergic receptors of asthmatic patients. *Chest 69*: 479-483.

Szentivanyi, A. (1968). The beta adrenergic theory of the atopic abnormality in bronchial asthma. *J. Allergy 42*: 203-232.

Tashkin, D. P., Conolly, M. E., Deutsch, R. I., Hui, K. K., Littner, M., Scarpace, P., and Abrass, I. (1982). Subsensitization of beta-adrenoceptors in airways and lymphocytes of healthy and asthmatic subjects. *Am. Rev. Respir. Dis. 125*: 185-193.

Taylor, S. M. and Downes, H. (1982). Bronchodilator mechanisms in bullfrog lung: Difference in response to isoproterenol, theophylline and papaverine. *J. Pharmacol. Exp. Ther. 233*: 359-367.

Taylor, W. F., and Heimlick, E. M. (1965). Ephedrine and theophylline in asthmatic children: quantitative observations on the combination and ephedrine tachyphylaxis. *Ann. Allergy 23*: 437-440.

Torda, T., Yamaguchi, I., Hirata, F., Kopin, I. N., and Axelrod, J. (1981). Quinacrine-blocked desensitization of adrenoceptors after immobilization stress or repeated injection of isoproterenol in rats. *J. Pharmacol. Exp. Ther. 236*: 334-338.

Torphy, T. J. (1984). Differential relaxant effects of isoproterenol on methacholine versus leukotriene D_4-induced contraction in the guinea pig trachea. *Eur. J. Pharmacol. 102*: 549-553.

Torphy, T. J. (1985). Biochemical regulation of airway smooth muscle tone. Current knowledge and therapeutic implications. *Rev. Clin. Basic Pharmacol. 6*: in press.

Torphy, T. J., Rinard, G. A., Rietou, M. G., and Mayers, S. E. (1983). Functional antagonism in canine tracheal smooth muscle: Inhibition by methacholine of the mechanical and biochemical responses to isoproterenol. *J. Pharmacol. Exp. Ther. 227*: 694-699.

Torphy, T. J., Zheng, C., Peterson, S. M., Fiscus, R. R., Rinard, G. A., and Mayer, S. E. (1985). Inhibitory effect of methacholine on drug induced relaxation, cyclic AMP accumulation, and cyclic AMP dependent protein kinase activation in canine tracheal smooth muscle. *J. Pharmacol. Exp. Ther. 233*: 409-417.

Van Arsdel, P. P., Schaffrin, R. M., Rosemblatt, J., Sprenkle, A. C., and Altman, L. C. (1978). Evaluation of oral fenoterol in chronic asthmatic patients. *Chest* (Suppl)*73*: 997-998.

Van den Berg, W., Leferink, J. G., Fokkens, J. K., Kreukmiet, J., Maes, R. A. A., and Bruynzeel, P. L. B. (1982). Clinical implications of drug-induced desensitization of the beta receptor after continuous oral use of terbutaline. *J. Allergy Clin. Immunol. 69*: 410-417.

Van den Brink, F. G. (1973). The model of functional interaction. I. Development and first check of a new model of functional synergism and antagonism. *Eur. J. Pharmacol. 22*: 270-278.

Van Metre, T. E. (1968). Adverse effects of inhalation of excessive amounts of nebulized isoproterenol in status asthmaticus. *J. Allergy 43*: 110.

Ward, M. J., and Tomlinson, D. R. (1976). On the question of tachyphylaxis to isoproterenol in guinea pigs. *Eur. J. Pharmacol. 36*: 283-288.

Watanabe, M., Olivo, Y., and Kasuga, Y. (1976). Desensitization of guinea-pig tracheal smooth muscle preparation to beta-adrenergic stimulants by a proceeding exposure to a high dose of catecholamines. *Jpn. J. Pharmacol. 26*: 191-199.

Weber, R. W., Smith, K. A., and Nelson, H. S. (1982). Aersolized terbutaline in asthmatics: Development of subsensitivity with long-term administration. *J. Allergy Clin. Immunol. 70*: 417-422.

Williams, J. C., Strausser, H. R., and Giles, R. E. (1983). Physiological consequences of beta adrenoceptor desensitization in guinea pigs. *Eur. J. Pharmacol. 88*: 347-356.

Wilson, A. F., Novey, H. F., Cloninger, P., Davis, J., and White, D. (1976). Cardiopulmonary effects of long-term bronchodilator administration. *J. Allergy Clin. Immunol. 58*: 204-212.

8

Physiology and Pharmacodynamics of the Xanthines

JOHN W. JENNE

Loyola-Stritch School of Medicine,
Maywood, and Edward Hines, Jr. Veterans
Administration Hospital
Hines, Illinois

I. Introduction

The xanthines are a class of compounds sharing a dioxypurine nucleus. Well-known naturally occurring methylated xanthines are caffeine (1,3,7 trimethyl-xanthine), theobromine (3,7-dimethylxanthine), and theophylline (1,3-dimethyl-xanthine), the latter synthesized as the common bronchodilator. Less well known synthetic modifications are diphylline (7-2,3 dihydroxypropyl theophylline) proxyphylline (7-hydroxypropyl theophylline), and now enprofylline (3-propylxanthine).

The xanthines share many common actions in variable proportions. These include stimulation of the central nervous system, heart, skeletal muscle, cilia, gastric secretion and urine output, elevation of blood sugar, free fatty acids and insulin, and inhibition of bronchial, uterine, and vascular smooth muscle and mediator release. Four major cellular mechanisms have been considered wholly or in part to play a role in each of them: (1) elevation of cyclic nucleotides, particularly cAMP, through inhibition of cyclic nucleotide phosphodiesterases; (2) translocation of calcium independently of cAMP; (3) antagonism of adenosine A_1 and A_2 receptors; and (4) stimulation of the adrenergic nervous system

Theophylline Enprofylline

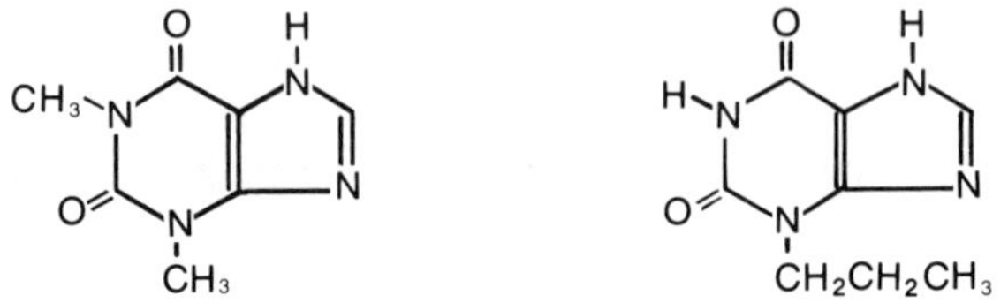

Antagonizes adenosine Lacks adenosine antagonism

Figure 1 Theophylline (1,3-dimethylxanthine) and enprofylline (3-propylxanthine). Note that enprofylline is not a methylxanthine.

(Rall, 1980). The problem is to identify which one or more mechanisms could operate at the relatively low therapeutic levels in patients (up to 50 μM unbound theophylline in plasma) and distinguishing between them. In some cases, they may overlap, such as in the stimulation of norepinephrine release through antagonism of adenosine inhibition.

A valuable tool in deciphering the role of adenosine has been the synthesis and testing of 3-propylxanthine, or enprofylline, developed by AB Draco of

Table 1 Actions of Theophylline

Adenosine inhibition likely	Adenosine inhibition unlikely
(Theophylline+ enprofylline−)	(Theophylline+ enprofylline+)
CNS activity	Bronchodilation
Gastric secretion (volume and acidity)	Cardiovascular stimulation
Tremor	Nausea and vomiting
Diuresis	Headache
Lipolysis	Relaxation of lower esophageal sphincter
Diaphragm contractility	Antipermeability

Actions are classified according to shared activity with enprofylline, and hence whether adenosine inhibition is likely to be involved. Enprofylline lacks adenosine-inhibitory qualities.

Sweden (Fig. 1). This xanthine is apparently nearly devoid of adenosine antagonistic qualities. Yet it is five times as potent as theophylline in relaxing smooth muscle, both in vitro and in vivo, and is three times as potent as an inhibitor of cyclic AMP phosphodiesterase enzyme from guinea pig lung (Bergstrand, 1980). Strictly speaking, while lack of adenosine antagonistic qualities precludes this mechanism for enprofylline, *it does not necessarily do so for theophylline.* Yet, it is strong negative evidence. Table 1 lists actions investigated to date in which adenosine antagonism is considered the likely principal mechanism (enprofylline ineffective) and those actions in which both theophylline and enprofylline are effective and therefore unlikely to involve adenosine antagonism as the major mechanism. Andersson and Persson have edited an extensive review (1985).

In the following discussion, we will use theophylline as the prototype xanthine, since this is the most effective xanthine currently approved for use in the United States, and the one for which we have the most investigative and clinical experience. The limited pharmacodynamic information available for other xanthines will be discussed at the end of the chapter.

II. Physiology

A. Smooth Muscle

Calcium contracts smooth muscle by combining with calmodulin to activate myosin light chain kinase, thus phosphorylating myosin to combine with actin and undergo crossbridge cycling. This process is modulated by cyclic-AMP-dependent protein kinase. A second calcium-dependent pathway involves phosphatidylinositol breakdown and protein kinase C activation without cyclic nucleotide involvement (see Chap. 3). Relaxation occurs with myosin dephosphorylation. Once contracted with a calcium spike, certain smooth muscles have the ability to maintain their tone in a "latched" state, with very little energy expenditure and at lower calcium levels (see Chap. 1).

As studied in vascular smooth muscle, dephosphorylation of cross-bridges partially relaxes muscle, but a slower relaxation phase then follows from the nonphosphorylated latched state, which is greatly accelerated by various muscle relaxants. This process may depend on calcium sequestration mechanisms, sometimes involving cyclic AMP, removing calcium from an unknown regulatory site. (Gerthoffer et al., 1984).

Studies with aequorin have helped elucidate the relationship of Ca^{2+} levels to the contraction-relaxation process. Aequorin is a bioluminescent protein that emits blue light when it combines with Ca^{2+}. Following aequorin injection into the sarcoplasm of either cardiac or smooth muscle, phasic shifts of Ca^{2+} and the effect of drugs can be correlated with tension changes (Morgan et al., 1984). There are stimulus-specific patterns of calcium behavior with contraction, suggesting that the same may hold for specific relaxants and for various relaxation-contraction pairs (Morgan and Morgan, 1984a). Remarkably, the first application of this technique to smooth muscle relaxation using ferret portal vein actually showed an *increase* in Ca^{2+} with isoproterenol suggesting an uncoupling of calcium from force production. Papaverine and forskolin behaved in a similar fashion (Morgan and Morgan, 1984b). Thus, relaxation is not simply a matter of altering Ca^{2+} levels.

Cyclic AMP

More than one mechanism may be involved in the relaxation of bronchial smooth muscle by theophylline and caffeine. The mechanism originally proposed, phosphodiesterase inhibition with consequent elevation of cAMP, has met with increasing skepticism. The IC_{50} (concentration required for 50% inhibition) of cyclic AMP and GMP phosphodiesterase (low Km) extracted from human bronchial smooth muscle is 100-200 μM, exceeded by a factor of 2 to 4 the unbound concentration of theophylline in plasma (Bergstrand, 1980). Yet some inhibition must occur. In guinea pig trachea, there is a disparity between the concentration of theophylline necessary to elevate whole muscle cAMP (1 mM) and the 10-20-fold lower concentration able to relax the muscle or produce detectable shifts in Ca^{2+} (Kolbeck et al., 1979). Several workers have emphasized the inconstant relationship between whole muscle cAMP and tension changes. The rise in cAMP associated with relaxation by theophylline or isoproterenol can be prevented using methacholine as the constrictant (Lohman et al., 1977). Discrepancies in effective concentration and timing of changes in cAMP (Polacek et al., 1971) and between cAMP and calcium efflux (Deth and Lynch, 1981) have been noted using several phosphodiesterase inhibitors. In bullfrog hemilung, a preparation with intrinsic tone, theophylline relaxation occurs with no change in whole muscle cAMP, while relaxation with isoproterenol and papaverine is associated with such changes but on a differing time scale between the drugs (Taylor and Downes, 1982). Moreover, relaxation by theophylline is more complete than by isoproterenol, a phenomenon also noted with guinea pig trachea (Karlsson and Persson, 1981) and some isolated human bronchi (Guillot et al., 1984), thus tending to discount a common cAMP-mediated mechanism.

Yet several indirect arguments favor the cAMP-phosphodiesterase inhibition mechanism, at least for a portion of theophylline's action. Some of them are discussed in Chapter 3. The regional nature of these changes in muscle and the lack of a simple relationship between tension and *whole muscle* cAMP and GMP content has been stressed (Andersson, 1975; Andersson et al., 1978). In rabbit colon and bovine mesenteric artery, there is appropriate timing of microsomal cAMP elevations and relaxation by various phosphodiesterase inhibitors including theophylline, both occurring in a matter of seconds (Andersson, 1972). With elevation of microsomal cAMP (by β-agonists), there is increased microsomal binding of Ca^{2+}. The potency of papaverine and theophylline for inhibition of the high-affinity phosphodiesterase and relaxation of canine bronchial strips is comparable (Triner et al., 1977). There is a strong correlation ($P < 0.001$) between the ability of seven cyclic AMP phosphodiesterase inhibitors, including caffeine and theophylline, to inhibit a high-affinity phosphodiesterase (one of five fractionated) and to relax canine tracheal smooth muscle (Polson et al., 1982). In fact, the molar ratios of K_i to ED_{50} are essentially unity, with constants in the "therapeutic range." In five species, a parallelism was found between calculated elevations in whole muscle and the relaxing ability of both theophylline and isoproterenol (Niewoehner et al., 1979). In human tracheal muscle, 50 μM theophylline, equivalent to about 10 μg/ml unbound drug, was found to inhibit phosphodiesterase about 40% (Svedmyr, 1977). Thus, changes in cAMP may well be occurring in human bronchial smooth muscle at plasma theophylline levels, at least in some discrete effector compartment.

In tracheal muscle, theophylline at 100 μM was shown to increase binding of cyclic AMP to an unknown protein fraction (Miech et al., 1979). With improved assays for cyclic AMP-dependent protein kinase, measurement of this activity can be a more sensitive indicator of cyclic-AMP-mediated changes than cyclic AMP itself (Torphy et al., 1985). Moreover, a current hypothesis is that cyclic GMP as well is involved in a negative feedback mechanism (Fiscus et al., 1984; Rapport, 1986). Its elevation (e.g., by theophylline) may actually contribute to smooth muscle relaxation. Theophylline could also potentiate the smooth muscle relaxing effect of β-agonists through its phosphodiesterase-inhibiting action, quite apart from its own mechanism of action. One is forced to withhold judgement until more is known.

Adenosine Antagonism and Catecholamines

Adenosine antagonism is receiving increasing prominence as at least one mechanism of action of theophylline on bronchial smooth muscle, having been originally proposed some time ago (Fredholm, 1980). Adenosine is released into the bloodstream with antigenic bronchoprovocation (Mann et al., 1983) and hypoxemia (Mentzer et al., 1975). Theophylline is a potent antagonist of both A_1 (cyclic-AMP-depressing) and A_2 (cyclic-AMP-stimulating) receptors at relevant concentrations, and many of theophylline's actions are believed to result through this action (Table 1). However, in vitro studies with bronchial smooth muscle tend to discount this mechanism for bronchodilation. While theophylline antagonizes the A_1 receptor-mediated contraction by adenosine, these receptors are sparse. In fact, adenosine is generally found to relax isolated tracheal smooth muscle from animals through its cyclic-AMP-stimulatory (A_2) receptors (Karlsson et al., 1982). Recent studies with isolated human airways from normals show little or no effect (Finney et al., 1985) although 10 μM adenosine did cause "threshold contractions" of airways from two patients allergic to birch pollen (Dahlen et al., 1983).

The strongest negative evidence comes from in vitro studies with enprofylline, a xanthine nearly lacking adenosine inhibitory qualities, yet five times as potent as theophylline as a smooth muscle relaxant. Figure 9 of Chapter 4 shows the relative smooth-muscle-relaxing activities (guinea pig trachea) and the CNS-stimulatory activities (ability to counter adenosine inhibition of electrically induced release of acetylcholine from mysenteric plexus of longitudinal muscle) of a number of xanthine derivatives. The 1-methyl group is essential for neurostimulatory qualities, but the 3-substitutions are more important for smooth muscle relaxation. Theophylline has both these groups, but enprofylline only the 3-substitutions (Fig. 1).

However, there is some very suggestive in vivo evidence that theophylline's bronchodilating action is due at least in part to an interaction with adenosine. In contrast to its lack of effect in normals, adenosine causes bronchoconstriction when inhaled by either allergic or nonallergic asthmatics (Cushley et al., 1983). Inhaled aminophylline shifts the subsequent dose-response curve to the right to a degree several times greater than it shifts the histamine dose-response curve (Cushley et al., 1984). Since adenosine is released into the synaptic cleft on nerve stimulation and is a presynaptic inhibitor of smooth muscle neurotransmission, both noradrenergic and cholinergic (Paton, 1981; Fredholm and Hedquist, 1980) theophylline could alter autonomic impulses to the intact lung by acting upon the nerve supply at its adenosine receptors. It is therefore disconcerting to find that the relative bronchodilating potency of enprofylline to theophylline is just as great in vitro (no nerve supply) as in vivo (Persson et al., 1981; Lunell et al., 1982) despite marked differences in their adenosine inhibitory qualities. Moreover, the adrenergic nerve supply to bronchial smooth muscle in humans is sparse at best (Richardson, 1979). Finally, an autonomic interaction by adenosine bronchoconstriction is blocked by anticholinergic and β-adrenergic drugs only to the same extent as bronchoconstriction produced by other stimuli (Mann et al., 1985), suggesting that prejunctional autonomic effects are not involved. An interaction between theophylline and adenosine on mediator release is another possibility, particularly since such an antagonism has been demonstrated in vitro with rat peritoneal mast cells (Marquardt et al., 1978). Theophylline could inhibit adenosine potentiation of the human lung allergic responses (Hughes et al., 1984). Somewhat against this hypothesis is the fact that there is no detectable mediator release to the circulation following adenosine challenge of allergic asthmatics (Cushley et al., 1985).

Catecholamine Stimulation

When an IV infusion of 5.6 mg/kg aminophylline was administered over 10 min to normal subjects, there was an abrupt rise in SG_{aw} peaking 5 min later, then declining slightly and leveling off (MacKay et al., 1983). This was paralelled by a rise in cAMP, including the early spike. Both could be blocked in a concentration-dependent manner with propranolol. This suggests that at least a part of theophylline's action is due to production of endogenous catecholamines, possibly by antagonizing adenosine inhibition of neurotransmitter release, in this case, release of catecholamines either from the adrenal or from tissue nerve endings. Since plasma catecholamines only rise slowly during loading and maintenance of aminophylline (Vestal et al., 1983; Higbee et al., 1982) it seems more likely that the early cAMP spike is being generated in the tissues although not necessarily in bronchial smooth muscle. The catecholamine mechanism for theophylline bronchodilation will require considerably more support.

In summary, the mechanism for theophylline's bronchodilator action is far from clear. There may well be multiple mechanisms, and there is some evidence supporting several at this time.

B. Cardiovascular System

In Vitro Studies

The actions of theophylline on the heart and the mechanisms are complex. In vitro studies have used unrealistically high theophylline concentrations to bring out drug actions, and these effects may not be relevant in vivo. For example, at 2.5 mM, theophylline increases both rate and force of myocardial contraction while prolonging time to peak tension and relaxation time (Marcus et al., 1972; Tsien, 1977; Morgan and Morgan, 1984). Part of theophylline's action on the heart is due to endogenous catecholamine release. Theophylline shifts the force-velocity curve of cat papillary muscle upwards and to the right (Marcus et al., 1972). Isometric tension experiments with theophylline show a progressive increase in peak tension and rate of tension development as theophylline is increased from 2.5 μM to 2.5 mM. This contrasts with β-adrenergic agonist action, in which time to peak tension is decreased. Yet, with prior reserpinization, the maximum inotropic effect of theophylline is reduced by 40%, indicating that theophylline's effect is likely to be a hybrid of direct effects, and indirect, catechol-mediated effects, probably through cyclic AMP. One might surmise that an adenosine-inhibitory effect might also play a major role in theophylline's action, since adenosine itself inhibits rate and force of contraction. This seems unlikely, since enprofylline, lacking adenosine-inhibitory qualities, is still three or more times as potent as theophylline in stimulating the guinea pig left atrium (Persson et al., 1981).

Table 2 Four Patterns of Light and Tension Responses Produced by Positive Inotropic Agents in the Cat Papillary Muscle

	Light			Tension		
Pattern w/Example	Peak	Time to peak	T 1/2	Peak	Time to peak	T 1/2
1. Isoproterenol	+3	-1	-2	+3	-2	-2
2. Theophylline	-1, +3	+2	+2	+3	+2	+2
3. Digitalis	+2	N.C.	N.C.	+2	N.C.	N.C.
4. Amrinone	+2	+1	-1	+2	N.C.	-1

T 1/2, half time for decline from peak; +, increase; –, increase; N.C., no change. Adapted from Morgan et al., 1984.

Calcium Movements and Drug Action

Calcium contracts cardiac muscle by removing the inhibition of troponin, a regulatory protein that restrains the natural tendency of actin and myosin to form crossbridges and contract. Calcium is released from sarcoplasmic reticulum to activate myofilaments, but the calcium release process is believed to be activated by a smaller influx of calcium during depolarization by the action potential (Fabiato and Fabiato, 1979). Relaxation occurs with reuptake of calcium by the sarcoplasmic reticulum (Tsein, 1977).

With aequorin, a bioluminescent indicator of Ca^{2+} levels, the action of inotropic drugs can be broken into four patterns, depending on their light and tension responses. These are listed in Table 2. Pattern 1 drugs include β-agonists, papaverine, cholera toxin, isobutylmethylxanthine, and dibuteryl cAMP. Pattern 2 drugs include theophylline and caffeine. Pattern 3 drugs include digitalis and vanadate, and pattern 4 amrinone (Morgan et al., 1984).

Examples of pattern 1 and patterns 2 responses are shown in Figure 2 with cat papillary muscle. It should be emphasized that lower concentrations of caffeine (e.g., 0.6 mM) can produce a marked pattern 2 tension effect without apparent change or even an increase in the aequorin signal. The flattening and prolongation of the latter occur at the higher caffeine concentration shown in Figure 2.

Caffeine and theophylline are thought to share the ability to inhibit calcium uptake by the sarcoplasmic reticulum and promote its release, without mediation of cAMP (Blinks et al., 1972). These xanthines actually increase calcium sensitivity of the myofilaments (Mope et al., 1980). Yet, at the high concentration of 2 mM, theophylline exerts an inotropic effect closely correlated

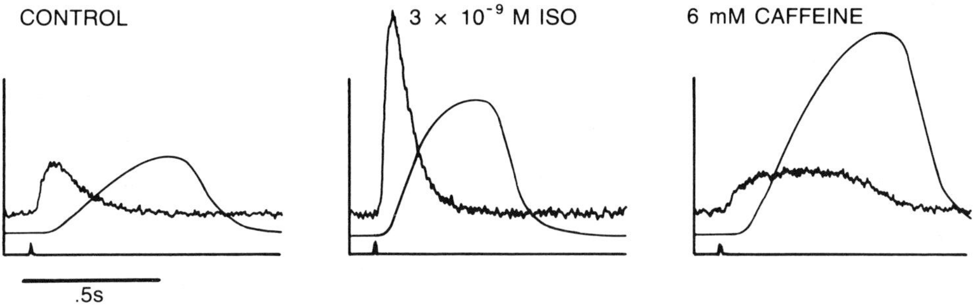

Figure 2 Comparative effect of 3×10^{-9} M isoproterenol and 6 mM caffeine on the time course of tension (smooth curve) and the aequorin light signal of the Ca^{2+} transient in cat papillary muscle. These are type I and type II patterns, respectively, as described in the text. At lower concentrations, the caffeine signal may increase in intensity. The intensity is a function of the Ca^{2+} level, but may increase simply through redistribution in the cell (modified from Morgan and Morgan, 1984c).

with changes in cAMP levels (Endoh et al., 1982; Tsein, 1977). With 6 mM caffeine there is a prolonged elevation of calcium levels corresponding to prolongation of the contractile phase contrasting with the effect of isoproterenol (Morgan et al., 1984).

Studies in the Intact Dog

The effects of theophylline in the dog depend somewhat on the state of anesthesia. In the anesthetized animal, there is a marked increase (25% over baseline) in the rate of increase of left ventricular pressure (dP/dt) at only 9 μg/ml theophylline when afterload is held constant. This action is blocked with verapamil (Dimarco et al., 1985). Coronary and systemic flow increase as vascular resistance falls, commensurate with a direct effect on the vessels (Dimarco et al., 1985). In the unanesthetized dog, however, while a loading dose of 10 mg/kg aminophylline over 10 min also increases dP/dt; this is blocked with propranolol (Rutherford et al., 1981). Coronary and systemic flow now decrease slightly with an increase in vascular resistance, and these changes are reversed with phentolamine. At 25 mg/kg aminophylline, coronary flow finally increases as vessels dilate with the increased work. These studies indicate that theophylline stimulates both α- and β-adrenergic systems in the dog, that pentobarbital anesthesia inhibits this nervous input, and that the slow inward channel calcium current is crucial to theophylline's action on the heart.

Table 3 Effect of Infused Theophylline on Pulse Rate and Several Metabolic Entities in Young Men

	0 μg/ml	5 μg/ml	10 μg/ml	15 μg/ml	20 μg/ml
Free fatty acids (mEq)	498	604	788	745	993
Insulin (μU/ml)	10	11	11	12	15
Glucose (mg/dl)	No change				
Epinephrine (pg/ml)	29	40	57	72	105
Norepinephrine (pg/ml)	190	197	244	264	312
Pulse	53-56	53	56	61	77

Adapted from Vestal et al., 1983

Cardiovascular Effects in Humans

To study the acute effects of theophylline on the cardiovascular system, a loading and maintenance dose of aminophylline was infused over 180 min into six normal young men on four different occasions (Vestal et al., 1983). At theophylline levels of 5, 10, 15, and 20 μg/ml, measurements were made of plasma catecholamines, plasma insulin, free fatty acids, sugar, and several cardiovascular noninvasive parameters (Table 3).

An increase in heart rate occurred only at the 15 and 20 μg/ml levels, with the supine rate gradually increasing from a mean of 52 to 77 beats/min at 20 μg/ml. Significantly, the rate increase paralleled the rise in plasma catecholamines, mean plasma epinephrine increasing from 29 to 105 pg/ml and norepinephrine increasing from 190 to 312 pg/ml. The authors surmised that norepinephrine originated partly from the adrenal and partly as spillover from much higher local tissue release. A slight but significant inotropic effect was observed at the 5 μg/ml theophylline level and above, manifested by a *shortening* of the duration of electromechanical systole adjusted for rate (QS_2 index). Somewhat similar cardiovascular effects were reported when theophylline was slowly infused up to a level of 10 μg/ml over 180 min to normals (Ogilvie et al., 1977). Mean heart rate increased from 54 to 67 beats/min. A slight shortening of systole was also noted, and 20% increase in forearm venous capacitance.

The effects of theophylline are more pronounced in the presence of impaired ventricular function or elevated pulmonary vascular resistance. When 1.0 g aminophylline was infused over 30 min into patients with chronic obstructive pulmonary disease (COPD), pulmonary vascular resistance decreased an average of 24% with a fall in mean pulmonary artery pressures from 19.7 to 14.8 mm (normal $\leq$ 20 mm), a drop in peripheral vascular resistance, a decrease in stroke

Table 4 Effect of Theophylline Acutely and After 16 Weeks on Cardiovascular and Pulmonary Indices

	Acute[a]		16 Weeks	
	Control	Short term (n = 15)	Control	Long term (n = 11)
RVEF (%)	42 ± 6	48 ± 6	43 ± 5[b]	48 ± 4 $(p < 0.005)$
LVEF (%)	64 ± 3	68 ± 6	61 ± 3	65 ± 3 $(p < 0.0025)$
HR	81 ± 5	95 ± 5	81 ± 6	95 ± 7
MAP (mm)	96 ± 2	96 ± 2	98 ± 2	97 ± 3
FEV_1 (L)	1.24 ± 0.10	1.46 ± 0.11	1.29 ± 0.12	1.63 ± 0.14

[a]Mean serum theophylline of 15 μg/ml.
[b]Seven of 11 patients had abnormally low RVEF before treatment. This normalized in five patients.
Adapted from Matthay et al., 1982.

work of both right and left ventricles, a rise in cardiac index, and a rise in heart rate from 85.1 to 109.8 (Parker et al., 1967). At this dosage, theophylline levels must have been in the 20 μg/ml range.

In cor pulmonale, an even more pronounced drop in mean pulmonary artery pressure was observed, from 39 to 25 mm (36%) (Parker et al., 1966). More recently, the acute and chronic effects of theophylline on right and left ventricular performance have been studied in COPD using noninvasive radionuclide first pass imaging techniques (Matthay et al., 1978, 1982). In all instances, there was an increase in right and left ventricular ejection fraction.

The cardiovascular parameters on 16 weeks of chronic therapy are shown in Table 4. These improvements are due, at least in part, to a reduction in afterload for both ventricles, with or without a direct inotropic action. The remarkable thing is that the improvement is maintained over 16 weeks. It seems unlikely to be due to elevated catacholamines since it has been shown that the rise in catecholamines from caffeine in the unadapted patient is largely a transient phenomenon.

In contrast to its effect on other systemic vessels, theophylline exerts a local vasconstricting effect on the cerebral vasculature (Gottstein and Paulson, 1972). This effect is independent of any effect secondary to hyperventilation since small doses infused directly into the carotid artery are effective without any effect on PCO_2.

C. Nervous System

Theophylline stimulates the central nervous system at many levels. A major mechanism is adenosine antagonism (Fredholm, 1985; Daly et al., 1981). Small doses of theophylline (1 mg/kg) antagonize the depressant actions of adenosine and reverse fluorazepam, diazepam, and lorazepam sedation, while enprofylline does not (Wangler and Fitzpatrick, 1985). In large doses, theophylline is able to produce generalized convulsions in many species (Persson and Erjefalt, 1981), while enprofylline does not, and in fact, is a depressant. 1-Alkylated xanthines antagonize adenosine-induced depression and increase spontaneous locomotor activity in mice (Persson et al., 1982b).

The neurostimulatory qualities of theophylline on the autonomic nervous system and its antagonism of adenosine can be studied in vitro in the mysenteric plexus-longitudinal muscle preparation (Paton, 1981). Adenosine inhibits electrically induced twitches caused by release of acetylcholine (Karlsson et al., 1982). It modulates both adrenergic and cholinergic neurotransmission (Hedquist et al., 1978; Visi and Knoll, 1976). Theophylline has a biphasic effect on the guinea pig ileum. At low concentrations (10-100 μM), it stimulates ileal contraction by counteracting adenosine inhibition of acetylcholine release but is without effect on phosphodiesterase activity. At higher concentrations (0.1 mM) it inhibits the contractile response and also inhibits phosphodiesterase (Gustafson et al., 1981).

Adenosine also inhibits the release of transmitter from rat phrenic nerve (Ginsberg and Hedquist, 1971). Therefore, theophylline should antagonize this activity while enprofylline should not. It has been postulated that theophylline potentiation of nervous input to the cat soleus muscle at high concentrations is due to phosphodiesterase inhibition and consequent elevation of cyclic AMP (Standaert and Dretchen, 1981). The action of theophylline in potentiating tremor and skeletal muscle contractility may be related to such motor nerve augmentation, as well as augmenting the action of beta agonists on muscle receptors.

D. Lower Esophageal Sphincter Pressure and Gastric Secretions

Theophylline is known to relax lower esophageal sphincter pressure (LESP) (Stein et al., 1980) and to increase gastric secretions (Foster et al., 1979). Since gastroesophageal reflux (GER) is believed to be an occasional cause of asthma (Mansfield and Stein, 1978), theophylline should be avoided in patients with overt GER and asthma. Further studies with both theophylline and enprofylline reveal that while theophylline increases both volume and acidity of gastric secretion, enprofylline does not (Johannesson et al., 1985). Neither stimulates gastrin. However, both drugs reduce LESP by about a third, and in the same potency ratio as their bronchodilator action.

E. Kidney

In the unadapted individual, theophylline is capable of producing a marked diuresis and loss of sodium and chloride while sparing potassium. Aminophylline is occasionally still used for this purpose in congestive heart failure. Diuresis and electrolyte loss is not seen with enprofylline (Johannesson et al., 1985), so that the effects of theophylline on the kidney appear to be mediated by adenosine, a substance causing vasoconstriction in renal afferent arterioles (Osswald et al., 1980).

F. "Metabolic" Actions

Plasma catecholamine changes after three hours of aminophylline are listed in Table 3 (Vestal et al., 1983). The authors hold out the possibility that blood volume reduction from the ensuing diuresis could also have been responsible for the gradual rise in catecholamines (Vestal, personal communication). A smaller catecholamine rise was recorded following an oral theophylline challenge at a plasma level of 7 μg/ml (Higbee et al., 1982) but not observed in another study at a theophylline level of about 10 μg/ml or at equipotent enprofylline levels (Andersson et al., 1975). The latter group also found no change in glucagon or renin, but confirmed the rapid rise in free fatty acids. Enprofylline did not elevate free fatty acids, suggesting that lipolysis is another process inhibited by adenosine.

G. Mucociliary Clearance

Mucociliary clearance depends upon both ciliary activity per se and the properties of the sol and gel phases of the mucus blanket. In vitro, theophylline has been shown to increase ciliary beat frequency, water flux into the lung, and mucous discharge from bronchial glands (Pavia et al., 1983). Using labeled particles, a modest increase in tracheobronchial clearance has been shown in chronic bronchitis during maintenance theophylline therapy (Sutton et al., 1981).

H. Mediator Release

The effect of therapeutic levels of theophylline on histamine release following antigen challenge is disputed despite in vitro evidence using sensitized human lung fragments (Orange et al., 1971). While in one study theophylline markedly inhibited immediate bronchospasm and release of histamine and neutrophilic chemotactic factor into the circulation, presumably a reflection of mediators released from perfused lung structure (Martin et al., 1980), a second and third study failed to confirm any appreciable effect on immediate bronchospasm (Nissen et al., 1980; Pauwels et al., 1985). Moreover, there is little or no effect of systemic theophylline on immediate skin test hypersensitivity, either alone or combined with a β agonist (Abramowitz et al., 1980). However, since histamine is only one component of the immediate bronchospastic response to an allergen, failure of theophylline to block the immediate response does not preclude inhibition of histamine release.

Although both theophylline and enprofylline produce only slight reduction of the immediate response at therapeutic levels in humans (serum levels of 10 μg/ml and 2.5 μg/ml, respectively) their principal effect is on the delayed response. The effectiveness of enprofylline virtually eliminates a significant adenosine inhibitory role for this action, while evoking other effects involved in the late response such as antipermeability effects (Pauwels et al., 1985).

The mechanism of in vitro xanthine inhibition of allergic mediator release is not clear. Early work suggests mediation by cyclic AMP (Orange et al., 1971; Bourne et al., 1972), possibly acting through inhibition of microtubular formation (Peters et al., 1982). Adenosine antagonism has been postulated, based on the fact that adenosine potentiates histamine release from rat peritoneal mast cells (Marquardt et al., 1978), and that theophylline antagonizes this potentiation at lower concentrations (10^{-5}–10^{-4} M) than required in the absence of adenosine (10^{-4}-10^{-3} M), (Fredholm, 1980). This seems rather weak evidence, added to the organ species differences in mast cell source.

At a dosage of only 3 mg/kg IV theophylline significantly reduces the bronchospastic response of guinea pigs to IV platelet-activating factor (PAF-acether) (Page et al., 1985). It is postulated that theophylline, cromolyn, and ketotifen, all of which share this property, do so by inhibiting its action on mediator release from activated platelets or other cells, particularly as involved in the late response to allergen (Morley et al., 1985).

I. Antipermeability Actions

A striking effect by both aminophylline and isoproterenol has been shown against production of pulmonary edema in rabbit lungs perfused in situ after acid aspiration (Mizus et al., 1985). The production is not due to a drop in pulmonary vascular pressure from these vasodilators, since it persists when perfusion pressures are maintained or even increased. This is a necessary control since, in the bacteremic sheep model, the major portion of the protective effect by these drugs is indeed due to the drop in perfusion pressure with vasodilation (Foy et al., 1979). Other studies, in guinea pig lung made edematous by histamine aerosol, also show the protective effect of aminophylline and beta agonists (Persson et al., 1979). The dosage of aminophylline used, 55 mg/kg orally, is consistent with the dosages required for bronchodilation in this species. When fluorescent dextran is used as a marker, topical application of isoproterenol also prevents vascular leakage from the hamster pouch after topical bradykinin (Svensko et al., 1979). From such experiments it is postulated that generated cyclic

AMP relaxes the contractile actimyosin filaments, producing the vascular endothelial gaps responsible for increased permeability (Mizus et al., 1985). The antipermeability effect of theophylline and β-agonists may be an important component in the prevention of the delayed phase of airway obstruction following therapeutic challenge (Pauwels, 1985).

J. Diaphragm Contractility and Fatigue

The ability of theophylline to enhance contractility of the diaphragm and other muscles of respiration, particularly in the fatigued state, may be one of its most important actions. Enprofylline may not share this quality, based on preliminary studies (Howell and Fitzgerald, 1985). This topic is covered in depth in Chapter 9.

III. Pharmacodynamics of Bronchodilation

Bronchodilation provides an excellent opportunity to explore a dose-response relationship. We can precisely grade drug action at concentrations virtually free of side effects. Our attempts to do this, however, illustrate the problems and limitations of devising a dose-response curve:

1. What errors are made in using plasma levels instead of effective tissue levels, both acutely and at steady state?
2. How should the pulmonary response be best expressed?
3. What is the nature of the dose-response curve? The slope? The V_{max}? Does the EC_{50} vary between individuals?
4. Does the response vary according to the nature and degree of bronchospasm?
5. Does the presence of other bronchodilators alter the theophylline response and vice versa?
6. Should we measure bronchial relaxation or prevention of bronchospasm?
7. What part of the airway should we look at: large or small?

We can deal with some of these questions from data already obtained in vivo. For other issues, there are clues from in vitro data.

A. Temporal Relationship of Plasma Levels to Effective Tissue Levels

Drug effects do not necessarily mirror plasma drug levels. They depend on levels in the relevant tissue compartment as it equilibrates with plasma levels. Thus, when 4 mg/kg IV aminophylline was administered over 5 min to asthmatic children and the rise in FEV_1 carefully monitored, there was about a 30 min delay between peak plasma levels and peak FEV_1 response (Maselli et al., 1970), although an effect began almost immediately. Moreover, the subsequent fall in FEV_1 lagged behind the plasma levels. When the same 4 mg/kg dose was infused slowly over an 8 hr period, the FEV_1 response rose in lock step with the rise in serum levels, with significant FEV_1 improvement at levels substantially below 5 μg/ml. The pharmacologic response to the drug was slightly different depending upon whether the patient was introduced abruptly or gradually to the drug.

Using the data of Maselli et al. and assuming a two-compartment model, the relationship of the "tissue" compartment levels (in direct contact with the bronchial receptors) to the central compartment was derived (Levy and Koysooko, 1975).

The calculated lag in *peak* tissue theophylline following bolus injection was nearly 1 hr. When theophylline was administered slowly, as by prolonged IV infusion or a slow-release tablet, there was no apparent lag. A similar lag in peak effect is evident in recent studies in adult asthmatics (Richer et al., 1982) but nevertheless the onset of effect is very rapid.

B. Expression of Pulmonary Response

When doing in vitro tissue studies, the response to a bronchodilator is customarily expressed as the "percent relaxation," usually against an imposed isometric tension but sometimes against intrinsic tone. The in vivo analogue of this is the *percent of achievable response* against the tone of existing bronchospasm.

$$\%\text{ of achievable response} = \frac{\Delta\,FEV_1}{FEV_1\,\text{max} - FEV_1\ \text{initial}}$$

The merits of using the "percent achievable" response can be seen if one considers how the more customary "percent increase" or "increase" in FEV_1 varies with baseline FEV_1. These two methods are useful providing the starting value is sufficiently less than normal, but as the starting value approaches normal, the response must rapidly decline. The "percent achievable" approach does not suffer from this problem. As the numerator declines, the denominator declines until one or both become zero when the formula collapses. The "percent achievable" is thus analogous to the "percent relaxation" used in vitro, and should follow a similar log-dose relationship.

Use of the customary method of expression may have unfairly influenced tests for so-called synergism between bronchodilators such as theophylline and a β-agonist. These drugs are generally considered to be additive, but the log-dose relationship has not been taken into account and the combined responses may be entering into an area of anatomical limitation as well. If synergism were

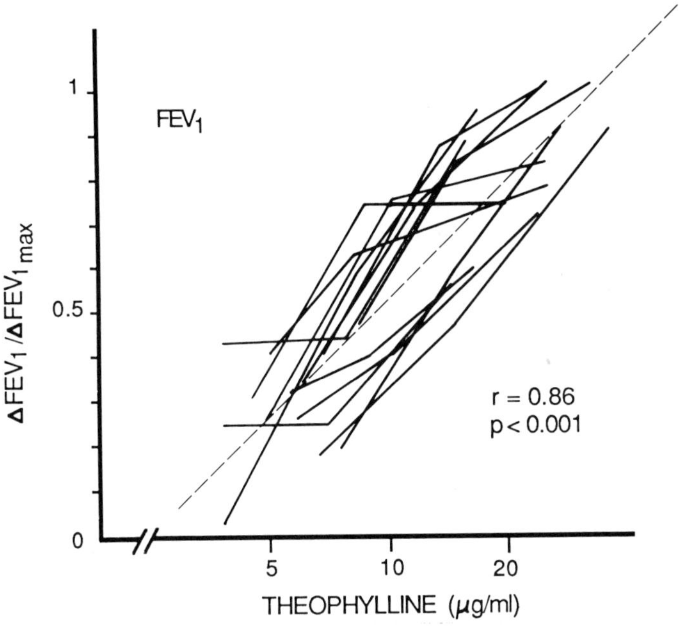

Figure 3 Effects of increasing concentrations of theophylline on the ratio of change in FEV_1 to the maximum increase obtained at any theophylline concentration to 20 μg/ml, or up to four puffs of albuterol. Aminophylline was infused to give levels of theophylline approximating 5, 10, 15, and 20 μg/ml (from Racineux et al., 1981).

judged on the basis of "percent achievable response" for both the individual and combined effects, a different picture could emerge.

C. Dose-Response Curve and Individual Variability

Fortunately, deliberate dose-response studies have been obtained utilizing some form of the "percent achievable" approach. Thus, Mitenko and Ogilvie (1973) loaded and maintained aminophylline in six asthmatics, expressing their response in terms of the "percent predicted." They concluded that the data fit a log-dose relationship. Racineux et al. improved on this approach by expressing the response in terms of the maximum obtainable response, either to the 5, 10, 15, and 20 μg/ml theophylline loaded and infused, *or* to up to four puffs of albuterol from a metered dose inhaler (Racineux et al., 1981). Again, expressed as $\Delta FEV_1/FEV_{1max}$, a fit to a log-dose relationship was obtained (Fig. 3).

With fewer than four points, it is difficult to distinguish between a log-dose relationship and a linear relationship. The necessity of doing so is apparent when one realizes that a log-dose relationship means that the response is proportional to the *ratios* of two concentrations rather than the difference between them as in a linear relationship response.

In the Mitenko and Ogilvie study, the mean log-dose relationship appeared to continue beyond 20 μg/ml. This was also true for the Racineux study, while the response to albuterol appeared to be leveling off at four puffs. This is a crucial distinction if true. It also introduces the question of whether additional bronchodilation can be obtained by combined therapy over that due to the beta agonist alone, as discussed later.

The so-called "therapeutic range" for theophylline respresents a compromise between effectiveness and an acceptable risk of toxicity. A disproportionate increase in pulmonary function occurs at low theophylline levels, but the advantage, or "therapeutic ratio," falls off rapidly as the levels rise into the potentially toxic rante (Jenne et al., 1972; Hendeles and Weinberger, 1983). The question arises as to whether the 10-20 μg/ml therapeutic range applies to all asthmatics equally, is true for all bronchoconstricting stimuli, true for both children and adults, and independent of the degree of asthma severity.

These questions have not been studied in detail. As one examines the individual dose-response curves of Mitenko and Ogilvie or Racineux et al., both of which are based on a "percent achievable" response concept, there is a spread of curves at approximately the same slope but at apparently different thresholds, with each curve corrected for that patient's reversibility. With fewer points, Billing et al. found a rather wide divergence of slopes, but used the more limited FEV_1 response, which ignores baseline FEV_1 differences (Billing et al., 1982). Considering all the available evidence, one can expect some response in all asthmatics, but there may be a difference in threshold. It is interesting that 3 of 22 stable asthmatics responded vigorously to theophylline addition after a very sluggish response to inhaled metaproterenol (Appel, 1984). We may be seeing here a response in those cases that have not proceeded far enough up their own dose-response curve with conventional β-agonist therapy.

D. Response as a Function of the Degree and Nature of Constricting Agent of Bronchospasm

While an FEV_1 response was found to low concentrations of theophylline in children—under 5 μg/ml (Masseli et al., 1970)—such a response was also seen in adults (Nicholson and Chick, 1973), although the latter authors' use of whole blood for theophylline slightly underestimated serum levels. In both studies responses commenced at levels in the neighborhood of 2 μg/ml. Furthermore, satisfactory clinical results have been shown for theophylline at levels in the 5-10 μg/ml range (Rachelefsky et al., 1978). It may be that asthmatics do show an adequate response to low levels in a mild ambulatory state but an inadequate response when their asthma worsens.

In a well controlled study dealing with asthmatic and COPD patients in an acute exacerbation treated with all drug modalities, a significant advantage was shown if theophylline was boosted to 20 μg/ml over those in whom it remained at 10 μg/ml (Voseh et al., 1982). These acutely ill patients may have had different dose-response curves to any bronchodilator than when in stable state, requiring a larger dose to achieve V_{max}.

There is an in vitro basis for such behavior. When guinea pig trachea is used, the log-dose response curve to either theophylline or isoproterenol shifts to the right with increasing tension produced by methacholine (Karlsson and Persson, 1981). Similar reductions in isoproterenol effectiveness with increasing constrictant have been shown in canine tracheal smooth muscle (Torphy et al., 1983, 1985) more so for cholinergic constriction than histamine or serotonin (Russell, 1984). We ourselves have found a marked loss of isoproterenol effectiveness with increasing doses of inhaled methacholine or histamine (but not IV serotonin) in a canine model (Jenne et al., 1985). Of considerable interest is that the in vitro shift was less pronounced for theophylline than for the β-agonist (Karlsson and Persson, 1981). In fact, the maximum relaxation produced by theophylline was three times the maximum for isoproterenol. The issue must be explored further with theophylline and other smooth muscle relaxants under physiological conditions, since the behavior with increasing constrictant concentration may depend upon the particular relaxant-constrictant pair. Thus, while relaxation of bovine tracheal muscle by theophylline and papaverine was complete whether contracted by histamine or cholinergic agents, isoproterenol was not able to completely relax the cholinergically contracted muscle (Andersson et al., 1978).

Recent studies with resected human bronchial muscle have shown a 100 times variation in EC_{50} for isoproterenol against acetylcholine contracted bronchi (Guillot et al., 1984). As the EC_{50} increased the maximum possible relaxation with isoproterenol decreased. Yet, these were completely relaxed with theophylline (Fig. 4). Furthermore, bronchi caused to become resistant to isoproterenol in vitro were still as sensitive to theophylline.

In acute asthmatics seen in the emergency room, the absolute PEFR response to injected aminophylline falls as the initial FEV_1 worsens (Appel and Shim, 1981) and, by itself, aminophylline is surprisingly less effective than a β-agonist (Rossing et al., 1980; Appel and Shim, 1981) although it lends added bronchodilation to subcutaneous epinephrine (Rossing et al., 1980). No advantage was shown by adding aminophylline to vigorously applied isoproterenol aerosol, out to one hour (Fanta et al., 1982), nor to metaproterenol, out to three hours (Siegel et al., 1985) despite severe bronchospasm. However, the preexisting mean theophylline level of 8 μg/ml complicates interpretation. Aminophylline may have a role in the most severely obstructed asthmatics, and those responding poorly. An emerging rationale is its potential role in combating dia-

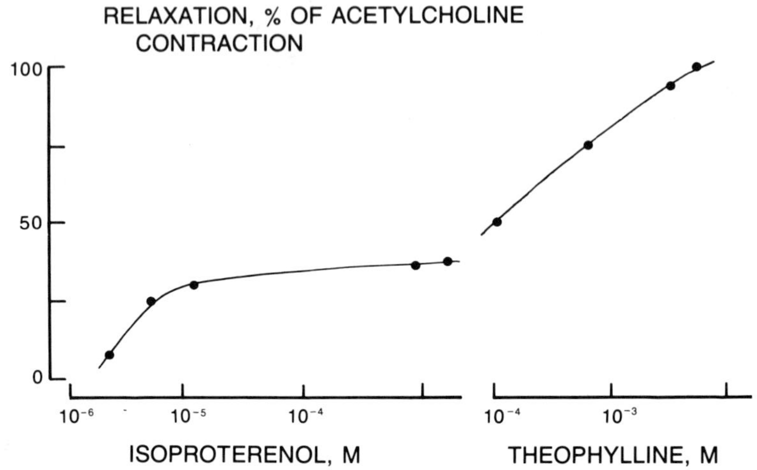

Figure 4 Dose-response curves for isoproterenol and theophylline for a group of 22 human bronchi (out of 74 lungs examined) that relaxed suboptimally to isoproterenol against submaximal constriction with acetylcholine. Note complete sensitivity to theophylline at 10^{-2} M (from Guillot et al., 1984).

phragm fatigue and forestalling respiratory failure (Aubier et al., 1982), discussed in Chapter 9. Proof of this in ill patients is still lacking, however.

E. Site of Bronchial Relaxation

Dose-response curves have been compared for relaxation by theophylline of small airways (1.0 mm diameter, n = 7) and larger airways (4-8 mm diameter, n = 90) (Persson, 1980; Svedmyr, 1977). The EC_{50}'s fall in the same range for the two sizes, although there is about a 10-fold range of individual responses. From this, one is inclined to conclude that theophylline is effective throughout the entire airway.

In asthmatics, theophylline, like terbutaline, produces changes in the density dependence of flow consistent with bronchodilator action at the predominant site of constriction, whether proximal or peripheral. Those patients with a high ΔV_{Emax50}, indicating relative proximal constriction, undergo a smaller increase posttheophylline, indicating proximal dilation. Those patients with a low ΔV_{Emax50} indicating more distal constriction, undergo a larger increment post theophylline indicating distal dilation (Fairshter et al., 1983).

F. Tailoring Levels to the Stimulus: Nocturnal Bronchospasm

While past efforts have concentrated on maintaining constant theophylline levels around the clock, this approach ignores the fact that bronchial caliber may fluctuate on a predictable pattern that calls for a greater bronchodilator level at that time. Thus, nocturnal asthma is an accepted indication here and abroad for a dose of theophylline at bedtime, for example, the 600 mg dose of a slow-release preparation (Barnes et al., 1982). Another study has now shown more even bronchodilation with a "24 hr" theophylline administered at bedtime in such patients than with a conventional b.i.d. dose (Neuenkirchen et al., 1985).

G. Combination with β-Agonists

Among the possible benefits of adding theophylline to a beta agonist are (1) more bronchodilation than possible by a reasonable increase in the dose of the beta agonist alone, (2) smoother control (reduced peak-trough fluctuations) when combined with inhaled β-agonist, (3) higher therapeutic ratio (fewer side effects), (4) access to obstructed airways, (5) benefits not directly involving the airway smooth muscle, such as respiratory muscle enhancement, effects on mediator release, and others.

Enhancement of Bronchodilation

Although the conventional wisdom has been to consider the combination of theophylline and a β-agonist only additive on pulmonary function (Wolfe et al., 1978), there is a need for caution if this analysis is based upon customary methods of expressing the result rather than "% of achievable response." The dose-response curve to either drug begins to plateau as the FEV_1 values improve and the "additive" effect may actually be an underestimate.

Further evidence of more than additivity would be that appreciably more bronchodilation results from further increase in β-agonist alone, once the plateau point is reached. This would depend upon the mechanism of the plateau. If it is due to the bronchi having reached the maximal dilation possible (i.e., an anatomical artifact), then no amount of added bronchodilator would increase the response. However, if the plateau were due to a pharmacologic limit against that particular constrictant, or a combination of the two, then bronchodilation by another mechanism might still produce more net effect.

The data of Billing et al. with IV aminophylline added to IV terbutaline are at least suggestive that aminophylline "breaks through" the terbutaline plateau at both 7.3 and 15.1 μg/ml mean theophylline levels, providing an increment of FEV_1 that would only be reached by prohibitively higher concentrations of terbutaline, if at all (Billing et al., 1982). Oral data suggest that the combination of 5.0 mg terbutaline and 400 mg aminophylline is at least twice as effective as either drug alone when the increments are added (Wolfe et al., 1978), and, by inference, synergistic, if a plateau of effect might be commencing at this dose (Wolfe et al., 1978; Fagerberg and Tegner, 1982).

In chronic bronchitis, individual dose-response curves have been created by infusing aminophylline to levels of 5, 10, 15, 20, and 25 μg/ml or to toxicity, and then adding inhaled salbutamol (Barclay et al., 1981). In 10 of 12 patients at their apparent theophylline plateau, 400 μg inhaled salbutamol provided a significant further increase in FVC. Later, in 10 patients apparent salbutamol plateaus were reached with 200 μg in two, 500 μg in four, 1,400 μg in three, and 3,200 μg in one. Infused aminophylline provided a further FVC increase in four of these, three being those patients requiring the most salbutamol (Barclay et al., 1982). These findings suggest that the benefits of adding theophylline vary with the individual and are most likely to occur in those not responding maximally to conventional doses of the β-agonist. Such incomplete responses are being further documented. Studies comparing the effectiveness of large doses of inhaled salbutamol and atropine methonitrate in COPD reveal a surprising further response to the latter evidently due to a strong cholinergic tone in this disease (Gross and Skorodin, 1984).

In 16 stable COPD patients, a recent crossover study measured airway responses to a large dose of salbutamol (800 μg) by inhalation, followed by a loading dose of theophylline to 25 μg/ml in serum, and vice versa (Filuk et al., 1985). Those patients responding poorly to salbutamol also responded poorly to theophylline. An additive effect was shown between the two drugs in both "nonresponders" and "responders." When relative effect on SG_{aw} and FEV_1 were compared, salbutamol appeared more effective on SG_{aw} than FEV_1 while theophylline had a greater effect on peripheral airways relative to salbutamol, whether due to the drug or the systemic route. The authors question the risk-benefit value of high doses of theophylline in stable COPD patients responding poorly to salbutamol, and this feeling is shared by others (Dull et al., 1982). Certainly, however, in acute exacerbations, vigorous attempts should be made to treat bronchospasm with both drugs.

Finally, low levels of theophylline, by themselves ineffective, may enhance the response to a beta agonist. In vitro parallels for this are the effect of low levels of papaverine when added to isoproterenol against supramaximally constricting doses of methacholine (Van den Brink et al., 1977) and the effect of only 2 μg/ml theophylline on the dose-response curve for isoproterenol against human bronchi (Svedmyr, 1977), and effect equivalent to a fourfold increase in the latter despite the ineffectiveness of theophylline alone at this concentration.

In asthmatics, the relatively low dose of 150 mg theophylline, when combined with ephedrine after 2 weeks on both, had an effect not apparent for either drug alone (Sims et al., 1978) and a 250 mg infusion of aminophylline markedly shifted the dose-response curve for IV salbutamol (Leopold and Handslip, 1979). Such low-dose effects of theophylline are obviously difficult to document, but, if present, might be very important clinically.

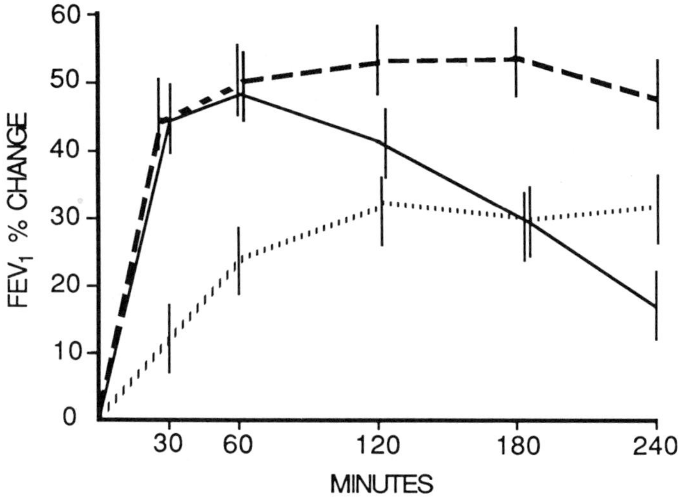

Figure 5 Effect of FEV_1 of 400 mg rapidly absorbed aminophylline (. . . . . . .), 200 μg albuterol by metered dose inhaler (———), and their effect combination (– – – – –) in asthmatic children. The effect of theophylline is more pronounced at the trough than the peak of albuterol action (from Lee and Evans, 1982).

In intact mongrel dogs, we have unequivocal evidence that theophylline potentiates the protective effect of isoproterenol against methacholine-induced bronchospasm (Jenne et al., 1986).

Smoothness of Control

For some reason, most investigators studying drug combinations focus on peak effects rather than trough responses, or area under the curve. This minimizes the ability to detect combined effects because of the log-dose factors entering into the peak responses. Yet, on a multiple dose schedule, asthmatics and other patients using bronchodilators experience discomfort during the *troughs* of response to their inhaled β-agonist, and the effect of combined theophylline is to smooth out and minimize these adverse fluctuations (Kemp et al., 1984). A simple single dose study illustrates the principle (Fig. 5) (Lee and Evans, 1982). Assessments of combined therapy are more profitably made at these troughs.

Reduction in Side Effects

When asthma severity worsens, the dosage of a single systemic bronchodilator can be raised only a limited extent due to the ceiling imposed by side effects, and another bronchodilator must be added. Lower dosages of both agents in combination may give fewer side effects than a large dosage of either one alone. While low dosages of theophylline may not add significantly to measured tremor from terbutaline, higher dosages do (Billing et al., 1982). Low dosages of theophylline and terbutaline together yield a lower tremor ratio but enhanced bronchodilation over twice the dosage of terbutaline alone (Svedmyr and Svedmyr. 1980). Unfortunately, there are few such quantitative studies to rely on.

Access to Obstructed Airways

Other putative benefits cited for combining a systemic bronchodilator such as theophylline are (1) systemic dilation of obstructed airways, and (2) enhancement of access to inhaled agents. The latter factor is considered responsible for an apparent synergism in the response to terbutaline aerosol produced by preceding theophylline (Svedmyr and Svedmyr, 1982). There is evidence of a more peripheral deposition of labeled aerosol when terbutaline is first administered subcutaneously (Tashkin et al., 1980). Yet, whether a systemic bronchodilator is of practical importance compared to simply increasing the inhaled dose has been argued, even in treating the acute attack. My own inclination in the most

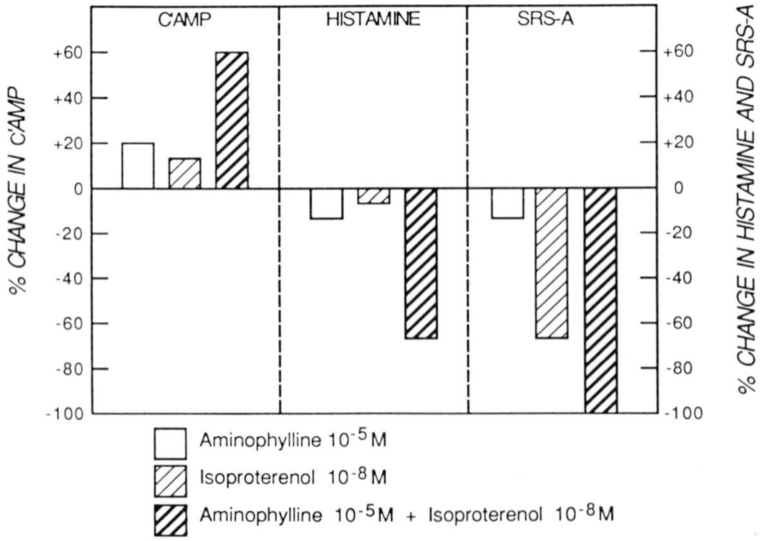

Figure 6 True synergism demonstrated between only 10^{-5} M aminophylline and 10^{-8} M isoproterenol on histamine and leukotriene release in sensitized human lung (from Orange et al., 1971).

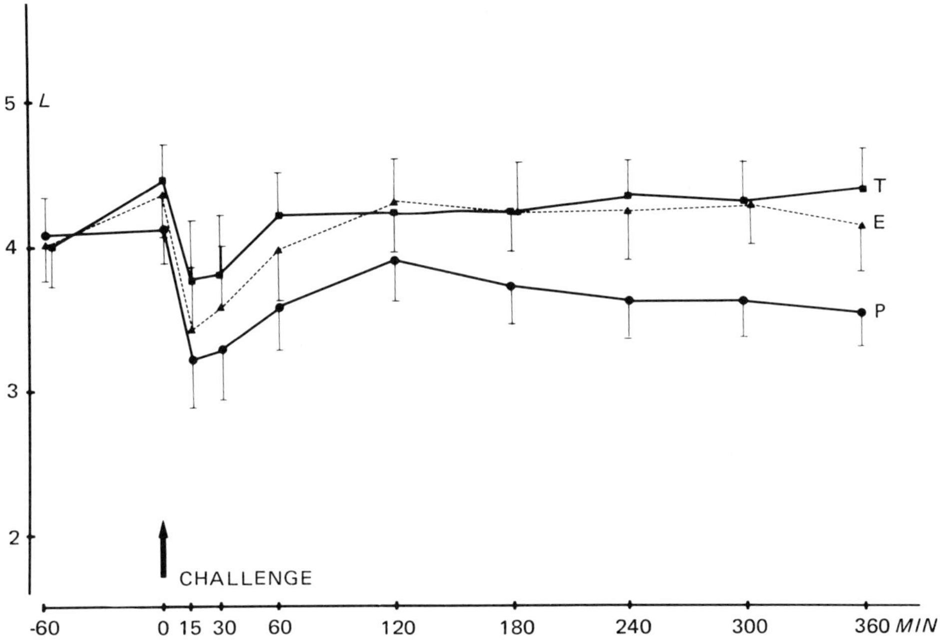

Figure 7 Mean absolute values of FEV_1 (± SE) in nine patients with asthma challenged with allergen at time 0 and treated with placebo (—— ● ——), theophylline (—— ■ ——), enprofylline (– – – ▲ – – –) from time -60 to 360 min. The effect of xanthines is principally on the late response (from Pauwels et al., 1985).

severe acute attacks is to use a combined systemic-aerosol route if only because of the problem of obstructed airways.

Benefits Not Directly Involving Airway Smooth Muscle

As with bronchospasm, there is a paucity of studies exploring the combined effects of xanthines and β-adrenergic agonists on phenomena such as mediator release or microvascular hyperpermeability. One would expect synergistic effects for those responses dependent on cyclic AMP, in view of its synergistic elevation with these agents. Thus at 10^{-3} M, theophylline produces an enormous synergism with 5×10^{-5} M isoproterenol in cyclic AMP production by perfused rat lung (Collins et al., 1973). More pertinent still, theophylline at 10^{-5} M and isoproterenol at 10^{-8} M show strong synergism in inhibiting histamine and SRS-A release and elevating cyclic AMP following antigen challenge of sensitized human lung (Orange et al., 1971) (Fig. 6).

H. Bronchodilation vs. Prevention of Bronchospasm

Some inconsistencies exist between improvement in FEV_1 and the effectiveness of a bronchodilator in preventing bronchospasm. Stable asthmatics with virtually normal spirometry may still have a high degree of bronchial reactivity. In general, however, the two are correlated.

On a different basis, lack of parallelism between the FEV_1 response and protection against methacholine challenge has been reported in mild asthmatic children after metaproterenol inhalation (Ahrens et al., 1984). The "activity-ratio" that is, the ratio of PC_{20} with bronchodilator to PC_{20} on placebo aerosol, peaks and falls off rather rapidly while the FEV_1 is slower to peak and decline. This is probably explainable by a log-dose relationship between drug concentration and FEV_1 response but a linear relationship when employing the methacholine reactivity expressed as the "dose-ratio." Theophylline also reduces methacholine reactivity (McWilliams et al., 1984) and there is a rough correlation between prevention of exercise-induced bronchospasm and the theophylline level in children, with a maximum effect at about 15 μg/ml (Pollack et al., 1977). Theophylline appears to be more effective in preventing the late phase of airway obstruction following antigen challenge than the early phase (Fig. 7) (Pauwels et al., 1985).

IV. Other Xanthines as Bronchodilators

Other xanthine derivatives having potential interest as bronchodilators are listed in Table 5.

Theobromine has recently been shown to have equivalent potency to theophylline in children at equal serum levels (Simons et al., 1985) and to have a similar half-life. Studies in adults also show a similar half-life (Tarka et al., 1983), but a tendency for prolongation on a methylxanthine-containing diet or on previous xanthine medication (Drouillard et al., 1978). The lack of a methyl group at the 1-position should eliminate CNS toxicity. Enprofylline is also a serious competitor to theophylline, particularly since a satisfactory slow-release preparation has been developed (Lunell et al., 1982, 1984). While lacking the seizure potential of theophylline, it retains the minor side effects of nausea, vomiting, and headache.

Proxyphylline has been shown to have only one-eighth the potency of theophylline in vivo and in vitro, and is considered by some to be unsuitable because of the high dosage required (Svedmyr et al., 1972). Yet its use continues. In a recent crossover comparison, 900 mg proxyphylline b.i.d. in a slow-release form produced a mean serum level of 37.1 μg/ml and a 26% increase in FEV_1 compared to a mean theophylline level on 250 b.i.d. of 12.4 μg/ml and a 41% increase in FEV_1 (Rasmussen et al., 1984). The reduction in inhaler use was equivalent.

Table 5 Xanthine Derivatives for which Commercial Preparations are Available

Compound	Half-life (mean, hr)	Elimination	Potency relative to theophylline
Theobromine (3,7 dimethylxanthine)	6.1 ± 0.7	Metabolic	Similar
Caffeine (1,3,7 trimethylxanthine)	3.9 ± 1.4	Metabolic	Slightly less
Enprofylline (3-propylxanthine)	1.6	Renal	Greater (5:1)
Proxyphylline (7-hydroxypropyl) theophylline	8-12	Metabolic	Much less (1:8)
Diphylline (7-2,3-dihydroxypropyl) theophylline	1.8	Renal	Less

With its short half-life and lower potency the dosage of diphylline is about six times that of theophylline. It has found limited use for IV injection in patients allergic to the ethylene diamine moiety of aminophylline (Lawyer et al., 1980).

There is renewed interest in caffeine because of the recent demonstration that a loading dose of 10 mg/kg peaking at 13.5 μg/ml gave essentially equivalent bronchodilation in children as 5 mg/kg aminophylline peaking at 8.1 μg/ml (Becker et al., 1984). Like theophylline, caffeine also increased diaphragm contractility and reduces fatigue, in contrast to methylxanthines lacking the methyl group at the one position (see Chap. 9).

VI. Implications for the Clinical Use of Theophylline

By itself, theophylline provides adequate and constant bronchodilation in the mildly asthmatic adult and child, and is largely successful even in the moderately severely asthmatic child (Weinberger, 1984). While better bronchodilation is obtainable if levels are maintained near the maximum recommended limits of 20 μg/ml, most clinicians prefer to keep mean levels in the 10-15 μg/ml range to provide a cushion of safety and to add other modalities as needed. However, if a predictable circadian pattern of bronchospasm exists, a more logical approach is to tailor theophylline levels to peak at the time of greatest need. This has been successful in severe nocturnal asthma (Barnes et al., 1985; Neuenkirchen et al., 1985).

In stable asthmatics, the effect of adding theophylline to conventional doses of an inhaled β-2 agonist is to raise the PEFR by 25 to 50 liters/min. The benefits are most evident in the early morning values (Appel, 1984; Smith et al., 1980). In acute asthma, while many clinicians have routinely used aminophylline in the emergency room, partly for its postacute effects, a plausible role exists only in the more severe cases, and those responding poorly to vigorously applied inhaled β-agonists, both for its augmentation of the β-adrenergic bronchodilator effect and its effectiveness in resisting fatigue and enhancing respiratory muscle action.

A new role for theophylline may be its apparent ability to prevent the delayed bronchial response to inhaled antigen (Pauwels et al., 1985) with the implications this has for better long-term control.

In stable COPD, while studies of maintenance theophylline alone are generally indicative of a 10-15% improvement in spirometry, it has been difficult for placebo-controlled trials to demonstrate either significant subjective preference or improved work performance in the group as a whole (Alexander et al., 1980; Eaton et al., 1982), although a minority of patients show distinct improvement. More recently, using a newly devised dyspnea scale, a significant overall subjective improvement has been shown despite a lack of bronchodilation (Mahler et al., 1985). Less elaborate series have reported a subjective preference over placebo (Murciano et al., 1983; Jenne et al., 1984). Most recently theophylline has been reported to stabilize and add objective benefit to chronic bronchitics already treated with salbutamol by inhalation (Taylor et al., 1985). Clearly, more such studies are needed. One of the confounding aspects in documenting subjective relief in COPD is the depressed sensitivity of these patients to changes in airway resistance (Gottfried et al., 1978) and the fact that improved dyspnea may depend on a multiplicity of factors such as reduction in lung volume (Druz and Sharp, 1982), reduced work of breathing (Jenne et al., 1984), enhanced diaphragm performance (Murciano et al., 1983), cardiovascular benefits (Matthay et al., 1982), or protection against bronchospastic episodes (Ramsdell et al., 1982; McWilliams et al., 1984). These difficult areas are a continuing challenge in evaluating the exact role of this drug in COPD.

References

Abramowitz, P. W., Perez, M. M., Johnson, C. E., and McLean, J. W. (1980). Effect of theophylline, terbutaline and their combination on the immediate hypersensitivity skin test reaction. *J. Allergy Clin. Immunol. 66*: 123-126.

Alexander, M. R., Dutl, W. L., and Kasik, J. E. (1980). Treatment of chronic obstructive pulmonary disease with orally administered theophylline. *JAMA 244*: 2280-2290.

Ahrens, R. C., Bonham, A. C., and Maxwell, G. A. (1984). A method for comparing the peak intensity and duration of action of aerosolized bronchodilators using bronchoprovocation with methacholine. *Am. Rev. Respir. Dis. 129*: 903-906.

Anderson, K-E., and Persson, C. G. A. (Eds.) (1985). *Anti-asthma Xanthines and Adenosine.* Excerpta Medica, Amsterdam.

Andersson, R., Nilsson, K., Wikberg, J., et al. (1975). Cyclic nucleotides and the contraction of smooth muscle. *Adv. Cyclic Nucl. Res. 5*: 491-518.

Andersson, R. G. (1972). Cyclic AMP and calcium ions in mechanical and metabolic response of smooth muscle: Influence of some hormones and drugs. *Acta Physiol. Scand.* (Suppl) *382*: 1-59.

Andersson, R. G., Kovesi, G., and Ericsson, E. (1978). Beta-adrenoceptor stimulation and cyclic AMP levels in bovine tracheal muscle of old and young animals. *Acta Pharmacol. Toxicol. (Kbh) 43*: 323-327.

Appel, D. W. (1984). Effect of aminophylline when added to metaproterenol sulfate and beclomethasone diproprionate aerosol. *J. Allergy Clin. Immunol. 73*: 291-297.

Appel, D., and Shim, C. (1981). Comparative effect of epinephrine and aminophylline in the treatment of acute asthma. *Lung 159*: 243-254.

Aubier, M., Marciano, D., Viiers, N., Lecocquie, Y., Fieury, B., Pariente, R. (1982). *Am. Rev. Respir. Dis.* (abstr) *125*: 206.

Barclay, J., Whiting, B., Merideth, P. A., et al. (1981). Theophylline-salbutamol interaction: Bronchodilator response to salbutamol at maximally effective plasma theophylline concentrations. *Br. J. Clin. Pharmacol. 11*: 203-208.

Barclay, J., Whiting, B., Addis, G. J. (1982). *Eur. J. Clin. Pharmacol. 22*:389-393.

Barnes, P. J., Greening, A. P., Neville, L., Timmers, J., and Poole, G. W. (1982). Single-dose slow release aminophylline at night prevents nocturnal asthma. *Lancet 1*: 299-301.

Becker, A. B., Simons, K. J., Gillespie, C. A., and Simons, F. E. R. (1984). The bronchodilator effects and pharmacokinetics of caffeine in asthma. *N. Engl. J. Med. 310*: 743-746.

Bergstrand, H. (1980). Phosphodiesterase inhibition and theophylline. *Eur. J. Respir. Dis.* (Suppl 109) *61*: 37-44.

Billing, B., Dahlquist, R., Garl, M., et al. (1982). Separate and combined use of terbutaline and theophylline in asthmatics. *Eur. J. Respir. Dis. 63*: 399-409.

Blinks, J. R., Olson, C. B., Jewell, B. R., and Braveny, P. (1972). Influence of caffeine and other methylxanthines on mechanical properties of isolated mammalian heart muscle. *Circ. Res.* 361-392.

Bourne, H. R., Lichtenstein, L. M., and Melmon, K. L. (1972). Pharmacological control of allergen histamine release. In vitro evidence from inhibitory role of 3′:5′-adenosine monophosphate in human leukocytes. *J. Immunol. 108*: 695-705.

Collins, M., Palmer G. C., and Baca, G. (1973). Stimulation of cyclic AMP in the isolated perfused rat lung. *Res. Commun. Chem. Pathol. Pharmacol. 6*: 805-812.

Cushley, M. J., Tattersfield, A. E., and Holgate, S. T. (1983). Inhaled adenosine and guanosine on airway resistance in normal and asthmatic subjects. *Br. J. Clin. Phrarmacol. 15*: 161-165.

Cushley, M. J., Tattersfield, A. E., and Holgate, S. T. (1984). Adenosine-induced bronchoconstriction in asthma. Antagonism by inhaled theophylline. *Am. Rev. Respir. Dis. 129*: 380-384.

Cushley, M. J., Church, M. K., Pao, G. J.-K., and Holgate, S. T. (1985). The role of mast cell mediation release in adenosine-induced bronchoconstriction. *J. Allergy Clin. Immunol. 75*: 272-278.

Dahlen, S., Hansson, G., Hedqvist, P., Bjorck, T., and Granstrom, E. (1983). Allergen challenge of lung tissue from asthmatics elicits bronchial contraction that correlates with the release of leukotrienes C_4, D_4, and E_4. *Proc. Natl. Acad. Sci. 80*: 1712-1716.

Daly, J. W., Bruns, R. F., and Snyder, S. H. (1981). Adenosine receptors in the central nervous system: Relationship to the central actions of methylxanthines. *Life Sci. 28*: 2083-2097.

Deth, R. C., and Lynch, C. J. (1981). Mobilization of a common source of smooth muscle Ca^{++} by norepinephrine and methylxanthines. *Am. J. Physiol. (Cell Physiol). 240*: C239-C247.

Dimarco, A. F., Nochomontz, M., Dimarco, M. S., Altase, M. D., and Nelson, S. G. (1985). Comparative effects of aminophylline on diaphragm and cardiac contractility. *Am. Rev. Respir. Dis. 132*: 800-805.

Drouillard, D. D., Vesell, E. S., and Dvorchik, B. H. (1978). Studies on theobromine disposition in normal subjects. Alterations induced by dietary abstention from or exposure to methylxanthines. *Clin. Pharmacol. Ther. 23*: 296-302.

Druz, W. S., and Sharp, J. T. (1982). Electrical and mechanical activity of the diaphragm accompanying body position in severe chronic obstructive pulmonary disease. *Am. Rev. Respir. Dis. 125*: 275-280.

Dull, W. L., Alexander, M. R., Adoul, P., and Uvalsa, R. F. (1982). The efficacy of isoproterenol inhalation for predicting the response to oral theophylline therapy in chronic obstruction disease. *Am. Rev. Respir. Dis. 126*: 656-659.

Eaton, M. L., MacDonald, F. M., and Church, T. R. (1982). Effects of theophylline on breathlessness and exercise tolerance in patients with chronic airflow obstruction. *Chest 82*: 538-542.

Endoh, M., Yamashita, S., and Taira, N. (1982). Positive inotropic effect of aminophylline in relation to cyclic nucleotide metabolism in the canine ventricular muscle. *J. Pharmacol. Exp. Ther. 221*: 775-783.

Fabiato, A., and Fabiato, F. (1979). Calcium and cardiac excitation contraction coupling. *Annu. Rev. Physiol. 41*: 473-484.

Fagerberg, E., and Tegner, K.-B. (1972). Effects of oral terbutaline in asthmatic patients. A dose response study. *Scand. J. Respir. Dis. 53*: 3.

Fairshter, R. D., Lowe, J. E., and Wilson, A. F. (1983). *Br. J. Clin. Pract. Symp.* Suppl. no. 23.

Fanta, C. H., Rossing, T. H., and McFadden, E. R., Jr. (1982). Emergency room treatment of asthma; relationships among therapeutic combinations, severity of obstruction and time course of response. *Am. J. Med. 72*: 416-422.

Filuk, R. B., Easton, P. A., and Antonisen, N. R. (1985). Responses of large doses of salbutamol and theophylline in patients with chronic obstructive pulmonary disease. *Am. Rev. Respir. Dis. 132*: 871-874.

Finney, M. J. B., Karlsson, J.-A., and Persson, C. G. A. (1985). *Br. J. Pharmacol. 85*: 29-36.

Fiscus, R. R., et al. *Biochim. Biophys. Acta 805*: 382-392.

Foster, L. H., Trudeau, W. L., and Goldman, A. L. (1979). Bronchodilator effects on gastric acid secretion. *JAMA 241*: 2613-2615.

Foy, T., Marrion, J., Brigham, K. L., and Harris, T. R. (1979). Isoproterenol and aminophylline reduce lung capillary filtration during high permeability. *J. Appl. Physiol. 46*(1): 146-151.

Fredholm, B. B. (1980). Are the actions of methylxanthines due to antagonism of adenosine? *Trends Pharmacol. Sci. 1*: 129-131.

Fredholm, B. B. (1985). In *Antiasthma Xanthines and Adenosine.* Edited by K.-E. Andersson and C. G. A. Persson. Excerpta Medica, Amsterdam, pp. 291-308.

Fredholm, B. B., and Hedquist, P. (1980). Modulation of neurotransmission by purine nucleotides and nucleosides. *Biochem. Pharmacol. 29*: 1635-1643.

Gerthoffer, W. T., Trevethick, M. A., and Murphy, (1984). Myosin phosphorylation and cyclic adenosine 3′,5′-monophosphate in relaxation of smooth muscle by vasodilators. *Circ. Res. 54*: 83-89.

Gottfried, S. B., Altose, M. D., Kelson, S. G., Fogarty, C. M., and Cherniak, N. S. (1978). The perception of changes in airflow resistance in normal subjects and patients with chronic airways obstruction. *Chest 73*(2): 286-288.

Gottstein, V., and Paulson, O. B. (1972). The effect of intracarotid aminophylline infusion on the cerebral circulation. *Stroke 3*: 560-565.

Gross, N. J., and Skorodin, M. (1984). Role of the parasympathetic system in airway obstruction due to emphysema. *N. Engl. J. Med. 311*: 421-425.

Guillot, G., Fornaris, M., Bedier, M., and Orehek, J. (1984). Spontaneous and provoked resistance to isoproterenol in isolated human bronchi. *J. Allergy Clin. Immunol. 74*: 713-718.

Gustaffson, L. E. (1984). *Acta. Physiol. Scand. 122*: 191-198.

Hendeles, L., and Weinberger, M. M. (1983). Theophylline. A 'state of the art' review. *Pharmacotherapy 3*: 2-44.

Higbee, M. D., Kumar, M., and Galant, S. P. (1982). Stimulation for endogenous catecholamine release by theophylline: a proposed additional mechanism of action for theophylline. *J. Allergy Clin. Immunol. 70*: 377-382.

Howell, S., and Fitzpatrick, R. S. (1985). Comparison of the effects of theophylline and enprofylline on fatigued diaphragm. *Am. Rev. Respir. Dis. 131* (No 4), part 2 (A322).

Hughes, P. J., Holgate, S. T., and Church, M. K. (1984). Adenosine inhibits and potentiates IgE-dependent histamine release from human lung mast cells by an A_2 purinoceptor mediated mechanism. *Biochem. Pharmacol. 33*: 3847-3852.

Jenne, J. W., Shaughnessy, T-K., and Druz, W. J. (1986). *Am. Rev. Respir. Dis. 133*(4): A58.

Jenne, J. W., Wyze, E., Rood, F. S., and MacDonald, F. M. (1972). Pharmacokinetics of theophylline. Application to adjustment of the clinical dose of aminophylline. *Clin. Pharmacol. Ther. 13*: 349-360.

Jenne, J. W., Siever, J. R., Druz, W. S., and Sharp, J. T. (1984). The effect of maintenance theophylline on lung work in severe emphysema while standing and walking. *Am. Rev. Respir. Dis. 130*: 600-605.

Jenne, J. W., Shaughnessy, T. K., Manfredi, S., and Druz, W. S. (1985). Bronchodilation by isoproterenol depends on both dose and nature of the constricting stimulus in the dog. *Am. Rev. Respir. Dis. 131*, part 2, No. 4, A280.

Johannesson, N., Andersson, K.-E., Joelsson, B., and Persson, C. G. A. (1985). Relaxation of lower esophageal sphincter and stimulation of gastric secretion and diuresis by antiasthmatic xanthines. *Am. Rev. Respir. Dis. 131*: 26-31.

Karlsson, J.-A., and Persson, C. G. A. (1981). Influences of tracheal contraction on relaxant effects *in vitro* of theophylline and isoproterenol. *Br. J. Pharmacol. 74*: 73-79.

Karlsson, J.-A., Kjellin, G., and Persson, C. G. A. (1982). Effects on tracheal smooth muscle of adenosine and methylxanthines and their interaction. *J. Pharm. Pharmacol. 34*: 788-793.

Kemp, J. P., Chevinsky, P., Orgel, H., et al. (1984). Concomitant bitolterol mesylate aerosol and theophylline for asthma therapy with 24 hour electrocardiographic monitoring. *J. Allergy Clin. Immunol. 73*: 32-43.

Kolbeck, R. C., Speir, W. A., Jr., Carrier, G. O., and Bransome, E. D. Jr. (1979). Apparent irrelevance of cyclic nucleotides in the relaxation of tracheal smooth muscle induced by theophylline. *Lung 156*: 173-183.

Lawyer, C. H., Bardana, E. J., Rodgers, R., and Gerber, N. (1980). Utilization of intravenous dihydroxypropyl theophylline (diphylline) in an aminophylline-sensitive patient and its pharmacokinetic comparison with theophylline. *J. Allergy Clin. Immunol. 65*: 353-357.

Lee, H. S., and Evans, H. E. (1982). Albuterol by aerosol and orally administered theophylline in asthmatic children. *J. Pediatr. 101*: 632-635.

Leopold, D., and Handslip, P. (1979). Additive interaction of aminophylline and salbutamol in asthma: An *in vivo* study using dose-response curves. *J. Int. Med. Res. 7* (Suppl 1): 52-55.

Levy, G., and Koysooko, R. (1975). Pharmacokinetic analysis of the effect of theophylline on pulmonary function in asthmatic children. *J. Pediatr. 86*: 789-793.

Lohman, S. M., Miech, R. P., and Butcher, F. R. (1977). Effects of isoproterenol, theophylline and carbachol on cyclic nucleotide levels and relaxation of bovine tracheal smooth muscle. *Biochim. Biophys. Acta 499*: 238-250.

Lunell, E., Svedmyr, N., Andersson, K.-E., and Persson, C. G. (1982). Effects of enprofylline, a xanthine lacking adenosine receptor antagonism, in patients with chronic obstructive lung disease. *Eur. J. Clin. Pharmacol. 22*: 395-402.

Lunnell, E., Andersson, K.-E., Persson, C. G. A., and Svedmyr, N. (1984). Intravenous enprofylline in asthma patients. *Eur. J. Respir. Dis. 65*: 28-34.

MacKay, A. D., Baldwin, C. J., and Tattersfield, A. E. (1983). Action of intravenously administered aminophylline on normal airways. *Am. Rev. Respir. Dis. 127*: 609-613.

Mahler, D. A., Matthay, R. A., Snyder, P. E., et al. (1985). Sustained release theophylline reduces dyspnea in non-reversible obstructive airway disease. *Am. Rev. Respir. Dis. 131*: 22-25.

Mann, J. S., Renwick, A. G., and Holgate, S. T. (1983). Antigen bronchial provocation causes an increase in plasma adenosine levels in asthma. *Clin. Sci. 65*: 220.

Mann, J. S., Cushley, M. J., and Holgate, S. T. (1985). Adenosine-linked bronchoconstriction in asthma. Role of parasympathetic stimulation and adrenergic inhibition. *Am. Rev. Respir. Dis. 132*: 1-6.

Mansfield, L. E., and Stein, M. R. (1978). Gastroesophageal reflux and asthma. A possible reflex mechanism. *Ann. Allergy 41*: 224-226.

Marcus, M. L., Skelton, C. L., Grauer, L. E., and Epstein, S. E. (1972). Effects of theophylline on myocardial mechanics. *Am. J. Physiol. 222*: 1361-1365.

Marquardt, D. L., Parker, C. W., and Sullivan, T. J. (1978). Potentiation of mast cell mediator release by adenosine. *J. Immunol. 120*: 871.

Martin, G. L., Atkins, P. C., and Dunsky, T. (1980). Effects of theophylline, terbutaline and prednisone on antigen-induced bronchospasm and mediator release. *J. Allergy Clin. Immunol. 66*: 204-212.

Maselli, R., Casal, G. L., and Ellis, E. F. (1970). Pharmacologic effects of intravenously administered aminophylline in asthmatic children. *J. Pediatr. 76*: 777-782.

Matthay, R. A., Berger, H. J., Davies, R., Loke, J., Gottschalk, A., and Zaret, B. L. (1978). Effects of aminophylline upon right and left ventricular performance in chronic obstructive pulmonary disease. *Am. J. Med. 65*: 904-910.

Matthay, R. A., Berger, H. J., Davies, R., Loke, J., Gottschalk, A., and Zaret, B. L. (1982). Improvement in performance by oral long-acting theophylline in chronic pulmonary disease. *Am. Heart J. 104*: 1022-1026.

McWilliams, B. C., Menendez, R., Kelly, H. W., and Howick, J. (1984). Effects of theophylline on inhaled methacholine and histamine in asthmatic children. *Am. Rev. Respir. Dis. 130*: 193-197.

Mentzer, M. R., Rubio, R., and Bern, R. M. (1975). *Am. J. Physiol. 229*: 1625-1631.

Miech, R. P., Niedzwicki, J. G., and Smith, I. R. (1979). Effect of theophylline on the binding of cAMP to soluble protein from tracheal smooth muscle. *Biochem. Pharmacol. 28*: 3687-3688.

Mitenko, P. A., and Ogilvie, R. I. (1973). Rational intravenous doses of theophylline. *N. Engl. J. Med. 289*: 600-603.

Mizus, I., Summer, W., Farrukh, I., Michael, J. R., and Gurtner, G. H. (1985). Isoproterenol or aminophylline attenuate pulmonary edema after acid lung injury. *Am. Rev. Respir. Dis. 131*: 256-259.

Mope, L., McClellan, G. B., and Winegard, S. (1980). Calcium sensitivity of the contractile system and phosphorylation of troponin in hyperpermeable cardiac cells. *J. Gen. Physiol. 75*: 271-282.

Morgan, J. P., and Morgan, K. G. (1984a). Stimulus specific patterns of intracellular calcium levels in smooth muscle of ferret portal vein. *J. Physiol. (Lond) 351*: 155-167.

Morgan, J. P., and Morgan, K. G. (1984b). Alteration of cytoplasmic ionized calcium levels in smooth muscle by vasodilators in the ferret. *J. Physiol. (Lond) 357*: 339-351.

Morgan, J. P., and Morgan, K. G. (1984c). *Am. J. Med. 77*(5A): 33-46.

Morgan, J. P., Chesebro, J. H., Ploth, J. R., Puga, F. J., and Schaff, H. V. (1984). Intracellular calcium transients in human working myocardium as detected with aequorin. *J. Am. Coll. Cardiol. 3*: 410-418.

Morley, J., Page, C. P., and Sanjar, S. (1985). Pharmacology of the late response to allergen and its relation to asthma prophylaxis. *Int. Arch. Allergy. Appl. Immunol. 77*: 73-78.

Murciano, D., Aubier, M., Lecocquic, Y., and Pariente, R. (1983). Effects of aminophylline on diaphragmatic strength and fatigue in patients with chronic obstructive pulmonary disease. *N. Engl. J. Med. 311*: 349-353.

Neuenkirchen, H., Wilkens, J. H., Dellerich, M., and Sybrecht, N. (1985). Nocturnal asthma: effects of a once per evening dose of sustained release theophylline. *Eur. J. Respir. Dis. 66*: 196-204.

Nicholson, D. P., and Chick, T. W. (1973). A re-evaluation of parenteral aminophylline. *Am. Rev. Respir. Dis. 108*: 241-247.

Niewoehner, D. E., Campe, H., Duane, S., et al. (1979). Mechanisms of airway smooth muscle response to isoproterenol and theophylline. *J. Appl. Physiol. 47*(2): 330-336.

Ogilvie, Ri, Fernande, P. G., and Winsberg, F. (1977). Cardiovascular response to increasing theophylline concentrations. *Eur. J. Clin. Pharmacol. 12*: 409-414.

Orange, R. P., Kaliner, M. A., and Leraia, P. J. (1971). Immunological release of histamine and slow reacting substance of anaphylaxis from human lung. Influence of cellular levels of cyclic AMP. *Fed. Proc. 30*: 1725-1729.

Osswald, H., Nabarovski, G., and Hermes, H. (1980). Adenosine as a possible mediator of metabolic control of glomerular filtration. *Int. J. Biochem. 12*: 263-267.

Page, C. P., Tomak, R. H. H., Senjar, S., et al. (1985). Suppression of PAF-acether responses: An antiinflammatory effect of anti-asthma drugs. *Agents Actions 16*.

Parker, J. O., Kelkar, K., and West, R. O. (1966). Hemodynamic effects of aminophylline in cor pulmonale. *Circulation 33*: 17.

Parker, J. O., Ashekian, P. B., Di Giorgi, S., and West, R. O. (1967). Hemodynamic effects of aminophylline in chronic obstructive pulmonary disease. *Circulation 35*: 365-372.

Paton, D. M. (1981). Structure activity relations for presynaptic inhibition of noradrenergic and cholinergic transmission by adenosine. Evidence for action on A_1 receptors. *J. Autonom. Pharmacol. 1*: 287-290.

Pauwels, R., Van Renterghem, D., Van Der Straeten, M., Johannesson, N., and Persson, C. G. A. (1985). The effect of theophylline and enprofylline on allergen-induced bronchoconstriction. *J. Allergy Clin. Immunol. 76*: 583-590.

Pavia, D., Sutton, P. P., Lapez-Vidriero, M. D., Agnew, J. E., and Clarks, S. W. (1983). Drug effects on mucociliary function. *Eur. J. Respir. Dis. 64*: (Suppl 28) 304-317.

Persson, C. G. A. (1980). Some pharmacological aspects on xanthines in asthma. *Eur. J. Respir. Dis. Suppl. 109*: 61:7-16.

Persson, C. G. A., Ekman, M., and Erjfält, I. (1979). Vascular anti-permeability effects of β-receptor agonists and theophylline in the lung. *Acta Pharmacol. Toxicol. 44*: 216-220.

Persson, C. G. A., Ekman, M., Persson, C. G. A., and Kjellin, G. (1981). Enprofylline, a principally new antiasthmatic xanthine. *Acta Pharmacol. Toxicol. 49*: 313-316.

Persson, C. G. A., and Erjfält, I. (1981). Convulsive effects of theophylline in conscious and anesthetized guinea pigs. *Acta Pharmacol. Toxicol. 48*: 32-38.

Persson, C. G. A., Karlsson, J.-A., and Erjefält, I. (1982). *Life Sci. 30*: 2181.

Peters, S. P., Schulman, E. S., Schleimer, R. P., Macglashen, D. W., Newball, H. H., and Lichtenstein, L. M. (1982). Dispersed human lung mast cells. Pharmacological aspects and comparison with human lung tissue fragments. *Am. Rev. Respir. Dis. 126*: 1034-1039.

Pierce, R. J., Payne, C. R., Williams, S. J., et al. (1981). Comparison of intravenous and inhaled terbutaline in the treatment of asthma. *Chest 79*: 506.

Polacek, I., Bolan, J., and Daniel, E. E. (1971). Accumulation of adenosine 3′,5′-monophosphate and relaxation in the rat uterus *in vitro. Can. J. Physiol. Pharmacol. 49*: 999-1004.

Pollack, J., Kiechel, F., Cooper, D., and Weinberger, M. (1977). Relationship of serum theophylline concentration to inhibition of exercise-induced bronchospasm and comparison with cromolyn. *Pediatrics. 60*: 840-844.

Polson, J. B., Krzanowski, J. J., Anderson, W. H., et al. (1979). Analysis of the relationship between pharmacological inhibition of cyclic nucleotide phosphodiesterease and relaxation of canine tracheal smooth muscle. *Biochem. Pharmacol. 28*: 1391-1395.

Polson, J. B., Krzanowski, J. J., and Szentivanyi (1982). Inhibition of high-affinity cyclic AMP phosphodiesterase and relaxation of canine tracheal smooth muscle. *Biochem. Pharmacol. 31*: 3403-3406.

Rachelefsky, G., Katz, R., and Siegel, S. C. (1978). A sustained release theophylline preparation: Efficacy in childhood asthma with low serum theophylline levels. *Ann. Allergy 40*: 252-257.

Racineux, J. L., Troussier, J., Turcant, A., et al. (1981). Comparison of bronchodilation effects of salbutamol and theophylline. *Bull. Eur. Physiopathol. Respir. 17*: 799-806.

Rall, T. W. (1980). The xanthines. In *The Pharmacological Basis of Therapeutics.* Edited by A. G. Gilman, L. S. Goodman and A. Gilman, New York, Macmillan, pp. 592-607.

Ramsdell, J. W., Nachtwey, F. J., and Moser, K. M. (1982). Bronchial hyperreactivity in chronic bronchitis. *Am. Rev. Respir. 126*: 829-832.

Rapaport, R. M. (1986). *Circ. Res. 58*: 407-410.

Rasmussen, F. V., Waldorff, S., and Madsen, L. (1984). Pharmacokinetics and bronchodilatory effect of proxyphylline and theophylline. *Eur. J. Respir. Dis. 65*: 20-27.

Richardson, J. B. (1979). Nerve supply to the lungs. *Am. Rev. Respir. Dis. 119*: 785-809.

Richer, C., Mathieu, M., Bah, H., Thuillez, C., Duroux, P., and Diudiclli, J.-F. (1982). Theophylline kinetics and ventilatory flow in bronchial asthma and chronic airflow obstruction: Influence of erythromycin. *Clin. Pharmacol. Ther. 31*: 579-586.

Robertson, D., Wade, D., Workman, E., Woosley, R. L., and Oates, J. A. (1981). Tolerance to the humoral and hemodynamic effects of caffeine in man. *J. Clin. Invest. 67*: 1111-1117.

Rossing, T. H., Fanta, C. H., Goldstein, D. H., Snapper, J. R., and McFadden, E. R., Jr. (1980). Emergency therapy of asthma: Comparison of the acute effects of parenteral and inhaled sympathomimetics and infused aminophylline. *Am. Rev. Respir. Dis. 122*; 365-371.

Russell, J. A. (1984). Differential inhibitory effect of isoproterenol on contractions of canine airways. *J. Appl. Physiol. 57*: 801-807.

Rutherford, J. D., Vatner, S. E., and Braunwald, E. (1981). Effects and mechanisms of action of aminophylline on cardiac function and regional blood flow distribution in conscious dogs. *Circulation 63*: 378-387.

Siegel, D., Sheppard, D., Gelb, A., and Weinberg, P. F. (1985). *Am. Rev. Respir. Dis. 132*: 283-286.

Simons, F. E. R., Becker, A. B., Simons, K. J., and Gillespie, C. A. (1985). The bronchodilator effect and pharmacokinetics of theobromine in young patients with asthma. *J. Allergy Clin. Immunol. 76*: 703-707.

Sims, J. A., do Pico, G. A., and Reed, C. E. (1978). Bronchodilating effect of oral theophylline-ephedrine combination. *J. Allergy Clin. Immunol. 62*: 15-21.

Smith, J. A., Weber, R. W., and Nelson, H. S. (1980). Theophylline and aerosolized terbutaline in the treatment of bronchial asthma. Double-blind comparison of optimal doses. *Chest 78*: 816-818.

Stein, M. R., Towner, T. G., Weber, R. W., et al. (1980). The effect of theophylline on the lower esophageal sphincter pressure. *Ann. Allergy 45*: 238-241.

Sutton, P. P., Pavia, D., Bateman, J. R. M., and Clark, S. W. (1981). The effect of oral aminophylline on lung mucociliary clearance in man. *Chest 80* (Suppl) 889-892.

Svedmyr, N. (1977). The role of theophyllines in asthma therapy. *Scand. J. Respir. Dis. Suppl. 101*: 125-137.

Svedmyr, K., and Svedmyr, N. (1982). Does theophylline potentiate inhaled β_2-agonists? *Allergy 37*: 101-110.

Svedmyr, N. E., and Svedmyr, K. (1980). *Eur. J. Respir. Dis.* 109 (Suppl): 67-68.

Svedmyr, K., Mellstrand, T., and Svedmyr, N. (1977). Comparison between effects of aminophylline, proxyphylline and terbutaline in asthmatics. *Scand. J. Respir. Dis. Suppl. 101*: 139-146.

Svenskjo, E., Artos, K.-E., Raymond, R. M., and Grega, G. J. (1979). Morphological and physiological correlation of bradykinin induced macromolecular flux. *Am. J. Physiol. 236* (4) 600-606.

Tarka, S. M., Arnaud, M. J., Dvorchik, B. H., and Vessel, E. S. (1983). Theobromine kinetics and metabolic disposition. *Clin. Pharmacol. Ther. 34*: 546-555.

Tashkin, D. P., Trevor, E., Chopra, S. K., and Taplin, G. V. (1980). Sites of airway dilatation in asthma following inhaled vs subcutaneous terbutaline. Comparison of physiological tests with radionuclide lung images. *Am. J. Med. 68*: 14-25.

Taylor, S. M., and Downes, H. (1982). Bronchodilator mechanisms in bullfrog lung: Differences in response to isoproterenol, theophylline and papaverine. *J. Pharmacol. Exp. Ther. 223*: 359-367.

Taylor, D. R., Buick, B., Kinney, C., Lowry, R. C., and McDevitt, D. G. (1985). Efficacy of orally administered theophylline, inhaled salbutamol and a combination of the two as chronic therapy in the management of patients with chronic obstructive airways disease. *Am. Rev. Respir. Dis. 131*: 747-751.

Torphy, T. J., Rinard, G. A., Rictow, M. G., et al. (1983). Functional antagonism in canine tracheal smooth muscle and inhibition by methacholine of the mechanical and biochemical response to isoproterenol. *J. Pharmacol. Exp. Ther. 227*: 694-699.

Torphy, T. J., Zheng, C., Peterson, S. M., Fiscus, R. R., Rinerd, G. A., and Mayer, S. E. (1985). Inhibitory effect of methacholine on drug-induced relaxation, cyclic AMP accumulation and cyclic AMP-dependent protein kinase activation in canine tracheal smooth muscle. *J. Pharmacol. Exp. Ther. 233*: 409-417.

Triner, L., Vulliemoz, Y., and Verosky, M. (1977). Cyclic 3′5′-adenosine monophosphate and bronchial tone. *Eur. J. Pharmacol. 41*: 37.

Tsein, R. W. (1977). Cyclic AMP and contractile activity in heart. *Adv. Cyclic Nucleotide Res. 8*: 365.

Van den Brink, F. G., Offermeier, J., and Griessel, H. J. (1977). Sensitization of contracted tracheal smooth muscle to β-adrenergic spasmolysis by subthreshold doses of papaverine. *Scand. J. Respir. Dis. Suppl. 98*: 48-50.

Vestal, R. E., Ericksson, C. E., Musser, B., Ozaki, L. K., and Halter, J. B. (1983). Effect of intravenous aminophylline on plasma levels of catecholamines and related cardiovascular and metabolic responses in man. *Circulation 67*: 162-171.

Voseh, S., Kewito, G., and Perruchoud, A. (1982). Theophylline serum concentrations effect in severe bronchial obstruction. The optimal use of intravenously administered aminophylline. *Am. Rev. Respir. Dis. 125*: 181-184.

Weinberger, M. (1984). Pharmacology and therapeutic use of theophylline. *J. Allergy Clin. Immunol. 73*; 525-540.

Whiting, B., Kelman, A. W., and Struthers, A. D. (1984). Prediction of response to theophylline in chronic bronchitis. *Br. J. Clin. Pharmacol. 17*: 9-14.

Wolfe, J. D., Tashkin, D. P., Calvarese, B., et al. (1978). Bronchodilator effects of terbutaline and aminophylline alone and in combination in asthmatic patients. *N. Engl. J. Med. 298*: 363-367.

9

Effects of Methylxanthines on Respiratory Skeletal Muscle and Neural Drive

GERALD S. SUPINSKI

Case Western Reserve University
School of Medicine
Cleveland, Ohio

It has been suggested (Roussos and Macklem, 1977, 1982) that respiratory muscle dysfunction (i.e., weakness and fatigue), may be the proximate cause of hypercapnia, dyspnea, exercise intolerance, and acute respiratory failure in patients with lung disease.

Recent work has shown that the methylxanthine drugs (e.g., theophylline) can augment respiratory muscle contractility, thereby preventing or reversing respiratory muscle fatigue and its consequences (Aubier et al., 1981, 1983a; Howell and Roussos, 1984; Supinski and Kelsen, 1984; Rochester, 1981). Some authors have even speculated that the effect of the methylxanthines on the respiratory muscles may constitute their major, clinically relevant, action (Aubier et al., 1981). In keeping with this concept, investigators (Rossing et al., 1980) have found that theophylline produces virtually no increase in the expiratory airflow of some asthmatics, despite the striking clinical improvement often elicited by this drug when it is administered to asthmatic patients.

This chapter will review the effect of the methylxanthines on respiratory muscle strength, respiratory muscle endurance, the respiratory muscles during acute respiratory failure, and the mechanism of action of the methylxanthines on skeletal muscle. In addition, a closely related topic, the effect of methylxanthines on respiratory neural drive, will be discussed.

I. Effect of Methylxanthines on Respiratory Muscle Strength

The methylxanthine drugs increase the force of contraction of both limb and respiratory skeletal muscles. For example, caffeine, the most extensively studied methylxanthine, potentiates the force output of skeletal muscles in response to low-frequency stimulation and, in particular, increases the height of the muscle twitch (i.e., the force produced in response to a single electrical stimulus) (Wittman and Kelsen, 1982; Jones et al., 1982). The in vitro response of skeletal muscle to caffeine appears to be a function of muscle length and fiber type, with a greater response for slow, oxidative fibers and at short lengths (Brust, 1976; Lopez et al., 1981).

In the past, this effect of the methylxanthines to augment muscle force was utilized primarily as an in vitro probe, permitting investigators to manipulate the intracellular processes involved in muscle contraction (Nassar-Gentina et al., 1981; Katz et al., 1977).

Recent studies have suggested, however, that these agents may also be effective in vivo in augmenting muscle force and, as a result, may provide a pharmacologic approach to the treatment of respiratory muscle dysfunction. Aubier and co-workers (1983a) were the first to investigate the effect of theophylline on diaphragm contractility in humans. These authors determined transdiaphragmatic pressure, a measure of diaphragm force-generating ability, before and after theophylline administration. Because diaphragm pressure-generating ability is a function of diaphragm fiber length, all measurements were made at the same, fixed diaphragm length. Because pressures also vary with the level of diaphragm excitation, pre- and postdrug data were expressed as a function of phrenic neural excitation as assessed from the magnitude of the integrated, rectified diaphragm electromyogram. They found that theophylline increased transdiaphragmatic pressure by an average of 15%, an effect seen at all levels of diaphragm excitation (Fig. 1). More importantly, this increase was achieved at a therapeutic plasma concentration (13 ± 1 mg/liter).

Subsequent studies have extended this initial work, examining (1) the ability of methylxanthines to produce a sustained, as well as an acute effect, on diaphragm strength; (2) the effect of this drug on other respiratory muscles, such as the intercostals; and (3) the effect of methylxanthines other than theophylline, such as caffeine, on respiratory muscle function (Aubier et al., 1983a; Supinski and Kelsen, 1984; Murciano et al., 1984; Sigrist et al., 1982).

To the extent that the response of skeletal muscle to the methylxanthines is similar to that of other tissues, one might expect that their effect on the res-

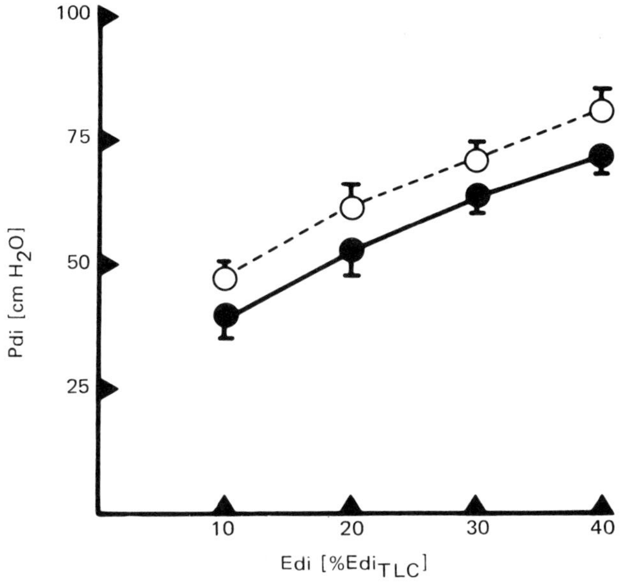

Figure 1 Relationship between transdiaphragmatic pressure (Pdi) and diaphragm electromyographic activity (Edi) before (solid symbols) and after (open circles) theophylline administration. Theophylline increased transdiaphragmatic pressure at all levels of electromyographic activity (from Aubier et al., 1981).

piratory muscles would diminish with chronic administration. For example, although caffeine has pronounced acute effects on blood pressure, heart rate, and adrenal catecholamine release, there is rapid tachyphylaxis to each of these effects with chronic administration (Robertson et al., 1981). Murciano and colleagues (1984) have found, however, that administration of theophylline for 30 days produces an increase in diaphragmatic muscle strength that is maintained over the entire period of study. On the average, theophylline (13.5 ± 4 mg/liter) increased the transdiaphragmatic pressure produced during a maximal inspiratory effort by 16%, while subjects treated with a placebo demonstrated no improvement.

As outlined above, the effects of the methylxanthines also appear to vary, at least in vitro, from muscle to muscle, depending upon fiber composition (Brust, 1976). Since the fiber composition of the different inspiratory muscles may vary, the response to methylxanthines may also vary from muscle to muscle. Sigrist et al. (1982) have shown, however, that theophylline significantly increases inspiratory pleural pressure swings even after the diaphragm is paralyzed by phrenicotomy. They found that the magnitude of the increase in

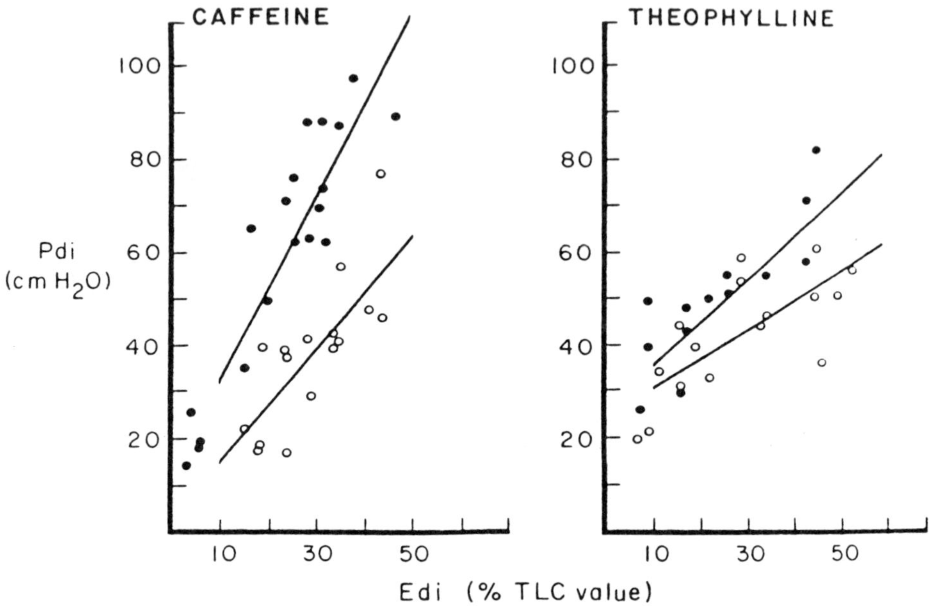

Figure 2 Effect of caffeine (left panel) and theophylline (right panel) on the relationship between transdiaphragmatic pressure (Pdi) and electromyographic activity (Edi) in a single subject. Edi is expressed as a percentage of the diaphragm electromyographic activity achieved with a maximum inspiratory effort with the airway open (i.e., at TLC). Both caffeine and theophylline increased Pdi at all levels of Edi (from Supinski and Kelsen, 1984).

pleural pressure generated by the intercostal muscles in response to theophylline (20%) was roughly comparable to the increase in transdiaphragmatic pressure reported by Aubier and co-workers (1983a) with similar plasma levels of theophylline (20 mg/liter), suggesting that the diaphragm and intercostal muscles have a qualitatively and quantitatively similar response to this drug.

Both in vitro and in vivo studies have indicated that the various methylxanthine analogues differ from one another in their relative potencies. Kramer and Wells (1980) and Jeppson and colleagues (1982) have shown in vitro that caffeine is threefold more potent than theophylline and, in addition, that the 1-methyl, 3-isobutyl, 8-methoxy methylxanthine derivatives are even more potent than caffeine. In keeping with these data, Aubier et al. (1983a) and Supinski and Kelsen (1984) have shown that caffeine increases the force generated by the diaphragm at a given submaximal level of muscle excitation in vivo, and that caffeine is of the same or greater potency than theophylline (Fig. 2). Although caffeine may be greater than theophylline in its effects on the respiratory muscles, it is known to be a weaker bronchodilator, to have less effect on the heart, and to have a lesser affinity for central nervous system adenosine receptors than does theophylline (Becker et al., 1984; Starr et al., 1937; Boulanger et al., 1982).

Howell and Fitzgerald (1985) have recently compared the effects of theophylline and enprofylline (not strictly a methylxanthine) on the force of contraction of the fatigued diaphragm. While theophylline increased twitch and tetanic tension by 20% and 18-29%, respectively, enprofylline only increased twitch tension by 5% and tetanic tension by 4-13%. As a result, although enprofylline is reported to be more effective as a bronchodilator, these data suggest it may be less potent than theophylline in treating or preventing respiratory muscle fatigue.

This evidence that the relative potencies of theophylline, caffeine, and enprofylline differ from organ to organ suggests that different mechanisms underlie the actions of the various methylxanthines on different tissues.

II. Effect of Methylxanthines on Respiratory Muscle Endurance

While it seems clear that the methylxanthines possess the ability to augment respiratory muscle strength, a more important action is their effect on the ability of the respiratory muscles to withstand fatigue. While the endurance of a given muscle is related to its strength, these two aspects of muscle function are not synonymous. Muscle strength is largely a function of muscle bulk, with hypertrophied muscles generating greater tensions. Muscle endurance, on the other hand, appears to depend both upon the ability of muscle metabolism to provide adequate levels of high energy phosphate compounds and upon the ability of the sarcoplasmic reticulum to provide sufficient intracellular calcium flux to activate the contractile proteins during rhythmic muscle excitation (Nadel, 1985; Edwards et al., 1977).

An increase in muscle strength might not, a priori, increase muscle endurance. In fact, training regimens designed to improve respiratory muscle strength have little effect on endurance and, conversely, regimens affecting endurance do not change strength (Leith and Bradley, 1976). It even seems possible that, providing other factors remain constant, an effect of pharmacologic agents to increase muscle force output might result in an increase in the rate at which energy supplies are depleted and might impair, rather than improve, muscle endurance.

The effect of methylxanthines on respiratory muscle endurance is, however, even more impressive than their effects on muscle strength. Methylxanthines have a pronounced ability both to retard and to reverse the development of inspiratory muscle fatigue, a finding confirmed by several independent studies

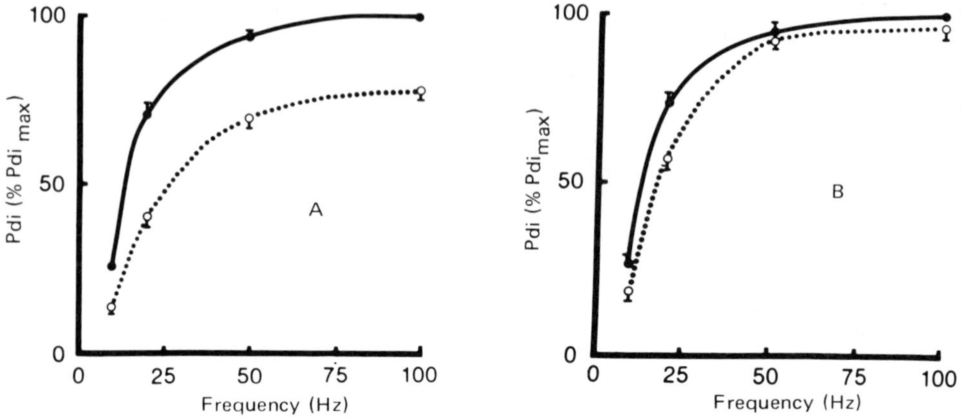

Figure 3 Effect of resistive breathing on the diaphragm force-frequency curve. Transdiaphragmatic pressure was elicited by transcutaneous stimulation of the phrenic nerve before (solid lines) and after (dashed lines) resistive loading. Panel A gives results without theophylline administration while panel B shows the effect of resistive loading after theophylline administration. Theophylline markedly diminished the effect of resistive loading on the force-frequency curve, that is, this drug preserved muscle force-generating ability (Aubier et al., 1981).

using a variety of methods to detect and quantitate respiratory muscle fatigue (Aubier et al., 1981; Murciano et al., 1984; Supinski et al., 1984b). Aubier and co-workers measured the transdiaphragmatic pressure elicited by transcutaneous stimulation of the phrenic nerve before and after diaphragm fatigue was produced by resistive loading of inspiration. In the absence of theophylline, resistive breathing significantly reduced transdiaphragmatic pressure at all levels of phrenic stimulation and, in particular, reduced the pressure generated in response to 20 Hz electrical stimulation by approximately 50%. In contrast, in the presence of theophylline, the same period of resistive breathing resulted in only small (i.e., $< 20\%$) reductions in transdiaphragmatic pressure (Fig. 3). When administered after the induction of fatigue, theophylline rapidly (30 min) doubled transdiaphragmatic pressure (20 Hz electrical stimulation). In the absence of theophylline, transdiaphragmatic pressure failed to show any appreciable recovery over the same time period. Theophylline therefore both prevented fatigue, as measured by this technique, and reversed fatigue once it was present.

Power spectral density analysis of the diaphragm electromyogram has also been used to study the effects of the methylxanthines on respiratory muscle endurance. The power spectrum is an extensively used index of muscle fatigue, with progressive shifts of the spectrum to lower frequencies as fatigue becomes more severe (Cohen et al., 1982). Both caffeine and theophylline reduce the rate at which this shift occurs when inspiration is loaded, signifying an improvement in diaphragm endurance (Murciano et al., 1984; Supinski et al., 1984b). In the case of theophylline, Murciano and colleagues (1984) have shown that a serum concentration of 13.5 mg/liter entirely prevents a change in diaphragm spectral densities at a level of load that produces pronounced decrements in the power spectrum when no theophylline is administered. In the case of caffeine, a 600 mg oral dose doubles the time required for a given shift in the power spectrum (Supinski et al., 1984b).

Finally, in a double-blind controlled study, caffeine markedly increased the time that a given external inspiratory load could be sustained, that is, caffeine increased the time to respiratory muscle exhaustion (Supinski et al., 1984b).

Taken together, these studies suggest that the methylxanthines have a substantial effect on endurance even though their effects on strength are quite modest (i.e., 12-16% increments with plasma concentrations of 10-20 mg/liter). The seemingly greater effects of these drugs on muscle endurance, as compared to strength, may be related to the mechanisms by which these drugs influence muscle contractility.

It is now thought that respiratory muscle fatigue is primarily the result of the development of an impairment in respiratory muscle excitation-contraction coupling: there is inadequate activation of the muscle actin-myosin contractile filaments in response to muscle membrane excitation by neural stimulation (Edwards, 1979). Though the precise site and manner in which repetitive muscle contraction results in this impairment are not entirely clear, it appears that calcium release and reuptake by the sarcoplasmic reticulum is involved. Calcium ions regulate muscle force output by interacting with the troponin moiety of the contractile protein complex (Fuchs et al., 1970). Several authors have suggested that fatigue may represent an impairment of calcium release and interaction with troponin (Edwards, 1979; Moxham et al., 1981).

It is also thought that the primary mechanism by which the methylxanthines produce their effects on muscle contractility is via an increase in intracellular calcium levels during contraction (Endo, 1975). While an increase in calcium release during muscle excitation would be expected to augment muscle force output of both fresh and fatigued muscles, troponin calcium-binding sites should quickly become saturated in fresh muscle (since basal calcium release is unimpaired) and, as a result, only small increments in force output would be possible.

In contrast, in fatigued muscle, intracellular calcium concentrations during contraction should be far from maximal, and a methylxanthine-mediated increment in sarcoplasmic calcium concentration might be expected to produce large effects on muscle force output. In essence, the methylxanthines may specifically reverse the biophysical impairment that is likely to be responsible for clinically relevant forms of respiratory muscle fatigue.

III. Effect of Methylxanthines on Respiratory Muscles During Acute Respiratory Failure

This chapter has focused on reports detailing the effects of methylxanthines on muscle function in normal subjects. The response of the respiratory muscles to methylxanthines might be expected to differ significantly, however, in the presence of acute respiratory failure. Hypercapnia and hypoxia, for example, may alter intracellular hydrogen ion concentrations which, in turn, are known to affect sarcoplasmic reticulum calcium release and reuptake (Schnader et al., 1983; Nakamura and Schwartz, 1972; Fabiato and Fabiato, 1978). Since the actions of the methylxanthines on skeletal muscle are mediated, at least in part, by an effect on sarcoplasmic reticulum calcium flux, the responsivity of respiratory muscle to the methylxanthines might be altered by hypoxia and/or hypercapnia. In addition, alterations in respiratory muscle length due to changes in lung volume may result from respiratory failure and may alter the response of skeletal muscles to the methylxanthines. Fortunately, the response of the respiratory muscles to methylxanthines appears to be preserved and even enhanced in the presence of many of these factors.

The effect of alterations in fiber length on the response of skeletal muscles to the methylxanthines has been studied both in vitro and in vivo. Caffeine produces relatively greater effects in vitro on muscle contractility when fiber length is shortened (Lopez et al., 1981). In vivo, the response of the diaphragm to theophylline is unaltered when fiber length is acutely reduced by lung inflation (Supinski et al., 1984a).

The response of the diaphragm to theophylline is also maintained in the presence of hypoxia and hypercapnia. Viires and co-workers (1984) have examined the effect of theophylline on diaphragm contractility during asphyxia using an animal model of respiratory failure in which hypoxic, hypercapnic ventilatory failure was produced with inspiratory resistive loading. These authors found that theophylline reduced the rate at which respiratory muscle fatigue developed, and, when administered after fatigue was well established, produced substantial increments in transdiaphragmatic pressure despite the presence of arterial carbon dioxide tensions of 67 ± 4 mmHg, and oxygen tensions of 45 ± 4 mmHg (Fig. 4). In fact, the effect of theophylline in the presence of respiratory failure (30% increase in transdiaphragmatic pressure) was quantitatively more impressive than in its absence (a 14% increase).

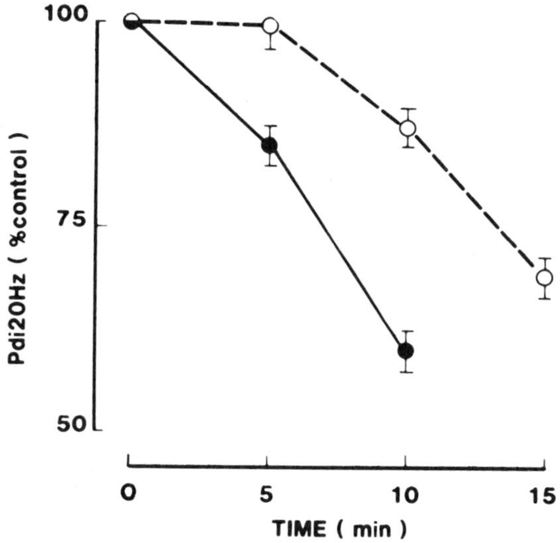

Figure 4 Transdiaphragmatic pressure elicited by electrophrenic stimulation (20 Hz) as a function of the duration of loaded breathing. Loaded breathing trials were performed with (open circles) and without (closed circles) prior administration of theophylline. Theophylline reduced the rate at which respiratory muscle fatigue developed (Viires et al., 1984).

Murciano et al. (1984) have examined the effect of theophylline on the strength and endurance of the diaphragm of patients with chronic obstructive lung disease who were hypoxic (PaO_2 57 ± 8 mmHg), hypercapnic $PaCO_2$ 53 ± 3 mmHg), and hyperinflated (total lung capacity 135% predicted). Theophylline significantly increased the transdiaphragmatic pressure generated by these patients during maximal inspiratory efforts against a closed airway while no such increase was observed during placebo administration. Theophylline also prevented changes in the power spectrum of the diaphragm electromyogram during loaded breathing in these patients.

These data suggest that the effect of theophylline is preserved and may even be enhanced in the presence of hypoxemia, hypercarbia, and/or hyperinflation. As a result, this drug would be expected to be of benefit in improving respiratory muscle performance in acutely ill patients with chronic obstructive lung disease.

IV. Mechanism of Action of Methylxanthines on Skeletal Muscle

The primary mechanism by which the methylxanthines are currently thought to augment muscle contractility is via an effect on muscle excitation-contraction coupling (Endo, 1975; Sandow, 1965). Although it was once thought that these drugs produced their effects principally by inhibiting intracellular phosphodiesterase enzymes, recent data suggest that this is unlikely. Not only are the drug concentrations associated with clinically relevant actions of these agents far below the drug levels required to inhibit cellular phosphodiesterase enzymes, but also the relative ability of the various methylxanthine analogues to increase skeletal muscle contractility and to relax airway smooth muscle bears no relationship to their respective potencies as phosphodiesterase inhibitors (Kramer and Wells, 1980; Jeppson et al., 1982).

Of the different methylxanthines, caffeine is the analogue for which an effect on excitation-contraction coupling is most firmly established as the probable mechanism of its action (Endo, 1975). This drug has been shown to potentiate the release and inhibit the reuptake of calcium ions by the sarcoplasmic reticulum of whole muscle preparations in which caffeine is added to the extracellular medium, of single cells into which caffeine is injected, and of suspensions of isolated cell fractions containing sarcoplasmic reticulum (Endo, 1975; Huddart, 1969; Caldwell, 1964; Weber and Herz, 1968). The calcium so released by this drug increases the level of actin-myosin protein activation during muscle excitation, thereby enhancing tension development.

The mechanism(s) by which other methylxanthine analogues, such as theophylline, exert their effects on skeletal muscle may vary somewhat from that of caffeine. For theophylline, in particular, two additional possible sites of action have been proposed (Aubier et al., 1983a; Varagic and Kentera, 1978; Connett, 1978).

Aubier and co-workers (1983a) found that verapamil, a drug known to block the movement of calcium ions through cell surface membranes, blocked the effect of theophylline on skeletal muscle in vivo. This evidence suggests that transport of calcium ions across the outer cell membrane may play a role in the action of theophylline on diaphragmatic skeletal muscle.

It has also been reported that theophylline activates a cation exchange channel in the outer cellular membrane that pumps hydrogen ions out of, and potassium ions into, the interior of the cell (Connett, 1978). As a result of this exchange, intracellular pH rises substantially following theophylline administration (increasing from a pH of 6.83 to 7.24 with 2 mM theophylline). In turn, intracellular pH strongly influences contractile protein function. When pH fails, hydrogen ions compete with calcium for attachment to the troponin unit of the actin-myosin subunit, reducing contractile protein activation (Nakamura and

Schwartz, 1972; Fabiato and Fabiato, 1978). In addition, acidosis reduces sarcoplasmic reticulum release of calcium. This action of theophylline to increase intracellular pH may, therefore, act to augment contractile protein activation and muscle force output. In addition, intracellular pH is thought to influence muscle velocity of shortening, which decreases when intracellular pH falls (Edman and Mattiazzi, 1981; Edman, 1979). Theophylline has recently been reported to increase muscle-shortening velocity, an action that may be accounted for by the effects of this drug on intracellular pH (Supinski and Kelsen, 1983).

In addition to these direct actions on skeletal muscle contractility the methylxanthines produce significant systemic effects that may influence skeletal muscle contractility. Both caffeine and theophylline increase catecholamine release from the adrenal medulla (Poisner, 1973; Berkowitz and Spector, 1971). Catecholamines, in turn, can act directly on skeletal muscle to augment contractility, an action that appears to be important in preserving diaphragm function during shock (Scharf and Bark, 1984). It seems possible, therefore, that methylxanthine-induced catecholamine release from the adrenal medulla may augment respiratory muscle contractility.

The methylxanthines increase cardiac output by augmenting cardiac contractility and reducing systemic vascular resistance (Matthay et al., 1978; Vestal et al., 1983). These drugs also increase plasma levels of glucose and free fatty acids by increasing lipolysis and glycogenolysis (Vestal et al., 1983; Rizza et al., 1982). By increasing plasma concentrations of key metabolic substrates and increasing the blood flow to exercising muscles, the methylxanthines may prolong the time required to deplete intracellular energy stores, thereby enhancing muscle endurance. In keeping with this hypothesis, Ivy et al. (1979) found that caffeine both increased endurance and reduced the rate of depletion of muscle glycogen stores in athletes performing submaximal isokinetic cycling exercise.

The relative importance of these various direct and systemic actions of the methylxanthines in improving respiratory muscle performance has not been established. It seems likely that the direct actions of these drugs on skeletal muscle ion fluxes are of primary importance in modulating their effects on muscle strength. The systemic effects of these drugs may, however, contribute to their effects on muscle endurance.

V. Effect of Methylxanthines on Respiratory Neural Drive

Caffeine and theophylline have long been recognized as respiratory stimulants, increasing ventilation in adult and newborn humans and animals (Eldridge et al., 1983; Richmond, 1949; Aubier et al., 1983b; Trippenbach et al., 1980; Rall, 1974). While the effect of these drugs on respiratory muscle strength would be expected to increase the level of ventilation resulting from a given level of res-

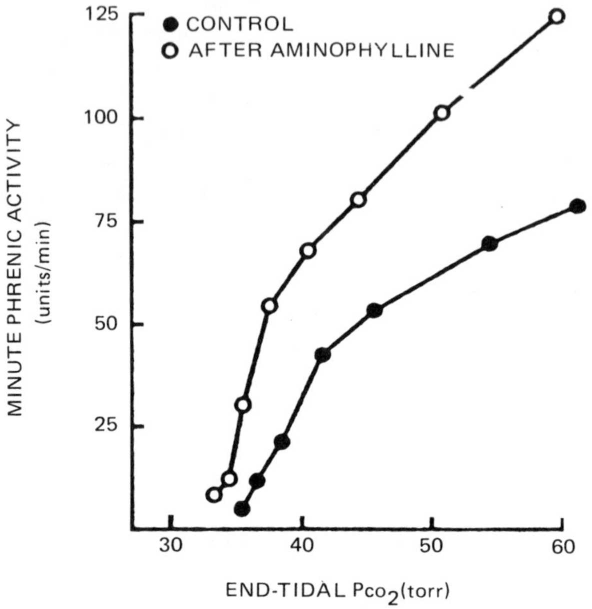

Figure 5 Relationship between phrenic nerve activity and end-tidal PCO_2 with (open circles) and without (closed circles) theophylline administration. Theophylline increased phrenic activity at all levels of PCO_2 (Eldridge et al., 1983).

piratory motor output, the methylxanthines have also been shown to augment respiratory drive at the level of the central nervous system (Eldridge et al., 1983; Aubier et al., 1983b). Eldridge and colleagues (1983) have demonstrated that theophylline increases phrenic neural activity at any given level of chemical ventilatory drive (Fig. 5). In particular, an intravenous dose of 4-8 mg/kg theophylline more than doubled phrenic nerve activity. Increases in respiratory neural output were not altered by vagotomy, carotid body removal, spinal section, adrenalectomy, or by suprapontine decerbration. This response was, however, attenuated by α-methyltyrosine, an inhibitor of dopamine biosynthesis. These results suggest that the action of the methylxanthines on respiratory neural drive occurs at the level of the midbrain and involves the action of the neurochemical dopamine.

The central ventilatory effects of the methylxanthines have several therapeutic applications. For example, aminophylline increases minute ventilation in patients with Cheyne-Stokes respiration (Dowell et al., 1963). Theophylline and caffeine are also currently used to treat premature infants with idiopathic apnea (Gerhardt et al., 1979). Although the precise cause of the apneic episodes seen in these infants is controversial, it is known that they have an elevated end-tidal PCO_2 at rest, indicating alveolar hypoventilation. Aminophylline increases the level of ventilation for any given tension of arterial carbon dioxide in these infants, shifting the carbon dioxide response curve so as to decrease the threshold of the hypercapneic ventilatory response. In theory, decreases in the ventilatory threshold to carbon dioxide should reduce respiratory center instability, preventing ventilatory oscillations and apneic episodes (Bulow, 1963). In keeping with this concept, theophylline both increases resting minute ventilation and significantly reduces apneic episodes in these infants (Gerhardt et al., 1979; Kuzemko and Paala, 1973).

Recent studies have suggested that fatigue of the respiratory muscles may result, in part, from the failure of the central nervous system to provide adequate levels of motor drive to activate the muscles, so-called "central" fatigue (Bellemare and Bigland-Ritchie, 1984). The ability of the methylxanthines to augment respiratory neural drive in the presence of hypoxia and hypercapnea (Stroud et al., 1955; Julich, 1957) may play an important role in reversing or preventing the development of such "central fatigue," and may constitute an additional mechanism by which these drugs may augment respiratory muscle endurance in patients with lung disease.

In summary, the effect of the methylxanthines on respiratory muscle performance may constitute an important therapeutic action. Further research is needed to define more fully the structure-activity relationships of the various methylxanthine derivatives in the hope of identifying an analogue with a greater therapeutic efficacy than the methylxanthines currently used in clinical settings.

VI. Addendum

Moxham et al. (1983) have recently challenged the view that theophylline increases the strength of the diaphragm. These authors were unable to detect any effect of aminophylline administration on the magnitude of the transdiaphragmatic twitch elicited by unilateral transcutaneous phrenic nerve stimulation. In subsequent work, however, a positive inotropic effect of theophylline was demonstrated by Aubier et al. (1985) when this same experiment was repeated using bilateral phrenic nerve stimulation with needle electrodes. In addition, Nochomovitz et al. (1984), have reported that theophylline increases diaphragmatic contractility in paralyzed patients who have implanted phrenic nerve stimulators. In this latter study, theophylline increased the transdiaphragmatic pressure generated at a given frequency of phrenic nerve stimulation.

It seems likely that the technique of assessing diaphragm strength by measuring transdiaphragmatic pressure during unilateral phrenic stimulation via surface electrodes is too insensitive to detect the effects of theophylline. Studies that have employed more stable stimulation techniques (e.g., implanted electrodes, bilateral stimulation, etc.) have invariably shown that theophylline increases diaphragmatic contractility.

References

Aubier, M., Detroyer, A., Sampson, M., Macklem, P. T., and Roussos, C. (1981). Aminophylline improves diaphragmatic contractility. *N. Engl. J. Med. 305*: 249-252.

Aubier, M., Murciano, D., Viires, N., Lecocguic, Y., and Pariente, R. (1983a). Diaphragmatic contractility enhanced by aminophylline: role of extracellular calcium. *J. Appl. Physiol. 54*: 460-464.

Aubier, M., Murciano, D., Viires, N., Lecocguic, Y., Palacios, S., and Pariente, R. (1983b). Increased ventilation caused by improved diaphragmatic efficiency during aminophylline infusion. *Am. Rev. Respir. Dis. 129*: 148-154.

Aubier, M., and Roussos, C. (1985). Effect of theophylline on respiratory muscle function. *Chest 88*: 915-975.

Becker, A. B., Simons, K. J., Gillespie, C. A., and Simons, F. E. R. (1984). The bronchodilator effects and pharmacokinetics of caffeine in asthma. *N. Engl. J. Med. 310*: 743-746.

Bellemare, F., and Bigland-Ritchie, B. (1984). Activity of the diaphragm, intercostals, and accessory muscles in respiratory muscle fatigue. *Am. Rev. Respir. Dis. 129*: 268.

Berkowitz, B. A., and Spector, S. (1971). Effect of caffeine and theophylline on peripheral catecholamines. *Eur. J. Pharmacol. 13*: 193-196.

Boulanger, J. P., Patel, J., and Marangos, (1982). Effects of caffeine and theophylline on adenosine and benzodiazepine receptors in human brain. *Neurosci. Lett. 30*: 161-166.

Brust, M. (1976). Fatigue and caffeine effects in fast-twitch and slow twitch muscles of the mouse. *Pflugers Arch. 367*: 189-200.

Bulow, K. (1963). Respiration and wakefulness in man. *Acta Physiol. Scand. 59*: 209-215.

Caldwell, P. C. (1964). Calcium and the contraction of Maia muscle fibers. *Proc. R. Soc. Ser. B. 160*: 512.

Cohen, C. A., Zagelbaum, G., Cross, D., Roussos, C., and Macklem, P. T. (1982). Clinical manifestations of inspiratory muscle fatigue. *Am. J. Med. 73*: 308.

Connett, R. J. (1978). Association of increased pH with calcium ion release in skeletal muscle. *Am. J. Physiol. 3*: 110-114.

Dowell, A. R., Hayman, A., Sieker, H. D., and Tripathy, K. (1963). Effect of aminophylline on respiratory center sensitivity in Cheyne-Stokes respiration and in pulmonary emphysema. *N. Engl. J. Med. 273*: 1447-53.

Edman, K. A. P. (1979). The velocity of unloaded shortening and its relation to sarcomere length and isometric force in vertebrate muscle fibers. *J. Physiol. 24*: 143-159.

Edman, K. A. P., and Mattiazzi, A. R. (1981). Effects of fatigue and altered pH on isometric force and velocity at zeroload in frog muscle fibres. *J. Muscle Res. Cell. Motil. 2*: 321-334.

Edwards, R. H. T. (1979). The diaphragm as muscle: Mechanisms underlying fatigue. *Am. Rev. Respir. Dis. 119*: 81-84.

Edwards, R. H. T., Hill, D. K., Jones, D. A., and Morton, P. A. (1977). Fatigue of long duration in human skeletal muscle after exercise. *J. Physiol. 272*: 764-778.

Eldridge, F. L., Millhorn, D. E., Waldrop, T. G., and Kiley, J. P. (1983). Mechanism of respiratory effects of methylxanthines. *Respir. Physiol. 53*: 239-261.

Endo, M. (1975). Mechanism of action of caffeine on the sarcoplasmic reticulum of skeletal muscle. *Proc. Jpn. Acad. 57*: 479-484.

Fabiato, A., and Fabiato, F. (1978). Effects of pH on the myofilaments of skinned cells from cardiac and skeletal muscle. *J. Physiol. 276*: 233-255.

Fuchs, F., Reddy, V., and Briggs, F. N. (1970). The interaction of cations with the calcium binding site of troponin. *Biochim. Biophys. Acta 221*: 407-409.

Gerhardt, T., McCarthy, J., and Bancalori, E. (1979). Effect of aminophylline on respiratory center activity and metabolic rate in premature infants with idiopathic apnea. *Pediatrics 63*: 537-542.

Howell, S., and Fitzgerald, R. S. (1985). Comparison of the effects of theophylline and enprophylline on fatigued diaphragm. *Am. Rev. Respir. Dis. 131*: A322.

Howell, S., and Roussos, C. (1984). Isoproterenal and aminophylline improve contractility of fatigued canine diaphragm. *Am. Rev. Respir. Dis. 129*: 118-124.

Huddart, H. (1969). Caffeine activation of crab skeletal muscle. *Comp. Biochem. Physiol. 29*: 1031-1038.

Ivy, J. L., Dostill, D. L., Fink, W. J., and Lowar, R. W. (1979). Influence of caffeine and carbohydrate feedings on endurance performance. *Med. Sci. Sports 11*: 6-11.

Jeppsson, A. B., Johansson, U., and Waldeck, B. (1982). Dissociation between the effects of some xanthine derivatives on the tracheal smooth muscle and on skeletal muscle. *Acta Pharmacol. Toxicol. 51*: 115-121.

Julich, H. (1957). Effects of theophylline derivatives on respiration. *Z. Gesamte Inn Med. 12*: 835-840.

Jones, D. A., Howell, S., Roussos, C., and Edwards, R. H. T. (1982). Low-frequency fatigue in isolated skeletal muscles and the effects of methylxanthines. *Clin. Sci. 63*: 161-167.

Katz, A. M., Repke, D. I., and Hasselbach, W. (1977). Dependence of ionophore- and caffeine-induced calcium release from sarcoplasmic reticulum vesicles on external and internal calcium ion concentrations. *J. Biol. Chem. 252*: 1938-1949.

Kramer, G. L., and Wells, J. N. (1980). Xanthines and skeletal muscle: Phosphodiesterase inhibition and increased twitch tension in rat diaphragms. *Mol. Pharmacol. 17*: 73-78.

Kuzemko, J. A., and Paala, J. (1973). Apnoeic attacks in the newborn treated with aminophylline. *Arch. Dis. Child. 48*: 404.

Leith, D. E., and Bradley, M. (1976). Ventilatory muscle strength and endurance training. *J. Appl. Physiol. 41*: 508-516.

Lopez, J. R., Wanek, L. A., and Taylor, S. R. (1981). Skeletal muscle: Length dependent effects of potentiating agents. *Science 214*: 79-82.

Mattay, R. A., Berger, H. J., Lake, J., Gottschalk, A., and Zaret, B. L. (1978). Effects of aminophylline upon right and left ventricular performance in chronic obstructive pulmonary disease. *Am. J. Med. 65*: 903-909.

Moxham, J., Wiles, C. M., Newham, D., and Edwards, R. H. T. (1981). Contractile function and fatigue of the respiratory muscles in man. In *Human Muscle Fatigue: Physiological Mechanisms.* Ciba Foundation Symposium Edited by R. Porter and J. Whelan. London, Pitman Medical, Vol. 82, pp. 197-205.

Moxham, J., Miller, J. M., Wiles, C. M., Newham, D., Edwards, R. H. T., and Green, M. (1983). The effect of aminophylline on human diaphragm and limb muscle contractility. *Thorax 38*: 232.

Murciano, D., Aubier, M., Lecocguic, Y., and Pariente, R. (1984). effects of theophylline on diaphragmatic strength and fatigue in patients with chronic obstructive pulmonary disease. *N. Engl. J. Med. 311*: 349-353.

Nadel, E. R. (1985). Physiological adaptations to aerobic training. *Am. Scientist 73*: 334-344.

Nakamura, Y., and Schwartz, S. (1972). The influence of hydrogen ion concentration on calcium binding and release by skeletal muscle sarcoplasmic reticulum. *J. Gen. Physiol. 59*: 22-32.

Nassar-Gentina, V., Passonneau, J. V., and Rapaport, S. I. (1981). Fatigue and metabolism of frog muscle fibers during stimulation. *Am. J. Physiol. 241*: C160-166.

Nochomovitz, M., Hopkins, M., Brodkey, J., Montenegro, H., Mortimer, J., and Cherniack, N. (1984). Conditioning of the diaphragm with phrenic nerve stimulation after prolonged disease. *Am. Rev. Respir. Dis. 130*: 685-688.

Poisner, A. M. (1973). Direct stimulant effect of aminophylline on catecholamine release from the adrenal medulla. *Biochem. Pharmacol. 22*: 469-475.

Rall, T. W. (1974). Central nervous system stimulants: the xanthines. In *The Pharmacologic Basis of Therapeutics,* ed. 4. Edited by Goodman and Gilman, New York, MacMillan.

Richmond, G. H. (1949). Action of caffeine and aminophylline as respiratory stimulants in man. *J. Appl. Physiol. 2*: 16-23.

Rizza, R. A., Haymond, M. W., and Gerich, J. E. (1982). Theophylline potentiates glucogen-induced hepatic glucose production in man but does not prevent hepatic downregulation to glucogen. *Metabolism 31*: 205-208.

Robertson, D., Wade, E., Workman, R., Woosley, R. L., and Oates, J. A. (1981). Tolerance to the humoral and hemodynamic effects of caffeine in man. *J. Clin. Invest. 67*: 1111-1120.

Rochester, D. F. (1981). Is diaphragmatic contractility important? *N. Engl. J. Med. 305*: 278-279.

Rossing, T. H., Fanta, C. H., Goldstein, D. H., Snapper, J. R., and McFadden, E. R. (1980). Emergency therapy of asthma: comparison of the acute effects of parenteral and inhaled sympathomimetics and infused aminophylline. *Am. Rev. Respir. Dis. 122*: 365-371.

Roussos, C., and Macklem, P. T. (1977). Diaphragmatic fatigue in man. *J. Appl. Physiol. 42*: 189-197.

Roussos, C., and Macklem, P. T. (1982). The respiratory muscles. *N. Engl. J. Med. 307*: 786-798.

Sandow, A. (1965). Excitation-contraction coupling in skeletal muscle. *Pharmacol. Rev. 17*: 265-320.

Scharf, S. M., and Bark, H. (1984). Function of canine diaphragm with hypovolemic shock and α-adrenergic blockade. *J. Appl. Physiol. 56*: 648-655.

Schnader, J. Y., Juan, G., Howell, S., and Roussos, C. (1983). Effects of acute changes in pCO_2 on the contractility of the diaphragm in dog. *Am. Rev. Respir. Dis. 127*: 232-238.

Sigrist, S., Thomas, D., Howell, S., and Roussos, C. (1982). The effect of aminophylline on inspiratory muscle contractility. *Am. Rev. Respir. Dis. 126*: 46-50.

Starr, I., Gamble, C. J., Margolias, A., Donal, J. S., Joseph, N., and Eagle, E. (1937). A clinical study of the action of ten commonly used drugs on cardiac output, work and size, on respiration, on metabolic rate, and on the electrocardiogram. *J. Clin. Invest. 16*: 799-823.

Stroud, M. W. III, Lambertson, C. J., Ewing, J. H., Kough, R. H., Gould, R. A., and Schmidt, C. F. (1955). The effect of aminophylline and meperidine alone and in combination on the respiratory response to carbon dioxide inhalation. *J. Pharmacol. Exp. Ther. 114*: 461-469.

Supinski, G. S., and Kelsen, S. G. (1983). Effect of aminophylline on diaphragmatic force and shortening velocity. *Fed. Proc. 42*: 1011.

Supinski, G. S., and Kelsen, S. G. (1984). Comparison of aminophylline and caffeine effects on diaphragm contractility in man. *Am. Rev. Respir. Dis. 130*: 429-433.

Supinski, G. S., Deal, E. C., Norcia, M., and Kelsen, S. G. (1984a). Effect of hypoxemia and hyperinflation on the diaphragmatic muscle response to aminophylline. *Am. Rev. Respir. Dis. 129*: 270.

Supinski, G. S., Levin, S., Nochomovitz, M. L., and Kelsen, S. G. (1984b). Effect of caffeine on respiratory muscle endurance in normal subjects. *Fed. Proc. 43*(4): 897.

Trippenbach, T., Zinman, R., and Milic-Emili, J. (1980). Caffeine effect on breathing pattern and vagal reflexes in newborn rabbits. *Respir. Physiol. 40*: 211-225.

Varagic, V., and Kentera, D. (1978). Interactions of calcium, dibutyryl cyclic AMP, isoprenaline, and aminophylline on the isometric contraction of the isolated hemidiaphragm of the rat. *Arch. Pharmacol. 303*: 47-53.

Vestal, R. E., Eriksson, C. E., Musson, B., Ozaki, L. K., and Hattor, J. B. (1983). Effect of intravenous aminophylline on plasma levels of catecholamines and related cardiovascular and metabolic responses in man. *Circulation 67*: 162-171.

Viires, N., Aubier, M., Murciano, D., Fleury, B., Talamo, C., and Pariente, R. (1984). Effect of aminophylline on diaphragmatic fatigue during acute respiratory failure. *Am. Rev. Respir. Dis. 129*: 396-402.

Weber, A., and Herz, R. (1968). The relationship between caffeine contractive and intact muscle and the effect of caffeine on reticulum. *J. Gen. Physiol. 52*: 750-759.

Wittman, T. A., and Kslsen, S. G. (1982). The effect of caffeine on diaphragmatic muscle force in normal hamsters. *Am. Rev. Respir. Dis. 126*: 499-504.

10

Theophylline
Pharmacokinetics and Clinical Applications

STANLEY J. SZEFLER

National Jewish Center
for Immunology and Respiratory Medicine, and
University of Colorado Health Sciences Center
Denver, Colorado

I. Introduction

Theophylline, a xanthine derivative, is considered one of several first-line drugs for the treatment of asthma. It is a potent bronchodilator useful in the management of acute exacerbations of asthma, as well as chronic reactive airway disease. The bronchodilator properties of theophylline were first described in the early 1920s; however, it was not until the mid-1930s that the application of theophylline for the treatment of asthma came into general use (May, 1974).

For a period of time during the mid-1950s to early 1960s, concern was raised over the incidence of severe adverse reactions, including death, associated with the use of theophylline, especially in infants and children (Ellis, 1978). With the ability to measure serum theophylline concentrations, it became apparent that patients differ in their ability to eliminate theophylline (Jenne et al., 1972). It was recognized that the resultant pharmacologic effect was not only dose-related within a given patient, but could be correlated to the serum theophylline concentration (Mitenko and Ogilvie, 1973). Dosage guidelines were developed (Mitenko and Ogilvie, 1973) and refined (Hendeles and Weinberger, 1983) to their present status.

Recognition of the fact that certain patients required frequent administration to maintain adequate serum theophylline concentrations prompted development of sustained-release delivery systems. This new technology was designed to decrease the rate of absorption sufficiently to offset rapid elimination. Initial formulations were suitable for every 8-hr administration followed by products intended for 12-hr dosing intervals. More recent developments include systems that facilitate once-daily administration. With the availability of these systems, new questions are raised about the consistency of theophylline absorption.

This discussion will focus on the approach to individualizing theophylline dosage regimens for patients. This goal is possible through the measurement of serum theophylline concentrations. Information will be provided on the nature of this measurement, with its application and limitations. In most cases periodic measurements are sufficient, however, more detailed evaluations of theophylline absorption and elimination may be necessary in some patients to identify a satisfactory dosing regimen. An approach to these investigations will be provided in the framework of recent observations regarding theophylline absorption from sustained-release theophylline (SRT) formulations. Principles of pharmacology and pharmacokinetics will be emphasized; understanding these principles will be extremely useful in assessing therapeutic agents with similar low margins of safety.

II. Pharmacokinetics

A. Serum Theophylline Concentration: What Does It Represent?

Essential to the proper interpretation of serum theophylline concentration (STC) measurements is an appreciation of conditions that influence drug disposition. These consist of drug absorption, distribution to tissue sites, and elimination either by metabolic pathways or renal excretion. At any one time, the measured STC represents a balance between the amount of drug absorbed and that being eliminated (Fig. 1). The measured concentration is dependent on the formulation (liquid, tablet, sustained-release) and the time of the blood sample in relation to the dose administered. Host factors control the rate of drug removal from the body. In most circumstances, the intrinsic release of drug from the dose formulation is the rate-limiting step for drug absorption; however, host factors can also affect the rate and extent of drug absorption.

Clinical response improves with increasing STC; however, this is accompanied by an increased risk for adverse effects. The desired range for STC is recognized as 10-20 μg/ml. This is not to suggest that all patients receiving dosages within this range will have optimal clinical effect or remain free from un-

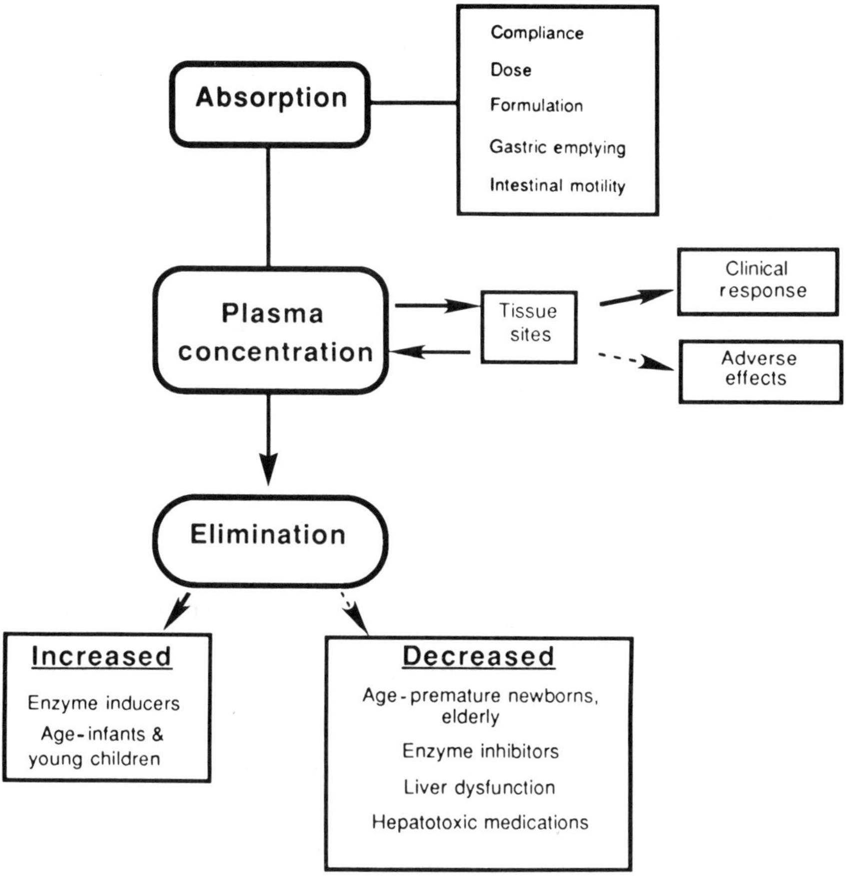

Figure 1 Schematic summary of conditions affecting the measured serum theophylline concentration.

desirable effects. Risks for severe toxicity, such as seizures and theophylline-related deaths, are considered high when STC exceeds 30 μg/ml. Less severe effects such as nausea, headache, insomnia, and irritability occur with, but are not limited to, STCs exceeding 20 μg/ml.

Several studies indicate that pulmonary function varies with fluctuations in STC (Mitenko and Ogilvie, 1973; Richer et al., 1982). Therefore, it would appear desirable to maintain the STC at a level that results in optimal clinical response with minimal variation in STC. This is most easily obtained with a constant intravenous infusion. With rapidly absorbed formulations this goal is difficult to accomplish, especially in patients in whom the drug has a short half-life.

Sustained-release delivery systems were designed to assist in minimizing the variation in STC. Theoretically, these formulations should not only maintain the desired response but also facilitate improved compliance by reducing the necessity for frequent dose administration. It is highly desirable to maintain a designated STC with a selected dose; however, the STC varies with time and is a function of conditions that affect theophylline absorption, distribution, and elimination.

B. Elimination

First-Order Elimination

Theophylline is eliminated from the body primarily through biotransformation of the active form to inactive metabolites. Less than 15% of an administered dose is excreted unchanged in the urine and is dependent on the urine flow rate (Jenne et al., 1976; Levy and Koysooko, 1976). The elimination of theophylline can be described by pharmacokinetic parameters, specifically half-life and clearance. Half-life (t 1/2) is the more familiar term and indicates the time necessary to reduce the amount of drug in the body by 50%. This can be derived clinically by measuring STCs before and after an intravenous dose of aminophylline. Graphic representation of the data as logarithmic serum theophylline concentration versus time allows calculation of the t 1/2 as well as the elimination rate constant (Fig. 2a).

The initial curvilinear phase, following completion of the intravenous dose represents the distributive phase during which the drug is undergoing distribution to sites peripheral from the circulation. The linear phase of elimination in this plot occurs after complete equilibration of theophylline between the circulation and peripheral tissue sites. The terminal slope is used to calculate the elimination rate constant (Kel or β). This parameter can be considered to represent the fraction of drug eliminated from the body per time unit. Kel sufficiently describes elimination when the mathematical model assumes elimination from one compartment. This model incorporates an assumption of rapid equilibration to tissue sites. For a more precise description of elimination, a distribution parameter (α) is included in the calculations. In this situation, referred to as a two-compartment model, β represents an elimination parameter derived from a computer fit of the logarithmic concentration-time plot (Fig. 2B). For purposes of this discussion, theophylline disposition can be described adequately by a simple one-compartment model. Since theophylline distributes rapidly to tissue sites, this is an acceptable assumption.

Theophylline's half-life can be determined directly from the graphic representation or from the relationship:

$$t\ 1/2 = 0.693/\text{Kel} \qquad (1)$$

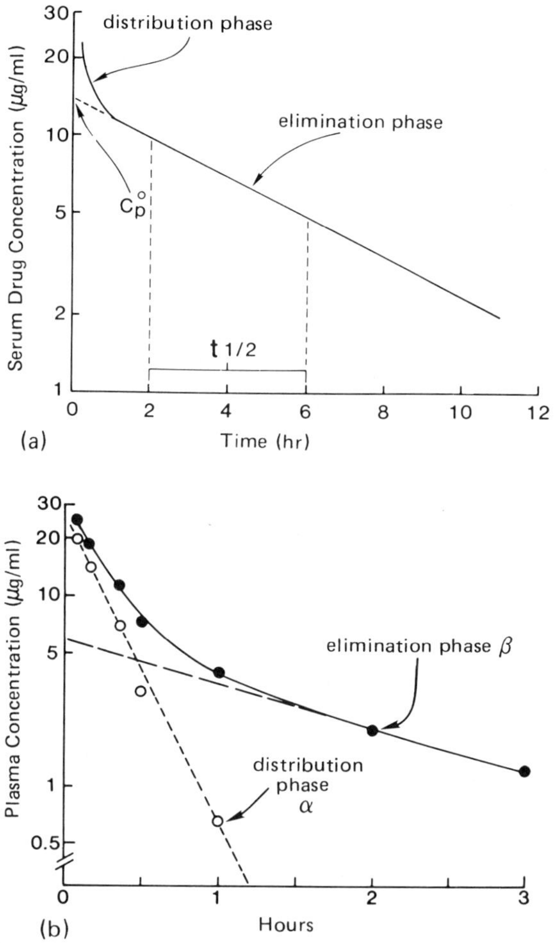

Figure 2 (a) Graph of serum drug concentration versus time after an intravenous study dose. The initial curvilinear pattern is a result of rapid drug distribution to tissue sites. The linear phase is primarily related to drug elimination. C_p^o is the extrapolated serum drug concentration for time 0 hr, assuming a one-compartment model. (b) derivation of pharmacokinetic parameters, distribution, (α), and elimination, (β), with a two-compartment model (adapted from data presented by Gibaldi and Perrier, 1975).

A more precise analysis of theophylline elimination is described by the clearance parameter. Clearance (Cl) represents the volume of plasma from which the drug is removed per unit time. It can be derived from:

$$Cl = (DOSE)(F)/AUC \qquad (2)$$

where AUC is the area under the serum theophylline concentration-time graph attributed to the administered dose. This determination usually follows serial blood sampling after an intravenous dose of aminophylline and therefore assumes that 100% of the dose is bioavailable (F). Cl is also equal to the product of Kel and Vd, the volume of drug distribution (Eq. 3).

Clearance is an important parameter since it can be utilized to determine the dosage necessary to obtain a desired plasma concentration (C_p^{SS}):

$$C_p^{SS} = \frac{(DOSE)\,(F)}{(Cl)\,(\tau)} = \frac{(DOSE)\,(F)}{(Vd)\,(Kel)\,(\tau)} \qquad (3)$$

C_p^{SS} represents the mean plasma concentration resulting from a specific dose administered over a certain time period (τ) or dosage interval. This equation is only valid if the system is at steady state (SS). Steady state is present when the amount of drug eliminated is equal to the amount of drug absorbed into the system. This occurs when a specific dose is regularly administered for at least five drug half-lives.

Half-life is an equally important pharmacokinetic parameter since it represents the period of time necessary to reduce the amount of drug in the body or the STC at equilibrium by 50%. Theophylline elimination measured by Cl or t 1/2 varies significantly between patients and even within individual patients over time. This may be related to age, concomitant medications, diet, or other disease states.

Theophylline elimination is dependent on metabolic biotransformation, and as a consequence, is highly related to hepatic function. In general, theophylline elimination varies with age and is slowest in premature newborns with immature metabolic capacities (Aranda et al., 1976; Giacoia et al., 1976; Baird-Lambert, et al., 1984). In relation to clearance measurements normalized for body weight, theophylline elimination is fastest, although highly variable, in children aged 1-9 years (Ellis et al., 1976; Loughnan et al., 1976; Nassif et al., 1981). With increasing age clearance decreases such that adolescents' rates are similar to those of healthy nonsmoking young adults (Ginchansky and Weinberger, 1977). In the elderly, theophylline metabolism apparently decreases and is most likely related to the development of other diseases affecting hepatic function, such as congestive heart failure, alcoholic cirrhosis and others.

Other medications should always be considered for their potential effect on theophylline metabolism. Certain medications are known to inhibit (erythromycin, troleandomycin, cimetidine) or accelerate (phenytoin, phenobarbital,

Table 1 Theophylline Half-Life and Clearance Values Related to Age

Age	Half-life (hr)	Clearance (ml/hr/kg)
Premature newborn	25	28
Term infants less than 6 months	10	48
6 months to 1 year	4	120
Children: 1-4 years	3.4	100
4-12 years	not available	100
12-17 years	3.7	60
Adults: healthy nonsmoking	8	45
Elderly: nonsmokers	8.6	35

Modified from data compiled by Hendeles and Weinberger (1983).

carbamazepine) theophylline metabolism. However, any medication that has the potential to alter hepatic function can affect theophylline elimination.

Similarly, any disease that has an effect directly (viral hepatitis, alcoholic cirrhosis) or indirectly (congestive heart failure, pneumonia) on liver function, will impair theophylline disposition. In addition, prolonged high fever has been associated with impairment of metabolism. Cigarette smoking (tobacco and marijuana) enhances theophylline metabolism significantly. A detailed account of conditions affecting theophylline metabolism has recently been summarized in several excellent reviews (Jusko et al., 1979; Hendeles and Weinberger, 1983; Bukowskyj et al., 1984; Jonkman and Upton, 1984). Table 1 summarizes average clearance values in relation to age, disease, and smoking status.

Zero-Order Elimination

With first-order elimination, a fraction of drug in the body is removed per unit time. This occurs when the capacity of the drug-metabolizing enzymes significantly exceeds the amount of drug in the body. In the situation where drug metabolizing enzymes are functioning at full capacity, there is a fixed amount of drug metabolized per unit time. This phenomenon is referred to as zero-order or dose-dependent kinetics. In most patients receiving theophylline therapy, this occurs with concentrations far exceeding 20 μg/ml. With a certain proportion of patients this may occur even with STCs within the therapeutic range (Weinberger and Ginchansky, 1977).

As shown in Figure 2, graphic representation of a logarithmic serum concentration-time plot is linear during first-order elimination. Figure 3a depicts

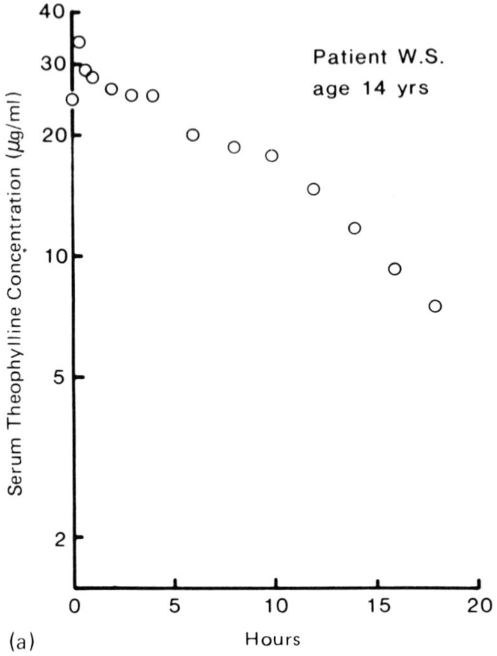

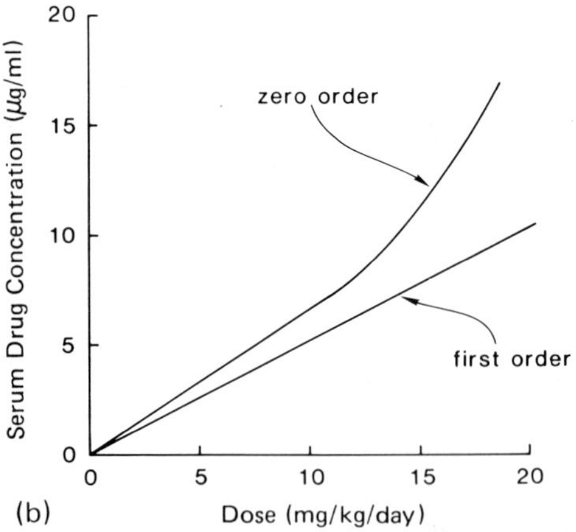

Figure 3 (a) Serum theophylline concentration-time plot after an intravenous dose of aminophylline. The nonlinear pattern is consistent with dose-dependent or enzyme-capacity-limited elimination (data compiled with the assistance of Robert J. Rogers, M.D.). (b) Dose-serum drug concentration relationship for a patient with first-order kinetics and another with dose-dependent or zero-order kinetics. At lower doses, the elimination is first-order for both situations.

the logarithmic STC-time plot for a patient with enzyme-capacity limited or dose-dependent elimination. As compared to the linear plot in Figure 2, a curvilinear pattern is present (Lesko, 1979).

This condition also has a significant effect on the resultant increase in STC obtained following an increase in theophylline dosage. With first-order elimination, the increase in C_p^{SS} is proportionate to the increase in dosage (Figure 3B). With the onset of dose-dependent kinetics at higher doses, the resultant increase in STC is proportionately greater than the increase in dose.

C. Distribution

Following an intravenous dose, theophylline is rapidly distributed to tissue sites. The extent of distribution is characterized by the pharmacokinetic parameter, volume of distribution (Vd). This is a mathematical parameter rather than a true volume. It represents the ratio of the amount of drug in the body to the concentration of drug in the plasma. The volume of distribution is calculated from the relationship of:

$$Vd = \frac{DOSE}{C_p o} \quad (4)$$

where C_p^o is the intercept extrapolated from the log linear elimination phase to the time of the administered dose (Fig. 2). This represents the theoretical STC if the drug were instantaneously distributed. In the situation where the patient has received previous doses of theophylline, C_p^o is equal to the extrapolated STC minus the STC measured prior to administering the study dose. Another method of calculating Vd is by dividing clearance by Kel.

The average Kd is 0.4-0.45 liters/kg with a range of 0.3-0.7 liters/kg. Vd is highest in the premature newborn, probably due to a higher proportion of the body water. The higher the Vd, the lower the STC obtained from a given dose.

The Vd is an important determinant in the identification of an appropriate loading dosage for the acute treatment of respiratory distress. In the absence of previous theophylline therapy, this is achieved with an intravenous aminophylline dose of 6 mg/kg (1 mg aminophylline = 0.79 mg theophylline). This is based on the assumption that 1 mg/kg theophylline will increase the STC by 2 μg/ml, as determined by altering Equation 4 to the following:

$$C_p = \frac{DOSE}{V_d} \quad (5)$$

where Cp is the STC desired and Vd the average volume of distribution, approximately 0.5 liters/kg. If the patient is receiving theophylline therapy, a partial loading dose (in mg/kg body weight) can be administered to achieve the desired concentration:

$$\text{Dose} = (C_p^{\text{desired}} - C_p^{\text{measured}})\,(0.5\ \text{L/kg}) \tag{6}$$

In each situation, the dosage should be based on the patient's ideal body weight. As previously discussed, the Vd may vary between 0.3 to 0.7 liters/kg for individual patients. Therefore, a follow-up STC measured 30 min after the infusion dose is helpful in assessing the need for an additional theophylline loading dose.

D. Absorption

Two aspects of theophylline absorption that affect the resultant STC at any time are the rate and extent of absorption from the dosage administered. Most studies performed to characterize theophylline absorption are related to analysis after single doses in normal adult volunteers. Information from these studies are used to project STC profiles during the multiple-dose theophylline administration.

Single-Dose Studies

Studies to characterize the rate and extent of absorption are usually conducted under ideal conditions. Subjects remain fasting for 8 hr before and 4 hr after the study dose. The dose is administered with a fixed volume of liquid and serial blood samples are collected for a designated period of time sufficient to describe the total period of absorption. The following equation can be applied to calculate the percent of an oral dose absorbed at various times after the dose is administered (Wagner and Nelson, 1963):

$$\text{percent absorbed} = \frac{A_T}{A\infty} \cdot 100 = \frac{C_T + \text{Kel} \int_{t=0}^{t=T} \text{Cdt}}{\text{Kel} \int_{t=0}^{t=\infty} \text{Cdt}} \cdot 100 \tag{7}$$

where A_T is the amount of drug absorbed to a specific time T, $A\infty$ is the total of drug absorbed, C_T the plasma concentration at time T, Kel the first order elimination rate constant, and $\int_{t=0}^{t=T} \text{Cdt}$ and $\int_{t=0}^{t=\infty} \text{Cdt}$ the respective areas under the plasma concentration-time curves from t = 0 to t = T and t = ∞. This equation is applicable with the assumption that theophylline is eliminated from the body according to a simple one-compartment model.

Figure 4 summarizes information obtained from an evaluation of theophylline absorption from two sustained-release delivery systems intended for administration every 12 hr (Pollack et al., 1984). It is apparent from this evaluation that the two products differ in absorption rates over the first 12 hr. On the average, product A is absorbed faster over the first 6 hr than over the remaining 6 hr. Product B is absorbed at a relatively constant rate over the entire 12 hour period. Utilizing mean absorption parameters, computer simulations are developed to project STC during multiple dose regimens. A closer evaluation of

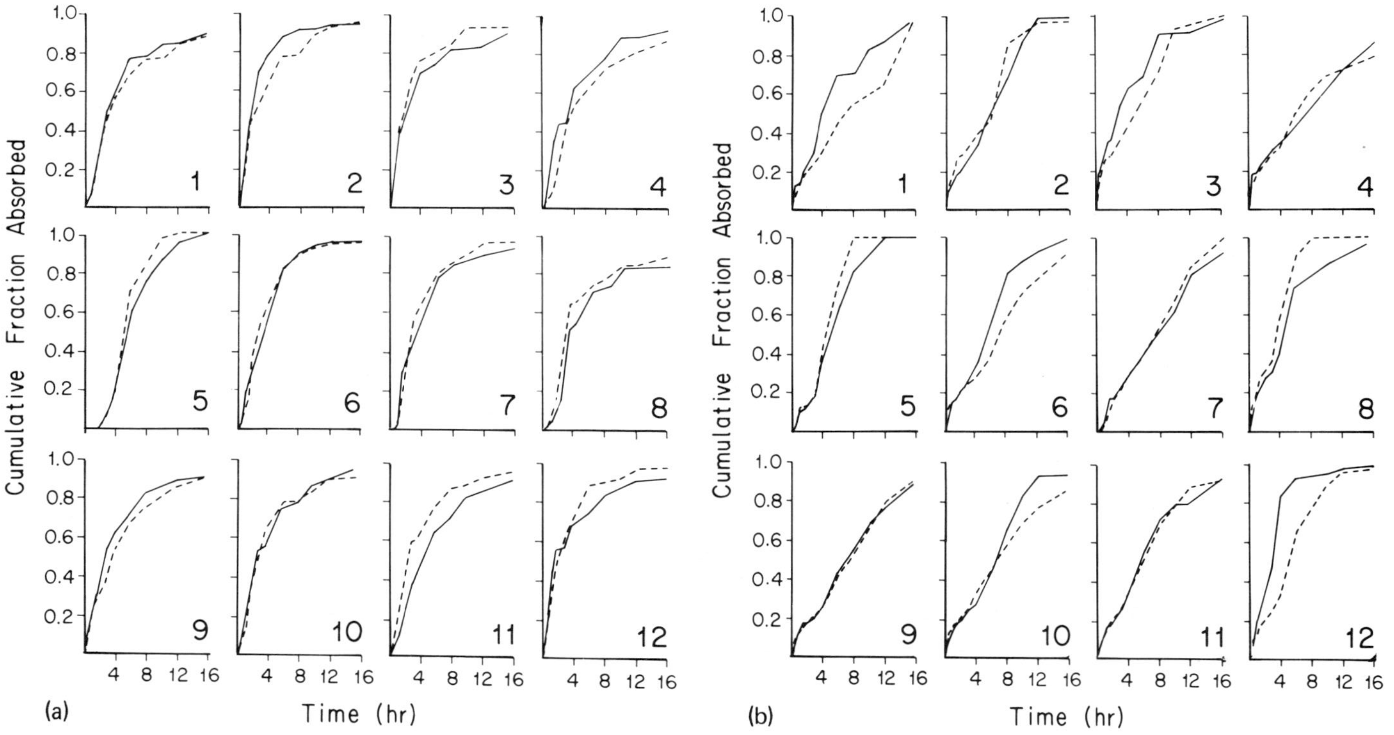

Figure 4 Compilation of data representing cumulative fraction of theophylline absorbed over time from two separate sustained-release theophylline products. Solid and dotted lines represent data from trials 1 and 2, respectively. Theophylline was administered in a crossover study to 12 normal volunteers. Each volunteer received two separate single doses of each formulation, a and b, separated by 1-week intervals (reprinted from data presented by Pollack et al., 1984).

Figure 4 also shows the wide variability in absorption within the study population, which includes an assessment of variability between and within subjects. Multiple-dose computer simulation data routinely do not include an estimate of adsorption variability.

Multiple-Dose Studies

Most multiple dose studies are limited to single dosage intervals, for example, a 12 hr period, and presented as mean STC from a population of study patients. This tends to minimize inter- and intrasubject variability. Recently, several investigators began to evaluate STC over a 24-hour period. In one report a diurnal pattern of STC was described with higher STC during the day and lower STC during the evening (Scott et al., 1981; Taylor et al., 1984). Unfortunately, the cause of this variation was not evaluated. This diurnal pattern could be related to either relatively slow absorption or fast elimination during the evening hours.

It appears from recent studies conducted in adolescent asthmatic patients that theophylline clearance is relatively constant over a 24-hr period (Rogers et al., 1985). Similar studies in adult volunteers support these observations (Taylor et al., 1983). In the same group of adolescent asthmatic patients, STC-were monitored over a 48-hr period while the patients received a sustained-release theophylline formulation administered every 12 hr. These patients were selected for close evaluation because of observed variability in STC during routine therapeutic drug monitoring. Four of eight patients demonstrated the previously described diurnal pattern (Fig. 5A). This was attributed to relatively increased theophylline absorption during the day compared to slower absorption during the evening hours. The remaining four patients had no identifiable pattern of STC (Fig. 5B).

In order to calculate the amount absorbed over time, a modification of the previously described Wagner-Nelson equation is useful (Wagner, 1983). The following equation is applied to analyze theophylline absorption within a dosage interval during multiple dose therapy:

$$A_T = Vd\,(C_n^T + Kel \int_{t=0}^{t=T} Cndt - C_n^o) \qquad (8)$$

where A_T represents the amount of drug absorbed from the beginning of the dosage interval to some time T in the dosage interval, Vd the volume of distribution, C_n^o the STC prior to the administered dose, C_n^T the STC at time T, Kel the elimination rate constant, and $\int_{t=0}^{t=T}$ Cndt the area under the STC-time curve for the time interval t=0 to t=T.

Applying this method of analysis facilitates the evaluation of individual patients. Several interesting features have been identified in certain patients. For

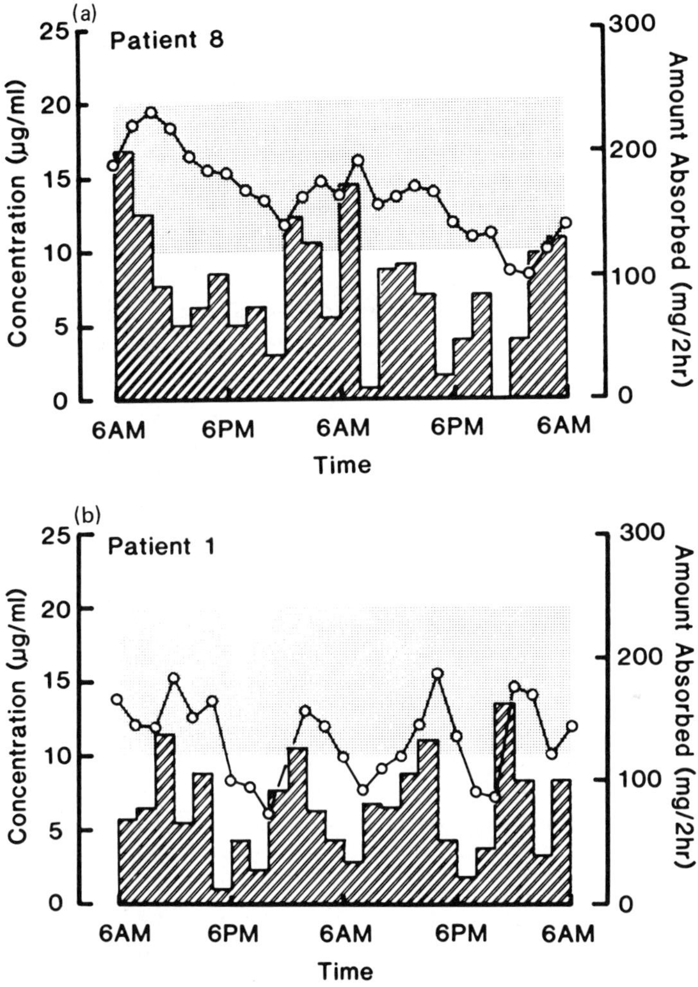

Figure 5 Serum theophylline concentrations (o——o) and calculated amount of theophylline absorbed (bar graph) for two patients during continuous treatment with a sustained-release theophylline preparation. All doses were administered at 6 AM and 6 PM. Shaded area represents the recognized therapeutic range for theophylline. Patient 8 is representative of a diurnal pattern. Patient 1 demonstrates an inconsistent pattern of concentration and amount absorbed (reprinted from Rogers et al., 1985).

example, in some patients with a diurnal variation in STC, absorption is not only delayed during the evening hours, but appears negligible between the hours of 12 midnight to 4 AM (Fig. 5a); then before the time of awakening, absorption again increases. One possible explanation is reduced intestinal motility during these hours with a subsequent increase shortly before awakening. Since STC is usually monitored before or several hours after the morning dose, this observation raises questions regarding information derived from our routine methods for theophylline monitoring.

In other patients (Fig. 5b), there is no consistent pattern for STC or the estimated amount of drug absorbed within the dosage interval. It is apparent from evaluating these patients that absorption is inconsistent and may be related to unidentified variations in gastrointestinal physiology. In patients with this degree of inconsistency in absorption, the patients at risk for wide variations in STC seem to be those in whom the drug has a short half-life, for example, less than 4 hr. In these patients, a decrease in absorption for a short period of time results in a significant decrease in STC. From this evaluation, it appears that absorption may cease not only after total absorption of the administered dose, but also during the dosage interval relative to changes in such factors as gastrointestinal motility.

Ideally, sustained-release theophylline preparations should be particularly useful in young children because therapy in this age group is complicated by rapid elimination and long sleep periods. Despite the frequent use of these preparations in children less than 6 years of age, there is very little information on the reliability of absorption in this age group. Haltom and Szefler (1985) examined theophylline absorption over a 24-hr period in eight children ages 2-6 years using two different SRT preparations: Slo-Phyllin Gyrocaps (William H. Rorer, Inc., Fort Washington, PA), intended for every 8-hr administration, and Slo-Bid Gyrocaps (William H. Rorer, Inc.), formulated for twice-daily dosing.

As compared to previous observations in STC in older children receiving a twice-daily formulation, Theo-Dur (Key Pharmaceuticals, Miami, FL), a different STC-time pattern was observed in children less than 6 years of age. In a group of children aged 6-13 years, Scott et al. (1981) reported a diurnal STC-time profile with the lowest STC occurring at approximately midnight. A definitive peak-trough pattern, however, was observed for both morning and evening doses of Slo-Bid in young children. The pre-dose and peak STC of the morning dose were both higher than those observed with the dose administered in the evening (Fig. 6B). Application of the modified Wagner-Nelson equation (Eq. 8) suggested that theophylline absorption following the evening dose was slower compared to the morning dose. The extent of absorption averaged approximately 98% for both doses.

In contrast to the relatively consistent STC-time profile and absorption with Slo-Bid administered twice daily, the STC-time pattern with the 8-hr prep-

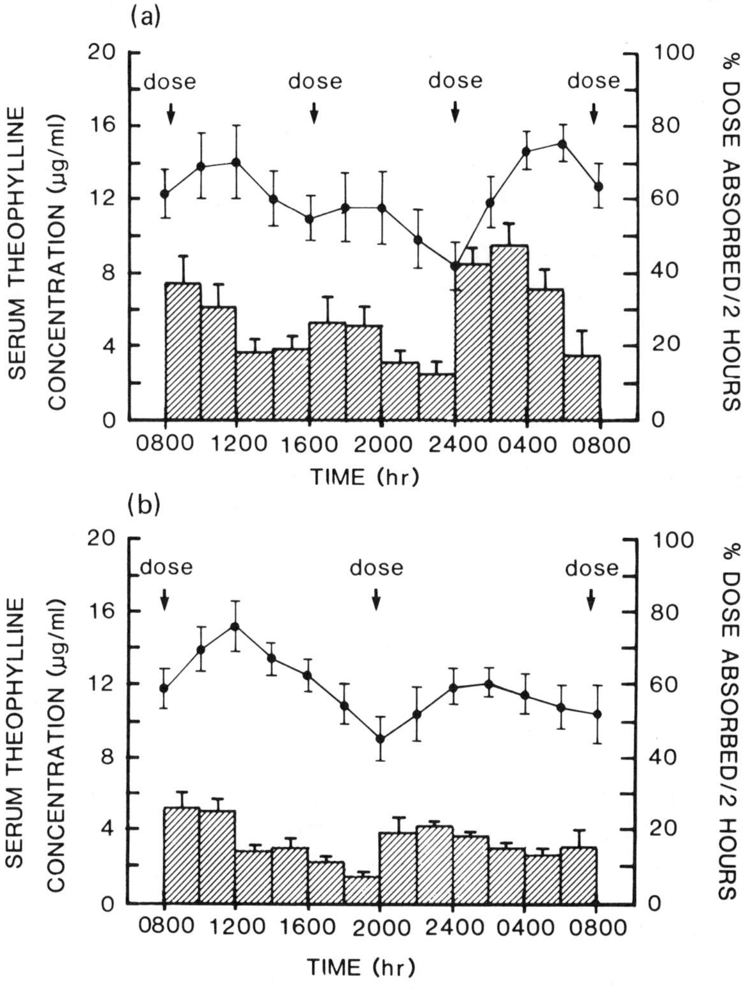

Figure 6 Summary (mean ± SEM) of serum theophylline concentrations (STCs) and absorption for eight patients during continuous therapy with Slo-Phyllin (a) and Slo-Bid (b) Gyrocaps. Points represent STC measured every 2 hr. Bar graphs indicate calculated percent of each dose absorbed over each 2 hr. Percent dose absorbed represents (calculated amount absorbed/dose) X 100 (reprinted from Haltom and Szefler, 1985).

aration, Slo-Phyllin, was significantly different (Fig. 6a). Slo-Phyllin was given at 8 AM, 4 PM, and midnight. Following the 8 AM dose, a true peak-trough pattern was observed with average fluctuation of 60% and calculated bioavailability of 102%. Of interest, following the 4 PM dose, the STC fell continuously during the dosing interval in five of eight patients. The mean bioavailability for this dosing interval was 77%. With the midnight dose, a very large and rapid rise in STC was observed. The fluctuation in STC exceeded 100% in five of eight patients between midnight and 8 AM, and the calculated bioavailability averaged 141% for the study population. It is apparent from these studies that analysis of a single daytime dosing interval is inadequate to characterize STC-time patterns and absorption throughout the day. Furthermore, there appear to be significant differences in theophylline absorption in young children compared to children over 6 years of age.

Application of the modified Wagner-Nelson equation to analyze absorption has certain limitations. In order to derive information on absorption, it is necessary to determine an accurate estimate of Kel and Vd. A separate study performed after an intravenous dose of aminophylline is occasionally conducted to derive the essential pharmacokinetic parameters. While it is likely that Kel and Vd remain constant over short periods of time, such as 24 hr, there is conflicting evidence regarding the feasibility of this assumption for longer periods of time (Ginchansky and Weinberger, 1977; Leung et al., 1977; Walson et al., 1977; Upton et al., 1982). It is, therefore, necessary to obtain these kinetic parameters as close as possible to the oral studies (Wagner, 1984) or else simultaneously using a double isotope technique (Vestel et al., 1983). The intravenous study should be conducted over a sufficiently long period of time to analyze whether there is any potential for dose-dependent or enzyme-capacity limited elimination with STC less than 20 μg/ml. The accurate analysis of STC is, without question, an essential variable to control.

III. Clinical Application

While research investigations utilize multiple concentration determinations over a designated time period, clinical applications are often limited to one or two STC measurements. With this restricted number of determinations, certain precautions must be considered for proper interpretation.

A. Indications

The greatest benefits of therapeutic drug monitoring are derived when a specific question is addressed. The clinician may question the patient's compliance, the adequacy of a selected dosage, the risk for toxicity, or confirm a suspected alteration in absorption or elimination secondary to other medications or a disease state. Once the specific question is identified and the patient carefully examined in relation to past history and present status, the appropriate time for blood sampling is determined.

If the purpose is to assess the risk for toxicity then it would be beneficial to determine the highest STC. For patients receiving twice-daily sustained-release theophylline formulations, a sample obtained 4-6 hr after the morning dose is usually representative of the peak STC for the day. It is important to recognize, however, that for once-daily preparations administered every 24 hr, the peak STC usually occurs between 8 and 12 hr after the dose (Szefler, 1985). For rapidly absorbed preparations, such as oral liquids or tablets, the peak STC occurs within 1-2 hr after the dose. If the question centers around the adequacy of the dose, it may also be useful to determine the lowest STC obtained. It is assumed that the lowest STC occurs just prior to an administered dose. To interpret the resultant STC and answer the specific question, it is therefore essential to understand the characteristics of the formulation administered.

B. Interpretation

Proper interpretation of an STC measurement requires the identification of the sample conditions including: the dose and formulation (oral tablet, liquid, or sustained-release), the time of the previous dose and the sampling time, the patient's age and weight, and concomitant medications or diseases. If the result is higher or lower than expected, a systematic evaluation should be conducted before further dosage adjustments are recommended.

Serum Concentrations Lower than Expected

In this situation, it is necessary to be certain that the dose, sampling time, and compliance are satisfactory. If these are considered adequate, then the possibility of accelerated theophylline elimination and/or impaired absorption should be examined. Rapid metabolism frequently occurs in young children, ages 1-9 years, and adolescents and young adults who smoke cigarettes or marijuana (Ellis et al., 1976; Powell et al., 1977; Jusko et al., 1978; Gardner et al., 1983). Other medications, such as anticonvulsant therapy (phenytoin, carbamazepine, phenobarbital) have the potential to accelerate theophylline metabolism (Piafsky et al., 1977a; Landay et al., 1978; Marquis et al., 1982; Rosenberry et al., 1983). A dietary change, such as from a low protein-high carbohydrate to a high protein-low carbohydrate, high to low methylxanthine, or significant addition of charcoal-broiled foods, has the potential to induce theophylline-metabolizing enzymes (Kappas et al., 1976, 1978; Caldwell et al., 1977; Thompson et al., 1983).

Before increasing the dosage, it is important to evaluate these patients. In patients with rapid theophylline metabolism, a low predose concentration is expected, especially in patients receiving rapidly absorbed formulations. In these situations, an STC at the estimated peak time could provide information on the expected range of STC.

Serum Concentrations Higher than Expected

Consistent concentrations approaching or exceeding 20 μg/ml are particularly worrisome since there is an increased risk for theophylline toxicity. Once again, the prescribed dosage and sampling time should be reviewed. Another possibility relates to excessive use of the prescribed medication either by self-medication or the use of several medications containing theophylline. Once these considerations are excluded, the patient should be evaluated for conditions that impair theophylline metabolism.

Theophylline elimination is reduced in the presence of diseases that directly or indirectly affect liver function such as liver disease, congestive heart failure, or certain medications (Mangione et al., 1978; Jenne et al., 1974; Piafsky et al., 1977b; Powell et al., 1978). Cimetidine can abruptly and substantially decrease theophylline metabolism (Reitberg et al., 1981). Macrolide antibiotics, such as troleandomycin and erythromycin, also inhibit theophylline metabolism. While troleandomycin consistently reduces theophylline elimination in all patients (Weinberger et al., 1977), the effect of erythromycin is highly variable between individual patients. On the average, theophylline elimination is reduced by 25% in the presence of erythromycin therapy, however, the degree of change may be minimal in some patients and exceed 50% in others (Zarowitz et al., 1981; Prince et al., 1981; LaForce et al., 1981). In addition, any medication that has an associated risk for hepatotoxicity has the potential to alter theophylline metabolism. Falsely high theophylline concentrations may be a result of analytical errors or assay interference related to concomitant medications, such as the metabolites of certain antimicrobial agents.

Inconsistent Concentrations

Occasionally, STC measurements in certain patients are inconsistent despite a fixed dosage regimen. This is a situation of particular concern in patients with inadequate symptom control. Decisions regarding dosage adjustments are difficult when certain measurements are below and others exceed the therapeutic range. Potential explanations include poor or erratic compliance, inconsistency in sampling times, errors in laboratory analysis, or assay interference.

Another source of variability, which is seldom appreciated, is the inherent variability related to theophylline absorption from sustained-release delivery systems. Studies conducted over 24-48 hr have identified the potential for significant variations in STC from dose-to-dose and day-to-day in certain patients (Rogers et al., 1985). Since theophylline clearance is relatively consistent over at least 24-hr periods, this variability in STC is attributed to inconsistent absorption. From other reports and from our own studies, it appears that variability in STC is more likely to occur in patients with a theophylline half-life less than 4 hr (Pollack et al., 1984). Therefore, STC measurements in young children and patients with conditions associated with the potential for accelerated theophylline metabolism should be interpreted with caution.

D. Detailed Evaluation

With STC measurements higher or lower than expected, the clinician must decide whether a dosage adjustment is indicated. Guidelines are available to assist in decisions regarding the specific change (Weinberger, 1984). However, it is important to assess fully the patient's clinical response, which should be the primary determinant in this decision. If the accuracy of the measurement is in question, either due to laboratory analysis or sampling time, it may be useful to repeat the STC with proper attention to the necessary conditions.

Occasionally, it is difficult to individualize theophylline dosage regimens in certain patients with multiple measurements of STC obtained under apparently optimal conditions. The STC may be persistently low despite continued dosage adjustments to total daily doses twice as high as recommended. Another situation is that of inconsistent STC. There may be a history of repeated dosage adjustments or frequent attempts at changing formulations in an effort to provide consistent STC in the therapeutic range. Questions may be raised regarding compliance, unusual theophylline metabolism, or inadequate or inconsistent absorption in these patients. In these cases, it may be useful to perform specific pharmacokinetic studies to identify the cause of the problem and to assist in the design of appropriate dosage regimens. Studies may be conducted during oral or intravenous administration. The benefits and limitations of each procedure will be discussed.

Intravenous Study

An evaluation of theophylline STC after an intravenous dose of aminophylline allows one to compute specific pharmacokinetic parameters including total clearance, half-life, elimination rate constant, and volume of distribution (Georgitis et al., 1984). A comparison of these values to available data from various age groups assists in the identification of patients with unusually fast or slow metabolism or those with high or low tissue distribution (Table 1). As described in Equation 3, both $t\,1/2$ and V_D affect the dosage necessary to attain a desired STC.

The purpose of administering an intravenous dose is to assure full and rapid systemic availability for accurate determination of pharmacokinetic parameters. To remove any potential interference from previously administered doses, patients should be placed on a rapidly absorbed formulation for at least

24 hr before the intravenous study dose. An additional precaution is selection of the study dose. In the transfer to rapidly absorbed preparations, it may be necessary to reduce the oral dosage or administer doses at frequent intervals, for example, every 4 hr, if incomplete absorption or rapid metabolism is suspected. These adjustments may be essential in reducing the risk of adverse effects while maintaining satisfactory clinical response.

An adequate study dose should provide STCs well within the therapeutic range. The STC measurements should be obtained before and at timed intervals for at least 12 hr. An example of a sample scheme includes STC prior to the administered dose, immediately postinfusion, 0.5, 1, 1.5, 2, 3, 4, 6, 8, 10, and 12 hr after beginning the infusion. It is desirable to sample for a period of at least two half-lives. A 12-hr interval may therefore be adequate in children; however, a longer interval may be necessary in patients with longer half-lives. A sufficiently long sampling time may also provide insight into the presence of dose-dependent or enzyme capacity-limited elimination. In this situation, a curvilinear pattern will be evident on a graphic presentation of the logarithmic STC-time data (Fig. 3A).

Oral Study

An oral study in itself provides limited information; however, when combined with an intravenous study, it facilitates a more comprehensive analysis of total bioavailability and absorption during a dosing interval. Without a complementary intravenous study, it is not possible to derive information specifically related to rapid metabolism and/or impaired absorption.

To perform this procedure, it is recommended that the patient receive his or her usual dose over at least 2 days prior to the scheduled study day. This is to ensure steady-state conditions. On the morning of the study dose, a predose sample is collected. Following this sample, the theophylline dose is administered, and samples for STC collected serially, for example, every 2 hr over 24 hr. The regularly scheduled doses are administered throughout the study period.

In the absence of a concomitant intravenous aminophylline study, it is only possible to evaluate the STC pattern over the study period; this in itself may be helpful. For example, this study was performed in a 4-year-old boy with severe steroid-dependent asthma. During routine monitoring, STCs were recorded at various times ranging from 5 to 15 μg/ml. The STC profile obtained over a 24 hr period during administration of a commonly prescribed sustained-release theophylline preparation (Theo-Dur Sprinkle, Key Pharmaceuticals) every eight hours is presented in Figure 7. The results obtained were completely unexpected. The STC was 16 μg/ml in the morning and continued to decrease to 4 μg/ml in the evening despite administration of regularly scheduled doses. Of greater concern, however, was the subsequent rise in STC to 30 μg/ml during

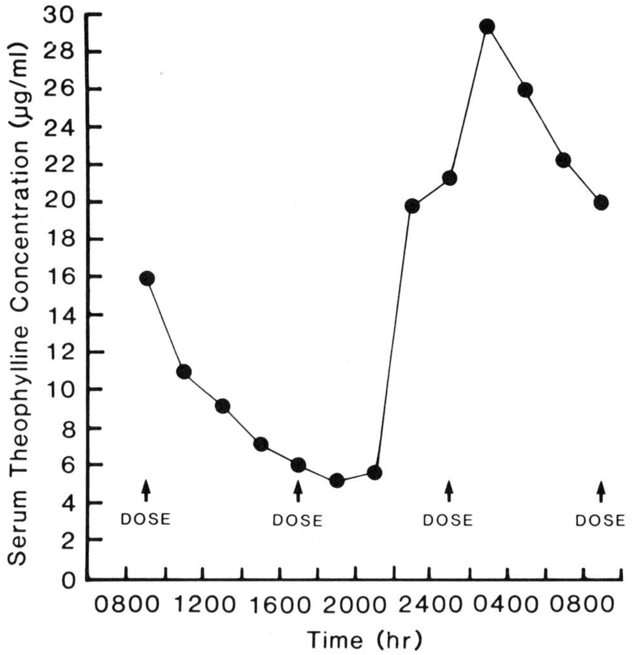

Figure 7 Serum theophylline concentration-time profile in a 4-year-old asthmatic patient. Theophylline was administered as Theo-Dur Sprinkle (Key Pharmaceuticals) 150 mg every 8 hr (data compiled with the assistance of Betty Mitchell, C.H.A.).

the night, when we seldom monitor STC. With this information, an alternative SRT preparation was administered and provided more consistent STC over a 24-hr study period with improved bioavailability.

With additional information obtained from an intravenous aminophylline study, a more extensive interpretation of the oral study can be provided. Equation (8) can be incorporated to calculate the amount of theophylline absorbed per sampling interval, for example each 2-hr interval in the 24-hr study period. In addition, bioavailability (F) can be determined over the entire study period or an individual dosage interval:

$$F = \frac{AUC_{oral}}{AUC_{I.V.}} \times \frac{Dose_{I.V.}}{Dose_{oral}} \times 100 \qquad (9)$$

A significant decrease in bioavailability may prompt trial with another SRT formulation or consideration of an absorption abnormally related to factors such as food, concomitant medications, disease, age, or gastrointestinal physiology. The limitations of this approach were described previously.

IV. Sustained-Release Delivery Systems

With the significant advances in pharmaceutical technology, many SRT preparations are now available for clinical use. Over 20 different preparations are now routinely prescribed. The original formulations permitted every 8 hr dosing. These innovations were soon followed by preparations that allowed twice daily dosing. Recently, the opportunity to administer once daily was provided with several new products. Criticisms have been raised over the reliability of systems intended for single daily administration. These concerns are primarily related to the total bioavailability and also the consistency of the release characteristics, especially in relation to meals. It has become apparent that similar questions can be raised for all controlled-release delivery systems. After a brief summary of the ideal characteristics of an SRT preparation below, an overview of the present concerns regarding the adequacy of available formulations is presented.

A. Ideal Characteristics

The main advantages of SRT are to minimize fluctuations in STC and reduce the number of doses required per day. A reduction in the dosing interval should theoretically improve compliance. Based on several clinical studies, the theory has been developed that STC should be maintained in the therapeutic range, commonly recognized as 10-20 μg/ml. To accomplish this goal at all times, it would be necessary to avoid fluctuations in STC exceeding 100%, based on the definition that % Δ STC is equal to the highest STC minus the lowest STC divided by the lowest STC. With rapidly absorbed theophylline products, this would require dosage administration at least every half-life. If we recognize that the average half-life in children is approximately 4 hr, and as low as 2 hr in some patients, it is obvious that dosage administration every half-life would be impractical.

Reducing the availability of drug for absorption, by altering the rate of drug release, decreases the fluctuation in STC. The goal we all seek is to design an oral system that would mimic the delivery rate of a constant intravenous infusion, the so-called "zero-order" rate or a constant amount of drug absorbed per unit time. Unfortunately, this is difficult and potentially impossible goal to reach. A reliable system would allow the clinician to titrate carefully dosage regimens based on STC obtained at any time. While this may be feasible with available preparations for patients in whom the drug has a relatively long half-life, it is doubtful that SRT formulations fulfill the need of the patients they were primarily intended for, namely young children and rapid theophylline metabolizers.

If the intention is to maintain STC in the therapeutic range at all times, a % Δ STC greater than 100% is not acceptable. Furthermore, the rate and extent of absorption must be consistent from dose to dose and from day to day within patients to provide reliability in the interpretation of STC. Recent evidence about the effect of food on the release characteristics of certain preparations has resulted in the review of all available SRT delivery systems. Questions have been raised regarding the proper time of dose administration in relation to meals.

B. Present Concerns

Characterization of SRT relative to absorption rate is usually performed during single dose administration, often in fasting patients. Simulations of single dose data during multiple-dose administration are useful in the analysis of potential changes in STC relative to varying elimination parameters. Information on absorption characteristics of various formulations and the potential effect on STC profiles is provided in several excellent detailed reviews (Hendeles et al., 1984; Weinberger, 1984). Use of this information on a clinical basis must include an appreciation of conditions that may affect both elimination and absorption of theophylline. Considerable information is now available on conditions affecting theophylline elimination. Relatively little is known regarding physiological variables that may affect the rate and extent of theophylline absorption.

Dederich and co-workers (1981) demonstrated the potential for dose to dose variability in STC profiles following administration of two separate single doses of several SRT preparations. Subsequently, several studies identified the effect of food on delaying the absorption rate of theophylline from two SRT formulations, Nuelin Retard (Riker) and Theo-Dur 100 and 300 mg tablets (Key Pharmaceuticals), following single doses administered with and without a meal (Pedersen, 1981; Leeds et al., 1982). There was no effect of food on the extent of absorption. For Somophyllin (Fisons Pharmaceutical Division), a reduction in the rate of absorption was observed in the first 2 hr after a meal as compared to the fasting state with no effect on the extent of absorption (Pedersen and Moller-Petersen, 1985).

Lagas and Jonkman (1983) demonstrated that for another SRT formulation, Theograd 250 mg tablets (Abbott Laboratories), the extent of absorption was significantly lower in the absence of food (64%) than in the nonfasting state (90%). The rate of absorption, however, was faster in the fasting state in relation to nonfasting conditions. Pedersen and Moller-Petersen (1984), on the other hand, demonstrated that for Theo-Dur Sprinkle (Key Pharmaceuticals), the absorption pattern and bioavailability were severely affected by concomitant food intake. In this case, bioavailability was reduced from 91% in the fasting state to 44% in the presence of food. The rate of absorption was also delayed with a meal. In addition, the type of meal may have a significant effect on the absorption characteristics of Theo-Dur Sprinkle (Pedersen, 1984). The extent of absorption was greater, and the rate of absorption faster, for a "wet" meal (applesauce and milk) than that determined with a "dry meal" (cornflakes, rye bread, and milk). Apparently, the absorption anomalies with Theo-Dur sprinkle observed in single-doses can be overcome by administering the drug 5 min prior to the meal (Pedersen and Moller-Petersen, 1984). Whether this is true during multiple-dose chronic therapy with Theo-Dur sprinkle is not known.

The most troubling development in this series is the observation that theophylline absorption from several once-daily SRT formulations is significantly altered in the presence of food. Bioavailability of Theo-24 (G.D. Searle and Co.) after an overnight fast was 71%, compared to 111% when administered with a meal (Hendeles et al., 1985). Food also affected the rate of theophylline absorption from Theo-24. After an initial delay in absorption, approximately one-half of the dose was absorbed within a 4-hr period beginning 6-8 hr after the dose administered with a breakfast of bacon, eggs, muffins, potatoes, and milk. With another once-daily SRT preparation, Uniphyl (Purdue-Frederick Co.), the bioavailability was 53% under fasting conditions compared to 96% when administered with a similar meal (Karim et al., 1985).

While the effect of food on single-dose SRT absorption characteristics is important in eliciting information, far too little information is available on theophylline absorption during multiple-dose administration. Using sampling for a 24-hr period and individual patient data, Kelly and Murphy (1979 and 1980) and Scott et al. (1981) identified significant variations in STC. While some patients may demonstrate diurnal patterns, with higher STC during the day than at night, other patients may have unpredictable fluctuations in STC (Rogers et al., 1985). This is attributed to the potential for considerable inconsistency in theophylline absorption in certain patients receiving SRT therapy.

An additional variable that may influence the rate of theophylline absorption from SRT formulations is the effect of posture. Warren et al. (1985) demonstrated that STCs were significantly lower when study subjects remained supine than when they remained standing 6 hr after a dose of Phyllocontin (Napp Laboratories).

The mechanisms affecting theophylline absorption must be identified. These may be related to the formulation (pH dependency, solubility), or the effect of food, posture, or concomitant medications on gastric physiology (Toothaker and Welling, 1980). Although specific information is not available for theophylline, absorption for most drugs is relatively poor in the stomach (Nimmo, 1976). Therefore, even with optimal dissolution of theophylline from the SRT preparation, the limiting step for absorption may be the rate of transfer of theophylline from the stomach to the relevant sites of absorption in the intestine. Numerous factors control the gastric emptying rate, including the type of food (solids, liquids, fats), medications (anticholinergic agents, beta-adrenergic agonists) and disease states (reflux, viral gastroenteritis) (Nimmo,

1976, Minami and McCallum, 1984). In addition, the rate and extent of absorption may be affected by the time of exposure to the absorption sites (Hirtz, 1984). It is obvious that SRT with prolonged absorption rates should be more susceptible to conditions affecting intestinal transit time and the stability of the epithelial absorption sites.

It is possible, but often inconvenient, to control the fasting state for doses administered in the morning. It is even more difficult to control these conditions for subsequent doses administered in the afternoon or evening, since most patients do not maintain regular or consistent meal schedules. It will be necessary to identify formulations resistant to these variables or at least identify patients at risk for significant variations in STC. In these patients, alternative forms of therapy may be considered.

V. Alternative Preparations

Theophylline is without doubt a significant bronchodilator in the treatment of acute and chronic obstructive respiratory disease. Its disadvantages include a relatively low margin of safety, numerous factors altering its elimination, and the risk for serious adverse effects. To minimize these concerns, attempts have been made to develop xanthine derivatives with a more selective bronchodilator effect and a much lower risk for adverse effects. Initial attempts date back to the 1950s with dyphylline and have continued with the most recent development, enprofylline.

It would appear desirable to develop a compound with equal or greater potency to theophylline, complete and consistent bioavailability, a relatively long elimination time, correlation of serum concentrations to therapeutic effect, and selective activity. Information on the structure-activity relationship of these various compounds was recently summarized by Persson (1982) and is presented in Figure 8.

Dyphylline, 7-(2,3-dihydroxypropyl)-theophylline, one of the first synthetic compounds, differs from theophylline in several features. Unlike theophylline, it is primarily eliminated by renal excretory pathways, and consequently has a half-life of approximately 2 hr (Simons et al., 1975; Simons and Simons, 1979). To facilitate compliance and maintain consistent plasma dyphylline concentrations, sustained-release formulations were developed and bioavailability measured as 68% with a range of 36.8-86.0% (Simons et al., 1977). Single-dose studies identified the bronchodilator properties of dyphylline; however, it was significantly less potent than theophylline (Hudson et al., 1973). The incidence of adverse effects related to dyphylline was minimal in this comparative evaluation. Since dyphylline is not dependent on biotransformation, dosage adjustments are not necessary in patients with liver abnormalities. Renal dysfunction, however, contributes to impaired dyphylline elimination (Lee et al., 1981).

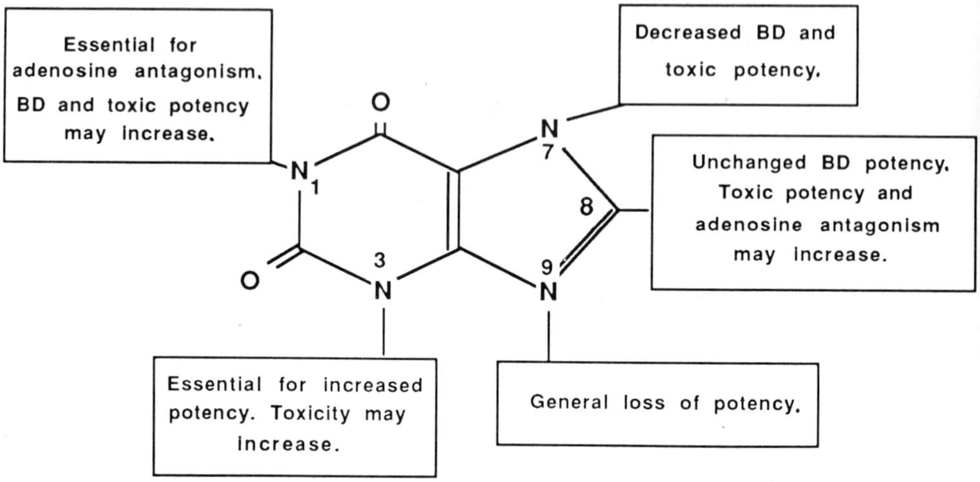

Figure 8 Some main features of alkyl substitution of various positions in the xanthine molecule (BD, bronchodilator; theophylline, 1,3 dimethylxanthine; enprofylline = 3-propyl-xanthine) (reprinted with permission from Persson, 1982).

Far too little information is available on the individualization of dyphylline dose to optimize clinical response and minimize adverse effects. Dyphylline is not converted to theophylline and is chemically distinct. Utilization of serum theophylline concentration measurements during dyphylline therapy provides misleading information and has the potential to result in severe adverse effects (Bussey, 1981).

Acephylline (theophylline-7-ylacetic acid) is eliminated very rapidly by active renal excretion with a half-life of 47 min. In addition, absorption is very poor and information on its bronchodilator effect in humans is not available (Zuidema and Merkus, 1979). Similarly, insufficient information is available regarding etophylline (B-hydroxyethyl-theophylline).

Proxyphylline (B-hydroxypropyl theophylline) was developed in 1956. In adults, half-life ranges between 8 and 12 hr, with the major route of elimination being biotransformation (Selvig, 1981). Single-dose studies identified evidence of saturation kinetics (Rasmussen et al., 1984). Preliminary studies indicate that the incidence of adverse effects is lower with proxyphylline than theophylline. This may be related to lower potency or differences in central nervous system distribution.

Enprofylline (3 propylxanthine), in contrast to the previously described agents, offers considerable potential as an alternative to theophylline. It may also be a useful probe to examine the mechanism of action of theophylline. It is extremely doubtful that the traditional mechanism of action for theophylline, namely phosphodiesterase inhibition, is operative at therapeutic concentrations (Bergstrand, 1980). Alternatively, theophylline is an antagonist of the endogenous purine nucleotide, adenosine (Persson, 1982). Adenosine may potentiate histamine release from mast cells with resultant bronchoconstriction.

Clinical studies with enprofylline demonstrate greater potency than theophylline as a bronchodilator, with significantly less incidence of adverse effects (Lunnell et al., 1982). Concentration-dependent bronchodilation occurs in the range of 1-4 μg/ml. In several systems enprofylline has minimal adenosine antagonist potency (Persson et al., 1982) and this property may not be an important aspect of xanthine bronchodilating effects (Lunnell et al., 1983). One disadvantage of enprofylline is its rapid elimination half-life of 2 hr (Lunnell et al., 1984). With concentration-dependent beneficial effects, it would be necessary to administer it frequently or derive a controlled-release delivery system. Further clinical studies are necessary to establish adequate dosage regimens and characterize the incidence of adverse effects.

VI. Future Developments

Most asthmatic patients can be managed very effectively with theophylline. Dosage guidelines are selected from standard regimens with adjustments incorporated for conditions that affect theophylline elimination. For patients with an inadequate response, STCs are monitored and dosage adjustments individualized as needed.

A proportion of patients will not receive an adequate response with theophylline therapy. In some patients, addition of beta-adrenergic agonists, cromolyn, and corticosteroids may be necessary. Improved response to theophylline may be derived from future developments in the theophylline delivery system or the expansion of monitoring techniques to identify patients with unusual patterns of theophylline elimination or absorption.

A. Delivery Systems

With the identification of conditions affecting theophylline absorption, improvements in the delivery system may be possible. Basic features such as the appropriate times to administer medications and the conditions of administration, such as meals and volume of fluid, must be answered. While it may be possible to limit the effect of certain variables, such as pH, on the dissolution rate of the formulation, other variables affecting absorption, such as gastric emptying time and intestinal transit time, may be impossible to compensate for. In these circumstances, it may be useful to identify appropriate delivery systems for individual patients.

For some patients, formulations designed for once-daily dosing may be adequate. For other patients, these formulations might be contraindicated due to unacceptable variations in STC. Furthermore, it may not even be feasible to administer theophylline preparations intended for twice-daily administration in certain patients. Erratic absorption in these patients may result in unpredictable inconsistencies in STC, necessitating the use of rapidly absorbed preparations or alternative medications. Methods to identify these patients must be improved.

B. Monitoring Techniques

Routine monitoring is usually performed during the day and most often at times when clinical control is satisfactory. Since STC may change rapidly in certain patients due to rapid elimination combined with inconsistent absorption, the ready accessibility of sampling and analytical techniques could provide significant clinical information. This would be particularly useful for STC assessment at the time of respiratory distress or signs of potential adverse effects. It would be most convenient if the sample could be collected at home. The potential also to analyze the STC at home would offer even greater benefits.

Collection of blood samples with sufficient volume for standard techniques is extremely difficult and psychologically distressing for the family. An alternative that initially provided a significant benefit was measuring theophylline concentration in saliva samples (Levy et al., 1974). The original reports were very promising; however, subsequent studies were not supportive. Major criticisms centered around assay reliability. However, with the obvious need to obtain samples under the conditions described, this area merits reevaluation.

Another very attractive alternative is the development of new monitoring systems that will preclude the necessity for instrumental analysis. Promising techniques with adequate reliability are on the horizon to facilitate analysis of theophylline concentration from fingerstick blood samples (Zuk et al., 1985). The analysis does not require an instrument and the technique may be feasible for a patient or parent who has received basic instructions. The potential advantages of this system are numerous.

Great strides have been made in improving our ability to utilize theophylline in a safe and effective manner. Theophylline is indeed a model drug for understanding all medications: in many ways, the information derived from clinical observations and research with theophylline has improved our approach to clinical medicine, in general. This chapter has focused on the principles of pharmacology essential in understanding important aspects of individualized dosage regimens. While it is intended to focus on theophylline, it is anticipated that these same principles can be applied to other medications used in the treatment of respiratory disorders.

Acknowledgments

This work was supported in part by Grant HL-30513 from the National Heart, Lung and Blood Institutes. The secretarial assistance of Helga Cole is greatly appreciated.

References

Aranda, J. V., Sitar, D. S., Parsons, W. D., Loughnan, P. M., and Neims, A. H. (1976). Pharmacokinetic aspects of theophylline in premature newborns. *N. Engl. J. Med. 295*: 413-416.

Baird-Lambert, J., Doyle, P. E., Thomas, D., Jager-Roman, E., Cvejic, M., and Buchanan, N. (1984). Theophylline metabolism in preterm neonates during the first weeks of life. *Dev. Pharmacol. Ther. 7*: 239-244.

Bergstrand, H. (1980). Phosphodiesterase inhibition and theophylline. *Eur. J. Respir. Dis. 61*: 37-44.

Bukowskyj, M., Nakatsu, K., Munt, P. W. (1984). Theophylline reassessed. *Ann. Intern. Med. 101*: 63-73.

Bussey, H. I. (1981). Theophylline toxicity after dyphylline therapy. *Am. Rev. Respir. Dis. 124*: 504.

Caldwell, J., Lancaster, R., Monks, T. J., and Smith, R. L. (1977). The influence of dietary methylxanthines on the metabolism and pharmacokinetics of intravenously administered theophylline. *Br. J. Pharmacol. 4*: 637-638.

Dederich, R. A., Szefler, S. J., and Green, E. R. (1981). Intrasubject variation in sustained-release theophylline absorption. *J. Allergy Clin. Immunol. 67*: 465-471.

Ellis, E. F. (1978). Theophylline and derivatives. In *Allergy Principles and Practice.* Edited by E. Middleton, Jr., C. E. Reed, and E. F. Ellis. St. Louis, C. V. Mosby, pp. 434-453.

Ellis, E. F., Koysooko, R., and Levy, G. (1976). Pharmacokinetics of theophylline in children with asthma. *Pediatrics 58*: 542-547.

Gardner, M. J., Tornatore, K. M., Jusko, W. J., and Kanarkowski, R. (1983). Effects of tobacco smoking and oral contraceptive use on theophylline disposition. *Br. J. Clin. Pharmacol. 16*: 271-280.

Georgitis, J. W., Szefler, S. J., Baswell, B., and Shen, D. D. (1984). Use of pharmacokinetic profile in evaluating patients with repeatedly low theophylline concentrations. *Ann. Allergy 53*: 231-235.

Giacoia, G., Jusko, W. J., Menke, J., and Koup, J. R. (1976). Theophylline pharmacokinetics in premature infants with apnea. *J. Pediatr. 89*: 829-832.

Gibaldi, M., and Perrier, D. (1975). Multicompartmental models. In *Pharmacokinetics.* New York, Marcel-Dekker, p. 54.

Ginchansky, E., and Weinberger, M. (1977). Relationship of theophylline clearance to oral dosage in children with chronic asthma. *J. Pediatr. 91*: 655-660.

Haltom, J. R., and Szefler, S. J. (1985). Theophylline absorption in young asthmatic children receiving sustained-release formulations. *J. Pediatr. 107*: 805-814, 1985.

Hendeles, L., and Weinberger, M. (1983). Theophylline: A "state of the art" review. *Pharmacotherapy 3*: 2-44.

Hendeles, L., Iafrate, R. P., and Weinberger, M. (1984). A clinical and pharmacokinetic basis for the selection and use of slow release theophylline products. *Clin. Pharmacokinet. 9*: 95-135.

Hendeles, L., Weinberger, M., Milavetz, G., Hill, M., and Vaughan, L. (1985). Food-induced "dose-dumping" from a once-a-day theophylline product as a cause of theophylline toxicity. *Chest 87*: 758-765.

Hirtz, J. (1984). The absorption window: Fact or fiction? *Pharm. Int. 7*: 175-178.

Hudson, L. D., Tyler, M. L., and Petty, T. L. (1973). Oral aminophylline and dihydroxypropyl theophylline in reversible obstructive airway disease: A single-dose, double-blind, crossover comparison. *Curr. Ther. Res. 15*: 367-372.

Jenne, J. W., Wyze, E., Rood, F. S., and MacDonald, F. M. (1972). Pharmacokinetics of theophylline: Application to adjustment of the clinical dose of aminophylline. *Clin. Pharmacol. Ther. 13*: 349-360.

Jenne, J. W., Nagasawa, H. T., and Thompson, R. D. (1976). Relationship of urinary metabolites of theophylline to serum theophylline levels. *Clin. Pharmacol. Ther. 19*: 375-381.

Jenne, J. W., Chick, T. W., Miller, B. A., and Strickland, R. D. (1977). Apparent theophylline half-life fluctuations during treatment of acute left ventricular failure. *Am. J. Hosp. Pharm. 34*: 408-409.

Jonkman, J. H. G., and Upton, R. A. (1984). Pharmacokinetic drug interactions with theophylline. *Clin. Pharmacokinet. 9*: 309-334.

Jusko, W. J., Schentag, J. J., Clark, J. H., Gardner, M., and Yurchak, A. M. (1978). Enhanced biotransformation of theophylline in marihuana and tobacco smokers. *Clin. Pharmacol. Ther. 24*: 406-410.

Jusko, W. J., Gardner, M. J., Mangione, A., Schentag, J. J., Koup, J. R., and Vance, J. W. (1979). Factors affecting theophylline clearances: Age, tobacco, marijuana, cirrhosis, congestive heart failure, obesity, oral contraceptives, benzodiazepines, barbiturates, and ethanol. *J. Pharm. Sci. 68*: 1358-1366.

Kappas, A., Anderson, K. E., Conney, A. H., and Alvares, A. P. (1976). Influence of dietary protein and carbohydrate on antipyrine and theophylline metabolism in man. *Clin. Pharmacol. Ther. 20*: 643-653.

Kappas, A., Alvares, A. P., Anderson, K. E., Pantuck, E. J., Pantuck, C. B., Chang, R., and Conney, A. H. (1978). Effect of charcoal-broiled beef on antipyrine and theophylline metabolism. *Clin. Pharmacol. Ther. 23*: 445-450.

Karim, A., Burns, T., Wearley, L., Streicher, J., and Palmer, M. (1985). Food-induced changes in theophylline absorption from controlled-release formulations. Part I. Substantial increased and decreased absorption with Uniphyl tablets and Theo-Dur Sprinkle. *Clin. Pharmacol. Ther. 38*: 77-83.

Kelly, H. W., and Murphy, S. (1979). Serum theophylline levels in asthmatic children receiving sustained-release theophylline tablets. *Am. J. Hosp. Pharm. 36*: 1698-1701.

Kelly, H. W., and Murphy, S. (1980). Efficacy of a 12-hour sustained-release preparation in maintaining therapeutic serum theophylline levels in asthmatic children. *Pediatrics 66*: 97-102.

LaForce, C. F., Miller, M. F., and Chai, H. (1981). Effect of erythromycin on theophylline clearance in asthmatic children. *J. Pediatr. 99*: 153-156.

Lagas, M., and Jonkman, J. H. G. (1983). Greatly enhanced bioavailability of theophylline on postprandial administration of a sustained release tablet. *Eur. J. Clin. Pharmacol. 24*: 761-767.

Landay, R. A., Gonzalez, M. A., and Taylor, J. C. (1978). Effect of phenobarbital on theophylline disposition. *J. Allergy Clin. Immunol. 62*: 27-29.

Lee, C. C., Wang, L. H., Majeske, B. L., and Marbury, T. C. (1981). Pharmacokinetics of dyphylline elimination by uremic patients. *J. Pharmacol. Exp. Ther. 217*: 340-344.

Leeds, N. H., Gal, P., Purohit, A. A., and Walter, J. B. (1982). Effect of food on the bioavailability and pattern of release of a sustained-release theophylline tablet. *J. Clin. Pharmacol. 22*: 196-200.

Lesko, L. J. (1979). Dose-dependent elimination kinetics of theophylline. *Clin. Pharmacokinet. 4*: 449-459.

Leung, P., Kalisker, A., and Bell, T. D. (1977). Variation in theophylline clearance rate with time in chronic childhood asthma. *J. Allergy Clin. Immunol. 59*: 440-444.

Levy, G., and Koysooko, R. (1976). Renal clearance of theophylline in man. *J. Clin. Pharmacol. 16*: 329-335.

Levy, G., Ellis, E. F., and Koysooko, R. (1974). Indirect plasma-theophylline monitoring in asthmatic children by determination of theophylline concentration in saliva. *Pediatrics 53*: 873-876.

Loughnan, P. M., Sitar, D. S., Ogilvie, R. I., Eisen, A., Fox, Z., and Neims, A. H. (1976). Pharmacokinetic analysis of the disposition of intravenous theophylline in young children. *J. Pediatr. 88*: 874-879.

Lunell, E., Svedmyr, N., Andersson, K. E., and Persson, C. G. A. (1982). Effects of enprofylline, a xanthine lacking adenosine receptor antagonism, in patients with chronic obstructive lung disease. *Eur. J. Clin. Pharmacol. 22*: 395-402.

Lunell, E., Svedmyr, N., Andersson, K. E., and Persson, C. G. A. (1983). A novel bronchodilator xanthine apparently without adenosine receptor antagonism and tremorogenic effect. *Eur. J. Respir. Dis. 64*: 333-339.

Lunell, E., Andersson, K. E., Persson, C. G. A., and Svedmyr, N. (1984). Intravenous enprofylline in asthma patients. *Eur. J. Respir. Dis. 65*: 28-34.

Mangione, A., Imhoff, T. E., Lee, R. V., Shum, L. Y., and Jusko, W. J. (1978). Pharmacokinetics of theophylline in hepatic disease. *Chest. 73*: 616-622.

Marquis, J. F., Carruthers, S. G., Spence, J. D., Brownstone, Y. S., and Toogood, J. H. (1982). Phenytoin-theophylline interaction. *N. Engl. J. Med. 307*: 1189-1190.

May, C. D. (1974). History of the introduction of theophylline into the treatment of asthma. *Clin. Allergy 4*: 211-217.

Minami, H., and McCallum, R. W. (1984). The physiology and pathophysiology of gastric emptying in humans. *Gastroenterology 86*: 1592-1610.

Mitenko, P. A., and Ogilvie, R. I. (1973). Rational intravenous doses of theophylline. *N. Engl. J. Med. 289*: 600-603.

Nassif, E. G., Weinberger, M. M., Shannon, D., Guiang, S. F., Hendeles, L., Jiminez, D., and Ekwo, E. (1981). Theophylline disposition in infancy. *J. Pediatr. 98*: 158-161.

Nimmo, W. S. (1976). Drugs, diseases and altered gastric emptying. *Clin. Pharmacokinet. 1*: 189-203.

Pedersen, S. (1981). Delay in the absorption rate of theophylline from a sustained release theophylline preparation caused by food. *Br. J. Clin. Pharmacol. 12*: 904-905.

Pedersen, S. (1984). Food and fasting intake of sustained-release theophylline preparations. *Br. J. Clin. Pract. 38* (Suppl. 35): 37-39.

Pedersen, S., and Moller-Petersen, J. (1984). Erratic absorption of a slow-release theophylline sprinkle product. *Pediatr. 74*: 534-538.

Pedersen, S., and Moller-Petersen, J. (1985). Influence of food on the absorption of theophylline from a sustained-release formulation (Somophyllin). *Clin. Allergy 15*: 253-259.

Persson, C. G. A. (1982). Xanthines for asthma—present status. *Trends Pharmacol. Sci. 3*: 312-313.

Persson, C. G. A., Karlsson, J. A., and Erjefölt, I. (1982). Differentiation between bronchodilation and universal adenosine antagonism among xanthine derivatives. *Life Sci. 30*: 2181-2189.

Piafsky, K. M., Sitar, D. S., and Ogilvie, R. I. (1977a). Effect of phenobarbital on the disposition of intravenous theophylline. *Clin. Pharmacol. Ther. 22*: 336-339.

Piafsky, K. M., Sitar, D. S., Rangno, R. E., and Ogilvie, R. I. (1977b). Theophylline kinetics in acute pulmonary edema. *Clin. Pharmacol. Ther. 21*: 310-316.

Pollack, G. M., Baswell, B., Szefler, S. J., and Shen, D. D. (1984). Comparison of inter- and intra-subject variation in oral absorption of theophylline from sustained-release products. *Int. J. Pharmaceut. 21*: 3-16.

Powell, J. R., Theircelin, J. F., Vozeh, S., Sansom, L., and Riegelman, S. (1977). The influence of cigarette smoking and sex on theophylline disposition. *Am. Rev. Respir. Dis. 116*: 17-23.

Powell, J. R., Vozeh, S., Hopewell, P., Costello, J., Sheiner, L. B., and Riegelman, S. (1978). Theophylline disposition in acutely ill hospitalized patients. *Am. Rev. Respir. Dis. 118*: 229-238.

Prince, R. A., Wing, D. S., Weinberger, M. M., Hendeles, L. S., and Riegelman, S. (1981). Effect of erythromycin on theophylline kinetics. *J. Allergy Clin. Immunol. 68*: 427-431.

Rasmussen, F. V., Waldorff, S., and Madsen, L. (1984). Pharmacokinetics and bronchodilatory effect of proxyphylline and theophylline. *Eur. J. Respir. Dis. 65*: 20-27.

Reitberg, D. P., Bernhard, H., and Schentag, J. J. (1981). Alteration of theophylline clearance and half-life by cimetidine in normal volunteers. *Ann. Intern. Med. 95*: 582-585.

Richer, C., Mathieu, M., Bah, H., Thuillez, C., Duroux, P., and Giudicelli, J-F. (1982). Theophylline kinetics and ventilatory flow in bronchial asthma and chronic airflow obstruction: Influence of erythromycin. *Clin. Pharmacol. Ther. 31*: 579-586.

Rogers, R. J., Kalisker, A., Wiener, M. B., and Szefler, S. J. (1985). Inconsistent absorption from a sustained-release theophylline preparation during continuous therapy in asthmatic children. *J. Pediatr. 106*: 496-501.

Rosenberry, K. R., Defusco, C. J., Mansmann, H. C., and McGeady, S. J. (1983). Reduced theophylline half-life by carbamazepine therapy. *J. Pediatr. 102*: 472-474.

Scott, P. H., Tabachnik, E., Mac Leod, S., Correia, J., Newth, C., and Levison, H. (1981). Sustained-release theophylline for childhood asthma: Evidence for circadian variation of theophylline pharmacokinetics. *J. Pediatr. 99*: 476-479.

Selvig, K. (1981). Pharmacokinetics of proxyphylline in adults after intravenous and oral administration. *Eur. J. Clin. Pharmacol. 19*: 149-155.

Simons, K. J., and Simons, F. E. R. (1979). Urinary excretion of dyphylline in humans. *J. Pharm. Sci. 68*: 1327-1328.

Simons, F. E. R., Simons, K. J., and Bierman, C. W. (1975). The pharmacokinetics of dihydroxypropyltheophylline: A basis for rational therapy. *J. Allergy Clin. Immunol. 56*: 347-355.

Simons, K. J., Simons, F. E. R., and Bierman, C. W. (1977). Bioavailability of a sustained-release dyphylline formulation. *J. Clin. Pharmacol. 4*: 237-242.

Szefler, S. J. (1985). Theophylline and its fickle unpredictability of absorption. *Ann. Allergy 55*: 580-583.

Taylor, D. R., Duffin, D., Kinney, C. D., and McDevitt, D. G. (1983). Investigation of diurnal changes in the disposition of theophylline. *Br. J. Clin. Pharmac. 16*: 413-416.

Taylor, D. R., Duffin, D., Kinney, C. D., and McDevitt, D. G. (1984). Circadian variation in plasma theophylline concentrations during maintenance therapy with a sustained-release preparation in patients with obstructive airways disease. *Br. J. Clin. Pharmacol. 18*: 27-30.

Thompson, P. J., Skypala, I., Dawson, S., McAllister, W. A. C., and Turner Warwick, M. (1983). The effect of diet upon serum concentrations of theophylline. *Br. J. Clin. Pharmacol. 16*: 267-270.

Toothaker, R. D., and Welling, P. G. (1980). The effect of food on drug bioavailability. *Annu. Rev. Pharmacol. Toxicol. 20*: 173-199.

Upton, R. A., Thiercelin, J-F., Guentert, T. W., Wallace, S. M., Powell, J. R., Sansom, L., and Riegelman, S. (1982). Intraindividual variability in theophylline pharmacokinetics: Statistical verification in 39 of 60 healthy young adults. *J. Pharmacokinet. Biopharm. 10*: 123-134.

Vestel, R. E., Thummel, K. E., Musser, B., and Mercer, C. D. (1983). Cimetidine inhibits theophylline clearance in patients with chronic obstruction pulmonary disease: a study using stable isotope methodology during multiple dose administration. *Br. J. Clin. Pharmacol. 15*: 411-418.

Wagner, J. G. (1983). Modified Wagner-Nelson absorption equations for multiple-dose regimens. *J. Pharm. Sci. 72*: 578-579.

Wagner, J. G. (1984). Estimation of drug absorption kinetics with emphasis on theophylline. In *Sustained-Release Theophylline in the Treatment of CRAO.* Edited by J. H. G. Jonkman, J. W. Jenne, and F. E. R. Simons. Amsterdam, Excerpta Medica, pp. 113-120.

Wagner, J. G., and Nelson, E. (1963). Per cent absorbed time plots derived from blood level and/or urinary excretion data. *J. Pharm. Sci. 52*: 610-611.

Walson, P. D., Strunk, R. C., and Taussig, L. M. (1977). Intrapatient variability in theophylline kinetics. *J. Pediatr. 91*: 321-324.

Warren, J. B., Cuss, F., and Barnes, P. J. (1985). Posture and theophylline kinetics. *Br. J. Clin. Pharmacol. 19*: 707-709.

Weinberger, M. (1984). The pharmacology and therapeutic use of theophylline. *J. Allergy Clin. Immunol. 73*: 525-540.

Weinberger, M., and Ginchansky, E. (1977). Dose-dependent kinetics of theophylline disposition in asthmatic children. *J. Pediatr. 91*: 820-824.

Weinberger, M., Hudgel, D., Spector, S., and Chidsey, C. (1977). Inhibition of theophylline clearance by troleandomycin. *J. Allergy Clin. Immunol. 59*: 228-231.

Zarowitz, B. J. M., Szefler, S. J., and Lasezkay, G. M. (1981). Effect of erythromycin base on theophylline kinetics. *Clin. Pharmacol. Ther. 29*: 601-605.

Zuidema, J., and Merkus, F. W. H. M. (1979). Chemical and biopharmaceutical aspects of theophylline and its derivatives. *Curr. Med. Res. Opin.* 6(Suppl. 6): 14-25.

Zuk, R. F., Ginsberg, V. K., Houts, T., Rabbie, J., Merrick, H., Ullman, E. F., Fischer, M. M., Sizto, C. C., Stiso, S. N., and Litman, D. J. (1985). Enzyme immunochromatography—a quantitative immunoassay requiring no instrumentation. *Clin. Chem. 31*: 1144-1150.

11

Aerosol Dynamics and Delivery Systems

ARCHIE WILSON

University of California Irvine Medical Center
Orange, California

I. General Principles

Aerosols are airborne suspensions of fine particles. The particles may be liquids or solids. By their nature, aerosols are unstable; they tend to settle (sedimentation), adhere to each other (coagulation), and adhere to structures such as tubing and mucosa (deposition). The bronchodilator activity of therapeutic aerosols is determined by not only their pharmacologic properties but also the pattern of distribution of their deposition in the airways. The airway deposition of inhaled aerosols is affected by the physical properties of the aerosols and the technique of inhalation utilized. Aerosols may be generated by a number of devices. The physical properties of aerosols are, in large part, controlled by the use and operating characteristics of the generating devices. These and other related subjects will be discussed in some detail in this chapter.

Aerosol particles may be all virtually the same size (monodispersed) or they may vary considerably in size (poly- or heterodispersed). It is convenient to characterize aerosol particles on the basis of their aerodynamic behavior (Mercer, 1973; Morrow, 1974; Lourenco and Cotromanes, 1982; Swift, 1985), defined as mass median aerodynamic diameter (MMAD). A particle with MMAD of 1 μm

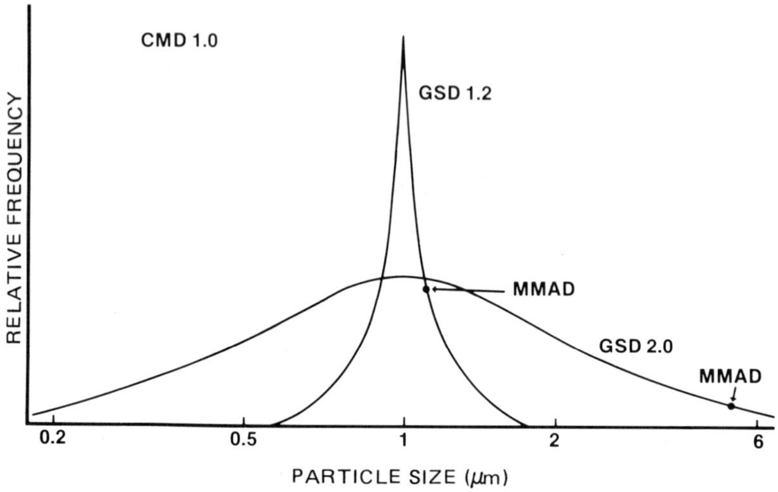

Figure 1 Frequency distribution of two aerosols with CMD of 1.0 and GSD of 1.20 and 2.00. Note that the curve is symmetrical only when frequency is plotted against the logarithm of particle diameter. Also note the marked effect of GSD on MMAD (for GSD 1.20, MMAD is 1.10 and for GSD 2.0, MMAD is 4.23 μm).

has the same rate of settling as a droplet of unit density and 1 μm diameter. Because therapeutic aerosols are almost always quite heterodisperse and have a distribution of particle sizes skewed towards larger particles, aerosol distribution is best described by a log normal distribution. Log normal distribution is related to the familiar gaussian distribution by the use of the natural logarithm of the standard deviation, that is, the geometric standard deviation (GSD) (Fig. 1), to quantify the dispersion of particles around the mean. Particle ranges are described by a predictable relationship between GSD and count median diameter (CMD), which is that size at which half of particles are larger and half smaller; CMD is identical to geometric mean diameter. Ninety-five percent of particles lie between the limits of the antilogs of ln CMD - 2 ln GSD and ln CMD + 2 ln GSD. Since ln 1 = 0, it should be understood that GSD of 1 represents perfectly monodisperse particles. Larger values of GSD are associated with more heterodispersion. Usually, GSD of 1.22 or less is considered functionally monodisperse. The relationship between CMD, GSD, and range of particle sizes is shown in Figure 1 and Table 1. Note not only the increasingly large effects of increments of GSD upon skewness, but also the effect of GSD upon total range (heterodispersion). The implications of this large degree of heterodispersion will

Table 1 Aerosol Size Characteristics (μM)

CMD	GSD	Range (67% Particles)	Range (95% Particles)	MMAD
1	1	1	1	1
1	1.2	0.83-1.2	0.69-1.44	1.10
1	1.4	0.71-1.4	0.51-1.96	1.40
1	1.6	0.63-1.6	0.39-2.56	1.94
1	1.8	0.56-1.8	0.31-3.24	2.82
1	2	0.6-2	0.25-4	4.23
1	2.2	0.45-2.2	0.21-4.84	6.46
1	2.4	0.42-2.4	0.17-5.76	9.97
1	2.6	0.38-2.6	0.15-6.76	15.47
1	2.8	0.36-2.8	0.13-7.84	24.06
2	1	2	2	2
2	1.2	1.67-2.4	1.39-2.88	2.21
2	1.6	1.25-3.2	0.78-5.12	3.38
2	2	1-4	0.5-8	8.45
2	2.4	0.83-4.8	0.34-11.52	19.94
2	2.8	0.71-5.6	0.26-15.68	48.11
4	1.2	3.33-4.8	2.78-5.76	4.47
4	2.	2-8	1-16	16.91
4	2.8	1.43-0.96	0.51-31.36	96.22

CMD, count median diameter; GSD, geometric standard deviation; MMAD, mass median aerodynamic diameter.

become more evident when airway deposition and physiological response are discussed below.

MMAD is accurately estimated from log normal distributions of particles by the equation:

$$\ln \text{MMAD} = \ln \text{CMD} + 3 \ln^2 \text{GSD}$$

Because mass is equal to volume multiplied by density and volume is equal to the cube of diameter multipled by $\pi/6$, mass and volume are heavily affected by the presence of large particles. For instance, in Table 1, note that for particles with CMD of 1 μm and GSD varying from 1 to 2.8, MMAD increases drastically with larger values of GSD. For CMD of 1 μm and GSD of 2, 95% of particles are in the range of 0.25-4 μm; however, MMAD of these particles is 4.23 μm, indicating that the combined weight of the about 96% of particles less than 4.23 μm is equal to the combined weight of the approximately 4% of particles greater than 4.23 μm. At even larger values of GSD, the effect is even more pronounced. Again, the implications of these facts will become clearer in later sections. As can also be seen from Table 1, while the effect of increasing GSD is profound and alinear upon range of particle size and MMAD, the effect of increasing CMD is one of simple multiplication; doubling CMD doubles both the range limits and MMAD.

Particle size may be affected by evaporation of liquids such as water, ethanol, or chlorofluorocarbons (freons, propellants) from particle surface or by uptake of water by hygroscopic aerosols. Such dynamic changes in particle size are particularly prevalent with therapeutic aerosols.

II. Aerosol Generation

Therapeutic aerosols are commonly produced by atomization of liquids within jet nebulizers or by rapid vibration of a standing pool of liquid (ultrasonic nebulization). Other forms of administration of therapeutic aerosols use preformed aerosols. Examples of the latter include metered-dose inhalers and powder dispensers. For experimental purposes, a number of monodisperse generators, such as the spinning top, have been utilized; these research tools will not be discussed further here.

A. Jet Nebulizer

All jet nebulizers have a similar design, represented by the familiar perfume atomizer (Fig. 2). A liquid is placed in the bottom of a closed container. A small tube extends from near the bottom of the container (in the liquid) to above the surface of the liquid. A stream of air is passed through another tube placed near the upper opening of the liquid feed tube, thereby drawing liquid upward by the Bernoulli effect. The resulting column of updrawn liquid is spread into a sheet by the airstream and scatters into particles of many sizes. Larger particles are collected on baffles or the walls of the container and drain back into the liquid reservoir for recycling. Smaller particles continue with the airstream and escape from the nebulizer as potentially usable aerosol. In some devices, depending upon the baffling, as much as 99.9% of the aerosol is recycled and, hence, only a small fraction of the aerosolized liquid escapes. Of course, with time, much of the liquid leaves the nebulizer container and becomes potentially usable aerosol.

Several operating characteristics of jet nebulizers limit the total amount of liquid aerosolized (Mercer et al., 1968; Ferron et al., 1976; Lewis et al., 1981; Clay et al., 1983a,b; Lewis, 1984). First, because of evaporation from particles

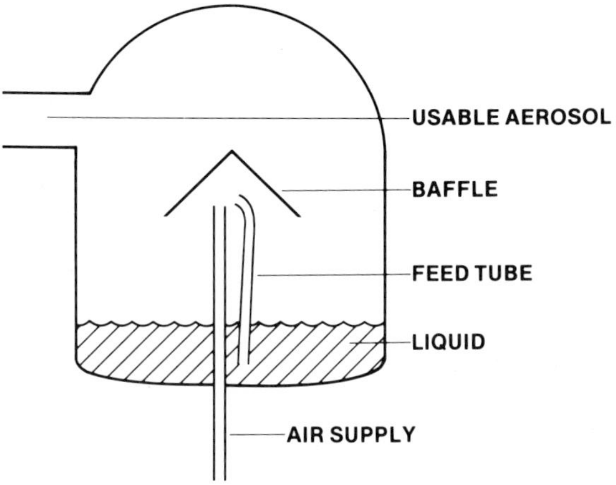

Figure 2 Schematic representation of a jet nebulizer. Aerosol output is dependent upon not only design but also fill volume and airflow rate.

within the nebulizer container and the constant recycling, the solid content of the liquid in the reservoir slowly increases, that is, the solution becomes more concentrated. Second, because there is, at any time, a large quantity of liquid adhering to the walls of the nebulizer container, nebulization may sputter and stop with a significant quantity of concentrated solution still remaining on the container walls. Estimates of adherent fluid range up to 65% of the original medication depending upon nebulizer design and volume fill (Clay et al., 1983a; Lewis, 1984). In one study, increasing volume fill in four different types of commercial nebulizers from 2 to 6 ml increased the amount nebulized from a mean of about 45 to 72% of the original volume (Clay et al., 1983a). Of course, duration of nebulization will increase with larger fill volume. In the study just cited, 2 ml fill volumes were associated with approximately 4 min duration of nebulization while 6 ml fills required about 15 min. The great increase in duration associated with the larger volume was primarily caused by the increase in volume of nebulized liquid; with a 2 ml fill, only about 0.9 ml was nebulized, while with a 6 ml fill about 4.3 ml was nebulized (an increase of 4.8 times). It should also be recognized that the nebulization rate begins to decline when the driving liquid reservoir has been reduced to about 2 ml; at this volume, nebulization rate decreased from about 0.4 mg/min to much lower values. Incidentally, this study (Clay et al., 1983a) indicated that 4 and 6 ml fills had similar emptying efficiencies and that the duration of nebulization was 10 min with the 4 ml fill (vs. 15 min for the 6 ml fill). Tapping the nebulizer will often cause droplets to fall from the container walls into the reservoir and can speed up or reinstitute nebulization when it has slowed down or stopped (Lewis, 1984).

Nebulizers progressively cool, dropping 8-12°C, during operation (Mercer et al., 1968; Clay et al., 1983a; Lewis, 1984). This cooling is due to the evaporation of liquid from the particle surfaces. Whether this phenomenon has much clinical significance, such as the production of bronchospasm, is not clear (Lewis, 1984); however, if such an effect occurs, it is seen only in a small subgroup of patients. With increasing air flow rates, the rate of nebulization increases, decreasing the time for apparent emptying of the nebulizer reservoir (Mercer et al., 1968; Clay et al., 1983; Lewis, 1984). Increasing air flow rates also decreases the size of the aerosol particles; in several commercial nebulizers, MMAD decreased from 4.5 to 12 μm at 4 liters/min to 2-4 μm at 8 liters/min. (Clay et al., 1983a). It is interesting that GSD increased as MMAD became smaller; at 4 μm MMAD, GSD was about 2; at lower values of MMAD, GSD is much greater. Hence, from Table 1 it is evident that CMD must be much less than 1 μm with MMAD of 4 μm and GSD of 2 for these nebulizers.

From the published data, it is also clear that the output of nebulizers is greatly affected not only by design, fill volume, and airflow rate but also by several other factors such as environmental temperature and presence of organic materials in the reservoir (Davis, and Bubb, 1978); these other factors will not be discussed further here. All parameters of the variables noted above should be specified when nebulizers are utilized in studies. Jet nebulizers continue to operate during expiration, hence a major fraction of the generated aerosol can be lost. This potential problem can be overcome by placing a large hole in the driving airstream tube, which will shunt the air from the nebulizer, except when it is covered by a thumb during inspiration. Similarly, intermittent positive pressure breathing devices (IPPB) nebulize only during inspiration. However, neither of these devices is clinically more efficacious than the continuously operating nebulizer (Chang and Levison, 1972; Shenfield et al., 1974; Webber et al., 1974). It is also unknown what effect intermittent nebulization has upon the size characteristics of the generated aerosol.

B. Ultrasonic Nebulizers

Ultrasonic nebulizers produce aerosol by vibrating liquid lying above a transducer at speeds of about 1 mHz (1,000 Hz = 1,000 cycles/sec) (Mercer, 1973; Lourenco and Cotromanes, 1982; Swift, 1985). This produces a cloud of particles that is carried out of the device to the patient by a stream of air; greater aerosol output can be accomplished by higher frequencies. A limit is reached at about 5 mHz; at that frequency water begins to boil (Swift, 1985). The MMAD and GSD do not seem to change much as frequencies are changed in ultrasonic nebulizers. Greater airflow causes greater aerosol output. Higher airflow will also cause more rapid solvent evaporation and, hence, more concentration of liquid in the nebulizer reservoir. Aerosol produced by ultrasonic nebulizers is heterodisperse, with MMAD values varying from 1 to 10 μm depending upon operating conditions (Mercer, 1973; Lourenco and Cotromanes, 1982; Swift, 1985).

Ultrasonic nebulizers have not been extensively used for delivery of bronchodilators. Presumably, this relative lack of use is due to the fact that the reservoir chamber of ultrasonic nebulizers usually must contain at least 10 ml for atomization to be continuous. This type of nebulizer also is capable of very high aerosol output. Because of the high water content of ultrasonic nebulizer, it is important to avoid the use of hypotonic solutions, particularly in asthmatics, to prevent development of bronchospasm (Cheney and Butler, 1968).

In summary, it is clear that aerosols varying in quantity, size, and distribution may be produced by nebulizers depending upon the latter's design and how they are operated.

C. Metered-Dose Inhalers

Metered-dose inhalers (MDI), because of their convenience and effectiveness, are probably the most widely used form of therapeutic aerosol administration, particularly for outpatients. In many countries they are also the mainstay of asthma treatment (Paterson et al., 1979).

Metered-dose inhalers are of two types: (1) suspension aerosols, in which the drug is suspended in the propellant, and (2) solution aerosols, in which the drug is dissolved in the propellants and a cosolvent such as ethanol. Most MDI in current use are of the suspension aerosol type (Weiner, 1958; Hayton, 1976; Moren, 1985).

There are two major components of MDI (Fig. 3): the canister: a closed plastic or metal cylinder that contains propellant, active medication, and the metering chamber; and the actuator: a molded plastic container that holds the canister and directs the released aerosol towards the patient's airways.

The propellants usually consist of three constituents, all chlorofluorocarbons, usually, freons 11, 12, and 114. The pressure inside the canister depends upon the exact mixture and amounts of propellants utilized. The resulting pressure within the canister is usually 3-4 atm. Finely divided particles of drug usually less than 1 μm are suspended in the pressurized (liquified) propellant (Weiner, 1958; Hayton, 1976; Moren, 1985). To prevent the drug particles from coagulating, a surface active agent such as sorbitan oleate, lecithin, or oleic acid is added; the amount of added surfactant is often quite large and may account for much of the taste of aerosols administered by MDI (Moren, 1985).

Metering chambers ordinarily contain 25-100 μl. The contents of the metering chamber are released when the canister is depressed into the actuator. Almost instantaneously, the propellants begin to evaporate, producing disintegration of the discharged liquid into myriad particles that are propelled forward

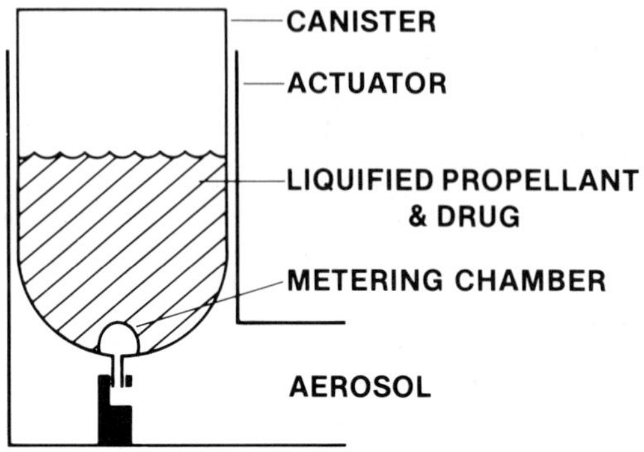

Figure 3 Schematic representation of a pressurized metered-dose inhaler (MDI).

with great momentum. The initial MMAD has been estimated to be about 45 μm and the initial velocity of the particles as close to 100 mph. Particle velocity quickly reduces because of air resistance but still is estimated to be about 25 mph at 4-5 inches from the actuator. At this distance, MMAD has been reduced, because of continued propellant evaporation from the particle surface, to about 12 μm (Newman and Pavia, 1985). The reader can easily confirm, by actuating an MDI and viewing the resultant aerosol against a dark background with side lighting, that the aerosol cloud extends at least 10 inches beyond the MDI. At greater distances and after more time, particle size is reduced to an MMAD of 2.8-5.5 μm and a GSD of 1.5-2.3, depending upon the MDI and the technique used in measuring particle size (Newman and Pavia, 1985; Hiller et al., 1980a). The size of the particles after evaporation of the propellant is complete is determined by the number and size of bronchodilator submicronic particles plus surfactant (the solid content) originally suspended in the propellant incorporated into the initial particles formed at the actuator orifice. It is evident from GSD values as high as 2.3 in the evaporated particles that quantities of bronchodilators and surfactant vary considerably in the particles initially formed; the CMD of the final particles is near 1 μm (Table 1).

There has been concern that propellants are potentially toxic and may cause cardiac arrhythmias. Careful investigation has indicated that propellants are not toxic to humans when MDI are used appropriately (Stewart et al., 1978; Thiessen and Pedersen, 1980).

In solution aerosols, bronchodilator substance is dissolved; solution is accomplished by cosolvents, such as ethanol, and use of more soluble salts of the bronchodilators, such as the hydrochlorides (Moren, 1985). Obviously, no surfactant is necessary in solution aerosols. Particle formation is similar: when the contents of the metering chamber are released, rapid evaporation of propellant (flashing) takes place and particles are simultaneously formed and propelled forward. It is thought that because of the presence of cosolvent, evaporation is retarded and particles stay larger longer. Additionally, ethanol may be irritating to mucosa. Because of their nature, solution aerosols do not require shaking prior to use. However, dissolved bronchodilators are probably less chemically stable than small suspended particles and may deteriorate more rapidly (Moren, 1985).

Certain bronchodilators, such as sympathomimetics, are hygroscopic; other antiasthma drugs, such as steroids and cromolyn, are not particularly hygroscopic. When hygroscopic particles enter the humid atmosphere of the airway they may absorb great quantities of water and increase their volume severalfold (Scherer et al., 1979; Hiller et al., 1980b; Brain et al., 1985). However, it should be noted that the potential swelling of the hygroscopic particles will be retarded by the presence of nonhygroscopic substances on the particle surfaces such as cosolvents and propellants (Moren, 1985). However, in one study in an humid atmosphere, MMAD increased 5.7-11.4 times for liquid-based MDI aerosols and 1.6-3.1 times for suspension aerosols (Hiller et al., 1980). Hence, it is difficult to predict how much swelling will occur in inhaled sympathomimetic particles during passage through the airways.

As discussed below, airway deposition of MDI bronchodilator aerosols is much more dependent upon how they are inhaled than is the case with nebulized bronchodilators. In some cases, special inhalation aids are required to ensure adequate airway deposition of MDI bronchodilator.

D. Powder Inhalers

Powder inhalers have been devised for the inhalation of insoluble materials required in quantities of 1 mg or greater, such as cromolyn (20 mg). In contrast, MDI typically delivers single doses in the range of tenths of a milligram. Another use of powder inhalers is to deliver agents usually placed in MDI, such as sympathomimetics and corticosteroids, to patients who have difficulty in properly using an MDI.

The successful use of powder inhalers requires attention to several technical problems such as ease of handling, quantification of dosage, means of delivery, and prevention of coagulation (Moren, 1985). In general, in most systems, the appropriate dosage is placed in a capsule along with a flow aid or filler such as large lactose or glucose particles. Inside the device, the capsule is initially either pierced by needles (Spinhaler) (Bell et al., 1971) or sheared in half (Rotohaler). During inhalation the capsule rotates or a propeller is turned, creating conditions that cause the contents of capsule to enter the inspired air and be broken up into small particles suitable for airway deposition. The minimum airflow required for successful aerosol inhalation with the Spinhaler is 35 liters/

min (Moren, 1985). The Spinhaler has primarily been used for inhalation of cromolyn. The Rotohaler has been used with both corticosteroids and sympathomimetics.

Direct comparisons between Rotohaler and MDI have been made for sympathomimetics. The dosages required for similar therapeutic response are either the same or twice as much drug as required with Rotohaler (Hetzel and Clark, 1977; Svedmyr et al., 1982). Powder inhaler devices are clearly much more difficult to prepare for use, but many patients still prefer these devices because coordination between inhalation and drug release is automatic, while with MDI this can be accomplished only with careful use. Powder inhalers may be very useful particularly for small children and some adults. Potential problems associated with powder inhalers include irritation and consequent cough due to direct effect of powder on airways; and coating of the walls of the capsule with drug with consequent nonrelease of drug or failure of the aggregated powder to break up, leading to deposition of virtually all drug in the mouth.

III. Airway Deposition of Aerosol

Bronchodilator aerosols are effective only when they deposit on airways. Though there is some absorption of drug from mucosa, the slowness of the rate and the small amounts of drug released during actuation of MDI indicate clearly that the major therapeutic response to inhaled drugs is not due to mucosal absorption of drug (Paterson et al., 1979; Pauwels, 1985). Sympathomimetics have been placed onto the buccal mucosa and the response compared to similar amounts inhaled from MDI; there was much less response from direct buccal mucosa application compared to MDI inhalation (Ruffin et al., 1978; Rodenstein and Stanescu, 1982). Blood levels of sympathomimetics have been measured following inhalation: there is usually an early blood level, presumably associated with alveolar and mucosal absorption, followed by a larger blood level appearing up to 5 hr later (Paterson et al., 1979; Pauwels, 1985; Walker et al., 1972; Laros et al., 1977; Davies, 1982). This latter peak is probably due to gastrointestinal absorption, since it can be blocked with activated charcoal ingestion (Davies, 1982). The blood levels following inhalation are much lower than the blood levels associated with equipotent but much larger (20-30 times) oral doses of the same drug. Not surprisingly, the systemic side effects of inhaled drugs are proportionally lower than those of the same drugs administered orally in larger amounts (Larsson and Svedmyr, 1977).

Several general principles apply to airway deposition of aerosols (Table 2). In general, particles should be smaller than 10 μm, and possibly smaller than 5 μm, but larger than 0.5 μm, if they are not hygroscopic (Morrow, 1974; Newman et al., 1985; Brain et al., 1985; Rees and Clark, 1982). Aerosols should be

Table 2 Principles of Aerosol Deposition

The nose efficiently traps particles; hence mouth breathing of aerosol is preferred.
Large particles (> 10 μm) are not inhaled beyond the upper airway. Very small particles (< 0.5 μm) tend to behave like gases and may be exhaled.
Rapid inspiratory airflow rates increase upper airway loss of aerosol.
Low lung volumes increases lung aerosol deposition.
Breathholding increases lung aerosol deposition.
Localized airway diseases tend to increase local aerosol deposition.

inhaled slowly through the mouth and breath-holding should be prolonged (Newman et al., 1981c; Dolovich et al., 1981; Newman et al., 1982); small hygroscopic particles may grow in a humid atmosphere (Scherer et al., 1979; Brain et al., 1985; Hiller et al., 1980). Low lung volumes may be preferred but this is not clear (Newman et al., 1985; Dolovich et al., 1981; Riley et al., 1976). These principles apply well to inhalation of aerosols that are uniformly present throughout inspiration, such as those generated by nebulizers or MDI combined with reservoirs (see below). Under these conditions, normal tidal breathing would seem likely to be more efficacious. However, studies with nebulizers have yielded conflicting results; one study reported a major increase over tidal breathing by deep inhalation and breathholding (Gottschalk et al., 1978). Other studies have found no difference in deposition between these two patterns of breathing (Dolovich et al., 1977). One study reported that 12% of nebulized aerosol was deposited in the thorax while most of the rest was either exhaled (20%) or remained in the nebulizer or tubing (67%) (Lewis et al., 1982). Other studies indicate lung (alveoli plus airway) deposition of 1-23% (Newman and Pavia, 1985). Presumably, numerous technical factors account for this great divergence in findings.

For aerosols inhaled as a bolus during inspirations, such as MDI and powder inhaler, many of the methodologic principles of inhalation noted for nebulizer apply but others, such as tidal breathing pattern, may not. Additionally, the large initial particle size and velocity associated with MDI, create new problems requiring other techniques. It has been clearly demonstrated that aerosol deposition from MDI is greater when MDI is activated during a slow inspiration (0.3-0.75 liters/sec air flow rate) followed by breathholding of 10 sec (Newman et al., 1981b; Newman and Clarke, 1983). Some data indicate that MDI is most efficacious when activation occurs at low (Newman et al., 1981b), medium (FRC) (Dolovich et al., 1981), and high (80% TLC) (Riley

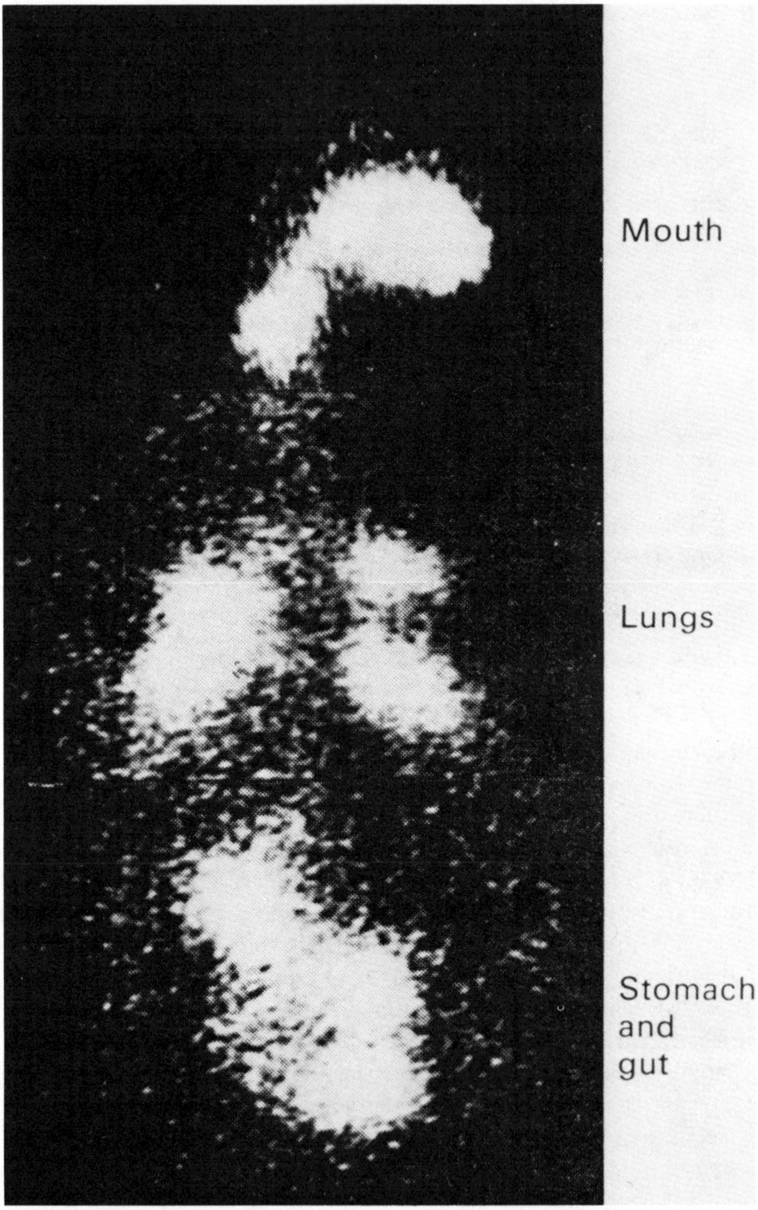

Figure 4 Deposition pattern from an MDI used correctly. Note that the bulk of the aerosol has deposited in the mouth and much of that was swallowed and appears in the stomach and gut. Only about 10% of the original dose has deposited in the lungs (reproduced with permission from Newman et al., 1981b).

et al., 1976) lung volumes. An additional point of contention is the position of actuator with reference to the mouth; though the data indicate greater lung deposition when the actuator is 2-4 cm from the (open) mouth compared to placement of actuator in either an open or closed mouth (Dolovich et al., 1981), other studies suggest that placement of MDI outside the mouth may lead to misdirection of spray and therefore should perhaps not be recommended (Newman and Clarke, 1983). In general, there is similar lung deposition with both nebulizer and MDI (mean of about 10% of original dose) with considerable individual variation for both techniques. The major difference between nebulizer and MDI is the major site of deposition; with MDI, 80% of aerosol deposits in the mouth and is swallowed (Fig. 4); the remaining 10% deposits in the MDI actuator. With nebulizers, about 90% remains within the nebulizer and attached tubing (Table 3) (Lewis, 1984; Newman et al., 1985).

Increasing propellant pressure from 3.5 to 5.5 atm actually causes increased lung deposition (Moren, 1978). Presumably, though the smaller particles, which are associated with higher pressure, have greater velocity, they apparently have less momentum than the larger but slower particles associated with lower pressure; hence, there is less deposition in the mouth with the higher pressure.

Because of difficulties in coordinating MDI actuation with slow inhalation, many patients do not use MDI properly and hence derive less than maximal benefit from MDI use. Several inhalation aids have been designed to improve MDI effectiveness (Dolovich et al., 1983; Newman et al., 1981; Tobin et al., 1982) (Fig. 5), particularly in patients who are unable to use MDI properly. These devices may assist inhalation in three possible ways: (1) directing aerosol straight into the mouth and thereby avoiding unnecessary external losses; (2) acting as an aerosol reservoir which, as discussed above, allows tidal breathing, uncoordinated with MDI activation, to be effective; (3) providing some feedback to patients as to their inspiratory flow rates. Devices such as short tubes act primarily as aerosol directors while longer and wider devices (cones, spheres, and collapsible bags; Fig. 5) also act as reservoirs. Flow rate monitors are available with some devices (Tobin et al., 1982). Another type of device developed to improve MDI response is a breath-activated MDI (Coady et al., 1976); this device, however, does not clearly produce better results.

Careful study has indicated that MDI inhalation aids do not increase bronchodilator effectiveness in patients who use MDI properly (Weeke, 1982). Inhalation aids, however, will considerably reduce aerosol deposition in the mouth and oropharynx from MDI in all patients (Dolovich et al., 1983) (from 81% to 9% in one study (Newman et al., 1985). Deposition patterns for nebulizer, and MDI with tube, cone, and rebreathing bag are compared in Table 3. Larger particles, because of their great initial momentum, instead of contacting and depositing in the mouth and oropharynx, settle out in the reservoirs and are hence not inhaled. This reduction in mouth and oropharyngeal aerosol

Table 3 Fate of Aerosol Leaving Nebulizer (%)

	Nebulizer[a]	MDI[b,c] (usual technique)	MDI[b] (correct technique)	MDI[c] + 10-cm tube	MDI[c] + 22-cm cone	MDI[b] + 700-ml bag
Equipment	67	10	(8)	26	29	75
Oropharynx	1	81	81	61	57	9
Exhaled	20	1	(0)	1	1	1
Lung	12	8	11	12	13	15

[a]Lewis et al., 1982.
[b]Newman et al., 1985.
[c]Newman et al., 1981b.
Values in parentheses were not specified in original reference but are assumed to be reasonable based on other data.

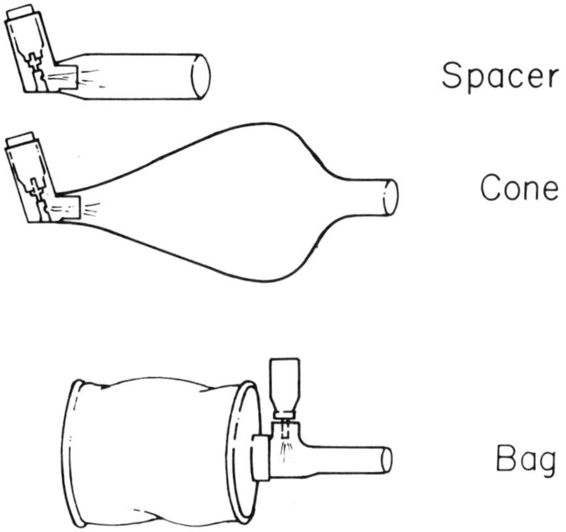

Figure 5 Devices used to improve delivery of aerosols from metered dose inhalers.

deposition is particularly important with use of inhaled corticosteroids, because of the high incidence of oral candidiasis and dysphonia associated with these agents (British Thoracic and Tuberculosis Association, 1976).

IV. Therapeutic Use of Aerosols

As noted above, in many countries, aerosolized sympathomimetics, particularly MDI, are the treatment of choice for acute intermittent asthma as well as many cases of moderate asthma. Many clinicians also believe that β_2 agonists delivered by MDI are the best means of preventing exercise-induced asthma (Anderson et al., 1979). Other agents that have been used successfully by aerosolization for treatment of asthma include anticholinergics (atropine sulfate, atropine methonitrate, ipatroprium hydrobromide), mast cell stabilizers (cromolyn and ketotifen), and corticosteroids (beclomethasone, budesonide, dexamethasone, betamethasone, and triamcinolone). Inhaled methylxanthines (theophylline) have not been very successful because of their relatively low potency and unpleasant taste (Cushley and Holgate, 1983; Bohadana et al., 1980).

Inhaled sympathomimetics have been investigated considerably more thoroughly than other types of agents. With relatively small but important changes in substitutions on the parent phenylethanolamine molecule, greater β-adrenergic specificity (isoproterenol), greater β_2 specificity (albuterol, terbutaline, and fenoterol), and perhaps greater duration of action (bitolterol) have been developed.

A. Log Dose-Response Curves

Many of the therapeutic and pharmacologic properties of aerosol generators are best studied by use of log dose/pharmacologic response curves. A number of these studies have been elegantly performed by Svedmyr and his colleagues in Sweden (Svedmyr et al., 1972, 1982; Thiringer and Svedmyr, 1974; Larsson and Svedmyr, 1977). The characteristic log dose response of physiological systems to increasing amounts of drugs is a result of drug-receptor interaction and the consequent gradual removal of free receptors (Goldstein et al., 1974). Such curves are difficult to demonstrate in humans with any form of bronchodilator administration other than inhaled because of the relatively early development of toxic side effects with other forms (oral, intravenous) forms of therapy (Thiringer and Svedmyr, 1974). Because of local deposition of bronchodilators with aerosol therapy, much smaller doses are required to produce bronchodilation than with systemic administration, thereby limiting total dosage and consequent side effects. In general, about 25 times more oral sympathomimetic must be given orally to produce the same bronchodilatation produced by the same drug with MDI. While some of the dose difference may be explained by sulfation and other chemical changes that take place in intestinal mucosa along with incomplete absorption, thereby causing reduced bioavailability of oral sympathomimetics, it is clear that direct airway deposition of aerosol is most important. There is less tremor and tachycardia with MDI than with either oral or intravenous therapy (Thiringer and Svedmyr, 1974; Larsson and Svedmyr, 1977).

Comparison has also been made between nebulized and MDI sympathomimetic administration. As noted above, 10-15% of inhaled aerosol is deposited in the lung when either nebulizers or MDIs are properly used (Table 3) (Lewis, 1984; Newman et al., 1985). Hence, it can be predicted that clinical results might be similar. Similar log dose response results for MDI and nebulizer have been reported with sympathomimetics (Cushley et al., 1983); another study found an approximately seven times greater effectiveness of MDI over either nebulizer or IPPB (Weber et al., 1979); it is likely that nebulizer technique was not optimal in the second study. Our experience is that log dose response curves with nebulizer, MDI, or MDI with extension are quite similar. Presumably the differences between studies can be accounted by differences in operation of both types of aerosol devices. Blood levels following nebulization of similar amounts of bronchodilator from nebulizer and MDI are similar (Cushley et al., 1983). Finally, bronchodilator response is directly related to lung deposition of bronchodilator.

B. Subsensitivity

Subsensitivity, or a diminished response to repeated administration, to a drug is a well-known phenomenon with sympathomimetics. Controversy also exists about the potential role of subsensitivity with inhaled sympathomimetics. When all sympathomimetics are withdrawn for 2 weeks and physiological response to inhaled bronchodilator is measured and compared to values obtained after several weeks of continuous sympathomimetic therapy, usually both peak and duration of response are moderately reduced (Steen et al., 1977; Repsher et al., 1978; Weber et al., 1982). However, it should be noted that subsensitivity is not progressive; major bronchodilation is still noted after chronic aerosol use. Others have noted subsensitivity in normal subjects, but not asthmatics, who have used MDI over several weeks (Harvey and Tattersfield, 1982). Hence subsensitivity to aerosol sympathomimetics probably does not form a major limitation to inhaled bronchodilator effectiveness (Svedmyr et al., 1976).

C. Site of Bronchoconstriction and Bronchodilator Effect

Recently, it has been shown that asthma may affect both large and small airways (the division is usually made at airway diameters of 2-3 mm, i.e., 10th order bronchi) (Fairshter and Wilson, 1980). In general, with greater degrees of obstruction, the likelihood of predominantly small-airway obstruction increases (Fairshter and Wilson, 1980). As detailed above, most clinical aerosol generators produce heterodisperse particles ranging from large to small. Hence, if bronchoconstriction affects both large and small airways, there may be a theoretical advantage of heterodisperse particles that can potentially deposit in airways of various sizes. It has been reported that, following use of MDI, the predominant site of bronchodilation is dependent upon the predominant site of bronchoconstriction before use of the bronchodilator. Predominantly large airway constriction is followed by large airway dilation, small airway constriction by small airway dilation (Fairshter and Wilson, 1980).

However, it should be noted that in one study utilizing slightly different methods, it was concluded that subcutaneous sympathomimetic produced small airway dilation while nebulized sympathomimetic caused a predominantly large airway response (Tashkin et al., 1980). A possible related finding is that in patients with chronic obstructive lung disease, bronchodilator therapy normally causes greater volume (FVC) than flow (FEV) response, presumably due to the combination of small airway dilation, which reduces airway closure at low lung volumes, and more large airway collapse, thereby reducing potential flow response (Healey et al., 1984).

D. Duration of Activity

Sympathomimetics given intravenously are relatively short-acting but are effective virtually immediately. Sympathomimetics given orally are slowly absorbed

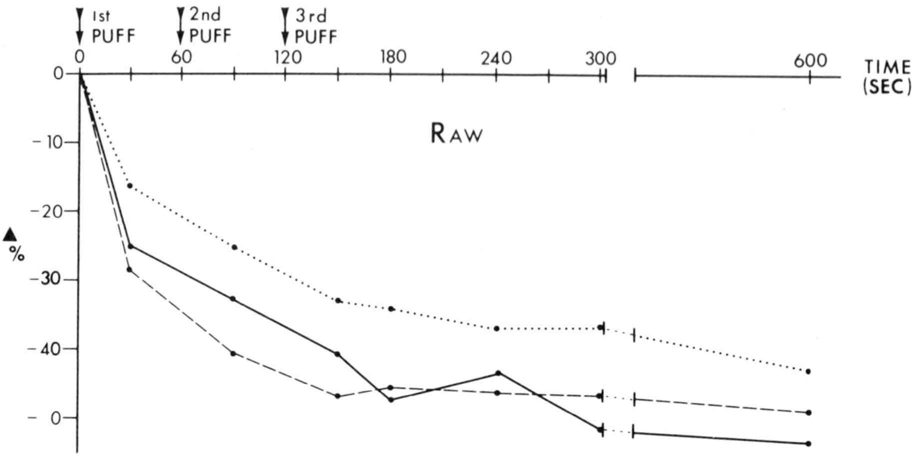

Figure 6 An example of the rapidity of action of three inhaled sympathomimetics from MDI. Significant bronchodilation had occurred within seconds of the first puff and peak effect occurred 3-8 min after the third puff. Though the duration of bronchodilation was longer for terbutaline (solid line) than metaproterenol (dotted line) and shortest for isoproterenol (dashed line), onset of activity was similar (adapted from Roth et al., 1977).

and reach a peak only after a few hours but then tend to act for a fairly long time (Clark, 1979). It is curious that inhaled sympathomimetics, like intravenous drugs, are fast-acting and, are yet, like oral drugs, long-acting (Clark, 1979; Roth et al., 1977). Figure 6 shows the speed of response to three different inhaled sympathomimetics. Even though the duration of activity varied greatly between the three drugs (due to differing rates of enzymatic degradation), rapid onset of action marked all drugs. Because of these differences between intravenous and oral agents and the fact that the bronchodilator effects of oral and inhaled sympathomimetics are additive (Svedmyr and Svedmyr, 1980), inhaled drug may either have different kinds of receptor response on the airway than on the blood side of bronchial muscle or be subject to different rates of drug removal.

References

Anderson, S., Searle, J. P., Ferris, L., Schoeffel, R., and Lindsay, D. A. (1979). An evaluation of pharmacotherapy for exercise-induced asthma. *J. Allergy Clin. Immunol. 64*: 612-624.

Bell, J. H., Hartley, P. S., and Cox, J. S. G. (1971). Dry powder aerosols I: A new powder inhalation device. *J. Pharm. Sci. 60*: 1559-1564.

Bohadana, A. B., Peslin, R., Teculescu, D., Polu, J. M., Belleville, F., and Massin, N. (1980). The bronchodilator action of theophylline aerosol in subjects with chronic airflow obstruction. *Bull. Eur. Physiopathol. Respir. 16*: 13-24.

Brain, J. D., Valberg, P. A., and Sneddon, S. (1985). Mechanisms of aerosol deposition and clearance. In *Aerosols in Medicine.* Edited by F. Moren, M. T. Newhouse, and M. B. Dolovich. Amsterdam, Elsevier, pp. 123-149. 123-149.

British Thoracic and Tuberculosis Association (1976). A controlled trial of inhaled corticosteroids in patients receiving prednisone tablets for asthma. *Br. J. Dis. Chest 70*: 95-101.

Chang, N., and Levison, H. (1972). The effect of a nebulized bronchodilator administered with or without intermittent positive pressure breathing on ventilatory function in children with cystic fibrosis and asthma. *Am. Rev. Respir. Dis. 106*: 867-872.

Cheney, F. W., Jr., and Butler, J. (1968). The effects of ultrasonically-produced aerosols on airway resistance in man. *Anesthesiology 6*: 1099-1106.

Clark, T. J. H. (1979). Factors influencing route of administration of airway therapy. In *Small Airways in Health and Disease.* Edited by P. Sadoul, J. Milic-Emili, B. G. Simonsson, and T. J. H. Clark. Amsterdam, Excerpta Medica, pp. 170-179.

Clay, M. M., Pavia, D., Newman, S. P., Lennard-Jones, T. S., and Clarke, S. W. (1983a). Assessment of jet nebulizers for lung aerosol therapy. *Lancet 2*: 592-594.

Clay, M. M., Pavia, D., Newman, S. P., and Clarke, S. W. (1983b). Factors influencing the size distribution of aerosols from jet nebulizers. *Thorax 38*: 755-759.

Coady, T. J., Davies, H. J., and Barnes, P. (1976). Evaluation of a breath actuated pressurized aerosol. *Clin. Allergy 6*: 1-6.

Cromptom, G. K. (1982). Clinical use of dry powder systems. *Eur. J. Respir. Dis.* Suppl. 122 *63*. 96-99.

*Cu*shley, M. J., and Holgate, S. T. (1983). Efficacy of inhaled methylxanthines as bronchodilators in asthma. *Thorax 38*: 223.

Cushley, M. J., Lewis, R. A., and Tattersfield, A. E. (1983). Comparison of three techniques of inhalation on the airway response to terbutaline. *Thorax 38*: 908-913.

Davies, D. S. (1982). Pharmacokinetic studies with inhaled drugs. *Eur. J. Respir. Dis.* Suppl. 119 *63*: 67-72.

Davis, S. S., and Bubb, M. D. (1978). Physico-chemical studies on aerosol solutions for drug delivery. III The effect of relative humidity on the particle size of inhalation aerosols. *Int. J. Pharm. 1*: 303-314.

Dolovich, M. B., Killian, D., Wolff, R. K., Obminski, G., and Newhouse, M. T. (1977). Pulmonary aerosol deposition in chronic bronchitis: Intermittent positive-pressure breathing versus quiet breathing. *Am. Rev. Respir. Dis.* *115*: 397-402.

Dolovich, M. B., Ruffin, R. E., Roberts, R., and Newhouse, M. T. (1981). Optimal delivery of aerosols from metered dose inhalers. *Chest* Suppl. *80:* 911-915.

Dolovich, M., Ruffin, R., Corr, D., and Newhouse, M. T. (1983). Clinical evaluation of a simple demand inhalation MDI aerosol delivery service. *Chest 84*: 36-41.

Fairshter, R. D., and Wilson, A. F. (1980). Relationship between the site of airflow limitation and localization of the bronchodilator response in asthma. *Am. Rev. Respir. Dis. 122*: 27-32.

Ferron, G. H., Kerrebijn, K. F., and Weber, J. (1976). Properties of aerosols produced with three nebulizers. *Am. Rev. Respir. Dis. 114*: 899-908.

Goldstein, A., Aronow, L., and Kalman, S. N. (1974). *Principles of Drug Action,* 2nd ed. New York, John Wiley, pp. 82-110.

Gottschalk, B., Leupold, W., and Woller, P. (1978). Deponierung von aerosolen in den oberen and unteren atemwegen. *Atemwegs Lungenkrank 4*: 378-380.

Harvey, J. E., and Tattersfield, A. E. (1982). Airway response to salbutamol: Effect of regular salbutamol inhalations in normal, atopic and asthmatic subjects. *Thorax 37*: 280-287.

Hayton, W. L. (1976). Propellant-powered nebulizers. *J. Am. Pharm. Assoc. (Sci. Ed.) 16*: 201-207.

Healey, F., Wilson, A. F., and Fairshter, R. D. (1984). Physiological correlates of airway collapse in chronic airflow obstruction. *Chest 85*: 476-481.

Hetzel, M. R., and Clark, T. J. H. (1977). Comparison of salbutamol Rotohaler with conventional pressurized aerosol (1977). *Clin. Allergy 7*: 563-568.

Hiller, F. C., Mazumder, M., Smith, G. M., and Bone, R. C. (1980a). Physical properties, hyproscopicity and estimated pulmonary retention of various therapeutic aerosols. *Chest 77*(2) (Suppl): 318-321.

Hiller, F. C., Mazumder, M. K., Wilson, J. D., and Bone, R. C. (1980b). Effect of low and high relative humidity on metered-dose bronchodilator solution and powder aerosols. *J. Pharm. Sci. 69*: 334-337.

Laros, C. D., Van Urk, P., and Rominger, K. L. (1977). Absorption, distribution and excretion of the tritium-labelled beta 2 stimulator fenoterol hydrobromide following aerosol administration and instillation into the bronchial tree. *Respir. 34*: 131-140.

Larsson, S., and Svedmyr, N. (1977). Bronchodilating effect and side effects of beta 2-adreno receptor stimulants by different modes of administration (tablets, metered aerosol, and combinations thereof). *Am. Rev. Respir. Dis. 116*: 861-869.

Lewis, R. A. (1984). Inhalation drugs in asthma management: State of the art, factors affecting delivery and clinical response to inhaled drugs. *NER Allergy Proc S*: 23-33.

Lewis, R., Fleming, J. S., Balanchandian, W., and Tattersfield, A. E. (1981). Particle size distribution and deposition from a jet nebulizer: Influence of humidity and temperatures. *Clin. Sci. 62*: 5.

Lewis, R. R., Cushley, M. J., Fleming, J. S., and Tattersfield, A. E. (1982). Is a nebulizer less efficient than a metered dose inhaler and do pear-shaped extension tubes work? *Am. Rev. Respir. Dis. (pt. 2) 125*: 94.

Lourenco, R. V., and Cotromanes, E. (1982). Clinical aerosols I. Characterization of aerosols and their diagnostic use. *Arch. Intern. Med. 142*: 2163-2172.

Mercer, T. T. (1973). Production and characterization of aerosols. *Arch. Intern. Med. 131*: 39-50.

Mercer, T. T., Tillery, M. I., and Chow, H. Y. (1968). Operating characteristics of some compressed-air nebulizers. *Am. Ind. Hyg. Assoc. J. 29*: 66-78.

Moren, F. (1978). Drug deposition of pressurized inhalation aerosols. II. Influence of vapor pressure and metered volume. *Int. J. Pharm. 1*: 213-218.

Moren, F. (1985). Aerosol dosage forms and formulations. In *Aerosols in Medicine.* Edited by F. Moren, M. T. Newhouse, and M. B. Dolovich. Amsterdam, Elsevier, pp. 261-288.

Morrow, P. E. (1974). Aerosol characterization and deposition. *Am. Rev. Respir. Dis. 110*: 88-99.

Newman, S. P., and Clarke, S. W. (1983). Inhalation technique with aerosol bronchodilators: Does it matter? *Pract. Cardiol. 9*: 157-164.

Newman, S. P., and Pavia, D. (1985). Aerosol deposition in man. In *Aerosols in Medicine.* Edited by F. Moren, M. T. Newhouse, and M. B. Dolovich. Amsterdam, Elsevier, pp. 193-219.

Newman, S. P., Moren, F., Pavia, D., Little, F., and Clarke, S. W. (1981a). Deposition of pressurized suspension aerosols inhaled through extension devices. *Am. Rev. Respir. Dis. 124*: 317-320.

Newman, S. R., Pavia, D., and Clarke, S. W. (1981b). Improving the bronchial deposition of pressurized aerosols. *Chest Suppl. 80*: 909-911.

Newman, S. P., Pavia, D., Garland, N., and Clarke, S. W. (1982). Effects of various inhalation modes on deposition of radioactive pressurized aerosols. *Eur. J. Resp. Dis. Suppl. 119 63*: 57-65.

Newman, S. P., Pavia, D., Moren, F., Sheahan, N. F., and Clarke, S. W. (1981c). Deposition of pressurized aerosols in the human respiratory tract. *Thorax 36*: 52-55.

Newman, S. P., Woodman, G., Clarke, S. W., and Sackner, M. A. (1985). Enhanced drug delivery from metered dose inhalers with the InspirEase. *Am. Rev. Respir. Dis. 131*: A96.

Paterson, J. W., Woolcock, D. J., and Shenfield, G. (1979). Bronchodilator drugs. *Am. Rev. Respir. Dis. 129*-1149-1188.

Pauwels, R. Pharmacokinetics of inhaled drugs. (1985). In *Aerosols in Medicine.* Edited by F. Moren, M. T. Newhouse, and M. B. Dolovich. Amsterdam, Elsevier, pp. 219-224.

Rees, P. J., and Clark, T. J. H. (1982). The importance of particle size in response to inhaled bronchodilators. *Eur. J. Respir. Dis. Suppl. 119 63*: 73-78.

Repsher, L. H., Anderson, J. A., Bush, R. K., Falliers, C. K., Kass, I., Kemp, J. P., Reed, C., Siegel, S. and C. K., Kass, I., Kemp, J. P., Reed, C., Siegel, S., and Webb, D. R. (1984). Assessment of tachyphylaxis following prolonged therapy of asthma with inhaled albuterol. *Chest 85*: 34-38.

Riley, D. J., Weitz, B. W., and Edelman, N. H. (1976). The responses of asthmatic subjects to isoproterenol inhaled at different lung volumes. *Am. Rev. Respir. Dis. 114*: 509-515.

Rodenstein, D., and Stanescu, D. C. (1982). Mouth spraying versus inhalation of fenoterol aerosol in healthy subjects and asthmatic patients. *Br. J. Dis. Chest 76*: 365-373.

Roth, M. J., Wilson, A. F., and Novey, H. S. (1977). A comparative study of the aerosolized bronchodilators, isoproterenol, metaproterenol and terbutaline in asthma. *Ann. Allergy 38*: 16-21.

Ruffin, R. E., Montgomery, J. M., and Newhouse, M. T. (1978): Site of beta-adrenergic receptors in the respiratory tract. *Chest 74*: 256-260.

Scherer, P. W., Haselton, F. R., Hanna, J. M., and Stone, D. R. (1979). Growth of hygroscopic aerosols in a model of human airways. *J. Appl. Physiol. 4*: 544-550.

Shenfield, G. M., Evans, M. E., and Paterson, J. W. (1974). The effect of a nebulized bronchodilator with and without intermittent positive pressure breathing on the absorption and metabolism of salbutamol. *Br. J. Clin. Pharmacol. 1*: 295-300.

Steen, S. N., Smith, R., Kuo, J., Ziment, I., and Beall, G. N. (1977). Comparison of bronchodilator effects of aerosol fenoterol and isoproterenol. *Chest 72*: 724-730.

Stewart, R. D., Newton, P. E., Baretta, E. D., Hermann, A. A., Forster, H. V., and Soto, R. J. (1978). Physiological response to aerosol propellants. *Environ. Health Perspect. 26*: 275-285.

Svedmyr, N., and Svedmyr, K. (1980). In-vitro and in-vivo effects of theophylline and beta 2 adrenostimulants in combination. *Eur. J. Respir. Dis.* Suppl. 109 *61*: 83-91.

Svedmyr, N., Malmberg, R., and Thiringer, G. (1972). The effect of a new adrenergic beta 2-receptor stimulating agent (rimiterol, R 798) in patients with chronic obstructive lung disease. *Eur. J. Respir. Dis. 53*: 302-313.

Svedmyr, N., Larsson, S. A., and Thiringer, G. K. (1976). Development of "resistance" in adrenergic receptors of asthmatic patients. *Chest 69*: 479-482.

Svedmyr, N., Lofdahl, C-G., and Svedmyr, K. (1982). The effect of powder aerosol compared to pressurized aerosol. *Eur. J. Respir. Dis.* Suppl. 119 *63*: 81-88.

Swift, D. L. (1985). Aerosol characterization and generation. In *Aerosols in Medicine.* Edited by F. Moren, M. T. Newhouse, and M. B. Dolovich. Amsterdam, Elsevier, pp. 53-76.

Tashkin, D. P., Trevor, E., Chopra, S. K., and Taplin, G. V. (1980). Sites of airway dilatation in asthma following inhaled versus subcutaneous terbutaline. *Am. J. Med. 68*: 14-26.

Thiessen, B., and Pedersen, O. F. (1980). Effect of freon inhalation on maximal expiratory flows and heart rhythm after treatment with salbutamol and ipratropium bromide. *Eur. J. Respir. Dis. 61*: 156-161.

Thiringer, G., and Svedmyr, N. (1974). Comparison of i.v. administered and inhaled terbutaline with dose-effect curves in patients with chronic obstructive lung disease. *Scand. J. Respir. Dis.* Suppl. 88: 56-67.

Tobin, M. J., Jenouri, G., Danta, I., Kim, C., Watson, H., and Sackner, M. A. (1982). Response to bronchodilator drug administration by a new reservoir aerosol delivery system and a review of other auxiliary delivery systems. *Am. Rev. Respir. Dis. 126*: 670-675.

Walker, S. R., Evans, M. E., Richards, A. J., and Paterson, J. W. (1972). The clinical pharmacology of oral and inhaled salbutamol. *Clin. Pharmacol. Ther. 13*: 861-867.

Webber, B. A., Shenfield, G. M., and Paterson, J. W. (1974). A comparison of three different methods for giving nebulized albuterol to asthmatic patients. *Am. Rev. Respir. Dis. 109*: 293-295.

Weber, R. W., Petty, W. W., and Nelson, H. S. (1979). Aerosolized terbutaline in asthmatics. Comparison of dosage strength, schedule and method of administration. *J. Allergy Clin. Immunol. 63*: 116-121.

Weber, R. W., Smith, J. A., and Nelson, H. A. (1982): Aerosolized terbutaline in asthmatics: Development of subsensitivity with long-term administration. *J. Allergy Clin. Immunol. 70*: 417-422.

Weeke, E. R. (1982). Reported clinical experiences with inhaled terbutaline aerosol via spacer devices. *Am. J. Respir. Dis.* Suppl. 119 *63*: 105-109.

Weiner, M. V. (1958). How to formulate aerosols to obtain the desired spray pattern. *J. Soc. Cosmet. Chem. 9*: 389-397.

12

Drug Actions on Mediators

ADAM WANNER

University of Miami School of Medicine
Miami, Florida

TAHIR AHMED and WILLIAM M. ABRAHAM

University of Miami School of Medicine
Miami, and Mount Sinai Medical Center
Miami Beach, Florida

I. Introduction

Since the discovery that mast cells and basophils contain histamine (Riley, 1959), attempts have been made to interfere with the actions of this and other inflammatory mediators by pharmacologic agents. This has led to the development of several classes of drugs capable of opposing the effects of inflammatory mediators by various mechanisms. According to the scheme depicted in Figure 1, drugs may exert effects on (1) the generation of chemical mediators by leukocytes and possibly other cells present in the airways, (2) the release of chemical mediators from those cells, and (3) the binding of the chemical mediators to their specific receptor sites on the target cell. The latter effect may be due to receptor antagonism or to modification of the number and distribution of the receptors and their subtypes by the drug.

The following discussion reviews the currently known actions of pharmacologic agents on these different steps of mediator generation and action from the leukocyte to the target cell.

Bronchial asthma is characterized by the pathophysiological triad of airway smooth muscle contraction, mucociliary dysfunction, and edema, all of

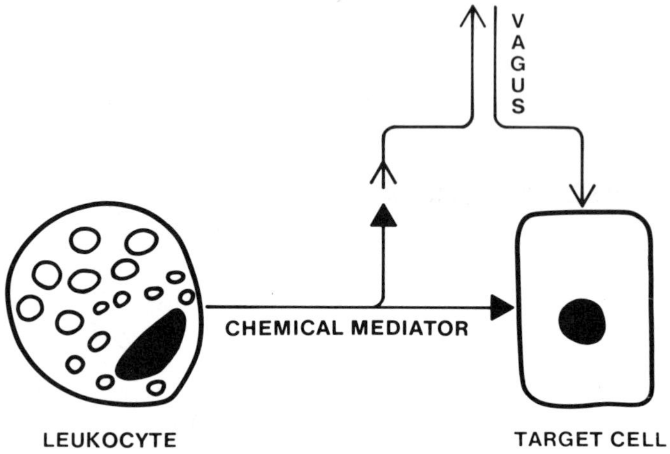

Figure 1 Conventional schema for the generation and release of chemical mediators from leukocyte (e.g., mast cell) and action on target cell (e.g., airway smooth muscle cell, autonomic neuron). The chemical mediators exert their effect directly by stimulation of receptors on target cells or indirectly by stimulation of receptors on cholinergic nerve fibers.

which are thought to contribute to the clinical manifestations of airflow obstruction, excessive airway secretions, and cough. This indicates that the targets of chemical mediators in asthma are airway and bronchial vascular smooth muscle, airway epithelium including its mucus-producing structures, and the bronchial capillary bed. The actions of the chemical mediators on these tissues may be direct or indirect by stimulation of autonomic neural pathways resulting in reflex vagal effects. The assumption made that if autonomic reflex mechanisms are involved, the same principles of mediator generation, secretion, and receptor binding (at afferent autonomic nerve ending or autonomic ganglia) are operative as with the direct end-organ effects of mediators.

II. Inhibition of Mediator Generation

The greatest potential for the inhibition of mediator generation is for "newly" formed and secondarily formed mediators. Most of the available information in this regard deals with the products of arachidonic acid and involves both the cyclooxygenase and lipoxygenase pathways. The biosynthesis of prostaglandins, thromboxanes, and leukotrienes from polyunsaturated fatty acids involves a

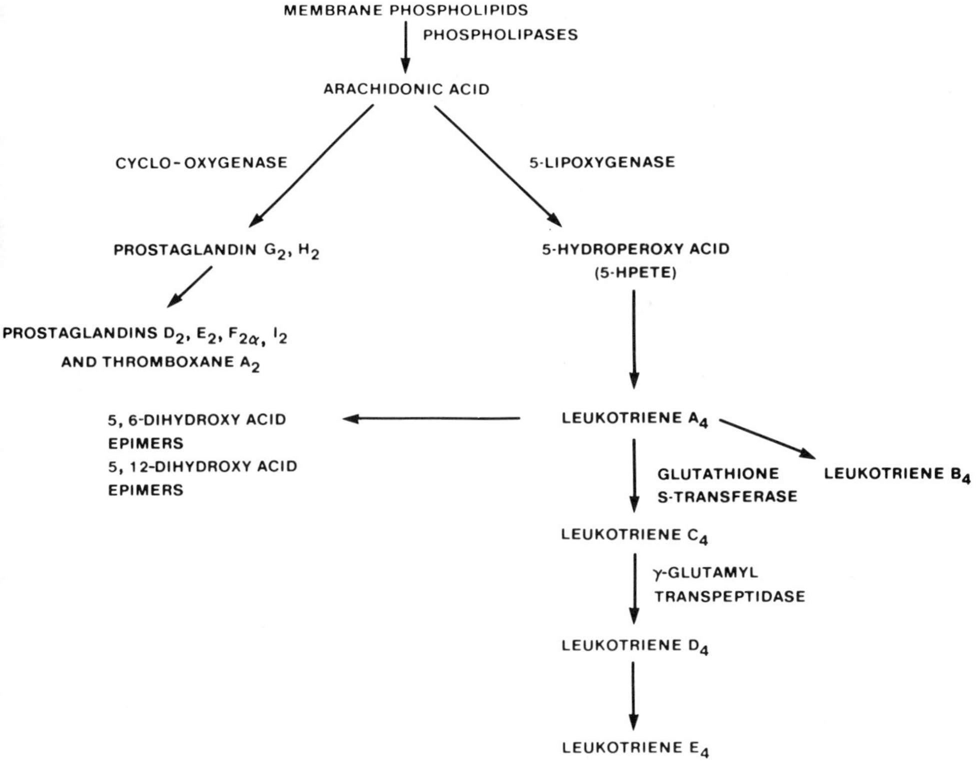

Figure 2 Biosynthetic pathways for the synthesis of prostaglandins and leukotrienes.

complex multienzyme system (Samuelsson et al., 1978, 1981; Granstrom, 1981; Maas et al., 1982). Because the products of arachidonic acid play an important role in the pathophysiology of airway disease, compounds that inhibit their synthesis have, understandably, received considerable attention.

Arachidonic acid (AA), after being liberated from phospholipids by phospholipase A_2, is metabolized either by the lipoxygenase or cyclooxygenase pathway (Fig. 2). Free AA is the substrate for a number of lipoxygenases giving rise to hydroperoxyeicosatetraenoic acids (HPETE). These can be reduced to corresponding hydroxy acids (HETE), and transformed into leukotrienes. On the other hand, oxygenation of AA, catalyzed by the enzyme cyclooxygenase or cyclooxygenation of 11-HPETE, leads to the formation of prostaglandin endoperoxide (PGG_2). Changes of the hydroperoxy group of PGG_2, catalyzed by the enzyme peroxidase, lead to 15-hydroxy-prostaglandin endoperoxide (PGH_2). PGH_2 in turn is isomerized to PGE_2 and other primary prostaglandins. PGH_2 is also the substrate for the enzyme thromboxane-synthetase, which forms thromboxane A_2 (TxA_2). The enzyme prostacyclin synthetase isomerizes PGH_2 to prostacyclin (PGI_2).

A. Inhibition of Phospholipase A_2

In order to be metabolized by oxidative tissue enzymes, AA has to be liberated from the cellular phospholipids by phospholipase A_2 (Blackwell et al., 1977). In certain cells, such as platelets, phospholipase requires calcium ions for its optimal biochemical activity, and therefore Ca^{2+} ionophores activate the AA cascade (Pickett et al., 1977). Thus, drugs that sequester Ca^{2+}, with or without raising levels of intracellular cyclic adenosine monophosphate (c-AMP), inhibit AA liberation and its subsequent metabolism. Mepacrine and bromophenacetyl are direct inhibitors of phospholipase A_2 (Vargaftig, 1977). Similarly, it has been demonstrated that glucocorticosteroids, by inducing the endogenous synthesis of a phospholipase A_2-inhibitor, hinder the release of AA (Gryglewski et al., 1975; Flower and Blackwell, 1979). While the phospholipase A_2 inhibitors have not been tested clinically, the antiinflammatory effect of glucocorticosteroids may well be partially due to the generation of an endogenous phospholipase A_2 inhibitor (Flower and Blackwell, 1979). Although Ca^{2+} is very important for the activity of phospholipase A_2, it is not known whether calcium antagonists have an inhibitory effect on the activity of this enzyme.

B. Inhibition of Cyclooxygenase

The best known route for further enzymatic transformation of AA is through cyclooxygenation of 11-HPETE to the prostaglandin endoperoxide PGG_2. The activity of cyclooxygenase is selectively and irreversibly inhibited by aspirin, indomethacin, and other nonsteroidal anti-inflammatory agents (Flower, 1974; Vane, 1971). However, the role played by the cyclooxygenase products in the pathophysiology of airway disease is the subject of controversy. Indeed, cyclooxygenase products may be as important in modulating as they are in mediating airway dysfunction. For example, an enhancement of bronchospasm has been recently observed after the administration of a cyclooxygenase inhibitor in patients with allergic asthma (Fish et al., 1981).

C. Inhibition of Prostaglandin Peroxidases and Isomerases

Peroxidases sequentially convert PGG_2 to PGH_2, which is then converted to primary prostaglandins by an isomerase. The inactivity of peroxidases is stimulated by phenol, its isomer aminobutyl-idophenol (MK447), as well as by chloropromazine (Kuehl et al., 1977; Lee, 1974; Gryglewski, 1981), whereas the activity of the isomerases is stimulated by albumin (Hamberg and Fredholm, 1976). However, no known inhibitors of these enzymes are available for clinical use.

D. Thromboxane and Prostaglandin Synthetase Inhibition

In contrast to primary prostaglandins, thromboxane A_2 (TxA_2) and prostacyclin (PGI_2) are generated from PGH_2 only in the presence of corresponding synthetases. Thromboxane-synthetase is located mainly in blood platelets and prostacyclin-synthetase mainly in vascular tissues.

A selective thromboxane-synthetase inhibitor interferes with the conversion of PGH_2 to TxA_2, without influencing the activity of cyclooxygenase and prostacyclin-synthetase. The currently known thromboxane-synthetase inhibitors are chemically and pharmacologically a heterogeneous group of compounds of variable selectivity and specificity. Nictindole (Gryglewski et al., 1977), imidazole (Moncada et al., 1977), and imidazole derivatives such as burimamide (Allan and Eakins, 1978) all have some thromboxane-synthetase-inhibiting activity; however they are irritants in mammalian tissue and are nonselective, and therefore of no use in vivo. Nicotinic acid, extracts from onion (*Allium cepa*) and extracts from garlic (*Allium sativum*) also have some thromboxane-synthetase-inhibiting activity (Gryglewski, 1981). A new approach to the selective inhibition of thromboxane-synthetase was initiated by the synthesis of substrate analogues of this enzyme including U-81606, and U-63557A (Fitzpatrick and Gorman, 1978). These or similar compounds may be important in vascular disorders; however, so far they have not been clinically tested in humans, and their role in airway disease is not likely to be of major importance.

Prostacyclin, in addition to being a potent vasodilator, is an important physiological inhibitor of platelet aggregation. A number of lipid peroxides and nicotine in vitro inhibit the activity of prostacyclin-synthetase (Salmon et al., 1978). Again, these agents are of uncertain clinical value.

E. Inhibition of Leukotriene Synthesis

Theoretically, leukotriene production can be inhibited at a number of steps, including inhibition of phospholipase A_2, 5-lipoxygenase, and glutathione-s-transferase (Jakschik et al., 1982; Bach et al., 1982).

Ca^{2+} enhances the activity of phospholipase A_2 and 5-lipoxygenase; this differentiates these enzymes from cyclooxygenase and 12-lipoxygenase, which do not require Ca^{2+} (Jakschik et al., 1980). Theoretically, therefore, it is possible that calcium antagonists may inhibit the activity of phospholipase A_2 and 5-lipoxygenase, without inhibiting cyclooxygenase. However, no such information is available in vitro or in vivo.

Table 1 Stimuli Associated with Mediator Release

Immunologic
Antigen
Anti-IgE
Nonimmunologic
Chemical
Compound 48/80
Calcium ionophore A-23187
Concanavalin A
Polymyxin B
Peptides (substance P)
Endogenous opiates (endorphins)
Noxious agents (ozone, sulfur dioxide)
Physical
Cold
Altered osmolality
Altered pH

Most of the lipoxygenase pathway inhibitors available for experimental use appear to interfere with both lipoxygenases and cyclooxygenases in vitro and are therefore not very selective. None of these compounds has been tested in vivo in humans or in animal models of airway disease. The development of a safe and selective lipoxygenase inhibitor for use in humans will be of great importance.

III. Prevention of Mediator Secretion

It has been well established both in vivo and in vitro that stimulation of IgE receptors on mast cells, basophils, and macrophages elicits the release of a variety of inflammatory mediators. Chemical and physical stimuli can also induce the generation and secretion of these mediators. These mediators, such as histamine and various products of arachidonate metabolism, constrict airway smooth muscle, stimulate mucus secretion, and increase vascular permeability, all of which factors contribute to airway disease. Other mediators of inflammation include neutrophil and eosinophil chemotactic factors, proteolytic enzymes, and proteoglycans (e.g., heparin), which also contribute to the overall inflammatory process (Wasserman, 1983). The following discussion focuses on what is known about the control of mediator secretion and the potential role of pharmacologic agents in modulating mediator release.

A. Process of Mediator Secretion

The mechanisms by which mediators are released from mediator-containing cells (primarily mast cells and basophils) are dependent on the stimulus and the cell type being stimulated. Table 1 lists some of the stimuli that elicit mediator release. Although the airway pathophysiology resulting from these stimuli is similar, it has been shown in vitro that they induce secretion via different mechanisms. Ishizaka and Ishizaka (1968) demonstrated that when antigen bridged two or more IgE molecules on the cell membrane, histamine release occurred. Subsequent studies showed that receptor aggregation alone, in the absence of IgE, was a sufficient trigger for mediator release (Ishizaka and Ishizaka, 1978; Ishizaka et al., 1980). The process of mediator release under conditions of receptor aggregation includes the methylation of phospholipids in the cell membrane to produce phosphatidylcholine; this changes the normal distribution of lipids in the membrane leading to changes in the microviscosity and fluidity of the cell membrane (Hirata and Axelrod, 1978, 1980). This process is followed by an increased Ca^{2+} uptake via open Ca^{2+} channels in the membrane, after which granular secretion (histamine release) occurs. That phospholipid methylation is an important step in antigen-induced mediator release is supported by experiments in which inhibition of methylation with adenosine derivatives prevented Ca^{2+} influx and subsequent mediator release (Morita et al., 1981; Morita and Sivaganian, 1981; Chiang et al., 1977).

A similar sequence of events has been shown to occur with concanavalin A (Con A), which binds to carbohydrate moieties of the IgE receptor. This binding results in the bridging of receptors, the formation of methylated lipids, Ca^{2+} influx, and mediator release (Hirata et al., 1979).

Phospholipid methylation is not, however, a necessary prerequisite for mediator release. Other agents such as the Ca^{2+} ionophore A-23187, polymyxin B, or compound 48/80 release histamine in some systems without being preceded by phospholipid methylation (Morita et al., 1981; Hirata et al., 1979). With these agents, protein phosphorylation occurs resulting in the production of phosphatidyl inositol and phosphatidic acid, and diacylglycerol formation; all of these substances can then be metabolized to arachidonic acid (see below). The production of these phospholipids (especially phosphatidic acid, which is an endogenous Ca^{2+} ionophore) precede the influx of Ca^{2+} and mediator release. Thus, depending on the stimulus (immunologic/nonimmunologic) the mechanism of stimulus secretion coupling may differ (Anderson, 1985).

Further evidence that the secretory pathways initiated by various stimuli differ comes from studies examining the time course of histamine release. Rat peritoneal mast cells stimulated in vitro with antigen showed a peak histamine release 30 sec after challenge; as might be expected, a similar response was observed after challenge with Con A. Compound 48/80 however, elicited a maximal response within 10 sec, whereas stimulation with the Ca^{2+} ionophore A-23187 resulted in peak histamine release after 60 sec (White and Pearce, 1981). Similar results have been obtained in vivo. Bronchial contraction (presumably via histamine release) began 40 sec after the injection of antigen into the bronchial artery of dogs, whereas contraction was elicited within 9 sec after injection of compound 48/80 (Garrity et al., 1983).

As indicated above, an important component of the secretory process is dependent on the influx of Ca^{2+}. Although in vitro experiments have identified several sources of Ca^{2+} that can be utilized for mediator secretion (White and Pearce, 1981), the influx of extracellular Ca^{2+} through open Ca^{2+} channels in the cell membrane is probably the most likely mechanism operating in vivo (Foreman, 1981).

The metabolism of arachidonic acid via the lipoxygenase/cyclooxygenase pathway is important not only because of the production of leukotrienes and prostaglandins but also because arachidonic acid and its metabolites might modulate histamine release. In rat mast cells and human basophils, IgE-mediated histamine release was prevented in a dose-dependent fashion by eicosatetraynoic acid (ETYA), a competitive antagonist of arachidonic acid (Peters et al., 1982). The cyclooxygenase inhibitor indomethacin enhanced histamine release, as did increasing concentrations of arachidonic acid. Subsequent experiments indicated that possibly an early metabolite of the 5-lipoxygenase pathway of arachidonate metabolism (5-hydroxyperoxyeicosatetraenoic acid [5-HPETE]) can induce the release of histamine (Peters et al., 1982).

Cyclic nucleotides must also be considered in the regulation of mediator secretion. Binding of IgE receptors by antigen stimulates membrane-bound adenylate cyclase to convert adenosine triphosphate (ATP) to cyclic adenosine monophosphate (c-AMP), which then activates c-AMP-dependent protein kinases. Utilizing ATP, these protein kinases phosphorylate specific proteins within the cell, which leads to granular secretion. Documentation of this pathway could seemingly contradict earlier studies indicating that increased intracellular levels of c-AMP (as occurs after stimulation with β-adrenergic agents) inhibit mediator release, whereas decreased levels of c-AMP (via α-adrenergic stimulation) increased mediator release. More recent studies have shown that two distinct increases in c-AMP occur upon immunologic stimulation, and that the initial rapid increase (15 sec) in c-AMP coincides with methyl transferase activation and therefore may be important for the secretory events described above (Winslow and Austen, 1982). From these observations it follows that inhibition of mediator release in vivo can be accomplished by (1) membrane stabilization, (2) prevention of Ca^{2+} influx and mobilization, and (3) prevention of arachidonic acid production. Therefore, pharmacologic agents that prevent mediator release should act on one of these sites.

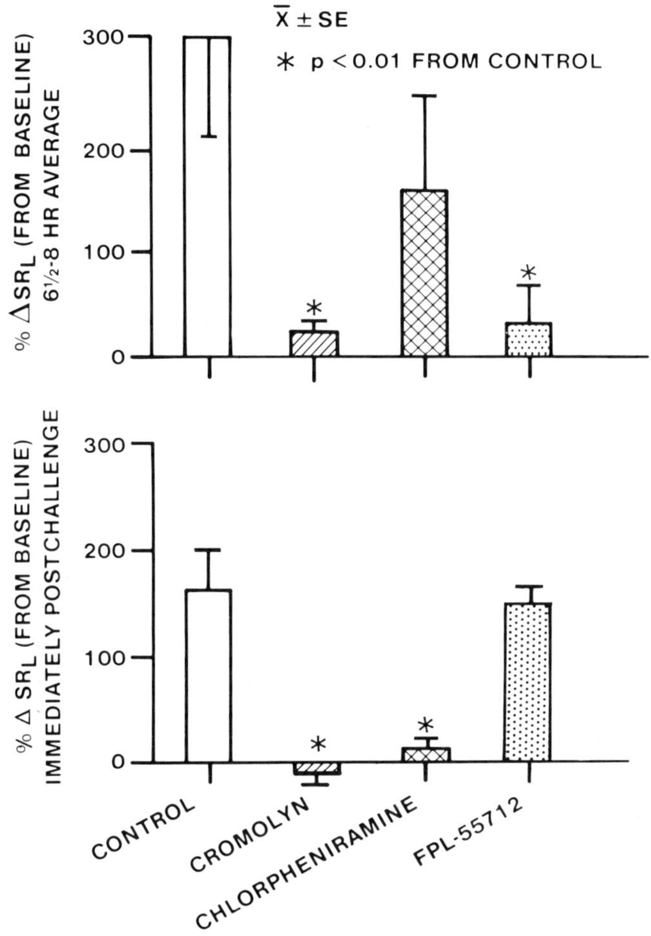

Figure 3 Effects of the inhibition of mediator secretion (cromolyn), H_1-histamine receptor blockade (chlorpheniramine), and sulfidopeptide-leukotriene receptor blockade (FPL-55712) on immediate (bottom) and late-phase (top) responses to inhaled antigen in allergic sheep. SR_L, specific pulmonary resistance. Controls depict response to antigen challenge without pretreatment. The pharmacologic agents were given either before antigen challenge (bottom) or at 5½ hr postchallenge (before the expected late-phase response; top). While chemical mediators appear to play an important role in both the immediate and late-phase response (blocked by cromolyn), histamine (through H_1-receptor stimulation) is the putative mediator of the immediate response and sulfidopeptideleukotriene (SRS-A) of the late-phase response (based on data reported by Delehunt et al., 1984; Abraham et al., 1981).

B. Drug Effects on Mediator Secretion

The therapeutic agents known to influence mediator release both in vivo and in vitro include disodium cromoglycate (and related compounds), Ca^{2+} antagonists, β-adrenergic agonists, methylxanthines, and glucocorticosteroids. The efficacy of these agents in modifying mediator release in vivo varies, as does their mode of action.

Cromolyn

It has long been recognized that disodium cromoglycate (cromolyn) could prevent antigen-induced bronchoconstriction in both animal models of allergic airway disease (Abraham et al., 1981, 1983) and asthmatic patients (Booij-Noord et al., 1971; Pepys and Hutchcroft, 1975; Atkins et al., 1978) (Fig. 3). Furthermore, cromolyn has been shown to be an effective agent in preventing nonimmunologic mast cell degranulation both in vivo (Russi et al., 1984) and in vitro (Ennis et al., 1981). Originally, it was suggested that cromolyn stabilizes mast cell membranes. More recent evidence, however, indicates that cromolyn may act by interfering with Ca^{2+} influx into the cells via its action on Ca^{2+} channels (Pearce et al., 1979; Dixon et al., 1980).

Calcium Channel Blockers

Since the influx of extracellular Ca^{2+} into the cell is required for mediator release, Ca^{2+} antagonists such as nifedipine and verapamil, which act as competitive antagonists of Ca^{2+} influx, should be capable of preventing antigen-induced mediator secretion. These agents, however, are only effective against antigen-induced histamine release from human basophils (Middleton et al., 1981), not against ionophore-induced histamine release (Bedard and Busse, 1983). These contrasting results may be dependent on different mechanisms of Ca^{2+} influx into the cells after antigen and ionophore stimulation or on different intracellular pools of Ca^{2+} being stimulated by these agents. Two types of Ca^{2+} channels have been described: voltage-dependent channels and receptor-operated or pharmacomechanical channels (Meisheri et al., 1981; Somlyo and Somlyo, 1968; Farley and Miles, 1977). The aforementioned Ca^{2+} antagonists are most effective inhibitors of voltage-dependent channels, suggesting that there may be different routes of Ca^{2+} entry into the cell with immunologic and nonimmunologic stimuli. Such a hypothesis is consistent with the observation that Ca^{2+} antagonists are consistently effective in protecting against exercise-induced bronchoconstriction (Cerrina et al., 1981; Henderson et al., 1983; Patel, 1981) but only partially effective against antigen-induced bronchoconstriction (Russi et al., 1985; So et al., 1982; Patel et al., 1983; Ahmed et al., 1985).

β-Adrenergic Agonists

β-Adrenergic agonists have been shown to inhibit mediator release; this action is thought to occur via the drugs' ability to increase intracellular levels of c-AMP. Increased levels of c-AMP have been shown to inhibit the turnover of phospholipids and the phospholipase-related release of arachidonic acid in many cell types (Winslow and Austen, 1982). This inhibition of arachidonate metabolism thereby limits phospholipid metabolism and subsequent alterations in the cell membrane necessary for mediator release. Increased intracellular levels of c-AMP have also been shown to increase the incorporation of ^{32}P into intracellular proteins, which may modulate mediator release (Sieghart et al., 1981; Theoharides et al., 1980).

That β-adrenergic agonists can inhibit allergen-induced mediator release is supported by studies in the skin as well as the airways. Atopic subjects treated by intradermal (i.d.) injection of 1 μg terbutaline followed 5 min later by i.d. injections of specific antigen had significantly reduced wheal and flare responses compared to control challenges (Gronneberg and Starndberg, 1981). Evidence that this protective effect resulted from inhibition of mediator release was provided by studies correlating antigen-induced wheal and flaring, histamine release, and histopathologic examination of mast cells at the injection site (Ting et al., 1983). In these experiments terbutaline produced a dose-dependent decrease in the skin response (wheal and flare) and histamine release to antigen injection. Electron micrographs of skin biopsy specimens from these injection sites indicated that the mast cells were intact in the areas treated with terbutaline, unlike those injected with ragweed alone where there was marked mast cell degranulation (Ting et al., 1983).

Similar observations have been made in the airways. Injection of compound 48/80 into an in situ isolated segment of dog trachea resulted in mast cell degranulation, as evidenced by tracheal contraction and elevated levels of plasma histamine (Brown et al., 1982). When the dogs were pretreated with 10 μg/kg isoproterenol, cyclic AMP levels tripled and subsequent injections of compound 48/80 elicited no tracheal contraction or elevation in plasma histamine. Pretreatment with terbutaline has also been shown to prevent acute antigen-induced bronchoconstriction and decreased tracheal mucus transport in allergic sheep (Weissberger et al., 1981).

In sensitive patients, oral terbutaline suppresses the postantigen rise in plasma histamine and neutrophil chemotactic factor and sharply curtails bronchospasm (Martin et al., 1980). Similar results are reported with inhaled salbutamol (Howarth et al., 1985). Yet, when the dose of antigen is increased so that bronchospasm returns despite terbutaline, plasma mediators remain suppressed, thus defying a simple relationship between the two (Martin et al., 1980).

In some asthmatic patients and certain animal models of allergic airway disease late bronchial obstruction can follow the resolution of acute antigen-induced bronchoconstriction (Pepys and Hutchcroft, 1974; Abraham et al., 1983; Delehunt et al., 1984). Although the pathogenesis of the late response is not completely understood, there is good evidence that these late responses are dependent on mediator release as are acute antigen-induced responses (Abraham et al., 1983; Delehunt et al., 1984). Figure 4 provides support for this argument. In these studies, inhalation of 25 mg metaproterenol prior to the onset of the late bronchial response completely inhibited this response (Perruchoud et al., 1984a). This same dose of metaproterenol, when given after the onset of the late response, failed to reverse the bronchial obstruction. These results suggest that the protective effect of the metaproterenol was probably the result of mediator release inhibition rather than bronchodilation. When this dose of metaproterenol is administered prior to antigen challenge both early and late bronchial responses

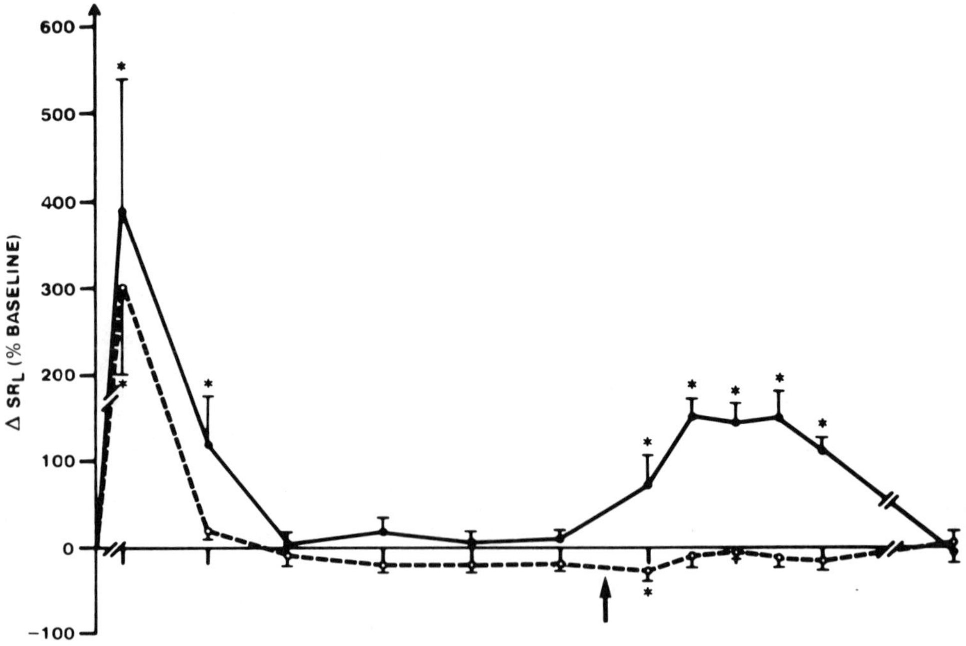

Figure 4 Effect of inhaled metaproterenol (25 mg total dose) on antigen-induced late responses in allergic sheep. Metaproterenol was administered 5½ hr after antigen challenge, before the onset of the late response. Specific lung resistance (SR_L) values are mean ± SE for 7 sheep; *$P < 0.05$ with respect to baseline (based on data from Perruchoud et al., 1984a).

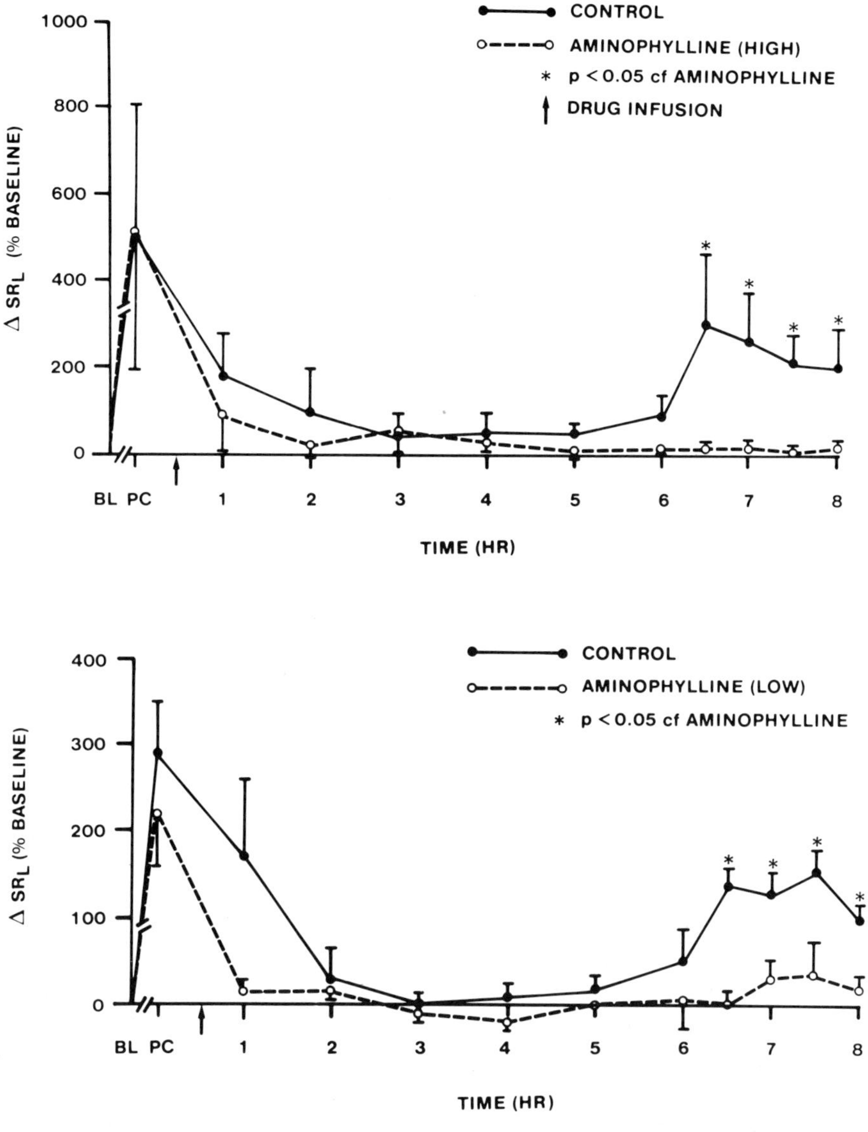

Figure 5 Effect of aminophylline on antigen-induced late responses in allergic sheep. In these experiments aminophylline infusion was initiated (↑) immediately after antigen challenge and maintained throughout the 8-hr experiment. In the top panel, aminophylline levels (mean ± SE) at 2.5 and 8 hr after antigen challenge were 0.8 ± 0.7; 11.99 ± 0.64 and 12.87 ± 1.09 μg/ml, respectively. In the lower panel, aminophylline levels were 4.66 ± 0.44; 4.54 ± 0.49, and 5.19 ± 0.49 μg/ml, respectively. Where aminophylline levels were < 3 μg/ml the late response was not blocked. Specific lung resistance (SR_L) values are mean ± SE for seven sheep (based on data from Perruchoud et al., 1984b).

are prevented (Perruchoud et al., 1984a). Pretreatment with cromolyn sodium produces similar results (Pepys et al., 1975; Abraham et al., 1983).

Methylxanthines

As with cromolyn, corticosteroids, and β-adrenergic agents, pretreatment of patients with theophylline prevents acute antigen-induced bronchoconstriction, elevations in plasma histamine, and increases in neutrophil chemotactic activity (Martin et al., 1980). Slow-release theophyllines have also been reported to inhibit late asthmatic responses to toluendiisocyanate (Crescio et al., 1985). Likewise, aminophylline has been shown to inhibit late asthmatic responses in allergic sheep (Fig. 5). As with the β-adrenergic agents, prevention of the late response by aminophylline is thought to result from mediator release inhibition since these same dosages of aminophylline when given prior to antigen challenge prevent both the early and late bronchial responses (Perruchoud et al., 1984b).

Methylxanthines have traditionally been thought to prevent mediator secretion by the increase of intracellular c-AMP levels through phosphodiesterase inhibition. However, methylxanthine concentrations required for such action are higher than those achieved clinically. Recently, methylxanthines have been shown to competitively antagonize adenosine, a biological modulator (Holgate et al., 1984). This antagonism, unlike that of phosphodiesterase, occurs in the clinically effective dosage range. It is not known if adenosine antagonism relates to the blocking of mediator release.

Glucocorticosteroids

Finally, large numbers of studies have tried to elucidate the mechanism of action of glucocorticosteroids. Among other actions, glucocorticosteroids have been shown to inhibit phospholipase A_2, thereby preventing arachidonate metabolism and hence mediator release. Pharmacologic studies showing that an inhibitor of phospholipase A_2 (P-bromophenacyl-bromide) blocks histamine release support this concept (Peters et al., 1982).

In summary, the beneficial effects of certain pharmacologic agents on mediator release from inflammatory cells are well established and of recognized clinical utility. Some of the underlying mechanisms remain to be elucidated.

IV. Antagonists of Mediators

The next site for possible drug action on mediators includes the specific receptors on target cells in the airway. These receptors are located in different tissues with different functions that have an influence on the pathophysiology of asthma and other forms of bronchial disease. It is therefore useful to consider separately the pharmacologic and physiological effects exerted by antagonists of chemical mediators on the various manifestations of airway disease (Fig. 6). Among the large number of chemical mediators with recognized actions in the airways, end-organ antagonists with clear in vitro and in vivo activity have only been described for histamine and slow reactive substance of anaphylaxis.

The biological role of chemical mediators can be assessed in two ways. One approach involves the application of a stimulus capable of liberating chemical mediators with defined end-organ effects. By observing the modifying actions of specific end-organ antagonists, the putative mediator can be identified. Such experiments tend to simulate tissue concentrations of mediators encountered in "real life." On the other hand, the assumption has to be made that the antagonists are specific for the agonist in question. The other approach is based on the administration of "pure" chemical mediators. While this ensures a high degree of specificity, the tissue concentrations of the exogenous agonists may bear no relationship to tissue concentrations in naturally occuring airway disease.

With these basic considerations in mind, the following discussion is limited to the antagonism of the bronchospasmogenic, mucosal, and vascular effects of histamine and slow reacting substances and includes observations with exogenous agonists only to confirm the experiments involving antagonists.

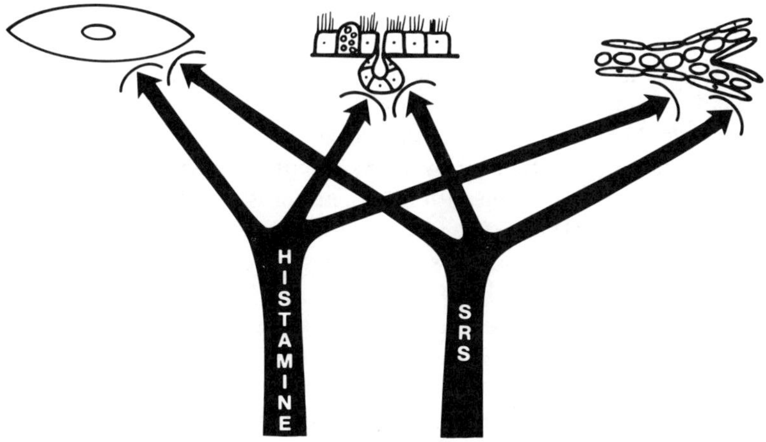

Figure 6 Proposed site of action for antagonists of histamine and slow reacting substance (sulfidopeptideleukotrienes): airway smooth muscle, airway epithelium including mucus-producing structures, and bronchial-vascular bed.

A. Histamine Antagonists

At least two subtypes of histamine receptors have been postulated, based on the ability of certain pharmacologic agents to block some but not all of the actions of histamine, or to reverse or enhance its actions. Most of these observations were made with the guinea pig ileum preparation that exhibits reproducible contractions to histamine. In 1944, Bovet et al. described mepyramine, the first potent histamine antagonist. Almost 30 years later, Black et al. (1972) found that burimamide antagonized histamine effects that were not blocked by the conventional antihistamines, including mepyramine. This led to the pharmacologic classification of histamine receptors into H_1-receptors blocked by mepyramine, and H_2-receptors blocked by burimamide. The list of H_1 and H_2 antagonists has become quite long and most of these compounds have gained wide clinical acceptance for the treatment of many disorders, but not for bronchial asthma. The reasons for the poor therapeutic effects of histamine antagonists in lower airway disease are not quite clear, since both H_1- and H_2-receptors exist in the lung (Ganellin, 1982), and the principal sources of histamine (i.e., the mast cell and basophil) are also present in airway tissues. The potential exists therefore for histamine effects in the airways. However, histamine is usually released transiently in response to a stimulus and rapidly metabolized by histaminase (or diamine oxidase) and histamine methyl transferase within the tissue where it is released. Thus, the role of histamine in the more prolonged (and clinically significant) manifestations of asthma may be limited.

Airway Smooth Muscle

H_1-receptor stimulation causes contraction and H_2-receptor stimulation causes relaxation of airway smooth muscle (Eyre, 1977). Thus, the contractile response to histamine would be expected to be enhanced by an H_2-receptor antagonist, and reversed to a relaxant response by an H_1-receptor antagonist. This has been demonstrated in conscious sheep with histamine-aerosol-induced bronchoconstriction (Ahmed et al., 1980). The increase in pulmonary resistance after inhalation of a 5% histamine solution was potentiated by pretreatment with the H_2-antagonist metiamide, blocked by pretreatment with both metiamide and the H_1-antagonist chlorpheniramine, and converted to a decrease in pulmonary resistance by pretreatment with chlorpheniramine (Fig. 7).

The distribution of H_1 and H_2 receptors in the tracheobronchial tree seems to vary among different species. In the sheep, for instance, Eyre (1969, 1973) reported a preponderance of H_1-receptors in strips of large airways and parenchymal lung strips, whereas H_2-receptors predominated in intermediate size airways. In vivo, the physiological effects of histamine antagonists also de-

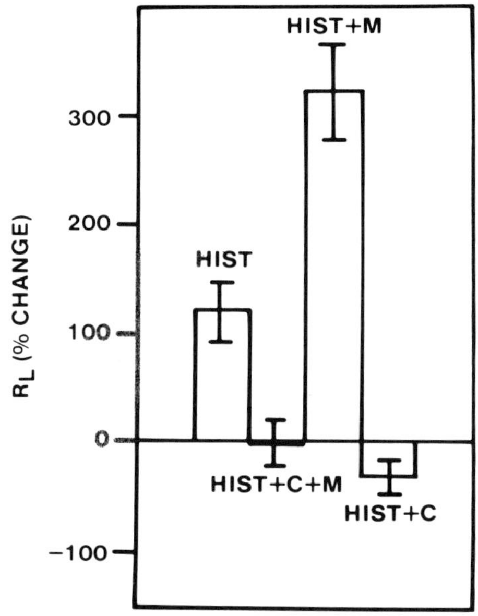

Figure 7 Characterization of H_1- and H_2-histamine receptor function in the airways of conscious sheep. R_L, pulmonary resistance; HIST, histamine aerosol; C, pretreatment with the H_1-receptor antagonist chlorpheniramine (intravenous administration) prior to histamine challenge; M, pretreatment with the H_2-receptor antagonist metiamide (intravenous administration) prior to histamine challenge. Note complete blockade of histamine-induced bronchoconstriction by combined pretreatment with C + M, enhanced histamine-induced bronchoconstriction by pretreatment with M (selective H_1-receptor stimulation), and histamine-induced bronchodilation after pretreatment with C (selective H_2-receptor stimulation) (constructed from data reported by Ahmed et al., 1980).

pend on the dosage and route of administration of the drugs. Thus, the observations of Hartmann et al. (1983) suggest that the H_2-receptor-blocking agent cimetidine produces the expected potentiation of histamine-induced bronchoconstriction at lower doses, but blocks the histamine effects at a high dosage, indicating H_1-receptor antagonism as well (Fig. 8). Such paradoxic actions of histamine antagonists have also been reported in humans (Hartmann et al., 1981; Nathan et al., 1979).

H_1-receptor blockade with chlorpheniramine has been shown to inhibit the immediate response to antigen challenge in allergic sheep (Abraham et al.,

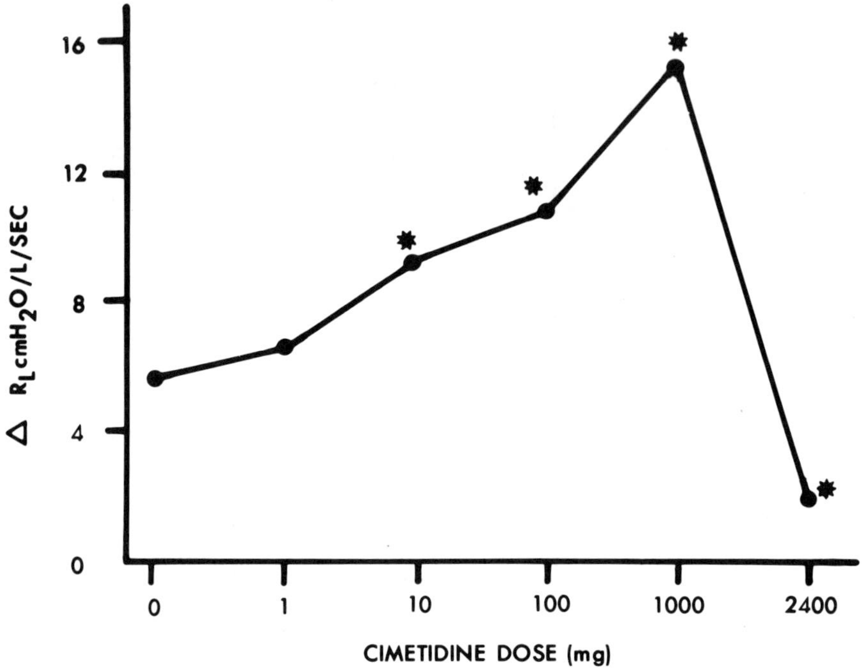

Figure 8 Modification of histamine-induced changes in pulmonary resistance (ΔR_L) with intravenous cimetidine in conscious sheep. Data shown as mean *, different from histamine alone ($P < 0.05$). The dosage-dependent enhancement of histamine-induced bronchoconstriction by the H_2-receptor-blocking agent cimetidine is converted to a blockade at the highest dose, indicating combined H_1- and H_2-receptor blockade (from Hartmann et al., 1983).

1981) (Fig. 3). This suggests that the previously demonstrated histamine release in the lung after antigen challenge is not only a marker of the allergic response but also plays a role in the associated early bronchoconstriction (Chiesa et al., 1975; Lazarus et al., 1979; Patterson et al., 1976a; Bhat et al., 1976). In contrast, when chlorpheniramine was given after resolution of the early antigen-induced response, the drug failed to prevent the late phase response in both asthmatic patients and allergic sheep (Booij-Noord et al., 1971; Delehunt et al., 1984); one might conclude from these findings that histamine is the putative mediator of the immediate, but not late phase response to antigen challenge.

In human subjects with asthma, H_1-receptor blocking agents would be expected to have the greatest potential for success in preventing induced bronchoconstriction rather than reducing baseline bronchomotor tone. Nathan et al.

(1979) observed, after pretreatment with the H_2-receptor blocker cimetidine, a decrease in the provocation dosage of histamine that produced a predetermined degree of bronchospasm, while they observed an increase after pretreatment with the H_1-receptor blocker chlorpheniramine in patients with asthma. This confirms the presence of two histamine receptors in human airways as well. Also in analogy to the observations in allergic animals, chlorpheniramine is capable of blunting the immediate bronchoconstrictor response to antigen in patients with allergic asthma (Popa, 1980). Augmentation of antigen-induced bronchoconstriction by H_2-blocking agents is generally not seen, presumably because of a functional depression of H_2-receptors in the allergic host (Tashkin et al., 1982; Abraham et al., 1981; Ahmed et al., 1983).

The available information therefore suggests that H_1-receptor antagonists can blunt or block the immediate bronchospastic response to antigen in allergic asthma. The protective effect of the agents on bronchospasm induced by exercise, cold air, and air pollutants, or other naturally occurring forms has thus far not been critically evaluated.

Airway Mucociliary Function

The clearly demonstrated impairment of lower airway mucociliary function in patients with asthma and in allergic animals after inhalation of antigen seems to be related, in part, to chemical mediators of anaphylaxis (Wanner, 1979). Theoretically, mucociliary interaction and hence clearance can be disrupted by destruction or dyskinesia of cilia, and alterations in the quantity and quality (rheologic properties) of mucus and periciliary fluid. There is mounting evidence that the abnormal production of mucus and periciliary fluid plays an important role in airway-disease-associated mucociliary dysfunction. Histamine, however, appears to be a weak mediator in this regard. Histamine is a relatively modest stimulator of mucus secretion and of ciliary beat frequency (Shelhamer et al., 1980; Wanner et al., 1983), and augments net ion and water transport toward the airway lumen (Nadel and Davis, 1978). This latter action of histamine appears to be mediated by H_1-receptors. Mucociliary clearance, the end-product of the interaction between cilia and respiratory secretions, is enhanced by histamine thereby eliminating this mediator as a significant contributor to asthma associated mucociliary dysfunction. For this reason, the evaluation of the effects of histamine antagonists on this manifestation of airway disease has not met with much interest.

Bronchial Circulation

Histamine has been clearly shown to influence bronchial vascular smooth muscle tone and permeability. Histamine receptor-blocking agents might therefore be of benefit in asthma associated bronchial vascular congestion and airway wall

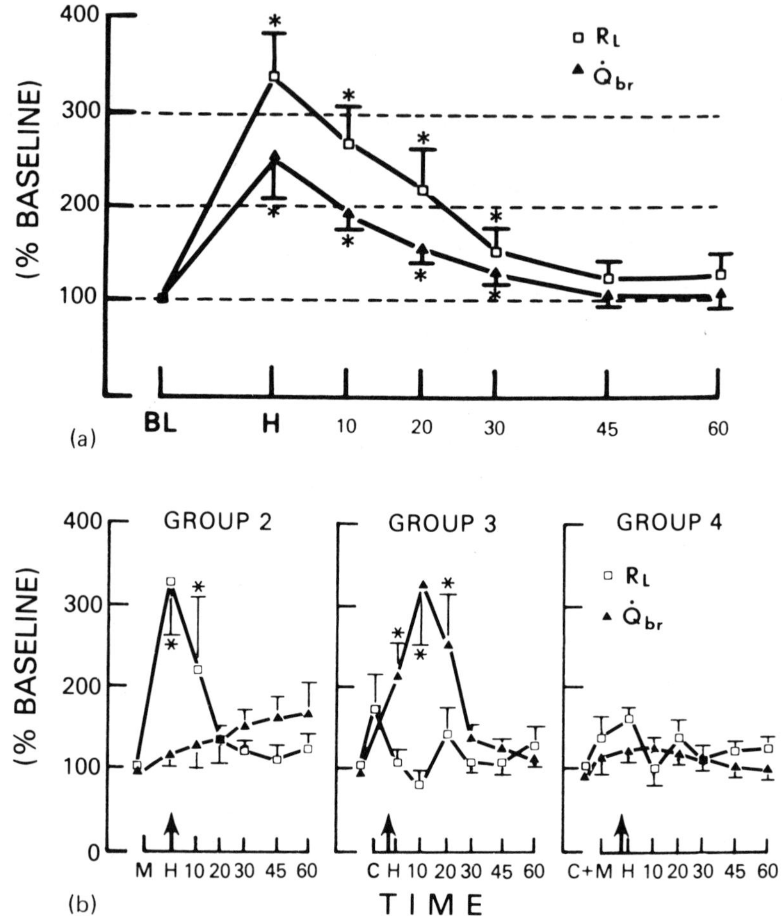

Figure 9 Effect of inhaled histamine on pulmonary resistance (R_L) and bronchial blood flow ($\dot{Q}_{br}$) in sheep. Mean values with S.E. represented by the brackets. *, significantly different from baseline; BL, baseline; H, immediately post-histamine challenge. Time is expressed in minutes. (a) Shows effects of histamine alone. (b) Shows modifying effects of the H_2-receptor antagonist metiamide (M) (group 2), the H_1-receptor antagonist chlorpheniramine (C) (group 3), and combined pretreatment (C + M) (group 4) on histamine-induced changes (from Long et al., 1985).

edema (Dunnill, 1960). Histamine increases bronchial blood flow, presumably by reducing bronchial vascular resistance, and Long et al. (1985) have shown that this is mediated predominantly by H_2-receptors (Fig. 9). The role of histamine in the control of microvascular permeability in the conducting airways has not been studied. In other vascular beds (e.g., pulmonary capillaries, skin capillaries), histamine clearly increases permeability and causes edema (Eyre and Chand, 1982). The respective roles of H_1- and H_2-receptors in the mediation of this effect are controversial. While most investigators agree that H_1-receptors are involved in the increased vascular permeability produced by histamine, the modifying effect of H_2-receptor stimulation is less clear (Chang et al., 1979; Harvey and Schocket, 1980; Nathan et al., 1981; Marks and Greaves, 1977; Ahmed et al., 1983). It appears, however, that in the normal skin, both H_1- and H_2-receptors mediate vascular permeability and have additive effects. In the allergic host, H_2-receptors seem to play a minor role.

B. Antagonists of Slow Reacting Substance

Leukotrienes C_4, D_4, and E_4 (sulfidopeptideleukotrienes) constitute slow reacting substance of anaphylaxis (SRS-A) which has now been shown to play a significant role in the pathogenesis of bronchial asthma. Leukotrienes are generated by mast cells, macrophages, eosinophils, neutrophils, basophils, mononuclear leukocytes, and possibly by various noninflammatory cells in various species including humans (Creticos et al., 1984; Lewis, 1984; Patterson et al., 1976b). The half-life of leukotrienes in lung tissue probably varies among the leukotrienes C_4 (LTC_4), D_4 (LTD_4), and E_4 (LTE_4), which are derived from each other in alphabetical order. In guinea pig lung, the half-life of LTD_4 has been shown to approximate 50 min (Sirois and Brousseau, 1983). To date, LTC_4 and LTD_4 receptors have been demonstrated in cell membranes obtained from guinea pig lungs, but it can be expected that these receptors will soon be found in more specific tissues and in other species as well (Hogaboom et al., 1983).

Since SRS-A is liberated during inflammatory processes in the airways and has profound effects on airway smooth muscle, mucociliary function and microvascular permeability, end-organ antagonists of SRS-A are of potential benefit in bronchial asthma. Several substances with leukotriene receptor blocking effect have been tested or are undergoing testing. A group of chemically related compounds, the first representative of which (FPL-55712) was originally described by Augstein et al. (1973), has been most extensively studied. The competitive receptor-blocking effect of FPL-55712 has been demonstrated by its ability to produce a parallel shift of the contractile response curve of guinea pig ileum to SRS-A without reducing the maximum response (Sheard et al., 1982). However, a Schild plot did not suggest true antagonism, probably due to the impurity of the SRS-A, which was obtained from biological sources. When FPL-55712 was used to antagonize LTC_4- and LTD_4-induced contractions, true competitive inhibition was demonstrated. This specificity of FPL-55712 for LTC_4 and LTD_4 receptors in several tissues (including lung) have been confirmed by other investigators (Holme et al., 1980; Mong et al., 1984). FPL-55712 is a weak antagonist of LTB_4, but appears to have effects on LTE_4-induced contractions as well (Welton et al., 1981a; Sirois et al., 1983; Bray, 1983). Recent work suggests the presence of at least two subtypes of LTD_4 receptors, one with a high affinity, one with a low affinity for FPL-55712 (Fleisch et al., 1982; Krell et al., 1983). Thus, subtypes of leukotriene receptors may exist in the airways. The physiological significance of these remains to be established.

In addition to the antagonism of SRS-A, FPL-55712 has other weak pharmacologic effects. These include inhibition of 5-lipoxygenase (leukotriene generation), mediator release (antiallergic), and phosphodiesterase (Buckle et al., 1979; Casey et al., 1983; Welton et al., 1981b; Chasin and Scott, 1978). Newer derivatives of FPL-55712, such as FPL-57231 and FPL-59257, seem to be more specific SRS-A antagonists with fewer additional actions (Sheard et al., 1982).

Airway Smooth Muscle

Leukotriene C_4 and LTD_4 have been shown to produce dosage-dependent bronchoconstriction in animals and humans, after both intravenous and aerosol administrations (Hamel et al., 1982; Bisgaard et al., 1983; Griffin et al., 1983). Leukotriene C_4 and LTD_4 are more potent bronchoconstrictors than histamine (Barnes et al., 1984; Weiss et al., 1982). In contrast to LTC_4 and LTD_4, LTE_4 may have more pronounced effects on central airways (Drazen et al., 1982). The duration of bronchoconstriction following a single administration of LTC_4 and LTD_4 inhalation challenge is 60-90 min (Holroyde et al., 1981). Whether SRS-A has direct or indirect (via activation of cyclooxygenase) smooth muscle effects, the actions are believed to be mediated by leukotriene receptors (Weichman et al., 1982; Leitch et al., 1983; Zijlstra et al., 1983).

With the exception of a few incidental in vivo observations in humans, the influence of leukotriene antagonists on airway smooth muscle has only been studied in vitro and in intact animal models (Holroyde et al., 1982). For example, FPL-55712 antagonizes SRS-A-induced contractions of human bronchial and parenchymal strips, and reverses the antigen-induced prolonged contraction (Adams and Lichtenstein, 1979; Ghelani et al., 1980).

Leukotriene antagonists have also been used to determine the role of SRS-A in the immediate and late phase responses to inhalation challenge with antigen. In allergic sheep, the principal mediator of the immediate response is histamine, while SRS-A seems to play an important role in the late phase response

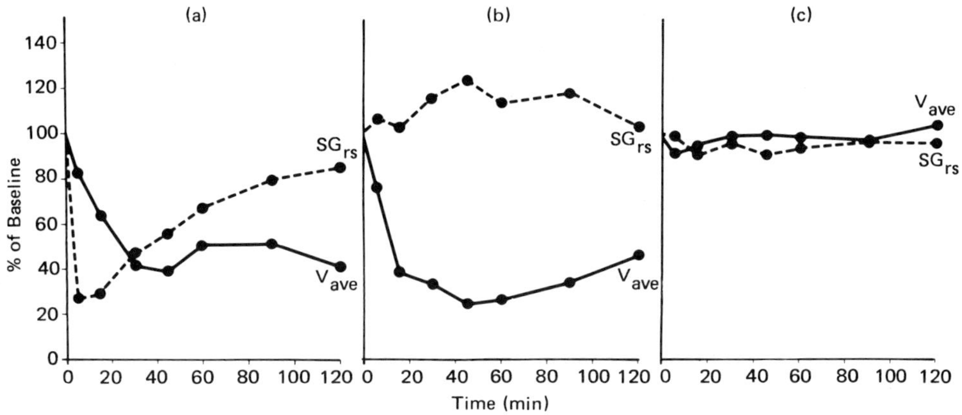

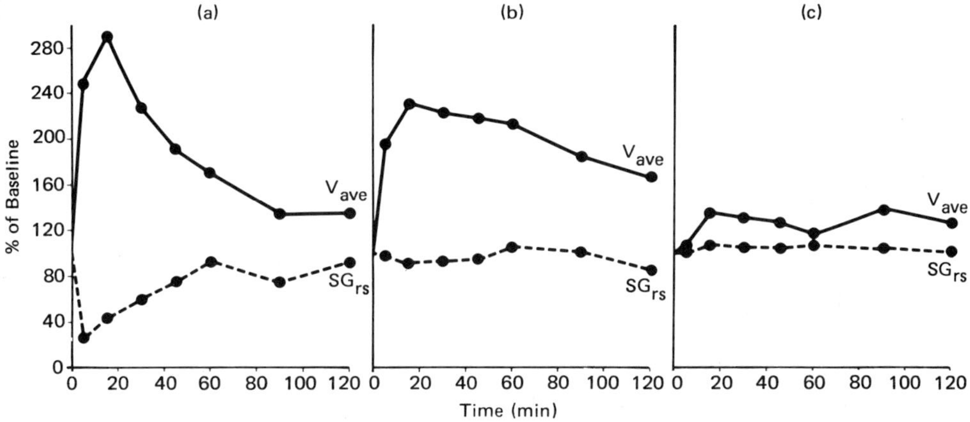

Figure 10 Relative changes in respiratory system conductance (SG_{rs}) and average tracheal mucus velocity (V_{ave}) after *Ascaris suum* challenge in dogs sensitized to *Ascaris suum* but not ragweed extract. Time 0 represents baseline values. (Top) depicts *Ascaris suum* challenge alone: dogs who responded to *Ascaris suum* challenge with bronchospasm (a); dogs with no bronchospastic response to *Ascaris suum* challenge (b); control dogs who inhaled ragweed extract (c). (Bottom). Effects of combined *Ascaris suum* antigen and FPL-55712 (SRS-A antagonist) challenge: dogs who responded with bronchospasm (a); dogs with no bronchospastic response (b); control dogs who inhaled FPL-55712 alone (c) (from Wanner et al., 1975).

(Abraham et al., 1981; Delehunt et al., 1984) (Fig. 3). In those experiments, the administration of cromolyn sodium (inhibition of mediator secretion) or of FPL-55712 after resolution of the immediate response prevented the late phase response, whereas chlorpheniramine was ineffective when given at the same time. It remains to be shown if these relationships are also present in other animal models and patients with bronchial asthma.

Airway Mucociliary Function

Patients with bronchial asthma have an impaired mucociliary clearance in the lower airways (Mezey et al., 1978; Bateman et al., 1979; Santa Cruz et al., 1974). In patients with allergic asthma, inhalation challenge with specific antigen causes a further depression in mucociliary clearance that can be prevented by the prior administration of cromolyn sodium (Mezey et al., 1978). This suggests an involvement of chemical mediators in antigen-induced mucociliary dysfunction which, in allergic sheep, has been shown to last 7-14 days after a single challenge (Allegra et al., 1983). A series of animal studies involving allergic dogs and sheep demonstrated that SRS-A rather than histamine is responsible for the depression of mucociliary clearance after antigen challenge (Wanner et al., 1975; Russi et al., 1983). FPL-55712 converted the antigen-induced depression of tracheal mucociliary transport into a stimulation, presumably due to the unopposed stimulatory effect of histamine when the depressant effect of SRS-A was antagonized by the FPL compound (Fig. 10). Similar observations have been made in patients with allergic asthma (Ahmed et al., 1981) (Fig. 11).

All of the component functions of mucociliary interaction, that is, ciliary activity, mucus secretion, and the production of periciliary fluid, are influenced by SRS-A. However, alterations of respiratory secretions by SRS-A seem to be more relevant to airway disease than changes in ciliary function. Leukotriene C_4 causes dosage-dependent ciliostimulation in vitro, and the transient ciliostimulatory effects of antigen-induced mediator secretion can be blocked by cromolyn sodium as well as FPL-55712 (but not H_1- and H_2-receptor blockers), suggesting a putative role of SRS-A (Maurer et al., 1982a,b). This transient increase in ciliary activity is unlikely to depress mucociliary clearance. In contrast, SRS-A-related quantitative and possibly qualitative alterations of mucus and periciliary fluid may well explain the impairment of mucociliary function. By using IgE-sensitized human airway fragments, Shelhamer et al. (1980) found a 35% increase in radiolabeled glycoprotein secretion after the administration of antigen to the preparation. In subsequent experiments, the same group of investigators showed that the anaphylactic release of glycoproteins is mediated primarily by lipoxygenase products of arachidonic acid including monohydroxyeicosatetraenoic acid, LTC_4 and LTD_4 (Marom et al., 1981, 1982). Similar observations were made by Phipps et al. (1983a) who studied the effects of purified

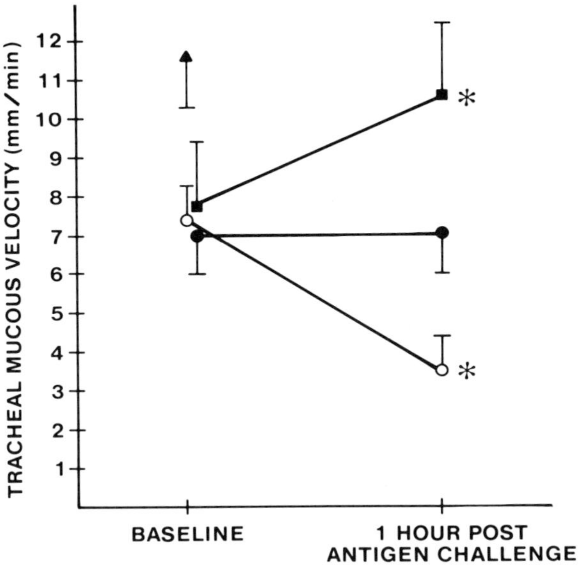

Figure 11 Effect of inhalation challenge with ragweed aerosol on tracheal mucus velocity in asymptomatic patients with ragweed asthma. Mean values with SE represented by bracket. *, significantly different from baseline; o, antigen-chllenge alone; ●, antigen challenge after cromolyn pretreatment; ■, antigen challenge after pretreatment with the SRS-A antagonist FPL-55712. The dosage of antigen was the same with or without pretreatment, and was defined as that required to decrease specific airway conductance by 35% after control antigen challenge (o). Note prevention of the antigen-induced depression of tracheal mucus velocity by cromolyn, and its conversion to a stimulation by FPL-55712. Also note depressed baseline tracheal mucus velocity in patients compared to normal age-matched non-smokers (▲) (constructed from data published by Mezey et al., 1978; Ahmed et al., 1981).

Ascaris suum antigen on tracheal glycoprotein secretion in vitro by using pieces of trachea obtained from allergic sheep who had previously responded with bronchospasm to inhaled *Ascaris suum* extract. *Ascaris suum* antigen increased the secretion of radiolabeled glycoprotein by about 60%. Both cromolyn and FPL-55712 blocked this effect. Recent work has suggested that the receptors mediating the secretagogue and spasmogenic actions of LTC_4 and LTD_4 may be stereochemically different (Coles et al., 1983). The changes in airway fluid observed after antigen challenge seem to relate more to SRSA than histamine (Phipps et al., 1983b).

These data assign a considerable importance to SRS-A in the pathogenesis of mucociliary dysfunction, primarily by excessive production of mucus. Therefore, the contribution of SRS-A to mucociliary dysfunction in airway disease offers new therapeutic approaches in the form of leukotriene antagonists.

Bronchial Circulation

The effects of SRS-A on bronchial blood flow and microvascular permeability have not been evaluated. In the skin, LTC_4, LTD_4, and LTE_4 have all been shown to produce vasodilation and increase microvascular permeability (Soter et al., 1983; Peck et al., 1981; Camp et al., 1982). Similar observations have been made in the vascular bed of the hamster cheek pouch (Dahlen et al., 1981). The SRS-A-induced hyperpermeability appears to be located primarily at the level of the postcapillary venules (Soter et al., 1983). Leukotriene C_4 and LTD_4 are more potent than LTE_4 in this regard; in comparison to histamine, the potency of SRS-A is greater by several orders of magnitude. The vascular smooth muscle effect of SRS-A seems to be species-specific. For example, SRS-A may cause vasoconstriction in the guinea pig skin while it is a vasodilator in human skin (Soter et al., 1983; Peck et al., 1981).

The role of SRS-A in the bronchial hyperemia and edema formation of bronchial asthma is currently being investigated. This will require the use of SRS-A antagonists.

V. Modification of Receptor Function

A. Abnormal Receptor Function in Airway Disease

The proposed mechanisms underlying airway hyperreactivity of bronchial asthma include diminished β-adrenergic responsiveness (Szantivanyi, 1968), increased cholinergic responsiveness (Simonsson et al., 1967), increased α-adrenergic activity (Henderson et al., 1979), and suppressed H_2-histamine receptor function (Ahmed et al., 1983). Before we discuss the pharmacologic modification of these receptor functions, it is important to evaluate the nature of their dysfunction in airway disease.

β-Adrenergic Suppression

The evidence for this concept has been extensively reviewed by Szantivanyi (1968) who proposed the theory of "β-adrenergic blockade" as the pathogenetic mechanism in asthma. Malfunction of the β-adrenergic receptors in other tissues has also been postulated to account for a variety of related conditions that often precede or accompany asthma, such as atopic dermatitis and allergic rhinitis. A number of studies have examined the possibility that bronchial asthma might be associated with partial β-adrenergic blockade similar to that observed in pertussis-sensitized animals (Kind, 1958; Parfentjev and Goodline, 1948). Several approaches have been used: (1) estimation of metabolic responses to exogenous catecholamine, such as changes in plasma concentration of glucose, lactate, pyruvate, and free fatty acids (Lockey et al., 1967; Kirkpatrick and Keller, 1967; Middleton and Finke, 1968); (2) measurements of cardiovascular responses to exogenous catecholamines (Cookson and Reed, 1963; Grieco et al., 1968; Grieco and Pierson, 1969); (3) eosinopenic responsiveness (Reed et al., 1970); (4) determining the effect of β-adrenergic blocking drugs in patients with asthma (Richardson and Sterling, 1969); and (5) determining the activity of adenyl-cyclase and ATPase in isolated leukocytes (Parker and Smith, 1973). Although there are some discrepancies, the data generally suggest that asthmatic patients indeed have abnormal responses to administered sympathomimetic amines and that some of the alterations mirror the responses observed in normal subjects treated with the β-adrenergic blocking agent propranolol.

Isoproterenol has been reported to produce a smaller rise in blood glucose, lactate, and pyruvate concentration (Lockey et al., 1967; Kirkpatrick and Keller, 1967; Middleton and Finke, 1968), a smaller vasodilator response (Cookson and Reed, 1963; Grieco et al., 1968; Grieco and Pierson, 1969), and a smaller eosinopenic response in asthmatic patients than in normal subjects (Reed et al., 1970). Recent investigations have also suggested that the lymphocytes of asthmatic children exhibited less isoproterenol-induced suppression of DNA synthesis, a finding consistent with blockade of lymphocyte β-adrenergic receptors (Smith et al., 1971). Similarly, leukocytes of asthmatic subjects show reduced isoproterenol stimulated synthesis of cyclic AMP (Parker and Smith, 1973). However, most of these studies were conducted in extrapulmonary tissues and direct evidence for suppressed β-receptors in airway smooth muscle is still lacking.

The pathogenesis of β-receptor blockade in bronchial asthma is not known (however, see Chapter 7). Circulating autoantibodies specific for the β_2-adrenergic receptor have been demonstrated in subjects with allergic airway disease (Venter et al., 1980). In subsequent studies it was observed that the presence of β-receptor autoantibodies correlated with abnormalities of the autonomic nervous system, particularly β-adrenergic hyporesponsiveness (Fraser et al., 1981). Furthermore, these autoantibodies also seem to inhibit the β-receptor activation of adenylate cyclase. However, the relevance of these antibodies to asthma, their correlation with disease and its severity, and their overall incidence is not well understood at present (Parker, 1981).

Cholinergic Hyperreactivity

Several lines of evidence suggest a potentially important role for the parasympathetic nervous system in the pathophysiology of allergic asthma. It has been observed that cholinergic agents greatly enhance the immunologic release of chemical mediators from human lung tissue in vitro, and attenuate the inhibitory effects of β-adrenergic stimuli (Kaliner et al., 1972). Chemical mediators, either released by antigen challenge or directly inhaled, may stimulate afferent cholinergic pathways via irritant receptors with resultant efferent vagal discharges producing bronchospasm in experimental animals and man (Simonsson et al., 1967; Karczewski and Widdicombe, 1969; Nadel, 1968). Thus, asthmatic subjects are more sensitive to the bronchoconstrictive effects of acetylcholine and other cholinergic agonists (Curry, 1946). Furthermore, bronchoconstriction produced by inhalation of antigen, sulfur dioxide, ozone, and other pollutants may be prevented by vagotomy in animals or by atropine blockade in humans (Boushey et al., 1980). All of these studies have pointed to a fundamental abnormality in the parasympathetic nervous system, and cholinergic hyperreactivity is considered a hallmark of bronchial asthma (Simonsson et al., 1967). The demonstration by Kaliner (1976) that patients with allergic rhinitis alone or in combination with asthma display a hyperresponsiveness of eccrine sweat responses to cholinergic agents suggests that the cholinergic hyperreactivity may also be a generalized defect and, along with suppressed β-receptors, may be part of an overall autonomic imbalance.

α-Adrenergic Hyperreactivity

Several observations lend support to the hypothesis that there is hyperresponsiveness of α-adrenergic receptors in reversible obstructive airway disease. First, Kneussel and Richardson (1978) demonstrated α-receptor responsiveness in human bronchial smooth muscle obtained at autopsy from patients with chronic bronchitis but not from normal control subjects. Second, the administration of α-adrenergic receptor agonists has been reported to increase airflow resistance in asthmatics but not in normal subjects (Snasshall et al., 1978). Third, increased vascular and pupillary α-receptor responsiveness has been found in allergic asthmatics, thus suggesting that, like the β-receptor hyperresponsiveness, α-receptor hyperresponsiveness may also be a generalized defect (Henderson et al., 1979). However, these findings have not been confirmed by others. Thus, Barnes et al. (1981) have shown that prazosin, a potent and selective α_1-antagonist, produces no changes in airway resistance in asthmatic subjects who respond to albuterol with bronchodilatation. Similarly, Thompson et al. (1982), using phenylephrine, were unable to demonstrate any α_1-adrenergic activity in the airway of asthmatics.

The presence of α-receptor sites has not been convincingly demonstrated in normal human subjects. However, it is possible that these receptors may be unmasked in disease states, such as bronchial asthma. Of particular interest is the finding by Simonsson et al. (1972) that endotoxin treatment could greatly enhance the responsiveness of human bronchi to an α agonist. The mechanism responsible for the unmasking of α-receptors in disease states, however, is not known.

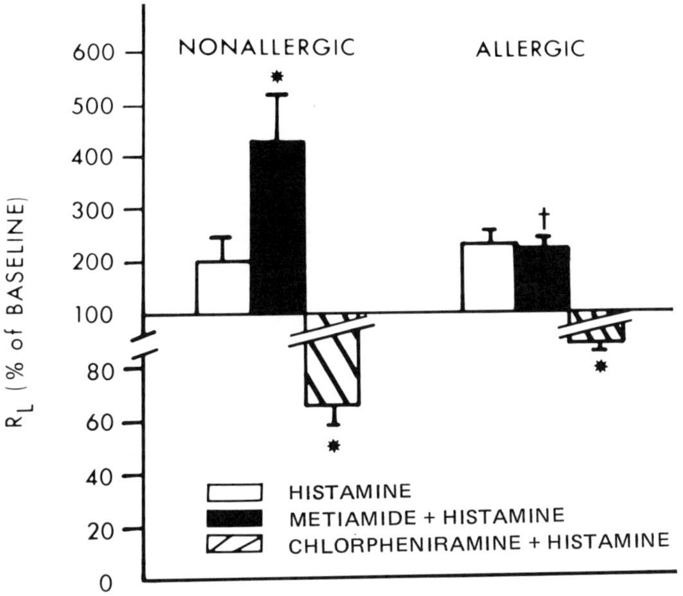

Figure 12 Comparative effect of histamine on pulmonary resistance (R_L) in nonallergic and allergic sheep, without and with antihistamine pretreatment. Histamine alone (open bars); histamine followed by metiamide pretreatment (closed bars); histamine after chlorpheniramine pretreatment (hatched bars). Data are shown as mean with SE. *, different from histamine alone ($P < 0.05$); †, different from the nonallergic group ($P < 0.05$) (from Ahmed et al., 1983).

Depression of H_2-Histamine Receptors

Increased bronchial reactivity to histamine is of special interest in view of its role in IgE-mediated allergic asthma. In allergic sheep, airway hyperreactivity to histamine seems to be related to a functional depression of H_2-receptors (Ahmed et al., 1983). This conclusion was based upon the absence of H_2-mediated bronchodilator effects of histamine in the airway of sheep allergic to *Ascaris suum* antigen (Fig. 12). Such a defect was also observed in extrabronchial and extrapulmonary sites such as the skin, and the pulmonary and systemic vasculature (Ahmed et al., 1983; Ahmed and King, 1983b).

In contrast to these data in allergic sheep, no study has thus far demonstrated the suppression of airway H_2-receptor function in subjects with allergic bronchial asthma. In fact, the data on airway H_1- and H_2-receptors in normals and subjects with bronchial asthma are quite conflicting. Using oral cimetidine as the H_2-antagonist, protection, enchancement or no effect against histamine-induced bronchoconstriction has been reported (Eiser et al., 1979; Maconochie et al., 1979; Nathan et al., 1981). The reason for these inconsistent findings in human subjects is not clear. Variations in the dosage of cimetidine, route of administration, and type of H_2-receptor antagonist may be some of the factors responsible.

The evidence for suppression of H_2-histamine receptors in human subjects with allergic bronchial asthma comes from extrapulmonary sites: white blood cells and stomach (Busse and Sosman, 1977; Beer et al., 1982; Ahmed and Gonzalez, 1985). Busse and Sosman (1977) have demonstrated a suppression of H_2-receptors on polymorphonuclear neutrophils of human asthmatics. Those investigators observed that inhibition by histamine of serum-activated, zymosan-induced lysosomal enzyme release was an H_2-receptor response that paralleled the increases in intracellular cyclic AMP. As compared to normal subjects, the H_2-histamine response of granulocytes from patients with asthma was decreased. Beer and associates (1982) have observed that atopic subjects were less able to produce histamine-induced suppression of T-cell activity, which correlated with decreased phenotypic expression of histamine H_2-receptors. The results of a recent study have suggested that patients with allergic bronchial asthma also exhibit suppressed gastric H_2-receptor function as assessed by the analysis of stimulated gastric acid output (Ahmed and Gonzalez, 1985). Peak acid output (PAO) was used as an indicator of stimulated gastric acid output following histalogue administration. Although no difference was observed in the basal acid output between the two groups, the asthmatic group had a significantly lower PAO. Pretreatment with the H_2-antagonist cimetidine suppressed PAO both in normals and asthmatics; however, the degree of suppression was greater in the normals. Thus the gastric acid secretion mediated by selective H_2-stimulation was lower in the asthmatic group. Although H_2-receptor defect has not been demonstrated in the airways of asthmatic subjects, it is of interest that cimetidine has no known adverse effect on clinical bronchial asthma, an effect one would expect if H_2-receptor function was intact.

B. Pharmacologic Modification of Receptor Function

A number of drugs used for the treatment of bronchial asthma modify the function of various receptors, either by causing down-regulation of the same receptor or by interfering with the function of other receptors.

β-Adrenergic Receptor Function

There is mounting evidence that glucocorticosteroids modify β-adrenergic receptor function. The generally accepted model of glucocorticosteroid action is via DNA-dependent, RNA-mediated protein synthesis. However, how this action ultimately interferes with the pathogenesis of bronchial asthma has not been conclusively elucidated. The mechanism of action of glucocorticosteroids in allergic airway disease is perhaps multifactorial, involving the generation and release of various mediators and the responsiveness of their receptor sites (Morris, 1985). The effects of glucocorticosteroids on β-adrenergic receptors have been studied in detail. It has been observed that within 4 hr of in vivo administration, glucocorticosteroids increase the density of β-adrenergic receptors in neutrophils and decrease those in lymphocytes (Davies and Lefkowitz, 1980). By 24 hr, the receptor density is increased in both types of cells due to enhanced receptor synthesis. Similarly, β-receptor affinity and coupling to adenylcyclase also increased, as demonstrated by an agonist-promoted high affinity state of β-adrenergic receptors in human neutrophils (Davies and Lefkowitz, 1981). Such studies are of clinical importance. Chronic therapy with β-adrenergic agonist, either in vivo or in vitro, causes desensitization or down-regulation of β-receptor function as assessed by diminished cyclic AMP responses to adrenergic stimulation (Morris et al., 1977). A variable degree of β-receptor desensitization also occurs in other tissues. Glucocorticosteroids have been shown to attenuate this agonist-induced desensitization of β-receptors (Davies and Lefkowitz, 1983). Pharmacologic concentrations of glucocorticosteroids increase β-adrenergic responsiveness in human tracheal muscle preparation exposed to propanolol (Townley et al., 1970). In vivo human studies are consistent with this concept, and glucocorticosteroids have been shown to potentiate or restore the bronchodilator responses to β-adrenergic agonists. Apart from their effects on the adrenergic receptors, other mechanisms may also contribute to the synergism between glucocorticosteroids and adrenergic agents (Morris, 1985). These include the influence of glucocorticosteroids on a cyclic AMP dependent protein-kinase that may enhance the effectiveness of cyclic AMP even when the quantity is unchanged. Glucocorticosteroids also prolong the action of endogenous catecholamines by interfering with their extraneuronal uptake and inactivation. Synthetic β-adrenergic agonists, however, are not influenced by this glucocorticosteroid action.

Other drugs that do not directly affect the β-adrenergic receptor function may alter the responsiveness of airway smooth muscle by modifying the activity of adenyl-cyclase and thus affecting the production of cyclic AMP. Diminished cyclic AMP responsiveness to β-adrenergic agonist in the leukocytes and lymphocytes of asthmatic individuals is a selective phenomenon, as the cyclic AMP response to prostaglandin E_1 (PGE_1) is normal (Parker et al., 1973a,b). Whereas glucocorticosteroids demonstrate a synergistic effect with β-adrenergic agonists, the effects of PGE_1 and β-adrenergic agonists are simply additive. Thus, PGE_1 per se does not alter β-adrenergic receptor function, but may alter the response by independently stimulating cyclic AMP. These observations are also supported by the finding that adenyl-cyclase in human leukocytes is stimulated by separately located beta-adrenergic and prostaglandin receptors (Bourne and Melmon, 1971). This may be of therapeutic importance in individuals with resistant asthma, especially those with resistance or tolerance to β-adrenergic agonists and a contraindication to therapy with glucocorticosteroids.

Muscarine Receptors

Muscarine agonists (e.g., acetylcholine) produce their effects through the activation of postganglionic muscarine receptors in the airways. Cholinergic hyperreactivity is a characteristic feature of bronchial asthma (Simonsson et al., 1967), and a temporary enhancement of cholinergic bronchial reactivity has been observed during pollen season (Sotomayor et al., 1984) or following an upper respiratory tract infection (Empey et al., 1976). This temporary enhancement of cholinergic bronchial reactivity can be prevented by glucocorticosteroids (Sotomayor et al., 1984). However, the data concerning the effects of oral glucocorticosteroids on basal bronchial reactivity remain controversial. Tiffeneau and Dunoyen (1956) have reported that the administration of oral glucocorticosteroids does not change airway hyperreactivity to inhaled cholinergic agonists in patients with asthma. Similar observations were recently made by Wolfe et al. (1979) and Easton (1981), using oral and inhaled glucocorticosteroids, respectively. In contrast, Arkins et al. (1968) have demonstrated an increase in methacholine reactivity in 7 of 11 asthmatic subjects after 2 weeks of daily oral glucocorticosteroid administration. The reason for this enhanced methacholine reactivity is unclear. In sheep, pharmacologic dosages of methylprednisolone (30 mg/kg) are unable to block or enhance carbachol-induced bronchoconstriction (Ahmed and King, 1983a). Thus the mechanism whereby glucocorticosteroids prevent the temporary enhancement of cholinergic reactivity during pollen season is unlikely to be related to any modification of muscarine receptor function. A recent study lends further support to this hypothesis, by demonstrating the failure of atropine, an antimuscarinic agent, to prevent this temporary enhancement of muscarinic hyperreactivity (Phillipe-Boudet et al., 1984).

Whether chronic glucocorticosteroid therapy alters the muscarine receptor density in the airways of asthmatic subjects is not known. The muscarine receptor density in rat lung membranes, chronically treated with glucocorticosteroids, is significantly increased (Marquardt et al., 1982). However, the significance of such a finding is presently unknown.

Histamine Receptor Function

The effects of glucocorticosteroids or other pharmacologic agents on histamine receptor function in humans are, to our knowledge, not known. In sheep, a single injection of methylprednisolone (30 mg/kg) 30 min before histamine challenge has the ability to suppress the airway responsiveness to histamine (Ahmed and King, 1983a) (Fig. 13). After pretreatment with methylprednisolone, histamine increased mean pulmonary airflow resistance (R_L) in that study to

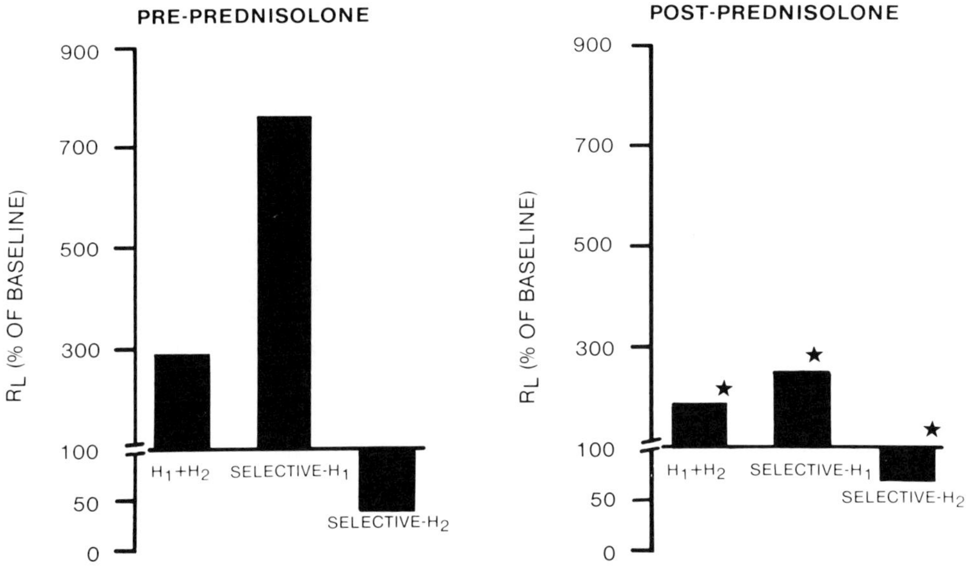

Figure 13 Modification of histamine receptor function with methylprednisolone succinate (30 mg/kg) administered as a single intravenous bolus 30 min before histamine aerosol challenge in allergic sheep. R_L, pulmonary resistance. Data expressed as mean and SE. *, different from preprednisolone value ($P < 0.05$). Selective H_1- and H_2-receptor stimulation was accomplished by pretreatment with the appropriate histamine antagonist (from Ahmed et al., 1983).

186% of baseline, which was significantly lower than the 290% increase in R_L without glucocorticosteroid pretreatment. This suppression of histamine responsiveness with methylprednisolone may have resulted from (1) a blunted H_1-receptor-mediated bronchoconstrictor action of histamine, or (2) enhanced H_2-receptor-mediated bronchodilator action. The data suggested that the blunted histamine responsiveness after methylprednisolone was entirely accounted for by a suppression of H_1-receptor function, without an enhancement of H_2-receptor function. Selective stimulation of H_1-receptors without methylprednisolone pretreatment increased R_L to 760% of baseline, whereas after methylprednisolone pretreatment selective H_1-stimulation increased R_L to 248% of baseline, thus demonstrating a marked suppression of H_1-receptor function. The mechanism whereby methylprednisolone suppressed H_1-receptors is not clear; as biochemical or radioligand studies have not been performed. A decreased activity of H_1-receptors, a lowered binding or affinity of receptors, an actual decrease in the number of H_1-receptors, or a combination thereof may be involved in the glucocorticosteroid-induced suppression of H_1-receptor function.

α-Adrenergic Receptors

The effects of glucocorticosteroids on airway α-adrenergic receptors are not known. This is partly due to the fact that the exact role of α-adrenergic receptors (whether masked or unmasked) in human airway disease has not been well established. However, in extrapulmonary tissues (i.e., aorta) hydrocortisone has been shown to potentiate the vascular responses mediated by both α- and β-adrenergic agonists (Kalsner, 1969).

VI. Conclusions

This review suggests that several pharmacologic agents are capable of interfering with the generation, secretion and actions, of inflammatory mediators under experimental conditions. However, the role of drugs with well-defined, selective effects on the different steps of the mediator cascade in the prevention and treatment of bronchial asthma and other types of bronchial disease is limited. Glucocorticosteroids, cromolyn, β-adrenergic agonists, and methylxanthines, while clinically effective, have been shown to possess the ability to act on more than one site in the mediator pathway. It is therefore often difficult to determine which effect predominates in a patient with airway disease. On the other hand, pharmacologic agents with a unique site of action are either clinically ineffective or weakly effective (e.g., histamine receptor antagonists), or have not been released for clinical use. However, the wealth of basic information accumulated in vitro and in vivo both in animal models and human subjects is expected to lay the foundation for the development of exciting new drugs for the management of patients with airway disease.

References

Abraham, W. M., Oliver, W. Jr., King, M. M., Yerger, L., and Wanner, A. (1981). Effect of pharmacologic agents on antigen-induced decreases in specific lung conductance in sheep. *Am. Rev. Respir. Dis. 124*: 554-558.

Abraham, W. M., Delehunt, J. C., Yerger, L., and Marchette, B. (1983). Characterization of a late phase pulmonary response after antigen challenge in allergic sheep. *Am. Rev. Respir. Dis. 128*: 839-844.

Adams, G. K., and Lichtenstein, L. (1979). *In vitro* studies of antigen-induced bronchospasm: Effect of antihistamine and SRS-A antagonist on response of sensitized guinea pig and human airways to antigen. *J. Immunol. 122*: 555-562.

Ahmed, T., and King, M. M. (1983a). Modification of airway histamine receptor function with methylprednisolone succinate. *J. Allergy Clin. Immunol. 71*: 224-229.

Ahmed, T., and King, M. (1983b). Functional depression of pulmonary and systemic vascular H_2-histamine receptors in allergic sheep. *Am. Rev. Respir. Dis. 127*(4): 302 (abstract).

Ahmed, T., Eyre, P., Januszkiewicz, A. J., and Wanner, A. (1980). Role of H_1- and H_2-receptors in airway reactions to histamine in conscious sheep. *J. Appl. Physiol. 49*: 826-833.

Ahmed, T., Greenblatt, D. W., Birch, S., Marchette, B., and Wanner, A. (1981). Abnormal mucociliary transport in allergic patients with antigen-induced bronchospasm: Role of slow reacting substances of analphylaxis. *Am. Rev. Respir. Dis. 124*: 110-114.

Ahmed, T., Krainson, J. P., and Yerger, L. D. (1983). Functional depression of H_2 histamine receptors in sheep with experimental allergic asthma. *J. Allergy Clin. Immunol. 72*: 310-320.

Ahmed, T., Russi, E., Kim, C. S., and Danta, I. (1985). Comparative effects of oral and inhaled verapamil on antigen-induced bronchoconstriction. *Chest 88*: 176-180.

Allan, G., and Eakins, K. E. (1978). Burimamide is a selective inhibitor of thromboxane A_2 biosynthesis in human platelet microsomes. *Prostaglandins 15*: 659-661.

Allegra, L., Abraham, W. M., Chapman, G. A., and Wanner, A. (1983). Duration of mucociliary dysfunction following antigen challenge in allergic sheep. *J. Appl. Physiol. 55*: 726-730.

Anderson, W. H. (1985). Biochemical mediators: release, chemistry, and function. In *Bronchial Asthma: Mechanisms and Therapeutics.* Edited by E. B. Weiss, M. S. Segal, and M. Stein. Boston/Toronto, Little, Brown, pp. 57-87.

Arkins, J. A., Schleuter, D. P., and Fink, J. N. (1968). The effect of corticosteroids on methacholine inhalation in symptomatic bronchial asthma. *J. Allergy 41*: 209-216.

Atkins, P. C., Norman, M. E., and Zweiman, B. (1978). Antigen-induced neutrophil chemotactic activity in man: Correlation with bronchospasm and inhibition by disodium cromoglycate. *J. Allergy Clin. Immunol. 62*: 149-155.

Augstein, J., Farmer, J. B., Lee, T. B., Sheard, P., and Tattersall, M. L. (1973). Selective inhibition of slow-reacting substance of anaphylaxis. *Nature 245*: 215-216.

Bach, M. K., Brashler, J. R., Morton, D. R., Steel, L. K., Kaliner, M. A., and Hugh, T. E. (1982). Formation of leukotriene C and D and pharmacologic modulation of their synthesis. In *Leukotrienes and Other Lipoxygenase Products,* Vol. 9. Edited by B. Samuelsson and R. Paoletti (Eds.). New York, Raven Press, pp. 103-114.

Barnes, N. C., Piper, P. J., and Costello, J. F. (1984). Comparative effects of inhaled leukotriene C_4, leukotriene D_4, and histamine in normal human subjects. *Thorax 39*: 500-504.

Barnes, P. J., Ind, P., and Dollery, C. T. (1981). Inhaled prazosin in asthma. *Thorax 36*: 378-381.

Bateman, J. R. M., Pavia, D., Sheahan, N. F., Agnew, J. E., and Clarke, S. W. (1979). Tracheobronchial clearance in asthma. *Thorax 34*: 418.

Bedard, R. M., and Busse, W. W. (1983). Nifedipine inhibition of human basophil histamine release. *Am. Rev. Respir. Dis. 127*: 70.

Beer, D. J., Osband, M. E., McCaffrey, R. P., Soter, N. A., and Rocklin, P. E. (1982). Abnormal histamine-induced suppressor-cell function in atopic subjects. *N. Engl. J. Med. 306*: 454-458.

Bhat, K. N., Arroyave, C. M., Marney, S. R., Stevenson, D. D., and Tan, E. M. (1976). Plasma histamine changes during provoked bronchospasm in asthmatic patients. *J. Allergy Clin. Immunol. 58*: 647-656.

Bisgaard, H., Groth, S., and Dirksen, H. (1983). Leukotriene D_4 induces bronchoconstriction in man. *Allergy 38*: 441-443.

Black, J. W., Duncan, W. A. M., Durant, G. J., et al. (1972). Definition and antagonism of histamine H_2-receptors. *Nature 236*: 385-390.

Blackwell, G. J., Duncombe, W. G., Flower, R. J., Parsons, M. F., and Vane, J. R. (1977). The distribution and metabolism of arachidonic acid in rabbit platelets during aggregation and its modification by drugs. *Br. J. Pharmacol. 59*: 353-366.

Booij-Noord, H., Orie, N. G. M., and de Vries, K. (1971). Immediate and late bronchial obstructive reactions to inhalation of house dust and protective effects of disodium cromoglycate and prednisolone. *J. Allergy Clin. Immunol. 48*: 344-354.

Bourne, H. R. N., and Melmon, K. L. (1971). Adenyl cyclase in human leukocytes: Evidence for activation by separate beta adrenergic receptors and prostaglandin receptors. *J. Pharmacol. Exp. Ther. 178*: 1-7.

Boushey, H. A., Holtzman, M. J., Sheller, J. R., and Nadel, J. A. (1980). Bronchial hyperreactivity. *Am. Rev. Respir. Dis. 121*: 389-413.

Bovet, D., Horclois, R., and Walthert, F. (1944). Propertes anti-histaminique de la N-p-methoxybenzyl-N-dimethylaminoethyl-α-amino-pyridine. *C. R. Soc. Biol. (Paris) 138*: 99-100.

Bray, M. A. (1983). The pharmacology and pathophysiology of leukotriene B_4. *Br. Med. Bull. 39*: 249-254.

Brown, J. K., Leff, A. R., Frey, M. J., Reed, B. R., Lazarus, S. C., Shields, R., and Gold, W. M. (1982). Characterization of tracheal mast cell reactions *in vivo*: Inhibition by a beta-adrenergic agonist. *Am. Rev. Respir. Dis. 126*: 342-346.

Buckle, D. R., Outred, D. J., Ross, J. W., Smith, H., Smith, R. J., Spicer, B. A., and Gasson, B. C. (1979). Aryloxyalkyloxy- and aralkyloxy-4-hydroxy-3-

nitrocoumarins which inhibit histamine release in the rat and also antagonise the effects of a slow reacting substance of anaphylaxis. *J. Med. Chem. 22*: 158-168.

Busse, W. W., and Sosman, J. (1977). Decreased H_2-histamine response of granulocytes of asthmatic patients. *J. Clin. Invest. 59*: 1080-1087.

Camp, R. D. R., Coutts, A. A., Greaves, M. W., Kay, A. B., and Walport, M. J. (1982). Responses of human skin to intradermal injection of leukotrienes C_4, D_4, and B_4. *J. Invest. Dermatol. 78*: 329.

Casey, F. B., Appleby, B. J., and Buck, D. C. (1983). Selective inhibition of the lipoxygenase metabolic pathway of arachidonic acid by the SRS-A antagonist, FPL 55712. *Prostaglandins 25*: 1-11.

Cerrina, J., Denjean, A., Alexandre, G., Lockhart, A., and Duroux, P. (1981). Inhibition of exercise-induced asthma by a calcium antagonist, nifedipine. *Am. Rev. Respir. Dis. 123*: 156-160.

Chasin, M., and Scott, C. (1978). Inhibition of cyclic nucleotide phosphodiesterase by FPL 55712, an SRS-A antagonist. *Biochem. Pharm. 27*: 2065.

Cheng, H. C., Reavis, O. K., Munro, N. L., and Woodward, J. K. (1979). Cutaneous vascular histamine H_1 and H_2 receptors in the guinea pig: the histamine skin wheal as a cutaneous vascular model. *Arch. Int. Pharmacodyn. Ther. 240*: 214-219.

Chiang, P. K., Richards, H. H., and Canteri, G. L. (1977). S-adenosyl-L-homocysteine hydrolase: Analogous of S-adenosyl-L-homocysteine as potential inhibitors. *Mol. Pharmacol. 13*: 939-947.

Chiesa, A., Dain, A., Meyers, G. L., Kessler, G. F., and Gold, W. M. (1975). Histamine release during antigen inhalation in experimental asthma in dogs. *Am. Rev. Respir. Dis. 111*: 148-156.

Church, M. K., Howarth, P. H., Durham, S. R., Lee, T. H., Kay, A. B., and Holgate, S. T. (1985). Influence of salbutamol and sodium cromoglycate on mast cell mediator release *in vivo*. *J. Allergy Clin. Immunol. 75*: 195 (abstract).

Coles, S. J., Neill, K. H., Reid, L. M., Austen, K. F., Nii, Y., Corey, E. J., and Lewis, R. A. (1983). Effects of leukotrienes C_4 and D_4 on glycoprotein and lysozyme secretion by human bronchial mucosa. *Prostaglandins 25*: 155-170.

Cookson, D. U., and Reed, C. E. (1963). A comparison of the effects of isoproterenol in the normal and asthmatic subject. *Am. Rev. Respir. Dis. 88*: 636-643.

Cresciole, S., Dal Vecchio, L., Zocca, E., Paleari, D., Pozzan, M., Mapp, C., and Fabbri, L. M. (1985). Slow-release theophylline inhibits the late asthmatic reaction to toluendiisocyanate in sensitized subjects. *J. Allergy Clin. Immunol. 75*: 129 (abstract).

Creticos, P. S., Peters, S. P., Adkinson, N. F. Jr., Naclerio, R. M., Hayes, E. C.,

Norman, P. S., and Lichtenstein, L. M. (1984). Peptide leukotriene release after antigen challenge in patients sensitive to ragweed. *N. Engl. J. Med. 310*: 1626-1630.

Curry, J. J. (1946). Action of histamine on respiratory tract in normal and asthmatic subjects. *J. Clin. Invest. 25*: 785-791.

Dahlen, S-E., Bjork, J., Hedqvist, P., Arfors, K-E., Hammarstrom, S., Lindgren, N-A., and Samuelsson, B. (1981). Leukotrienes promote plasma leakage and leukocyte adhesion in postcapillary venules: *In vivo* effects with relevance to the acute inflammatory response. *Proc. Natl. Acad. Sci. USA 78*: 3887-3891.

Davies, A. O., and Lefkowitz, R. J. (1980). Corticosteroid-induced differential regulation of beta-adrenergic receptors in circulating human polymorphonuclear leukocytes and mononuclear leukocytes. *J. Clin. Endocrinol. Metab. 51*: 599-605.

Davies, A. O., and Lefkowitz, R. J. (1981). Agonist-promoted high affinity state of the B-adrenergic receptor in human neutrophils: Modulation by corticosteroids. *J. Clin. Endocrinol. M etab. 53*(73): 703-708.

Davies, A. O., and Lefkowitz, R. J. (1983). *In vitro* desensitization of beta-adrenergic receptors in human neutrophils: Attentuation by corticosteroids. *J. Clin. Invest. 71*: 565-571.

Delehunt, J. C., Perruchoud, A. P., Yerger, L., Marchette, B., Stevenson, J. S., and Abraham, W. M. (1984). The role of slow-reacting substance of anaphylaxis in the late bronchial response after antigen challenge in allergic sheep. *Am. Rev. Respir. Dis. 130*: 748-754.

Dixon, M., Jackson, D. M., and Richards, I. M. (1980). The action of sodium cromoglycate on "C" fibre endings in the dog lung. *Br. J. Pharmacol. 70*: 11-13.

Drazen, J. M., Venugopalan, C. S., Austen, K. F., Brion, F., and Corey, E. J. (1982). Effect of leukotriene E on pulmonary mechanics in the guinea pig. *Am. Rev. Respir. Dis. 125*: 290-294.

Dunnill, M. S. (1960). The pathology of asthma, with special reference to changes in the bronchial mucosa. *J. Clin. Pathol. 13*: 27-33.

Easton, J. G. (1981). Effect of an inhaled corticosteroid on methacholine airway reactivity. *J. Allergy Clin. Immunol. 67*: 388-390.

Eiser, N. M., McRae, K. D., and Guz, A. (1979). Bronchial histamine receptors in normal, atopic and asthmatic subjects. *Thorax 34*: 703.

Empey, D. W., Laitinen, L. A., Jacobs, L., Gold, W. M., and Nadel, J. A. (1976). Mechanism of bronchial hyperreactivity in normal subjects after upper respiratory tract infection. *Am. Rev. Respir. Dis. 113*: 131-139.

Ennis, M., Truneh, A., White, J. R., and Pearce, F. L. (1981). Inhibition of histamine secretion from mast cells. *Nature 289*: 186-187.

Eyre, P. (1969). The pharmacology of sheep tracheo-bronchial muscle. A re-

laxant effect of histamine on the isolated bronchi. *Br. J. Pharmacol. 36*: 409-417.
Eyre, P. (1973). Histamine H_2-receptor in the sheep bronchus and cat trachea. The action of burimamide. *Br. J. Pharmacol. 48*: 321-323.
Eyre, P. (1977). Pulmonary histamine H_1 and H_2 receptor studies. In *Asthma: Physiology, Immunopharmacology and Treatment.* Edited by L. M. Lichtenstein and K. F. Austen. New York, Academic Press, pp. 169-180.
Eyre, P., and Chand, N. (1982). Histamine receptor mechanisms of the lung. In *Pharmacology of Histamine Receptors.* Edited by C. R. Ganellin and M. E. Parsons. Bristol, England. Wright-PSG, pp. 298-322.
Farley, J. M., and Miles, P. R. (1977). Role of depolarization in acetylcholine-induced contractions of dog trachealis. *J. Pharmacol. Exp. Ther. 201*: 199-205.
Fish, J. E., Ankin, M. G., Adkinson, N. F., and Peterman, V. I. (1981). Indomethacin modification of immediate-type immunologic airway responses in allergic asthmatic and non-asthmatic subjects. *Am. Rev. Respir. Dis. 123*: 609-614.
Fitzpatrick, F. A., and Gorman, R. R. (1978). A comparison of imidazole and 9, 11-azaprosta-5, 13-dienoic acid: Two selective thromboxane-synthetase inhibitors. *Biochim. Biophys. Acta 539*: 162-172.
Fleisch, J. H., Rinkema, L. E., and Baker, S. R. (1982). Evidence for multiple leukotriene D_4 receptors in smooth muscle. *Life Sci. 31*: 577-581.
Flower, R. J. (1974). Drugs which inhibit prostaglandin biosynthesis. *Pharmacol. Rev. 26*: 33-67.
Flower, R. J., and Blackwell, G. J. (1979). Anti-inflammatory steroids induce the biosynthesis of a phospholipase A_2 inhibitor which prevents prostaglandin generation. *Nature 278*: 456-459.
Foreman, J. C. (1981). Calcium and histamine secretion from mast cells and leukocytes. In *Biochemistry of the Acute Allergic Reactions.* Edited by E. L. Decker, A. S. Simon, and K. F. Austen. Alan R. Liss, New York, pp. 315-328.
Fraser, C. M., Venter, J. C., and Kaliner, M. (1981). Autonomic abnormalities and autoantibodies to beta-adrenergic receptors. *N. Engl. J. Med. 305*: 1165-1170.
Ganellin, C. R. (1982). Chemistry and structure-activity relationships of drugs acting at histamine receptors. In *Pharmacology of Histamine Receptors.* Edited by C. R. Ganellin and M. E. Parsons. Bristol, England. Wright-PSG, pp. 10-102.
Garrity, E. R., Stimler, N. P., Munoz, N. M., Fried, R., and Leff, A. R. (1983). Response of bronchial smooth muscle to mast cell degranulation in situ. *J. Appl. Physiol. 55*: 1803-1810.
Ghelani, A. M., Holroyde, M. C., and Sheard, P. (1980). Response of human

isolated bronchial and lung parenchymal strips to SRS-A and other mediators of asthmatic bronchospasm. *Br. J. Pharmacol. 71*: 107-112.

Granstrom, E. (1981). Biosynthesis of prostaglandins and thromboxanes. In *The Prostaglandin System: Endoperoxides, Prostacyclins, and Thromboxanes.* Edited by F. Berti and G. P. Velo. New York, Plenum Press, pp. 15-25.

Grieco, M. H., Pierson, R. N. Jr., and Pi-Sunyer, F. X. (1968). Comparison of circulatory and metabolic effects of isoproterenol, epinephrine and methoxanthine in normal and asthmatic subjects. *Am. J. Med. 44*: 863-872.

Grieco, M. H., and Pierson, R. N. Jr. (1969). The effects of isoproterenol and methacholine on pulmonary blood volume in asthmatic and normal subjects. *J. Allergy 43*: 177.

Griffin, M., Weiss, J. W., Leitch, A. G., et al. (1983). Effects of leukotriene D on the airways in asthma. *N. Engl. J. Med. 308*: 436-439.

Gonzalez, H., and Ahmed, T. (1986). Suppression of gastric H_2-receptor mediated function in patients with bronchial asthma and ragweed allergy. *Chest 89*: 491-496.

Gronneberg, R., and Strandberg, K. (1981). Effect of terbutaline on cutaneous responses in man to rechallenge with allergen and compound 48/80. *Allergy 36*: 33-38.

Gryglewski, R. J. (1981). Pharmacological interference in arachidonic acid cascade. In *The Prostaglandin System: Endoperoxides, Prostacyclins, and Thromboxanes.* Edited by F. Berti and G. P. Velo. New York, Plenum Press, pp. 85-92.

Gryglewski, R. J., Panezenko, B., Korbut, R., Grodzinska, L., and Cetkiewicz, A. O. (1975). Corticosteroids inhibit prostaglandin release from perfused lungs of sensitized guinea pigs. *Prostaglandins 10*: 343.

Gryglewski, R. J., Zmuda, A., Korbut, R., Krecioch, E., and Bieron, K. (1977). Selective inhibition of thromboxane A_2 biosynthesis in blood platelets. *Nature 267*: 627-628.

Hamberg, M., and Fredholm, B. B. (1976). Isomerization of prostaglandin H_2 into prostaglandin D_2 in the presence of serum albumin. *Biochim. Biophys. Acta 431*: 189.

Hamel, R., Masson, P., Ford-Hutchinson, A. W., Jones, T. R., Brunet, G., and Piechuta, H. (1982). Differing mechanisms for leukotriene D_4-induced bronchoconstriction in guinea pigs following intravenous and aerosol administration. *Prostaglandin 24*: 419-432.

Hartmann, V., Magnussen, H., Holle, J. P., and Schuler, E. (1981). Modulation of histamine-induced bronchoconstriction with inhaled, oral, and intravenous clemastine in normal and asthmatic subjects. *Thorax 36*: 737-740.

Hartmann, V., Magnussen, H., Oliver, W. Jr., Abraham, W. M., Wanner, A., and Ahmed, T. (1983). Histamine receptor blocking effects of cimetidine in the airways. *Agents Actions 13*: 16-20.

Harvey, R. P., and Schocket, A. L. (1980). The effect of H_1 and H_2 blockade on cutaneous-histamine response in man. *J. Allergy Clin. Immunol. 65*: 136-139.

Henderson, W. R., Shelhamer, J. H., Reingold, D. B., Smith, L. J., Evans, R., and Kaliner, M. (1979). Alpha-adrenergic hyperresponsiveness in asthma: Analysis of vascular and pupillary responses. *N. Engl. J. Med. 300*: 642-647.

Henderson, A. F., Heaton, R. W., and Costello, J. F. (1983). Effect of nifedipine on bronchoconstriction induced by inhalation of cold air. *Thorax 38*: 512-515.

Hirata, F., and Axelrod, J. (1978). Enzymatic methylation of phosphatidylethanolamine increases erythrocyte membrane fluidity. *Nature 275*: 219-220.

Hirata, F., and Axelrod, J. (1980). Phospholipid methylation and biological signal transmission. *Science 209*: 1082-1090.

Hirata, F., Axelrod, J., and Crews, F. T. (1979). Concanavalin A stimulates phospholipid methylation and phosphatdiylserine decarboxylation in rat mast cells. *Proc. Natl. Acad. Sci. USA 76*: 4813-4816.

Hogaboom, G. K., Mong, S., Wu, H-L., and Crooke, S. T. (1983). Peptidoleukotrienes: Distinct receptors for leukotriene C_4 and D_4 in the guinea-pig lung. *Biochem. Biophys. Res. Commun. 116*: 1135-1143.

Holgate, S. T., Mann, J. S., and Cushley, M. J. (1984). Adenosine as a bronchoconstrictor mediator in asthma and its antagonism by methylxanthines. *J. Allergy Clin. Immunol. 74*: 302-306.

Holme, G., Brunet, G., Piechuta, H., Masson, P., Girard, Y., and Rokach, J. (1980). The activity of synthetic leukotriene C-1 on guinea-pig trachea and ileum. *Prostaglandins 20*: 717-728.

Holroyde, M. C., Altounyan, R. E. C., Cole, M., Dixon, M., and Elliot, E. V. (1981). Bronchoconstriction produced in man by leukotrienes C and D. *Lancet 2*: 17-18.

Howarth, P. H., Durham, S. R., Lee, T. H., Kay, A. B., Church, M. K., and Holgate, S. T. (1985). Influence of albuterol, cromolyn sodium, and ipratropium bromide on the airway and circulating mediator responses to allergen provocation in asthma. *Am. Rev. Respir. Dis. 132*: 986-992.

Ishizaka, K., and Ishizaka, T. (1968). Induction of erythema-wheal reactions by soluble antigen-Ig-E antibody complexes in man. *J. Immunol. 101*: 68-78.

Ishizaka, T., and Ishizaka, K. (1978). Triggering of histamine release from rat mast cells by devalent antibodies against IgE receptors. *J. Immunol. 120*: 800-805.

Ishizaka, T., Hirata, F., Kishizaka, K., and Axelrod, J. (1980). Stimulation of phospholipid methylation, Ca^{++} influx and histamine release by binding of IgE receptors on rat mast cells. *Proc. Natl. Acad. Sci. USA 77*: 1903-1906.

Jakschik, B. A., Sun, F. F., Lee, L. H., and Steinoff, M. M. (1980). Calcium stimulation of a novel lipoxygenase. *Biochem. Biophys. Res. Commun. 95*: 103-110.

Jakschik, B. A., Disantis, D. M., Sankarappa, S. K., and Sprecker, H. (1982). Modulation of leukotriene formation by various acetylenic acids. In *Leukotrienes and Other Lipoxygenase Products*, Vol. 9. Edited by B. Samuelsson and R. Paoletti. New York, Raven Press, pp. 127-136.

Kaliner, M. (1976). The cholinergic nervous system and immediate hypersensitivity. I. Eccrine sweat responses in allergic patients. *J. Allergy Clin. Immunol. 58*: 308-315.

Kaliner, M., Orange, R. P., and Austen, K. F. (1972). Immunological release of histamine and slow reacting substance of anaphylaxis from human lung. IV. Enhancement by cholinergic and alpha adrenergic stimulation. *J. Exp. Med. 136*: 556-567.

Kalsner, S. (1969). Mechanism of hydrocortisone potentiation of responses to epinephrine and nor-epinephrine in rabbit aorta. *Circ. Res. 24*: 383-395.

Karczewski, W., and Widdicombe, J. G. (1969). The role of the vagus nerve in the respiratory and circulatory reactions to anaphylaxis in rabbits. *J. Physiol. 201*: 293-304.

Kind, L. S. (1958). The altered reactivity of mice after inoculation with pertussis vaccine. *Bacteriol. Rev. 22*: 173.

Kirkpatrick, C. H., and Keller, C. (1967). Impaired responsiveness to epinephrine in asthma. *Am. Rev. Respir. Dis. 96*: 692-699.

Kneussl, M. P., and Richardson, J. B. (1978). Alpha-adrenergic receptors in human and canine tracheal and bronchial smooth muscle. *J. Appl. Physiol. 45*: 307-311.

Krell, R. D., Tsai, B. S., Berdoulay, A., Barone, M., and Giles, R. E. (1983). Heterogeneity of leukotriene receptors in guinea-pig trachea. *Prostaglandins 25*: 171-178.

Kuehl, F. A., Humes, J. L., Egan, R. W., Ham, E. A., Beveridge, G. C., and Van Arman, C. G. (1977). Role of prostaglandin endoperoxide PGG_2 in inflammatory processes. *Nature 265*: 170-173.

Lazarus, S. C., Chersown, S. E., Frey, M. J., Reed, B. R., Mjorndal, T. O., and Gold, W. M. (1979). Experimental canine anaphylaxis: cyclic nucleotides histamine and lung function. *J. Appl. Physiol. 46*: 919-925.

Lee, R. W. (1974). The influence of psychotropic drugs on prostaglandin biosynthesis. *Prostaglandins 5*: 63-68.

Leitch, A. G., Corey, E. J., Austen, K. F., and Drazen, J. M. (1983). Indomethacin potentiates the pulmonary response to aerosol leukotriene C_4 in the guinea pig. *Am. Rev. Respir. Dis. 128*: 639-643.

Lewis, R. A. (1984). The leukotrienes and other mediators of asthma: Newer concepts. *Immunol. Allergy Prac. 6*: 31-36.

Lockey, S. D., Glennon, J. A., and Reed, C. E. (1967). Comparison of some metabolic responses in normal and asthmatic subjects to epinephrine and glucagon. *J. Allergy 40*: 349-354.

Long, W. M., Sprung, C. L., Fawall, H. E., Yerger, L. D., Eyre, P., Abraham, W. M., and Wanner, A. (1985). Effects of histamine on bronchial artery blood flow and bronchomotor tone. *J. Appl. Physiol. 59*: 254-261.

Maas, R. L., Brash, A. R., and Oates, J. A. (1982). Novel leukotrienes and lipoxygenase products from arachidonic acid. In *Advances in Prostaglandin Thromboxane Research,* Vol. 9. Edited by B. Samuelsson, P. W. Ramwell, and R. Paoletti. New York, Raven Press, pp. 29-44.

Maconochie, J. G., Woodings, E. P., and Richards, D. A. (1979). Effects of H_1 and H_2 receptor blocking agents on histamine-induced bronchoconstriction in non-asthmatic subjects. *Br. J. Clin. Pharmacol.* 7: 231-236.

Marks, R., and Greaves, W. M. (1977). Vascular reaction to histamine and compound 48/80 in human skin: Suppression by a histamine H_2 receptor blocking agent. *Br. J. Clin. Pharmacol. 4*: 367-369.

Marom, Z., Shelhamer, J. H., and Kaliner, M. (1981). Effects of arachidonic acid, monohydroxyeicosatetraenoic acid and prostaglandins on the release of mucous glycoproteins from human airways. *in vitro. J. Clin. Invest. 67*: 1695-1702.

Marom, Z., Shelhamer, J. H., Bach, M. K., Morton, D. R., and Kaliner, M. (1982). Slow-reacting substances, leukotrienes C_4 and D_4, increase the release of mucus from human airways *in vitro. Am. Rev. Respir. Dis. 126*: 449-451.

Marquardt, D. L., Motulsky, H. J., and Wasserman, S. I. (1982). Rat lung cholinergic receptor: characterization and regulation by corticosteroids. *J. Appl. Physiol. 53*: 731-736.

Martin, G. L., Atkins, P. C., Dunsky, E. H., and Zweiman, B. (1980). Effects of theophylline, terbutaline, and prednisone on antigen-induced bronchospasm and mediator release. *J. Allergy Clin. Immunol. 66*: 204-212.

Maurer, D. R., Schor, J., Sielczak, M., Wanner, A., and Abraham, W. M. (1982a). Ciliary motility in airway anaphylaxis. *Cell Motil. (Suppl.) 1*: 67-70.

Maurer, D. R.. Sielczak, M., Oliver, W., Jr., Abraham, W. M., and Wanner, A. (1982b). Role of ciliary motility in allergic mucociliary dysfunction. *J. Appl. Physiol. 52*: 1018-1023.

Meisheri, K. D., Hwang, O., and van Breemen, C. (1981). Evidence for two separate Ca pathways in smooth muscle plasmalemma. *J. Membrane Biol. 59*: 19-25.

Mezey, R. J., Cohn, M. A., Fernandez, R. J., Januszkiewicz, A. J., and Wanner, A. (1978). Mucociliary transport in allergic patients with antigen-induced bronchospasm. *Am. Rev. Respir. Dis. 118*: 677-684.

Middleton, E. Jr., and Finke, S. R. (1968). Metabolic responses to epinephrine in bronchial asthma. *J. Allergy 42*: 288-299.

Middleton, E., Jr., Drzewiecki, G., and Triggle, D. (1981). Effects of smooth muscle calcium antagonists on human basophil histamine release. *Biochem. Pharmacol. 30*: 2867-2869.

Moncada, S., Bunting, S., Mullane, K., Thorogood, P., and Vane, J. R. (1977). Imidazole: A selective inhibitor of thromboxane synthetase. *Prostaglandins 13*: 611-618.

Mong, S., Wu, H-L., Hogaboom, G. K., Clark, M. A., Crooke, S. T. (1984). Characterization of the leukotriene D_4 receptor in guinea-pig lung. *Eur. J. Pharmacol. 102*: 1-11.

Morita, Y., and Siraganian, R. P. (1981). Inhibition of IgE mediated histamine release from rat basophilic leukemia cells and rat mast cells by inhibitors of transmethylation. *J. Immunol. 127*: 1339-1344.

Morita, Y., Chiang, P. K., and Siraganian, R. P. (1981). Effect of inhibitors of transmethylation on histamine release from human basophils. *Biochem. Pharmacol. 30*: 785-791.

Morris, H. G. (1985). Mechanisms of action and therapeutic role of corticosteroids in asthma. *J. Allergy Clin. Immunol. 75*: 1-13.

Morris, H. G., Rusnak, S. A., Selner, J. C., Barzens, K., and Barnes, J. (1977). Adrenergic desensitization in leukocytes of normal and asthmatic subjects. *J. Cyclic Nucleotide Res. 3*: 439-446.

Nadel, J. A. (1968). Mechanisms of airway response to inhaled substances. *Arch. Environ. Health 16*: 171-174.

Nadel, J. A., and Davis, B. (1978). Autonomic regulation of mucus secretion and ion transport in airways. In *Asthma: Physiology, Immunopharmacology and Treatment.* Edited by L. M. Lichtenstein and K. F. Austen (Eds.). Academic Press, New York, pp. 197-210.

Nathan, R. A., Segall, N., Glover, G. C., and Schocket, A. L. (1979). The effects of H_1 and H_2 antihistamines on histamine inhalation challenges in asthmatic patients. *Am. Rev. Respir. Dis. 120*: 1251-1258.

Nathan, R. A., Segall, N., and Schocket, A. (1981). A comparison of the actions of H_1 and H_2 antihistamines on histamine-induced bronchoconstriction and cutaneous wheal responses in asthmatic patients. *J. Allergy Clin. Immunol. 67*: 171-177.

Parfentjev, I. A., and Goodline, M. A. (1948). Histamine shock in mice sensitized with hemophilus pertussis vaccine. *J. Pharmacol. Exp. Ther. 92*: 411-413.

Parker, C. W. (1981). Autoantibodies and beta-adrenergic receptors. *N. Engl. J. Med. 305*: 1212-1213.

Parker, C. W., and Smith, J. W. (1973). Alterations in cyclic adenosine monophosphate metabolism in human bronchial asthma. I. Leukocyte responsiveness to B-adrenergic agents. *J. Clin. Invest. 52*: 48-59.

Parker, C. W., Baumann, M. L., and Huber, M. G. (1973a). Alterations in cyclic

AMP metabolism in human bronchial asthma: II. Leukocyte and lymphocyte responses to prostaglandins. *J. Clin. Invest. 52*: 1336-1341.

Parker, C. W., Huber, M. G., and Baumann, M. L. (1973b). Alterations in cyclic AMP metabolism in human bronchial asthma: III. Leukocyte and lymphocyte responses to steroids. *J. Clin. Invest. 52*: 1342-1348.

Patel, K. R. (1981). Calcium antagonists in exercise-induced asthma. *Br. Med. J. 282*: 932-933.

Patel, K. R., Al Shama, M. R., and Kerr, J. W. (1983). The effect of inhaled verapamil on allergen-induced asthma. *Clin. Allergy 13*: 119-122.

Patterson, R., Harris, K., Suszko, I. M., and Roberts, M. (1976a). Reagin-mediated asthma in rhesus monkeys and relation to bronchial cell histamine release and airway reactivity to carbocholine. *J. Clin. Invest. 57*: 586-593.

Patterson, R., Chakrin, L. W., Suszko, I. M., Mengel, J., and Wardell, J. R. Jr. (1976b). IgE-mediated histamine and RS-A release from respiratory cells and peripheral blood leukocytes of rhesus monkeys. *J. Lab. Clin. Med. 87*: 1016-1024.

Pearce, F. L., Atkinson, G., Ennis, M., Truneh, A., Weston, P. M., and White, J. R. (1979). Effect of anti-allergic compounds on histamine release induced by basic agents, antigen and the calcium ionophore A23187. In *The Mast Cell.* Edited by J. Pepys, and A. M. Edwards. Kent, England, Pitman Medical, pp. 69-75.

Peck, M. J., Piper, P. J., and Williams, T. J. (1981). The effect of leukotrienes C_4 and D_4 on the microvasculature of guinea-pig skin. *Prostaglandins 21*: 315-321.

Pepys, J., and Hutchcroft, B. J. (1975). Bronchial provocation tests in etiologic diagnosis and analysis of asthma. *Am. Rev. Respir. Dis. 112*: 829-859.

Perruchoud, A. P., Yerger, L., Russi, E., Stevenson, J. S., and Abraham, W. M. (1984a). Prevention of allergic late bronchial obstruction by metaproterenol. *Am. Rev. Respir. Dis. 129*: A5 (abstract).

Perruchoud, A. P., Yerger, L., and Abraham, W. M. (1984b). Differential effects of aminophylline on the early and late antigen-induced bronchial obstruction in allergic sheep. *Am. Rev. Respir. Dis. 129*: A282 (abstract).

Peters, S. P., Schleimer, R. P., Marone, G., Kagey-Sobotka, A., Siegel, M. I., and Lichtenstein, L. M. (1982). Lipoxygenase products of arachidonic acid: Role in modulation of IgE-induced histamine release. In *Leukotrienes and Other Lipoxygenase Products.* Edited by B. Samuelsson, and R. Paoletti. New York, Raven Press, pp. 315-324.

Phillipe-Boudet, L., Latimer, K. M., Roberts, R. S., et al. (1984). The effect of atropine on allergen induced increases in bronchial responsiveness to histamine. *Am. Rev. Respir. Dis. 130*: 368-372.

Phipps, R. J., Denas, S. M., and Wanner, A. (1983a). Antigen stimulates glycoprotein secretion and alters ion fluxes in sheep trachea. *J. Appl. Physiol. 5*: 1593-1602.

Phipps, R., Denas, S., and Wanner, A. (1983b). Leukotriene D_4 stimulates secretion of glycoproteins, ions and water in sheep trachea. *Fed. Proc. 42*: 461.

Pickett, W. C., Jesse, R. L., and Cohen, P. (1977). Initiation of phospholipase A_2 activity in human platelets by the calcium ion ionophore A-23187. *Biochim. Biophys. Acta 486*: 209-213.

Popa, V. T. (1980). Effect of an H_1 blocker, chlorpheniramine, on inhalation tests with histamine and allergen in allergic asthma. *Chest 78*: 442-451.

Reed, C. E., Cohen, M., and Enta, T. (1970). Reduced effect of epinephrine on circulating eosinophils in asthma and after beta-adrenergic blockade or Bordetella pertussis vaccine. *J. Allergy 46*: 90-102.

Richardson, P. S., and Sterling, G. M. (1969). The effects of beta-adrenergic receptor blockade on airway conductance and lung volume in normal and asthmatic subjects. *Br. Med. J. 3*: 143-145.

Riley, J. F. (1959). *The Mast Cells.* London, Livingstone.

Russi, E., Abraham, W. M., Chapman, G. A., J. S. Stevenson, E. Codias, and Wanner, A. (1985). Effects of leukotriene D_4 on mucociliary function and respiratory function in allergic sheep and nonallergic sheep. *J. Appl. Physiol. 59*: 1416-1422.

Russi, E. W. Perruchoud, A. P., Yerger, L. D., Stevenson, J. S., Tabak, J., Marchette, B., and Abraham, W. M. (1984). Late phase bronchial obstruction following nonimmunologic mast cell degranulation. *J. Appl. Physiol. 57*: 1182-1188.

Russi, E., Danta, I., and Ahmed, T. (1985). Comparative modification of antigen induced bronchoconstriction by the calcium antagonists nifedipine and verapamil. *Chest 88*: 74-78.

Salmon, J. A., Smith, D. R., Flower, R. J., Moncada, S., and Vane, J. R. (1978). Further studies on the enzymatic conversion of prostaglandin endoperoxide into prostacyclin by porcine aorta microsomes. *Biochim. Biophys. Acta 523*: 250.

Samuelsson, B., Goldyne, M., Granstrom, E., Hamberg, M., Hammarstrom, S., and Malmsten, C. (1978). Prostaglandins and thromboxanes. *Annu. Rev. Biochem. 47*: 997-1029.

Samuelsson, B., Borgeat, P., Hammarstrom, S., and Murphy, R. C. (1981). In *Advances in Prostaglandin Thromboxane Research,* Vol. 6. Edited by B. Samuelsson, P. W. Ramwell and R. Paoletti (Eds.). Raven Press, New York, pp. 1-18.

Santa Cruz, R., Landa J., Hirsch, J., and Sackner, M. A. (1974). Tracheal mucous velocity in normal men and patients with obstructive lung disease: Effects of terbutaline. *Am. Rev. Respir. Dis. 109*: 458-463.

Sheard, P., Holroyde, M. C., Ghelani, A. M., Bantick, J. R., and Lee, T. B. (1982). Antagonists of SRS-A and leukotrienes. In *Leukotrienes and Other Lipoxygenase Products.* Edited by B. Samuelsson and R. Paoletti. New York, Raven Press, pp. 229-235.

Shelhamer, J. H., Marom, Z., and Kaliner, M. (1980). Immunologic and neuropharmacologic stimulation of mucous glycoprotein release from human airways *in vitro*. *J. Clin. Invest. 66*: 1400-1408.

Sieghart, W., Theoharides, T. C., Douglas, W. W., and Greengard, P. (1981). Phosphorylation of a single mast cell protein in response to drugs that inhibit secretion. *Biochem. Pharmacol. 30*: 2737-2738.

Simonsson, B. G., Jacobs, F. M., and Nadel, J. A. (1967). Role of autonomic nervous system and the cough reflex in the increased responsiveness of airways in patients with obstructive airway disease. *J. Clin. Invest. 46*: 1812-1818.

Simonsson, B. G., Svedmyr, N., Skoogh, B. E., Anderson, and Bergh, N. P. (1972). *In vivo* and *in vitro* studies on alpha receptors in human airways potentiation with bacterial endotoxin. *Scand. J. Respir. Dis. 53*: 227-236.

Sirois, P., Roy, S., and Borgeat, P. (1983). Specificity of receptors for leukotrienes A_4, B_4, C_4, D_4, E_4, and histamine on the guinea-pig lung parenchyma. Effect of FPL-55712 and desensitization of the myotropic activity. *Prostaglandins 26*: 91-101.

Sirois, P., and Brousseau, Y. (1983). Leukotriene transformation by guinea-pig lungs. *Prostaglandins Leukotrienes Med. 10*: 133-143.

Smith, J. W., Steiner, A. L., Newberry, W. M. Jr., and Parker, C. W. (1971). Cyclic adenosine 3,5 monophosphate in human lymphocytes: Alterations after phytohemagglutinin stimulation. *J. Clin. Invest. 50*: 432-441.

Snashall, P. D., Boother, F. A., and Sterling, G. M. (1978). The effect of alpha-adrenoreceptor stimulation on the airways of normal and asthmatic man. *Clin. Sci. Mol. Med. 54*: 283-289.

So, S. Y., Lam, W. K., and Yu, D. Y. (1982). Effect of calcium antagonists on allergen-induced asthma. *Clin. Allergy 12*: 595-600.

Somlyo, A. P., and Somlyo, A. V. (1968). Electromechanical and pharmacomechanical coupling in vascular smooth muscle. *J. Pharmacol. Exp. Ther. 159*: 129-145.

Soter, N. A., Lewis, R. A., Corey, E. J., and Austen, F. K. (1983). Local effects of synthetic leukotrienes (LTC_4, LTD_4, LTE_4 and LTB_4) in human skin. *J. Invest. Dermatol. 80*: 115-119.

Sotomayor, H., Badier, M., Vervloet, D., and Orehek, J. (1984). Seasonal increase of carbachol airway responsiveness in patients allergic to grass pollen: Reversal by corticosteroids. *Am. Rev. Respir. Dis. 130*: 56-58.

Szantivanyi, A. (1968). The beta-adrenergic theory of the atopic abnormality in bronchial asthma. *J. Allergy 42*: 203-232.

Tashkin, D. P., Ungerer, R., Wolfe, R., Mendoza, G., and Calvarese, B. (1982). Effect of orally administered cimetidine on histamine- and antigen-induced bronchospasm in subjects with asthma. *Am. Rev. Respir. Dis. 125*: 691-695.

Theoharides, T. C., Sieghart, W., Greengard, P., and Douglas, W. W. (1980). Antiallergic drug cromolyn may inhibit histamine secretion by regulating phosphorylation of a mast cell protein. *Science 207*: 80-82.

Thompson, N. C., Daniel, E. E., and Hargreave, F. E. (1982). Role of smooth muscle $alpha_1$-receptors in nonspecific bronchial responsiveness in asthma. *Am. Rev. Respir. Dis. 126*: 521-525.

Ting, S., Szeiman, B., and Lavker, R. (1983). Terbutaline modulation of human allergic skin reactions. *J. Allergy Clin. Immunol. 71*: 437-441.

Tiffeneau, R., and Dunoyer, P. (1956). Action de la cortisone sur l'hypersensibilité cholinérgique pulmonaire de l'asthmatique. *Presse Med. 64*: 719-721.

Townley, R. G., Reeb, R., Fitzgibbons, T., and Adolphson, R. L. (1970). The effects of corticosteroids on the beta-adrenergic receptors in bronchial smooth muscle. *J. Allergy 45*: 118 (abstract).

Vane, R. J. (1971). Inhibition of prostaglandin synthesis as a mechanism of aspirin-like drugs. *Nature 231*: 232-235.

Vargaftig, B. B. (1977). Carrageenan and thrombin trigger prostaglandin-synthetase independent aggregation of rabbit platelets: Inhibition by phospholipase A_2 inhibitors. *J. Pharm. Pharmacol. 29*: 222-228.

Venter, J. C., Fraser, C. M., and Harrison, L. C. (1980). Autoantibodies to $beta_2$-adrenergic receptors: A possible cause of adrenergic hyporesponsiveness in allergic rhinitis and asthma. *Science 207*: 1361-1363.

Wanner, A. (1979). The role of mucociliary dysfunction in bronchial asthma. *Am. J. Med. 67*: 477-485.

Wanner, A., Zarzecki, S., Hirsch, J., Epstein, S. (1975). Tracheal mucous transport in experimental canine asthma. *J. Appl. Physiol. 39*: 950-957.

Wanner, A., Maurer, D., Abraham, W. M., Szepfalusi, Z., and Sielczak, M. (1983). Effects of chemical mediators of anaphylaxis on ciliary function. *J. Allergy Clin. Immunol. 72*: 663-667.

Wasserman, S. I. (1983). Mediators of immediate hypersensitivity. *J. Allergy Clin. Immunol. 72*: 101-115.

Weichman, B. M., Muccitelli, R. M., Osborn, R. R., Holden, D. A., Gleason, J. G., and Wasserman, M. A. (1982). *In vitro* and *in vivo* mechanisms of leukotriene-mediated bronchoconstriction in the guinea pig. *J. Pharmacol. Exp. Ther. 222*: 202-208.

Weiss, J. W., Drazen, J. M., Coles, N., McFadden, E. G. Jr., Weller, P. F., Corey, E. J., Lewis, R. A., and Austen, K. F. (1982). Bronchoconstrictor effects of leukotriene C in humans. *Science 215*: 196-198.

Weissberger, D., Oliver, Jr., W., Abraham, W. M., and Wanner, A. (1981). Impaired tracheal mucous transport in allergic bronchoconstriction: Effect of terbutaline pretreatment. *J. Allergy Clin. Immunol. 67*: 357-362.

Welton, A. F., Crowley, H. J., Miller, D. A., and Yaremko, B. (1981a). Biological activities of a chemically synthesized formo of leukotriene E_4. Prostaglandins 21: 287-296.

Welton, A. F., Hope, W. C., Tobias, L. D., and Hamilton, J. G. (1981b). Inhibition of antigen-induced histamine release and thromboxane synthase by FPL 55712, a specific SRS-A antagonist? *Biochem. Pharm. 30*: 1378-1382.

White, J. R., and Pearce, F. L. (1981). Role of membrane bound calcium in histamine secretion from rat peritoneal mast cells. *Agents Actions 11*: 324-329.

Winslow, C. M., and Austen, K. F. (1982). Enzymatic regulation of mast cell activation and secretion by adenylate cyclase and cyclic AMP-dependent protein kinases. *Fed. Proc. 41*: 22-29.

Wolfe, J. D. (1979). The effect of corticosteroids on cholinergic hyperreactivity. *J. Allergy Clin. Immunol. 63*: 162 (abstract).

Zijlstra, F. J., Vincent, J. E., and Bonta, I. L. (1983). Separation of the two components of the contractile activity of leukotriene C_4 on the guinea pig lung parenchymal strip. *Prostaglandins Leukotrienes Med. 11*: 385-389.

13

Pharmacokinetics and Pharmacodynamics of Glucocorticosteroids

ROGER ELLUL-MICALLEF

University of Malta
Msida, Malta

I. Development of Therapy with Glucocorticosteroids

A. Systemic

The isolation, characterization of structure, synthesis, and understanding of the mode of action of glucocorticosteroids proved to be a slow process, mainly because of the initial need to handle large amounts of starting material and because of the limited available technology. Cortisone, originally termed Compound E, along with a number of other adrenocortical hormones, was first isolated in crystalline form in Kendall's laboratory in December 1933, following nearly 20 years of painstaking work (Mason et al., 1936). In 1946, Sarrett announced his successful synthesis of cortisone, while hydrocortisone was synthesized a few years later (Wendler et al., 1950).

The first clinical use of cortisone is associated with rheumatoid arthritis (Hench et al., 1949). A number of other clinical trials were quickly reported (Hench et al., 1950; Freyburg et al., 1950). Work in patients with rheumatoid arthritis was soon followed by the investigation of the effects of intramuscular cortisone in patients with bronchial asthma (Carryer et al., 1950; Randolph and Rollins, 1950).

Following the introduction of prednisone and prednisolone (Herzog et al., 1955) under the names of metacortandracin and metacortandrolone, Barach and his colleagues demonstrated their therapeutic value in asthma in the same year, and pointed out their decreased mineralocorticoid effects. Hydrocortisone was first administered intravenously to asthmatic patients by Burrage and Irwin (1955). In an attempt to potentiate the anti-inflammatory effects and to diminish unwanted systemic effects, a number of other glucocorticosteroids have been subsequently synthesized and studied. These include methylprednisolone (Spero et al., 1956), dexamethasone (Bernstein et al., 1956), triamcinolone (Peak et al., 1979), and cloprednol (Ortega et al., 1976; Ellul-Micallef et al., 1978). They do not appear to possess any marked advantages and prednisolone remains the standard oral preparation.

B. Inhalational

As glucocorticosteroids became more readily available they rapidly gained a prominent place in the management of a wide variety of clinical conditions. There followed a quick appreciation of their serious side effects and potential hazards, subsequently emphasized in a number of review articles (David et al., 1970; Lieberman et al., 1972; Rimsza, 1978). Because of their systemic side effects, efforts were made, as early as 1950, to deliver glucocorticosteroids locally to the airways in an attempt to achieve a higher local concentration with a lower dosage than would be needed by systemic administration (Reeder & Mackey, 1950). For a long time these efforts proved to be unsuccessful (Cotes et al., 1956; Uhde, 1957; Crepea, 1963; Toogood and Lefcoe, 1965; Novey and Beall, 1965).

The breakthrough came with betamethasone valerate and beclomethasone dipropionate, which were the first topical glucocorticosteroids administered in aerosol form to be devoid of any marked systemic effects and to achieve clinical success in the management of asthma (Clark, 1972; Brown et al., 1972; Smith et al., 1973; Godfrey and Konig, 1973; Frears et al., 1973). Beclomethasone dipropionate is today probably the most widely used inhaled glucocorticosteroid in asthma. Triamcinolone acetonide, a nonpolar, water-insoluble fluorinated corticosteroid, was developed a little later in the United States. Several studies attest to its usefulness in bronchial asthma both in adults and children (Williams, 1975; Chervinsky, 1977; Grieco et al., 1978; Bernstein et al., 1982). A more recently introduced synthetic polar, fluorinated glucocorticosteroid is flunisolide (Chaplin et al., 1980b). The efficacy and safety of this aerosol appear to be established (Lowell et al., 1976; Shapiro et al., 1981; Meltzer et al., 1982). As the search continues for newer compounds with greater topical anti-inflammatory activity and decreased systemic effects, other glucocorticosteroids make their appearance. The latest in the series is budesonide (Thalen and Brattsand,

1979), an epimeric mixture of a nonhalogenated glucocorticosteroid shown to be two to three times more potent than beclomethasone dipropionate in dermal vasoconstriction tests in humans (Johansson et al., 1982). A large number of clinical studies have shown it to compare very favorably with other inhaled glucocorticosteroids (Ellul-Micallef et al., 1980; Willey et al., 1982; Ellul-Micallef and Johansson, 1983).

II. Relation of Structure to Function of Glucocorticosteroids

The glucocorticosteroids are a group of C_{21} steroids (Fig. 1). Structurally they are characterized by:

1. A double bond at C-4 and an oxo group at C3
2. A side chain at C-17
3. A hydroxyl or oxo group at C-11
4. A hydroxyl group at C-17
5. A C-21 hydroxyl group with an oxo group at C-20

The circled areas on the molecule shown in Figure 2 are the sites that cannot be altered without significant loss of glucocorticosteroid activity. The structure of the molecule is so delicate that if the 11-hydroxyl group is in the α- instead of the natural β-position the steroid is completely inactivated (Rogers et al., 1952). Substitutions at various sites have resulted in the synthesis of a number of compounds with enhanced anti-inflammatory and diminished miner-

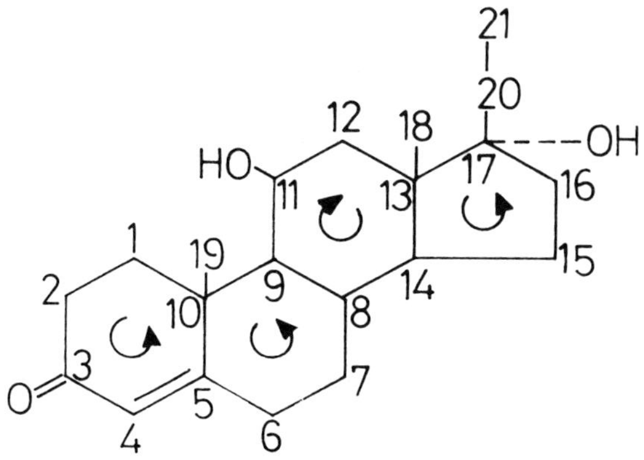

Figure 1 Basic structure of glucocorticosteroids.

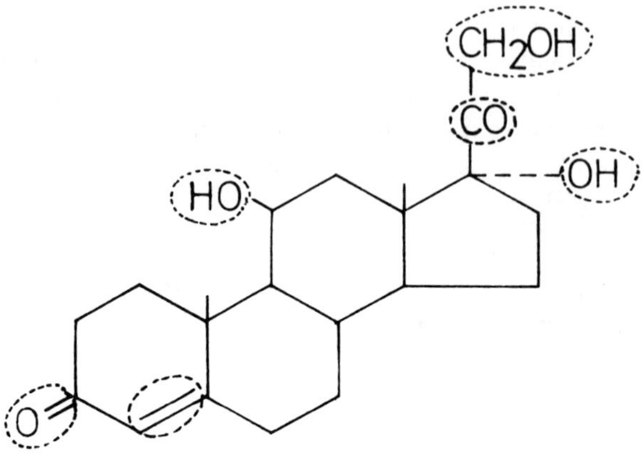

Figure 2 Sites thought essential for glucocorticosteroid activity.

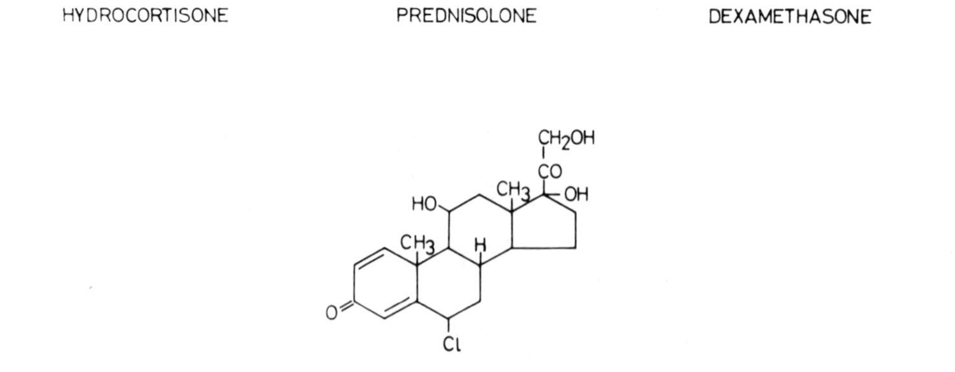

Figure 3 Structure of different glucocorticosteroids used systemically.

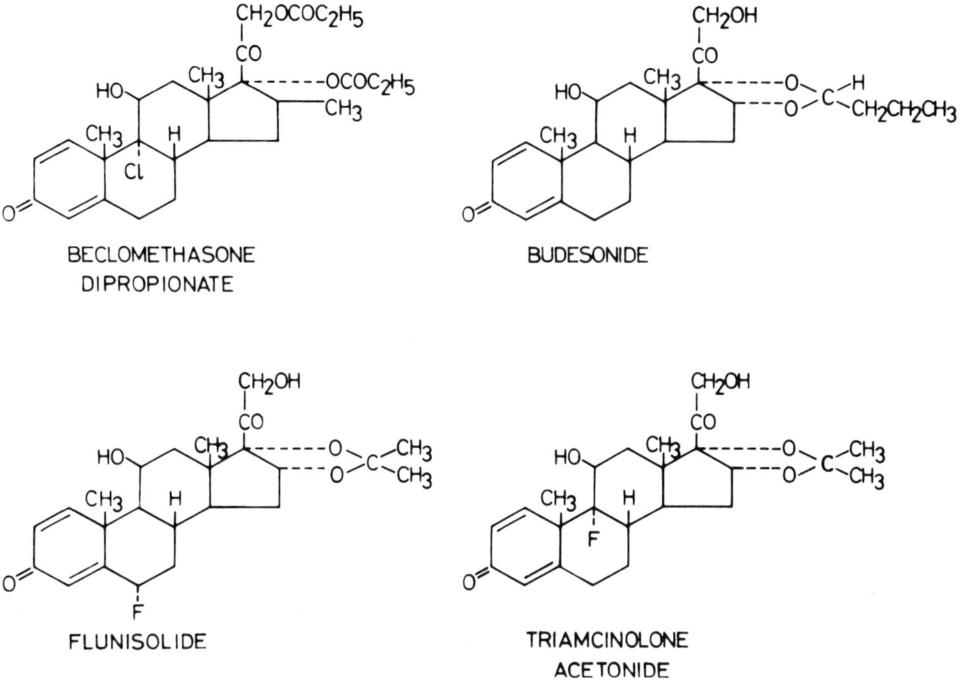

Figure 4 Structure of different glucocorticosteroids administered by inhalation.

alocorticoid activities compared to hydrocortisone. For example, the introduction of a 1,2 double bond resulted in prednisolone, a glucocorticosteroid with a fourfold enhancement of anti-inflammatory activity. Furthermore, the modification on the basic hydrocortisone structure also altered steroid metabolism, producing glucocorticosteroids with different half-lives. Structural alterations resulting in different synthetic glucocorticosteroids may be readily appreciated in Figure 3. Dexamethasone was synthesized as a result of introducing a methyl group on the 16-carbon atom (Arth et al., 1958). To arrive at a compound with marked topical activity, some of the hydroxyl groups in the hydrocortisone molecule were substituted with acetonide or ester groups, such as beclomethasone dipropionate (Fig. 4). Triamcinolone acetonide and flunisolide were obtained by substituting asymmetrical 16α and 17α acetal groups and the introduction of a halogen atom (Bernstein et al., 1956; Fried et al., 1958; Demos et al., 1960). The introduction of halogen substituents (a chlorine or fluorine atom) in the 6α or 9α position, while enhancing glucocorticosteroid activity, need not necessarily increase topical activity. Steroid nucleus fluorination in the 6α or 9α

Table 1 Relative Potencies of Various Glucocorticosteroids

Systemically administered

	Anti-inflammatory effect	Salt-retaining effect	Equivalent dose (mg)	Relative affinity for receptor
Hydrocortisone	1	1	20	1
Cortisone	0.8	0.8	25	0.01
Prednisone	4	0.8	5	0.05
Prednisolone	4	0.8	5	2.2
Methylprednisolone	5	0.5	4	11.9
Triamcinolone	5	0	4	1.9
Betamethasone	25	0	0.6	5.4
Dexamethasone	30	0	0.75	7.1

Inhaled (after Johansson, 1980)

	Topical anti-inflammatory effect (vasoconstriction test)	Ratio of topical to systemic potency
Dexamethasone isonicotinate	0.02	—
Triamcinolone acetonide	0.2	0.05
Beclomethasone dipropionate	0.3-0.5	0.11
Flucinolone acetonide	0.05	—
Betamethasone valerate	0.3	—
Budesonide	1.0	1

or both 6α and 9α positions (Singer and Borman, 1956; Sarett et al., 1963) seems to enhance systemic activity more than it does topical activity because it appears to decrease systemic metabolism and transcortin binding (Brattsand et al., 1982).

Recent structure-activity investigations from the group at Lund, Sweden, have demonstrated that it is more important to optimize the 16α, 17α-acetal substitution than to introduce fluorine atoms in the 6α, 9α or 6α and 9α positions to achieve marked topical anti-inflammatory activity (Thalen and Brattsand, 1979). The acetonide or ester modifications of glucocorticosteroids appear to increase local activity, presumably by improving their penetration of cells to reach intracellular cytoplasmic receptors (Rousseau et al., 1972).

Budesonide is a new 16α, 17α-acetal glucocorticosteroid without halogen atoms in this structure, while beclomethasone dipropionate is a 17α, 21-diester with a chlorine atom in the 9α position (Fig. 4). The topical activity of beclomethasone dipropionate is somewhat reduced after hydrolysis of the 21-propionate group and even more so after cleavage of the 17α-ester bond. Lung esterases begin to hydrolyze beclomethasone dipropionate soon after inhalation (Martin et al., 1974), while cleavage of the 17α-ester bond probably occurs mainly in the liver. The high local activity of budesonide is produced by the asymmetrical alkyl chain in the acetal group. This compound has been shown to have a very high glucocorticosteroid-receptor affinity (Dahlberg et al., 1984). Budesonide is not metabolized locally in the lung but is extensively biotransformed in the liver via oxidative and reductive steps (Andersson et al., 1982). Table 1 shows the relative potencies of various glucocorticosteroids.

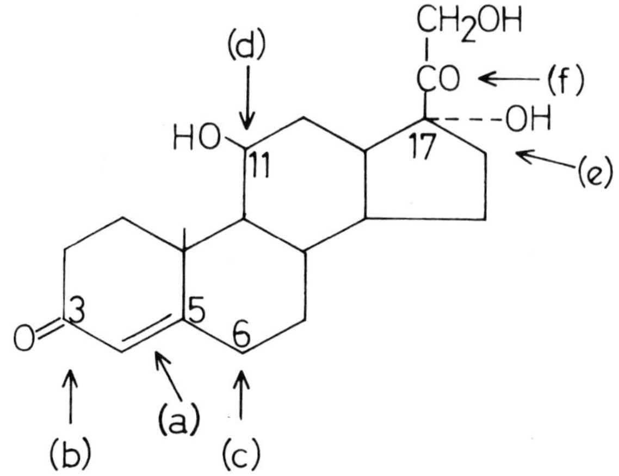

Figure 5 Different ways in which glucocorticosteroids may be metabolized.

Glucocorticosteroids are metabolized via a number of pathways (Seutter, 1975) as may be readily seen in Figure 5. Reduction in activity results from the following metabolic transformations: (a) reduction of the double bond at C-4; (b) reduction of the C-3 oxo group to a secondary alcohol group; (c) hydroxylation of C-6; (d) oxidation of the 11-hydroxyl group, which is a slow process; (e) oxidation of the 17β-hydroxyl group with the loss of a two carbon fragment; and (f) reduction of the C-20 oxo group to a secondary alcohol group. Glucocorticosteroid biotransformation occurs mainly in the liver, but to a lesser extent in other tissues such as the kidney and is excreted in the urine. Conjugation as glucuronides or sulfides renders these agents more water-soluble. The rate of metabolic degradation is diminished by the inclusion of a double bond at C-1, C-2 or by the addition of a fluorine atom in the molecule (Sarett et al., 1963).

III. Clinical Pharmacokinetics of Glucocorticosteroids

A. General Considerations

A large number of studies on the clinical pharmacokinetics of both naturally occurring glucocorticosteroids and their synthetic analogues, in both normal subjects and in patients, were undertaken soon after the various compounds became available (Vermeulen, 1959; Peterson, 1959, 1960; Berliner and Dougherty, 1961). Table 2 summarizes some pharmacokinetic parameters of different glucocorticosteroids.

The pharmacokinetics of glucocorticosteroids do not appear to be influenced by age or by smoking (Rose et al., 1981c). There is some disagreement in the literature as to whether the pharmacokinetics of glucocorticosteroids differ between asthmatics and normal subjects. Most studies carried out with oral prednisolone indicate that the half-lives, total plasma clearances, and steady-state volumes of distribution of this steroid in asthmatic and normal subjects were similar (Rose et al., 1980; May et al., 1980; McAllister et al., 1981). One report, however, shows irregular prednisolone serum concentration profiles following oral doses of 20 mg prednisolone in asthmatics (Wilson et al., 1975). Hydrocortisone has also been investigated in a number of studies but the findings differ. In two studies by Collins and his colleagues (Collins et al., 1960, 1975), no change was reported in the metabolic clearance of hydrocortisone when this was given intravenously in dosages of 2-8 mg/kg to healthy volunteers, asthmatics not previously given glucocorticosteroids, and asthmatics receiving more than 10 mg prednisone daily. Early workers (Dwyer et al., 1967; Schwartz et al., 1968), on the other hand, had found that when hydrocortisone was administered to steroid-dependent asthmatics, its metabolic clearance was greater than in healthy volunteers or asthmatics not on glucocorticosteroids. It has been suggested that as glucocorticosteroids induce the oxidative metabolism of many drugs they may

Table 2 Pharmacokinetic Parameters of Various Glucocorticosteroids

	Plasma half-life ($t_{1/2}$, min)	Peak plasma levels (t_{max} hr)	Serum protein binding (%)	Systemic bioavailability (F, %)	Clearance (Clp, ml/min)
Systemic					
Hydrocortisone	90-120	0.5	90	80	230
Cloprednol	90-120	0.5	N.K.	100	N.K.
Methylprednisolone	150	1-2	N.K.	95	400
Prednisolone	150-210	1-2	85-90	75-100	125
Dexamethasone	240	1-1.5	84	80	200
Betamethasone	420	N.K.	87	95	200
Inhaled					
Beclomethasone dipropionate	900	N.K. (5 hr when given orally)	87	N.K.	N.K.
Budesonide	150	0.20 ± 0.13	86-90	73	1450
Flunisolide	96-120	0.03 (0.25 when given intranasally)	N.K.	20	960
Triamcinolone acetonide	60-120	N.K. (3 hr when given intramuscularly)	N.K.	N.K.	N.K.

N.K., not known

well be able to stimulate their own metabolism (Araki et al., 1964). The balance of evidence, however, seems to swing away from this, and such a self-induction certainly does not seem to occur with prednisolone (May et al., 1980; Rose et al., 1981a).

The rate and extent of drug absorption from the intestinal tract are known to depend, among other factors, on the gastrointestinal transit time, the permeability and vascularity of the intestinal mucosa, the degree of activity of the villi, the pH, and the mucus content of the lumen (Gibaldi, 1977). The presence of inflammatory bowel disease would thus be expected to result in alterations in glucocorticosteroid absorption profiles.

However, most of the studies carried out both in adults (Elliot et al., 1980; Tanner et al., 1981), and in children and adolescents (Mislap et al., 1983), show that although there is some initial delayed absorption of orally administered prednisone or prednisolone in patients with active ulcerative colitis or Crohn's disease, their bioavailability is complete. Conversion of prednisone to prednisolone is also unimpaired in these patients whether they are in remission or in the active phase of the disease. The fractional binding of prednisone to plasma proteins was, however, found to be decreased in the active stage of inflammatory bowel disease (Mislap et al., 1983). On the other hand, Schaffer and his colleagues (1983) have shown that compared with a normal group, absorption of orally administered prednisolone was reduced in seven patients with Crohn's disease. Differences between the studies reported may have resulted from the fact that the extent of involvement of the small and large bowel in these patients with Crohn's disease differed. Prednisolone is thought to be predominantly absorbed in the jejunum. Other disease states, particularly hepatic disorders, may also alter glucocorticosteroid pharmacokinetics (Gambertoglio et al., 1980).

Powell and Axelsen (1972) found that in patients with liver disease there was a significant correlation between the extent of plasma binding of prednisolone and the serum albumin concentration. Patients with chronic active liver disease have been recently reported to have higher concentrations of serum free prednisolone (Uribe et al., 1978) and to have abnormal prednisolone pharmacokinetics with a lower prednisolone clearance (Powell-Jackson et al., 1984). The conversion of prednisone to prednisolone is claimed to be impaired in patients with acute viral hepatitis, chronic active hepatocellular disease (Powell and Axelsen, 1972) and hepatic cirrhosis (Madsbad et al., 1980). Other workers have, however, shown that impaired liver function need not necessarily result in a significant impairment of the conversion of prednisone to prednisolone (Schalm et al., 1976; Uribe et al., 1978). Indeed, in chronic active hepatitis the bioavailability of both prednisolone and prednisone has been reported to be similar (Davies et al., 1978).

Except for some earlier studies, most of the work on the bioavailability and pharmacokinetics of glucocorticosteroids in patients with renal disease (Englert et al., 1958; Nugent et al., 1959) has been done in hemodialysis patients (Sherlock and Letteri, 1977; Bergrem, 1983) or in those who have received a transplant and were also on immunosuppressive therapy (Park et al., 1974; Gambertoglio et al., 1979). The metabolism of hydrocortisone has been reported to be reduced and, with deterioration of renal function, hydrocortisone conjugates are said to accumulate in the blood (Englert et al., 1958; Roseman et al., 1982). However, other workers have not found that the half-life of hydrocortisone was increased (Nugent et al., 1959; Feldman and Singer, 1975) or that the pharmacokinetics of prednisolone were altered (Coburg et al., 1970; Park et al., 1974; Bergrem, 1983).

Even in patients with the nephrotic syndrome after both oral and intravenous prednisolone, the unbound concentrations, the mean residence time, and the volume of distribution of unbound prednisolone were reported to be no different from those in normal subjects (Bergrem, 1983; Frey and Frey, 1982, 1985). Obviously, although the increase in the unbound fraction of a glucocorticosteroid may lead to intensified biological effects, the impaired binding may result in enhanced drug elimination. It is, therefore, difficult to predict accurately the clinical consequences of decreased protein binding in any individual patient, even though attempts at adjusting dosage in such circumstances have been made (Centeno et al., 1978). It thus seems unlikely that the administration of a uniform glucocorticosteroid dosage will lead to similar clinical responses in individual patients. Future development of more accessible techniques will make monitoring of the plasma levels and the degree of protein binding, at least in instances where therapeutic problems are anticipated, result in better clinical control.

There are many reports in the literature of drugs that influence glucocorticosteroid metabolism and of other drugs that interact with them (Jubiz and Meikle, 1970; Lofdahl et al., 1984). Early reports showed that diphenylhydantoin (phenytoin) enhanced microsomal hydroxylation enzyme activity and resulted in an increased clearance rate of glucocorticosteroids in both rats and humans (Werk et al., 1964, 1969; Haque et al., 1972). Phenobarbital has also been shown to decrease the half-life and increase the metabolic clearance rate of dexamethasone in asthmatic subjects (Brooks et al., 1972). Other drugs that have been reported to increase glucocorticosteroid metabolism and enhance their clearance include primidone (Hancock and Levell, 1978), rifampin (Edwards et al., 1974), and ephedrine (Brooks et al., 1977). Macrolide antibiotics, in particular troleandomycin (TAO), have been reported to have a glucocorticosteroid-sparing effect (Spector et al., 1974). This action appears to be specific for methylprednisolone, and TAO has been found to inhibit methylprednisolone elimination and hence increase its half-life (Szefler et al., 1980) but precisely how this is done is not yet known (Szefler et al., 1982). Oral contraceptives are reported to increase transcortin levels and to reduce the clearance of both hydrocortisone and prednisolone (Briggs and Briggs, 1979; Boekenoogen et al., 1983).

B. Pharmacokinetics of Systemically Administered Glucocorticosteroids

Hydrocortisone

Like all the other glucocorticosteroids, hydrocortisone is carried in the body partly bound to transcortin, an α_1 glycoprotein (Doughaday, 1956; Slaunwhite and Sandberg, 1959), partly bound to albumin (Westphal, 1957; Ballard, 1979) and partly as the free drug. This unbound form is considered to be the biologically active form of the drug (Burton and Westphal, 1972). Transcortin has a high affinity for glucocorticosteroids but a relatively low plasma concentration (approximately 10^{-7} M). Albumin, in spite of a lower affinity constant, has a greater steroid-binding capacity than transcortin because of its greater plasma concentration (approximately 10^{-4} M). Transcortin has a much higher affinity for hydrocortisone and prednisolone than for other synthetic glucocorticosteroids. Although various studies are available on the pharmacokinetics of orally administered hydrocortisone (Toothaker et al., 1982a,b), it is the pharmacokinetics of intravenous hydrocortisone that are of immediate relevance to the treatment of bronchial asthma. It has been shown that the distribution and elimination characteristics of hydrocortisone in healthy male volunteers were independent of dosage size at low intravenous dosages up to 20 mg, but were dosage-dependent after an intravenous dose of 40 mg (Toothaker and Welling, 1982). The peak level achieved with a 40-mg dose was reported to be 1,854 μg/ml. It is perhaps worth noting that at levels below 200 μg/ml, hydrocortisone is tightly bound to transcortin and the free fraction of the circulating drug is only 5%, while at plasma hydrocortisone concentrations higher than 200 μg/ml, a greater fraction is more loosely bound to albumin and the free fraction increases to about 25%. There seems to be a variation in the rate of disappearance of hydrocortisone from the plasma after its intravenous administration. The apparent half-life of exogenous hydrocortisone was reported to be higher in the morning (8 A.M.), when endogenous hydrocortisone levels were also at their peak, than in the afternoon (4 P.M.). This could indicate the possible existence of a different metabolic rate at various times of the day (Morselli et al., 1970). The hydrocortisone-binding capacity of transcortin has also been described to show a diurnal variation, the binding capacity being highest at night (Angeli et al., 1978).

Prednisone and Prednisolone

Prednisone is a biologically inert glucocorticosteroid that seems to be mainly absorbed from the upper jejunum by passive diffusion (Hulme et al., 1975), and needs to be converted to the active form, prednisolone, in the liver via the reduction of the 11-keto group, primarily by 11 β-hydroxydehydrogenase (Jenkins and Sampson, 1967; Pickup, 1979). Conversion of prednisone to prednisolone occurs rapidly and seems to be consistent with a first-pass and/or presystemic type of biotransformation (Rose et al., 1981b). Numerous studies in normal subjects (Lee et al., 1978; Rose et al., 1981b; Legler et al., 1982; Bergrem et al., 1983), as well as in a mixed group of patients and normals (Pickup et al., 1977) and in asthmatic patients (Rose et al., 1981; McAllister et al., 1981a,b) have indicated that prednisone and prednisolone exhibit dosage-dependent, nonlinear kinetics over the range of dosages used in clinical practice. With the administration of increasingly larger dosages the values for total plasma clearance increase. The progressive increase in the dosage administered will, therefore, not result in a proportionate increase in the plasma concentration of prednisolone. No significant increase in half-life with increasing dosage has been reported with intravenous prednisolone (Pickup et al., 1977; McAllister et al., 1981a; Bergrem et al., 1983) and any changes in half-life reported following oral prednisolone are marginal (Collins et al., 1985). Both the distribution volume and the systemic clearance of prednisolone increase with an increase in dose (McAllister et al., 1981b; Rose et al., 1981b).

A recent study has investigated the pharmacokinetics of prednisone and prednisolone under steady-state conditions by continuously infusing prednisolone, at two different concentrations, in 10 normal subjects (Legler et al., 1982). Previous studies had all been carried out using single doses of prednisone or prednisolone. The results of this study confirm that prednisolone exhibits dosage- and concentration-dependent kinetics and that this is mainly due to its nonlinear protein binding over the therapeutic concentration range, caused by the saturation of the binding sites on transcortin. Although it appears that the clearance of free prednisolone is increased with increasing concentrations, the interpretation of this observation is complicated by insufficient knowledge about the degree of interconversion of prednisone and prednisolone. Thus, the reported increase (30%) in the apparent clearance of free prednisolone may or may not reflect a change in the body's ability to eliminate it (Legler et al., 1982). Legler's (1982) study reports a 12% unbound plasma prednisolone concentration with a low-dosage (5.5 μg/kg/hr) infusion and double this concentration with a high-dosage (64 μg/kg/h) administration of prednisolone. Nonlinear protein binding, therefore, appears to be the main reason for prednisolone's nonlinear kinetics (Bergrem et al., 1983; Meffin et al., 1984).

Dexamethasone

The pharmacokinetics of dexamethasone has been the subject of study of several investigators (Hichens and Hogans, 1974; English et al., 1975; Duggan et al., 1975; Hare et al., 1975). These studies have often reported wide intersubject and interstudy variations in a number of pharmacokinetic parameters of dexamethasone. The development of a high-performance liquid chromatographic technique has made the more accurate study of dexamethasone disposition possible (Tsuei et al., 1978). Unlike oral prednisolone, which has a nearly 100%

bioavailability (Al-Habet and Rogers, 1980), the bioavailability of oral dexamethasone is only about 80% (Duggan et al., 1975). This has been confirmed in a further study in which dexamethasone was administered both orally and intravenously to the same subjects (Rose et al., 1981c). A comparison of the area under the plasma concentration-time curve showed incomplete systemic availability of dexamethasone. Dexamethasone has a greater ability to bind to plasma proteins than betamethasone (Peets et al., 1969) but both are mainly bound to albumin and do not seem to compete with hydrocortisone for binding sites on transcortin. Knowledge about the metabolic pathways of dexamethasone is still incomplete (Rose et al., 1981c).

C. Pharmacokinetics of Inhaled Glucocorticosteroids

Beclomethasone Dipropionate

It is now widely recognized that glucocorticosteroid aerosols have become one of the principal forms of maintenance therapy in bronchial asthma. This is mainly because of their high bioavailability resulting from their topical administration to the airways and the greatly reduced risk of side effects due to the relatively low dosage requirements. The greater part of any inhaled drug is deposited in the mouth and pharynx and swallowed. In fact, only a small proportion (less than 10%) of the dose enters the small airways and is absorbed from there (Davies, 1975). Topically active glucocorticosteroids are known to be rapidly absorbed into the lung; this has been shown in studies with beclomethasone dipropionate (Martin et al., 1975) as well as with flunisolide (Chaplin et al., 1980a). Beclomethasone dipropionate is readily but slowly absorbed when given orally and it has been estimated that more than 90% of a 4-mg dose of the tritium-labeled drug given as a microfine suspension was absorbed (Martin et al., 1975). Beclomethasone dipropionate is hydrolyzed by fecal esterases to beclomethasone-17-propionate and beclomethasone (Martin et al., 1974). Since this glucocorticosteroid is only sparingly soluble in water (Levy, 1967), it is absorbed rather slowly from the gastrointestinal tract, maximum plasma concentration is said to occur after about 5 hr. Most of it is probably immediately hydrolyzed to beclomethasone-17-α-propionate (BMP). The vasoconstriction potency of BMP is almost as high as that of beclomethasone dipropionate and thus hydrolysis does not represent an inactivation step (Harris, 1975). Further hydrolysis of BMP to beclomethasone and biotransformation by oxidative or reductive pathways results in inactive polar metabolites which are excreted via the bile (Andersson and Ryerfeldt, 1984). In vitro studies have shown that beclomethasone dipropionate is strongly bound to plasma proteins; 87% binding to human plasma proteins has also been reported in an in vivo investigation (Martin et al., 1975).

Beclomethasone dipropionate when administered intravenously to humans is as powerful a systemic glucocorticosteroid as dexamethasone (Harris et al., 1973) yet when given by inhalation or orally at doses up to 1 mg it is said not to suppress the hypothalamic-pituitary-adrenal (HPA) axis. However, the drug given by inhalation affects HPA function at a lower dosage than that required after oral administration (Harris, 1975). It follows then that the portion absorbed from the lungs is mainly responsible for any systemic effects. The specific activity of tritium-labeled beclomethasone dipropionate is not high enough to allow the study of pulmonary absorption and metabolism of an inhaled dose of the drug in humans (Martin et al., 1975). Lung esterases are known to hydrolyze beclomethasone dipropionate rapidly to BMP and then more slowly to beclomethasone (Martin et al., 1974; Hartiala et al., 1979; Andersson and Ryrfeldt, 1984). It is, therefore, probable that both unchanged drug and BMP are readily absorbed from the lung into the bloodstream.

Triamcinolone Acetonide

This is a highly potent, nonpolar, water-insoluble, halogenated glucocorticosteroid developed in the United States. It is a fluorinated ester, aerosolized with freon-12 as propellant and alcohol 1% w/v. Its aerosol unit is designed to minimize deposition of the drug in the mouth (Sly et al., 1978). Studies in both children and adults have demonstrated a marked beneficial effect on asthma symptoms (Henry et al., 1974; Spector and Farr, 1975a; Bernstein et al., 1982) and to have a significant steroid-sparing effect (Chervinsky, 1977). Earlier studies with triamcinolone showed that this glucocorticosteroid is bound to plasma albumin to a lesser extent than hydrocortisone (Florini and Buyske, 1961). Like most other synthetic glucocorticosteroids, triamcinolone acetonide is mainly biotransformed by oxidative pathways by hydroxylation of the 6 β-position (Kupfer and Partridge, 1970; Gordon and Morrison, 1978). Loss of the acetal group, however, has never been conclusively demonstrated to be a metabolic pathway for such glucocorticosteroids. Although the fluorine atom in the 9 α-position slows down its metabolism, triamcinolone acetonide is still rapidly metabolized in the liver, as shown by a number of in vitro studies (Ryrfeldt et al., 1982). As with other topical glucocorticosteroids negligible biotransformation occurs in the skin (Andersson et al., 1982).

Flunisolide

This synthetic, topical, polar glucocorticosteroid is fluorinated in the 6α position. Clinical studies have shown it to be effective in the management of asthma in both children (Meltzer et al., 1982) and adults (Slavin et al., 1980). Pharmacokinetic studies in normal subjects have shown that the drug is readily absorbed through the lung as well as from the alimentary tract and nasal mucosa (Chaplin et al., 1980a). The bioavailability of flunisolide after a single 1-mg inhaled dose was 30-40%, the peak plasma concentration being achieved in

2 min and maintained at this level for about 1 hr. When administered via the nose the bioavailability was calculated to be 49%, the peak plasma concentration being reached 15 min after administration. An oral dose of 1 mg ^{14}C-labeled flunisolide resulted in a systemic availability of only 21%, peak levels being achieved after 20 min. Rapid hepatic degradation occurs by extensive first pass 6α-hydroxylation (Chaplin et al., 1980b). The elimination rate of flunisolide is apparently similar after administration by oral, inhaled, and intravenous routes.

Budesonide

Budesonide is an epimeric mixture of a new synthetic nonhalogenated glucocorticosteroid. Of the topical glucocorticosteroids, budesonide's pharmacokinetics have been best characterized. In animal models it has a better ratio between topical and systemic effects than either beclomethasone dipropionate or triamcinolone (Brattsand et al., 1982b). The topical anti-inflammatory potency of budesonide, as judged by vasoconstriction tests in normal subjects, was twice that of beclomethasone dipropionate, three times that of flunisolide, and more than 1,000 times either prednisolone or hydrocortisone. However, budesonide has a significantly lower effect in depressing plasma cortisol levels and changing the total or differential white blood cell count than beclomethasone dipropriionate (Johannson et al., 1982). The plasma protein binding of budesonide was found to be around 90% with negligible binding to transcortin (Ryrfeldt et al., 1982). After oral dosing, the first-pass metabolism of budesonide was reported to be about 90% (Ryrfeldt et al., 1982). In vitro studies have shown that budesonide was rapidly biotransformed in the liver (two to four times more rapidly than BMP) to the relatively inactive metabolites 6β-hydroxybudesonide and 16α hydroxyprednisolone (Andersson and Ryrfeldt, 1984). The key role of the liver is also supported by in vitro studies with lung, kidney, and skin in which no biotransformation of budesonide occurs (Brattsand et al., 1982a; Andersson et al., 1982). Budesonide is a 1:1 mixture of two epimers with [22R] and [22S] configuration (Albertsson et al., 1978. Epimer [22R] has a somewhat higher (two to three times) topical anti-inflammatory potency (Brattsand et al., 1981) and is more susceptible to liver biotransformation as shown in in vitro studies (Andersson et al., 1982). Kinetic studies with the two epimers have also been carried out in normal volunteers (Ryrfeldt et al., 1984). Following inhalation administration, 32% of the radioactive drug was excreted in the urine and 15% in the feces, while with an oral dose, 45% was recovered in the urine and 30% in the feces (Ryrfeldt et al., 1982).

IV. Pharmacodynamics of Glucocorticosteroids

A. Glucocorticosteroid Action at a Subcellular Level

The currently accepted model of glucocorticosteroid action is shown in Figure 6. Glucocorticosteroids are thought to pass through the cell membrane by pas-

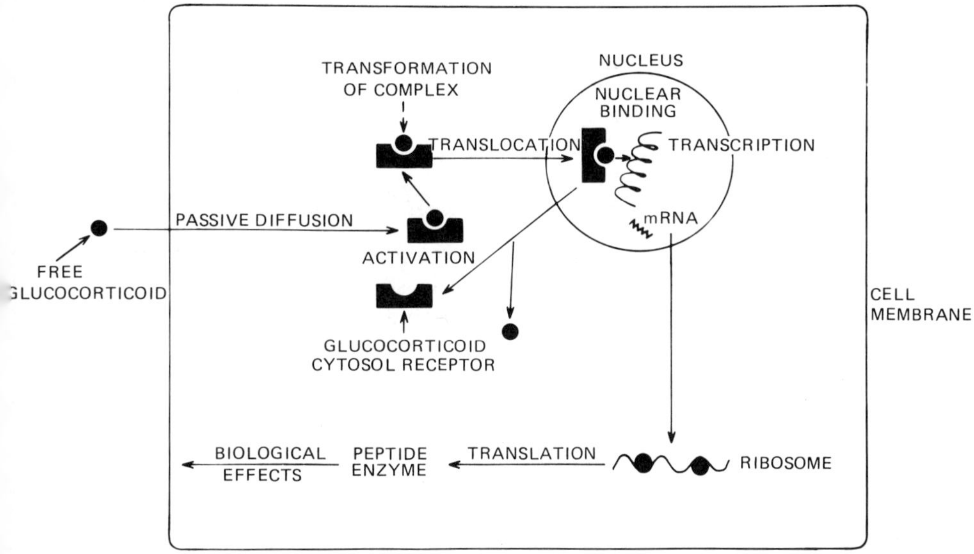

Figure 6 Glucocorticosteroid action at a subcellular level.

sive diffusion into the cytoplasm, where they bind to specific receptor proteins thought to be located initially in the cytoplasm (Lan et al., 1984). The glucocorticosteroid receptor (GR) is an intracellular oligomeric phosphoprotein with multiple domains (Sherman and Stevens, 1984). The receptor is currently thought to have a molecular weight of 94,000 and may have two subunits, a 94K and a 72K unit. As with other steroid receptors, the GR has been described to consist of three domains; domain A contains the steroid-binding site, domain B has the DNA-binding site, and domain C is the immunogenic part to which antibodies bind (Nordeen et al., 1981; Carlstedt-Duke et al., 1984).

The binding of glucocorticosteroids to the receptor seems to promote the dissociation and probably the dephosphorylation of its subunits, a process that has at times been referred to as "activation" (Schmidt and Litwack, 1982) and sometimes as "transformation" (Sherman and Stevens, 1984). The glucocorticosteroid stabilizes its receptor in a high-affinity state.

Further conformational changes in the receptor-steroid complex cause it to acquire a higher affinity for the nucleus and DNA (Rousseau et al., 1973; Higgins et al., 1973). The mechanism of activation of the steroid-receptor complex is not known. Some workers have suggested retaining the term "activation" for the change that occurs when the receptor acquires the hormone-binding form while using the term "transformation" to refer to the change of the glucocorticosteroid-receptor complex to a form with a higher affinity toward nuclear components (Liao and Hiipakka, 1984). The glucocorticosteroid-receptor complex is then translocated to the nucleus, where it interacts with specific receptor-binding regions on the DNA. Glucocorticosteroids thereby control the expression of a small number of transcriptionally active genes (Hager and Palmiter, 1981; Evans et al., 1982) probably by stimulating the induction of mRNA. Glucocorticosteroids are thought to be able to regulate between five to ten genes.

It is not known how the hormones are able to find these genes among so many. The mechanism by which the glucocorticosteroid-receptor complexes increase the specific transcription has also not been defined (Baulieu, 1984). The ultimate step is the translation of mRNA into specific proteins, which brings about the phenotypic response. Although many cells and tissues contain these specific glucocorticosteroid receptors the phenotypic response to these hormones differs, as expected, from one tissue type to another.

Little is known with any degree of certainty about the fate of the glucocorticosteroid-receptor complex after its induction of RNA synthesis. The receptor or the hormone or both may undergo such modifications that they are no longer capable of binding tightly together, resulting in the release of the receptor from the genomic structure (Liao and Hiipakka, 1984). Other possible mechanisms may of course come into play; there are indications that the replenishment of the receptors may be achieved through a process of resynthesis rather than one of recycling (Jungblut et al., 1979). The picture is still necessarily incomplete and there are a number of controversial issues such as whether the glucocorticosteroid receptors are really cytoplasmic (King and Greene, 1984; Welshons et al., 1984; Schrader, 1984), and whether DNA recognition by the receptor may involve a receptor-associated RNA molecule (Economidis and Rousseau, 1985). Other areas requiring further elucidation include the mechanism of receptor regulation (McIntyre and Samuels, 1985), the actual nature of the activation step, the possibility of both transcriptional and posttranscriptional control mechanisms, the way in which transcription is stimulated (Lan et al., 1984), as well as the existence and nature of endogenous inhibitors of inactivation, transformation, and translocation (Dahmer et al., 1984).

B. Mechanisms of Action of Glucocorticosteroids in Asthma

Anti-inflammatory Role

Although a number of different mechanisms are thought to be involved in the action of glucocorticosteroids in bronchial asthma, our knowledge of them is still incomplete. Glucocorticosteroids are believed to play a major anti-inflammatory role. It has been known for a long time that these drugs suppress the signs and symptoms of inflammation through their actions on the various features of the inflammatory reaction.

The link between the way glucocorticosteroids exert their anti-inflammatory effects and their general mechanism of action (described in the previous section) has been provided by the elegant studies of the effect of glucocorticosteroids on arachidonic acid metabolism (Hong and Levine, 1976; Blackwell et al., 1978; Danon and Assouline, 1978). A number of workers have described the ability of these anti-inflammatory steroids to reduce markedly the synthesis of prostaglandins both in intact cells (Tashjian et al., 1975; Parente et al., 1978) and isolated organs (Floman and Zor, 1976; Bonilla and Dupont, 1976) by inhibiting the release of polyunsaturated fatty acid precursors (arachidonic acid) for both the cyclooxygenase and lipoxygenase pathways (Grglewski et al., 1975; Nijkamp et al., 1976). Gryglewski's group in Krakow (1975) showed that glucocorticosteroids blocked prostaglandin release from perfused lungs but had no effect on the direct conversion of arachidonic acid to prostaglandins. This implied that glucocorticosteroids reduced the supply of arachidonic acid substrate for prostaglandin synthesis by interfering with the enzyme phospholipase A_2, which is responsible for the enzymatic cleavage of arachidonic acid from membrane phospholipids. Their work was subsequently confirmed and extended by Levine and his group in the United States (Hong and Levine, 1976; Tam et al., 1977). This inhibitory action of glucocorticosteroids was later shown to be abolished by the addition of exogenous arachidonic acid, reconfirming the antiphospholipase A_2 activity of glucocorticosteroids (Russo-Marie and Duval, 1982). This antiphospholipase effect has been shown to be brought about by "second messenger" proteins synthesized by and released from cells under glucocorticosteroid action. The synthesis of such proteins has been demonstrated in rat peritoneal macrophages and called "macrocortin" (Carnuccio et al., 1980; Blackwell et al., 1980) as well as in rabbit neutrophils, and called "lipomodulin" (Hirata et al., 1980). It is important to keep in mind that both neutrophils and macrophages have prominent inflammatory roles. Blackwell and co-workers (1982) later demonstrated that both macrocortin and lipomodulin are released into rat pleural and peritoneal cavities following the systemic administration of glucocorticosteroids or ACTH.

Macrocortin was first reported to have a 15 k molecular weight (Blackwell et al., 1980), while lipomodulin was said to have a 40 k molecular weight (Hirata et al., 1980). It is now generally accepted that at least part of the acute anti-inflammatory effect of glucocorticosteroids is mediated by the synthesis and release of these proteins with antiphospholipase A_2 activity. The formation of such important mediators as prostaglandins, thromboxanes, and leukotrienes may thus be inhibited by glucocorticosteroids since arachidonic acid is the starting point of these mediators. The role of Paf-acether (platelet-activating factor) in asthma is still undefined but its formation may also be reduced, since generation of this factor can be dependent upon phospholipase A_2 activation (Parente and Flower, 1985).

Besides their effects on the arachidonic acid pathway, glucocorticosteroids have also been shown to effect histamine release in humans (Morr and Bornemann, 1980). The inhibition of histamine release has been shown to be time-dependent in a study on human basophils (Schleimer et al., 1981) and mouse mast cells (Daëron et al., 1982). This time-dependency of glucocorticosteroid action has been shown in their ability to inhibit the immediate response to challenge (Burge, 1982; Dahl and Johansson, 1982).

Glucocorticosteroids affect the vascular aspects of the inflammatory response not only through their inhibition of the release of various mediators (Altura, 1966) but also through a direct vasoconstrictor action (Ebert and Barclay, 1952; Angelo-Khattar and Thulesius, 1983) preventing an increase in vascular permeability and consequent edema formation (Tsurufuji and Sugio, 1978). Glucocorticosteroids appear to regulate local blood flow by modulating vascular responsiveness to other substances, such as histamine, bradykinin, and catecholamines. This action on the macromolecular permeability of the microvasculature has been shown both when the drugs were administered systemically as well as when they were applied topically (Svensjö and Roempke, 1985). It has been hypothesized that the action of glucocorticosteroids on vascular tone is mediated by the inhibition of prostacyclin produced by the vascular endothelium and possibly elsewhere in the lung (Axelrod, 1983).

A further feature of inflammation on which glucocorticosteroids appear to have some effect is mucus. Mucus plugging is widespread in patients with severe asthma and may reflect both an increase in secretion and a decrease in mucus clearance rates (Hogg, 1982), but may persist within peripheral airways even during clinical remission. It has been shown that histamine, a number of HETE compounds, as well as the leukotrienes C_4 and D_4 enhance the secretion of mucus glycoproteins (Marom et al., 1982, 1983). Glucocorticosteroids have been shown to reduce mucus glycoprotein secretion from human airways in vitro (Marom et al., 1984) and to decrease sputum production in patients with stable asthma (Agnew et al., 1983) as well as to improve mucus clearance from peripheral lung zones but not from intermediate and inner lung zones (Agnew et al., 1984). Glucocorticosteroids may well affect the properties of mucus as well as exert an action on the physicochemical properties of the periciliary fluid on which ciliary activity appears to depend (Luk and Dulfano, 1983).

Action of Glucocorticosteroids on Function and Kinetics of Cells Involved in Development of the Asthmatic Condition

It is now being increasingly accepted that bronchial mast cells play a prominent role in initiating the inflammatory responses and airway narrowing that are characteristic features of bronchial asthma. A number of cells, including eosinophils and neutrophils, appear to be the targets of mast cell-derived mediators (Robinson and Holgate, 1985). The activation of these cells is thought to be particularly important in the development of the late asthmatic reaction. Glucocorticosteroids are known to influence both the function and the kinetics of various cells.

Mast Cells and Basophils

There is no evidence that pharmacologic dosages of glucocorticosteroids have any effect in inhibiting the degranulation of mast cells (Schleimer et al., 1983). It appears that glucocorticosteroids may have a somewhat weak inhibitory effect on leukotriene secretion in vitro but have certainly no effect on histamine secretion. Basophils are often considered to resemble mast cells functionally and are often thought of as the circulating counterparts of the mast cell, in spite of the fact that the two types of cell have distinct progenitors and important morphological differences (Lagunoff, 1985). In contrast to mast cells, basophils are susceptible to inhibition by glucocorticosteroids but not by cromolyn sodium. The incubation of basophils for a number of hours with glucocorticosteroids will impair the ability of these cells to respond to allergen challenge by releasing preformed mediators.

Eosinophils

Eosinopenia is one of the earliest recognized effects of glucocorticosteroids. This eosinopenic effect seems to be the result of a combination of factors: a rapid tissue sequestration of eosinophils (Anderson and Bro-Rasmussen, 1968) and inhibition of the leaving of mature cells from the bone marrow (Hudson, 1966). Zweiman and colleagues (1976) have also indicated that there is a dampening of the rate of eosinophil migration in the tissues following glucocorticosteroid administration. Glucocorticosteroids are also thought to reduce eosinophil adherence and, together with the chemotaxis inhibitory effect, will result in a diminished recruitment of these cells to inflammatory sites (Altman et al., 1981). In spite of this, some workers have described a marked deposition of eosinophil-derived material in chronic bronchial asthmatics despite prolonged glucocorticosteroid therapy (Filley et al., 1982).

Neutrophils

Glucocorticosteroid administration in humans results in a neutrophil leukocytosis, probably as a result of an increase in the release of these cells from the bone marrow and their reduced migration from the intravascular space (Bishop et al., 1968). Glucocorticosteroids have been shown to inhibit neutrophil adherence in both in vitro and in vivo studies (Clark et al., 1979; Venezio et al., 1982). Other glucocorticosteroid effects on neutrophil functions that have been reported include the inhibition of degranulation, reduced phagocytosis, and O_2 generation (Klebanoff and Clark, 1978), but these effects are generally seen at suprapharmacologic dosages; hence none of them may be very relevant to the beneficial effects of these drugs on the asthmatic condition. It appears that the main effect of glucocorticosteroids on neutrophils is the prevention of their accumulation at sites of inflammation, thereby inhibiting possible interactions between them and endothelial cells (Mishler, 1977). Some workers have reported that in dogs, neutrophil depletion inhibited airway hyperresponsiveness to ozone (O'Byrne et al., 1984), possibly by preventing the production of neutrophil-derived prostaglandins or thromboxane (O'Byrne et al., 1984). It is perhaps apt to point out that ozone-induced hyperresponsiveness may not necessarily reflect faithfully what actually happens in asthma.

Lymphocytes

Transient lymphopenia following glucocorticosteroid therapy has been reported in normal volunteers (Yu et al., 1974) as well as in steroid-dependent asthmatic children (Chai and Gilbert, 1973). The lymphopenia is thought to be due to a redistribution of circulating lymphocytes, especially the T_M subset (Haynes and Fauci, 1978), migrating back to the bone marrow but not the spleen (Fauci, 1975; Beardsley and Cohen, 1978), and possibly some involution of lymphoid tissues. The number of circulating helper-inducer lymphocytes (T_4) have been said to be more markedly reduced than the suppressor-cycotoxic (T_8) subset (Slade and Hepburn, 1983). On the other hand other workers claim that prednisone does not change the T_4/T_8 ratio (Schuyler et al., 1984). Unfortunately, both studies did not account for the atopic status of their subjects and this could explain the discrepancy in results. In a recent study, oral prednisone was shown to result in a decrease in T_4/T_8 ratio in a group of atopic asthmatics but not in a nonatopic normal group (Gerblich et al., 1985). A possible way in which glucocorticosteroids exert their effects is through the inhibition of the producion of interleukin 1 and the expression of Ia antigens by macrophages (Snyder and Unanue, 1982) which stimulate T-helper cells, as well as the inhibition of lymphocyte-produced interleukin 2, which induces the proliferation of responsive T-lymphocytes (Larsson, 1980; Smith, 1980).

The nature of glucocorticoid-induced modulation of human B lymphocytes responses is complex. There have been previous reports of both a marked fall in circulating B cells (Yu et al., 1974; Beardsley and Cohen, 1978) and of no definite response to oral prednisone (Slade and Hepburn, 1983). More information has recently become available on the sequential events in the human B cell activation cascade (Butler et al., 1983) allowing studies on the direct effects of glucocorticosteroids on human lymphocytes at different states of activation. A recent study from Fauci's laboratory (Cupps et al., 1985) demonstrates the graded effect of in vitro hydrocortisone on cell activation, proliferation, and differentiation on lymphocytes obtained from healthy volunteers. To be effective, hydrocortisone had to be present in culture during the first 24 hr, suggesting the drug-induced modulation of an early event. Early events such as activation and proliferation were profoundly suppressed but the final events in the B cell cycle; the differentiation to the immunoglobulin-producing state were unaffected. Immunoglobulin secretion was either not affected or indeed enhanced, depending on the system used. Others have also reported that the addition of dexamethasone to lymphocyte cultures resulted in a further increase of IgE production where spontaneous in vitro IgE synthesis was occurring, and that this was partly due to a direct effect on B cells (Hemady et al., 1985). However, relatively high dosages of glucocorticosteroids are required in vivo to suppress immunoglobulin production (Butler and Rossen, 1973) and there is no interference at pharmacologic dosages (Claman, 1975; Chiang et al., 1980).

Monocytes and Macrophages

Glucocorticosteroids produce a marked monocytopenia and reduce the migration of these cells to sites of inflammation through as yet ill-defined mechanisms (Thompson and Van Furth, 1970; Dale et al., 1974). It is generally accepted that macrophages play a key role in inflammation and secrete products that have either a direct local action or recruit other cell types. Macrophages help to regulate cellular immunity by secreting interleukin 1, an indispensible cofactor for secretion of the mitogenic lymphokine, interleukin 2. The cell membrane of macrophages, unlike that of lymphocytes, contains substantial amounts of phospholipase A_2 and since the predominant unsaturated fatty acid component of their membrane phospholipids is arachidonic acid, the macrophage may well be a major source of arachidonate metabolites. An early and important step in lymphocyte activation seems to be the insertion of arachidonic acid into phospholipids by acetyl CoA: acetyltransferase. The source of arachidonic acid and phospholipase A_2 for lymphocytes may thus be associated macrophages. Glucocorticosteroids are, however, known to inhibit not only phospholipase A_2 but also the actions of acetyl CoA:acyltransferase in cultured lymphocytes (Morley et al., 1984). Glucocorticosteroids, by inhibiting the migration of these cells to sites of inflammation, preventing the formation and secretion of interleukin 1 necessary for lymphocyte activation, and blocking the formation of various products of phospholipid metabolism, exert beneficial anti-inflammatory effects (Werb et al., 1978).

Restoration of Diminished Responsiveness to β-2-Adrenoreceptor Agonists

There is a certain amount of controversy as to whether β-2-adrenoreceptor agonists administration ever results in clinically relevant subsensitivity or in tachyphylaxis in the lungs (Jenne, 1982), producing a decreased effect or a reduction in duration of effect or both. Reports in the literature both support (Nelson et al., 1977; Jenne et al., 1977; Conolly et al., 1982; Weber et al., 1982) and deny the production of subsensitivity (Larsson et al., 1977; Peel and Gibson, 1980; Harvey et al., 1981; Repsher et al., 1984). Some workers, for unexplained reasons, have also been able to induce tachyphylaxis in normal human airways

(Holgate et al., 1977) but not in those of asthmatics or nonasthmatic atopic subjects (Harvey and Tattersfield, 1982). It is now becoming increasingly accepted that, when used in conventional therapeutic dosages, β-2-adrenoreceptor agonists do not generally result in clinically significant subsensitivity. However, the real clinical situation may be surprisingly different from studies carried out under carefully monitored conditions. It is a common experience among those who have large numbers of asthmatics in their care that a number of these patients abuse β agonists, particularly the inhaled forms, in spite of increasing attempts at patient education. Among these patients the phenomenon of tachyphylaxis or subsensitivity appears to arise most frequently and numbers may well increase in future through the indiscriminate use of nebulizers from which the dosage delivered is much greater. A clinical impression is that there seem to be wide individual differences in susceptibility to the development of subsensitivity, and there appear to be subsets of these patients in whom it may be possible to predict the development of tachyphylaxis at an early stage (Clauzel et al., 1985).

Lymphocytes obtained from asthmatics and incubated with isoprenaline have been shown to have a diminished production of cyclic AMP compared to lymphocytes from normal volunteers. This diminished β-adrenoreceptor responsiveness or desensitization in lymphocytes from asthmatics was reversed following high-dosage glucocorticosteroid administration or incubation of the lymphocytes with glucocorticosteroids (Parker et al., 1973; Hui et al., 1982). Most in vitro studies have been carried out using lymphocytes but there seems to be a difference in susceptibility between various tissues to the development of desensitization of β-adrenoreceptors (Hasegawa and Townley, 1983). These in vitro studies have been supported by a number of in vivo investigations (Ellul-Micallef and Fenech, 1975a; Holgate et al., 1977; Arnaud and Charpin, 1982).

Figure 7 shows the restoration of responsiveness to inhaled isoprenaline by a single intravenous injection of 40 mg prednisolone in a group of asthmatics with β-adrenoreceptor subsensitivity. The molecular basis of subsensitivity is thought to be a diminished number of cell surface β receptors (down-regulation) and a decrease in the proportion of receptors in the high-affinity state (Wessels et al., 1979). It is currently thought that subsensitivity involves agonist-induced internalization of the receptors (Toews et al., 1984). It has been suggested that the sensitivity of β-adrenoreceptors is regulated by the synthesis and subsequent degradation of phospholipids, mainly phosphatidylcholine via transmethylation (Hirata, 1984). Quinacrine and glucocorticosteroids, which are known to block the development of subsensitivity, may do so by inhibiting the activity of phospholipase A_2. Glucocorticosteroids are known to increase markedly β-adrenoreceptor density in normal and transformed cultured human lung cells (Mano et al., 1979); the appearance of the new β-adrenoreceptors occurs within 12 hr of exposure (Fraser and Venter, 1980) and promote the coupling between

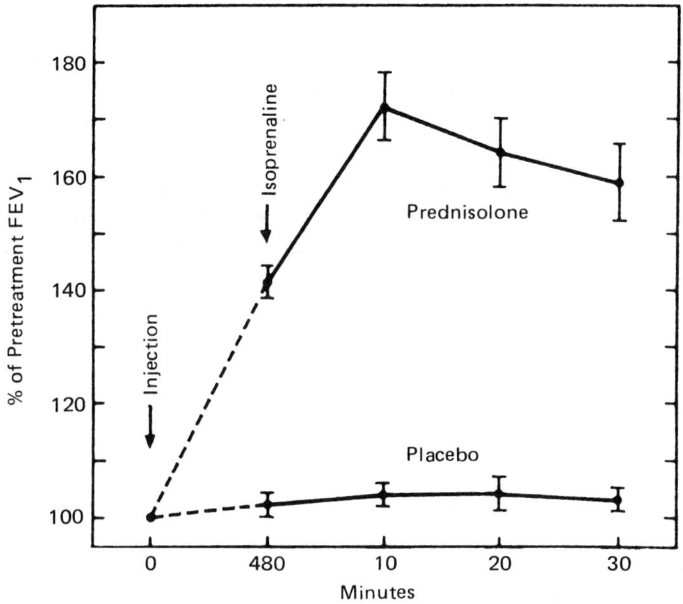

Figure 7 Effect of isoprenaline aerosol 8 hr after intravenous injection of 0.11 mmol (40 mg) prednisolone or placebo.

the agonist-receptor complex and adenyl cyclase (Davies and Lefkowitz, 1981). Although both in vitro and in vivo studies clearly demonstrate that β-2-adrenoreceptor subsensitivity can be reversed by glucocorticosteroids, this mode of action does not appear to be particularly significant in the average asthmatic requiring glucocorticosteroid therapy. It may, however, assume clinical relevance in those patients, admittedly not the majority, in whom subsensitivity to β agonists does develop.

Effects of Glucocorticosteroids on Airway Smooth Muscle

Glucocorticosteroids have been said to have both a direct relaxing effect on airway smooth muscle (Aviado and Carillo, 1970) and potentiate β-2-adrenoreceptor-mediated relaxation (Townley et al., 1970; Geddes et al., 1974). Lefcoe (1956) was the first to report that hydrocortisone produced relaxation of guinea pig tracheal muscle in vitro. Anderson and Kövesi (1974) claimed that hydrocortisone reduces the basal tone of the guinea pig, rat, and human airway. Other workers have, however, failed to detect any in vitro effect on guinea pig tracheal smooth muscle tone (Brink et al., 1977). Doubts have been cast on earlier studies, since it has been shown that the direct relaxing effects shown might well have been produced by the paraben preservatives present in the glucocorticosteroid preparations (Geddes and Lefcoe, 1973). In spite of there being no real evidence to support the view that these drugs have a direct relaxant effect on airway smooth muscle, this mechanism of action is still being listed in recent review articles (Spector, 1985).

Various studies on animals and humans show that glucocorticosteroids potentiate the β-2-adrenoreceptor effects of catecholamines on airway smooth muscle, both in vitro (Foster et al., 1983) and in vivo (Pun et al., 1973; Shenfield et al., 1975). The mechanisms involved have not been really defined. This glucocorticosteroid effect may be the result of a number of actions including adenyl cyclase activation (Logsdon et al., 1972), β-adrenoreceptor sensitization (Besse and Bass, 1966), inhibition of catecholamine uptake, and inhibition of catechol-0-methyl transferase (Pun et al., 1973; Foster et al., 1983). Glucocorticosteroids may also bring about such potentiation by increasing the fluidity of cell membranes sufficient to increase the rate of coupling between the β-adrenoreceptor and adenyl-cyclase (Rimon et al., 1978).

Effects of Glucocorticosteroids on Bronchial Hyperresponsiveness and the Late Reaction

Bronchial hyperresponsiveness is a phenomenon in which the airways respond in an exaggerated manner to both specific and nonspecific stimuli. It is now generally accepted as a cardinal feature of bronchial asthma and regarded by many as the primary pathogenetic event in the acquisition of this condition (McFadden, 1984). Bronchial hyperresponsiveness is probably a multifactorial phenomenon resulting from a number of possible causes, including inflammation as the probable major cause (Hogg, 1981; Boushey and Holtzman, 1985), and, possibly, disorders of autonomic regulation of the airways and alterations in the nature of bronchial smooth muscle (Ellul-Micallef, 1985). The increase in nonspecific bronchial hyperresponsiveness has been reported to occur only if exposure to a sensitizing agent has induced a late asthmatic response (Cockroft et al., 1977), although recently some doubts have been cast on this association (Boyd et al., 1984).

It has been known for some time that glucocorticosteroids block the development of the late reaction very effectively (Booij-Noord et al., 1971). Although glucocorticosteroids block the late reaction more effectively than cromolyn sodium, it has been claimed that they are less effective than cromolyn sodium in reducing bronchial hyperresponsiveness (Altounyan, 1979). Reports in the literature on the effect of glucocorticosteroids on nonspecific bronchial hyperresponsiveness have resulted in conflicting data. Some have shown that both oral (Spector and Farr, 1975b; Wolfe et al., 1979) and inhaled glucocorti-

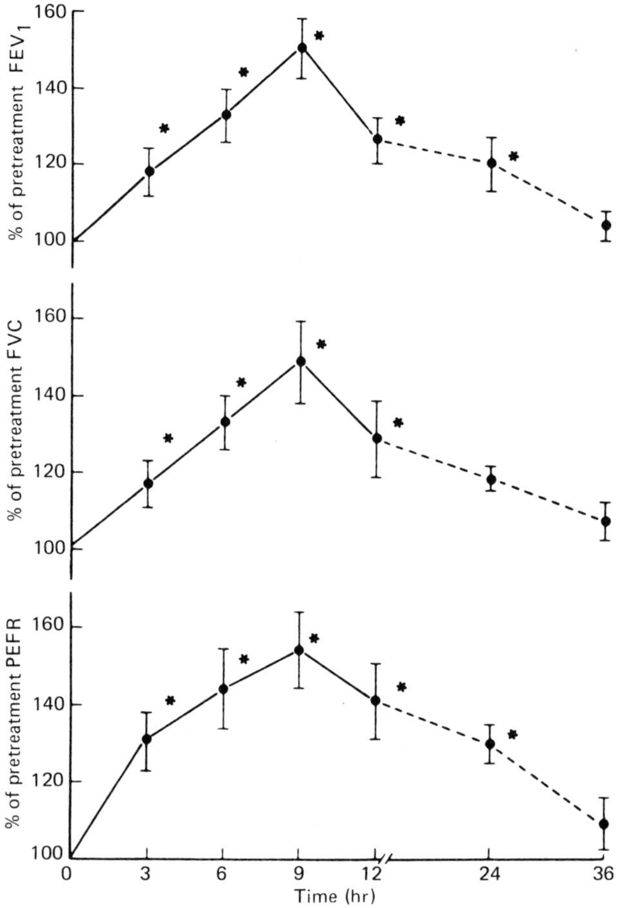

Figure 8 Effect of a single oral dose of 0.11 mmol (40 mg) prednisolone on FEV_1, FVC, and PEFR in six asthmatic patients. *, Points significantly different from control ($P < 0.05$).

costeroids, even when administered for prolonged periods of time (Easton, 1981) had no effect on nonspecific bronchial hyperresponsiveness. On the other hand, other workers have shown these drugs to have a positive effect in reducing hyperresponsiveness (Juniper et al., 1980; Clarke, 1982; Israel et al., 1984; Sotomajor et al., 1984; Hartley, 1985; Ellul-Micallef, 1985). Nonstandardization of factors involved in performing bronchial challenge tests as well as initial patient selection and compliance are possible reasons for the conflicting results.

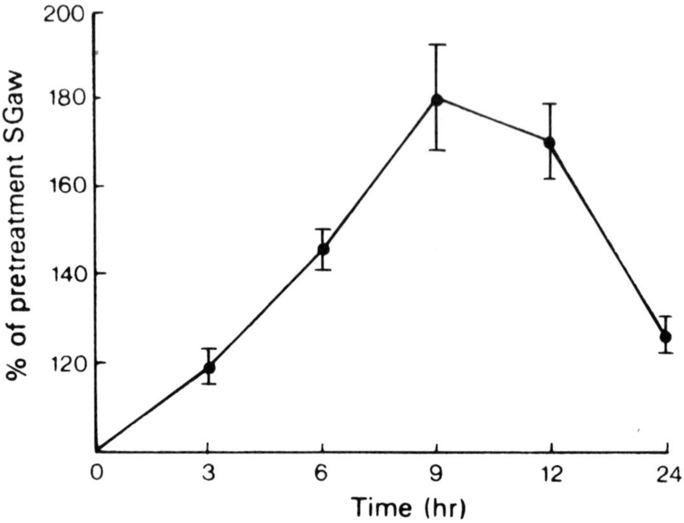

Figure 9 Effect of a single oral dose of 0.11 mmol (40 mg) of prednisolone on specific airway conductance (SGaw). Group mean values ± S.E. mean are shown for eight asthmatic patients.

C. Physiological Changes and Sites of Action in Bronchial Asthma

Walsh and Grant (1966) were the first to introduce the idea of a trial with glucocorticosteroids in bronchial asthma. The acute effects of these drugs in bronchial asthma have been recently reviewed (Ellul-Micallef, 1982). Prior to the studies of Ellul-Micallef and colleagues there was no objective physiological evidence showing that glucocorticosteroids produced an improvement in lung function in asthmatic patients (Feldman and McFadden, 1977; Jenne, 1979). A number of studies by other workers quickly followed (Arnaud et al., 1975; Dugue, Orehek, Arnaud et al., 1977; Di Marzo et al., 1980). In patients with stable chronic bronchial asthma the administration of glucocorticosteroids resulted in a significant improvement in measurements of dynamic and static lung volumes, body plethysmography, and maximum flow-volume curves (Ellul-Micallef et al., 1971, 1974) (Figs. 8 and 9).

It is generally recognized that airway narrowing in asthma is widespread and unevenly distributed throughout the lung. The relative contributions by central and peripheral airways to the resistance to airflow may also change with alterations in the severity of the condition. There is evidence to suggest that the

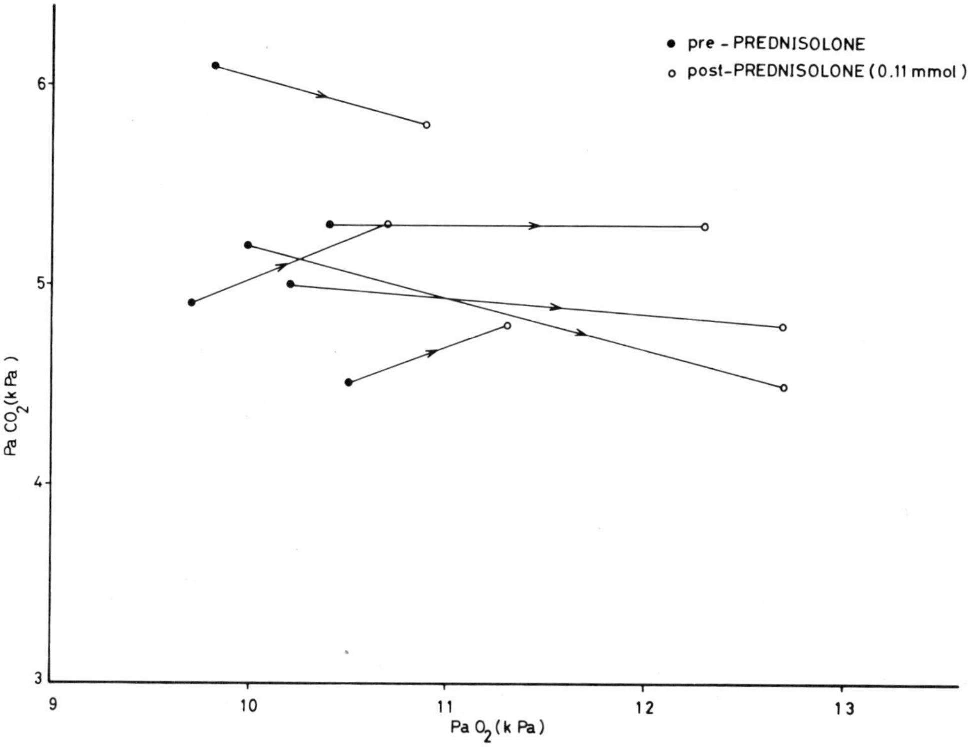

Figure 10 Arterial blood gases in six chronic asthmatic patients 1 hr before and 9 hr after a single dose of 0.11 mmol (40 mg) prednisolone phosphate.

site of airflow may become progressively more peripheral as asthma worsens (Fairshter and Wilson, 1980). Glucocorticosteroids appear to act on both the large as well as the small airways when administered both orally (Ellul-Micallef, 1972) and intravenously (Klaustermayer and Hale, 1976). In adult chronic asthmatics, the administration of oral prednisolone resulted in a decrease in airway resistance and, in contrast to what may occur with methylxanthines and sympathomimetic drugs, in an improvement in arterial oxygen tension (Fig. 10). In these patients there was also a reduction of the alveolar-arterial oxygen tension gradient Pa/PAO_2 and venous admixture effect, but there was little change in the ratio of dead space to tidal volume (V_D/V_T) (Ellul-Micallef, 1972; Ellul-Micallef et al., 1980a). A similar lack of change in V_D/V_T ratio despite a marked difference in Pa/PAO_2 had been previously reported in chronic asthmatics treated with isoprenaline and aminophylline (Tai and Read, 1967).

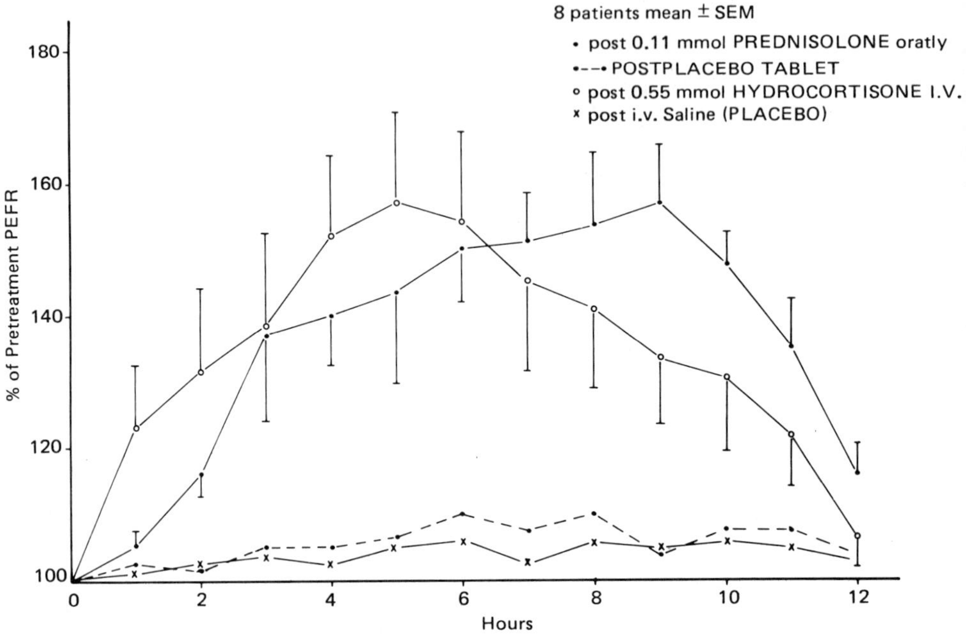

Figure 11 Percentage increase in PEFR after a single dose of 0.11 mmol (40 mg) prednisolone orally, 0.55 mmol (200 mg) hydrocortisone intravenously, and placebo orally and intravenously to eight patients with chronic stable asthma.

In acute adult asthmatics, on the other hand, it appears that the relief of arterial hypoxemia lags behind changes in airflow obstruction (Rebuck and Read, 1971; Arnaud et al., 1977; Fanta et al., 1983). However, in children with severe asthma the addition of glucocorticosteroids to the therapeutic regime produced significant improvement in arterial oxygen tension with little change in the rate and degree of improvement in the forced expiratory volume in 1 sec (FEV_1), which suggests that the drugs may have acted on the peripheral airways (Pierson et al., 1974). These different results emphasize the fact that pathophysiology differs in various states of asthma and between different groups of patients. The beneficial effect of glucocorticosteroids on blood-gas exchange in asthma may have also partially occurred from their action on sites other than the airways. It has been shown that in patients with chronic stable asthma, an intravenous injection of prednisolone resulted in an increase in "effective" pulmonary blood flow (Winfield et al., 1980).

Since the introduction of these drugs for the treatment of asthma there has been considerable controversy as to their usefulness in both the chronic

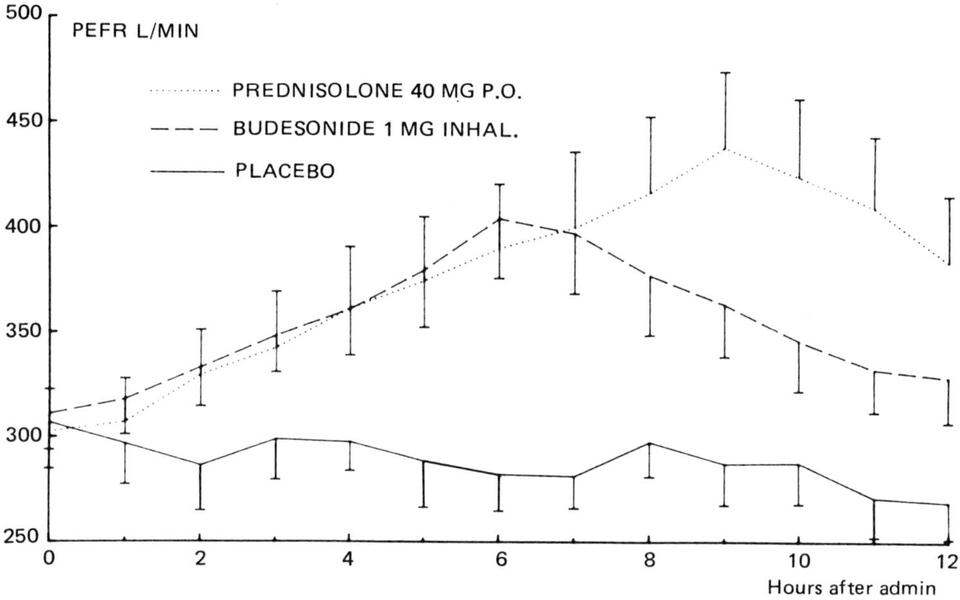

Figure 12 Effect of a single oral dose of 40 mg prednisolone, 1 mg budesonide given by inhalation and placebo tablets on PEFR. Group mean values ± S.E. mean are shown for 12 asthmatic patients.

(Medical Research Council Report, 1956) and acute (Kattan et al., 1980; Luksza, 1982) forms of the condition. There is, however, no lack of evidence in the literature proving the importance of glucocorticosteroids in the management of bronchial asthma (Ellul-Micallef, 1982; Grant, 1982). Objective evidence of the usefulness of intravenous hydrocortisone in improving the FEV_1 in patients with acute asthma has been provided by a well controlled clinical trial (Fanta et al., 1983).

D. Time Course of Response to Glucocorticosteroids

Soon after the introduction of these drugs in the treatment of bronchial asthma (Carryer et al., 1950; Randolph and Rollins, 1950) it became clinically obvious that there is a time lag between their administration and the onset of improvement. Various time intervals had been suggested (Schwartz, 1951; Saperia, 1966; Herxheimer, 1966) but these were often based on subjective impressions.

The first systematic physiological studies were carried out in chronic asthmatic patients in the early 1970s. In these patients, in whom previous bronchodilator therapy was withheld, a single oral morning dosage of 0.11 mmol (40 mg) prednisolone resulted in significant improvement in a number of physiological variables 3 hr after administration. The maximum effect was detectable within 9-12 hr after which there was a return towards pretreatment values over a period of 36 hr (Figs. 8 and 9) (Ellul-Micallef et al., 1974). Studies with intravenous preparations have resulted in a quicker onset of action, but in the case of prednisolone a similar time course of response. A single intravenous injection of 0.11 mmol (40 mg) prednisolone phosphate resulted in significant changes being observed after 1 hr, a maximum change after 8 hr, the effect being still significant after 30 hr (Ellul-Micallef and Fenech, 1975b). The intravenous use of 0.55 mmol (200 mg) hydrocortisone hemisuccinate resulted in a somewhat more rapid overall effect; a significant increase in peak expiratory flow rate (PEFR) was seen at the time of its first measurement, 1 hr after drug administration, the overall peak effect occurred after 5 hr, the change being no longer significant after 12 hr (Fig. 11) (Ellul-Micallef, 1972, 1982). Similar results with intravenous hydrocortisone were obtained later (Arnaud et al., 1975, 1977). Further studies with intravenous methylprednisolone showed an onset of response occurring after 2 hr, with a peak response varying between 4 and 6 hr (Klaustermeyer and Hale, 1976) or after 7 hr (Di Marzo et al., 1980).

Except in the case of status asthmaticus, the administration of glucocorticosteroids by inhalation has obvious advantages. The time-course of response to these inhaled drugs is, therefore, highly relevant. Studies were carried out with different inhaled dosages of budesonide in chronic asthmatic patients and its time course of action compared with oral prednisolone (Fig. 12). A statistically significant increase in PEFR was produced 1 hr after the inhalation of 1000 μg budesonide, peak effect occurred between 6 and 7 hr (Ellul-Micallef et al., 1980). Similar responses were obtained with 100 μg, 400 μg, and 1,600 μg of the drug (Ellul-Micallef and Johansson, 1983). There was a general trend for budesonide to produce a peak effect 1-3 hr earlier than oral prednisolone but to lose its effect sooner. The results reported refer to group mean values; there were, of course, individual variations.

The time taken by glucocorticosteroids to work in acute asthma has been reported to be even longer. In a number of studies the time taken for a detectable effect on pulmonary function was at least 6 hr (Fig. 13) and sometimes longer (Collins et al., 1975; McFadden et al., 1976; Fanta et al., 1983) and a maximum improvement might require as long as 6 days to occur (Shenfield et al., 1975). The differences in the speed of action of glucocorticosteroids reported to occur between chronic and acute asthmatics are probably due to differences in the pathophysiology underlying the two states of the condition. A double blind randomized trial of three regimens of I.V. methyl prednisolone in

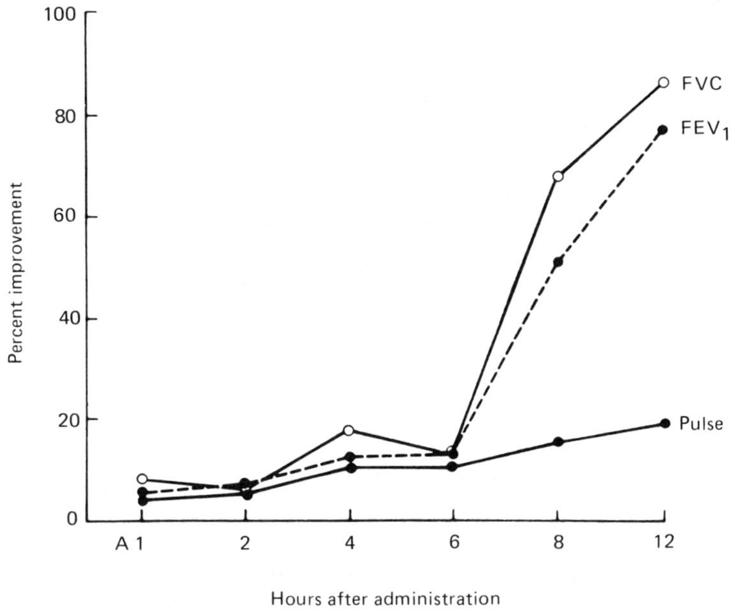

Figure 13 Rate of improvement after starting corticosteroid treatment in patients with severe acute asthma (Collins et al., 1975).

status asthmaticus has shown that low doses (15 mg every 6 hours) are inferior to medium doses (60 mg every 6 hours) or high doses (125 mg every 6 hours), the latter two doses achieving 50% improvement in FEV_1 at 36 and 24 hours, respectively, while only five of eight patients had done so by 72 hours with the low doses (Haskell et al., 1983).

The effects of these drugs on pulmonary function in bronchial asthma appears to follow a similar time course to that of other biological effects of glucocorticosteroids, such as blood glucose (West, 1958; Walton et al., 1970), and on leukocyte kinetics (Mishler, 1977; Slade and Hepburn, 1983). The time lag reported between the administration of glucocorticosteroids and their biological actions is now known to fit in with what is thought to be their cellular mechanism of action (Blackwell et al., 1980; Hirata et al., 1980). Certain effects such as the increase in leukocyte intracellular CAMP levels and the steroid inhibition of ACTH release are said to occur too rapidly to be explained by de novo transcriptional events and protein synthesis. Such effects could be explained by the fact that macrocortin is known to exist as a preformed intracellular store and its secretion is induced by glucocorticosteroids (Blackwell, 1983).

References

Agnew, J. E., Bateman, J. R. H., Sheahan, N. F., et al. (1983). Effect of oral corticosteroids on mucus clearance by cough and mucociliary transport in stable asthma. *Bull. Eur. Physiopathol. Respir. 19*: 37-41.

Agnew, J. E., Bateman, J. R. M., Pavia, D., et al. (1984). Peripheral airways mucus clearance in stable asthma is improved by oral corticosteroid therapy. *Bull. Eur. Physiopathol. Respir. 20*: 295-301.

Albertsson, J., Oskarsson, A., and Svensson, L. (1978). X-ray study of budesonide: Molecular structures and solid solutions of the (22S) and (22R) epimers of 11 β, 21 dihydroxy-16α-17α propylmethylenedioxy-1,4-prednadiene-3, 20-dione. *Acta Cryst. B34*: 3027-3036.

Al-Habet, S., and Rogers, H. J. (1980). Pharmacokinetics of intravenous and oral prednisolone. *Br. J. Clin. Pharmacol. 10*: 503-508.

Altman, L. C., Hill, J. S., Harfield, W. M., et al. (1981). Effects of corticosteroids on eosinophil chemotaxis and adherence. *J. Clin. Invest. 67*: 28-36.

Altounyan, R. E. C. (1979). Review of the clinical activity and modes of action of sodium cromoglycate. In *The Mast Cell, Its Role in Health and Disease.* Edited by J. Pepys and A. M. Edwards. Turnbridge Wells, Pitman Medical, pp. 199-216.

Altura, B. M. (1966). Role of glucocorticoids in local regulation of blood flow. *Am. J. Physiol. 211*: 1393-1397.

Anderson, V., and Bro-Rasmussen, F. (1968). The kinetics of cortisol-induced eosinopenia in the rat. Paper read at the 12th Congress of the International Society of Haematology, New York.

Andersson, P., Edsbacker, S., Ryrfeldt, A., et al. (1982). In vitro biotransformation of glucocorticoids in liver and skin homogenate fractions from man, rat and hairless mouse. *J. Steroid Biochem. 16*: 787-795.

Andersson, R. G. G., and Kövesi, G. (1974). The effect of hydrocortisone on tension and cyclic AMP metabolism in tracheal smooth muscle. *Experientia 30*: 748-785.

Andersson, P., and Ryrfeldt, A. (1984). Biotransformation of the topical glucocorticoids budesonide and beclomethasone 17 α-21-dipropionate in human liver and lung homogenate. *J. Pharm. Pharmacol. 36*: 763-765.

Angeli, A., Frajria, R., De Paoli, R., et al. (1978). Diurnal variation of prednisolone binding to serum corticosteroid binding globulin in man. *Clin. Pharmacol. Ther. 23*: 47-53.

Angelo-Khattar, M. M., and Thulesius, O. (1983). Vascular effects of glucocorticosteroids, with special reference to budesonide. *Gen. Pharmacol. 14*: 125-127.

Araki, Y., Yakota, O., Kato, T., et al. (1964). Dynamics of synthetic corticosteroids in man. In *Steroid dynamics.* Edited by T. Nakato and J. F. Tait. New York, Academic Press, pp. 463-480.

Arnaud, A., and Charpin, J. (1982). Interaction between corticosteroids and $beta_2$-agonists in acute asthma. *Eur. J. Respir. Dis. (Suppl 122) 63*: 126-131.

Arnaud, A., Orehek, J., Autran, P., et al. (1975). Etude du délai d'action d'un corticoide injecté sur l'obstruction bronchique de l'asthmatique. *Nouv. Presse Méd. 4*: 16.

Arnaud, A., Dugue, P., Orehek, J., et al. (1977). Traitment de l'attaque d'asthme: Efficacieté compareée des corticoides et d'une association corticoides-bêta-stimulant adrénergique. *Nouv. Presse Méd. 6*: 4183-4186.

Arth, G. E., Johnsston, D. B. R., Fried, J., et al. (1958). 16-Methylated steroids. I. 16α methylated analogs of cortisone, a new group of anti-inflammatory steroids. *J. Am. Chem. Soc. 80*: 3160-3161.

Aviado, D. M., and Carrillo, L. R. (1970). Anti-asthmatic action of corticosteroids: A review of the literature on their mechanisms of action. *J. Clin. Pharmacol. 10*: 3-11.

Axelrod, L. (1983). Inhibition of prostacyclin production mediates permissive effect of glucocorticosteroids on vascular tone. *Lancet 1*: 904-906.

Ballard, P. L. (1979). Delivery and transport of glucocorticoids to target cells. In *Glucocorticoid Hormone Action.* Edited by J. D. Baxter and G. G. Rousseau. Berlin, Springer Verlag, pp. 25-48.

Barach, A. L., Bickerman, H. A., and Beck, G. J. (1955). Clinical and physiological studies on the use of metacortandracin in respiratory disease. I. Bronchial asthma. *Dis. Chest 27*: 515-527.

Baulieu, E. E. (1984). Pharmacology of steroid receptors from molecular and cellular studies to efficient antihormonal drugs. *Biochem. Pharmacol. 33*: 905-912.

Beardsley, G. P., and Cohen, H. J. (1978). Corticosteroid-induced lymphocytopenia in man: Absence of splenic influence and effect of recipient serum. *Am. J. Hematol. 4*: 255-259.

Bergrem, H. (1983). Pharmacokinetics and protein binding of prednisolone in patients with nephrotic syndrome and patients undergoing hemodialysis. *Kidney Int. 23*: 876-879.

Bergrem, H., Grottum, P., and Rugstad, H. E. (1983). Pharmacokinetics and protein binding of prednisolone after oral and intravenous administration. *Eur. J. Clin. Pharmacol. 24*: 415-419.

Berliner, D. L., and Dougherty, T. F. (1961). Hepatic and extrahepatic regulation of corticosteroids. *Pharmacol. Res. 13*: 329-359.

Bernstein, S., Lenhard, R. H., Allen, W. S., et al. (1956). 16-Hydroxylated steroids. IV. The synthesis of the 16-alpha-hydroxy derivatives of 9-alpha-halosteroids. *J. Am. Chem. Soc. 78*: 5693-5697.

Bernstein, I. L., Chervinsky, P., and Falliers, C. J. (1982). Efficacy and safety of triamcinolone acetonide aerosol in chronic asthma. *Chest 81*: 20-26.

Besse, J. C., and Bass, A. D. (1966). Potentiation by hydrocortisone of responses to catecholamines in vascular smooth muscle. *J. Pharmacol. Exp. Ther. 154*: 224-238.

Bishop, C. R., Athens, J. W., Boggs, D. R., et al. (1968). Leukokinetic studies: XIII. A non steady-state evaluation of the mechanism of cortisone-induced granulocytosis. *J. Clin. Invest. 47*: 249-260.

Blackwell, G. J. (1983). Specificity and inhibition of glucocorticoid-induced macrocortin secretion from rat peritoneal macrophages. *Br. J. Pharmacol. 79*: 587-594.

Blackwell, G. J., Flower, R. J., Nijkamp, F. P., et al. (1978). Phospholipase A_2 activity of guinea pig isolated perfused lungs: stimulation and inhibition by anti-inflammatory steroids. *Br. J. Pharmacol. 62*: 79-89.

Blackwell, G. J., Carnuccio, R., Di Rosa, M., Flower, R. J., Parente, L., and Persico, P. (1980). Macrocortin: A polypeptide causing the anti-phospholipase effect of glucocorticoids. *Nature 287*: 147-149.

Blackwell, G. J., Carnuccio, R., Di Rosa, M., et al. (1982). Glucocorticoids induce the formation and release of anti-inflammatory and anti-phosphatase proteins into the peritoneal cavity of the rat. *Br. J. Pharmacol. 76*: 185-194.

Boekenoogen, S. J., Szefler, S. J., and Jusko, W. J. (1983). Prednisolone disposition and protein binding in oral contraceptive users. *J. Clin. Endocrinol. Metab. 56*: 702-709.

Bonilla, C. A., and Dupont, J. (1976). Fatty acid and prostaglandin composition of left ventricular myocardium from dexamethasone-treated dogs with severe low output syndrome. *Prostaglandins 41*: 935-942.

Booij-Noord, H., Orie, N. G. M., and de Vries, K. (1971). Immediate and late bronchial obstructive reactions to inhalation of house dust and protective effects of disodium cromoglycate and prednisolone. *J. Allergy Clin. Immunol. 48*: 344-354.

Boushey, H. A., and Holtzman, M. J. (1985). Experimental airway inflammation and hyperreactivity. *Am. Rev. Respir. Dis. 131*: 312-313.

Boyd, G., Gaffney, D., and Winter, J. (1984). Bronchial reactivity following antigen challenge in asthmatics. Paper read at Annual Meeting of the Societas Europea Physiologiae Clinicae Respiratoriae, Barcelona, 1984.

Brattsand, R., Thalen, A., Roempke, K., et al. (1981). Influence of steroid nucleus fluorination and type of 16α, 17α-acetal substition on the topical to systemic glucocorticoid activity ratio of 16α, 17α-acetal corticoids. *J. Steroid Biochem. 16*: 779-786.

Brattsand, R., Kallstrom, Nilsson, E., et al. (1982a). The lung disposition of budesonide in guinea pig and rat. *Eur. J. Respir. Dis. 63 (Suppl 122)*: 263-265.

Brattsand, R., Thalen, A., Roempke, K., et al. (1982b). Development of new corticosteroids with a very high ratio between topical and systemic activities. *Eur. J. Respir. Dis. 63 (Suppl 122)*: 62-73.

Briggs, M. H., and Briggs, M. (1979). Oral contraceptives and plasma protein metabolism. *J. Steroid Biochem. 11*: 425-428.

Brink, C., Ridgway, P., and Douglas, J. S. (1977). Modification of airway smooth muscle responses in the guinea pig by hydrocortisone, in vitro and in vivo. *J. Pharmacol. Exp. Ther. 203*: 1-11.

Brooks, S. M., Werk, E. E., Ackerman, S. J., et al. (1972). Adverse effects of phenobarbital on corticosteroid metabolism in patients with bronchial asthma. *N. Engl. J. Med. 286*: 1125-1128.

Brooks, S. M., Sholiton, L. J., Werk, E. E., and Altenau, P. (1977). The effects of ephedrine and theophylline on dexamethasone metabolism in bronchial asthma. *J. Clin. Pharmacol. 17*: 308-318.

Brown, H. M., Storey, G., and George, W. H. S. (1972). Beclomethasone dipropionate: A new steroid aerosol for the treatment of allergic asthma. *Br. Med. J. 1*: 585-590.

Burge, P. S. (1982). The effects of corticosteroids in the immediate asthmatic reaction. *Eur. J. Respir. Dis. 63* (Suppl 122): 163-166.

Burrage, W. S., and Irwin, J. W. (1955). Hydrocortisone in the therapy of asthma. *Ann. N.Y. Acad. Sci. 61*: 377-391.

Burton, R. M., and Westphal, U. (1972). Steroid hormone-binding proteins in blood plasma. *Metabolism 21*: 253-276.

Butler, J. L., Muraguchi, A., Lane, H. C., et al. (1983). Development of human T-T cell hybridoma secreting B cell growth factor. *J. Exp. Med. 157*: 60-68.

Butler, W. T., and Rossen, R. D. (1973). Effect of corticosteroids on immunity in man. I. Decreased serum IgG concentration caused by 3-5 days of high doses prednisolone. *J. Clin. Invest. 52*: 2629-2640.

Carlstedt-Duke, J., Wrange, O., Okret, S., et al. (1984). The glucocorticoid receptor in rat liver. *Biochem. Pharm. 33*: 913-916.

Carnuccio, R., Di Rosa, M., and Persico, P. (1980). Hydrocortisone induced inhibitor of prostaglandin biosynthesis in rat leucocytes. *Br. J. Pharmacol. 68*: 14-16.

Carryer, H. M., Prickman, L. E., Maytum, C. K., et al. (1950). Effects of cortisone on bronchial asthma and hay fever occurring in subjects sensitive to ragweed pollen. *Proc. Mayo Clinic 25*: 282-295.

Centeno, F., Robles, G., Uribe, M., et al. (1978). Nomogram for prednisone-prednisolone adjustment dose in patients with hypoalbuminaemia. *Rev. Invest. Chem. 30*: 35-39.

Chai, H., and Gilbert, A. (1973). The effect of alternate-day prednisolone on the white blood count in children with chronic asthma. *J. Allergy Clin. Immunol. 51*: 65-70.

Chaplin, M. D., Cooper, W. C., Segre, E. J., et al. (1980a). Correlation of flunisolide plasma levels to eosinopenic response in humans. *J. Allergy Clin. Immunol. 65*: 445-453.

Chaplin, M. D., Rooks, W., Swenson, E. W., et al. (1980b). Flunisolide metabolism and dynamics of a metabolite. *Clin. Pharmacol. Ther. 27*: 402-413.

Chervinsky, P. (1977). Treatment of steroid-dependent asthma with triamcinolone acetonide aerosol. *Ann. Allergy 38*: 192-197.

Chiang, J-L, Patterson, R., McGillen, J. J., Phair, J. P., Roberts, M., Harris, K. E., and Reising, K. S. (1980). Long-term corticosteroid effect on lymphocyte and polymorphonuclear cell function in asthmatics. *J. Allergy Clin. Immunol. 65*: 263-268.

Claman, H. N. (1975). How corticosteroids work. *J. Allergy Clin. Immunol. 55*: 145-151.

Clark, R. A. F., Gallin, J. I., and Fauci, A. S. (1979). Effects of in vivo prednisone on in vitro eosinophil and neutrophil adherence and chemotaxis. *Blood 53*: 633-641.

Clark, T. H. J. (1972). Effect of beclomethasone dipropionate delivered by aerosol in patients with asthma. *Lancet 1*: 1361-1364.

Clarke, P. S. (1982). The effect of beclomethasone dipropionate on bronchial hyperreactivity. *J. Asthma 19*: 91-93.

Clauzel, A. M., Bres, J., Benyounes, A., et al. (1985). Attempt of predicting beta-adrenergic tachyphylaxis. *J. Allergy Clin. Immunol. 75*: 180 (abst.).

Coburg, A. J., Gray, S. H., Katz, F. H., et al. (1970). Disappearance rates and immuno-suppression of intermittent intravenously administered prednisolone in rabbits and human beings. *Surg. Gynecol. Obstet. 131*: 933-942.

Cockcroft, D. W., Ruffin, R. E., Dolovich, J., and Hargreave, F. E. (1977). Allergen-induced increase in non-allergic bronchial reactivity. *Clin. Allergy 7*: 503-513.

Collins, J. V., Clark, T. J. H., Harris, P. W. R., et al. (1960). Intravenous corticosteroids in the treatment of acute bronchial asthma. *Lancet 1*: 1047-1050.

Collins, J. V., Clark, T. J. H., Brown, D., and Townsend, J. (1975). The use of corticosteroids in the treatment of acute asthma. *Q. J. Med. (New Series) 44*: 259-273.

Collins, J. V., McAllister, W. A. C., and Morley, J. (1985). Corticosteroids: Mechanisms and dosage schedules. In *Bronchial Asthma. Mechanisms and Therapeutics,* 2nd ed. Edited by E. B. Weiss, M. S. Segal and M. Stein. Boston/Toronto, Little, Brown, pp. 675-689.

Conolly, M. E., Tashkin, D. P., Hui, K. K. P., Littner, M. R., and Wolfe, R. N. (1982). Selective subsensitization of beta-adrenergic receptors in central airways of asthmatics and normal subjects during long-term therapy with inhaled salbutamol. *J. Allergy Clin. Immunol. 70*: 423-431.

Cotes, P. M., McLean, A., and Sayer, J. B. (1956). Absorption of inhaled hydrocortisone. *Lancet 2*: 807-808.

Crepea, S. B. (1963). Inhalation corticosteroid (dexamethasone PO_4) management of chronically asthmatic children. *J. Allergy 34*: 119-126.

Cupps, T. R., Gerrard, T. L., Falkoff, R. J. M., et al. (1985). Effects of in vitro corticosteroids on β cell activation, proliferation and differentiation. *J. Clin. Invest. 75*: 754-761.

Daëron, M., Sterk, A. R., Hirata, F., Ishizaka, T. (1982). Biochemical analyses of glucocorticoid induced inhibition of IgE-mediated histamine release from mouse mast cells. *J. Immunol. 129*: 1212-1218.

Dahl, R., and Johansson, S-Å. (1982). Importance of duration of treatment with inhaled budesonide on the immediate and late bronchial reaction. *Eur. J. Respir. Dis.* (Suppl 122): 167-175.

Dahlberg, E., Thalen, A., Brattsand, R., et al. (1984). Correlation between chemical structure, receptor binding and biological activity of some novel, highly active 16α, 17α-acetal substituted glucocorticoids. *Mol. Pharmacol. 25*: 70-78.

Dahmer, M. K., Housley, P. R., and Pratt, W. B. (1984). Effects of molybdate and endogeneous inhibitors on steroid-receptor inactivation, transformation and translocation. In *Annual Review of Physiology.* Edited by R. M. Berne. California, Annual Reviews Inc., pp. 67-81.

Dale, D. C., Fauci, A. S., and Wolff, S. M. (1974). Alternate-day prednisolone: Leukocyte kinetics and susceptibility to infection. *N. Engl. J. Med. 291*: 1154-1158.

Danon, A., and Assoutine, G. (1978). Inhibition of prostaglandin biosynthesis by corticosteroids requires RNA and protein synthesis. *Nature 273*: 552-554.

David, D. S., Grieco, M. H., and Cushman, P. (1970). Adrenal glucocorticoids after twenty years. *J. Chron. Dis. 22*: 637-711.

Davies, A. O., and Lefkowitz, R. J. (1981). Agonist promoted high affinity state of the β-adrenergic receptor in human neutrophils: modulation by corticosteroids. *J. Clin. Endocrinol. Metab. 53*: 703-708.

Davies, D. S. (1975). Pharmacokinetics of inhaled substances. *Postgrad. Med. J. 51 (Suppl. 7)*: 69-75.

Davies, M., Williams, R., Chakraborty, J., et al. (1978). Prednisone or prednisolone for the treatment of chronic active hepatitis? A comparison of plasma availability. *Br. J. Clin. Pharmacol. 5*: 501-505.

Demos, C. H., Place, V. A., and Ruesegger, J. H. (1960). Structure-function relationship of 16 α-hydroxylated steroids and their acetonide analogues. *Acta Endocrinol. (Kbh) 51 (Suppl)*: 759-763.

Di Marzo, A., Rosati, G., Gliozzi, F., et al. (1980). Ricerche sperimentali sull' attività dei corticosteroidi nell'asma bronchiale. *Fisiopatol. Respir. 1*: 431-443.

Doughaday, W. H. (1956). Binding of corticosteroids by plasma proteins. II. Paper electrophoresis and equilibrium paper electrophoresis. *J. Clin. Invest. 35*: 1434-1439.

Duggan, D. E., Yeh, K. C., Matalia, N., et al. (1975). Bioavailability of oral dexamethasone. *Clin. Pharmacol. Ther. 18*: 205-209.

Dugue, P., Orehek, J., Arnaud, A., and Charpin, J. (1977). Effet d'une injection d'hydrocortisone sur l'obstruction bronchique de l'asthme. *Bull. Eur. Physiopathol. Resp. 13*: 619-627.

Dwyer, J., Lazarus, L., and Hickie, J. B. (1967). A study of cortisol metabolism in patients with chronic asthma. *Aust. Ann. Med. 16*: 297-304.

Easton, J. G. (1981). Effect of an inhaled corticosteroid on metacholine airway reactivity. *J. Allergy Clin. Immunol. 67*: 388-390.

Ebert, R. H., and Barclay, W. R. (1952). Changes in connective tissue reaction induced by cortisone. *Ann. Intern. Med. 37*: 506-518.

Economidis, I. V., and Rousseau, G. G. (1985). Association of the glucocorticoid hormone receptor with ribonucleic acid. *FEBS Letters 181*: 47-52.

Edwards, O. M., Courtenay-Evans, E. J., Galley, J. M., et al. (1974). Changes in cortisol metabolism following rifampicin therapy. *Lancet 2*: 549-551.

Elliott, P. R., Powell-Tuck, J., Gillespie, P. E., et al. (1980). Prednisolone absorption in acute colitis. *Gut 21*: 49-51.

Ellul-Micallef, R. (1972). The time course of response to corticosteroids in bronchial asthma. Ph.D. Thesis, University of Edinburgh.

Ellul-Micallef, R. (1982). The acute effects of corticosteroids in bronchial asthma. *Eur. J. Respir. Dis. 63 (Suppl 122)*: 118-125.

Ellul-Micallef, R. (1985). Bronchial hyperresponsiveness and the late reaction. In *Glucocorticosteroids, Inflammation and Bronchial Hyperreactivity*. Edited by J. C. Hogg, R. Ellul-Micallef, and R. Brattsand. Amsterdam, Excerpta Medica, pp. 75-85.

Ellul-Micallef, R., and Fenech, F. F. (1975a). Effect of intravenous prednisolone on asthmatics with diminished adrenergic responsiveness. *Lancet 2*: 1269-1271.

Ellul-Micallef, R., and Fenech, F. F. (1975b). Intravenous prednisolone in chronic bronchial asthma. *Thorax 30*: 312-315.

Ellul-Micallef, R., and Johansson, S. A. (1983). Acute dose response studies in bronchial asthma with a new corticosteroid–Budesonide. *Br. J. Clin. Pharmacol. 15*: 419-422.

Ellul-Micallef, R., Borthwick, R. C., and McHardy, G. J. R. (1971). Time-course of response to corticosteroids in chronic airway obstruction. *Scot. Med. J. 16*: 534 (abst.).

Ellul-Micallef, R., Borhtwick, R. C., and McHardy, G. J. R. (1974). The time-course of response to prednisolone in chronic bronchial asthma. *Clin. Sci. 47*: 105-117.

Ellul-Micallef, R., Fenech, F. F., and Parrott, D. (1978). Comparison of clopred-nol and prednisolone in chronic asthmatic patients. *Br. J. Clin. Pharmacol. 6*: 91-93.

Ellul-Micallef, R., Borthwick, R. C., and McHardy, G. J. R. (1980a). The effect of oral prednisolone on gas exchange in chronic bronchial asthma. *Br. J. Clin. Pharmacol. 9*: 479-482.

Ellul-Micallef, R., Hansson, E., and Johansson, S. A. (1980b). Budesonide: A new corticosteroid in bronchial asthma. *Eur. J. Respir. Dis. 61*: 167-173.

Englert, E., Brown, H., Willardson, D. G., et al. (1958). Metabolism of free and conjugated 17-hydroxycorticosteroids in subjects with uraemia. *J. Clin. Endocrinol. 18*: 36-48.

Evans, R. M., Birnberg, N. C., and Rosenfeld, M. G. (1982). Glucocorticoid and thyroid hormones transcriptionally regulate growth hormone gene expression. *Proc. Natl. Acad. Sci. U.S.A. 79*: 7659-7663.

Fairshter, R. D., and Wilson, A. F. (1980). Relationship between the site of airflow limitation and localization of the bronchodilator response in asthma. *Am. Rev. Respir. Dis. 122*: 27-32.

Fanta, C. H., Rossing, T. H., and McFadden, E. R. (1983). Glucocorticoids in acute asthma. A critical controlled trial. *Am. J. Med. 74*: 845-851.

Fauci, A. S. (1975). Mechanisms of corticosteroid action on lymphocyte subpopulations. I. Redistribution of circulating T and B lymphocytes to bone marrow. *Immunology 28*: 669-680.

Feldman, H. A., and Singer, I. (1975). Endocrinology and metabolism in uraemia and dialysis: A clinical review. *Medicine 54*: 345-376.

Feldman, N. T., and McFadden, E. R. Jr. (1977). Asthma. Therapy old and new. *Med. Clin. North Am. 61*: 1239-1250.

Filley, W. V., Holley, K. E., Kephart, G. M., et al. (1982). Identification by immunofluorescence of eosinophil granule major basic protein in lung tissues of patients with bronchial asthma. *Lancet 2*: 11-15.

Flomay, Y., and Zor, U. (1976). Mechanism of steroid action in inflammation: Inhibition of prostaglandin synthesis and release. *Prostaglandins 12*: 403-413.

Florini, J. R., and Buyske, D. A. (1961). Plasma protein binding of triamcinolone-H3 and hydrocortisone-4-C14. *J. Biol. Chem. 236*: 247-251.

Foster, P. S., Goldie, R. G., and Paterson, J. W. (1983). Effect of steroids on β-adrenoceptor-mediated relaxation of pig bronchus. *Br. J. Pharmacol. 78*: 441-445.

Fraser, C. M., and Venter, J. C. (1980). The synthesis of β-adrenergic receptors in cultured human lung cells: Induction by glucocorticoids. *Biochem. Biophys. Res. Commun. 94*: 390-397.

Frears, J. F., Wilson, L. C., and Friedman, M. (1973). Betamethasone 17-valerate by aerosol in childhood asthma. *Arch. Dis. Child. 48*: 856-863.

Frey, B. M., and Frey, F. J. (1985). The effect of altered prednisolone kinetics in patients with the nephrotic syndrome and in women taking oral contraceptive steroids on human mixed lymphocyte cultures. *J. Clin. Endocrinol. Metab. 60*: 361-369.

Frey, F. J., and Frey, B. M. (1982). Altered prednisolone kinetics in patients with the nephrotic syndrome. *Nephron 32*: 45-48.

Freyburg, R. H., Traeger, C. T., Adams, C. H., et al. (1950). Effectiveness of cortisone administered orally. *Science 112*: 429-434.

Fried, J., Borman, A., Kessler, W. B., et al. (1958). Cyclic 16α, 17α-ketals and acetals of 9α-fluoro-16αhydroxycortisol and prednisolone. *J. Am. Chem. Soc. 80*: 2338-2339.

Gambertoglio, J., Amend, W., Vincenti, F., et al. (1979). The pharmacokinetics of prednisone in cushingoid and noncushingoid kidney transplant patients. *Clin. Res. 27*: 231A.

Gambertoglio, J. C., Amend, W. J. C., Jr., and Benet, L. Z. (1980). Pharmacokinetics and bioavailability of prednisone and prednisolone in healthy volunteers and patients: A review. *J. Pharmacokin. Biopharm. 8*: 1-52.

Geddes, B. A., and Lefcoe, N. M. (1973). Respiratory smooth muscle relaxing effect of commercial steroid preparations. *Am. Rev. Respir. Dis. 107*: 395-399.

Geddes, B. A., Jones, T. R., Dvorsky, R. J., and Lefcoe, N. M. (1974). Interaction of glucocorticoids and bronchodilators on isolated guinea pig tracheal and human bronchial smooth muscle. *Am. Rev. Respir. Dis. 110*: 420-427.

Gerblich, A., Urda, G., and Schuyler, M. (1985). Atopic asthma: T-cell response to corticosteroids. *Chest 87*: 44-50.

Gibaldi, M. (1977). Gastrointestinal absorption. In *Biopharmaceutics and Clinical Pharmacokinetics.* Edited by M. Gibaldi. Philadelphia, Lea and Febiger, pp. 15-41.

Godfrey, S., and Konig, P. (1973). Beclomethasone aerosol in childhood asthma. *Arch. Dis. Child. 48*: 665-670.

Gordon, S., and Morrison, J. (1978). The metabolic fate of triamcinolone acetonide in laboratory animals. *Steroids 32*: 25-35.

Grant, I. W. B. (1982). Are corticosteroids necessary in the treatment of severe acute asthma? *Br. J. Dis. Chest 76*: 125-129.

Grant, I. W. B., Crompton, G. K., Malone, D. N. S., et al. (1972). Treatment of asthma with beclomethasone aerosol. *Br. Med. J. 2*: 110-111.

Grieco, M. H., Dwek, J., Larsen, K., and Rammokan, G. (1978). Clinical effect of aerosol triamcinolone acetonide in bronchial asthma. *Arch. Int. Med. 135*: 1337-1341.

Gryglewski, R. J., Panczenko, B., Korbut, R., Grodzinka, L., and Cetkiewicz, A. O. (1975). Corticosteroids inhibit prostaglandin release from perfused mesenteric blood vessels of rabbit and from perfused lungs of sensitized guinea pigs. *Prostaglandins 10*: 343-355.

Hager, L. J., and Palmiter, R. D. (1981). Transcriptional regulation of mouse liver metallothionen-1 gene by glucocorticoids. *Nature 291*: 340-342.

Hancock, K. W., and Levell, M. J. (1978). Primidone/dexamethasone interaction. *Lancet 2*: 97-98.

Haque, N., Thrasher, K., Werk, E. E., et al. (1972). Studies on dexamethasone metabolism in man: Effect of diphenylhydantoin. *J. Clin. Endocrinol. Metab. 34*: 44-50.

Hare, L. E., Yeh, K. C., Ditzler, C. A., et al. (1975). Bioavailability of oral dexamethasone. II. Dexamethasone phosphate. *Clin. Pharmacol. Ther. 18*: 330-337.

Harris, D. M. (1975). Properties and therapeutic uses of some corticosteroids with enhanced topical potency. *J. Steroid. Biochem. 6*: 711-716.

Harris, D. M., Martin, L. E., Harrison, C., et al. (1973). The effect of oral and inhaled beclomethasone dipropionate on adrenal function. *Clin. Allergy 3*: 243-248.

Hartiala, J., Uotila, P., and Nienstedt, W. (1979). Absorption and metabolism of intratracheally instilled cortisol and beclomethasone dipropionate in isolated perfused rat lungs. *Med. Biol. 57*: 294-297.

Hartley, J. P. R. (1985). The effect of budesonide on bronchial hyperreactivity. In *Glucocorticosteroids, Inflammation and Bronchial Hyperreactivity*. Edited by J. C. Hogg, R. Ellul-Micallef, and R. Brattsand. Amsterdam, Excerpta Medica, pp. 110-115.

Harvey, J. E., Baldwin, C. J., Wood, P. J., Alberti, K. G., and Tattersfield, A. E. (1981). Airway and metabolic responsiveness to intravenous salbutamol in asthma: Effect of regular inhaled salbutamol. *Clin. Sci. Mol. Med. 60*: 579-585.

Harvey, J. E., and Tattersfield, A. E. (1982). Airway response to salbutamol. Effect of regular salbutamol inhalations in normal atopic and asthmatic subjects. *Thorax 37*: 280-287.

Hasegawa, M., and Townley, R. G. (1983). Difference between lung and spleen susceptibility of beta-adrenergic receptors to desensitization by terbutaline. *J. Allergy Clin. Immunol. 71*: 230-238.

Haskell, R. J., Wong, B. M., and Hansen, J. E. (1983). A double-blind, randomized clinical trial of methylprednisolone in status asthmaticus. *Arch. Int. Med. 143*: 1324-1327.

Haynes, B. F., and Fauci, A. S. (1978). The differential effect of in vivo hydrocortisone on the kinetics of subpopulations of human peripheral blood thymus-derived lymphocytes. *J. Clin. Invest. 61*: 703-707.

Hemady, Z., Gellis, S., Chambers, M., et al. (1985). Effect of dexamethasone on de novo IgE synthesis by human blood lymphocytes. *J. Allergy Clin. Immunol. 75*: 304-312.

Hench, P. S., Kendall, E. C., Slocumb, C. H., et al. (1949). The effect of a hormone of the adrenal cortex (17-hydroxy-11-dehydrocorticosterone: Compound E) and of pituitary adrenocorticotropic hormone on rheumatoid arthritis. *Proc. Staff Meet. Mayo Clinic 24*: 181-197.

Hench, P. S., Kendall, E. C., Slocumb, C. H., et al. (1950). Effects of cortisone acetate and pituitary ACTH on rheumatoid arthritis, rheumatic fever, and certain other conditions. A study in clinical physiology. *Arch. Intern. Med. 85*: 545-606.

Henry Williams, M. Jr., Kane, C., and Shim, C. S. (1974). Treatment of asthma with triamcinolone acetonide delivered by aerosol. *Am. Rev. Respir. Dis. 109*: 538-543.

Herxheimer, H. (1966). Steroids for asthmatic children. *Br. Med. J. 2*: 521.

Herzog, H. L., Nobile, A., Tolksdorf, S., et al. (1955). New anti-arthritic steroids. *Science 121*: 176.

Hichens, M., and Hogans, A. F. (1974). Radioimmunoassay for dexamethasone in plasma. *Clin. Chem. 20*: 266-271.

Higgins, S. J., Rousseau, G. G., Baxter, J. D., et al. (1973). Early events in glucocorticoid action: Activation of the steroid receptor and its subsequent nuclear binding studied on a cell-free system. *J. Biol. Chem. 248*: 5866-5872.

Hirata, F. (1984). Modulation of beta-adrenoreceptor function by phospholipids. In *Beta-adrenoreceptors of Asthma.* Edited by J. Morley, London, Academic Press, pp. 49-53.

Hirata, F., Schiffman, E., Venkatasubramanian, K., Salomen, D., and Axelrod, J. (1980). A phospholipase A_2 inhibitory protein in rabbit neutrophils induced by glucocorticoids. *Proc. Natl. Acad. Sci. U.S.A. 77*: 2533-2536.

Hogg, J. C. (1981). Bronchial mucosal permeability and its relationship to airway reactivity. *J. Allergy Clin. Immunol. 67*: 421-425.

Hogg, J. C. (1982). The pathophysiology of asthma. *Chest 82*: 85-128.

Holgate, S. T., Baldwin, C. J., and Tattersfield, A. E. (1977). β-Adrenergic agonist resistance in normal human airways. *Lancet 2*: 375-377.

Hong, S. C., and Levine, L. (1976). Inhibition of arachidonic acid release from cells as the biochemical action of anti-inflammatory steroids. *Proc. Natl. Acad. Sci. U.S.A. 73*: 1720-1734.

Hudson, G. (1966). Eosinophil granulocyte reactions. In *Bone Marrow Reactions.* Edited by J. M. Yoffey. Baltimore, William and Wilkins, pp. 86-99.

Hui, K. K. P., Conolly, M. E., and Tashkin, D. P. (1982). Reversal of human lymphocyte β-adrenoceptor desensitization by glucocorticoids. *Clin. Pharmacol. Ther. 32*: 566-571.

Hulme, B., James, V. H. T., and Rault, R. (1975). Absorption of enteric and non-enteric coated prednisolone tablets. *Br. J. Clin. Pharmacol. 2*: 317-320.

Israel, R. H., Poe, R. H., Wicks, C. M., Greenblatt, D. W., and Kalley, M. C. (1984). The protective effect of methylprednisolone on carbachol-induced bronchospasm. *Am. Rev. Respir. Dis. 130*: 1019-1022.

Jenne, J. W., Chick, T. W., Strickland, R. D., and Wall, F. J. (1977). Subsensitivity of beta responses during therapy with a long-acting beta-2 preparation. *J. Allergy Clin. Immunol. 59*: 383-390.

Jenne, J. W. (1979). Beta adrenergic agents—how much is enough? *J. Allergy Clin. Immunol. 63*: 74-75.

Jenne, J. W. (1982). Whither beta-adrenergic tachyphylaxis? *J. Allergy Clin. Immunol. 70*: 413-416.

Jenkins, J. S., and Sampson, P. A. (1967). Conversion of cortisone to cortisol and prednisone to prednisolone. *Br. Med. J. 2*: 205-207.

Johansson, S. A., Andersson, K. E., Brattsand, R., Gruvstad, E., and Hedner, P. (1982). Topical and systemic glucocorticoid potencies of budesonide, beclomethasone diproprionate and prednisolone in man. *Eur. J. Respir. Dis. 63 (Suppl 122)*: 74-82.

Jubiz, W., Hickle, A. W., Levinson, R. A., et al. (1970). Effect of diphenylhydantoin on the metabolism of dexamethasone. *N. Engl. J. Med. 238*: 11-14.

Jungblut, P. W., Hughes, A., Gaues, J., et al. (1979). Mechanisms involved in the regulation of steroid receptor levels. *J. Steroid Biochem. 11*: 273-278.

Juniper, E. F., Frith, P. A., and Hargreave, F. E. (1980). Long-term stability of non-specific airway responsiveness to histamine and effect of beclomethasone. *Am. Rev. Respir. Dis. 121*: 76 (abst).

Kattan, M., Gurwitz, D., and Levison, H. (1980). Corticosteroids in status asthmaticus. *J. Pediatr. 96*: 596-599.

King, W. J., and Greene, G. L. (1984). Monoclonal antibodies localize oestrogen receptor in nuclei of target cells. *Nature 307*: 745.

Klaustermeyer, W. B., and Hale, F. C. (1976). The physiologic effect of an intravenous glucocorticoid in bronchial asthma. *Ann. Allergy 37*: 80-86.

Klebanoff, S. J., and Clark, R. A. (1978). *The Neutrophil: Function and Clinical Disorders.* Amsterdam, North-Holland.

Kupfer, D., and Partridge, R. (1970). 6 β-Hydroxylation of triamcinolone acetonide by a hepatic enzyme system. *Arch. Biochem. Biophys. 140*: 23-28.

Lagunoff, D. (1985). The mast cell. In *Bronchial Asthma Mechanisms and Therapeutics* 2nd ed. Edited by E. B. Weiss, M. S. Segal, and M. Stein. Boston/Toronto, Little, Brown, pp. 236-249.

Lan, N. C., Karin, M., Nguyen, T., et al. (1984). Mechanisms of glucocorticoid hormone action. *J. Steroid Biochem. 20*: 71-88.

Larsson, E. L. (1980). Cyclosporin A and dexamethasone suppress T cell responses by selectively acting at distinct sites of the triggering process. *J. Immunol. 124*: 2828-2833.

Larsson, S., Svedmyr, N., and Thiringer, G. (1977). Lack of bronchial β-adrenoreceptor resistance in asthmatics during long term treatment with terbutaline. *J. Allergy Clin. Immunol. 59*: 93-100.

Lee, D. A. H., Taylor, G. M., Walker, J. G., et al. (1978). The effect of concurrent administration of antacids on prednisolone absorption. *Br. J. Clin. Pharmacol. 8*: 92-94.

Lefcoe, N. M. (1956). The effect of hydrocortisone hemisuccinate on the tracheal smooth muscle of the guinea pig and cat. *J. Allergy 27*: 352-358.

Legler, U. F., Frey, F. J., and Benet, L. Z. (1982). Prednisolone clearance at steady state in man. *J. Clin. Endocrinol. Metabl. 55*: 762-767.

Levy, G. (1967). Effect of dissolution rate on absorption, metabolism and pharmacologic activity of drugs. *J. Mond. Pharm. 3*: 237-254.

Liao, S., and Hiipakka, R. A. (1984). Mechanism of action of steroid hormones at the subcellular level. In *Biochemistry of Steroid Hormones* 2nd ed. Edited by H. L. J. Makin. Boston, Blackwell Scientific Publications, pp. 633-680.

Lieberman, P., Patterson, R., and Kunske, R. (1972). Complications of long-term steroid therapy for asthma. *J. Allergy Clin. Immunol. 49*: 329-336.

Lofdahl, C. G., Millstrand, T., and Svedmyr, N. (1984). Glucocorticoids and asthma. Studies of resistance and systemic effects of glucocorticoids. *Eur. J. Respir. Dis. 65 (Suppl 136)*: 69-77.

Logsdon, P. J., Middleton, E., and Coffey, R. G. (1972). Stimulation of leukocyte adenyl cyclase by hydrocortisone and isoproterenol in asthmatic and non-asthmatic subjects. *J. Allergy Clin. Immunol. 50*: 45-56.

Lowell, F. C., Ohman, J. L., and Williams, M. (1976). Double-blind trial of flunisolide aerosol in bronchial asthma. *J. Allergy Clin. Immunol. 57*: 257 (abstr.).

Luk, C. K., and Dulfano, M. J. (1983). Effect of pH, viscosity and ionic-strength changes on ciliary beating frequency of human bronchial explants. *Clin. Sci. 64*: 449-451.

Luksza, A. R. (1982). Acute severe asthma treated without steroids. *Br. J. Dis. chest 76*: 15-19.

Madsbad, S., Bjerregaard, B., Henriksen, J. H., et al. (1980). Impaired conversion of prednisone to prednisolone in patients with liver cirrhosis. *Gut 21*: 52-56.

Mano, K., Akbarzadeh, A., and Townley, R. G. (1979). Effect of hydrocortisone on beta-adrenergic receptors in lung membranes. *Life Sci. 25*: 1925-1930.

Marom, Z., Shelhamer, J. H., Bach, M. K., Morton, D. R., and Kaliner, M. (1982). Slow-reacting substances, leukotrienes C_4 and D_4, increase the release of mucus from human airways in vitro. *Am. Rev. Respir. Dis. 126*: 449-451.

Marom, Z., Shelhamer, J. H., Sun, F., et al. (1983). Human airway monohydroxyeicosatetraenoic acid generation and mucus release. *J. Clin. Invest. 72*: 122-127.

Marom, Z., Shelhamer, J. H., Alling, D., and Kaliner, M. (1984). The effects of corticosteroids on mucus glycoprotein secretion from human airways in vitro. *Am. Rev. Respir. Dis. 129*: 62-65.

Martin, L. E., Tanner, R. J. N., Clark, T. J. H., et al. (1974). Absorption and metabolism of orally administered beclomethasone dipropionate. *Clin. Pharmacol. Ther. 15*: 267-275.

Martin, L. E., Harrison, C., and Tanner, R. J. N. (1975). Metabolism of beclomethasone dipropionate by animals and man. *Postgrad. Med. J. 51* (Suppl. 4): 11-20.

Mason, H. L., Myers, C. S., and Kendall, E. C. (1936). The chemistry of crystalline substances isolated from the suprarenal gland. *J. Biol. Chem. 114*: 613-631.

May, C. S., Caffin, J. A., Halliday, J. W., et al. (1980). Prednisolone pharmacokinetics in asthmatic patients. *Br. J. Dis. Chest 74*: 91-92.

McAllister, W. A. C., Mitchell, D. M., and Collins, J. V. (1981a). Prednisolone pharmacokinetics compared between night and day in asthmatic and normal subjects. *Br. J. Clin. Pharmacol. 11*: 303-304.

McAllister, W. A. C., Winfield, C. R., and Collins, J. V. (1981b). Pharmacokinetics of prednisolone in normal and asthmatic subjects in relation to dose. *Eur. J. Clin. Pharmacol. 20*: 141-145.

McFadden, E. R., Kiser, R., de Groot, W. J., Holmes, B., Kikder, R., and Viser, G. (1976). A controlled study of the effects of single doses of hydrocortisone on the resolution of acute attacks of asthma. *Am. J. Med. 60*: 52-57.

McFadden, E. R. Jr. (1984). Pathogenesis of asthma. *J. Allergy Clin. Immunol. 73*: 413-424.

McIntyre, W. R., and Samuels, H. H. (1985). Triamcinolone acetonide regulates glucocorticoid-receptor levels by decreasing the half-life of the activated nuclear-receptor form. *J. Biol. Chem. 260*: 418-427.

Medical Research Council Report (1956). Controlled trial of effects of cortisone acetate in chronic asthma. *Lancet 2*: 798-806.

Meffin, P. J., Brooks, P. M., and Sallustio, R. (1984). Alterations in prednisolone disposition as a result of time of administration, gender and dose. *Br. J. Clin. Pharmacol. 17*: 395-404.

Meltzer, E. O., Kemp, J. P., Orgel, A., et al. (1982). Flunisolide aerosol for treatment of severe, chronic asthma in steroid dependent children. *Pediatrics 69*: 340-345.

Mishler, J. M. (1977). The effects of corticosteroids on mobilization and function of neutrophils. *Exp. Hematol. 5*: (Suppl.) 15-32.

Mislap, R. L., George, D. E., Szefler, S. J., et al. (1983). Effect of inflammatory bowel disease on absorption and disposition of prednisolone. *Dig. Dis. Sci. 28*: 161-168.

Morley, J., Hanson, J. M., and Youlten, L. J. F. (1984). Mediators of allergy. In *Allergy: Immunological and Clinical Aspects.* Edited by M. H. Lessof. New York, J. Wiley, pp. 45-72.

Morr, H., and Bornemann, G. (1980). Effect of glucocorticosteroids on histamine release from the human lung in vitro. *Allergologie 4*: 237-239.

Morselli, P. L., Marc, V., Garattini, S., et al. (1970). Metabolism of exogenous cortisol in humans. *Biochem. Pharmacol. 19*: 1643-1647.

Nelson, H. S., Rain, D. Jr., Doner, H. C., and Posey, W. C. (1977). Subsensitivity to bronchodilator action of albuterol produced by chronic administration. *Am. Rev. Respir. Dis. 116*: 871-878.

Nijkamp, F. P., Flower, R. J., Moncada, S., et al. (1976). Partial purification of rabbit aorta contracting substance-releasing factor and inhibition of its activity by anti-inflammatory steroids. *Nature 263*: 479-483.

Nordeen, S. I., Lan, N. C., Showers, M. O., et al. (1981). Photoaffinity labeling of glucocorticoid receptors. *J. Biol. Chem. 256*: 10503-10508.

Novey, H. S., and Beall, G. (1965). Aerosolized steroids and induced Cushing's syndrome. *Arch. Intern. Med. 115*: 602-605.

Nugent, C. A., Eik-nes, K., and Tyler, F. H. (1959). A comparative study of the metabolism of hydrocortisone and prednisolone. *J. Clin. Endocrinol. 19*: 526-534.

O'Byrne, P. M., Walters, E. H., Aizawa, H., et al. (1984). Indomethacin inhibits the airway hyperresponsiveness but not the neutrophil influx induced by ozone in dogs. *Am. Rev. Respir. Dis. 130*: 220-224.

Ortega, E., Rodriquez, C., Strand, E. J., et al. (1976). Metabolic effects of Cloprednol—a new systemic corticosteroid. *J. Clin. Pharmacol. 16*: 122-128.

Park, H. S., Greene, J. A., and Bacon, G. E. (1974). Disappearance of high dose prednisolone from plasma after renal transplantation. *Clin. Nephrol. 2*: 18-23.

Parker, C. W., Huber, M. G., and Baumann, M. L. (1973). Alterations in cyclic AMP metabolism in human bronchial asthma. III. Leukocyte and lymphocyte responses to steroids. *J. Clin. Invest. 52*: 1342-1348.

Parente, L., Ammendola, G., Persico, P., et al. (1978). Glucocorticosteroids and the inflammatory process. *Pol. J. Pharmacol. Pharm. 30*: 141-155.

Parente, L., and Flower, R. J. (1985). Hydrocortisone and "macrocortin" inhibit the zymosan-induced release of lyso-PAF from rat peritoneal leukocytes. *Life Sci. 36*: 1225-1228.

Peak, M. D., Cayton, R. M., and Howard, P. (1979). Triamcinolone in corticosteroid-resistant asthma. *Br. J. Dis. Chest 73*: 39-44.

Peel, E. T., and Gibson, G. J. (1980). Effects of long term inhaled salbutamol therapy on the provocation of asthma by histamine. *Am. Rev. Respir. Dis. 121*: 973-978.

Peets, E. A., Staub, M., and Symchowicz, S. (1969). Plasma binding of betamethasone-^{3}H, dexamethasone-^{3}H and cortisol-^{14}C—a comparative study. *Biochem. Pharmacol. 18*: 1655-1663.

Peterson, R. E. (1959). Metabolism of adrenocorticosteroids in man. *Ann. N.Y. Acad. Sci. 82*: 846-849.

Peterson, R. E. (1960). Adrenocortical steroid metabolism and adrenal cortical function in liver disease. *J. Clin. Invest. 39*: 320-331.

Pickup, M. E., Lowe, J. R., Leatham, P. A. et al. (1977). Dose dependent pharmacokinetics of prednisolone. *Eur. J. Clin. Pharmacol. 12*: 213-219.

Pickup, M. E. (1979). Clinical pharmacokinetics of prednisone and prednisolone. *Clin. Pharmacokin. 4*: 111-128.

Pierson, W. E., Bierman, C. W., and Kelley, V. C. (1974). A double-blind trial of corticosteroid therapy in status asthmaticus. *Pediatrics 54*: 282-288.

Powell, L. W., and Axelsen, E. (1972). Corticosteroids in liver disease: Studies on the biological conversion of prednisone to prednisolone and plasma protein binding. *Gut 13*: 690-696.

Powell-Jackson, B., English, J., and Williams, R. S. (1984). Prednisolone pharmacokinetics and autoimmune chronic active hepatitis: effects of cimetidine and spironolactone. *Gut 25*: A571 (abstr.).

Pun, L. Q., McCulloch, M. W., and Rand, M. J. (1973). The effect of hydrocortisone on the bronchodilator activity of sympathomimetic amines and on the uptake of isoprenaline in the isolated guinea pig trachea. *Eur. J. Pharmacol. 22*: 162-168.

Randolph, T. G., and Rollins, J. P. (1950). Effect of cortisone on bronchial asthma. *J. Allergy 21*: 288-293.

Rebuck, A. S., and Read, J. (1971). Assessment and management of severe asthma. *Am. J. Med. 51*: 788-798.

Reeder, W. H., and Mackey, G. S. (1950). Nebulized cortisone in bacterial pneumonia. *Dis. Chest. 18*: 528-534.

Repsher, L. H., Anderson, J. A., Bush, R. K., Falliers, C. J., Kass, F., Kemp, J. P., Reed, C., Siegel, S., and Webb, D. (1984). Assessment of tachyphylaxis following prolonged therapy of asthma with inhaled albuterol aerosol. *Chest 85*: 34-38.

Rimon, G., Hanski, E., Braun, S., et al. (1978). Mode of coupling between hormone receptors and adenylate cyclase elucidated by modulation of membrane fluidity. *Nature 276*: 394-396.

Rimsza, M. E. (1978). Complications of corticosteroid therapy. *Am. J. Dis. Child. 132*: 806-810.

Robinson, C., and Holgate, S. T. (1985). Mast cell-dependent inflammatory mediators and their putative role in bronchial asthma. *Cli. Sci. 68*: 103-112.

Rogers, E. F., Leanza, W. J., Conbere, C. P., et al. (1952). Aldehydes derived drom cortisone and hydrocortisone. *J. Am. Chem. Soc. 74*: 2947 (Letter).

Rose, J. Q., Nickelsen, J. A., and Middleton, E. (1980). Prednisolone disposition in steroid-dependent asthmatics. *J. Allergy Clin. Immunol. 66*: 366-373.

Rose, J. Q., Nickelsen, J. A., Ellis, E. F., Middleton, Jr. E., and Jusko, W. J. (1981a). Prednisolone disposition in steroid dependent asthmatic children. *J. Allergy Clin. Immunol. 67*: 188-193.

Rose, J. Q., Yurchak, A. M., and Jusko, W. J. (1981b). Dose dependent pharmacokinetics of prednisone and prednisolone in man. *J. Pharmacokin. Biopharm. 9*: 389-417.

Rose, J. Q., Yurchak, A. M., Meikle, A. W., et al. (1981c). Effect of smoking on prednisone, prednisolone and dexamethasone pharmacokinetics. *J. Pharmacokin. Biopharm. 9*: 1-14.

Roseman, P. M., Farag, A., Peckham, R., et al. (1982). Pituitary-adreno-cortical function in chronic renal failure: Blunted suppression and early escape of plasma cortisol levels after intravenous dexamethasone. *J. Clin. Endocrinol. Metab. 54*: 528-533.

Rousseau, G. G., Baxter, J. D., and Tomkins, G. M. (1972). Glucocorticoid receptors: Relations between steroid binding and biological effects. *J. Mol. Biol. 67*: 99-108.

Rousseau, G. G., Baxter, J. D., Higgins, S. J., et al. (1973). Steroid-induced nuclear binding of glucocorticoid receptors in intact hepatoma cells. *J. Mol. Biol. 79*: 539-554.

Russo-Marie, F., and Duval, D. (1982). Dexamethasone-induced inhibition of prostaglandin production does not result from a direct action on phospholipase activities but is mediated through a steroid-inducible factor. *Biochem. Biophys. Acta 712*: 177-185.

Ryrfeldt, A., Andersson, P., Edsbacker, S., et al. (1982). Pharmacokinetics and metabolism of budesonide, a selective glucocorticoid. *Eur. J. Respir. Dis. 63 (S122)*: 86-95.

Ryrfeldt, A., Edsbacker, S., and Pauwels, R. (1984). Kinetics of the epimeric glucocorticoid budesonide. *Clin. Pharmacol. Ther. 35*: 525-530.

Saperia, J. (1966). Steroids for asthmatic children. *Br. Med. J. 2*: 521.

Sarett, L. H., Patchett, A. Y., and Steelman, S. L. (1963). The effects of structural alteration on the antiinflammatory properties of hydrocortisone. In *Progress in Drug Research.* Edited by E. Jucker. Basel, Birkhayser Verlag, pp. 13-153.

Schaffer, J. A., Williams, S. E., Twinberg, L. A., et al. (1983). Absorption of prednisolone in patients with Crohn's disease. *Gut 24*: 182-186.

Schalm, S. W., Summerskill, W. H. J., and Go, V. L. W. (1976). Development of radioimmunoassays for prednisone and prednisolone: Application to studies of hepatic metabolism of prednisone. *Mayo Clin. Proc. 51*: 761-766.

Schleimer, R. P., Lichtenstein, L. M., and Gillespie, E. (1981). Inhibition of basophil histamine release by anti-inflammatory steroids. *Nature 292*: 454-455.

Schleimer, R. P., Schulman, E. S., MacGashan, D. W., et al. (1983). Effects of dexamethasone on mediator release from human lung fragments and purified lung mast cells. *J. Clin. Invest. 71*: 1830-1835.

Schmidt, T. J., and Litwack, G. (1982). Activation of the glucocorticoid-receptor complex. *Physiol. Rev. 62*: 1131-1192.

Schrader, W. T. (1984). New model for steroid hormone receptors? *Nature 308*: 17-18.

Schuyler, M., Gerblich, A., and Urda, G. (1984). Prednisone and T lymphocyte subpopulations. *Arch. Intern. Med. 144*: 973-975.

Schwartz, E. (1951). Oral cortisone in intractable bronchial asthma. *J. Allergy 22*: 1-3.

Schwartz, H. J., Lowell, F. N., and Melby, J. C. (1968). Steroid resistant bronchial asthma. *Ann. Intern. Med. 69*: 493-499.

Seutter, E. (1975). Metabolism of systemically given corticosteroids. *Dermatologica 151*: 129-134.

Shapiro, G. G., Izu, A. E., Furukawa, C. T., et al. (1981). Short-term double-blind evaluation of flunisolide aerosol for steroid-dependent asthmatic children and adolescents. *Chest 80*: 671-675.

Shenfield, G. M., Hodson, M. E., Clark, S. W., et al. (1975). Interaction of corticosteroids and catecholamines in the treatment of asthma. *Thorax 30*: 439-435.

Sherlock, J. E., and Letteri, J. M. (1977). Effect of hemodialysis on methylprednisolone plasma levels. *Nephron 18*: 208-211.

Sherman, M. R., and Stevens, J. (1984). Structure of mammalian steroid receptors: Evolving concepts and methodological developments. In *Annual Review of Physiology.* Edited by R. M. Berne. California, Annual Reviews, Inc., pp. 83-105.

Singer, F. M., and Borman, A. (1956). Anti-inflammatory activities of several 9 α-halo derivatives of adrenal steroids. *Proc. Soc. Exp. Biol. Med. 92*: 23-26.

Slade, J. D., and Hepburn, B. (1983). Prednisone-induced alterations of circulating human lymphocyte subsets. *J. Lab. Clin. Med. 101*: 479-487.

Slaunwhite, W. R., and Sandberg, A. A. (1959). Transcortin: A corticosteroid-binding protein of plasma. *J. Clin. Invest. 38*: 384-391.

Slavin, R. G., Izu, A. E., Bernstein, I. L., Blumenthal, M. N., Bolen, J. F., Ouellette, J. J., Reed, C. E., and Oren, J. Multicenter study of flunisolide aerosol in adult patients with steroid-dependent asthma. *J. Allergy Clin. Immunol. 66*: 379-385.

Sly, R. M., Imseis, M., Frazer, M., et al. (1978). Treatment of asthma in children with triamcinolone acetonide aerosol. *J. Allergy Clin. Immunol. 62*: 76-82.

Smith, A. P., Booth, M., and Davey, A. J. (1973). A controlled trial of beclomethasone dipropionate for asthma. *Br. J. Dis. Chest 67*: 208-214.

Smith, K. A. (1980). T-cell growth factor. *Immunol. Rev. 51*: 337-357.

Snyder, D. S., and Unanue, E. R. (1983). Corticosteroids inhibit murine Ia expression and IL1 production. *J. Immunol. 129*: 1803-1805.

Sotomajor, H., Badier, M., Vervloet, D., and Orehek, J. (1984). Seasonal increase of carbachol airway responsiveness in patients allergic to grass pollen. Reversal by corticosteroids. *Am. Rev. Respir. Dis. 130*: 56-58.

Spector, S. L. (1985). The use of corticosteroids in the treatment of asthma. *Chest 87*: 735-785.

Spector, S. L., and Farr, R. S. (1975a). Efficacy of inhaled triamcinolone vs. placebo in steroid dependent asthmatic patients. *Clin. Res. 23*: 352a.

Spector, S. L., and Farr, R. S. (1975b). A comparison of methacholine and histamine inhalation in asthmatics. *J. Allergy 56*: 308-316.

Spector, S. L., Katz, F. H., and Farr, R. S. (1974). Troleandomycin: Effectiveness in steroid-dependent asthma and bronchitis. *J. Allergy Clin. Immunol. 54*: 367-379.

Spero, G. B., Thompson, J. L., Magerlein, B. J., et al. (1956). Adrenal hormones and related compounds. IV. 6-Methyl steroids. *J. Am. Chem. Soc. 78*: 6213-6214.

Svensjö, E., and Roempke, K. (1985). Time-dependent inhibition of bradykinin and histamine-induced increase in microvascular permeability by local glucocorticosteroid treatment. In *Glucocorticosteroids, Inflammation and Bronchial Hyperreactivity*. Edited by J. C. Hogg, R. Ellul-Micallef, and R. Brattsand. Amsterdam, Excerpta Medica, pp. 136-144.

Szefler, S. J., Rose, J. Q., Ellis, E. F., Spector, S. L., Green, A. W., and Jusko, W. J. (1980). The effect of troleandomycin on methylprednisolone elimination. *J. Allergy Clin. Immunol. 66*: 447-451.

Szefler, S. J., Brenner, M., Jusko, W. J., Spector, S. L., Flesher, K. A., and Ellis, E. F. (1982). Dose- and time-related effect of troleandomycin on methylprednisolone elimination. *Clin. Pharmacol. Ther. 32*: 166-171.

Tai, E., and Read, J. (1967). Response of blood gas tensions to aminophylline and isoprenaline in patients with asthma. *Thorax 22*: 543-546.

Tam, S., Hong, S-C. L., and Levine, L. (1977). Relationships among the steroids of anti-inflammatory properties and inhibition of prostaglandin production and arachidonic acid release by transformed mouse fibroblasts. *J. Pharmacol. Exp. Ther. 203*: 162-168.

Tanner, A. R., Halliday, J. W., and Powell, L. W. (1981). Serum prednisolone levels in Crohn's disease and coeliac disease following oral prednisolone administration. *Digestion 21*: 310-315.

Tashjian, A. H. Jr., Voelkel, E. F., McDonough, J., et al. (1975). Hydrocortisone inhibits prostaglandin production by mouse fibrosarcoma cells. *Nature 258*: 739-741.

Thalen, A., and Brattsand, R. (1979). Synthesis and anti-inflammatory properties of budesonide, a new non-halogenated glucocorticoid with high local activity. *Arzn-Forsch/Drug Res. 29*: 1687-1690.

Thompson, J., and Van Furth, R. (1970). The effects of glucocorticosteroids on the kinetics of mononuclear phagocytes. *J. Exp. Med. 131*: 429-442.

Toews, M. L., Waldo, G. L., Harden, T. K., et al. (1984). Relationship between an altered membrane form and a low affinity form of the α-adrenergic receptor occurring during catecholamine-induced desensitization. *J. Biol. Chem. 259*: 11844-11850.

Toogood, J. H., and Lefcoe, N. M. (1965). Dexamethasone aerosol for the treatment of steroid-dependent bronchial asthmatic patients. *J. Allergy 36*: 321-322.

Toothaker, R. D., and Welling, P. G. (1982). Effect of dose size on the pharmacokinetics of intravenous hydrocortisone during endogenous hydrocortisone suppression. *J. Pharmacokin. Biopharm. 10*: 147-156.

Toothaker, R. D., Craig, W. A., and Welling, P. G. (1982a). Effect of dose size on the pharmacokinetics of oral hydrocortisone suspension. *Am. Pharmaceut. Assoc. 7*: 1182-1185.

Toothaker, R. D., Sundaresan, G. M., Hunt, J. P., et al. (1982b). Oral hydrocortisone pharmacokinetics: A comparison of fluorescence and ultraviolet HPLC assays for hydrocortisone in plasma. *J. Pharm. Sci. 71*: 573-576.

Townley, R. G., Reeb, R., Fitzgibbon, T., et al. (1970). The effect of corticosteroids on the beta-adrenergic receptors in bronchial smooth muscle. *J. Allergy 45*: 118 (Abstr.).

Tsuei, S. E., Ashley, J. J., Moore, R. G., et al. (1978). Quantitation of dexamethasone in biological fluids using high performance liquid chromatography. *J. Chromatogr. Biomed. Appl. 145*: 213-220.

Tsurufuji, S., and Sugio, K. (1978). Molecular mechanism in the manifestation of anti-inflammatory activity of glucocorticosteroids. *Eur. J. Rheum. Inflamm. 1*: 226-231.

Uhde, H. (1957). Aerosoltherapie mit Prednisolonlosung. *Munchen. Med. Wochenschr. 99*: 891-893.

Uribye, M., Schalm, S. W., Summerskill, W. H. J., et al. (1978). Oral prednisone for chronic active liver disease: Dose responses and bioavailability studies. *Gut 19*: 1131-1135.

Venezio, F. R., Westenfelder, G. O., and Phair, J. P. (1982). The adherence of polymorphonuclear leukocytes in patients with sepsis. *J. Infect. Dis. 145*: 351-357.

Vermeulen, A. (1959). The metabolism of 4-^{14}C prednisolone. *J. Endocrinol. 18*: 278-291.

Walsh, S. D., and Grant, I. W. B. (1966). Corticosteroids in treatment of chronic asthma. *Br. Med. J. 2*: 796-802.

Walton, J., Watson, B. S., and Ney, R. L. (1970). Alternate-day versus shorter-interval steroid administration. *Arch. Intern. Med. 126*: 601-607.

Weber, R. W., Smith, J. A., and Nelson, H. S. (1982). Aerosolized terbutaline in asthmatics: Development of subsensitivity with long-term administration. *J. Allergy Clin. Immunol. 70*: 417-422.

Welshons, W. V., Lieverman, M. E., and Gorski, J. (1984). Nuclear localization of unoccupied oestrogen receptors. *Nature 307*: 747-749.

Wendler, N. L., Graber, R. P., Jones, R. E., et al. (1950). Synthesis of 11-hydroxylated cortical steroids. 17 (α)-hydroxy-corticosterone. *J. Am. Chem. Soc. 72*: 5793-5794.

Werb, Z. R., Foley, R., and Munck, A. (1978). Interaction of glucocorticosteroids with macrophages: Identification of glucocorticoid receptors in monocytes and macrophages. *J. Exp. Med. 147*: 1684-1694.

Werk, E. E., Choi, Y., Sholiton, L., et al. (1969). Interference in the effect of dexamethasone by diphenyl-hydantoin. *N. Engl. J. Med. 281*: 32-34.

Werk, E. E., MacGee, J., and Sholiton, L. J. (1964). Effect of diphenylhydantoin on cortisol metabolism in man. *J. Clin. Invest. 43*: 1824-1835.

Wessels, M. R., Mullikin, D., and Lefkowitz, R. J. (1979). Selective alteration in high affinity binding: A mechanism for beta-adrenergic receptor desensitization. *Mol. Pharmacol. 16*: 10-20.

West, K. M. (1958). Relative eosinopenic and hyperglycaemic potencies of glucocorticoids in men. *Metabolism 7*: 441-444.

Westphal, V. (1957). Steroid protein interactions. III. Spectrophotometric demonstration of interaction between proteins and progesterone, desoxycorticosterone and cortisol. *Arch. Biochem. 66*: 71-78.

Willey, R. F., Godden, D. J., Carmichael, J., Preston, P., Frame, M., and Crompton, G. K. (1982). Comparison of twice daily administration of a new corticosteroid budesonide with beclomethasone dipropionate four times daily in the treatment of chronic asthma. *Br. J. Dis. Chest 76*: 61-68.

Williams, M. H. Jr. (1975). Treatment of asthma with triamcinolone acetonide aerosol. *Chest 68*: 765-768.

Wilson, C. G., Ssendagire, R., May, C. S., and Paterson, J. W. (1975). Measurement of plasma prednisolone in man. *Br. J. Clin. Pharmacol. 2*: 321-325.

Winfield, C. R., McAllister, W. A. C., and Collins, J. V. (1980). Changes in effective pulmonary blood flow with prednisolone. *Thorax 35*: 238 (abstr.).

Wolfe, J. D., Rosenthal, R. R., Bleecker, E., et al. (1979). The effect of corticosteroids on cholinergic hyperreactivity. *J. Allergy Clin. Immunol. 63*: 162 (abstr.).

Yu, D. T., Clements, P. J., Paulus, H. E., et al. (1974). Human lymphocyte subpopulations. Effects of corticosteroids. *J. Clin. Invest. 53*: 565-571.

Zweiman, B., Slott, R. I., and Atkins, P. C. (1976). Histologic studies of human skin test responses to ragweed and compound 48/80. III. Effects of alternate-day steroid therapy. *J. Allergy Clin. Immunol. 58*: 657-663.

14

Calcium Channel Blockers

PETER J. BARNES

Cardiothoracic Institute
Brompton Hospital, London, England

Movement of calcium ions (Ca^{2+}) into cells is fundamental to many cellular functions including muscle contraction and secretion. The development of drugs that interfere with this calcium entry has provided new insights into disease and provided powerful new therapeutic agents, particularly in cardiovascular medicine. The pathology of asthma is complex and airway obstruction is probably the result of several pathologic processes, including airway smooth muscle contraction, mucus gland secretion, increased microvascular permeability leading to bronchial wall edema, and secretion of mediators from mast cells and other inflammatory cells. Since all these pathologic events may involve cellular entry of Ca^{2+}, calcium channel blocking drugs might be useful in the treatment of asthma. Calcium antagonists might not only provide a novel addition to antiasthma therapy, but also throw light on the underlying pathogenesis of airway obstruction and bronchial hyperreactivity in asthma. It has even been suggested that increased cellular Ca^{2+} entry may be the basic defect of asthma (Middleton, 1980). It is not surprising that there has recently been considerable interest in the use of calcium channel blockers in asthma, and several reviews have recently been published (Barnes, 1983; Fanta and Drazen, 1983; Middleton, 1983; Russi and Ahmed, 1984).

This chapter will discuss recent advances in the understanding of calcium regulation, and, in particular, how this might relate to the various target cells involved in asthma. The clinical experience with currently available calcium antagonists will then be presented, followed by a discussion of possible directions for future drug development in this rapidly growing area.

I. Role of Calcium in Cell Function

A. Ca^{2+} Entry

All cells maintain a steep gradient between intracellular and extracellular Ca^{2+} concentration. The concentration of free extracellular Ca^{2+} is approximately 10^{-3} M, whereas recent estimates suggest a concentration of 10^{-7} M inside the cell. The cell membrane itself is impermeable to Ca^{2+}, and the low intracellular Ca^{2+} concentration is maintained by active extrusion of Ca^{2+} via specific pumps. With activation of the cell, Ca^{2+} enters through specific channels in the cell membrane. These channels are macromolecular structures which span the cell membrane and selectively permit the entry of Ca^{2+} down its concentration

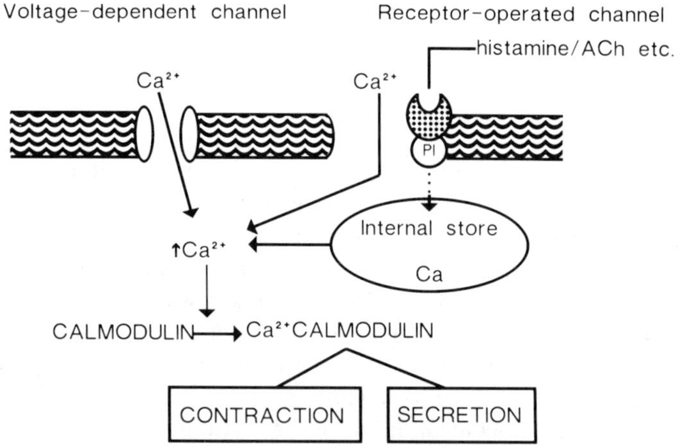

Figure 1 CA^{2+} entry into airway cells. External calcium ions (Ca^{2+}) may enter the cell via voltage-dependent channels or via receptor-operated channels, which are activated by several receptors (e.g., histamine, muscarinic), probably by stimulating the breakdown of phosphatidylinositol (PI) in the cell membrane. Intracellular Ca^{2+} may also increase by release from intracellular stores, such as endoplasmic reticulum and mitochondria, which may be triggered by a PI product. A rise in intracellular Ca^{2+} then activates calmodulin, which triggers contraction and secretion.

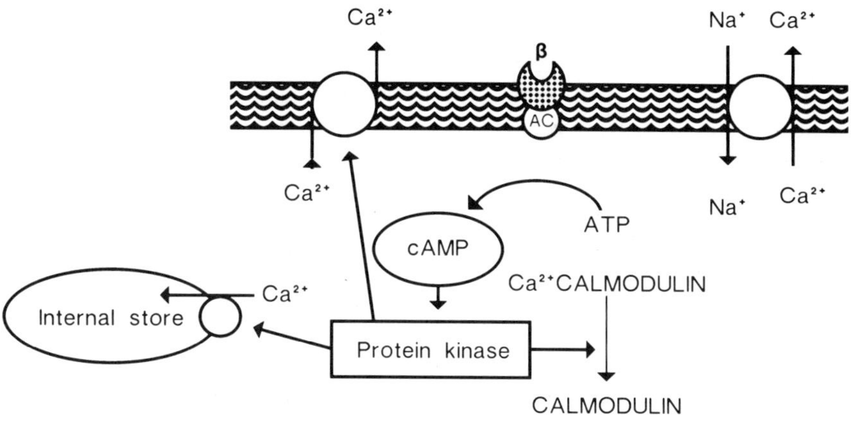

Figure 2 Removal of Ca^{2+} from airway smooth muscle cells. Ca^{2+} is removed from the cell by at least three mechanisms. Ca^{2+} is exchanged for Na^+, and there is also a specific Ca^{2+} stimulated by cyclic AMP via protein kinases. Protein kinases also stimulate Ca^{2+} removal into internal stores, and the dissociation of Ca^{2+} from calmodulin. Thus β-agonists, by stimulating cAMP production, lower internal Ca^{2+} and lead to relaxation of smooth muscle.

gradient. Recent studies with fluorescent markers of intracellular Ca^{2+} concentration indicate that Ca^{2+} entry is rapid, transient, and long outlived by the cellular response. When the concentration of Ca^{2+} within the cell reaches a critical level (approximately 10^{-6} M), Ca^{2+} binds to a specific calcium-binding protein, calmodulin. The Ca^{2+}-calmodulin complex then activates a specific kinase and enzyme cascade that brings about contraction or secretion. Thus Ca^{2+} couples the stimulus, which acts on the outside of the cell, to the response, thereby functioning as a second messenger.

B. Calcium Channels

There are at least two types of calcium channel (Fig. 1). One opens in response to cellular depolarization and is therefore termed a voltage-operated channel (VOC). It is estimated that there are at least 10,000 VOCs in each cardiac cell ter, 1983). The other channel opens in response to activation of specific receptors, such as muscarinic, histamine, or α-adrenergic receptors, and is therefore termed a receptor-operated channel (ROC) (Bolton, 1979). Current evidence suggests that receptor activation leads to Ca^{2+} entry by hydrolysis of a specific phospholipid in the cell membrane (phosphatidylinositol biphosphate). which leads to a membrane permeability change. This reaction also leads to the formation of inositol triphosphate, which then triggers the release of Ca^{2+} from internal stores (Rasmussen and Barrett, 1984). Indeed intracellular Ca^{2+} concentration may increase by release of calcium from stores, such as endoplasmic reticulum and mitochondria, within the cell. This indicates that some responses may be calcium-dependent, yet do not require the entry of Ca^{2+} into the cell from outside.

C. Removal of Ca^{2+}

In order to terminate a response, the intracellular Ca^{2+} concentration must be lowered. The mechanism for Ca^{2+} removal are therefore fundamental to an understanding of the molecular basis of bronchodilatation. There are several mechanisms for lowering intracellular Ca^{2+}. Ca^{2+} may be pumped out of the cell by an ATP-dependent Ca^{2+} pump, or may be exchanged for Na^+ by a specific Na^+-Ca^{2+} pump (Fig. 2). In addition, Ca^{2+} may be pumped back into endoplasmic reticulum or mitochondrial stores. The relationship between cyclic nucleotides and intracellular Ca^{2+} is complex because it differs in each type of cell. In smooth muscle a rise in intracellular cyclic AMP stimulates removal of Ca^{2+} from cytoplasm by all three mechanisms described above, and also speeds the dissociation of Ca^{2+} bound to calmodulin. Thus β-adrenoceptor agonists relax airway smooth muscle by lowering intracellular Ca^{2+} and by interfering with the Ca^{2+}-dependent contractile cascade.

II. Calcium Channel Blockers

Voltage-dependent channels are specific to calcium although cations of a similar size such as barium may also slip through. However larger cations such as manganese and lanthanum block these channels. Recently, organic compounds that specifically block these VOCs have been developed; these drugs include dihydropyridines (such as nifedipine, nicardipine, and nimodipine), verapamil, and diltiazem (Schwartz and Triggle, 1984). These drugs are effective at low concentrations, which suggests that they act at specific sites on the cell membrane, and since there are no apparent structural similarities between these classes of blocker, they probably interact with different sites on the calcium channel. Binding studies using radiolabeled derivatives indicate that these drugs bind with high affinity to different sites on the calcium channel, and that complex interaction between the different classes of calcium antagonist may occur (Murphy et al., 1983). There are also functional differences between the drugs, and verapamil appears to be more effective after tissues are repeatedly stimulated; this finding suggests that it may only bind to the calcium channel when it is in an open state. This might explain why verapamil is more effective than nifedipine against cardiac arrhythmias. Calcium antagonists are only effective at VOCs, and have no action at ROCs, at least at clinically relevant concentrations. Recently dihydropyridines, which have agonist activity, have been developed and, as expected, cause contraction of smooth muscle (Schramm et al., 1983).

Calcium channel blockers have now been used extensively in the treatment of cardiovascular diseases, particularly unstable angina and hypertension. They appear to be safe and do not have significant unwanted effects. Although they are relatively specific for VOCs, at higher dosages they may have other actions such as α-receptor blockade, phosphodiesterase inhibition and inhibition of Na-K-ATPase, and may not be as selective as previously believed (Smith, 1983). This means that caution must be applied in the interpretation of in vitro findings when high dosages of these drugs have been used to elicit effects.

III. Calcium and Airways

Although this subject has been less extensively studied than the cardiovascular system, there is now a considerable body of evidence on the calcium dependency of the various cells of the airway believed to be involved in asthma (Table 1).

A. Airway Smooth Muscle

The source of Ca^{2+} for contraction differs between muscle types. In skeletal muscle contraction depends on calcium stores in the sarcoplasmic reticulum and is therefore independent of extracellular Ca^{2+}. For this reason calcium channel blockers have no obvious effects on skeletal muscle contraction. By contrast contraction of vascular smooth muscle is very dependent on extracellular Ca^{2+}, which enters the cell mainly via VOCs, and is therefore very sensitive to calcium channel blockers. Airway smooth muscle appears to be dependent on both internal and external sources of calcium, however. The situation is complicated by the fact that the source of Ca^{2+} for contraction may vary not only with the stimulus, but also with the magnitude of the stimulus. Thus in dog tracheal smooth muscle verapamil is potent at inhibiting potassium chloride and serotonin-induced contraction, but is much less effective against comparable acetylcholine-induced contraction (Coburn, 1977). Furthermore, verapamil inhibits contractions due to low concentrations of acetylcholine but not those elicited by high concentrations (Farley and Miles, 1978). Similar results have been found in guinea pig trachea (Creese and Denborough, 1981). The implications of these studies are that calcium channel blockers may be effective against some stimuli, but not against others. In vitro calcium antagonists reduce the contractile effect of several spasmogens in airway smooth muscle from several species, including humans (Fanta et al., 1982; Drazen et al., 1983; Cheng and Townley, 1983; Advenier et al., 1984). Calcium antagonists differ in potency and in general the order of potency is nifedipine > verapamil > diltiazem. This rank order is similar

Table 1 Possible Effects of Calcium Antagonists in Airways

Cell type	Possible effect
Airway smooth muscle	Prevent contraction
Mast cell	Prevent mediator release
Airway submucosal gland	Reduce mucus secretion
Inflammatory cells	Reduce chemotaxis / mediator release
Autonomic nerves	Reduce cholinergic / increased nonadrenergic inhibitory nerve effects
Bronchial microvasculature	Reduce permeability

to that found in other smooth muscle preparations, but the effect of calcium antagonists in airway smooth muscle is much less than in vascular and uterine smooth muscle (Schwartz and Triggle, 1984). The reason for the lower potency of these agents in airway smooth muscle is uncertain, although it seems likely that Ca^{2+} entry is largely via ROCs, rather than via VOCs. Although calcium channel blockers are not very effective at preventing induced contraction of airway smooth muscle, they are potent at reversing established contraction (Cheng and Townley, 1983; Drazen et al., 1983). This suggests that the maintenance of airway tone may involve Ca^{2+} entry via VOCs, but that initiation of contraction occurs by Ca^{2+} entry through ROCs.

Similarly in vivo calcium antagonists attenuate the bronchoconstrictor response to methacholine and prostaglandins in normal dogs and guinea pigs (Malo et al., 1982; Fanta et al., 1982), and to citric acid in hyperreactive dogs (Brugman et al., 1983). It is interesting that calcium channel blockers have no effect on resting airway tone, even when given in a relatively high dosage by inhalation.

B. Mast Cells

It has been known for several years that extracellular calcium is necessary for antigen-induced release of mediators from mast cells (Mongar and Schild, 1958). Both the calcium ionophore A23187, which carries calcium across the cell membrane, and direct intracellular injection of calcium stimulate histamine release from rat peritoneal mast cells, the amount released being proportional to the calcium influx (Foreman et al., 1977). Bridging of IgE bound to the mast cell membrane may lead to increased phospholipid methylation of the cell membrane, resulting in Ca^{2+} influx (Ishizaka et al., 1980). Conversely, lanthanum and methoxyverapamil inhibit IgE-dependent histamine release from these cells (Suzuki et al., 1982).

Mediator release from human lung is also dependent on extracellular calcium, and both verapamil and nifedipine have been shown to inhibit secretion of slow-reacting substance of anaphylaxis (SRS-A) from passively sensitized human lung fragments (Cerrina et al., 1982; Lee et al., 1983), although the concentration required to show an effect has been very high, and there is little effect on histamine release. Calcium antagonists may have a preferential effect on SRS-A release because 5-lipoxygenase, a key enzyme in the synthesis of leukotrienes, is critically dependent on Ca^{2+} (Jakschik et al., 1980). Similarly, nifedipine and nicardipine have been found to have no significant inhibitory effect on histamine secretion from isolated human lung and tonsillar mast cells, at least in therapeutically relevant concentrations (Kim et al., 1985). Nifedipine inhibits secretion of SRS-A, and platelet-activating factor from human neutrophils, and the release of histamine from human basophils in vitro, but again the concentrations required are very high (Jouvin-Marche et al., 1983; Jensen et al., 1983). In vivo nifedipine reduces basal plasma histamine and blunts the rise in plasma histamine in asthmatics after exercise (Barnes et al., 1981), although this is likely to reflect an effect on basophils rather than on airway mast cells. In allergic sheep verapamil has no effect on methacholine- or histamine-induced bronchoconstriction, while significantly attenuating allergen-induced bronchospasm. This implies that the protective effect may be through inhibition of mast cell mediator release (Russi et al., 1983). In vitro studies of human airways passively sensitized to antigen however argue against this (Henderson et al., 1983b) and, taken with the in vitro evidence of mediator release, indicate that calcium antagonists are unlikely to have a significant effect on inflammatory mediator release at therapeutic concentrations.

C. Mucus Secretion

All secretory processes depend on Ca^{2+} but little is known of the role of extracellular Ca^{2+} in airway mucus secretion. In chicken trachea, both increasing and decreasing extracellular Ca^{2+} appear to increase mucus secretion (Balfre, 1978). In dogs, extracellular calcium is necessary for submucosal gland secretion (Coles et al., 1982), and in dog airway epithelium is necessary for stimulation of active ion transport (Martin and Zaremba, 1978). It has been postulated that in cystic fibrosis there may be an abnormally high intracellular Ca^{2+} concentration, which may lead to hypersecretion from all gland cells (Sorscher and Breslow, 1982).

D. Neurotransmission

Neurotransmission is dependent on extracellular Ca^{2+} (Reuter, 1983), and the autonomic nervous system is important in regulating airway tone in humans (Nadel and Barnes, 1984). Calcium antagonists might have effects on airway tone by modulation of autonomic neurotransmission. There is almost no information about this subject. Preliminary studies indicate that nifedipine has little effect on cholinergic neural contractile responses in isolated airway smooth muscle, but produces an unexpected enhancement of nonadrenergic inhibitory nerve responses (Cuss et al., 1985).

E. Chemotaxis

Chemotaxis of inflammatory cells such as neutrophils and eosinophils is calcium-dependent (Becker and Stossel, 1980), and therefore calcium antagonists might have an effect on the inflammatory response in the asthmatic airway. Furthermore, the release of inflammatory products from neutrophils and eosinophils is also calcium-dependent but there is almost no information about the effects of calcium antagonists.

F. Pulmonary Blood Vessels

Inflammatory mediators cause increased microvascular leakiness in the airways, leading to bronchial edema. There is evidence that verapamil may prevent the development of leakiness in some microvascular beds (Persson and Svensjö, 1984), and it is therefore possible that calcium antagonists might attenuate or prevent bronchial edema in asthma.

Calcium antagonists are potent vasodilators in the systemic circulation and also in the pulmonary circulation. Recently, nifedipine has been shown to attenuate acute hypoxic vasoconstriction in animals (Redding et al., 1984; Stanbrook et al., 1984) and in humans (Simonneau et al., 1981; Kennedy et al., 1983). The effect of calcium antagonists on the bronchial circulation has not been studied in detail. In anesthetized dogs, calcium channel blockers have a more potent effect on tracheal blood flow than on airway smooth muscle tone (Himori and Taira, 1980) but the clinical relevance of this finding is not yet certain.

IV. Clinical Studies

Several clinical studies on calcium antagonists have now been performed in asthma and these have recently been summarized (Barnes, 1985).

A. Effect on Airway Function

Many studies have now demonstrated that calcium antagonists have no significant effect on airway function in asthmatic or normal subjects, even when sensitive tests such as airway resistance have been used. Thus in a study of asthmatic patients given 20 mg nifedipine sublingually there was no evidence of bronchodilatation, yet all showed a significant bronchodilator response to an inhaled β-agonist (Williams et al., 1981). This is unlikely to be explained by too low a dosage of nifedipine since even when it is inhaled in high concentration (10 mg) no effect on baseline specific airway conductance has been found (Cuss and Barnes, 1985). In a few studies a statistically significant improvement in airway function has been recorded but the changes are so small as to be of no clinical relevance (Patakas et al., 1983). These studies imply that resting bronchomotor tone in asthma is probably not maintained through voltage-dependent calcium entry. These clinical findings are in agreement with the animal studies discussed above, in which no effect of calcium antagonists on resting bronchomotor tone has been found. The lack of bronchodilatation is somewhat surprising, since in vitro calcium antagonists are potent at reversing established contraction of airway smooth muscle. Recently this has been explored in vivo, and inhaled nifedipine rapidly reverses bronchoconstriction induced by inhaled histamine back to baseline values (Cuss and Barnes, 1985b). This might indicate that when there is marked bronchoconstriction as in acute severe asthma attacks, calcium antagonists might produce bronchodilatation.

B. Provoked Bronchoconstriction

Several reports have investigated the protective effect of calcium antagonists against various bronchoconstrictor challenges (Table 2). The first report of calcium antagonists in asthma showed that nifedipine (20 mg sublingually) completely prevented exercise-induced asthma in 10 patients with mild asthma (Cerrina et al., 1981) but subsequent studies have found less complete protection either with sublingual nifedipine (Barnes et al., 1981; Corris et al., 1983) or inhaled verapamil (Patel, 1981a). The stimulus for exercise-induced asthma is cooling of the upper airways and calcium antagonists have a small protective effect against cold-air-induced bronchoconstriction (Henderson et al., 1983b; Solway et al., 1984). Both nifedipine and verapamil attenuate the bronchoconstrictor effect of histamine, although the effect is rather small (Williams et al., 1981; Barnes et al., 1981; Corris et al., 1983) and occasionally no protective effect has been found (Patel, 1981b).

The attenuation of cholinergic bronchoconstriction is even less impressive (Popa et al., 1983; Patel, 1981b) which might be predicted from in vitro studies showing less protection against acetylcholine than against histamine-induced contraction of airway smooth muscle. In general, nifedipine is more potent than verapamil, and the few studies that have been done on diltiazem have shown it to be least effective (Magnussen et al., 1984). This order of potency is similar to that seen in vitro against airway smooth muscle. The dosage of nifedipine that may be given sublingually or orally is limited by cardiovascular side effects, so it is possible that a greater effect would be found if the concentration of nifedipine

Table 2 Clinical Effects of Calcium Antagonists in Asthma

Bronchodilatation	0
Exercise-induced bronchospasm	++
Cold-air-induced bronchospasm	+
Histamine-induced bronchospasm	++
Cholinergic-agonist-induced bronchospasm	+
Antigen-induced bronchospasm	+
Nonspecific bronchial hyperreactivity	?

could be increased. Recently nifedipine has been given by inhalation in a high dosage, but the protective effect against histamine-induced bronchoconstriction was no greater than when given sublingually (Cuss and Barnes, 1985a). This might indicate that the maximal effect of calcium antagonists in protecting against bronchoconstriction is limited.

The effects of calcium antagonists are disputed against antigen-induced bronchoconstriction, with some studies showing partial protection (Henderson et al., 1983b) while others have not been able to demonstrate protection (So et al., 1982; Patel et al., 1983). The protective effect against antigen is probably explained by an effect on airway smooth muscle rather than on mast cell mediator release, since no greater effect is achieved against antigen than against nonspecific bronchoconstrictors.

C. Combination Studies

Although calcium antagonists themselves do not appear to be very potent, their interaction with bronchodilators has not been fully explored. In vitro, calcium antagonists potentiate the relaxant effect of β-agonists and theophylline (Kitamura and Ishiihara, 1980). In vivo, the duration, but not the peak effect, of salbutamol and isoproterenol is prolonged by nifedipine (Lever et al., 1984; Cuss et al., 1984), and the bronchodilator dose-response to intravenous terbutaline is potentiated (Svedmyr et al., 1984). The magnitude of these effects is rather small, however, and probably does not have any clinical relevance.

D. Future Possibilities

The acute effects of calcium antagonists are disappointing in asthma, and there are several possible explanations for this. It seems unlikely that the dosage of calcium antagonist given is a limiting factor as discussed above. There is some tissue selectivity with calcium channel blockers so it is possible that calcium antagonists might be developed with a greater potency for airways and mast cells than for other cells. This seems unlikely on present evidence since the rank order of potency of available calcium antagonists is the same in all smooth muscle preparations (nifedipine > verapamil > diltiazem), all being less potent in airway smooth muscle than other smooth muscle preparations (Schwartz and Triggle, 1984). This means that any calcium antagonists developed with a greater potency will still have more effect on vascular than on airway smooth muscle. The different classes of calcium antagonist might interact, since binding studies indicate that diltiazem increases the affinity of dihydropyridine binding (Murphy et al., 1983). Whether such interaction has any functional significance is uncertain, but it may be possible in the future to investigate combinations of these drugs on airway function. The most likely explanation for the relatively weak effects of calcium antagonists in the airways is that VOCs do not play a major role in the regulation of intracellular Ca^{2+} in the airways and that other mechanisms of calcium entry such as ROCs or release of calcium from intracellular stores are more important.

The acute effects of calcium antagonists have been studied extensively but there is little information on the long-term effects of these drugs. It is conceivable that prolonged administration of calcium antagonists might reduce bronchial hyperreactivity, and there is some indication that, when administered over a few days, there is a reduction in early morning wheeze (Patakas et al., 1983).

E. Clinical Evaluation

The effects of calcium antagonists in asthma have been disappointing, and on present evidence they cannot be recommended in the treatment of asthma. The marginal benefits seen in acute challenge situations have to be set against the likelihood of side effects such as headache, flushing, and ankle edema, which may develop during treatment. Although calcium antagonists may prolong and potentiate the effects of other bronchodilators, these effects are small and therefore have no clinical value.

Close examination of the studies reported show that in some patients the effects of calcium antagonists are impressive. Thus nifedipine may completely protect against development of exercise-induced asthma in some patients. There is no obvious relationship between the completeness of protection and any index of severity of asthma and the reason why there should be such marked differences between individuals is not yet clear. Nevertheless, it may indicate that some patients could benefit clinically from these drugs.

An important clinical message from these studies in asthma is that calcium channel blockers are very safe to use. This means that they can be used to treat angina and hypertension in patients with airway obstruction in whom β-adrenoceptor antagonists are contraindicated.

F. Pulmonary Vascular Effects

Calcium antagonists have potent effects on pulmonary vessels and therefore might be of use in pulmonary hypertension. There is good evidence that nifedipine can inhibit acute hypoxic pulmonary vasoconstriction (Simonneau et al., 1981; Kennedy et al., 1984) and might therefore be useful in reducing raised pulmonary vascular resistance in acute exacerbations of chronic obstructive pulmonary disease (COPD). Furthermore, they may be useful in preventing the development of elevated pulmonary vascular resistance and cor pulmonale in COPD. However, the fact that nifedipine equally reduces systemic vascular resistance means that it may not be clinically useful and is unlikely to be of benefit in primary pulmonary hypertension since any reduction in systemic blood pressure might be dangerous.

In asthma the vasodilating effect on hypoxic vasoconstriction may prove to be deleterious, since it will result in the shunting of blood to poorly ventilated areas, leading to arterial hypoxemia. This could be a problem when there is marked ventilation perfusion mismatch as in acute severe asthma.

V. Future Developments

Although currently available calcium antagonists are not clinically useful, the fact remains that Ca^{2+} underlies many of the pathologic processes that contribute to the airway obstruction of asthma. In vitro studies indicate that Ca^{2+} entry in airway smooth muscle in response to various inflammatory mediators and in mast cells in response to IgE cross-linking may occur via ROCs rather than via VOCs. A drug that selectively blocks ROCs or interferes with phosphatidylinositol breakdown might therefore be of great value in the treatment of asthma. Unfortunately, no such drug is yet available.

Intracellular stores of calcium may be an important source of Ca^{2+} for contraction and secretion in the airways. Several drugs have recently been developed that appear to block intracellular calcium release. These drugs are obviously a long way from clinical application and may indeed be dangerous.

An alternative strategy might be antagonism of calcium binding to calmodulin, thereby interfering with the contractile and secretory processes. One such drug is trifluoperazine, which inhibits calmodulin effects in a tracheal smooth muscle preparation (Sparrow et al., 1984) but has many other pharmacologic actions that would make it unselective in intact cells. More selective calmodulin antagonists, such as calmidazolium, have more recently been developed and in the future such drugs could prove useful in the treatment of asthma, since they could be delivered by the aerosol route, thereby achieving tissue selectivity.

VI. Conclusions

Ca^{2+} entry is involved in many pathologic events relevant to asthma, namely contraction of airway smooth muscle, mast cell mediator release, mucus secretion, and possibly also microvascular permeability, autonomic neurotransmission, and inflammatory cell chemotaxis and secretion. Calcium antagonists, which block the entry of Ca^{2+} via voltage-dependent calcium channels, might therefore be of benefit in the treatment of asthma. In vitro calcium antagonists are less potent on airway smooth muscle than on other smooth muscle types, and have no effect on mast cell mediator release at therapeutically relevant concentrations. Clinical studies have shown that calcium antagonists have no bronchodilator effect in asthmatic subjects, but do have a small protective effect against bronchoconstriction provoked by exercise, cold air, antigen, and cholinergic agonists. They also prolong the action of bronchodilators. All these effects are small however, so that these drugs are not useful as antiasthma therapy. Whether there is any greater effect when given long-term is not known. The disappointing clinical results with calcium antagonists suggest that Ca^{2+} entry via voltage-dependent channels is not very important in the pathogenesis of airway obstruction, and blockers of receptor-operated calcium channels, or of calcium release from intracellular stores might be more effective. No such drugs are yet available for clinical use. Calcium antagonists have been shown to be safe in asthma, and are therefore useful in the treatment of angina and hypertension in patients with airway obstruction, in whom β-blockers are contraindicated.

References

Advenier, C., Cerrina, J., Duroux, P., Fluch, A., and Renier, A. (1984). Effects of five different calcium antagonists on guinea-pig isolated trachea. *Br. J. Pharmacol. 82*: 727-733.

Balfre, K. (1978). The effects of calcium and calcium ionophore A23187 on mucin secretion and potential difference in isolated chicken trachea. *J. Physiol. 275*: 80-81.

Barnes, P. J. (1983). Calcium channel blockers in asthma. *Thorax 38*: 481-485.

Barnes, P. J. (1985). Clinical studies with calcium antagonists in asthma. *Br. J. Clin. Pharmacol. 20*: 289-298S.

Barnes, P. J., Wilson, N. M., and Brown, M. J. (1981). A calcium antagonist, nifedipine, modifies exercise-induced asthma. *Thorax 36*: 726-730.

Becker, E. L., and Stossel, T. P. (1980). Chemotaxis. *Fed. Proc. 39*: 2949-2952.

Bolton, T. B. (1979). The mechanism of action of transmitters and other substances in smooth muscle. *Physiol. Rev. 59*: 606-718.

Brugman, T. M., Darnell, M. L., and Hirshman, C. A. (1983). Nifedipine aerosol attenuates airway obstruction in dogs with hyperreactive airways. *Am. Rev. Respir. Dis. 127*: 14-17.

Cerrina, J., Denjean, A., Alexandra, G., Lockhart, A., and Duroux, P. (1981). Inhibition of exercise-induced asthma by a calcium antagonist, nifedipine. *Am. Rev. Respir. Dis. 123*: 156-160.

Cerrina, J., Hadji, L., Marche, E., Duroux, P., and Benveniste, J. (1982). Effect of the Ca^{2+} antatonist nifedipine on histamine and SRS release from human lung tissue. *Am. Rev. Respir. Dis. 125*: 64 (abstract).

Cheng, J. B., and Townley, R. G. (1983). Pharmacological characterization of effects of nifedipine on isolated guinea-pig and rat tracheal smooth muscle. *Arch. Int. Pharmacodyn. 263*: 228-244.

Coburn, R. F. (1977). The airway smooth muscle cell. *Fed. Proc. 36*: 2692-2697.

Coles, S. J., Judge, J., and Reid, L. (1982). Differential effects of calcium ions on glycoconjugate secretion by canine tracheal explants. *Chest 81* (Suppl): 34-35.

Corris, P. A., Nariman, S., and Gibson, G. J. (1983). Nifedipine in the prevention of asthma induced by exercise and histamine. *Am. Rev. Respir. Dis. 128*: 991-992.

Creese, B. R., and Denborough, M. A. (1981). Sources of calcium for concentration of guinea-pig isolated tracheal smooth muscle. *Clin. Exp. Pharmacol. Physiol. 8*: 175-182.

Cuss, F. M. C., and Barnes, P. J. (1985a). The effect of inhaled nifedipine on bronchial reactivity to histamine. *J. Allergy Clin. Immunol. 76*: 718-723.

Cuss, F. M. C., and Barnes, P. J. (1985b). Inhaled nifedipine and histamine induced bronchoconstriction in man. *Am. Rev. Respir. Dis.* In press.

Cuss, F. M. C., Mannix, S. E., and Barnes, P. J. (1984). Nifedipine prolongs isoprenaline-induced bronchodilation in normal subjects. *Clin. Sci. 67*: 1P-79P.

Cuss, F. M. C., Palmer, J. D., and Barnes, P. J. (1985). Effect of nifedipine on autonomic control of airway smooth muscle in vitro. *Am. Rev. Respir. Dis. 131*: A283.

Drazen, J. M., Fanta, C. H., and Lacoutre, P. G. (1983). Effect of nifedpine on constriction of human tracheal strips in vitro. *Br. J. Pharmacol. 78*: 687-691.

Fanta, C. H., and Drazen, J. M. (1983). Calcium blockers and bronchoconstriction. *Am. Rev. Respir. Dis. 127*: 673-674.

Fanta, C. H., Venugopalan, C. S., Lacoutre, P. G., and Drazen, J. M. (1982). Inhibition of bronchoconstriction in the guinea pig by a calcium channel blocker, nifedipine. *Am. Rev. Respir. Dis. 125*: 61-66.

Farley, J. M., and Miles, P. R. (1978). The sources of calcium for acetylcholine-induced contractions of dog tracheal smooth muscle. *J. Pharmacol. Exp. Ther. 207*: 340-346.

Foreman, J. C., Hallett, M. B., and Mongar, J. L. (1977). The relationship between histamine secretion and ^{45}Ca uptake by mast cells. *J. Physiol. 271*: 193-214.

Henderson, A. F., Dunlop, L. S., and Costello, J. F. (1983a). Effect of nifedipine on antigen-induced bronchoconstriction. *Am. Rev. Respir. Dis. 127*: 549-593.

Henderson, A. F., Heaton, R. W., and Costello, J. F. (1983b). The effect of nifedipine on bronchoconstriction induced by inhalation of cold air. *Thorax 38*: 512-515.

Himori, N., and Tiara, N. (1980). Differential effects of the calcium antagonist vasodilators nifedipine and verapamil on the tracheal musculature of the dog. *Br. J. Pharmacol. 68*: 595-597.

Ishizaka, F., Hirata, F., Ishizaka, K., and Axelrod, J. (1980). Stimulation of phospholipid methylation Ca^{2+} influx and histamine release by bridging of IgE receptors on rat mast cells. *Proc. Nat. Acad. Sci. 77*: 1903-1910.

Jakschik, B., Sun, F. F., Lee, L., and Steinhoff, M. M. (1980). Calcium stimulation of a novel lipoxygenase. *Biochem. Biophys. Res. Commun. 95*: 103-110.

Jensen, C., Skov, P. S., and Norn, S. (1983). Inhibitory effect of calcium antagonists on histamine release from human leucocytes. *Allergy 38*: 233-237.

Jouvin-Marche, E., Cerrina, J., Coëffer, E., Duroux, P., and Benveniste, J. (1983). Effect of the Ca^{2+} antagonist nifedipine on the release of platelet-activating factor (PAF-ocether), slow-reverting substance and beta-glucuronidase from human neutrophils. *Eur. J. Pharmacol. 89*: 19-26.

Kennedy, T. P., Michael, J. R., Huang, C-K., Kallman, C. H., Zahka, K., Schlott, W., and Summer, W. (1983). Nifedipine inhibits hypoxic pulmonary vasoconstriction during rest and exercise in patients with chronic obstructive pulmonary disease. *Am. Rev. Respir. Dis. 129*: 544-551.

Kim, Y-Y., Holgate, S. T., and Church, M. K. (1985). Inhibition of histamine release from dispersed human lung and tonsillar mast cells by nicordipine and difedipine. *Br. J. Clin. Pharmacol.* In press.

Kitamura, S., and Ishihara, Y. (1980). Effect of calcium antagonist, etafenone hydrochloride, on isolated guinea pig trachea tissues. *Arzneim. Forsch. 30*: 1088-1091.

Lee, V. Y., Hughes, J. M., Seale, J. P., and Temple, D. M. (1983). Verapamil inhibits mediator release from human lung in vitro. *Thorax 38*: 386-387.

Lever, A. M. L., Corris, P. A., and Gibson, G. J. (1984). Nifedipine enhances the bronchodilator effect of salbutamol. *Thorax 39*: 576-578.

Magnussen, H., Hartmann, V., and Reuss, G. (1984). Influence of diltiazem on bronchoconstriction induced by cold air breathing during exercise. *Thorax 39*: 579-582.

Malo, P. E., Wasserman, M. A., and Griffin, R. L. (1982). Effect of intravenous and aerosol nifedipine on prostaglandin F_{2alpha} and histamine-induced bronchoconstriction in anesthetized dogs. *J. Pharmacol. Exp. Ther. 221*: 410-415.

Marin, M. G., and Zaremba, M. M. (1978). Effect of calcium on ion transport and electrical properties of tracheal epithelium. *J. Appl. Physiol. 44*: 900-904.

Middleton, E. (1980). Antiasthmatic drug therapy and calcium ions: Review of pathogenesis and role of calcium. *J. Pharmacol. Sci. 69*: 243-251.

Middleton, E. (1983). Role of calcium and calcium antagonists in airway function. *Eur. J. Respir. Dis. 64* (suppl 128): 123-132.

Mongar, J. L., and Schild, H. O. (1958). The effect of calcium and pH on the anaphylactic reaction. *J. Physiol. 140*: 272.

Murphy, K. M. M., Gould, R. J., Largent, B. L., and Snyder, S. H. (1983). A unitary mechanism of calcium antagonist drug action. *Proc. Natl. Acad. Sci. USA 80*: 860-864.

Nadel, J. A., and Barnes, P. J. (1984). Autonomic regulation of the airways. *Annu. Rev. Mech. 35*: 451-467.

Patakas, D., Vlachoianni, E., Tsara, V., Louridas, G., and Argiropoulou, P. (1983). Nifedipine on bronchial asthma. *J. Allergy Clin. Immunol. 72*: 269-273.

Pastel, K. R. (1981a). Calcium antagonists in exercise-induced asthma. *Br. Med. J. 282*: 932-933.

Patel, K. R. (1981b). The effect of verapamil on histamine and methocholine induced bronchoconstriction. *Clin. Allergy 11*: 441-447.

Patel, K. R., Al Shama, K. R., and Kerr, J. W. (1983). The effect of inhaled verapamil on allergen-induced bronchoconstriction. *Clin. Allergy 13*: 119-122.

Persson, C. G. A., and Svensjö, E. (1984). Vascular responses and their suppression: drugs interfering with vascular permeability. In: *Handbook of Inflammation,* vol. 5. Edited by I. L. Bonta, M. A. Bray, and M. J. Parnham. Amsterdam, Elsevier.

Popa, V. T., Somani, P., and Simon, V. (1983). The effects of inhaled verapamil on resting tone and reactivity to histamine or acetylcholine in normal or asthmatic subjects. *Am. Rev. Respir. Dis. 127*: 108 (abstract).

Rasmussen, H., and Barrett, P. Q. (1984). Calcium messenger system: An integrated view. *Physiol. Rev. 64*: 938-984.

Redding, G. R., Tuck, R., and Escourrou, P. (1984). Nifedipine attenuates acute hypoxic pulmonary vasoconstriction in awake piglets. *Am. Rev. Respir. Dis. 129*: 785-789.

Reuter, H. (1983). Calcium channel modulation by neurotransmitters, enzymes, and drugs. *Nature 301*: 569-574.

Russi, E. W., and Ahmed, T. (1984). Calcium and calcium antagonists in airway disease. *Chest 86*: 475-482.

Russi, E. W., Marchette, B., Yerger, L., Abraham, W. M., and Ahmed, T. (1983). Modification of allergic bronchoconstriction by a calcium antagonist: mode of action. *Am. Rev. Respir. Dis. 127*: 675-679.

Schramm, M., Thomas, G., Towart, R., and Franckowiak, G. (1983). Novel dihydropyridines with positive inotropic action through activation of Ca^{2+} channels. *Nature 303*: 535-537.

Schwartz, A., and Triggle, D. J. (1984). Cellular action of calcium channel blocking drugs. *Annu. Rev. Med. 35*: 325-339.

Simmoneau, G., Escourrou, P., Duroux, P., and Lockhart, A. (1981). Inhibition of hypoxic pulmonary vasoconstriction by nifedipine. *N. Engl. J. Med. 304*: 1582-1585.

Smith, R. D. (1983). Calcium entry blockers: Key issues. *Fed. Proc. 42*: 201-206.

So, S. W., Lam, W. K., and Yu, D. Y. C. (1982). Effect of calcium antagonists on allergen-induced asthma. *Clin. Allergy 12*: 595-600.

Solway, J., and Fanta, C. H. (1985). Differential inhibition of bronchoconstriction by the calcium channel blockers verapamil and nifedipine. *Am. Rev. Respir. Dis.* In press.

Sorscher, E. J., and Breslow, J. L. (1981). Cystic fibrosis: a disorder of calcium-stimulated secretion and transepithelial sodium transport. *Lancet 1*: 368-370.

Sparrow, M. P., Pfitzner, G., Gagelman, M., and Reugg, J. C. (1984). Effect of calmodulin, Ca^{2+} and CAMP protein kinase on skinned tracheal smooth muscle. *Am. J. Physiol. 246*: C308-C314.

Suzuki, T., Mori, K., and Uchida, M. (1982). Inhibition by calcium antagonists of histamine release and calcium influx of rat mast cells: differences between induction of histamine release by conanavalin A and compound 48/80. *Eur. J. Pharmacol. 85*: 155-161.

Svedmyr, K., Lofdahl, C-G., and Svedmyr, N. (1984). Nifedipine—a calcium channel blocker in asthmatic patients. Interaction with terbutaline. *Allergy 39*: 17-22.

Williams, D. O., Barnes, P. J., Vickers, H. P., and Rudolf, M. (1981). Effect of nifedipine on bronchomotor tone and histamine reactivity in asthma. *Br. Med. J. 283*: 348.

15

Measurement and Significance of the Bronchodilator Response

DONALD P. TASHKIN

UCLA School of Medicine
Los Angeles, California

The measurement of response to a bronchodilator compound (or combination of broncholytic agents) has importance for (1) diagnostic assessment in the office or laboratory of the presence and degree of reversible airflow obstruction; (2) monitoring the effectiveness of bronchodilator therapy in acutely and chronically ill patients with reversible airflow obstruction, in the emergency room, hospital, or outpatient facility; and (3) investigation of the therapeutic efficacy of experimental bronchodilator compounds as well as older agents (alone and in combination) in single- and multiple-dose clinical trials. Methods of measuring response to a bronchodilator usually require pulmonary function tests before and at various times after bronchodilator administration or initiation of a trial of bronchodilator therapy. Less commonly, the efficacy of a bronchodilator is judged by its protective effect against experimentally induced bronchospasm, its impact on objectively measured exercise performance, or its influence on arterial blood gases.

A number of factors influence the measured response to a bronchodilator and thus may confound interpretation: (1) the intrinsic responsiveness of airway smooth muscle and, when the effect of multiple doses is being assessed, the reversibility of other pathophysiological features of airflow obstruction (e.g., excessive and/or retained mucus, inflammation, edema); (2) the severity of the baseline obstruction; (3) the class of bronchodilator agent being evaluated (β_2-adrenergic, methylxanthine, or anticholinergic); (4) the dose is administered; (5) the route of administration and, if the inhaled route is used, the method of aerosol generation and technique of inhalation; (6) the timing of the test in relation to the peak action of the drug; (7) possible residual effects of previously administered bronchodilator drug(s) that have not yet "washed out"; and (8) the test(s) used for measuring the response.

Once a bronchodilator response has been measured, it needs to be interpreted. This interpretation is influenced by the factors noted above as well as the intertrial variability of the test, the method of expressing the response in quantitative terms (e.g., absolute or percentage change from baseline, percent of maximal achievable improvement), the question of what constitutes a "significant" response and the related problem of differentiating between statistically and clinically "significant" responses.

In this chapter we will discuss the methods of evaluating a bronchodilator response, the various factors influencing the response, methods of quantitatively expressing the response, and interpretation of "significance."

I. Methods of Evaluating Bronchodilator Response

A. Response Measures

Tests of Forced Exhalation: Timed Spirometry and Maximal Expiratory Flow-Volume (MEFV) Curves

Most commonly, response to a bronchodilator is determined by performing pulmonary function tests before and after bronchodilator administration. A test of forced exhalation is most commonly employed. Following inhalation to total lung capacity (TLC), the subject performs a maximally forced, complete exhalation down to residual volume (RV) into a volumetric or flow-sensing spirometer. The spirometer generates a forced expired volume-time curve (spirogram) or maximal expiratory flow-volume (MEFV) curve. From the spirogram, the forced vital capacity (FVC), or total volume expired, and the volume expired during the first second (FEV_1) are determined and forced expiratory flow (FEF) is calculated over different portions of the curve, such as the middle half ($FEF_{25-75\%}$) (Fig. 1). Vital capacity (VC) can also be determined from a slow (or unforced) complete exhalation from TLC to RV. From the MEFV curve peak expiratory flow is easily determined and FEF (or $\dot{V}_{max}$) is calculated at different instants corresponding to different percentages of the FVC, such as 25%, 50%, and 75% below TLC (FEF 25, 50, or 75 or $\dot{V}_{max\ 25,\ 50,\ \text{or}\ 75}$) (Fig.

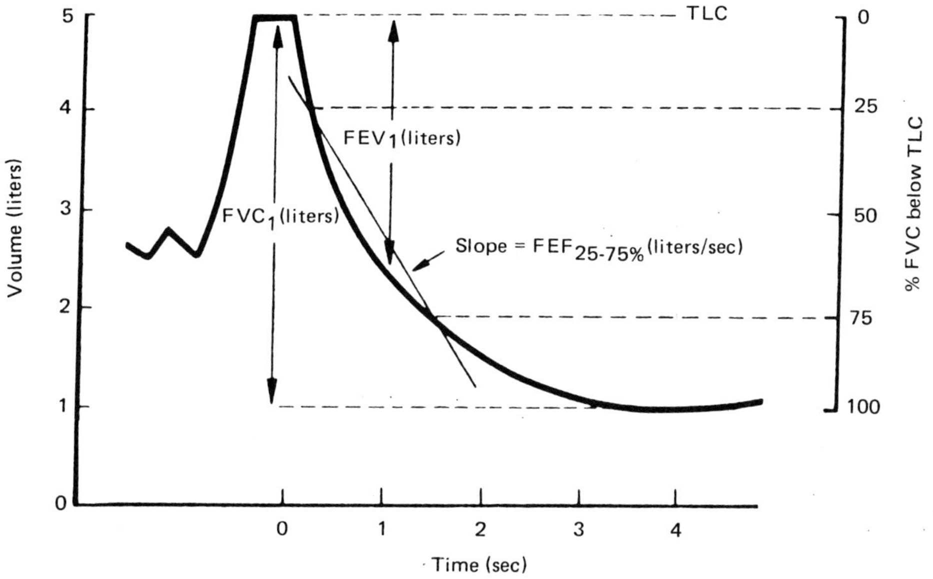

Figure 1 Forced expired volumes and flow rates derived from the forced expiratory volume-time curve. $FEF_{25-75\%}$ is the mean forced expiratory flow over the middle portion of the vital capacity.

2.) Peak expiratory flow rate (PEFR) can be read off the peak of the MEFV curve or it can be determined separately using a simple, portable hand-held spring-loaded rotary vane device (Wright and McKerrow, 1959).

Partial Flow-Volume Curves

The partial flow-volume technique (Fig. 3) can be used to obviate possible effects of the deep inspiration to TLC just prior to forced exhalation. The maximal inspiratory maneuver can cause either transient bronchoconstriction (Lloyd, 1963) or bronchodilation (Vincent et al., 1970; Green and Mead, 1974) which will affect FEF ($\dot{V}_{max}$) during the immediately subsequent forced exhalation (see below). A partial flow-volume curve is obtained after a partial, rather than deep, inspiratory maneuver, followed by a maximally forced exhalation to RV. From RV the subject then inhales fully to TLC from which he or she performs a maximally forced exhalation to RV. The full inspiratory maneuver establishes TLC as a reference point for calculating $\dot{V}_{max}$ from the corresponding partial expiratory flow-volume curve at a fixed percentage of the FVC from TLC.

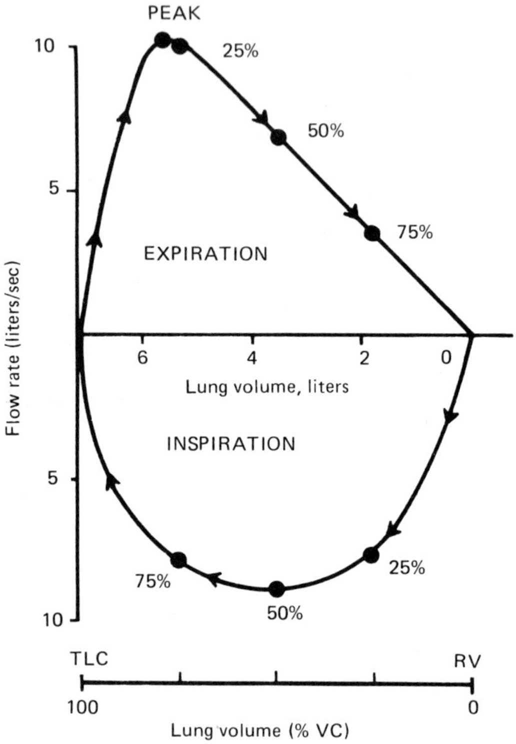

Figure 2 Maximal expiratory and inspiratory flow-volume curves. Instantaneous forced expiratory and inspiratory flow rates can be readily determined at 25, 50, and 75% of the expiratory and inspiratory vital capacity, respectively.

MEFV Curves Breathing Air and 80% He/20% O_2

Deductions concerning the predominant site(s) of bronchodilation within the airways are made from observations of the influence of a bronchodilator on the density dependence of maximal expiratory flow (see below). To evaluate the effect of gas density on $\dot{V}_{max}$, MEFV maneuvers are repeated after three maximal inhalations of an 80% helium/20% oxygen mixture (which is one-third as dense as air) or after several minutes of tidal breathing of the He/O_2 mixture to allow replacement of most of the resident nitrogen in the lungs by the less-dense helium, ascertained by an end-tidal nitrogen concentration less than 5% (Dosman et al., 1975) (Fig. 4). Density dependence of flow is usually quantitated by calculating the absolute increment in $\dot{V}_{max\ 50}$ (if any) during He/O_2 compared to air breathing and expressing this increment as a percentage of the $\dot{V}_{max\ 50}$

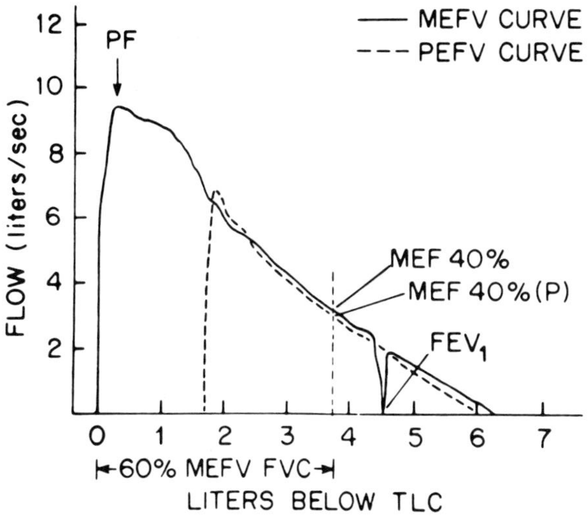

Figure 3 Maximal (solid line) and partial (dashed line) expiratory flow-volume curves. The MEF 40% is the flow rate measured at a lung volume 60% of the forced vital capacity below total lung capacity. From the partial expiratory flow-volume curve MEF 40% (P) is the flow rate measured at the same lung volume as the MEF 40% (from Littner et al., 1979, with permission).

breathing air ($\Delta\ \dot{V}_{max\ 50\%}$) or by calculating the ratio of $\dot{V}_{max\ 50}$ breathing He/O_2 to that breathing air. Also, the volume above RV at which $\dot{V}_{max}$ during He/O_2 breathing first becomes identical to $\dot{V}_{max}$ during air breathing can be calculated and expressed as a percent of VC (volume of isoflow, percent) (Hutcheon et al., 1974).

Airway Resistance and Thoracic Gas Volume

Response to a bronchodilator is sometimes assessed by plethysmographic measurement of changes in airway resistance (R_{aw}) and thoracic gas volume (V_{tg}) at functional residual capacity (FRC). The other subdivisions of lung volume (e.g., TLC and RV) can be calculated from plethysmographically determined FRC and measurements derived from an accompanying slow vital capacity maneuver. This technique provides a rapid means of assessing changes in static lung volumes in response to bronchodilator therapy, in contrast to the more time-consuming methods of determining lung volume using inert gas distribution or dilution. Plethysmographic measurements of R_{aw} and FRC are generally carried out using a technique of rapid, shallow painting (2/sec) which maximizes the glottic opening, thereby minimizing laryngeal resistance (DuBois et al., 1956a,b), although the tests can also be performed during slow tidal breathing (Miller and Simi,

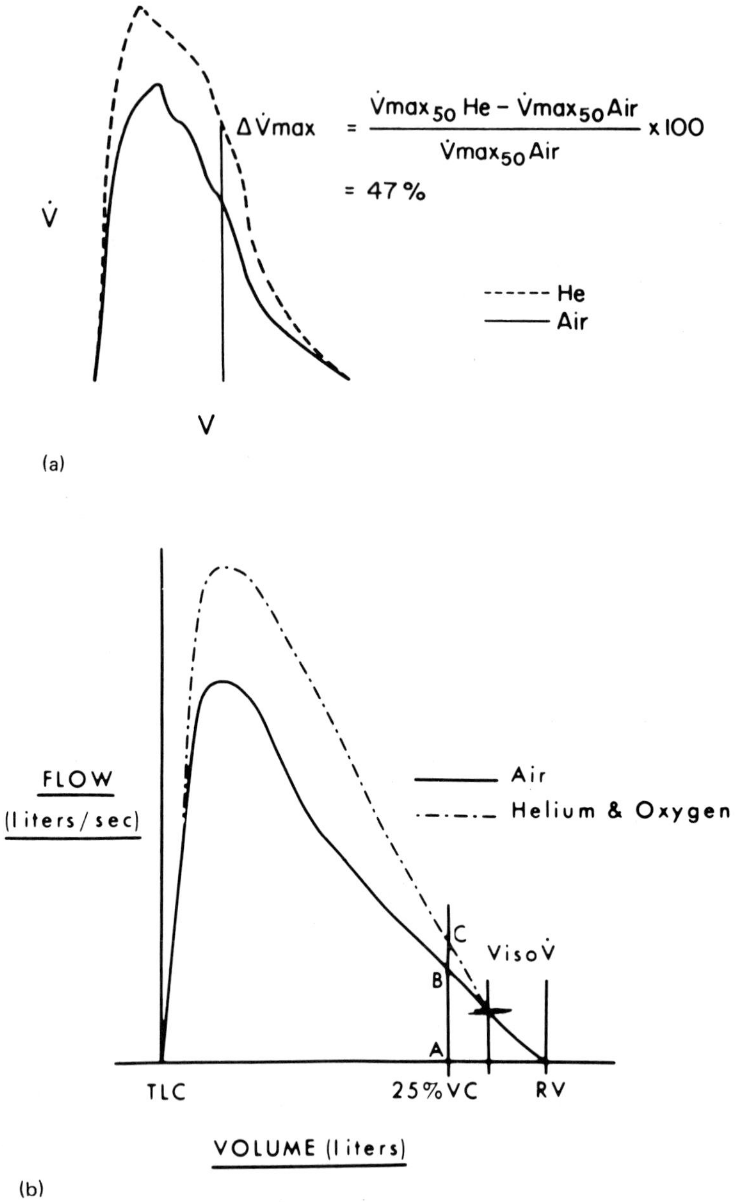

Figure 4 (a) Maximum expiratory flow volume curves on air (——), and 80% He, 20% O_2 (- - - -). Maximum expiratory flow is on the ordinate and volume on the abscissa. Volume decreases to the right (from Macklem, P. T., *Basics of RD*, 4:27, 1976, with permission). (b) Maximal expiratory flow-volume curves breathing air and He + O_2. The point where flows breathing air and He + O_2 are the same is identified, and Viso$\dot{V}$ is measured from this point to RV (from Hutcheon et al., 1974, with permission).

1976). The tests are performed in a whole-body plethysmograph either of constant volume ("pressure" box) (DuBois et al., 1956a,b) or with an attached spirometer or pneumotachograph at an outlet in the wall of the box ("volume" or "flow" box) (Mead, 1960; Bouhuys, 1969; Leith and Mead, 1974). In the "pressure" box, changes in thoracic gas volume are measured from changes in box pressure during panting against a closed shutter, whereas in the "flow" box changes in thoracic volume are measured with the attached spirometer or integrated pneumotachograph. The latter volume signal must be modified to compensate for transient increases in box pressure due to the impedance of the spirometer or pneumotachograph. Airway resistance (ratio of alveolar pressure to airflow) is determined by relating changes in mouth pressure to simultaneous changes in air flow measured by a pneumotachograph during rapid shallow panting. Mouth pressure is "converted" to alveolar pressure using the separately determined relationship between changes in box pressure and mouth pressure during panting against a closed shutter, under which condition mouth pressure reflects alveolar pressure.

Another clinically useful method of measuring resistance to breathing that does not require a body plethysmograph or esophageal balloon catheter utilizes a modification of the technique of forced oscillation originally described by Dubois et al. (1956c), which estimates total respiratory flow resistance (R_{rs}). This method involves the application of a sinusoidally oscillating airflow to the mouth at a frequency greater than the natural respiratory rate, using a loudspeaker and power amplifier. The resultant changes in mouth (or transthoracic) pressure are related to changes in flow at instants when the sum of the compliance and inertance of the respiratory system is zero so that the total change is due to flow resistance alone. Such conditions are met when the applied frequency equals the resonant frequency of the respiratory system (which can also be simulated using a subtraction technique) or at flow maxima and minima when volume acceleration is zero. This technique can be used as a practical alternative to body plethysmography to assess the effect of a bronchodilator (or bronchoconstrictor) on flow resistance. Advantages of this technique are that it does not require bulky equipment, it causes minimal subject inconvenience (a mouthpiece and nose clip), and requires little cooperation by the subject.

Inhalation Challenges with Bronchoconstrictor Stimuli

Bronchodilator drugs afford variable protection against bronchoconstriction experimentally induced by methacholine, histamine, exercise, cold air, hypotonic saline, or antigen. Therefore, bronchial inhalation challenge studies can be used to evaluate the effectiveness of different dosages of a bronchodilator (compared with placebo or another bronchodilator) in preventing induced bronchospasm. The methodology of bronchial challenge procedures has been reviewed elsewhere (Spector, 1983).

Arterial Blood Gases

Derangements in arterial blood gases, particularly a widened alveolar-arterial oxygen difference ($A\text{-}aDO_2$), are common in patients with chronic airflow obstruction. The widened $A\text{-}aDO_2$ is due mainly to regional impairment in ventilation in relation to pulmonary blood flow caused by irregularly diffuse airways narrowing. Administration of a bronchodilator can either have no effect on $A\text{-}aDO_2$ (Littner et al., 1983; Palmer, 1971; Conolly et al., 1971) or cause temporary worsening of arterial oxygenation even in the presence of a concomitant reduction in overall bronchomotor tone (Palmer, 1971; Knudson and Constantine, 1967; Gazioglu et al., 1971; Chick et al., 1973; Tai and Reed, 1967). The short-term widening of the $A\text{-}aDO_2$ sometimes noted after bronchodilator administration is presumably related to worsening of $\dot{V}/\dot{Q}$ relationships due to disproportionate regional increases in pulmonary blood flow resulting from the vasodilator and cardiodynamic effects of the bronchodilator (Palmer, 1971). On the other hand, chronic bronchodilator therapy can cause improvement in arterial oxygenation in the long run by lessening airflow obstruction and thereby improving $\dot{V}/\dot{Q}$ relationships. Thus, arterial blood gases may be one means of assessing the long-term efficacy of maintenance bronchodilator treatment.

Symptoms and Measures of Exercise Performance

In long-term bronchodilator therapy, a dissociation has been noted between improvement in pulmonary function tests and symptomatic benefit (McGavin et al., 1976, 1978; Alexander et al., 1980; Eaton et al., 1982). A closer parallel has been noted between subjective improvement and better performance on exercise tests such as the 12-min walk (12MW). A 12MW is performed by instructing patients to walk on level ground (e.g., in a hospital corrider) for 12 min at a pace of their choice. The total distance covered in the 12 min is noted. Subjective reporting of the level of daily physical activities can be related to oxygen consumption by the oxygen cost diagram. In this diagram, everyday activities are ranked along a 100-mm vertical scale that indicates the oxygen consumption corresponding to any given activity. Patients are asked to mark the line at the point best describing their activity capabilities at the present time. The 12MW and the oxygen cost diagram can be used as objective or semiquantitative subjective indicators of exercise performance and activity tolerance for assessing the impact of a bronchodilator therapeutic regimen in patients with disabling chronic airflow obstruction due to asthma or chronic bronchitis and emphysema with a reversible component (Alexander et al., 1980).

B. Bronchodilator Administration

For diagnostic evaluation, the bronchodilator usually administered is a β-adrenergic agonist aerosol inhaled via a freon-propelled metered-dose inhaler (MDI) or a compressed-gas-powered Venturi-type nebulizer. The advantages of using an inhaled over an oral bronchodilator for routine assessment of acute bronchodilator responsiveness are mainly the faster onset of action, shorter time to peak bronchodilation (usually within 15 min), and lower incidence of unwanted side effects. Although increasing attention is being paid to anticholinergic compounds, a β-agonist aerosol is still generally preferable for diagnostic purposes because of the shorter interval before maximal bronchodilation, which may be delayed for as long as 60-90 min following inhalation of an anticholinergic aerosol. However, there may be special circumstances in which evaluation of the bronchodilator response specifically to an anticholinergic compound can be useful (see below).

Therapeutic responses to bronchodilators administered by a variety of routes (inhaled, oral, subcutaneous, and/or intravenous) are more commonly measured in the emergency room or hospital setting or as part of an investigational drug evaluation program. In the course of emergency room or in-hospital management of severe acute asthma, *repeated* measurements of lung function before and shortly after an inhaled β-adrenergic agent administered at varying intervals provide clinically useful information on the magnitude and duration of acute bronchodilator effectiveness and the trend toward possible improvement in airway responsiveness (Rebuck and Read, 1971). During chronic maintenance therapy with oral and/or inhaled bronchodilators, periodic measurement of lung function allows objective assessment of the long-term utility of bronchodilators in improving baseline lung function, a major goal of therapy. Repeating the measurement shortly after a bronchodilator aerosol gives additional information concerning acute bronchodilator responsiveness. However, as will be pointed out below, the acute response is influenced by the baseline level of lung function and by the persistence of any short-term effects of the last dose(s) of maintenance medication.

II. Factors Influencing the Response to a Bronchodilator

A. Responsiveness of Airway Smooth Muscle

The responsiveness of airway smooth muscle (ASM) is related to the degree of bronchospasm (increased smooth muscle tone) present and the ability of the contracted smooth muscle to relax in response to pharmacologic manipulation (stimulation of membrane β-adrenoceptors, inhibition of muscarinic receptors, calcium antagonism). We are attempting to measure the responsiveness of ASM by quantitating the response to a bronchodilator, assuming that all other factors influencing bronchodilator effects are controlled. Bronchodilator responsiveness bears some relation to airway hyperreactivity to nonspecific constrictor stimuli. Nonspecific airway hyperreactivity may be due, at least partly, to (1) abnormal autonomic control of ASM (increased cholinergic and α-adrenergic responsiveness, decreased β-adrenergic responsiveness) (Szentivanyi, 1968; Tattersfield et al., 1973; Coleridge et al., 1976; Simonsson et al., 1967; Holtzman et al., 1980) and/or (2) increased contractile responsiveness of the smooth muscle itself unrelated to specific pharmacoreceptor activity (Boushey et al., 1980; Kepron et al., 1977; Antonissen et al., 1980; Souhrada and Dickey, 1976). Therefore, a bronchodilator could relax contracted ASM by counteracting defects in the activity of cell-surface autonomic receptors, in the smooth muscle cell's intrinsic electromechanical contractility, or in other non-receptor-mediated contractile mechanisms.

B. Severity of the Baseline Obstruction

Normal subjects show little improvement in FEV_1 or FVC when given bronchodilators (Watanabe et al., 1974). Similarly, asthmatics with no or only mild airflow obstruction at baseline exhibit a relatively modest (if any) increase in FEV_1 or FVC since they have little room for improvement in these parameters. As their airflow obstruction increases, so does their spirometric response to bronchodilator therapy, reflecting their greater degree of possible functional improvement. On the other hand, when obstruction becomes severe, response is again diminished, most likely reflecting factors other than bronchospasm (secretions, edema, inflammation) that are not readily reversible and are principally responsible for the severity of the obstruction. Thus, as noted by Hume and Gandevia (1957), the curve relating FEV_1 responses to varying baseline FEV_1 values is bell-shaped, the response being smallest when obstruction is very mild or very severe and greatest when obstruction is moderate.

C. Type of Bronchodilator(s) Used

The presence and degree of bronchodilator response in any individual patient may depend on the class of bronchodilator used and the mechanism(s) of reversible airflow obstruction in that particular patient. For example, many patients with chronic bronchitis respond well to atropine but not at all to isoproterenol (Klock et al., 1975; Marini and Lakshminarayan, 1980). This implies that cholinergic influences may play a more important role than adrenergic factors in the pathophysiology of reversible airflow obstruction in patients with chronic bronchitis. Therefore, inaccurate conclusions could be drawn regarding the presence or absence of a reversible bronchospastic component in such subjects if the bronchomotor response was assessed only in relation to a β-adrenergic agonist. In contrast, asthmatic subjects tend to exhibit a greater peak magnitude of response to a β-agonist than to anticholinergic medication (Bruderman et al., 1983; Elwood and Abboud, 1982; Ruffin et al., 1982), which suggests that adrenergic influences may be more important pathogenetically than cholinergic mechanisms in asthma. On the other hand, some asthmatics who respond poorly to an adrenergic bronchodilator respond well to an anticholinergic, possibly reflecting β-adrenergic tolerance (Burge et al., 1980).

Additive bronchodilation has been noted when bronchodilator compounds of different classes are administered together. For example, in asthmatic patients the combination of theophylline with either an oral (Wolfe et al., 1978) or inhaled (Smith et al., 1980) β-agonist has been found to produce greater bronchodilation than that achieved with either agent alone, even when both compounds were administered in high dosages (Wolfe et al., 1978). Similarly, the combination of anticholinergic and β-adrenergic agents can produce additive bronchodilation in patients with asthma or chronic bronchitis (Douglas et al., 1979). For example, in asthmatics, Ullah et al. (1981) found that the addition of either inhaled albuterol or ipratropium after maximal bronchodilation had been produced by the other agent caused a further increase in FEV_1. Douglas and associates (1979) reported similar results in patients with severe bronchitis. These findings suggest that the results of bronchodilator challenge studies employing a single agent, even when administered in maximally effective dosages, can underestimate the presence and/or degree of airway responsiveness.

Different classes of bronchodilators show varying efficacy against different bronchospastic stimuli, as indicated in Table 1 for inhaled β-agonist and anticholinergic drugs. Theophylline has also been shown to have prophylactic value in inhibiting bronchospasm induced by antigen (Falliers and Katsampes, 1976) and exercise (Bierman et al., 1977). However, its protective effect against non-nonspecific bronchoprovocation by histamine or methacholine is less clear. DeCotiis and co-workers (1980) failed to show any blocking effect of single doses of theophylline (mean serum theophylline concentration 13.4 μg/ml) on methacholine-induced bronchospasm. Spector (1978) was also unable to demonstrate any inhibiting effect of single-dose aminophylline (6 mg/kg; serum theophylline concentrations not measured) on bronchoprovocation with either methacholine or histamine. On the other hand, in children with moderately severe asthma, McWilliams et al. (1984) found that oral theophylline (average serum concentration 13 μg/ml), compared to placebo, led to a significant two- to threefold attenuation of the bronchoconstrictor responses to histamine and methacholine, respectively. The protective effect against nonspecific bronchoprovocation did not correlate with the degree of bronchodilation following theophylline.

D. Dosages of the Bronchodilator Administered

Clearly, the bronchodilator response to a pharmacologic agent is dependent on the dosage given. The relationship between ASM relaxation and dosage (or serum concentration) is log linear (Nelson et al., 1983; Mitenko and Ogilvie, 1973). The dosage chosen for clinical purposes is generally adjusted to produce maximal

Table 1 Summary of Comparative Efficacy of Anticholinergic and Beta-Adrenergic Bronchodilators Against Different Bronchospastic Stimuli

Stimulus	Efficacy of anticholinergic agents	Efficacy of adrenergic agents relative to anticholinergic agents
Cholinergic agents	Fully protective	
Histamine	Partially protective at most	More effective
Various mediators, $PGF_2\alpha$, serotonin, bradykinin	Partially protective at most	
Beta blockade	Effective reversal	Much less effective
Gases, dust, irritants	Variable, usually some protection	
Antigens	Variable, from none to excellent	More effective
Exercise, hyperventilation, cold air	Moderately effective, possibly more so in large doses	Invariably more effective
Psychogenic factors	Good protection	Probably less effective

From Gross, N. J., and Skorodin, M. S. (1984).

bronchodilation and minimal unwanted physiological effects and varies with the route of administration (see below). The inhaled route is generally preferred for β-adrenergic and anticholinergic bronchodilators because it is associated with fewer side effects than the systemic route for a given degree of bronchodilation. However, there is disagreement as to the optimal dosage of inhaled β-agonists and anticholinergics (Nelson et al., 1983; Gross, 1975; Wood and Paterson, 1975; Simonsson et al., 1975; Kamburoff and Günther, 1975). For metered-dosage inhalers, two inhalations are commonly administered as a standard "dose" both for therapy and for formal measurement of bronchodilator response. This practice is supported by the results of several investigators who have failed to demonstrate progressively greater bronchodilation with higher metered dosages of either a beta-agonist (Alliott et al., 1972; Ruffin et al., 1978; Heimer et al., 1980; Williams and Kane, 1975) or ipratropium, an anticholinergic bronchodilator (Gross, 1975; Yeager et al., 1976; Storms et al., 1975; Baigelman and Chodosh, 1977; Newcomb et al., 1985). On the other hand, others (Nelson et al., 1983) have shown a linear relationship between the increase in FEV_1 and the log dose of albuterol delivered via MDI in doses of from one to eight inhalations; the response to four to six inhalations was significantly greater than that to one inhalation ($P < 0.05$) and that to eight inhalations was significantly greater than the response to one or two inhalations ($P < 0.01$) (Fig. 5). For ipratropium delivered by MDI, some authors have demonstrated increasing bronchodilation up to a dosage of 60-80 μg (three to four puffs) (Wood and Paterson, 1975; Newcomb et al., 1985). Nelson et al. (1983) showed that the response to 15 mg isoproterenol administered by intermittent positive pressure breathing (IPPB) exceeded that to a standard therapeutic dose of isoproterenol of 1.25 mg ($P < 0.01$), as well as that to 2.5, 5, and 10 mg ($P < 0.05$) also administered by IPPB. These findings suggest, particularly for inhaled β-agonists, that the customarily administered "therapeutic dose" of two inhalations from an MDI or 1.25 mg isoproterenol (or the equivalent of other β-agonist solutions) via a compressed-gas-driven nebulizer may elicit less than a maximally attainable bronchodilator response and thus may underestimate the presence or degree of bronchodilator responsiveness.

With regard to theophylline, the log linear relationship between serum concentration and bronchodilator effect is well recognized (Mitenko and Ogilvie, 1973). A "therapeutic" range of serum levels (10-20 μg/ml) has been recommended, based on clinical observations that higher concentrations are associated with increasingly more frequent side effects in the face of increasingly limited gains in bronchodilator effectiveness, while lower concentrations are less efficacious (Mitenko and Ogilvie, 1973). Recently, however, the pendulum of clinical opinion has begun to shift in the direction of revising the therapeutic range downward to include lower serum concentrations (Rogers et al., 1985). This reassessment derives from increasing evidence of theophylline toxicity when serum

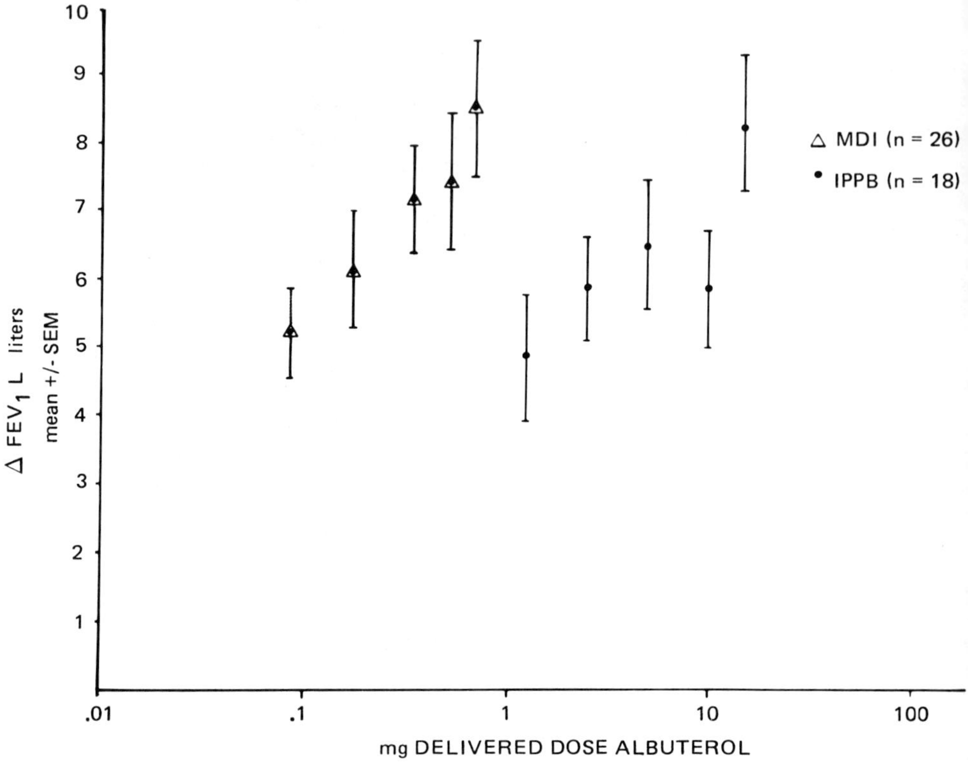

Figure 5 Maximum increases in FEV_1 are plotted against an aerosolized dose of albuterol by metered dose inhaler (MDI) (26 patients) and IPPB (18 patients). The correlation by each mode of administration between the log of the dose of albuterol and absolute improvement in FEV_1 is significant. The response to the highest three doses by metered dose inhaler is significantly greater than that to the lowest dose ($P < 0.05$), whereas the response to the highest dose by IPPB is significantly greater than that to any other dose ($P < 0.05$) (Note: The "delivered dose" from IPPB was the dose placed in the nebulizer) (from Nelson et al., 1983, with permission).

levels are "in range" (i.e., between 10 and 20 μg/ml) and the observation that less toxic levels of theophylline in the low "therapeutic" or even in the "subtherapeutic" range may be only slightly less effective than higher dosages due to the log linear relationship between the serum level and bronchodilation. This point becomes more obvious when the concentration-response curve for theophylline is plotted using linear rather than log-linear coordinates (Rogers et al., 1985 (Figs. 6 and 7).

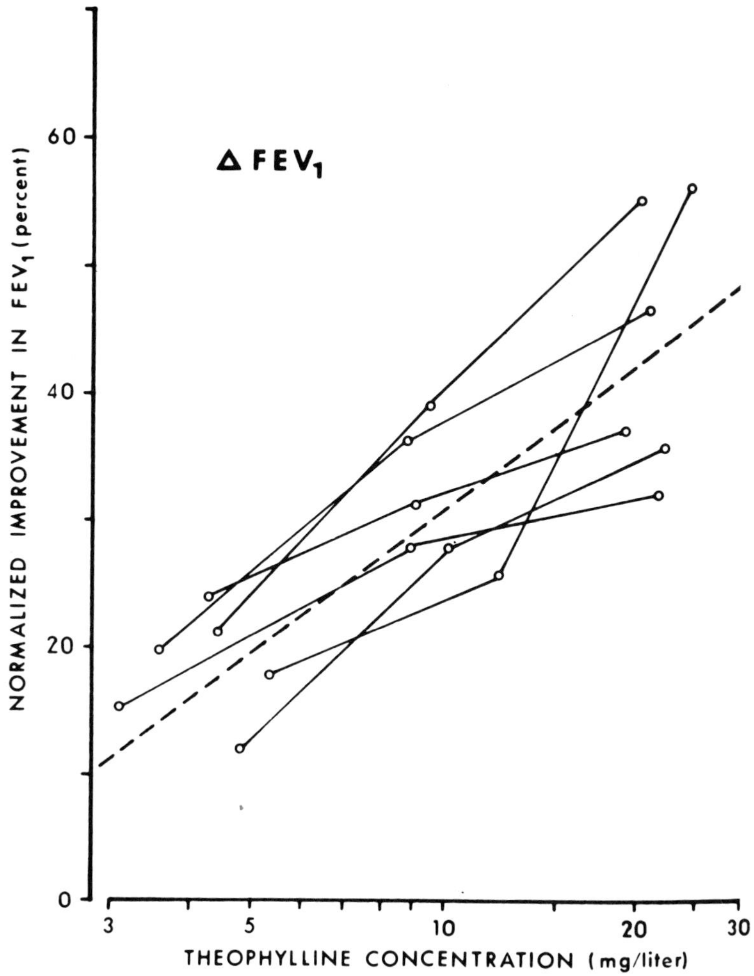

Figure 6 Dose-response relation for changes in forced expiratory volume in the first second (FEV_1) against the plasma theophylline concentration plotted semilogarithmically. Plots for each subject are presented individually (0–0–0) as well as the unweighted least-squares regression line for the whole group (- - - -). For each subject the FEV_1 is normalized by division of the mean difference from the placebo value at each drug concentration plateau by the predicted value minus the placebo value (from Mitenko and Ogilvie, 1973).

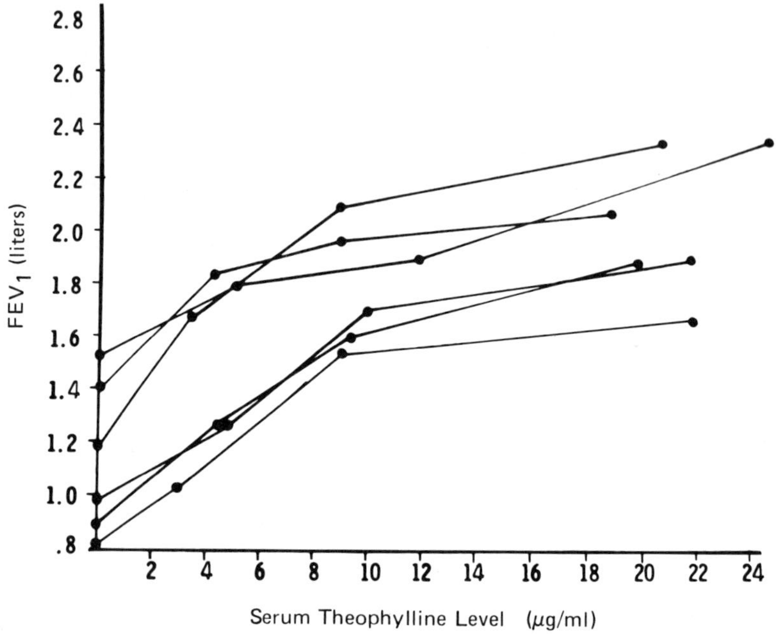

Figure 7 Data of Mitenko and Ogilvie (see Figure 6) replotted on a linear scale. Note that the dose-response relationship plateaus with relatively little improvement in FEV_1 above serum theophylline concentrations of 10-12 μg/ml. (From Rogers, R. M., Owens, G. R., and B. E. Pennock, 1985, with permission).

E. Route of Administration

The onset, magnitude, and duration of bronchodilation are influenced by the route of bronchodilator administration and, for inhaled agents, by the method of drug delivery. The predominant site(s) of dilator action within the airways may also be affected by the route of administration.

Aerosol Route

Beta-adrenergic agonists and anticholinergic bronchodilators (atropine, ipratropium) are most commonly administered as aerosols. The effectiveness of these aerosols in reducing bronchomotor tone is dependent on the actual dosage of the drug delivered to the lung, the site(s) of deposition within the lung (tracheobronchial, alveolar), and the degree of dispersion throughout the surface of the lower airways. An additional factor is the rate at which the deposited drug is removed from the sites of deposition within the lower respiratory tract by mucociliary clearance or absorption into the systemic circulation. These factors,

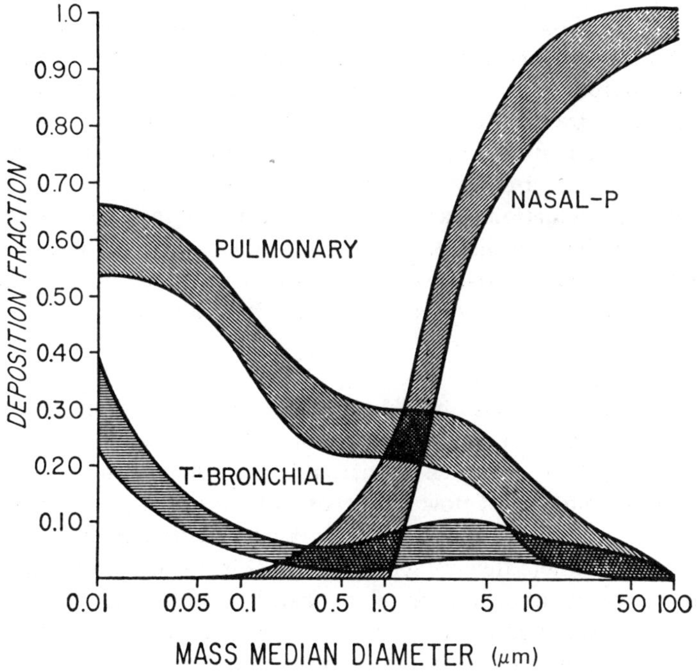

Figure 8 Regional deposition fractions for aerosols of specific mass (aerodynamic) diameters; shaded areas represent envelopes of curves for geometric standard deviations ranging from 1.2 (nearly homogeneous aerosols) to 4.5 (very heterodispersed aerosols) (from the Task Group on Lung Dynamics (1966), © 1966, Pergamon Press Ltd., with permission).

in turn, are influenced by (1) the aerodynamic properties of the nebulized particles, which are determined, in part, by the method of aerosol generation and delivery; (2) the pattern of inhalation of the aerosol, including the inspiratory flow rate, lung volume over which the aerosol is inhaled, and breathholding time at end-inspiration; (3) the geometry of the airways; (4) the responsiveness of the airways where the drug is actually deposited; and (5) the time sequence of aerosol administration.

Bronchodilator aerosols are most often generated by either cartridge-type metered-dose inhalers (MDIs) containing freon propellants or jet-type nebulizers powered by compressed air (hand-bulb, motor-driven compressor, or IPPB devices). Aerosols generated by these devices are polydispersed through a broad range of particle sizes, the larger particles ($> 10\ \mu m$) being trapped in the jet-type nebulizer or the actuator of the MDI. Only about 10% of the solution aerosolized by the jet-type device ever leaves the nebulizer, as opposed to approximately 85% of the aerosol generated by an MDI. Consequently the dosage of a β-agonist that must be added to a "wet" nebulizer is about 10 times the metered-dose output of an MDI producing an equivalent degree of bronchodilation (Fig. 5). The size range of the aerosol actually leaving the nebulizer depends on the time after actuation that the particle size measurements are made and the distance from the nebulizer at which the measurements are made. For example, immediately after actuation of a pressurized inhaler of terbutaline sulfate, the mass median aerodynamic diameter (MMAD) of the particles is 36 μm, which falls to about 12 μm at a distance of 10 cm (Moren and Andersson, 1980; Newman et al., 1982). The microcrystals of the drug itself are only ~ 2.8 μm in diameter after complete evaporation of the propellants, which may not occur for several seconds after actuation.

Aerosol particles deposit in the respiratory tract by three mechanisms: inertial impaction, gravitational sedimentation, and Brownian diffusion. Most particles > 5-10 μm are deposited by inertial impaction in the upper airway where the linear velocities of flow are highest, whereas 0.5-1 μm particles are mostly deposited by gravitational sedimentation and Brownian diffusion in peripheral airways where flow velocities are low (Fig. 8). The breathing patterns also influence the site of deposition of an inhaled aerosol. A rapid breathing pattern with a high inspiratory flow rate favors deposition by impaction in the upper and central airways, whereas lower inspiratory flow rates and longer transit times through any segment of the airway favor deposition by gravitational sedimentation at more peripheral sites within the lung (Landahl et al., 1951). A longer breathhold at end-inspiration also favors greater retention of very small particles in the lung by allowing more time for flow velocities to diminish sufficiently for such particles to settle out by gravity, thus reducing loss of inhaled particles in the exhaled air. Using submicronic aerosols labeled with ^{99m}Tc and comparable aerodynamically to bronchodilator aerosols generated by MDIs, Newman and co-workers (1982) found that a larger fraction of the particles (14%) deposited in the lung when patients with asthma or bronchitis inhaled the aerosol at low inspiratory flow rates (0.5 1/sec) with a long breathholding time (10 sec) than when inhaled flow rates were faster (1.33-1.5 l/sec) or breathholding time was shorter (4 sec). Each of the latter breathing patterns effectively halved the bronchial deposition rate to 7% (Fig. 9). For all breathing patterns, > 70% of the aerosol was deposited in the oral pharynx.

The lung volume at which an aerosol is inhaled also appears to influence its deposition in the lower respiratory tract. Riley and associates (1979) found that the effectiveness of both single and sequential slow (approximately 0.25 l/sec) inhalations of a bronchodilator aerosol was significantly enhanced when the inhalation was initiated at a high, compared to a low, lung volume (80% vs. 20% vital capacity). Presumably, the widened air passages at the higher lung volumes

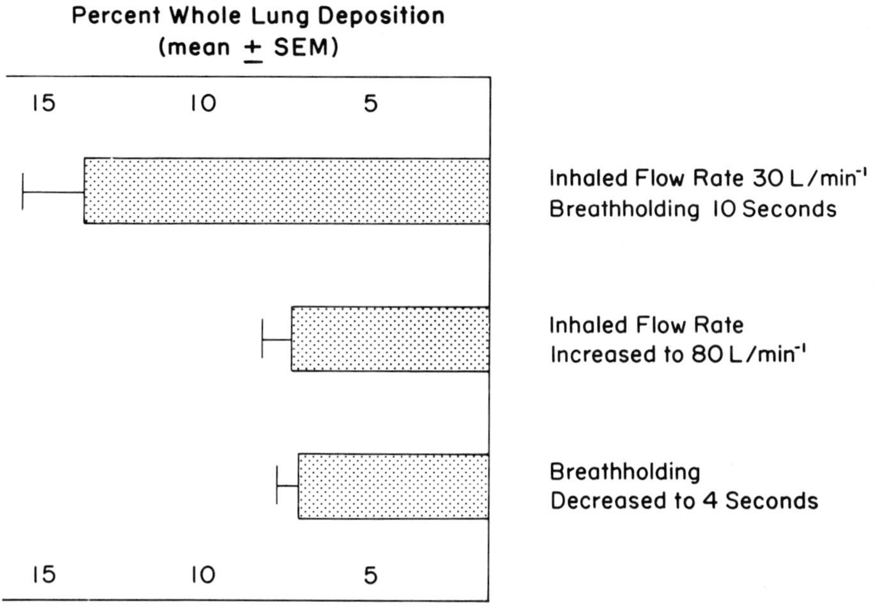

Figure 9 Effect of inhalation mode on the deposition of a pressurized suspension aerosol in the lungs. A mean 14% of the dose reached the lungs when the aerosol was inhaled slowly (30 l/min) followed by 10 sec breathholding. Deposition was reduced when the inhaled flow rate was increased to 80 l/min, or when breathholding was reduced to 4 sec (from Newman et al., 1982, with permission).

allow the aerosol to be dispersed over a larger bronchial surface to achieve greater penetration of distal airways. Since the major change in airway dimensions occurs at low transpulmonary pressures between RV and FRC with little further increase in airway diameter as lung volume increases above FRC to TLC (Hyatt and Flath, 1966), initiation of aerosol inhalation at FRC should be comparable to beginning the inhalation at higher lung volumes and has the added advantage of greater ease in coordinating the inhalation with actuation of the nebulizer. This expectation is supported by the findings of Dolovich and associates (1981). Using a radiolabeled pressurized solution aerosol, these workers found greater aerosol deposition in the lungs when the nebulizer was actuated at FRC than at either RV or close to TLC. Beginning the inhalation too close to TLC constrains the volume of aerosol inhaled and may thus reduce the total number of particles (and, therefore, the amount of drug) deposited. Landahl and associates (1951) have shown that deeper breathing with large tidal volumes increases particle deposition in the lung. When wet aerosols are administered during tidal breathing, particle deposition is dependent on the depth as well as the rate of inspiration; deposition in the lower respiratory tract is favored by slow, deep breathing (Pavia et al., 1977; Muir and Davies, 1967).

A number of recent studies have evaluated the possible advantages of extension-tube or aerosol-chamber attachments to MDIs in enhancing particle deposition in the lungs and improving the efficacy of bronchodilator aerosols. Theoretically, these attachment devices should improve aerosol delivery to the lung by allowing a longer time and distance before the aerosol reaches the mouth for the aerosol velocity to slow and particle size to diminish by evaporation. The slower velocity and smaller particle size of the aerosol entering the mouth should lessen the likelihood of inertial impaction on the oropharynx and favor penetration into the lower respiratory tract. Using radiolabeled particles, Newman et al. (1981) have demonstrated that extension devices (10-cm cylindrical tube, 22-cm cone) do increase deposition in the lung while decreasing deposition in the oropharynx due, in part, to trapping of larger particles in the device. Similar enhancement of lung deposition has been reported when the mouthpiece of the nebulizer was held a few centimeters in front of the open mouth (Newcomb et al., 1985). However, greater aerosol penetration of the lung with use of spacer attachments may not necessarily translate into superior bronchodilation. The results of several studies in asthmatics with mild to marked airflow obstruction do not demonstrate consistently significant differences in magnitude or duration of bronchodilation when MDIs with and without spacer attachments are compared (Lindgren et al., 1980; Bloomfield et al., 1979; Godden and Crompton, 1981; Spicer et al., 1980; Poppius, 1980; Gomm et al., 1980; Dolovich et al., 1983). On the other hand, significant improvement in bronchodilation following one actuation of a metaproterenol MDI has been reported with the adjunctive use of a reservoir aerosol delivery system containing a 700-ml collapsible bag and a reed in the mouthpiece to signal audibly when inspiratory flow rate exceeds 0.3 l/sec (Inspirease) (Tobin et al., 1982). However, incorrect MDI use was partly responsible for the observed difference in bronchodilation, and the use of a standard dose (two actuations) of the metaproterenol MDI might have narrowed this difference since response to a standard dose might be on the flat portion of the dose-response curve. Nonetheless, one of the advantages of an extension tube or aerosol reservoir attached to an MDI is to compensate partially for an uncoordinated technique of MDI use, leading to improved aerosol delivery and bronchodilation in some subjects.

With respect to the relative efficacy of different methods of bronchodilator aerosol generation (MDI, compressor-driven nebulizer, IPPB), recent studies have not shown any difference in the effectiveness of inhaled β-adrenergic bronchodilators delivered via an MDI with an aerochamber extender (Monoghan) and a hand-held compressed-gas-driven nebulizer in hospitalized patients with

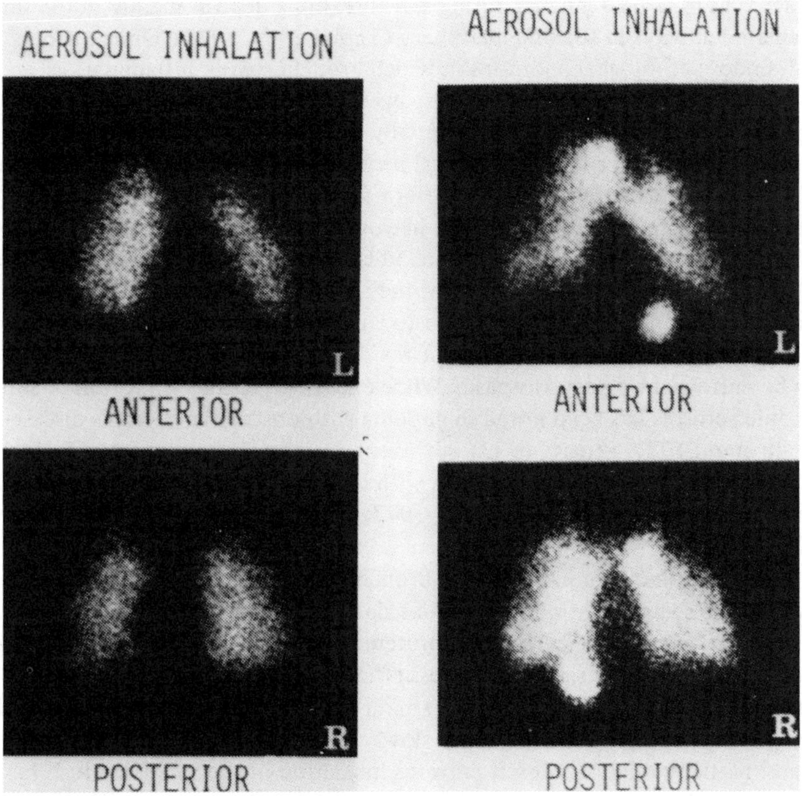

Figure 10 Normal radioaerosol lung images in a 57-year-old man with normal lung function tests (left panels). Note uniform distribution of the aerosol throughout the lung with minimal deposition in the airways. Grossly abnormal radioaerosol lung image pattern in a 58-year-old man with severe air flow obstruction (right panels). Note excessive deposition of aerosol in the central airways with regions of grossly diminished deposition in the periphery.

bronchospastic disease (Berenberg et al., 1985). Other studies have failed to demonstrate any differences in the effectiveness of aerosolized bronchodilators delivered by continuous-pressure-driven nebulizers and intermittent positive pressure breathing (IPPB) (Loren et al., 1977; Smelzer and Barnett, 1973; Chang and Levison, 1972; Intermittent Positive Pressure Breathing Trial Group, 1983).

The predominant site of deposition of nebulized particles is also dependent on the geometry of the airways. In the normal tracheobronchial tree, small-size aerosols (< 2 μm) inhaled during slow breathing deposit mainly in the small nonciliated airways in the lung periphery (Taplin et al., 1977). On the other hand, under pathologic conditions in which bronchospasm, inflammation, and increased secretions cause irregular narrowing of the larger airways, even submicronic aerosols can deposit preferentially at these sites of narrowing in the central airways with reduced peripheral penetration (Taplin et al., 1977; Stuart, 1973) (Fig. 10). Theoretically, the preferred sites of deposition of a bronchodilator aerosol are those airways most narrowed by bronchospasm and thus probably most responsive to the bronchodilator action of the locally deposited drug. On the other hand, deposition of the aerosol at sites of narrowing due to excessive retained mucus may not lead to any beneficial action in these areas while possibly retarding penetration of the drug to more peripheral airways that may be narrowed by bronchospasm. While excessive central deposition of submicronic aerosols has been noted in patients with obstructive airways disease (Taplin et al., 1977; Stuart, 1973), sufficient peripheral penetration of bronchodilator aerosols does occur in patients with bronchospastic disease to cause dilation of smaller airways (Ingram et al., 1977; Fairshter and Wilson, 1980; Pierce et al., 1981).

The response to inhalation of a bronchodilator from an MDI is also influenced by the sequential timing of the inhalations. Heimer and colleagues (1980) showed that three puffs from a metaproterenol MDI (0.6 mg per puff) inhaled in rapid sequence were significantly less effective than the same three puffs inhaled in a sequence of 1 puff every 10 min (Fig. 11). These findings may result from greater penetration of the more slowly sequenced aerosol into airways already partially dilated by each previous inhalation of the aerosol, which has had sufficient time to produce peak or near-peak levels of bronchodilation before the next dose. Inhalation of divided doses at only 2-min intervals was not shown to have advantages over administration of the same total dose as a single inhalation (Dulfano et al., 1977), possibly because this time interval between successive doses was too short to allow peak bronchodilation to occur between doses. The above findings imply that in cumulative dose-response studies of aerosolized bronchodilators, effects that some have attributed to higher cumulative dosages of the drug (Nelson et al., 1983) may be due, instead or in part, to the sequential method of administering the drug (Heimer et al., 1980). The benefits of delaying the second (or third) puff of a metered-dose bronchodilator to achieve greater overall bronchodilation must be weighed against the inconvenience of these delays and the possibility of forgetting to take the subsequent puff(s), causing reduced effectiveness.

Oral Route

Oral bronchodilators include methylxanthines and β-adrenergic stimulants. Compared to topically administered β-adrenergic aerosols, especially those generated

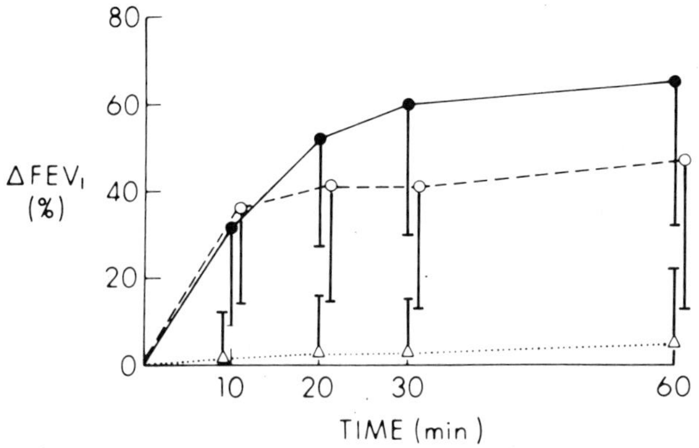

Figure 11 Percent change in FEV_1. Bars represent 1 SD in one direction only. Regimen of 1 puff of aerosolized metaproterenol (659 μg/puff) inhaled every 10 min for 30 min was used (solid line). FEV_1 increased significantly at 10, 20, and 30 min. On a regimen of 3 puffs of metaproterenol (650 μg/puff) inhaled in rapid sequence at time "0" (dashed line), FEV_1 increased significantly at 10 and 20 min. FEV_1 is significantly greater on the former than the latter regimen. On a regimen of placebo inhalations (dotted line), FEV_1 did not improve significantly (from Heimer et al., 1980, with permission).

by MDIs, the oral β-agonists (which are delivered to airway smooth muscle indirectly via the circulation) must be given in much larger dosages to achieve a comparable peak bronchodilator effect. The aerosol and oral routes also differ with respect to the time of onset and peak magnitude of bronchodilation. The onset of bronchodilation is generally rapid (from less than 1 to 5 min) following most β-agonists aerosols, slightly slower after anticholinergic aerosols, such as ipratropium, and slower still (approximately 30 min) after ingestion of an oral β-agonist, due to delay in gastrointestinal absorption. Oral methylxanthines have a variable onset of action depending on the absorption and release characteristics of the preparation, being most rapid (15-30 minutes) for hydroalcoholic solutions, other liquid preparations, and fast-acting tablet formulations and slowest (1-2 hr) for slow-release preparations. Furthermore, food may slow the absorption of all oral bronchodilators. *Peak* bronchodilation also begins sooner after a β-agonist aerosol (5-30 min) than an anticholinergic agent ($\geq$ 60 min) or an oral β-agonist (2-4 hr) or methylxanthine (2 hr, 4-6 hr, and 8-12 hr after short-, intermediate- and long-acting preparations, respectively).

Duration of action is highly variable, irrespective of the route of bronchodilator administration. Duration of action is shorter following the catecholamine aerosols (epinephrine, isoproterenol, and isoethrine) (1-3 hr) than newer β-agonist aerosols (metaproterenol, albuterol, terbutaline, bitolterol, and fenoterol) (4-6 hr). The duration of effectiveness of oral preparations of the latter compounds is comparable to their duration of action when given by inhalation. The length of action of theophylline compounds is quite variable and is a function not only of the absorption and release characteristics of the compound but also of metabolic clearance and the achievement of a "relatively steady" plasma concentration with multiple dosing following initiation of therapy. Bronchodilation lasts 4-6 hr after shorter-acting theophylline compounds and 8-24 hr following longer-acting sustained-release preparations.

The bronchodilator effect of an oral bronchodilator is likely to extend to a greater range of airways (both peripheral and central) than is reached by an aerosol, at least in patients with chronic airflow obstruction in whom peripheral penetration of the aerosol may be impeded by obstruction at central sites. In stable asthmatics, for example, Larsson and Svedmyr (1977) found that maximally tolerated doses of oral albuterol produced larger increases in FVC than maximal inhaled doses, despite the achievement of a greater increase in FEV_1 by the inhaled route. These findings suggest that the small airways were dilated to a greater extent by the oral compound as a result of greater reduction in air trapping and consequent decrease in residual volume. Conversely, compared to an oral agent, an aerosolized bronchodilator might exert a greater effect on the central airways of asthmatics with predominant obstruction in the larger airways where excessive deposition of the inhaled drug might be expected to occur due to inertial impaction. This possibility is illustrated by the greater protection against exercise-induced bronchospasm produced by an inhaled than an oral β-agonist when administered in dosages producing comparable overall bronchodilation to asthmatics with predominantly central airflow limitation (Anderson et al., 1976). On the other hand, aerosolized bronchodilators *can* cause dilation of the peripheral airways of both asthmatics and patients with chronic bronchitis and emphysema with a reactive airways component, as suggested by immediate effects on density-dependence of flow (Ingram et al., 1977; Fairshter and Wilson, 1980; Antic and Macklem, 1976; Douglas et al., 1979) and by increases in vital capacity due to decreases in residual volume (see below).

Subcutaneous and Intravenous Routes

Bronchodilators are sometimes given subcutaneously (epinephrine, terbutaline) or by slow intravenous infusion (aminophylline, albuterol, terbutaline, isoproterenol) to patients with severe asthma whose response to inhaled drugs is unsatisfactory. In these patients, the parenteral route may have the advantage of delivering the bronchodilator via the systemic circulation to sites in the airways distal to occlusive plugs and thus inaccessible to the aerosol. In support of this concept, Tashkin et al. (1980) found that both large and small airways of chronic asthmatics were dilated by terbutaline given subcutaneously (0.5 mg) but only large airways were dilated by terbutaline given by inhalation (0.5 mg). On the other hand, Pierce et al. (1981) found that administration of much larger dosages of inhaled terbutaline (2.5 mg) to asthmatics led to comparable effectiveness and sites of action as the intravenous route. The latter findings could be explained by (1) greater systemic absorption of the larger aerosol doses from sites of deposition in the upper and central airways with recirculation to more peripheral airways (DeTroyer et al., 1978) and/or (2) wider dispersion of the inhaled drug over a broader surface of the tracheobronchial tree due to the larger dosage and longer duration of inhalation. The bronchodilator action of even large dosages of inhaled terbutaline can be further enhanced by prior injection of either aminophylline or terbutaline, possibly due to greater penetration of the aerosol into the lower respiratory tract after the latter has already been partially dilated by a systemically administered agent (Svedmyr and Svedmyr, 1980).

F. Timing of the Test in Relation to the Peak Action of the Drug

Bronchodilator responsiveness is often assessed by performing measurements at only one time following administration of a bronchodilator rather than attempting to characterize the entire time course of the response. In the former circumstance, it is necessary to perform the postbronchodilator measurements at or close to the expected time of peak action; otherwise, the degree—and even the presence—of responsiveness may be underestimated. In view of the longer delay between the appearance of peak bronchodilation and inhalation of some of the longer-acting β-agonist aerosols (as long as 30-45 min) compared to isoproterenol (about 5 min), the common practice of waiting only 5 min following inhalation of the aerosol before performance of the postbronchodilator measurement could lead to false conclusions about true bronchodilator responsiveness. Similarly, the even longer time lag before peak bronchodilation after inhaled anticholinergic medication ($\geq$ 60 min) requires an even longer delay in the postbronchodilator measurement for accurate assessment of response to this class of bronchodilators.

G. Residual Effects of Previously Administered Bronchodilators

If some residual bronchodilation from previously administered bronchodilator(s) is present at baseline, the measured acute response to an administered bronchodilator is likely to underestimate the magnitude of possible response since the airways are already partially bronchodilated. In evaluating the acute bronchodilator response to inhaled isoproterenol in 38 patients with moderate to severe chronic obstructive pulmonary disease (COPD), Alexander et al. (1980) found that 22 (58%) of the patients exhibited a 15% improvement in FEV_1 and/or FVC when the test was performed after they had been "off" bronchodilator therapy for 4 weeks, whereas only 9 (24%) showed a similar acute bronchodilator response after they had taken theophylline daily for 4 weeks. These authors suggested that the common practice of omitting only the last scheduled dose of a maintenance bronchodilator prior to a diagnostic acute bronchodilator challenge may not be adequate. Unfortunately, their study did not address the question of how long a "wash out" period is required to avoid underestimating the potential response to a bronchodilator. For patients on maintenance therapy with a sustained-release theophylline agent, gastrointestinal absorption may continue for as long as 24 hr after the last dose was administered and metabolic degradation of absorbed drug may also be delayed to an extent depending on the activity of drug-metabolizing hepatic enzymes. Thus, at least 2 or 3 days may be required before plasma levels of theophylline decline to negligible levels.

Methylxanthines other than theophylline are commonly consumed as constituents of popular dietary beverages and foods, including coffee, tea, cocoa, and chocolate. Caffeine, a widely available drug in coffee, tea, soft drinks, and medications such as analgesics and cold preparations, can cause bronchodilation in asthmatics with a potency of $\sim$ 40% that of theophylline (Simmons et al., 1983). Although the content of caffeine in a cup of coffee varies considerably (Gilbert et al., 1976; Bunker and McWilliams, 1979), Simmons and others (1983) have shown that three cups of coffee (total of 464 mg caffeine) can increase the FEV_1 by $>$ 20% in asthmatic subjects. This caffeine-induced bronchodilation had its onset at 30 min with a peak effect at 2 hr and a duration of action of at least 3 hr, by which time the FEV_1 was still $>$ 15% above baseline (Fig. 12). These authors also showed a significant dose-response relationship between peak increases in serum caffeine concentration and increases in lung function. Moreover, caffeine is partially metabolized to theophylline (Sved et al., 1976; Midha et al., 1977), but the peak elevation in serum theophylline concentration from three cups of coffee, which occurs at $\sim$ 3 hr after ingestion, is only about 2 μg/ml. The potentially confounding effect of previous caffeine intake can be avoided by withdrawing all caffeine-containing products for at least 12 hr before bronchodilator challenge testing. Although theobromine has relatively weak physiological potency (Rall, 1980; Becker et al., 1984), theobromine-containing products (chocolate and cocoa) should probably be proscribed as well.

For patients receiving oral and/or inhaled β-agonists, a shorter wash-out period (approximately 12 hr) may be sufficient prior to a diagnostic bronchodilator challenge to avoid the confounding influence of residual drug-related bronchodilation. On the other hand, long-term administration of an inhaled and/or oral β-agonist (especially in larger doses) can lead to β-adrenergic subsensitization (tachyphylaxis, tolerance) (Holgate et al., 1977; Nelson et al., 1977; Jenne

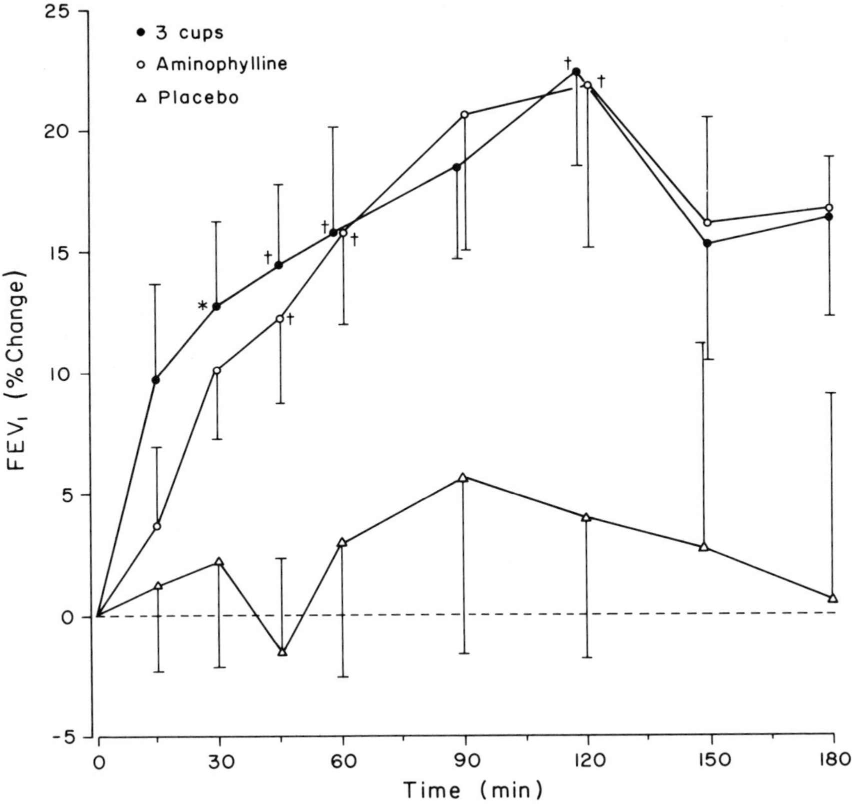

Figure 12 Percent change in FEV_1 from baseline over time following placebo, aminophylline (200 mg), and 3 cups of coffee (total of 464 mg caffeine). *P < 0.05; † P < 0.01 (from Gong et al. (1986), with permission).

et al., 1977; Plummer, 1978; Miller and Rice, 1980; Branscomb, 1978), recovery from which may require as long as 1 week (or even longer) of abstinence from β-adrenergic medication (Galant et al., 1978). If β-adrenergic subsensitivity is present, the maximal achievable response to a given dose of a β-agonist may be impaired and bronchodilator responsiveness thereby underestimated. Omitting β-adrenergic therapy for only 12-24 hr prior to testing may not be sufficient to reverse β-adrenergic tachyphylaxis. On the other hand, a single-dose of intravenous corticosteroids can lead to recovery of β-adrenergic responsiveness within several hours by up-regulating previously down-regulated β-adrenoreceptors and/or restoring the coupling of the receptor to activation of adenylate cyclase (Tashkin et al., 1982; Hui et al., 1982; Samuelson and Davies, 1984). This action of corticosteroids is of considerable value therapeutically in symptomatic asthmatics who are poorly responsive to β-adrenergic treatment.

H. Tests Used to Measure a Bronchodilator Response

The measured bronchodilator response is dependent on (1) the very tests used to measure the response, (2) the physiological determinants of these tests, (3) host factors (such as effort, motivation, learning, and the nature and severity of the underlying pulmonary disease process) that may interact with these physiological determinants, (4) the maneuvers required in performing the tests (which may themselves alter airway physiology, again depending on the nature of the underlying disease), and (5) normal intertrial test variability. In addition, certain tests may provide insight into the site(s) within the airways (e.g., small vs large airways) where the dilator response is predominant.

Physiological Determinants

Vital Capacity

Vital capacity, the maximal volume that can be exhaled from TLC to RV, is determined by the latter volumes. TLC is determined by the opposition to expansion of the respiratory system imposed by lung elasticity (which can be reduced in asthma) and chest wall stiffness (which is normally not limiting) and by both voluntary effort and the strength of the inspiratory muscles (mainly the diaphragm) in overcoming these elastic forces. RV is determined by closure of airways (usually peripheral airways), elastic opposition of the chest wall to compression, voluntary effort, and the strength of the expiratory muscles (mainly abdominal) in compressing the chest wall. In asthma, VC can be normal, supernormal, or reduced. A supernormal VC can result from an elevated TLC (due to decrease in lung and/or chest wall stiffness) in the presence of an RV which is either normal or increased to a lesser extent than the increase in TLC. In the absence of complications such as atelectasis, pneumothorax, or pneumonia, a reduced VC in asthma is generally due to an elevated RV due to trapping of gas behind airways narrowed by disease and closed prematurely. The VC can be statistically within predicted normal limits and still be associated with an elevated RV and/or TLC. In this situation, effects of bronchodilator therapy on RV could still lead to an appreciable change in VC.

Forced Expiratory Flow

Several investigators have examined the factors limiting forced expiratory flow (Fry and Hyatt, 1960; Mead et al., 1967; Pride et al., 1967; Dawson and Elliott, 1977). Forced expiratory flow at any lung volume is determined by (1) the recoil pressure of the lung at that lung volume (i.e., on the elastic properties of the lung), (2) the resistance of the airways upstream toward the alveoli from equal

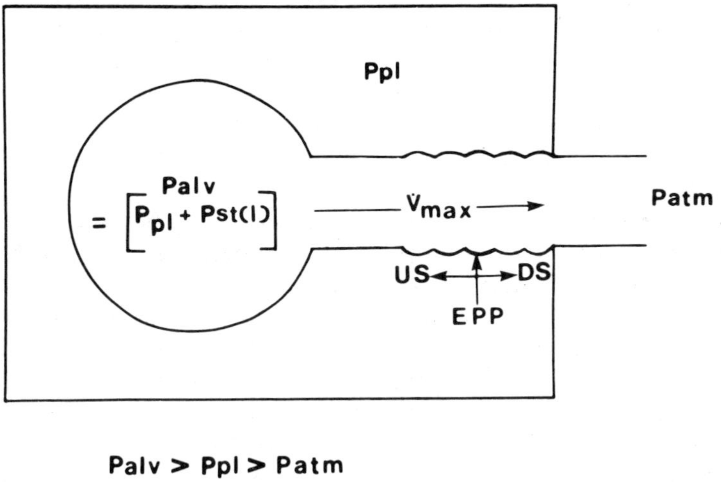

Figure 13 Simplified schema of the chest wall (box), lung (circle), and intrathoracic airways (tube) during a maximal exhalation. Pleural pressure (P_{pl}) is less than alveolar pressure (Palv) by an amount equal to the static-recoil pressure of the lung (Pst[1]) at any volume. During forced exhalation, Palv exceeds P_{pl}, which in turn exceeds atmospheric pressure (Patm). Thus, at a point within the airway, intrabronchial pressure equals P_{pl}. The driving pressure of airways upstream from this equal-pressure point (EPP) is the Pst(1), which equals the difference between Palv and P_{pl}. Therefore, upstream resistance equals Pst(1) divided by maximal expiratory-flow rate (V_{max}). Since downstream airways (DS) cannot produce more flow than is delivered by upstream airways (US), the geometry of the upstream airways and Pst(1) determines $\dot{V}_{max}$. The location of the EPP is determined by a complex interaction between distributed resistance, compliance of airways and Pst(1) (from Ingram and McFadden, 1977, with permission).

pressure points (points in the airways where the intraluminal pressure equals the pleural pressure, which is the lateral pressure applied to the outside of the airways (Fig. 13), (3) the compliance (compressibility) of the walls of the airways in the flow-limiting segment at or downstream from equal pressure points or "choke" points (Pride et al., 1967; Dawson and Elliott, 1977), (4) the density of the gas in the lungs (Dawson and Elliott, 1977; Schilder et al., 1963) and, to a variable extent, (5) effort which diminishes as lung volume decreases (Fry and Hyatt, 1960; Mead et al., 1967). After exhalation of the first 20 or 30% of the forced vital capacity, flow becomes essentially independent of effort. At lower lung volumes, the small airways contribute increasingly to the overall resistance of the airways. Air flow in this region is essentially independent of effort.

Forced expiratory flow may be reduced in asthma for any one or more of the following reasons: (1) reduced lung recoil due to reversible loss in lung stiffness; (2) increased airway resistance due to narrowing by inflammatory edema, mucous secretions, and/or bronchospasm; (3) increased compliance of airway walls due partly to the relaxing effect of bronchodilators on airway smooth muscle; and (4) decreased effort due to muscle fatigue, lack of motivation, or other factors.

The effect of a bronchodilator on forced expiratory flow is the net outcome of effects on each of the above-mentioned determinants of flow. For example, although bronchodilators can increase resting airway caliber by relaxing airway smooth muscle, at the same time they can increase airway wall compliance by reducing myogenic tone (Stamm et al., 1976; Bouhuys and van de Woestijne, 1971; Lonky and Tisi, 1980), and β-adrenergic bronchodilators can decrease lung elastic recoil (McFadden et al., 1970; Ayres et al., 1974), possibly due to a relaxant effect on contractile elements in alveolar ducts and air spaces in the lung (Colebatch, 1970; Laitinen et al., 1976). An increase in airway wall compliance predisposes to dynamic compression of airways downstream from equal pressure points by the high pleural pressures generated during a forced expiratory maneuver that are applied to the lateral walls of the airways. At the same time, a reduced recoil pressure lowers the driving pressure for forced expiratory flow and decreases the tethering effect that helps hold airways open. Thus, the effects of a bronchodilator on airway wall compliance and lung recoil can negate or blunt its beneficial effect on airway resistance, resulting in no or relatively little net increase in forced expiratory flow.

Airway Resistance

Plethysmographic airway resistance (R_{aw}) reflects resistance to air flow generally at or near FRC and at flow rates of ± 0.5 1/sec. Resistance measured by the forced oscillation technique also reflects mainly the resistance of the airways plus the additional resistance of the lung tissue and chest wall. Airway resistance measurements are not affected by the turbulence generated by high linear velocities of flow, by convective acceleration, or by dynamic airway compression that influence flow resistance during forced expiratory maneuvers. The major determinant of R_{aw} is the geometry of the airways (primarily that of the central airways and major bronchi) which in turn is influenced by lung volume, tracheobronchomotor tone, structural changes in and around the airway walls (inflammatory edema, fibrosis), and intraluminal material (mucus, organized exudate, etc.). The relation between lung volume and R_{aw} is exponential but that between lung volume and the reciprocal of R_{aw}, or airway conductance (G_{aw}), is more nearly linear (Briscoe and DuBois, 1958). Consequently, the effect of lung volume on R_{aw} is often adjusted by dividing G_{aw} by the lung volume at which it is determined to obtain the term G_{aw}/V_{tg}, or specific airway conductance (SG_{aw}). Alternatively, the reciprocal of SG_{aw}, or specific airway resistance ($SR_{aw} = R_{aw} \times V_{tg}$), may be used. These expressions, although useful, do not accurately adjust for the influence of volume on G_{aw} since the conductance-volume relationship is not linear in all individuals and, even when linear, the regression line does not usually pass through the origin (Sobol et al., 1969). A more valid method of volume adjustment involves determination of G_{aw} at different lung volumes (conductance-volume plot) so that values of G_{aw} measured before and after challenge with a bronchodilator or bronchoconstrictor agent can be compared at the same volume.

Functional Residual Capacity

Thoracic gas volume (V_{tg}) at functional residual capacity (FRC) is the resting volume of the respiratory system; it is normally determined by the relative recoil properties of the lung and chest wall which, at FRC, are equal and opposite. When lung recoil is reduced, as in emphysema or asthma, FRC increases as a new equilibrium between lung and chest wall recoil is established at a higher lung volume. In obstructive lung diseases, FRC may also be increased as a consequence of gas trapping behind airways that are functionally closed in the normal FRC range. The latter mechanism probably contributes substantially to the hyperinflation of asthma since bronchodilation very often is associated with a reduction in FRC, presumably due to a lessening of air trapping rather than an increase in lung recoil. In fact, the effect of a bronchodilator on the static elastic properties of the lung is, if anything, to reduce recoil in the FRC range (McFadden et al., 1970; McCarthy and Sigurdson, 1980).

The plethysmographic assessment of changes in lung volumes in asthma can be erroneous due to nonhomogeneous swings in alveolar pressure which are likely to be greater in regions supplied by closed airways; as a result, alveolar pressure swings measured at the mouth are underestimated, leading to an overestimation of thoracic gas volume. This source of error could account for an exaggerated apparent increase in lung volume during acute exacerbations of asthma and a reciprocal exaggerated reduction in lung volumes when severe bronchospasm is relieved by bronchodilator therapy (Brown et al., 1978). Rodenstein et al. (1981) found an apparent link between the error in plethysmographic measurement of lung volume and the severity of obstruction and noted errors as large as 1.9 liters. They conclude that the plethysmographic method is unsuitable for measuring lung volume in patients with airways obstruction, particularly when the obstruction is severe.

Isolated or Predominant Volume Responses to Bronchodilator Therapy

When the flow response to a bronchodilator is blunted by the factors noted previously, the vital capacity can still improve if the peripheral airways are dilated. This improvement is due to relief of air-trapping and reduction in residual volume. Since the relaxed peripheral airways are likely to be located upstream from equal pressure points, they are not susceptible to dynamic airway compression by the positive pleural pressure generated during exhalation to residual volume. Acute reductions in FRC are also common following bronchodilator therapy; the decreases in FRC are probably secondary to relief of air-trapping in the tidal volume range.

Ramsdell and Tisi (1979) noted an isolated volume response to a bronchodilator in a large proportion of patients with chronic airflow obstruction. Of 129 patients who exhibited a "significant" fall (mean 27%) in R_{aw} 10 min after inhalation of 2.25 mg isoproterenol, 46 (41%) had a "significant" increase in VC (mean 15%) and a "significant" decline in plethysmographically determined FRC (mean 13%) without any change in forced expiratory flow. It is interesting that those patients with an isolated volume response to the bronchodilator showed a mean reduction in R_{aw} similar to that noted in the patients whose forced expiratory flow increased following the bronchodilator. However, the isolated volume responders had a more marked degree of airway obstruction and hyperinflation compared to the flow responders, consistent with a decreased lung elastic recoil (Pel) in the former. The decreased Pel in these patients could have reduced the tethering support of their intrapulmonary airways, thereby predisposing them to more dynamic airway compression during a forced expiratory maneuver. This effect could be exaggerated by bronchodilator therapy if the latter is associated with a further reduction in Pel, as well as an increase in airway wall compliance due to a reduction in myogenic tone.

Girard and Light (1983) studied 17 patients with moderate to severe chronic airflow obstruction who exibited sizable increases in FVC (27 ± 8%) after a bronchodilator with little or no increase in FEV_1 (3.6 ± 3.8%). They noted two different types of response accounting for the increase in FVC. One was characterized by associated increases in FEV_3 and FEV_6 (seven patients), which they attributed to true bronchodilation involving peripheral airways that contribute to the latter portion of the timed spirogram. The other type of response was associated with no increase in FEV_3 or FEV_6 (10 patients); in these patients the improvement in FVC was attributed simply to an increase in the duration of expiration after bronchodilator administration, possibly due to learning to blow out longer after repetitive maneuvers. However, the possibility that the latter response also represents a bronchodilator effect cannot be excluded.

Ayres and co-workers (1974) noted a variable spirometric and plethysmographic response to isoproterenol in 134 patients with COPD. More than 90% of the patients showed a significant (> 15%) decrease in R_{aw} (mean decrease, approximately 40%), approximately 25% showed a significantly increased VC (mean increase, 22%), and a partially overlapping 25% showed an increase in forced expiratory flow (mean increase in peak expiratory flow rate, 36%). Thus,

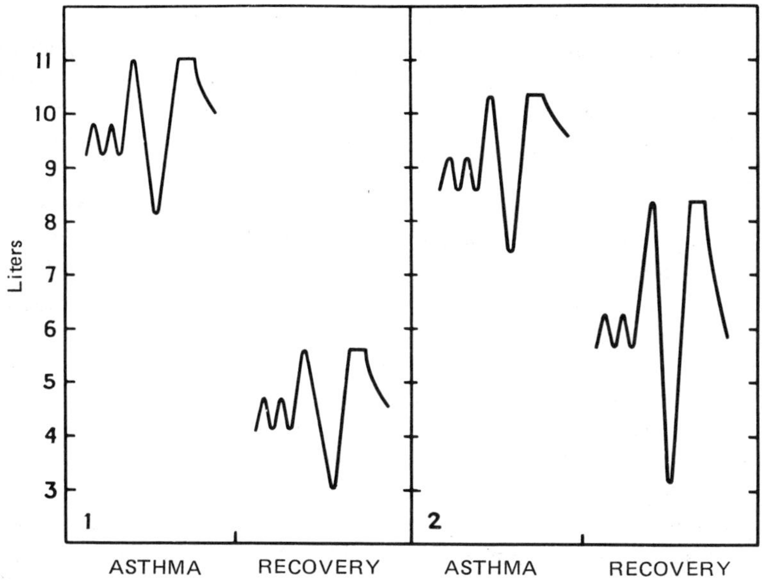

Figure 14 Diagrammatic representation of lung volume and FEV_1 in two patients (1 and 2) during episode of asthma and following clinical recovery. The resting level at the end of each tidal breath represents FRC. The points of maximal inspiration and expiration represent TLC and RV, respectively. The final segment of each tracing represents the FEV_1 (from Woolcock et al., 1965, with permission).

nearly all examined patients with chronic airflow obstruction appeared to respond to bronchodilator administration by reducing bronchomotor tone, while less than half responded by increasing VC and/or forced expiratory flow. The authors concluded that failure of forced expiratory flow to increase after inhalation of a β-agonist should not be interpreted as evidence of an unresponsive airway. In the absence of measurements of airway resistance and FRC, an increase in VC may be the only indication of bronchodilator responsiveness.

Occasional patients with severe asthma or COPD with an asthmatic component exhibit notable subjective improvement during therapy with no or disproportionately little increase in FEV_1. Woolcock and Read (1965, 1966) have pointed out that the subjective benefit reported by these patients may in fact represent true physiological improvement in airflow obstruction that is not reflected in the FEV_1 response. These authors serially measured subdivisions of lung volume (by helium dilution), in addition to FEV_1, in 30 patients at repeated intervals during recovery from episodes of severe asthma. In four patients in whom substantial clinical improvement was observed during treatment, the FEV_1 showed no or relatively little improvement. In all four patients, RV, TLC, and FRC were markedly elevated initially, the latter to a level higher than the postrecovery TLC, and these values all fell considerably during therapy (Fig. 14). The authors contend that the failure of FEV_1 to increase significantly during therapy in these patients masks a true improvement in airflow obstruction that is only evident when the corresponding changes in lung volume are taken into account. Before therapy, the FEV_1 was measured at a higher absolute lung volume at which the corresponding higher elastic recoil pressure pulled the airways wider open, thus reducing flow resistance. With treatment, the lung volume decreased, but FEV_1, now measured at lower lung volume, remained the same or increased only slightly, implying a true improvement in the obstructive changes that had made it impossible to generate any airflow at all at the lower lung volumes before treatment (Fig. 14). The relief of dyspnea in these patients was attributed to reduction in the FRC toward normal with a corresponding reduction in the markedly increased *elastic* work of inspiration associated with the very high FRC that had been present before treatment. In patients appearing to respond to treatment clinically in whom objective benefit cannot be demonstrated with simple measurements of FEV_1 or PEFR, determination of lung volumes may provide a more adequate physiological assessment of response to therapy.

Volume Dependence of Forced Expiratory Flow Rates

Forced expiratory flow is determined largely by lung elastic recoil pressure (Pel) and airflow resistance. Both Pel and airflow resistance are related to lung volume (Pel decreases and resistance increases as lung volume diminishes). Forced expiratory flow is therefore dependent on the volume at which it is measured. Consequently, in comparing pre- and postbronchodilator values of FEF it is important to use an isovolume technique, that is, to calculate forced expiratory flow at the same volume or over the same volume range from the pre- and postbronchodilator flow-volume or volume-time curves. Vital capacity is often increased by a bronchodilator as a result of a reduction in RV due to lessening of air trapping whereas TLC is generally not altered (Paré et al., 1983; McFadden et al., 1970). Therefore, the volume corresponding to any given percentage of the postbronchodilator FVC will represent a lower percentage of TLC (i.e., a lower absolute lung volume) than the volume corresponding to the same percentage of the prebronchodilator FVC. Similarly, the middle range of the postbronchodilator FVC may also span a lower range of absolute lung volume than the middle range of the prebronchodilator FVC. The isovolume method is easily accomplished by matching the pre- and postbronchodilator curves at the same volume or over the same range of volume used for calculating flow rates from the prebronchodilator curve (Sherter et al., 1978) (Fig. 15). Failure to use the isovolume method can result in an underestimation of any improvement in FEF

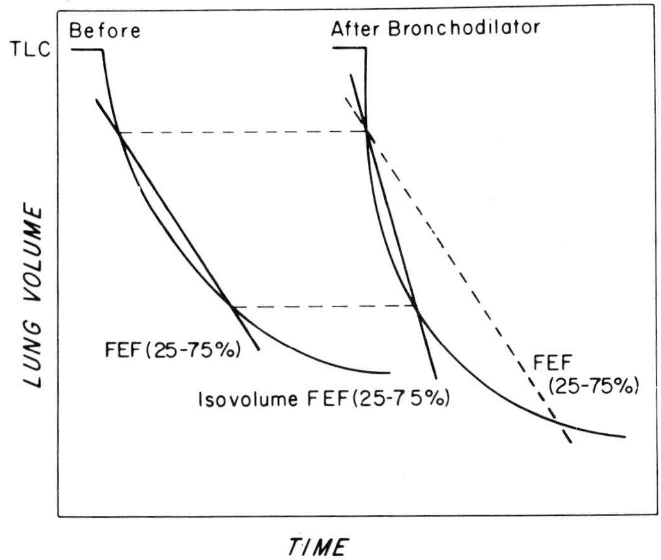

Figure 15 Isovolume $FEF_{25\text{-}75\%}$ is measured by matching maximal inspiratory points of tracings before and after bronchodilator therapy. Points at 25% and 75% of curves after bronchodilator therapy are matched to those measured on tracing before bronchodilator therapy. Thus, on tracing after bronchodilator therapy, one is not measuring flow in middle 50% of that breath, but during same segment of volume as on forced expiration before bronchodilator therapy (from Sherter et al., 1978).

after bronchodilator therapy. Use of FEV_1 to assess bronchodilator responsiveness avoids this problem because FEV_1 is always measured from the same absolute lung volume, namely TLC.

Influence of Test Maneuvers on Airway Physiology

The deep inspiration from FRC to TLC required for measurements of PEFR and forced expiratory volumes and flow rates derived from spirometry and MEFV curves can itself induce bronchomotor changes that influence the results of these measurements. In 40 asthmatic patients, Gayrard et al. (1975) found a transient (usually < 60 sec) increase in specific airway resistance (59% mean increase in SR_{aw}) accompanied by only a modest increase in V_{tg} immediately following a deep inspiration (Fig. 16). In 2 of the 40 patients, the deep inspiration provoked an attack of asthma. The increase in SR_{aw} was partly or completely blocked in most patients by prior inhalation of an anticholinergic or β-adrenergic broncho-

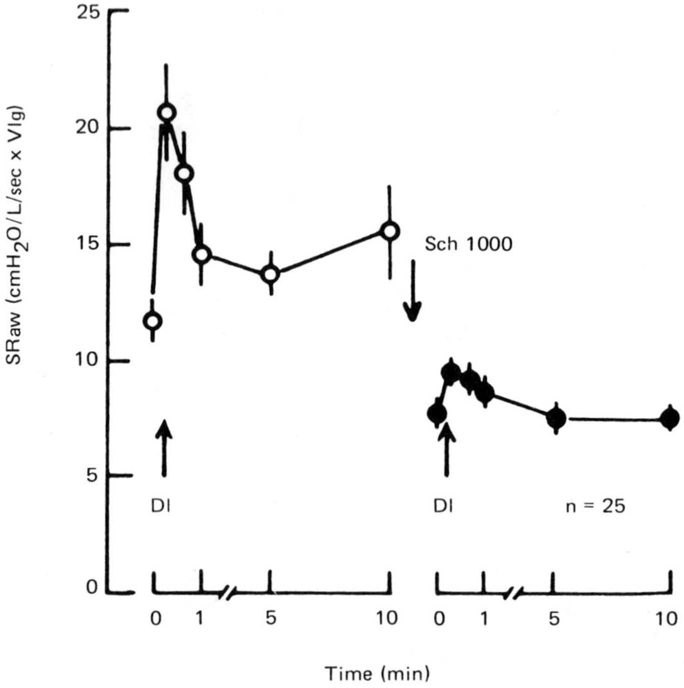

Figure 16 Effects of deep inspiration (DI) on specific airway resistance (SR_{aw}) in patients with asthma, before (open circles) and after (closed circles) inhalation of an anticholinergic drug, Sch 1,000. Mean values ± 1 SE (from Gayrard et al., 1975, with permission).

dilator, which suggested vagally mediated reflex bronchoconstriction as the mechanism for the increase in SR_{aw}. On the other hand, Colebatch and Greaves (1979), who observed a decrease in airway conductance in 11 of 17 asthmatics following a maximum inhalation, found that pretreatment with ipratropium or intravenous atropine blocked the bronchoconstriction in only two of the seven subjects studied, whereas a β-agonist abolished the bronchoconstrictor response to inflation in all of eight subjects examined. They concluded that in some asthmatics inflation-induced bronchoconstriction appears to involve a vagal reflex, while in others local airway mechanisms may be involved. Gayrard and associates found that deep expiration also induced bronchoconstriction, which was weaker (35% mean increase in SR_{aw}) than that provoked by deep inspiration. Others (Simonsson et al., 1967) have also reported a bronchoconstrictor effect of deep expiration in asthmatic subjects.

In contrast, in normal individuals and nonasthmatics with allergic rhinitis, deep inspiration does not induce bronchoconstriction but can cause transient bronchodilation, especially when the airways are first pharmacologically constricted (Nadel and Tierney, 1961; Fish et al., 1977). By comparing forced expiratory flow rates at 25% above residual volume calculated from partial and maximal expiratory flow volume curves, Zamel and co-workers (1983) observed that a few asthmatics (3 of 20) are also able to increase forced expiratory flow rates substantially after taking a deep breath; however, most of their asthmatic subjects exhibited no increase or a modest decrease in forced expiratory flow after a deep lung inflation.

A practical implication of the differing effects of deep inspiration on bronchomotor tone in normal and asthmatic subjects is that the difference in forced expiratory flow rates between these two groups at baseline may be exaggerated. Furthermore, interpretation of the spirometric response to a bronchodilator in asthmatics may be confounded by any reduction in the prebronchodilator forced expiratory flow rates resulting from inflation-induced constriction. Since a bronchodilator can block this effect, an increase in forced expiratory flow following a bronchodilator could represent, to a varying extent, inhibition of the constrictor effect of the preceding deep inspiration rather than a true increase in bronchial caliber over baseline.

When no or mild airflow obstruction is present, airway responsiveness may be assessed by determining the effect of graded dosages of a constrictor agent (rather than a bronchodilator) on forced expiratory flow. However, spirometric assessment of a bronchoprovocative stimulus is also confounded by the bronchomotor effect of deep inspiration (Orehek et al., 1981). In healthy individuals, the transient bronchodilator effect of deep inspiration is most evident after pharmacologically induced bronchoconstriction (Nadel and Tierney, 1961; Fish et al., 1977). Moreover, in asthmatics, after pharmacologic induction of bronchospasm, deep inspiration no longer causes bronchoconstriction in most and may even produce bronchodilation in some (Fish et al., 1977; Orehek et al., 1981). It has been postulated that the mechanism of bronchodilation after a maximal inspiration may be hysteresis of airway smooth muscle that exhibits a temporary reduction in tension after being maximally stretched (stress relaxation) (Fish et al., 1977). Augmentation of postinspiration bronchodilation by pharmacologic airway constriction may be due to a greater degree of stress relaxation of the airways in the contracted state, as has been shown in the lungs of rabbits (Hughes et al., 1959). That the same mechanism may apply to human airways is supported by the finding of a significant correlation between the bronchodilator effect of a deep inspiration in asthmatics and the degree of induced bronchoconstriction (Beaupré and Orehek, 1982). The latter correlation could also be explained, in part, by the hyperbolic relationship between airway resistance and airway diameter: a given change in airway diameter after lung inflation could lead to a greater change in airway resistance, the narrower the airway was before inspiration (Beaupré and Orehek, 1982).

Inspiration-induced bronchoconstriction in asthmatics does not appear to be correlated with sensitivity to methacholine-induced bronchospasm (Fish et al., 1977). Therefore, if this phenomenon is indeed due to vagally mediated reflex bronchoconstriction, it could be the result not of increased end-organ muscarinic responsiveness but of the increased sensitivity of asthmatics to stimulation of afferent bronchial epithelial irritant receptors during stretching of the intrapulmonary airways when lung volume increases to TLC. In contrast, in normal subjects mechanical stretching of the airways during deep inspiration may cause a hysteretic stress relaxation of airway smooth muscle with a consequent transient reduction in airway tone. If a similar phenomenon occurs in asthma, the consequent tendency for airway resistance to decrease can be counterbalanced by irritant receptor-mediated reflex bronchoconstriction. Alternatively, as suggested by Zamel and others (1983) airway hysteresis in asthmatics may simply be impaired. Interestingly, in most asthmatics with *spontaneous*, as opposed to pharmacologically induced, obstruction, deep inspiration appears to produce bronchoconstriction, and the degree of postinspiration bronchospasm seems to be related to the baseline level of obstruction (Orehek et al., 1980). Possibly, patients with more severe spontaneous asthma have a greater sensitivity to irritant receptor-mediated, postinspiration reflex bronchoconstriction, whereas *pharmacologically induced* bronchospasm enhances the opposing dilator effect of lung inflation by augmenting stress relaxation.

The inspiratory flow rate during full inhalation and the duration of the breathhold at TLC can modify the bronchomotor effect of deep inspiration (Beaupré and Orehek, 1982). In carbachol-bronchoconstricted asthmatics who exhibited bronchodilation after deep inspiration, a *slow* inspiration or a 10-sec breathhold at TLC caused significantly less bronchodilation than either a fast inspiration or no breathhold. The modifying effect of the long breathholding period is consistent with the time dependence of stress relaxation. The latter is a transient phenomenon, which may begin to wane after several seconds (Green and Mead, 1974). The enhanced bronchodilator effect of a fast inspiratory maneuver is consistent with more vigorous stretching of the airways with high inspiratory flow rates, thus increasing airway hysteresis. These considerations suggest that modification of the technique of spirometry to include a slow inhalation to TLC followed by a long breathhold before forced exhalation might obviate any appreciable dilator effect of deep inspiration. On the other hand, the influence of such maneuvers on the constrictor effect of a maximal inflation in patients with spontaneous asthma is not known.

To obviate the confounding effect of deep inspiration in measuring the dynamic response to a bronchodilator or bronchoconstrictor agent, it is probably best to rely on testing methods that do not require a deep inspiration.

Such methods include direct measurements of airway resistance (body plethysmography, forced oscillation technique), which involve shallow panting or tidal breathing maneuvers, and partial expiratory flow volume (PEFV) curves. With the PEFV curve technique (Bouhuys, 1974), forced expiratory flow rates are calculated during forced exhalation after only a partial, rather than a maximal, inspiration, thus obviating or blunting any bronchomotor effect of a full inspiration. The ensuing maximal inspiration serves only to fix the level of TLC to allow calculation of forced expiratory flow rates from the partial flow volume as a percentage of the full vital capacity. Use of the partial flow-volume technique also permits detection of the effect of deep inspiration on forced expiratory flow by isovolume comparison of the forced expiratory flow rates determined from the partial versus the maximal flow volume curve (Zamel et al., 1983; Fish et al., 1981). However, the disparity between isovolume maximal and partial flow rates could be due to more than one mechanism, including reflex bronchoconstriction, variable degrees of airway hysteresis, and differences in lung elastic recoil (the driving pressure for forced expiratory flow in the upstream segment), recoil pressure being greater during forced expiratory maneuvers that start at lower lung volumes (Zamel et al., 1983). By eliminating the confounding influence of deep inhalation, flow rates from PEFV maneuvers are probably more sensitive indicators than flow rates from MEFV curves in assessing the response to a bronchodilator (Barnes et al., 1981) or a bronchoconstrictor (Littner et al., 1979).

Test Validity and Reliability

The validity of assessments of bronchodilator response using tests of forced exhalation depends on the accuracy of measurements of forced expiratory volumes and flow rates. The latter, in turn, depends on the performance characteristics of the measuring instrument, the effort and cooperation of the patient, and the technical skill of the person performing the tests, including the ability to motivate the patient to perform maximally. It is clearly important that equipment be properly calibrated, that subjects be adequately instructed in the testing procedures, and that results be accurately calibrated and transcribed. The reader is referred elsewhere for a detailed discussion of pulmonary function testing methodology and quality control (Clausen, 1982; Intermountain Thoracic Society Pulmonary Function Task Force, 1984).

Performance criteria for diagnostic spirometry have been recommended by the American Thoracic Society (ATS Statement, 1979). Tests of forced exhalation are critically dependent on patient effort, motivation, and cooperation. Not only must the exhalation be maximally forced, but the patient must also inhale and exhale completely against the uncomfortable opposition of lung and/or chest wall elastance. At least three acceptable tracings are required to assure that maximal effort and cooperation have been obtained. FVC and FEV1 should each show agreement within ± 5% or 100 ml between the two best of three acceptable curves obtained prior to bronchodilator administration. A similar agreement is desirable between curves obtained following administration of the bronchodilator. If subject effort and cooperation are not optimal during prebronchodilator trials or wax or wane during the postbronchodilator period, an incorrect indication of "true" maximally achievable bronchodilation may result. The results of field spirometry routinely employing at least five trials and performed by well-trained, experienced technicians on approximately 15,000 participants in a population study (Detels, R., personal communication) indicated the best FEV_1 and FVC are usually achieved after two or more efforts. These results suggest that prior to administration of a bronchodilator, at least three (and possibly more) trials may be required (in untrained subjects) to achieve maximal reproducible values with which to compare postbronchodilator responses. On the other hand, an excessive number of expiratory maneuvers could lead to diminishing forced expiratory flow due to fatigue, loss of motivation, or reflex bronchoconstriction from the effects of repeated deep inspirations (spirometry-induced bronchospasm) (Gimeno et al., 1972; Gayrard et al., 1975). Once satisfactory efforts are obtained at baseline, fewer efforts are generally required during the postbronchodilator period to achieve maximal and reproducible results.

Test Variability

Assessment of the response to a bronchodilator is affected by the variability of the tests used to measure the response. Test variability is dependent on the particular type of measurement being performed, equipment accuracy, technician skill, and a number of factors relating to the subject performing the test. The latter include effort, ability to perform the test properly, diurnal variability, prior exposure to bronchodilator or constrictor influences (e.g., medication, aeroallergens, cigarette smoke, air pollution), and the presence or absence and magnitude of ventilatory abnormality.

Pennock et al. (1981) performed spirometry on 20 asthmatic subjects 9 times daily and found an individual within-day coefficient of variation (standard deviation/mean) of 6.7, 8.1, and 14% for FVC, FEV_1 and $FEF_{25\text{-}75\%}$, respectively. Assuming that a Gaussian distribution was applicable, they suggested that these values might be used to assess the significance of changes in spirometric indices after a bronchodilator. Since values more than 1.65 times the coefficient of variation would be expected in $< 5\%$ of the population due to "normal" variability, a significant change in FVC, FEV_1, and $FEF_{25\text{-}75\%}$ within a day's time in an asthmatic subject would be one that was greater than 11, 13, and 23%, respectively. Similar cut-points could be used to assess the significance of short-term changes in these spirometric indices after administration of a bronchodilator to obstructed individuals. Normal subjects were noted

Table 2 Mean Percent and Absolute Changes in Spirometric Indices After Placebo Inhalations in Asthmatic Subjects

Index	Mean % change	S.D.	Upper confidence limit[a]
PEFR[b]	-7.50	39.2%	71.7%
FVC	1.27	6.7%	14.9%
FEV_1	0.97	5.6%	12.3%
FEF_{25-75}	-0.14	22.4%	45.1%
	Absolute mean difference		Upper confidence limit[a]
PEFR	-7.6 L/s	32.9 L/s	58.9 L/s
FVC	0.025 L	0.156 L	0.340 L
FEV_1	0.011 L	0.083 L	0.178 L
FEF_{25-75}[c]	-0.039 L/s	—	

[a]Ninety-five percent of the population is defined by the mean ± 2.02 standard deviations of the mean.
[b]Not a normal distribution in form of percent change. Range: –28.2 to 37.9%. Confidence limits calculated by logarithmic transformation and then converted back to percent change form.
[c]Not a normal distribution range –2.04 to + 0.39 liters/sec.)
From Sourk and Nugent, (1983), with permission.

to have less individual variation; therefore, a significant acute response to a bronchodilator would require a greater than 5,5, or 13% change in FVC, FEV_1, or $FEF_{25-75\%}$, respectively, in a healthy individual. Since larger individual week-to-week coefficients of variation were observed, even greater changes in FVC, FEV_1, and $FEF_{25-75\%}$ (21, 23 and 30%, respectively, in asthmatic subjects) would have to occur 1 or more weeks following the initiation of a bronchodilator program before such changes could be considered significant.

Sourk and Nugent (1983) used a different approach to define confidence intervals for assessing statistically significant responses to an inhaled bronchodilator. They measured changes in spirometry following double-blind inhalation of a placebo aerosol in 40 patients referred to the pulmonary function laboratory for routine evaluation. Two-tailed 95% confidence intervals were then derived for *percent changes* in PEFR, FVC, FEV_1, FEF_1/FVC ratio, and $FEF_{25-75\%}$ from the baseline preplacebo values and for *absolute changes* in these indices from baseline. Table 2 shows the mean percent and absolute changes in spirometry after placebo inhalation as well as the upper 95% confi-

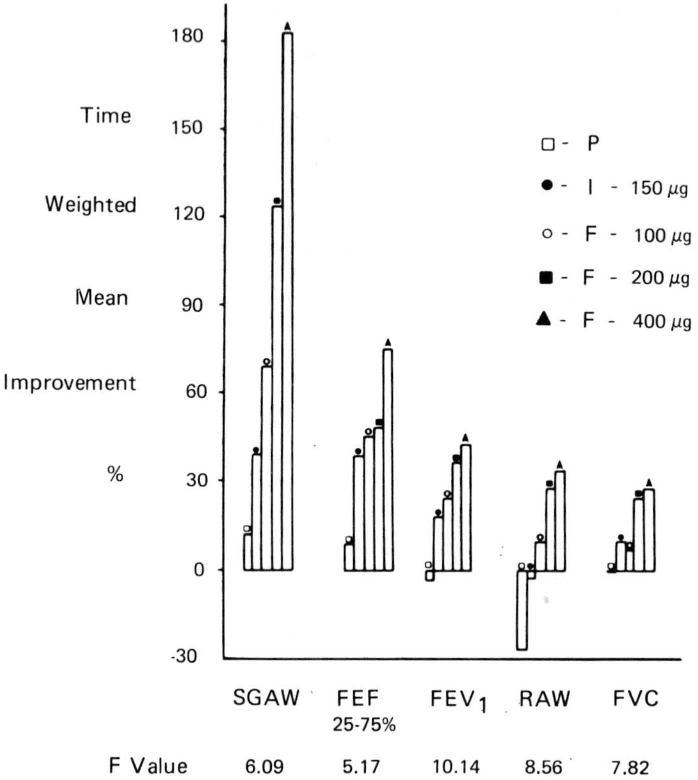

Figure 17 The mean time-weighted percent improvements after placebo (P), isoproterenol (I), and varying dosages of fenoterol (F) for the various tests and the associated F values. While the percentage of improvement after each drug is greatest when measured by R_{aw}, the F value is greatest for the FEV_1 (from George et al., 1978, with permission).

dence limits for a two-tailed population, defined as the mean plus 2 standard deviations of the mean, which would exclude 2.5% of normal responses to placebo. The upper limits of normal variability for FVC and FEV_1 are similar to those noted by Pennock and co-workers (1981), but the variation in $FEF_{25\text{-}75\%}$ is about twice as large. It is interesting that Sourk and Nugent (1983) found no correlation between the magnitude of the placebo response and baseline lung function or a history of smoking, in contrast to the findings of others (Hruby and Butler, 1975) of greater within-day variability in lung function in obstructed patients than healthy controls.

Table 3 Mean Plethysmographic and Spirometric Values Before and After Bronchodilator in 75 Normal Subjects

	Before bronchodilator (mean ± SD)	After bronchodilator (mean ± SD)	Percent change (mean ± SD)	P
R_{aw}	1.393 (0.368)	1.125 (0.270)	-18.4 (9.5)	<0.0001
G_{aw}	0.762 (0.180)	0.938 (0.220)	+24.3 (14.8)	<0.0001
V_{tg}	3059 (753)	3069 (743)	+0.3 (11.3)	NS
SG_{aw}	0.257 (0.065)	0.317 (0.083)	+23.6 (13.6)	<0.0001
FVC	4521 (1051)	4528 (1047)	+0.2 (2.5)	NS
FEV_1	3610 (856)	3692 (861)	+2.5 (3.9)	NS
$FEF_{25\text{-}75}$	3.78 (1.33)	4.37 (1.61)	+16.2 (16.4)	<0.02

R_{aw}, airway resistance (cm H_2O/liter/sec); G_{aw}, conductance = 1 R_{aw} (liter/sec/cm H_2O); V_{tg}, thoracic gas volume (ml); SG_{aw}, specific airway conductance = G/V_{tg} (liter/sec/cm H_2O/liter); FVC, forced expiratory vital capacity (ml); FEV_1, forced expiratory volume in 1 sec (ml); $FEF_{25\text{-}75}$, maximal midexpiratory flow (liter/min). NS = statistically not significant ($P > 0.05$).
From Wantanabe, S., et al., (1974) with permission.

Differing variability among the various physiological measures of a bronchodilator response will affect the sensitivity of these measures in detecting a true response (in comparison with placebo) and in distinguishing statistically between the responses to different bronchodilator agents. Light et al. (1977) analyzed the acute effect of different bronchodilator regimens on several tests of lung function (SG_{aw}, R_{aw}, FEV_1, FVC, $FEF_{25\text{-}75\%}$, FEV_1/FVC%) in 20 asthmatic subjects. They noted a disparity between the *magnitude* of improvement in lung function expressed as percent change from baseline, and the *level of significance* of the difference in improvement between different drug regimens, expressed as the F value derived from analysis of variance (ANOVA) (Fig. 17). The F value is a measure of the ratio of between-group separation to within-group variation and thus takes into account the inherent variability of the test. For example, although both SG_{aw} and $FEF_{25\text{-}75\%}$ showed a greater mean percent improvement following the active bronchodilator agents than did FEV_1, the latter measure yielded the highest F value of ANOVA and detected the largest number of statistically significant differences in pairwise comparisons of the various drug regimens. These findings suggest that the FEV_1 may be superior to plethysmographic airway resistance and other measures derived from spirometry in detecting a true bronchodilator response. In contrast, the FEV_1/FVC ratio yielded the lowest F value, indicating that it is a poor index of bronchodilator responsiveness. This finding is not surprising since the FVC often improves along with the FEV_1 in response to a bronchodilator, thus minimizing any change in FEV_1/FVC ratio.

In contrast to the above findings in patients with reversible airflow obstruction, Watanabe and others (1974) found that in 75 *normal* subjects of varying size the only measures that improved significantly in response to a bronchodilator aerosol were airway conductance indices (SG_{aw}, G_{aw}, R_{aw}) ($P < 0.001$) and $FEF_{25\text{-}75\%}$ ($p < 0.02$); FEV_1 and FVC showed no significant change (Table 3). Bouhuys and van de Woestijne (1971) and McFadden and associates (1970) also noted much greater changes in SG_{aw} than in forced expiratory flow rates in normal subjects after bronchodilator administration. This disparity between plethysmographic and spirometric responses to a bronchodilator challenge in normal subjects may be due to factors already mentioned that affect the spirometric response. The significant improvement in some measures following administration of a bronchodilator to healthy individuals reflects the bronchomotor tone that is normally present. The large standard deviations of the percent increases in some of these indices (Table 3) suggest that there is wide variation in resting bronchomotor tone among normal persons.

III. Assessing the Predominant Site of Action of a Bronchodilator Within the Airways

Several investigators have used maximal or partial flow-volume curves obtained during air and 80% He/20% O_2 breathing to examine the predominant site of airway dilation after administration of a bronchodilator (Fig. 4; see above). The physiological significance of density dependence of flow can be appreciated by reference to the equal pressure point theory of maximal expiratory flow limitation (Fry and Hyatt, 1960; Ingram and McFadden, 1977; Fig. 13). During maximal expiratory flow maneuvers, the major flow regime in larger airways is turbulent since the total cross-sectional area for flow in these airways is relatively small and linear velocities of flow are high. In addition, larger pressure losses occur in the larger airways due to convective acceleration of gas molecules to maintain the same bulk flow through a system of progressively diminishing cross-sectional area. Flow under these circumstances is density dependent and will increase if the density of the gas is decreased. Conversely, the predominant flow regime in smaller airways is laminar since the total cross-sectional area for flow in these airways is relatively large and linear velocities of flow are low; moreover, the pressure losses due to convective acceleration in this region are small. Flow in peripheral airways during maximal expiratory maneuvers is therefore independent of density. During the breathing of a low-density gas mixture such as 80% He/20% O_2, maximal expiratory flow will increase if the major component of resistance upstream from equal pressure points is due to turbulence and to convective acceleration but will not be affected appreciably when upstream resistance is due mainly to laminar flow. In normal individuals, over the upper half of the vital capacity, equal pressure points are in proximal airways (lobar or segmental bronchi) (Macklem and Wilson, 1965) where the total cross-sectional area is relatively small; upstream resistance therefore is due mainly to turbulence and convective acceleration and $\dot{V}_{max}$ over this volume range (including $\dot{V}_{max50}$) increases appreciably in response to He/O_2 breathing. On the other hand, in individuals with widespread obstruction involving small airways, static recoil pressure is more readily dissipated by the narrowed peripheral airways so that equal pressure points move upstream where the total cross-sectional area is relatively greater and laminar flow conditions are more likely to prevail. In the latter subjects, $\dot{V}_{max50}$ increases relatively little if at all during He/O_2 breathing (Dosman et al., 1975).

Despas et al. (1972) found that asthmatic subjects were almost evenly divided between those responding to He/O_2 breathing by significant increases in $\dot{V}_{max}$ ($\Delta\dot{V}_{max50} > 20\%$) and those not responding to He/O_2. These findings suggest that in reversible airways obstruction either the large or small airways may be the major site of obstruction, in contrast to chronic irreversible obstructive airway disease in which the small airways are principally involved (Dosman et al., 1975). On the other hand, Meadows and co-workers (1980) have observed normal density dependence of maximal expiratory flow in 11 of 22 patients with established COPD who had no evidence of asthma. These authors suggested that increased compliance of the central airways or dysanapsis between the growth of the lung and the airways might account for the normal density dependence observed in their COPD patients. Antic and Macklem (1976) noted that some asthmatics who were nonresponders to He/O_2 became responders after use of an aerosolized β-agonist (Fig. 18). They interpreted this finding to indicate relief of bronchospasm in peripheral airways since dilation at these sites would allow equal pressure points to move proximally to more central airways where a more turbulent flow and greater convective acceleration would tend to increase the density dependence of flow. The same authors noted that under some circumstances in which a bronchodilator does not cause any demonstrable increase in FEF during air breathing, it might be possible to detect an increase in FEF during the breathing of a low-density gas mixture (Fig. 19). If a bronchodilator causes dilation of small airways, less of the driving pressure for FEF is dissipated across these airways thus allowing equal pressure points to move mouthward. In this circumstance, the length and resistance of the upstream segment increase, thereby potentially offsetting the reduction in resistance accom-

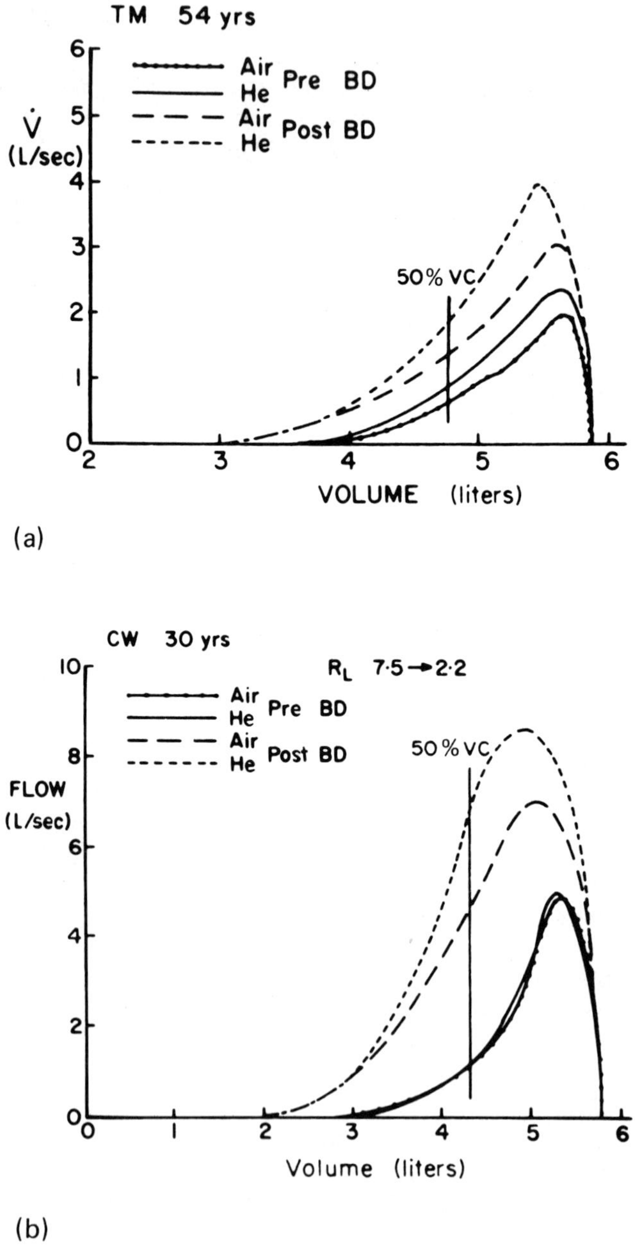

TM 54 yrs
Air
He
Pre BD
Air
He
Post BD
V̇
(L/sec)
50% VC
VOLUME (liters)
(a)
CW 30 yrs
R_L 7·5→2·2
Air
He
Pre BD
Air
He
Post BD
50% VC
FLOW
(L/sec)
Volume (liters)
(b)

Figure 18

panying dilation of the larger airways and leading to little net increase in FEF during air breathing if the larger airway were dynamically compressed due to an increase in their mural compliance. On the other hand, if the bronchodilated peripheral airways caused a reduction in the proportion of the driving pressure dissipated across these airways where flow is relatively independent of density, then density dependence of flow would increase and the dilation of these airways could be detected by an increased response to He/O_2 breathing during bronchodilator therapy.

A number of workers have used air and He/O_2 MEFV curves in normal or obstructed individuals to determine the sites of action within the airways of different classes of bronchodilator compounds. In young normal subjects, Ingram et al. (1977) found that aerosolized atropine sulfate (0.6 mg) caused a decrease in density dependence of maximal expiratory flow (decreased ratio of $\dot{V}_{max}$ He/O_2 to $\dot{V}_{max}$ air at isolung volume), whereas inhaled isoproterenol caused an increase in density dependence. They concluded that atropine caused a greater relative dilation of the larger upstream airways (resulting in a relatively greater contribution to total airflow resistance of the smaller airways where flow is less density dependent), whereas isoproterenol produced a preferential dilation of the smaller airways (causing equal pressure points to move into more proximal, larger airways where flow is more density dependent). These findings are consistent with earlier evidence that when the sympathetic nervous system is intact, the parasympathetic nervous system has a constructing influence predominantly on central airways, its effects on peripheral airways being modulated by adrenergic influences that could dominate at the latter site (Woolcock et al., 1969). On the other hand, Douglas et al. (1979) noted both decreases and increases in density dependence of flow in normal subjects following inhalation of ipratropium, a quarternary ammonium derivative of atropine. These results suggest that inhaled anticholinergic compounds can dilate both large and small airways in healthy individuals, thus implying the presence of vagally regulated bronchomotor tone at both sites within the normal tracheobronchial tree.

Figure 18 (a) Maximal expiratory flow-volume (MEFV) curves obtained in a 54-year-old, atopic, female nonsmoker (patient TM) who had recurrent, acute respiratory infections and was a responder both before and after use of bronchodilators (BD). (b) The MEFV curve obtained in a 30-year-old, nonatopic, female nonsmoker (patient CW) who had recurrent, acute respiratory infections and was a nonresponder before BD and a responder after BD. The solid vertical line in each figure is drawn at 50% of the pre-BD vital capacity (VC). yrs, years; $\dot{V}$, maximal expiratory flow in liters/sec (L/sec); He, helium (from Antic and Macklem, 1976, with permission).

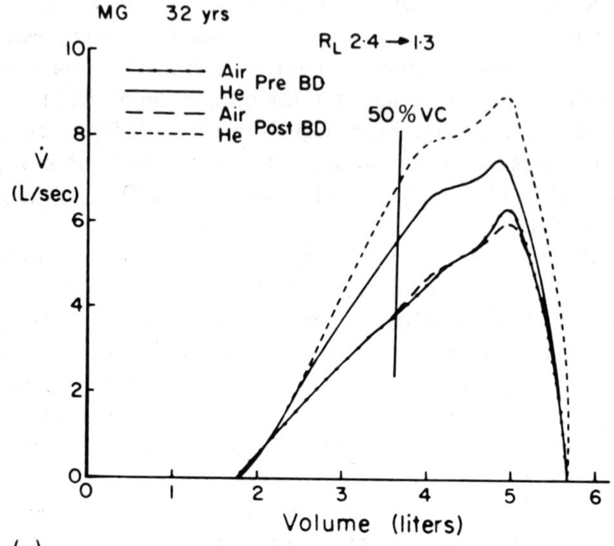
MG 32 yrs
R_L 2·4 → 1·3
Air
He
Pre BD
Air
He
Post BD
50% VC
V̇
(L/sec)
Volume (liters)

(a)

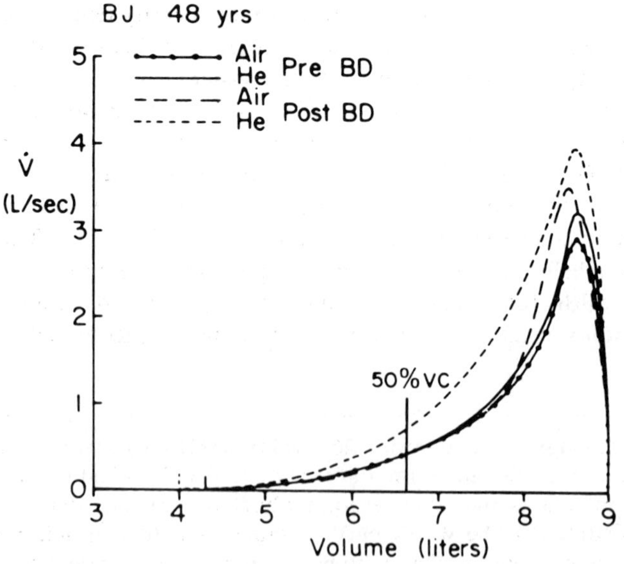
BJ 48 yrs
Air
He
Pre BD
Air
He
Post BD
V̇
(L/sec)
50% VC
Volume (liters)

(b)

Figure 19

Douglas and co-workers (1979) studied 19 patients with severe chronic bronchitis and emphysema who exhibited a bronchodilator response to ipratropium. At baseline, little or no density dependence of flow was noted, suggesting obstruction predominantly in smaller airways. Ipratropium caused modest increases in density dependence in 12 of these patients and decreases in 7, with no significant mean change overall. These findings suggest that in patients with chronic airflow obstruction an anticholinergic bronchodilator can act at sites in both large and small airways.

Wellman and associates (1976) studied 13 patients (11 with COPD) who showed little density dependence of flow at baseline, suggesting predominant small airways obstruction. An inhaled β-agonist (isoproterenol) caused a modest overall bronchodilator effect but no appreciable change in He/O_2 responsiveness. This implies that the predominant site of airflow limitation remained in the small airways even after treatment. However, the β-agonist also resulted in a shift in the maximum flow static recoil curve upward and to the left, indicating a reduction in the resistance of the upstream segment and dilation of the peripheral airways, albeit to an extent not sufficient to displace equal pressure points from small to large airways. These data suggest that in patients with COPD an inhaled beta-agonist exerts its action predominantly on the peripheral airways, in contrast to inhaled anticholinergic bronchodilators which can act diffusely throughout the tracheobronchial tree (Douglas et al., 1979).

In 21 asthmatics of whom 12 were initial responders to He/O_2 and 9 were initial nonresponders, Partridge and Saunders (1981) observed that inhaled ipratropium had no significant group effect on density dependence of flow, implying a generalized action of inhaled anticholinergic bronchodilators throughout the tracheobronchial tree in asthmatics, as has also been observed in chronic bronchitics (Douglas et al., 1979). In addition, the overall bronchodilator effect of ipratropium was not correlated with the initial major site of airflow limitation,

---

Figure 19 Two examples of lack of improvement of the maximal expiratory flow at 50% of vital capacity ($\dot{V}_{max50}$) breathing air after the use of bronchodilators (BD), but marked improvement of the $\dot{V}_{max50}$ while breathing helium-O_2 after BD, compared with the values obtained before BD, indicating a change in the mechanical properties of the lung not shown when breathing room air alone. A solid vertical line is drawn through the maximal expiratory flow-volume (MEFV) curve at 50% of the pre-BD vital capacity. (a) The MEFV curve in a 32-year-old, female atopic nonsmoker (patient MG) with recurrent, acute respiratory infections, who was asymptomatic at the time of the study. (b) The MEFV curve in a 48-year-old, male atopic smoker (patient BJ) with chronic bronchitis, who was receiving corticosteroids. yrs, years; $\dot{V}$, maximal expiratory flow, in liters/sec ; VC, vital capacity (from Antic and Macklem, 1976, with permission).

suggesting that anticholinergic bronchodilators do not have preferential effectiveness in patients with predominant large airway obstruction, in contrast to earlier findings in asthmatics with exercise-induced bronchospasm (McFadden et al., 1977).

In 17 patients (14 with asthma) with predominantly large-airways obstruction and a brisk response to an inhaled β-agonist, the latter was accompanied by a significant increase in density dependence of flow, a seemingly paradoxical increase in the resistance of the upstream segment with air and a decrease in upstream resistance with He/O_2 (Wellman et al., 1976). These changes could be explained by a mouthward movement of equal pressure points due to dilation of small airways by the β-agonist so that less driving pressure would be dissipated across these airways. As a result, the relative contribution to flow limitation of larger airways in the now longer upstream segment would increase, thus increasing density dependence of flow. Despite increases in upstream resistance, maximal expiratory flow breathing air could increase if the isovolume static recoil pressure (Pst) (i.e., the driving pressure for flow in the upstream segment) also increased in response to the bronchodilator. A rapid *increase* in Pst after the inhaled β-agonist was noted by the authors in three of their asthmatic patients (Wellman et al., 1976) and has also been reported after treatment of asthmatic attacks (McFadden and Lyons, 1969). On the other hand, a shift in the pressure volume curve of the lung in the opposite direction (i.e., toward a *lower* isovolume recoil pressure) has also been reported after treatment of asthmatics with bronchodilators (McFadden et al., 1970; McCarthy and Sigurdson, 1980). Since SG_{aw} also increased substantially following isoproterenol treatment in these patients with predominantly large airway obstruction, it is likely that the bronchodilator action of the beta agonist extended to both large and small airways.

Paré and associates (1983) considered that dilation of peripheral airways might preferentially increase FVC by reducing air trapping due to premature airway closure, whereas dilation of central airways would preferentially increase flow rates. They classified asthmatics into two groups based on their pattern of response to an inhaled bronchodilator: (1) flow responders who showed a predominant increase in expiratory flow rates characterized by $\Delta FEV_1/\Delta FVC > 1$, and (2) volume responders with a predominant increase in FVC indicated by $\Delta FEV_1/\Delta FVC < 1$. Reasoning that these two patterns of response might be related to the major site(s) of airflow limitation in asthmatics, as well as the major site(s) of action of a bronchodilator, they formulated the following hypotheses. First, asthmatics with predominant small airway narrowing ($\Delta\dot{V}_{max}$ after He/O_2 $< 20\%$ are mainly volume responders and those with predominant large airway obstruction ($\Delta\dot{V}_{max} > 20\%$) are mostly flow responders. Secondly, bronchodilators act mainly on peripheral airways in the volume responders and on the central airways in the flow responders, as indicated by a increase in density dependence of flow in the former and a decrease in the latter. And thirdly, the pattern of response to β-agonists differs from that to an anticholinergic bronchodilator since the former has been shown to act preferentially in small airways while the action of the latter extends to more central airways (Ingram et al., 1977; Hensley, 1978). None of these hypotheses could be proven, however. The pattern of response was not related to the initial density dependence of flow, (i.e., to the major site of airways narrowing initially) or to the change in density dependence after either a β-agonist or anticholinergic bronchodilator, suggesting that inhaled bronchodilators do not necessarily act preferentially at the predominant sites of airway narrowing. Moreover, neither the pattern of response nor the bronchodilator-induced changes in density-dependence of flow were related to the class of bronchodilator compound used, which implies that the action of an inhaled β-agonist or anticholinergic bronchodilator does not necessarily predominate at one site or the other within obstructed airways. These observations are consistent with other data in asthmatics (Partridge and Saunders, 1981) and chronic bronchitis (Douglas et al., 1979; Wellman et al., 1976) but not apparently in normals (Hensley et al., 1978).

It is interesting that Paré and associates (1983) noted a relationship between the *directional* change in density dependence of flow after a bronchodilator and both the pattern of response and baseline lung function: those whose density dependence *decreased* tended to be *volume* responders and have low expiratory flow rates and more hyperinflation and air trapping initially. These findings in the volume responders were attributed to diffuse dilatation of airways with opening of previously closed peripheral airways that had contributed very little to forced expiratory flow. The newly recruited peripheral airways could not contribute to flow limitation; if these recruited airways were still relatively narrow, a laminar flow would prevail and the effect of the contribution of these newly recruited airways would be to decrease density dependence. Conversely, in asthmatics with less severe disease, peripheral airways that were only modestly narrowed initially could be fully dilated, causing equal pressure points to move mouthward, thus increasing density dependence of flow.

The relationship between the site(s) of action of a bronchodilator within the airways and the route of administration has been investigated by several workers. Tashkin et al. (1980) compared the sites of airway dilation of 0.5 mg terbutaline administered to 12 asthmatics by wet aerosol inhalation vs. subcutaneous injection. They assumed that $> 20\%$ increases in SG_{aw} and PEFR indicated dilation of large airways and that $> 10\%$ increases in the ratio of $\dot{V}_{max50}$ breathing He/O_2 to that breathing air and $> 10\%$ decrease in the capacity of isoflow (sum of residual volume and volume of isoflow) reflected dilation of peripheral airways. They found that inhaled terbutaline caused large airway dilation in most subjects but not appreciable small airway dilation in any subject, whereas subcutaneous terbutaline caused dilation of both large and small airways

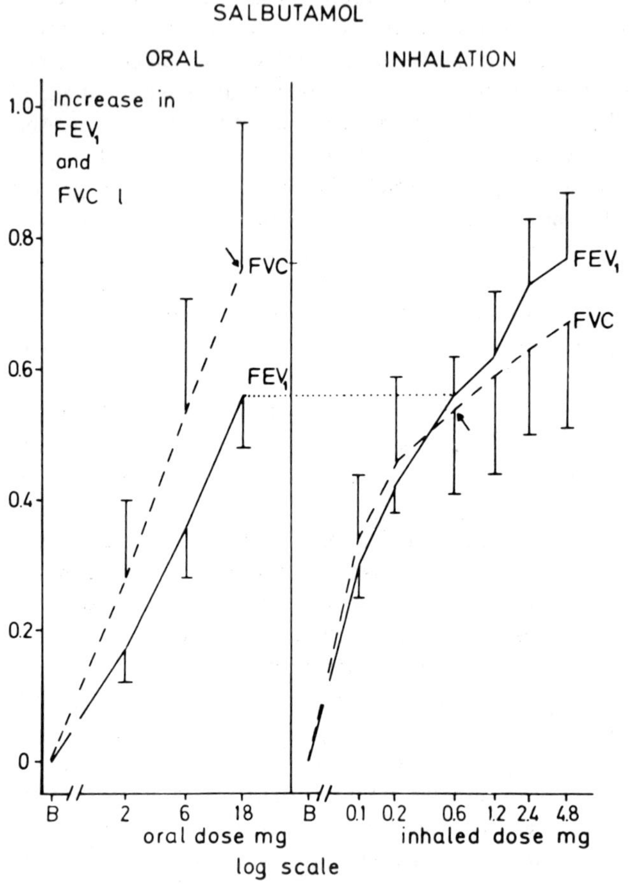

Figure 20 Effects on 1-sec forced expiratory volume (FEV_1) and forced vital capacity (FVC) of increasing inhaled and oral dosages of salbutamol. Arrows point to FVC values caused by oral and inhaled dosages giving the same effect on FEV_1. These identical FEV_1 values are connected by the dotted line. The mean ± SE baseline value for FEV_1 on the inhalation test day was 2.34 ± 0.39 l; that on the oral test day, 2.32 ± 0.39 l. Mean SE values (N = 7) are shown (from Larsson and Svedmyr, 1977, with permission).

in most subjects. In contrast, Pierce et al. (1981) found no significant or consistent effect of intravenous vs. inhaled terbutaline on He/O_2 responsiveness in eight asthmatics. Moreover, both intravenous and inhaled terbutaline caused significant increases in PEFR and FVC and a significant reduction in the slope of the alveolar argon plateau, which suggests that both routes of administration have similar sites of action. These authors (Pierce et al., 1981) employed five times the dosage of inhaled terbutaline used by Tashkin et al. (1980); therefore, a larger amount of the aerosolized β-agonist could have been absorbed into the systemic circulation leading indirectly to bronchodilation of peripheral airways not penetrated directly by the aerosol (DeTroyer et al., 1978).

Larsson and Svedmyr (1977) examined the effects on FEV_1 and FVC of increasing inhaled and oral doses of salbutamol in asthmatics (Fig. 20). A significantly higher FEV_1 was observed with maximally tolerated inhaled compared to oral medication, reflecting the selective action of a bronchodilator on the airways when administered topically by inhalation as opposed to orally. Conversely, the oral route was associated with a significantly greater increase in FVC (due to a reduction in RV as gas trapping behind obstructed peripheral airways is decreased when the latter are dilated) than the inhaled route at dosages corresponding to the same increase in FEV_1. These findings imply a relatively greater effect of oral than inhaled bronchodilators on peripheral airways. On the other hand, comparing oral terbutaline (5 mg) and conventional doses of two β-agonists administered by metered dose inhalers in asthmatics, Fairshter and Wilson (1980) found comparable overall bronchodilation and no difference between effects of the oral and inhaled routes of β-agonist administration on density dependence of flow. Their results suggest that inhaled β-agonists are capable of dilating peripheral airway in asthmatics.

In 65 asthmatics, Fairshter and Wilson (1980) noted a linear relationship between density dependence of flow and the prebronchodilator $\dot{V}_{max50}$ while they were breathing air. This suggests that the major site of airflow limitation moves peripherally with increasing severity of asthma. They also found a significant inverse relationship ($r = -0.59$; $P < 0.001$) between the prebronchodilator $\Delta\dot{V}_{max50}$ and the change in $\Delta\dot{V}_{max50}$ after a β-agonist bronchodilator regardless of the route of administration (oral or inhaled) of the bronchodilator (Fig. 21). Density dependence of flow increased in patients with initially low values of $\Delta\dot{V}_{max50}$ and decreased in those with initially high values. A similar inverse relationship between changes in $He\text{-}O_2$ responses after a β-agonist and initial density dependence of flow was noted by Meadows and colleagues (1980). These observations suggest that the predominant site of bronchodilator action of a β-agonist in asthmatics is not confined to the peripheral airways but is related to the prebronchodilator site of predominant airflow obstruction. The principal response of asthmatics with mainly small airway flow limitation appears to be dilation of peripheral airways and that of asthmatics with predominant central airflow limitation seems to be dilation of large airways.

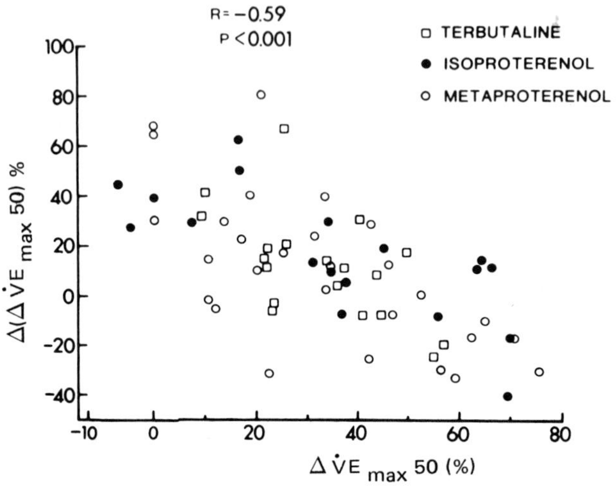

Figure 21 Relationship between bronchodilator values of $\Delta\dot{V}E_{max50}$ (abscissa) and $\Delta(\Delta\dot{V}E_{max50})$ where $\Delta(\Delta ME_{max50}) = \Delta\dot{V}E_{max50}$ after bronchodilators minus $\Delta\dot{V}E_{max50}$ before bronchodilators. The correlation is inverse and significant ($r = -0.59$; $P < 0.001$) indicating that subjects with low prebronchodilator values of $\dot{V}E_{max50}$ have the largest increments in this value after bronchodilator administration. Points are shown in terms of the bronchodilator eventually received, even though the values on the abscissa represent prebronchodilator results (From Fairshter and Wilson, 1980, with permission).

De Troyer and colleagues (1978) compared the effects of large doses of inhaled ipratropium (240 μg) and intravenous atropine (1.25 mg) on R_{aw} and on pressure-volume, flow-volume, and maximum flow-static recoil curves of normal subjects. Both routes of anticholinergic bronchodilator administration resulted in similar decreases in R_{aw} (~ 50%) and similar increases in maximal expiratory flow at high lung volumes, but only *intravenous* atropine increased maximal expiratory flow and upstream resistance at low lung volumes and decreased recoil pressures. The authors concluded that whereas the dilating action of the anticholinergic aerosol was confined to the large central airways, *intravenous* atropine dilated both large and small airways, including alveolar ducts. Since ipratropium is poorly absorbed, indirect effects of even large dosages of the aerosol via absorption into the systemic circulation were precluded.

Measurements of $\Delta\dot{V}_{max50}$ have been found to be associated with considerable within-subject variability, casting doubt on the reliability of this test in assessing changes in density dependence of flow in individual subjects (Berend et al., 1981). On the other hand, Zeck and associates (1981) found only a relatively small degree of variability in the ratio of $\dot{V}_{max50}$ breathing He/O_2 to that breathing air (6%), although the variability of the volume of isoflow was so great (coefficient of variation 105%) as to render the latter test unreliable.

IV. Expressing the Results

The method of expressing the bronchodilator response in quantitative terms can influence interpretation of the statistical as well as clinical "significance" of the response. Percent improvement of baseline is the most common method of expression. Other includes absolute improvement and percent of maximal achievable improvement; the latter is calculated as the difference between the post- and prebronchodilator values expressed as a percentage of the difference between the best value ever recorded for that subject (or the predicted value) and the prebronchodilator value:

$$\frac{\text{Postbronchodilator value} - \text{prebronchodilator value}}{\text{best value ever recorded} - \text{prebronchodilator value}} \times 100$$

Use of each of these methods can lead to problems in interpretation. Figure 22 graphically illustrates the percent improvement (A), percent of achievable improvement (B), and absolute improvement (C) in FEV_1 of a hypothetical patient studied on seven different occasions. At these different times the baseline FEV_1 varied from 0.5 l to 3.5 l, predicted being 4.0 l.

Although not shown in Figure 22, it should be noted that a bronchodilator response is still possible (and not infrequently observed in practice) when the baseline FEV_1 is within the limits of normal (4 liters in this case). Curve C illustrates a parabolic relationship between absolute response to a bronchodilator and baseline lung function, as previously noted by Hume and Gandevia (1957) in six asthmatic patients, each studied on numerous occasions. When lung function is near normal, relatively little absolute improvement is possible. As obstruction increases, more reversible bronchospasm is present and improvement is greater. However, with more severe obstruction acute bronchodilator responses decrease due to less readily reversible bronchial pathologic conditions, including secretions, inflammation, and edema. The small bronchodilator response noted when obstruction is severe (low baseline FEV_1) is indicated by the sloping down of *all* the curves on the left side of the figure. On the other hand, when obstruction is mild and there is relatively little room for improvement, full achievement of the small degree of possible improvement is reflected by a high level of percent achievable improvement (curve B) but only an intermediate level of absolute improvement (curve C) and a strikingly low level of percent improvement (curve A). The minimal percent improvement results from dividing a relatively small absolute change by a high baseline value. Curve A appears to be the

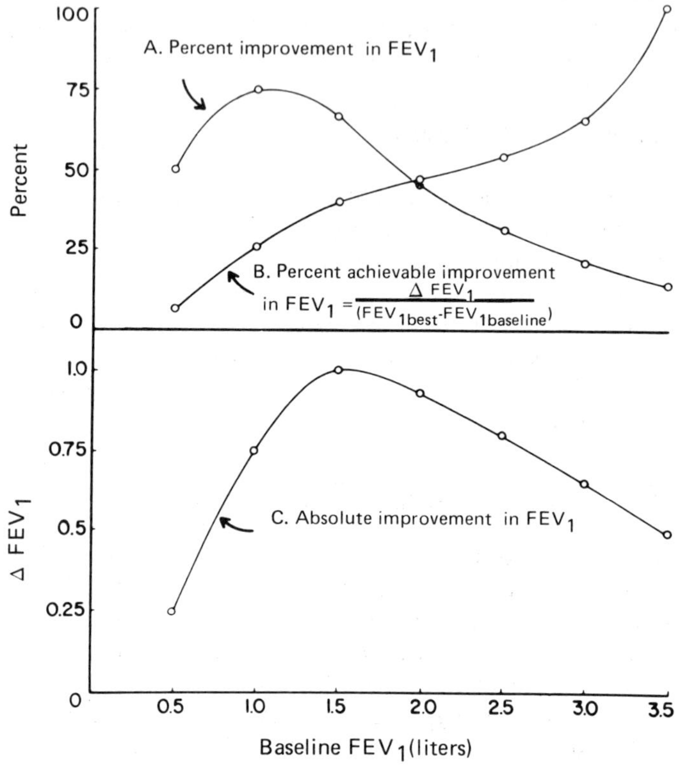

Figure 22 Three ways of representing the bronchodilator responses in a hypothetical patient studied on seven different occasions with seven different baseline values (FEV_1 ranging from 0.5 to 3.5) with arbitrary responses.

most misleading way of representing a bronchodilator response since it is most dependent on baseline lung function. However, as is apparent from inspection of all three curves, none of the methods of expressing a bronchodilator response obviates the confounding effect of the level of baseline function on the response. Consequently, in comparative studies of bronchodilator drugs, including different agents, different dosages of the same agent and/or placebo, it is important that each subject have fairly comparable baseline lung function at each testing session. Subjects should not be tested unless the prebronchodilator FEV_1 values fall within a predetermined range, usually within 20% of each other.

If measurements are made at serial times after a bronchodilator is administered, then we may be able to ascertain the time of onset, peak magnitude and duration of bronchodilation, and the time to peak action. The latter is an important consideration when postbronchodilator measurements are obtained at only one point. The duration of bronchodilation may be as important to a patient as the peak response since it determines the frequency of dosing required to prevent symptoms of "breakthrough" bronchospasm when the bronchodilator effect has worn off. Moreover, tachyphylaxis to a β-agonist may be manifested more by curtailment in the duration than in the peak magnitude of bronchodilation (Plummer, 1978). In analyzing postbronchodilator measurements over time, we can calculate the area under the response-time curve by the trapezoidal method, summing up the areas of a series of trapezoids at each measurement time. The areas obtained with one drug can then be compared with that obtained with another active agent or placebo.

Research studies of bronchodilator drugs might include (1) dose-response curves to determine the maximally effective dosage associated with acceptable side effects and (2) bronchoprovocation testing to determine the protective effect of a bronchodilator agent on experimentally induced bronchospasm (methacholine, histamine, exercise, cold air, hyperventilation, hypo-osmolar solutions). Dose-response studies should include measurements obtained at the time of expected peak action. Bronchoconstrictor challenge studies should also be timed so that the provocative stimulus is not applied until the peak bronchodilator effect of the drug has been achieved.

One advantage of the bronchoprovocation model for evaluating the efficacy of a bronchodilator is that the bronchospasm can be reproducibly provoked, thereby obviating problems in interpretation relating to variable degrees of spontaneous baseline airways obstruction (see above). However, most studies of the effect of a bronchodilator on induced bronchoconstriction provide information relating only to peak intensity and not the duration of this protective effect. Ahrens and co-workers (1984) recently examined the duration of the protective effect of nebulized metaproterenol against provocation by methacholine administered 3/4, 2-1/4, and 4-1/2 hr after the bronchodilator. At 2 1/4 hr, the bronchodilator effect of metaproterenol remained maximal but its protective effects against methacholine had declined by 50%. By 4 hr, the drug exhibited a significant bronchodilator effect but its effect on airway responsiveness to methacholine had disappeared. Eggleston and Beasley (1981) also noted that dosages of terbutaline and isoproterenol producing equivalent bronchodilation caused markedly different degrees of inhibition of exercise-induced bronchospasm. The reason for the disparity in the time-response relationships between the effect of a β-agonist on airway tone and its effect on nonspecific airways reactivity may be due either to different mechanisms for these two actions of a beta-agonist (Eggleston and Beasly, 1981) or to differences in the potency of the bronchoconstrictor stimuli involved in spontaneous bronchospasm (mild) vs. induced bronchospasm (marked) (Ahrens et al., 1984). In the latter case, a larger concentration of a β-agonist in the lung would be required to overcome induced bronchoconstriction compared to spontaneous bronchospasm. The clinical implications of these findings are that dosing intervals based on duration of bronchodilation may not be adequate for protection against naturally occurring spasmogenic stimuli, such as exercise, cold air, or exposure to physical or chemical irritants, among others.

V. Defining a Significant Response to a Bronchodilator

The significance of a bronchodilator response can be defined by the test(s) performed to quantitate the response and the variability of the particular tests used. A number of additional factors, previously discussed, can influence a bronchodilator response and need to be taken into consideration. As already noted, some tests are inherently more variable than others so that a greater degree of improvement is required for the response to be considered significant. Moreover, test variability is affected by the presence or absence (and probably degree) of dysfunction at baseline, so that obstructed individuals show more variable responses than do healthy people. Furthermore, intertrial variability in test results increases over time, so that tests separated by an interval of a week or a month, for example, will require a larger change than tests performed only minutes apart for differences in these results to be considered significant. For example, in the average obstructed patient, the FEV_1 or FVC would have to increase by 12% or more within the same day to be considered significant. On a chronic basis, however, an improvement of 20-25% would be necessary (Pennock et al., 1981).

When we are examining responses to a bronchodilator in a *group* of subjects rather than an individual patient, statistical tests can be applied to ascertain whether or not there has been a significant change in the mean group value following use of a bronchodilator and whether this change is statistically greater than that found after placebo; the confidence limit usually selected is 95% for a one-tailed test of significance or 97.5% for a two-tailed test. However, statistically significant responses to a bronchodilator are not necessarily correlated with clinical effectiveness. A bronchodilator response may be statistically significant and yet not be important clinically and vice versa. For example, a 15% improvement in FEV_1 in a patient with COPD may be statistically significant, but its clinical relevance can be argued. For this reason, other indices of effectiveness are often sought, such as improvement in symptoms and exercise tolerance. Systemically administered bronchodilators have effects on other organs such as the diaphragm (Aubier et al., Murciano et al., 1984) and the heart (Matthay et al., 1978), which need to be considered in evaluating their overall benefit.

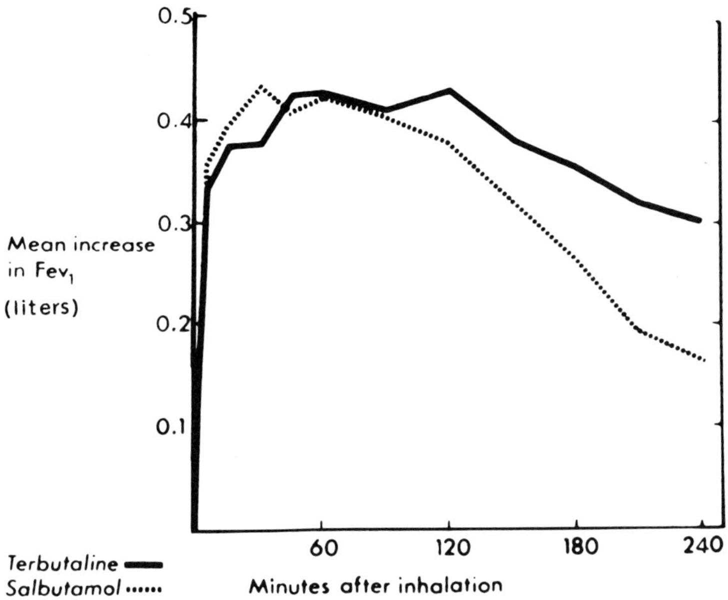

Figure 23 Response to inhalation of terbutaline and salbutamol aerosols given in matched doses (peak response) (from Freedman, 1972, with permission).

VI. Designing a Single-Dose Bronchodilator Study

Studies comparing two or more bronchodilators are routinely performed as part of the clinical evaluation of investigational new drugs. Most of these studies are placebo-controlled and use a randomly ordered, double-blind design. Nevertheless, errors in design still occur. The following recommendations have been made previously but warrant re-emphasis.

Dosages should be equipotent with respect to peak responses (Fig. 23) if different bronchodilator agents are being compared. Otherwise, the relative duration of action cannot be compared.

Dosages should be submaximal. If the dosage of one drug exceeds that required for a peak bronchodilator effect and the other does not, erroneous conclusions can be drawn concerning the relative duration of effectiveness (Fig. 24).

Baseline lung function should not vary by > 20% within any subject across study days (see discussion above) and should also be somewhat comparable between subjects (especially when a parallel group design is employed).

A *placebo* should be used to prevent subject and investigator biases; to control for the effect of suggestion, which can lead to appreciable bronchodilation in approximately 50% of asthmatics, probably mediated by vagal pathways

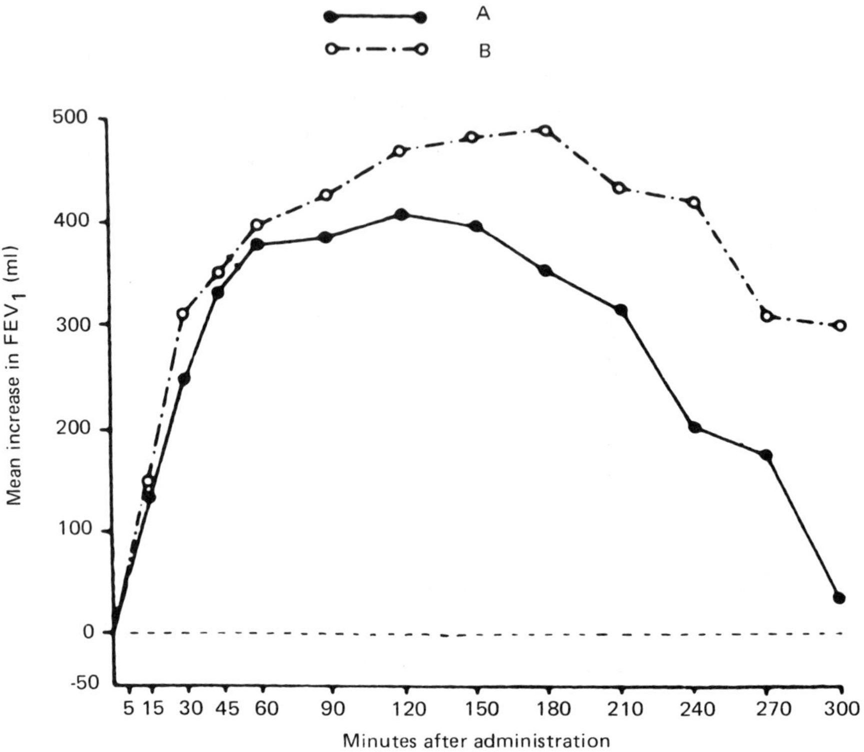

Figure 24 Mean increase in FEV_1 at intervals after administration of terbutaline at an oral dose of (A) 5 mg and (B) 10 mg illustrating the effect of dosage on apparent rate of decline of effect (from Freedman, 1971, with permission).

(Luparello et al., 1968); and to compensate for spontaneous changes due to diurnal variation and residual effects of previously administered bronchodilators.

Other bronchodilators should be withheld when possible. Long-acting theophylline preparations need to be discontinued at least 24-48 hr before testing. As already noted, COPD patients on maintenance theophylline therapy respond only about half as well to an inhaled β-agonist as patients not receiving theophylline, even when the last dosage was withheld (Eaton et al., 1982). Oral and longer-acting inhaled β-agonists should not be taken within at least 8 hr of testing, if possible. However, to eliminate the possibility of tachyphylaxis to a β-agonist, which can blunt the initial response to an experimental β-adrenergic bronchodilator, an initial "washout" period of as long as 2 weeks may be required (Nelson et al., 1977). Corticosteroids can enhance the effect of an adrenergic agent (especially if β-adrenergic tachyphylaxis has occurred) and should therefore be maintained at the same dosing level throughout the study in patients already receiving oral or inhaled corticosteroid therapy.

The order of the drugs should be randomized and the study should be double-blind, unless the intent is to test efficacy in severe or unstable patients or preliminary pilot data are desired. Otherwise, systematic biases can occur due to the order in which the drugs are administered, such as residual effects of recently discontinued medication, effects of the first day on response to the second, emotional effects related to the first day of testing, environmental effects, etc. Two kinds of randomization designs are commonly used: (1) a parallel-group design in which patients are randomly allocated to one or two or more treatment groups, and before and after measurements are taken; and (2) a crossover design. In the latter, each patient is assigned to receive all the treatments in a random order and thus serves as his or her own control. In crossover studies, successive testing sessions must be separated by enough time to remove all residual effects of the previous treatment.

Patients' conditions should be stable and not too severe unless the study is specifically designed to evaluate acutely or chronically severe asthmatics. Patients with severe asthma are less likely to respond favorably to bronchodilator therapy due to secretions and inflammation in their airways. Moreover, they do not tolerate withdrawal of concomitant bronchodilator medication, thus confounding interpretation of the results.

Patients should be tested at the same time of day to minimize effects of diurnal variation. If oral agents are being tested, patients should also fast to reduce variability in absorption rates.

Some patients may have marked bronchomotor responses to the deep breath preceding forced exhalation; it may be preferable to employ partial flow-volume curves or body plethysmography in such subjects. Some patients may always respond better to one drug than another despite a different response of the group as a whole (drug-patient interaction). Subjects may have different degrees of exposure to artifactual bronchospastic stimuli during the course of a testing session: coughing, exercise, additives in food or beverages, passive smoking, and others. Of course, informed consent and Institutional Review Board approval for human research are necessary.

VII. Analyzing Data from Clinical Trials of Bronchodilators

The goals of a clinical trial of a bronchodilator are usually clearly defined. The investigator will first want to compare the drug of interest to a placebo to determine if there is any bronchodilator effect. If there is, the new drug may also be compared to a known bronchodilator to see if its effect is great enough to warrant its use over other available drugs. Also, the dose-response relationship of the drug may be examined. For example, at what point does the dose-response curve plateau, that is, give much less of an effect for a given increment in dosage? What dosage will give maximal bronchodilation with minimal or acceptable side effects? Other questions requiring different approaches in the analysis include examination of the time of onset of significant clinical response, the magnitude of the peak response, the duration of response or the average response over a given time interval. The number and severity of adverse side effects, relative to other drugs in use, should also be examined.

Before proceeding with complex statistical tests, it is desirable to use other methods to examine the data. Chief among these is simply plotting the mean response of the subjects (the measured physiological parameters of interest) against time. The data can be plotted as the mean of the absolute or percent change from baseline or percent of maximal possible improvement (see above). When the baselines are highly variable, the results can be affected in undesirable ways, as already discussed. When the data are plotted, the time course of the response to several drugs can be shown on the same plot frame, making visual comparisons easy. Such plots can frequently suggest trends that may not be revealed by more sophisticated statistical tests designed to test specific hypotheses. Further analysis is frequently suggested by examination of such plots.

When statistical tests are applied to the data, it is important to keep in mind the nature of statistical analysis and the underlying assumptions on which the tests are made. These statistical tests are an application of probability theory. For example, if certain assumptions are made about the nature of the data, we can test the hypothesis that the populations of data for the different treatments have the same mean (the null hypothesis). However, even if the test indicates that the means are not equal, there is still a built-in probability that we may be wrong if we conclude that the means really are different. No absolute statements can be made, although we may feel confident in making statements about the data when the probabilities are extreme. If a number of tests examining the data in different ways give consistent results, our confidence is greater than if statistical significance were revealed by only one test. It must be remembered that a statistical test is designed to test some specific hypothesis related to the population that the data represents, not make sweeping statements about the drug in question. The assumptions underlying the test in use must be considered also. For most of the tests that we will consider, the data are expected to be a sample from a population of data normally distributed, and each observation used is expected to be independent of the others. There is frequently some difficulty with each of these assumptions, as discussed below.

The simplest study to analyze would be one in which some physiological measures were made just once before and once after the administration of a single test drug. In this case, one need only look at the differences between pre-

and postdrug measurements. A t-test can test whether or not these differences are equal to zero. If two drugs are tested, their relative efficacy can be determined by comparing the responses to each drug with each other. If the subjects taking the first drug are not the same as the subjects taking the second drug, an independent t-test (unpaired) will compare the mean responses for each group. If each subject took both drugs, a paired t-test is best used to compare the responses to each drug. The paired approach is usually more powerful than the unpaired, but the choice of which test to use is determined by the study design. Care must be taken to use the correct test in order to make valid conclusions based on the statistical results.

The t-tests provide a statistic with a known probability distribution; that is, the probability of getting a given t value just by chance is known. The probability (or P value) can be calculated or found in a table. However, there is still the question of one-tailed versus two-tailed tests. One may be interested in a difference in only one direction. For example, when looking at whether or not a drug is a bronchodilator compared to placebo, significant differences between the drug and placebo may be of interest only if the active drug produces a greater response than placebo. If the drug does not have a greater response than placebo, it does not matter if they are the same or the placebo has a greater response; all that matters is that the active drug is or is not better than placebo. In this situation, a one-tailed test would be appropriate. If the direction of whatever difference may be found is not important, or no particular direction can be expected, the proper test would be two-tailed.

When comparisons between several drugs are made, analysis of variance (ANOVA) is used (Winer, 1971; Dunn and Clark, 1974; Dixon and Massey, 1983). ANOVA compares the means of all the drugs simultaneously, although it does not, by itself, say which means are different. A one-way ANOVA comparing each drug with the other is equivalent to a two-sided unpaired t-test when there are only two drugs. If each subject is given each drug, a two-way randomized block design with drug and subject as the two factors can be performed. This type of analysis takes into account the paired nature of the data, thus allowing for the intersubject differences without the problems of transformed variables such as percent change (which may not be normally distributed, thus violating one of the assumptions of ANOVA).

One more modification of the ANOVA is important in analysis of this type of data. In order to adjust for variations in baseline values, an analysis of covariance (ANCOVA) can be performed. ANCOVA adjusts the observed postdrug treatment means linearly for the mean baseline of each treatment, rather than just subtracting the baseline as in the t-tests above. The adjusted group means are then compared to each other. A two-way ANCOVA can be used just as the two-way ANOVA would be, but a problem can develop if the baselines vary too much. If a subject's baseline is very much higher on one day than another, he or she may have less room for improvement, so that the postdrug values are closer to the baseline values. This can destroy the linear relationship on which the adjustment in the ANCOVA is based.

If analysis of variance shows that there is an overall difference across treatment categories, one can perform a multiple comparisons test to determine which treatments are different from each other. There are several different multiple comparisons tests, each with its own advantages (and disadvantages). Some test each pair of treatments chosen separately (e.g., linear contrasts from ANOVA, Fisher's LSD, Tukey, Scheffe, etc.), while others look for groups of treatments that are different from other groups of treatments (Duncan multiple range test, Newman-Keuls, etc.) (Winer, 1971, Milliken and Johnson, 1984). One of the simplest of these tests (and frequently one of the best) is a series of t-tests. These will suffice in most cases, as long as the number of t-tests performed is accounted for in the interpretation of the results, as described below.

In many clinical trials of bronchodilators, measurements are made serially after administration of the test drugs. This allows the investigator to determine the relative efficacy of the drugs at different times after treatment. One method is to perform the tests described above separately for the measurements at each time. When this is done, the number of tests performed must be considered when one is interpreting the results. The interpretation should be made with the visual aid of plots of the data against time. An analysis of variance with repeated measures would allow all of the data to be evaluated in one analysis, but care must be taken in the use of this method. If the response of each subject is roughly the same with time (i.e., the shape of the plot of the measurement vs. time is the same for all subjects) a repeated-measures ANOVA will probably by appropriate. The output from repeated-measures ANOVA programs (such as BMDP2V [Dixon, 1983]) will provide the information necessary to decide if this model is valid. If it is not, one method that still uses the time nature of the data is to perform a separate regression analysis for each subject and use statistical tests on the resulting regression parameters.

There are many ways in which the data can be reduced to one measurement per day for each subject, depending on the clinical questions of interest. For example, statistical analysis can be performed on the peak response to each drug. Also, the total time each drug causes a response above a chosen threshold, or greater than placebo, can be used. The sum of the responses at all times (a sort of "average" response for the day) or the area under each subject's time-response curve (which is simply the sum of the responses when the time intervals are equal) can be used. The sums can be restricted to only the time intervals of interest. These parameters will sometimes confirm trends noted on the initial examination of plots and other descriptive data even when statistical tests are negative. For example, the results from an ANOVA at each time may not indicate differences between drugs for a chosen variable despite the fact that one drug's mean time-response curve is consistently higher than the other's. The area under the curve may confirm the tendency detected by eye. Before using such summary variables, one must be sure that they are normally distributed. If they are not, some powerful nonparametric statistical methods can still be used.

When the data are not normally distributed, for example, for categorical data such as the occurrence of symptoms, the number of asthma attacks in a day, or the frequency of as-needed use of bronchodilators, nonparametric tests are required (Siegel, 1956; Snedecor and Cochran, 1980). The chi-square test for two-way tables is frequently used to test for differences in these measures between groups. The Kruskal-Wallis test is a nonparametric analysis of variance for independent observations. In crossover studies, the Friedman two-way analysis of variance (which ranks the treatments and tests for differences in the rank sums across subjects), blocking on subjects, may be used. These tests can also be applied to nonnormal parameters derived from the physiological data. Many tests are available for testing other specific hypotheses.

The dose-response relationship for new bronchodilators is often of interest. Again, the simplest initial approach is to plot the response vs. each dose of a drug given during the study. The response can be expressed as the peak percent change from baseline or some other parameter that will allow for intersubject differences and baseline variation. Regression analysis may help determine if a dose-response relationship exists. Inspection of the plot will allow one to determine the minimum dosage required for a significant clinical effect and the greatest useful dosage beyond which increasingly smaller improvement is attained for similar increases in dosage.

In choosing a statistical test and interpreting the results of the analysis, it is important to keep in mind several aspects of the statistical methods, to avoid some of the pitfalls that frequently trap the unwary investigator. One problem is not understanding the meaning of "significance." Because statistical tests are applications of probability theory, the results do not allow one to make absolute statements. Several tests, examining the data in different ways, help to give more confidence in the conclusions drawn from the results. This does not mean that different tests will actually find different "truths," but that the data may look different from different perspectives, and that the uncertainties in using these probability statements must be considered when evaluating the results. It is also important to remember that there is a difference between statistical and clinical significance. A statistically significant difference between the responses to two bronchodilators would not be important if the difference is clinically not meaningful.

In published trials of bronchodilator drugs, the results of statistical tests are frequently given with P values: probabilities for the test statistics. A P value of 0.05 is frequently used as a cutoff point for deciding if a test is significant. A different level can be used, depending on how sure one wants to be of the statements made. P values are often given as "< 0.05," "< 0.01," probably because tables provide the test statistics for only specific P levels. With computers now providing the exact P values, it would be more informative to state the exact values for the reader when the results are considered significant.

Because the P value is never zero, when many tests are performed simultaneously some of them would be expected to give significant results just by chance. Consequently, care must be taken when performing many comparisons, such as multiple t-tests or other multiple comparisons tests following analysis of variance. Some multiple comparisons tests adjust the reported P value to compensate for the number of tests, but others do not.

When one-sided t-tests are used, the P value used for significance is commonly adjusted by dividing by the number of tests (Milliken and Johnson, 1984; Dunn and Clark, 1974). For example, if three drugs are compared by ANOVA and multiple t-tests, the P level of the three t-tests (drug A vs. B, A vs. C, and B vs. C) would be adjusted from 0.05 to 0.017 (0.05/3). Because the choice of 0.05 is somewhat arbitrary (although traditional), this is a case of applying an exact rule to adjust an arbitrary number. Also, there is sometimes disagreement about how many tests must be allowed for in the adjustment, for example, should one adjust for all of the tests performed on all physiological parameters or adjust separately for each set of tests for each parameter. One alternative is simply to provide the test results without adjustment, inform the reader of the number of different tests, and suggest that care must be taken in their interpretation. This allows the reader to use his or her own criteria in drawing conclusions from the test results.

Of course, many important aspects of statistical data analysis cannot be discussed here. A biostatistician should usually be consulted, even for seemingly straightforward analyses, to insure that nothing is overlooked. There are many more ways to examine the data than those described here, and a creative statistician can help find these. It is also important that the investigator take an active part in the analysis rather than leave it entirely to the statistician, because the investigator is more familiar with the data and the methods of data collection. For instance, the statistician might not know when the data are not independent or when the data would not be expected to be normally distributed. For proper analysis and interpretation of the data, the investigator and statistician must work together as a team.

Acknowledgment

The author thanks Michael Simmons for assistance in discussing statistical approaches to analysis of data from bronchodilator trials.

References

Ahrens, R. C., Bonham, A. C., Maxwell, G. A., and Weinberger, M. M. (1984). A method for comparing the peak intensity and duration of action of aerosolized bronchodilators using bronchoprovocation with methacholine. *Am. Rev. Respir. Dis. 129*: 903-906.

Alexander, M. R., Dull, W. L., and Kasik, J. E. (1980). Treatment of chronic obstructive pulmonary disease with orally administered theophylline. *JAMA 244*: 2286-2290.

Alliott, R. J., Lang, B. D., Rawson, D. R. W., and Leckie, W. J. H. (1972). Effects of salbutamol and isoprenaline/phenylephrine in reversible airways obstruction. *Br. Med. J. 1*: 539-542.

Anderson, S. D., Seale, J. P., Rozea, P., Bandler, L., Theobald, G., and Lindsay, D. A. (1976). Inhaled and oral salbutamol in exercise-induced asthma. *Am. Rev. Respir. Dis. 114*: 493-500.

Antic, R., and Macklem, P. T. (1976). The influence of clinical factors on site of airway obstruction in asthma. *Am. Rev. Respir. Dis. 114*: 851-859.

Antonissen, L. A., Mitchell, R. W., Kroeger, E. A., Kepron, W., Stephens, N. L., and Bergen, J. (1980). Histamine pharmacology in airway smooth muscle from a canine model of asthma. *J. Pharmacol. Exp. Ther. 213*: 150-155.

ATS Statement (1979). Snowbird Workshop on standardization of spirometry. *Am. Rev. Respir. Dis. 119*: 831-838.

Aubier, M., De Troyer, A., Sampson, M., Macklem, P. T., and Roussos, C. (1981). Aminophylline improves diaphragmatic contractility. *N. Engl. J. Med. 305*: 249-252.

Ayres, S. M., Griesbach, S. J., Reimold, F., and Evans, R. G. (1974). Bronchial component in chronic obstructive lung disease. *Am. J. Med. 57*: 183-191.

Baigelman, W., and Chodosh, S. (1977). Bronchodilator action of the anticholinergic drug, ipratropium bromide (Sch 1000), as an aerosol in chronic bronchitis and asthma. *Chest 71*: 324-328.

Barnes, P. J., Gribbin, H. R., Osmanliev, D., and Pride, N. B. (1981). Partial flow-volume curves to measure bronchodilator dose-response curves in normal humans. *J. Appl. Physiol. 50*: 1193-1197.

Beaupré, A., and Orehek, J. (1982). Factors influencing the bronchodilator effect of a deep inspiration in asthmatic patients with provoked bronchoconstriction. *Thorax 37*: 124-128.

Becker, A. B., Simons, K. J., Gillespie, C. A., and Simons, F. E. R. (1984). The bronchodilator effects and pharmacokinetics of caffeine in asthma. *N. Engl. J. Med. 310*: 743-746.

Berenberg, M. J., Baigelman, W., Cupples, L. A., and Pearce, L. (1985). Comparison of updraft nebulizer versus metered dose inhaler attached to an aerochamber for the administration of metaproterenol to hospitalized patients. *Am. Rev. Respir. Dis.* (abstract) *131*: A95.

Berend, N., Nelson, N. A., Rutland, J., Marlin, G. E., and Woolcock, A. J. (1981). The maximum expiratory flow-volume curve with air and low-density gas mixture. An analysis of subject and observer variability. *Chest 80*: 23-30.

Bierman, C. W., Shapiro, G. G., Pierson, W. E., and Dorsett, C. S. (1977). Acute and chronic theophylline therapy in exercise-induced bronchospasm. *Pediatrics 60*: 845-849.

Bloomfield, P., Crompton, G. K., and Winsey, N. J. P. (1979). A tube spacer to improve inhalation of drugs from pressurised aerosols. *Br. Med. J. 2*: 1479.

Bouhuys, A. (1969). Recent applications of volume displacement body plethysmographs. *Prog. Respir. Res. 4*: 24-38.

Bouhuys, A. (1974). *Breathing.* 1st ed. New York, Grune and Stratton, p. 187.

Bouhuys, A., and van de Woestijne, K. P. (1971). Mechanical consequences of airway smooth muscle relaxation. *J. Appl. Physiol. 30*: 670-676.

Boushey, H. A., Holtzman, M. J., Sheller, J. R., and Nadel, J. A. (1980). Bronchial hyperreactivity. *Am. Rev. Respir. Dis. 121*: 389-413.

Branscomb, B. V. (1978). Efficacy and side effects of fenoterol compared with isoproterenol administered by metered dose inhalers in asthma. *Chest 73* (Suppl): 1002-1004.

Briscoe, W. A., and DuBois, A. B. (1958). The relationship between airway resistance, airway conductance and lung volume in subjects of different age and body size. *J. Clin. Invest. 37*: 1279-1285.

Brown, R., Ingram, R. H., Jr., and McFadden, E. R. Jr. (1978). Problems in the plethysmographic assessment of changes in total lung capacity in asthma. *Am. Rev. Respir. Dis. 118*: 685-692.

Bruderman, I., Cohen-Aronovski, R., and Smorzik, J. (1983). A comparative study of various combinations of ipratropium bromide and metaproterenol in allergic asthmatic patients. *Chest 83*: 208-210.

Bunker, M. L., McWilliams, M. (1979). Caffeine content of common beverages. *J. Am. Diet. Assoc. 74*: 28-32.

Burge, P. S., Harries, M. G., and I'Anson, E. (1980). Comparison of atropine with ipratropium bromide in patients with reversible airways obstruction unresponsive to salbutamol. *Br. J. Dis. Chest 74*: 259-262.

Chang, N., and Levison, H. (1972). The effect of a nebulized bronchodilator administered with or without intermittent positive pressure breathing on ventilatory function in children with cystic fibrosis and asthma. *Am. Rev. Respir. Dis. 106*: 867-872.

Chick, T. W., Nicholson, D. P., and Johnson, R. L. Jr. (1973). Effects of isoproterenol on distribution of ventilation and perfusion in asthma. (Note) *Am. Rev. Respir. Dis. 107*: 869-873.

Clausen, J. L. (ed.) (1982). *Pulmonary Function Testing. Guidelines and Controversies. Equipment, Methods, and Normal Values.* New York, Academic Press.

Colebatch, H. J. H. (1970). The humoral regulation of alveolar ducts. In *Airway Dynamics, Physiology and Pharmacology.* Edited by A. Bouhuys. Springfield, Charles C. Thomas, p. 169.

Coleridge, H. M., Coleridge, J. C. G., Ginzel, K. H., Baker, D. G., Banzett, R. B., and Morrison, M. A. (1976). Stimulation of 'irritant' receptors and afferent C-fibres in the lungs of prostaglandins. *Nature (Lond.) 264*: 451-453.

Conolly, M. E., Warrell, D. A., Newton Howes, J. A., Paterson, J. W., Beilin, L. J., Robertson, D. G., and Dollery, C. T. (1971). A comparison of the cardiorespiratory effects of isoprenaline and salbutamol in patients with bronchial asthma. *Postgrad. Med. J. 47*(Suppl): 77-81.

Dawson, S. V., and Elliott, E. A. (1977). Wave-speed limitation on expiratory flow–a unifying concept. *J. Appl. Physiol. 43*: 498-515.

DeCotiis, B. S., Braman, S. S., and Corrao, W. M. (1980). The protective effect of theophylline and terbutaline on a methacholine inhalation challenge. *Am. Rev. Respir. Dis. 121*(Suppl): 125.

Despas, P. J., Leroux, M., and Macklem, P. T. (1972). Site of airway obstruction in asthma as determined by measuring maximal expiratory flow breathing air and a helium-oxygen mixture. *J. Clin. Invest. 51*: 3235-3243.

De Troyer, A., Yernault, J. C., and Rodenstein, D. (1978). Influence of $beta_2$-agonist aerosols on pressure-volume characteristics of the lungs. *Am. Rev. Respir. Dis. 118*: 987-995.

Dixon, W. J. (Ed.) (1983). *BMDP Statistical Software.* Berkeley, University of California Press, pp. 359-386.

Dixon, W. J., and Massey, F. J. Jr. (1983). *Introduction to Statistical Analysis,* 4th edition. New York, McGraw-Hill Book Company.

Dolovich, M., Eng, P., Ruffin, R., Corr, D., and Newhouse, M. T. (1983). Clinical evaluation of a simple demand inhalation MDI aerosol delivery service. *Chest 84*: 36-41.

Dolovich, M. B., Ruffin, R. E., Roberts, R., and Newhouse, M. T. (1981). Optimal delivery of aerosols from metered dose inhalers. *Chest 80*(Suppl): 911-915.

Dosman, J., Bode, F., Urbanetti, J., Martin, R., and Macklem, P. T. (1975). The use of a helium-oxygen mixture during maximum expiratory flow to demonstrate obstruction in small airways in smokers. *J. Clin. Invest. 55*: 1090-1099.

Douglas, N. J., Davidson, I., Sudlow, M. F., and Flenley, D. C. (1979). Bronchodilatation and the site of airway resistance in severe chronic bronchitis. *Thorax 34*: 51-56.

DuBois, A. B., Botelho, S. Y., Bedell, G. N., Marshall, R., and Comroe, J. H. Jr. (1956a). A rapid plethysmographic method for measuring thoracic gas volume: a comparison with a nitrogen washout method for measuring functional residual capacity in normal subjects. *J. Clin. Invest. 35*: 322-326.

DuBois, A. B., Botelho, S. Y., and Comroe, J. H. Jr. (1956b). A new method for measuring airway resistance in man using a body plethysmograph: Values in normal subjects and in patients with respiratory disease. *J. Clin. Invest. 35*: 327-335.

DuBois, A. B., Brody, A. W., Lewis, D. H., and Burgess, B. F. Jr. (1956c). Oscillation mechanics of lungs and chest in man. *J. Appl. Physiol. 8*: 587-594.

Dulfano, M. J., Glass, P., and McPhillips, J. J. (1977). Comparison of the bronchodilator effects of the same amounts of terbutaline aerosol given as a single dose or in divided doses. *Ann. Allergy 39*: 266-271.

Dunn, O. T., and Clark, V. A. (1974). *Applied Statistics: Analysis of Variance and Regression.* New York, Wiley.

Eaton, M. L., MacDonald, F. M., Church, T. R., and Niewoehner, D. E. (1982). Effects of theophylline on breathlessness and exercise tolerance in patients with chronic airflow obstruction. *Chest 82*: 538-542.

Eggleston, P. A., and Beasley, P. P. (1981). Bronchodilation and inhibition of induced asthma by adrenergic agonists. *Clin. Pharmacol. Ther. 29*: 505-510.

Elwood, R. K., and Abboud, R. T. (1982). The short-term bronchodilator effects of fenoterol and ipratropium in asthma. *J. Allergy Clin. Immunol. 69*: 467-473.

Fairshter, R. D., and Wilson, A. F. (1980). Relationship between the site of airflow limitation and localization of the bronchodilator response in asthma. *Am. Rev. Respir. Dis. 122*: 27-32.

Falliers, C. J., and Katsampes, C. F. (1976). Pharmacologic modification of induced asthma. *Ann. Allergy 36*: 99-103.

Fish, J. E., Ankin, M. G., Kelly, J. F., and Peterman, V. (1981). Regulation of bronchomotor tone by lung inflation in asthmatic and nonasthmatic subjects. *J. Appl. Physiol. 50*: 1079-1086.

Fish, J. E., Peterman, V. I., and Cugell, D. W. (1977). Effect of deep inspiration on airway conductance in subjects with allergic rhinitis and allergic asthma. *J. Allergy Clin. Immunol. 60*: 41-46.

Fry, D. L., and Hyatt, R. E. (1960). Pulmonary mechanics. A unified analysis of the relationship between pressure, volume, and gasflow in the lungs of normal and diseased human subjects. *Am. J. Med. 29*: 672-689.

Galant, S. P., Duriseti, L., Underwood, S., and Insel, P. A. (1978). Decreased beta-adrenergic receptors on polymorphonuclear leukocytes after adrenergic therapy. *N. Engl. J. Med. 299*: 933-936.

Gayrard, P., Orehek, J., Grimaud, C., and Charpin, J. (1975). Bronchoconstrictor effects of a deep inspiration in patients with asthma. *Am. Rev. Respir. Dis. 111*: 433-439.

Gazioglu, K., Condemi, J. J., Hyde, R. W., and Kaltreider, N. L. (1971). Effect of isoproterenol on gas exchange during air and oxygen breathing in patients with asthma. *Am. J. Med. 50*: 185-190.

Gilbert, R. M., Marshman, J. A., Schwieder, M., and Berg, R. (1976). Caffeine content of beverages as consumed. *Can. Med. Assoc. J. 114*: 205-208.

Gimeno, F., Berg, W. C., Sluiter, H. J., and Tammeling, G. J. (1972). Spirometry-induced bronchial obstruction. *Am. Rev. Respir. Dis. 105*: 68-74.

Girard, W. M., and Light, R. W. (1983). Should the FVC be considered in evaluating response to bronchodilator? *Chest 84*: 87-89.

Godden, D. J., and Crompton, G. K. (1981). An objective assessment of the tube spacer in patients unable to use a conventional pressurized aerosol efficiently. *Br. J. Dis. Chest 75*: 165-168.

Gomm, S. A., Keaney, N. P., Winsey, N. J. P., and Stretton, T. B. (1980). Effect of an extension tube on the bronchodilator efficacy of terbutaline delivered from a metered dose inhaler. *Thorax 35*: 552-556.

Green, M., and Mead, J. (1974). Time dependence of flow-volume curves. *J. Appl. Physiol. 37*: 793-797.

Gross, N. J. (1975). Sch 1000: A new anticholinergic bronchodilator. *Am. Rev. Respir. Dis. 112*: 823-828.

Heimer, D., Shim, C., and Williams, M. H. Jr. (1980). The effect of sequential inhalations of metaproterenol aerosol in asthma. *J. Allergy Clin. Immunol. 66*: 75-77.

Hensley, M. J., O'Cain, C. F., McFadden, E. R. Jr., and Ingram, R. H. Jr. (1978). Distribution of bronchodilatation in normal subjects: beta-agonist versus atropine. *J. Appl. Physiol. 45*: 778-782.

Holgate, S. T., Baldwin, C. J., and Tattersfield, A. E. (1977). Beta-adrenergic agonist resistance in normal human airways. *Lancet 2*: 375-377.

Holtzman, M. J., Sheller, J. R., DiMeo, M., Nadel, J. A., and Boushey, H. A. (1980). Effect of ganglionic blockade on bronchial reactivity in atopic subjects. *Am. Rev. Respir. Dis. 122*: 17-25.

Hruby, J., and Butler, J. (1975). Variability of routine pulmonary function tests. *Thorax 30*: 548-553.

Hughes, R., May, A. J., and Widdicombe, J. G. (1959). Stress relaxation in rabbits' lungs. *J. Physiol. 146*: 85-97.

Hui, K. K. P., Conolly, M. E., and Tashkin, D. P. (1982). Reversal of human lymphocyte β-adrenoceptor desensitization by glucocorticoids. *Clin. Pharmacol. Ther. 32*: 566-571.

Hume, K. M., and Gandevia, B. (1957). Forced expiratory volume before and after isoprenaline. *Thorax 12*: 276-278.

Hutcheon, M., Griffin, P., Levison, H., and Zamel, N. (1974). A new test in detection of mild abnormalities of lung mechanics. *Am. Rev. Respir. Dis. 110*: 458-465.

Hyatt, R. E., and Flath, R. E. (1966). Influence of lung parenchyma on pressure-diameter behavior of dog bronchi. *J. Appl. Physiol. 21*: 1448-1452.

Ingram, R. H., Jr., and McFadden, E. R. Jr. (1977). Localization and mechanisms of airway responses. *N. Engl. J. Med. 297*: 596-600.

Ingram, R. H., Jr., Wellman, J. J., McFadden, E. R. Jr., and Mead, J. (1977). Relative contributions of large and small airways to flow limitation in normal subjects before and after atropine and isoproterenol. *J. Clin. Invest. 59*: 696-703.

The Intermittent Positive Pressure Breathing Trial Group (1983). Intermittent positive pressure breathing therapy of chronic obstructive pulmonary disease. A clinical trial. *Ann. Intern. Med. 99*: 612-620.

Intermountain Thoracic Society Pulmonary Function Task Force (1984). *Clinical Pulmonary Function Testing,* 2nd edition. Edited by A. H. Morris, R. E. Kanner, R. O. Crapo, and R. M. Gardner. Salt Lake City, Intermountain Thoracic Society.

Jenne, J. W., Chick, T. W., Strickland, R. D., and Wall, F. J. (1977). Subsensitivity of beta responses during therapy with a long-acting beta-2 preparation. *J. Allergy Clin. Immunol. 59*: 383-390.

Kamburoff, P. L., and Günthner, W. (1975). Dose-dependent effects of Sch 1000 MDI on the airways resistance indices in patients with chronic airways obstruction. *Postgrad. Med. J. 51*(Suppl 7): 97.

Kepron, W., James, J. M., Kirk, B., Sehon, A. H., and Tse, K. S. (1977). A canine model for reaginic hypersensitivity and allergic bronchoconstriction. *J. Allergy Clin. Immunol. 59*: 64-69.

Klock, L. E., Miller, T. D., Morris, A. H., Watanabe, S., and Dickman, M. (1975). A comparative study of atropine sulfate and isoproterenol hydrochloride in chronic bronchitis. *Am. Rev. Respir. Dis. 112*: 371-376.

Knudson, R. J., and Constantine, H. P. (1967). An effect of isoproterenol on ventilation-perfusion in asthmatic vs. normal subjects. *J. Appl. Physiol. 22*: 402-406.

Laitinen, L. A., Empey, D. W., Poppius, H., Lemen, R. J., Gold, W. M., and Nadel, J. A. (1976). Effects of intravenous histamine on static lung compliance and airway resistance in normal man. *Am. Rev. Respir. Dis. 114*: 291-295.

Landahl, H. D., Tracewell, T. N., and Lassen, W. H. (1951). On the retention of air-borne particulates in the human lung. II. *Arch. Ind. Hyg. Occup. Med. 3*: 359-366.

Larsson, S., and Svedmyr, N. (1977). Bronchodilating effect and side effects of beta$_2$-adrenoceptor stimulants by different modes of administration (tablets, metered aerosol, and combinations thereof). A study with salbutamol in asthmatics. *Am. Rev. Respir. Dis. 116*: 861-869.

Leith, D. E., and Mead, J. (1974). *Principles of Body Plethysmography.* Bethesda, MD, National Heart and Lung Institute.

Light, R. W., Conrad, S. A., and George, R. B. (1977). The one best test for evaluating the effects of bronchodilator therapy. *Chest 72*: 512-516.

Lindgren, S. B., Formgren, H., and Morén, F. (1980). Improved aerosol therapy of asthma: effect of actuator tube size on drug availability. *Eur. J. Respir. Dis. 61*: 56-61.

Littner, M. R., Schachter, E. N., and Bouhuys, A. (1979). Modification of induced airway constriction in healthy subjects. *Ann. Allergy 43*: 135-143.

Littner, M. R., Tashkin, D. P., Siegel, S. C., and Katz, R. (1983). Double-blind comparison of acute effects of inhaled albuterol, isoproterenol and placebo on cardiopulmonary function and gas exchange in asthmatic children. *Ann. Allergy 50*: 309-316.

Lloyd, T. C. Jr. (1963). Bronchoconstriction in man following single deep inspirations. *J. Appl. Physiol. 18*: 114-116.

Lonky, S. A., and Tisi, G. M. (1980). Determining changes in airway caliber in asthma: the role of submaximal expiratory flow rates. *Chest 77*: 741-748.

Loren, M., Chai, H., Miklich, D., and Barwise, G. (1977). Comparison between simple nebulization and intermittent positive-pressure in asthmatic children with severe bronchospasm. *Chest 72*: 145-147.

Luparello, T., Lyons, H. A., Bleecker, E. R., and McFadden, E. R. Jr. (1968). Influence of suggestion on airway reactivity in asthmatic subjects. *Psychosom. Med. 30*: 819-825.

Macklem, P. T., and Wilson, N. J. (1965). Measurement of intrabronchial pressure in man. *J. Appl. Physiol. 20*: 653-663.

Marini, J. J., and Lakshminarayan, S. (1980). The effect of atropine inhalation in "irreversible" chronic bronchitis. *Chest 77*: 591-596.

Matthay, R. A., Berger, H. J., Loke, J., Gottschalk, A., and Zaret, B. L. (1978). Effects of aminophylline upon right and left ventricular performance in chronic obstructive pulmonary disease. *Am. J. Med. 65*: 903-910.

McCarthy, D. S., and Sigurdson, M. (1980). Lung elastic recoil and reduced airflow in clinically stable asthma. *Thorax 35*: 298-302.

McFadden, E. R. Jr., Ingram, R. H. Jr., Haynes, R. L., and Wellman, J. J. (1977). Predominant site of flow limitation and mechanisms of postexertional asthma. *J. Appl. Physiol. 42*: 746-752.

McFadden, E. R. Jr., and Lyons, H. A. (1969). Serial studies of factors influencing airway dynamics during recovery from acute asthma attacks. *J. Appl. Physiol. 27*: 452-459.

McFadden, E. R. Jr., Newton-Howes, J., and Pride, N. B. (1970). Acute effects of inhaled isoproterenol on the mechanical characteristics of the lungs in normal man. *J. Clin. Invest. 49*: 779-790.

McGavin, C. R., Cupta, S. P., and McHardy, G. J. R. (1976). Twelve-minute walking test for assessing disability in chronic bronchitis. *Br. Med. J. 1*: 822-823.

McGavin, C. R., Artvinli, M., Naoe, H., and McHardy, G. J. R. (1978). Dyspneoea, disability and distance walked: Comparison of estimates of exercise performance in respiratory disease. *Br. Med. J. 2*: 241-245.

McWilliams, B. C., Menendez, R., Kelly, H. W., and Howick, J. (1984). Effects of theophylline on inhaled methacholine and histamine in asthmatic children. *Am. Rev. Respir. Dis. 130*: 193-197.

Mead, J. (1960). Volume displacement body plethysmograph for respiratory measurements in human subjects. *J. Appl. Physiol. 15*: 736-740.

Mead, J., Turner, J. M., Macklem, P. T., and Little, J. B. (1967). Significance of the relationship between lung recoil and maximum expiratory flow. *J. Appl. Physiol. 22*: 95-108.

Meadows, J. A. III, Rodarte, J. R., and Hyatt, R. E. (1980). Density dependence of maximal expiratory flow in chronic obstructive pulmonary disease. *Am. Rev. Respir. Dis. 121*: 47-53.

Midha, K. K., Sved, S., Hossie, R. D., and McGilveray, I. J. (1977). High performance liquid chromatographic and mass spectrometric identification of dimethylxanthine metabolites of caffeine in human plasma. *Biomed. Mass Spectrom. 4*: 172-177.

Miller, W. C., and Rice, D. L. (1980). A comparison of oral terbutaline and fenoterol in asthma. *Ann. Allergy 44*: 15-18.

Miller, W. C., and Simi, W. W. (1976). Clinical application of quiet breathing airway resistance. *J. Asthma Res. 13*: 137-141.

Milliken, G. A., and Johnson, D. E. (1984). *Analysis of Messy Data.* Belmont, CA, Lifetime Learning Publications.

Mitenko, P. A., and Ogilvie, R. I. (1973). Rational intravenous doses of theophylline. *N. Engl. J. Med. 289*: 600-603.

Morén, F., and Andersson, J. (1980). Fraction of dose exhaled after administration of pressurized inhalation aerosols. *Int. J. Pharmacol. 6*: 295-300.

Muir, D. C. F., and Davies, C. N. (1967). The deposition of 0.5 μm diameter aerosols in the lungs of man. *Ann. Occup. Hyg. 10*: 161-174.

Murciano, D., Aubier, M., Lecocguic, Y., and Pariente, R. (1984). Effects of theophylline on diaphragmatic strength and fatigue in patients with chronic obstructive pulmonary disease. *N. Engl. J. Med. 311*: 349-353.

Nadel, J. A., and Tierney, D. F. (1961). Effect of a previous deep inspiration on airway resistance in man. *J. Appl. Physiol. 16*: 717-719.

Nelson, H. S., Raine, D. Jr., Doner, H. C., and Posey, W. C. (1977). Subsensitivity to the bronchodilator action of albuterol produced by chronic administration. *Am. Rev. Respir. Dis. 116*: 871-878.

Nelson, H. S., Spector, S. L., Whitsett, T. L., George, R. B., and Dwek, J. H. (1983). The bronchodilator response to inhalation of increasing doses of aerosolized albuterol. *J. Allergy Clin. Immunol. 72*: 371-375.

Newcomb, R., Tashkin, D. P., Hui, K. K., Conolly, M. E., Lee, E., and Daupinee, B. (1985). Rebound hyperresponsiveness to muscarinic stimulation after chronic therapy with an inhaled muscarinic antagonist. *Am. Rev. Respir. Dis. 132*: 12-15.

Newman, S. P., Morén, F., Pavia, D., Little, F., and Clarke, S. W. (1981). Deposition of pressurized suspension aerosols inhaled through extension devices. *Am. Rev. Respir. Dis. 124*: 317-320.

Newman, S. P., Pavia, D., and Clarke, S. W. (1982). Kinetics of the inhaled route. In: *New Concepts in the Topical Treatment of Asthma and Related Disorders.* London, Cliggott Publishing Company, pp. 5-9.

Orehek, J., Charpin, D., Velardocchio, J. M., and Grimaud, C. (1980). Bronchomotor effect of bronchoconstriction-induced deep inspirations in asthmatics. *Am. Rev. Respir. Dis. 121*: 297-305.

Orehek, J., Nicoli, M. M., Delpierre, S., and Beaupré, A. (1981). Influence of the previous deep inspiration on the spirometric measurement of provoked bronchoconstriction in asthma. *Am. Rev. Respir. Dis. 123*: 269-272.

Palmer, K. N. V. (1971). Effect of bronchodilator drugs on arterial blood gas tensions in bronchial asthma. *Postgrad. Med. J. 47*(Suppl): 75-77.

Paré, P. D., Lawson, L. M., and Brooks, L. A. (1983). Patterns of response to inhaled bronchodilators in asthmatics. *Am. Rev. Respir. Dis. 127*: 680-685.

Partridge, M. R., and Saunders, K. B. (1981). Site of action of ipratropium bromide and clinical and physiological determinants of response in patients with asthma. *Thorax 36*: 530-533.

Pavia, D., Thomson, M. L., Clarke, S. W., and Shannon, H. S. (1977). Effect of lung function and mode of inhalation on penetration of aerosol into the human lung. *Thorax 32*: 194-197.

Pennock, B. E., Rogers, R. M., and McCaffree, D. R. (1981). Changes in measured spirometric indices. What is significant? *Chest 80*: 97-99.

Pierce, R. J., Payne, C. R., Williams, S. J., Denison, D. M., and Clark, T. J. H. (1981). Comparison of intravenous and inhaled terbutaline in the treatment of asthma. *Chest 79*: 506-511.

Plummer, A. L. (1978). The development of drug tolerance to beta$_2$-adrenergic agents. *Chest 73*(Suppl): 949-958.

Poppius, H. (1980). Inhalation of terbutaline spray through an extended mouthpiece. *Respiration 40*: 278-283.

Pride, N. B., Permutt, S., Riley, R. L., and Bromberger Barnea, B. (1967). Determinants of maximal expiratory flow from the lungs. *J. Appl. Physiol. 23*: 646.

Rall, T. W. (1980). Central nervous system stimulants. The xanthines. In: *The Pharmacological Basis of Therapeutics,* 6th ed. Edited by A. G. Gilman, L. S. Goodman and A. Gilman. New York, MacMillan, pp. 592-607.

Ramsdell, J. W., and Tisi, G. M. (1979). Determination of bronchodilation in the clinical pulmonary function laboratory. Role of changes in static lung volumes. *Chest 76*: 622-628.

Rebuck, A. S., and Read, J. (1971). Assessment and management of severe asthma. *Am. J. Med. 51*: 788-798.

Riley, D. J., Liu, R. T., and Edelman, N. H. (1979). Enhanced responses to aerosolized bronchodilator therapy in asthma using respiratory maneuvers. *Chest 76*: 501-507.

Rodenstein, D., Stanescu, D. C., Cauberghs, M., and van de Woestijne, K. P. (1981). Failure of body plethysmography to accurately measure lung volume in bronchial obstruction. *Am. Rev. Respir. Dis. 123* (abstract): 88.

Rogers, R. M., Owens, G. R., and Pennock, B. E. (1985). The pendulum swings again. Toward a rational use of theophylline (Editorial). *Chest 87*: 280-282.

Ruffin, R. E., McIntyre, E., Crockett, A. J., Zielonka, K., and Alpers, J. H. (1982). Combination bronchodilator therapy in asthma. *J. Allergy Clin. Immunol. 69*: 60-65.

Ruffin, R. E., Kenworthy, M. C., and Newhouse, M. T. (1978). Response of asthmatic patients to fenoterol inhalation: A method of quantifying the airway bronchodilator dose. *Clin. Pharmacol. Ther. 23*: 338-345.

Samuelson, W. M., and Davies, A. O. (1984). Hydrocortisone-induced reversal of beta-adrenergic receptor uncoupling. *Am. Rev. Respir. Dis. 130*: 1023-1026.

Schilder, D. P., Roberts, A., and Fry, D. L. (1963). Effect of gas density and viscosity on the maximal expiratory flow-volume relationship. *J. Clin. Invest. 42*: 1705-1713.

Sherter, C. B., Connolly, J. J., and Schilder, D. P. (1978). The significance of volume-adjusting the maximal midexpiratory flow in assessing the response to a bronchodilator drug. *Chest 73*: 568-571.

Siegel, S. (1956). *Nonparametric Statistics for the Behavioral Sciences.* New York, McGraw-Hill Book Company.

Simmons, M., Gong, H. Jr., Tashkin, D. P., Hui, K., and Lee. E. (1983). Bronchodilator effects of coffee in asthmatics. *Chest 84*: 332 (abstract).

Simonsson, B. G., Jacobs, F. M., and Nadel, J. A. (1967). Role of autonomic nervous system and the cough reflex in the increased responsiveness of airways in patients with obstructive airway disease. *J. Clin. Invest. 46*: 1812-1818.

Simonsson, B. G., Jonson, B., and Ström, B. (1975). Bronchodilatory and circulatory effects of inhaling increasing doses of an anti-cholinergic drug, ipratropium bromide (Sch 1000). *Scand, J. Respir. Dis. 56*: 138-149.

Smelzer, T. H., and Barnett, T. B. (1973). Bronchodilator aerosol. Comparison of administration methods. *JAMA 223*: 884-889.

Smith, J. A., Weber, R. W., and Nelson, H. S. (1980). Theophylline and aerosolized terbutaline in the treatment of bronchial asthma. Double-blind comparison of optimal doses. *Chest 78*: 816-818.

Snedecor, G. W., and Cochran, W. G. (1980). *Statistical Methods,* 7th edition, Iowa City, The Iowa State University Press.

Sobol, B. J., Emirgil, C., and Wadhwani, B. (1969). The uncertain relationship between airway conductance and lung volume. *Am. Rev. Respir. Dis. 100*: 350-356.

Souhrada, J. F., and Dickey, D. W. (1976). Mechanical activities of trachea as measured *in vitro* and *in vivo*. *Respir. Physiol. 26*: 27-40.

Sourk, R. L., and Nugent, K. M. (1983). Bronchodilator testing: Confidence intervals derived from placebo inhalations. *Am. Rev. Respir. Dis. 128*: 153-157.

Spector, S. L. ed. (1983). *Provocative Challenge Procedures: Bronchial, Oral, Nasal, and Exercise,* Vols. I and II. Boca Raton, FL, CRC Press, Inc.

Spector, S. L. (1978). Effect of beta-adrenergic agents on skin test responses and bronchial challenge responses. *Chest 73*(Suppl): 976-977.

Spicer, J. E., Cayton, R. M., Frame, M. H., and Winsey, N. J. P. (1980). Influence of tube-spacer on aerosol efficacy. *Lancet 2*: 1248.

Stamm, A. M., Clausen, J. L., and Tisi, G. M. (1976). Effect of aerosolized isoproterenol on resting myogenic tone in normals. *J. Appl. Physiol. 40*: 525-532.

Storms, W. W., DoPico, G. A., and Reed, C. E. (1975). Aerosol Sch 1000. An anticholinergic bronchodilator. *Am. Rev. Respir. Dis. 111*: 419-422.

Stuart, B. O. (1973). Deposition of inhaled aerosols. *Arch. Intern. Med. 131*: 60-73.

Sved, S., Hossie, R. D., and McGilveray, I. J. (1976). The human metabolism of caffeine to theophylline. *Res. Commun. Chem. Pathol. Pharmacol. 13*: 185-192.

Svedmyr, N., and Svedmyr, K. (1980). In-vitro and in-vivo effects of theophylline and β_2-adrenostimulants in combination. *Eur. J. Respir. Dis. 61* (Suppl 109): 83-91.

Szentivanyi, A. (1968). The beta adrenergic theory of the atopic abnormality in bronchial asthma. *J. Allergy 42*: 203-232.

Tai, E., and Read, J. (1967). Response of blood gas tensions to aminophylline and isoprenaline in patients with asthma. *Thorax 22*: 543-549.

Taplin, G. V., Tashkin, D. P., Chopra, S. K., Anselmi, O. E., Elam, D., Calvarese,

B., Coulson, A., Detels, R., and Rokaw, S. N. (1977). Early detection of chronic obstructive pulmonary disease using radionuclide lung imaging procedures. *Chest 71*: 567-575.

Tashkin, D. P., Conolly, M. E., Deutsch, R. I., Hui, K. K., Littner, M., Scarpace, P., and Abrass, I. (1982). Subsensitization of beta-adrenoceptors in airways and lymphocytes of healthy and asthmatic subjects. *Am. Rev. Respir. Dis. 125*: 185-193.

Tashkin, D. P., Trevor, E., Chopra, S. K., and Taplin, G. V. (1980). Sites of airway dilatation in asthma following inhaled vs. subcutaneous terbutaline: Comparison of physiologic tests with radionuclide lung images. *Am. J. Med. 68*: 14-26.

Tattersfield, A. E., Leaver, D. G., and Pride, N. B. (1973). Effects of β-adrenergic blockade and stimulation on normal human airways. *J. Appl. Physiol. 35*: 613-619.

Tobin, M. J., Jenouri, G., Danta, I., Kim, C., Watson, H., and Sackner, M. A. (1982). Response to bronchodilator drug administration by a new reservoir aerosol delivery system and a review of other auxiliary delivery systems. *Am. Rev. Respir. Dis. 126*: 670-675.

Ullah, M. I., Newman, G. B., and Saunders, K. B. (1981). Influence of age on response to ipratropium and salbutamol in asthma. *Thorax 36*: 523-529.

Vincent, N. J., Knudson, R., Leith, D. E., Macklem, P. T., and Mead. J. (1970). Factors influencing pulmonary resistance. *J. Appl. Physiol. 29*: 236-243.

Watanabe, S., Renzetti, A. D. Jr., Begin, R., and Bigler, A. H. (1974). Airway responsiveness to a bronchodilator aerosol. I. Normal human subjects. *Am. Rev. Respir. Dis. 109*: 530-537.

Wellman, J. J., McFadden, E. R., Jr., and Ingram, R. H., Jr. (1976). Density-dependence of maximal expiratory flow rates before and after bronchodilators in patients with obstructive airways disease. *Clin. Sci. Mol. Med. 51*: 133-139.

Williams, M. H., Jr., and Kane, C. (1975). Dose response of patients with asthma to inhaled isoproterenol. *Am. Rev. Respir. Dis. 111*: 321-324.

Winer, B. J. (1971). *Statistical Principles in Experimental Design.* New York, McGraw-Hill Book Company.

Wolfe, J. D., Tashkin, D. P., Calvarese, B., and Simmons, M. (1978). Bronchodilator effects of terbutaline and aminophylline alone and in combination in asthmatic patients. *N. Engl. J. Med. 298*: 363-367.

Wood, M. J., and Paterson, J. W. (1975). Evaluation of cumulative doses of Sch 1000 in asthmatics (abstract). *Postgrad. Med. J. 51*(Suppl 7): 100.

Woolcock, A. J., Macklem, P. T., Hogg, J. C., and Wilson, N. J. (1969). Influence of autonomic nervous system on airway resistance and elastic recoil. *J. Appl. Physiol. 26*: 814-818.

Woolcock, A. J., and Read, J. (1965). Improvement in bronchial asthma not reflected in forced expiratory volume. *Lancet 2*: 1323-1325.

Woolcock, A. J., and Read, J. (1966). Lung volumes in exacerbations of asthma. *Am. J. Med. 41*: 259-273.

Wright, B. M., and McKerrow, C. B. (1959). Maximum forced expiratory flow rate as a measure of ventilatory capacity. *Br. Med. J. 2*(2): 1041-1047.

Yeager, H. Jr., Weinberg, R. M., Kaufman, L. V., and Katz, S. (1976). Asthma: Comparative bronchodilator effects of ipratropium bromide and isoproterenol. *J. Clin. Pharmacol. 16*: 198-204.

Zamel, N., Hughes, D., Levison, H., Fairshter, R. D., and Gelb, A. F. (1983). Partial and complete maximum expiratory flow-volume curves in asthmatic patients with spontaneous bronchospasm. *Chest 83*: 35-39.

Zeck, R. T., Solliday, N. H., Celic, L., and Cugell, D. W. (1981). Variability of the volume of isoflow. *Chest 79*: 269-272.

16

Anticholinergic Agents

NICHOLAS J. GROSS and MORTON S. SKORODIN

Loyola-Stritch School of Medicine
Maywood, and Edward Hines, Jr.
Veterans Administration Hospital
Hines, Illinois

I. Introduction

Various plant preparations have been used for the treatment of respiratory disorders for many centuries. For the most part the plants belong to the *Datura* genus and the active ingredients are atropine and closely related alkaloids, which have potent and more or less specific antimuscarinic properties. Detailed descriptions and indications for their use exist in 17th century writings from the Indian subcontinent, but their use in other parts of the world goes back at least as far (Gandevia, 1975). Parts of the plant, typically the leaves of *Datura stramonium*, were smoked as a cigar or cigarette; in addition to the salutary affects of this practice on airways obstruction, not unpleasant psychotropic effects occurred which probably did not decrease its acceptability. In fact, stramonium smoking was as much recreational as medicinal.

The British in India took up its uses in the late 18th century and in 1802 a General Gent returned to England with some pulverized roots of *Datura ferox* which his physician friend, a Dr. Sims, found to be of dramatic benefit in his asthmatic relatives and patients. This appears to have been the introduction of this class of drugs to European medicine. The *Datura* genus grows in Europe and its use for respiratory purposes developed rapidly within and outside the medical profession. By the second half of the 19th century its use was widespread and endorsed by standard medical texts. Until well into the present century these agents, although somewhat crude in preparation, were the major and only effective bronchodilators available.

The discovery of epinephrine and the development of adrenergic agents in the first decades of the 20th century shifted attention away from the atropine-like preparations and their use all but disappeared. However, in the last 20 years interest in anticholinergic bronchodilators has revived. This is due in part to a clearer understanding of the role of the parasympathetic system in the control of airway tone, and in part to the development by the pharmaceutical industry of synthetic congeners of atropine that lack many of atropine's undesirable side effects.

II. Anatomy of the Parasympathetic System in the Lungs

A. Autonomic Nerves

The rationale for the use of anticholinergic agents as bronchodilators is based on the concept that bronchomotor activity in the human airways is largely due to cholinergic parasympathetic drive. Abolition of this parasympathetic drive by competition at muscarinic receptors results in bronchodilatation. The anatomy of the autonomic innervation of the lungs is complex and still not completely elucidated; the following is a simplification of our current understanding of its organization (Richardson and Ferguson, 1979; Richardson and Beland, 1976; Jeffery, 1981).

Parasympathetic innervation of the lungs is supplied by the vagus nerves. Branches of the vagus enter the lung at the hila and travel into the lung along the posterior walls of the airways. These preganglionic fibers end at peribronchial ganglia in the large and medium-sized airways where their terminals synapse with cell bodies of the postganglionic parasympathetic nerves. The axons of the postganglionic nerves travel a short distance to end at or close to effector cells in the airway wall, smooth muscle cells, mucus glands, possibly mast cells, and airway epithelial cells. These postganglionic terminals have been shown by histologic and histochemical studies to be cholinergic, and concentrated in the large and medium-sized airways. Activation of this vagal parasympathetic cholinergic system produces bronchoconstriction, mucus secretion, and ciliary activity among other effects. These effects are abolished by anticholinergic antimuscarinic agents such as atropine. Quantitatively, this is the predominant nerve supply to the airways in humans (Fig. 1).

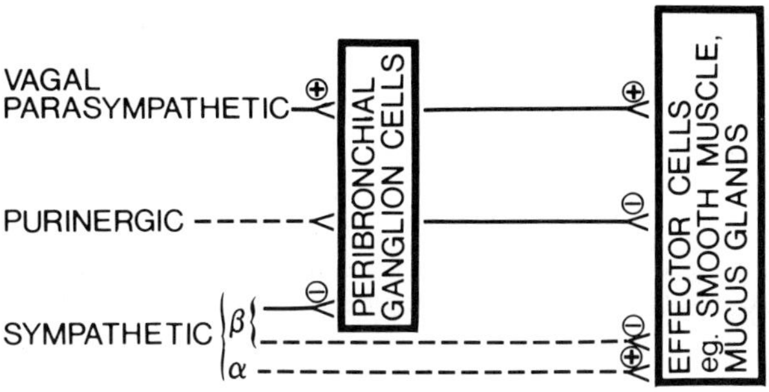

Figure 1 Diagrammatic representation of efferent autonomic innervation of human airways. +, excitatory; –, inhibitory; dashed lines, existence doubtful. (From Gross and Skorodin, 1984a, with permission.)

Beta-adrenergic nerves in the lung are present but sparse by comparison; they also enter the lungs at the hila and travel along the airways. Their terminals end on the ganglion cells of the peribronchial plexa. This affords one route by which the β-adrenergic system can influence airway tone, namely by modulating the activity of the parasympathetic system at the postganglionic cell. Beta-adrenergic nerves may also end directly on effector cells, smooth muscle, and others, but this is believed to be rare in the human.

Alpha-adrenergic nerves may also exist in the lung, although this is uncertain and based on indirect evidence. If present, their activation is presumed to result in smooth muscle contraction.

The third nervous system is probably the dominant inhibitor of smooth muscle contraction in humans and therefore of considerable clinical relevance (Richardson and Beland, 1976; Barnes, 1984). Its preganglionic fibers are believed to follow those of the vagal parasympathetic branches, and its postganglionic fibers terminate on smooth muscle cells where their activation results in long-lasting relaxation. This effect is not blocked by adrenergic or cholinergic blockade, hence the system is sometimes referred to as nonadrenergic noncholinergic (NANC). Such NANC nerves also stimulate mucus secretion (in the ferret trachea, at least), mediate relaxation of the pulmonary vasculature, and possibly inhibit mediator release from mast cells. The mediators of the third system are believed to be vasoactive intestinal peptide (VIP) and peptide histidine methionine (PHM).

Other neural pathways that affect airway function are known, such as collateral branches of afferent nerves that terminate on smooth muscle cells and release substance P and calcitonin gene-related peptide (CGRP), both of which are smooth muscle constrictors (Polak and Bloom, 1982; Pernow, 1983; Lundberg et al., 1983). The importance of these additional pathways in humans is uncertain.

The overall control of airway caliber by neural mechanisms in normal humans can be summarized as follows. Basal bronchomotor tone is due to parasympathetic cholinergic activity via the vagal efferents, acting on large and medium-sized airways. The α-adrenergic system, substance P terminals, and possibly other terminals that release bronchoactive substances may enhance bronchomotor tone from time to time, such as when irritant substances are inhaled. Bronchoconstrictor activity is opposed predominantly by the third NANC system acting directly on effector cells, and also to a lesser degree by the β-adrenergic system acting on the postganglionic cells of the parasympathetic system.

B. Autonomic Receptors in the Lungs

The neural pathways described above effect changes in airways by the liberation of mediators that bind to receptors on the effector cells. However, these receptors are also available for binding of circulating agents. Therefore, a description of the nerves in the lung, by itself, gives an incomplete picture of the autonomic control of airways function.

Autoradioligand studies of mammalian airways (Barnes et al., 1983a,b; Cheng and Townley, 1982) show that muscarinic receptors are found principally in the central airways, where they outnumber other receptors. In smaller airways and peripheral regions of the lung they are sparse and greatly outnumbered by other receptors. This corresponds to the distribution of cholinergic nerves (above) and to physiological evidence on the site of action of the parasympathetic system in the airways (below). As the mediator of the parasympathetic system, acetylcholine, is rapidly degraded by cholinesterases, which are ubiquitous, it is appropriate that muscarinic receptors are anatomically closely related to cholinergic terminals.

Alpha and β-adrenergic receptors are found mainly in the bronchioles where they are present in high density (Barnes et al., 1983a). Since the corresponding nerves are not found at this level, activation of these receptors presumably depends on circulating catecholamines. Less is known of the VIP receptors of the third system. Preliminary studies (Barnes, 1984) suggest that VIP receptors are widespread in the airways, where they are probably closely related to nerve terminals of this system.

There is evidence that in airway disease a relative increase in the number of α-adrenergic receptors is present (Barnes et al., 1980a,b). Analogous data for muscarinic receptors in humans with airways disease are not available at present. However active sensitization of guinea pigs does not affect either the density or affinity of lung muscarinic receptors (Cheng and Townley, 1983; Mita et al., 1983; Suzuki et al., 1985).

C. Muscarinic Receptor Biology

The nature of the muscarinic receptor is incompletely understood (Heilbronn and Bartfai, 1978); almost all the available information comes from tissues other than airways, which is unfortunate because the muscarinic receptor functions differently in different tissues. The affinity of the receptor for various antagonists in various tissues is high and constant (the dissociation constant is of the order of 10^{-10}M) suggesting a single binding site (Nathanson, 1982). However, its affinity for various agonists is lower and inconstant (dissociation constants are of the order of 10^{-5} to 10^{-7}M) suggesting either multiple binding sites or variable conformation. In the rat cerebral cortex there appear to be at least two binding sites which differ in affinity for agonists but not antagonists (Birdsall et al., 1978). Muscarinic receptor subtypes have been sought, but with little success until recently. It now appears that receptor subtypes may indeed exist, at least in the rat forebrain (Ellis and Lenox, 1985).

The receptor is regulated in ways that are common to other receptor systems; the receptor number can be reduced (down-regulated) by prolonged exposure to agonists (Noble et al., 1978; Siman and Klein, 1980), but not by antagonists (Shifrin and Klein, 1980). The kinetics of receptor loss and recovery suggest increased receptor breakdown; recovery follows over a period of hours or days and is blocked by inhibitors of protein synthesis. These features are typical of agonist-induced receptor endocytosis. In addition, other systems show a short-term decrease in responsiveness (desensitization) independent of receptor number that occurs and is reversed in minutes.

Relevant studies on the regulation of muscarinic receptors in the lung are sparse at present. Receptor number is highest in the first few weeks after birth in the rodent lung, and declines progressively through maturity and adult life (Suzuki et al., 1985). Parenteral administration of the muscarinic antagonist ipratropium for 10 days did not alter receptor density; but administration of a potent cholinesterase inhibitor decreased receptor density, and vagotomy increased receptor density. These findings, in lung, are entirely consistent with data from other tissues (above). Corticosteroids have been reported to have either no effect (Suzuki et al., 1985), or to increase the number of receptors (Marquardt et al., 1982). In none of these studies was receptor affinity altered.

The structure of the muscarinic receptor is under active study at present. Solubilization of membranes and ligand binding suggests that the receptor contains a single polypeptide of molecular weight 83,000-86,000 with a single binding site (Birdsall et al., 1979; Haga, 1980). Its biochemical action remains obscure; stimulation of cyclic GMP formation, stimulation of membrane phosphatidate and phosphatidyl inositol turnover, and calcium ion influx are observed cellular consequences of activation of the muscarinic receptor (Gold, 1980; Heilbronn and Bartfai, 1978; Salmon and Honeyman, 1980).

III. The Parasympathetic System in Airway Physiology

A. Cholinergic Control of Airway Smooth Muscle Tone

Normal airway caliber is determined by the level of bronchomotor tone: the degree of contraction of airway smooth muscle during resting or basal conditions. The level of bronchomotor tone can be altered in either direction in response to normal physiological requirements and various stimuli. A large body of evidence developed over the last two decades suggests that it is largely due to the level of tonic parasympathetic activity (Nadel, 1980; Widdicombe, 1977a). Much of this evidence is derived from animal experiments, which will be summarized below.

Electrical stimulation of the efferent vagi produces ipsilateral bronchoconstriction in a time scale of seconds (Colebatch and Halmagyi, 1963; Olsen et al., 1965; Woolcock et al., 1969), which suggests that it is due to smooth muscle contraction rather than some other mucosal effect. The bronchoconstriction is observed principally in the airways most abundantly innervated by cholinergic nerves: the large and medium-sized airways (Olsen et al., 1965; Nadel et al., 1971). It is associated with acetylcholine release (Carlyle, 1963), blocked by blocking vagal conduction distal to stimulation (Martinez et al., 1961; Colebatch and Halmagyi, 1963; Olsen et al., 1965; Karczewski and Widdicombe, 1969), or by atropine (Nadel and Widdicombe, 1963; Vincent et al., 1970), potentiated by cholinesterase inhibitors (Colebatch and Halmagyi, 1963; Olsen et al., 1965), and mimicked by acetylcholine analogues such as methacholine. By contrast, electrical stimulation of sympathetic fibers results in slow bronchodilatation (Dixon and Ransom, 1912) whose extent depends on the level of vagal tone; sympathetic stimulation has the most bronchodilator effect when vagal tone is present and little or no such effect when vagal activity is blocked (Cabezas et al., 1971). Moreover, β-adrenergic blockade has little bronchoconstrictor effect when vagal activity is normal (Zaid and Beall, 1966; DeKock, 1970; Tattersfield et al., 1973; Zuskin et al., 1974), or has been abolished by atropine (DeKock, 1970; MacDonald et al., 1967; Langer, 1967; Greico and Pierson, 1971), and results in significant bronchoconstriction only in conditions where vagal activity may be greater than normal (McNeill and Ingram, 1966; Richardson and Sterling, 1969). These findings suggest that the sympathetic system works through the parasympathetic system, that is, sympathetic bronchodilatation of normal airways depends on a level of parasympathetic tone. This scheme is in keeping with the anatomy of the autonomic innervation of the airways (above). It gives the parasympathetic system a central role in controlling airway caliber.

However, many additional factors complicate the picture. How important are nonparasympathetic bronchoconstrictor mechanisms, α-adrenergic nerves,

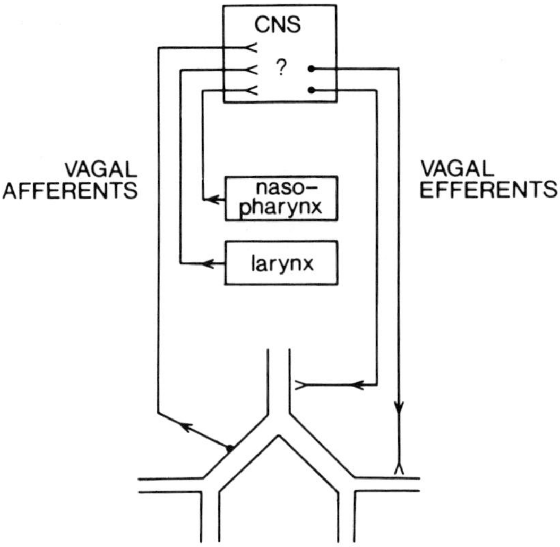

Figure 2 Diagrammatic representation of vagal reflex pathways from irritant receptors through vagal efferents, central nervous system (CNS), and vagal efferents to effector cells in the airway (from Gross and Skorodin, 1984a, with permission).

and substance P terminals, for example? or humoral factors that may act directly on effector cells? Most importantly, how is this scheme altered in disease states where airway obstruction may be due to numerous factors other than bronchomotor tone? Much uncertainty surrounds these issues.

Given that the vagal parasympathetic system exerts important effects on airways caliber we will consider ways in which its activity is controlled. Little is known of the function and connections of the vagal nuclei in the brain stem. Presumably they receive input from higher centers because "psychogenic asthma" appears to be mediated through vagal efferents (below). The vagal nuclei also receive input from the pulmonary vagal afferents which thus form the afferent limb of a reflex arc whose motor limb is the vagal efferent supply (Fig. 2).

B. Vagal Reflexes

Vagal afferents originate in a wide field that includes the entire respiratory tract and parts of the gastrointestinal tract. Reflex bronchospasm can result from stimuli originating anywhere in this territory: the nasopharynx (Nadel and Widdicombe, 1962; Tomori and Widdicombe, 1969; Allison et al., 1974), larynx (Nadel and Widdicombe, 1962; Boushey et al., 1972, 1974), the airways (Nadel et al., 1965; Widdicombe, 1954, 1977a; Sellick and Widdicombe, 1971; Mills et al., 1970), and probably the esophagus (Mansfield et al., 1981). At least two types of receptors of vagal afferent nerves are described: rapidly adapting "irritant receptors" located beneath the tight junctions between epithelial cells

(Widdicombe, 1954, 1977b), and nonmyelinated C fibers also in the epithelium (Colebatch and Halmagyi, 1963). Stimuli that act through these pathways include mechanical, physical, chemical, and immunologic stimuli are discussed below.

The experimental evidence supporting reflex bronchospasm via this vagal afferent and efferent arc is strong; it is set out in detail in reviews such as those by Widdicombe (1979) and Nadel (1980). For example, sulfur dioxide delivered to the isolated upper airways results in constriction of the lower airways (Nadel et al., 1965); allergen delivered to only one lung produces bilateral bronchoconstriction (Gold et al., 1972); histamine-produced bronchoconstriction is largely prevented by vagotomy (DeKock et al., 1966); or by atropine or the ganglion-blocking agent hexamethonium, but the effect of the muscarinic receptor agonist methacholine is blocked by atropine and not hexamethonium (Holtzman et al., 1980). While it is clear that reflex bronchospasm can be demonstrated in animal and human experiments, the question remains as to how important this reflex is in clinical situations.

C. Site of Anticholinergic-Mediated Bronchodilatation

Tests of small vs. large airways function, respiratory dead space, and static lung recoil have been used to determine the site of anticholinergically mediated bronchodilatation in normal humans and subjects with airway disease. Some investigators have found that anticholinergic agents produce effects throughout the tracheobronchial system down to the terminal lung units in normal subjects (De Troyer et al., 1979) and patients with airway disease (Partridge and Saunders, 1981; Douglas et al., 1979). Others have found their effects to be concentrated on the central airways in both normal (Ingram et al., 1977; Hensley et al., 1978) and asthmatic subjects (Ashutosh et al., 1980; McFadden et al., 1977). However, the route of administration is obviously important, since it determines where and in what concentration the agent is able to act. Inhaled atropine has its greatest effect on central airways; after intravenous administration its effect is more uniform than when inhaled (De Troyer et al., 1979; Weiss et al., 1982; Holzman et al., 1983; Sheppard et al., 1983) but possibly still not as marked on small airways as that of β-adrenergic agents, whose effect is concentrated on small airways.

IV. Pharmacology of Anticholinergic Agents

A. Structure

The anticholinergic bronchodilators are antagonists of the muscarinic effects of acetylcholine. The prototype is atropine whose action is regarded as highly specific for muscarinic receptors. Both agonists and antagonists of muscarinic receptors have an ammonium group and an ester linkage 4.3-4.4 Å apart that are

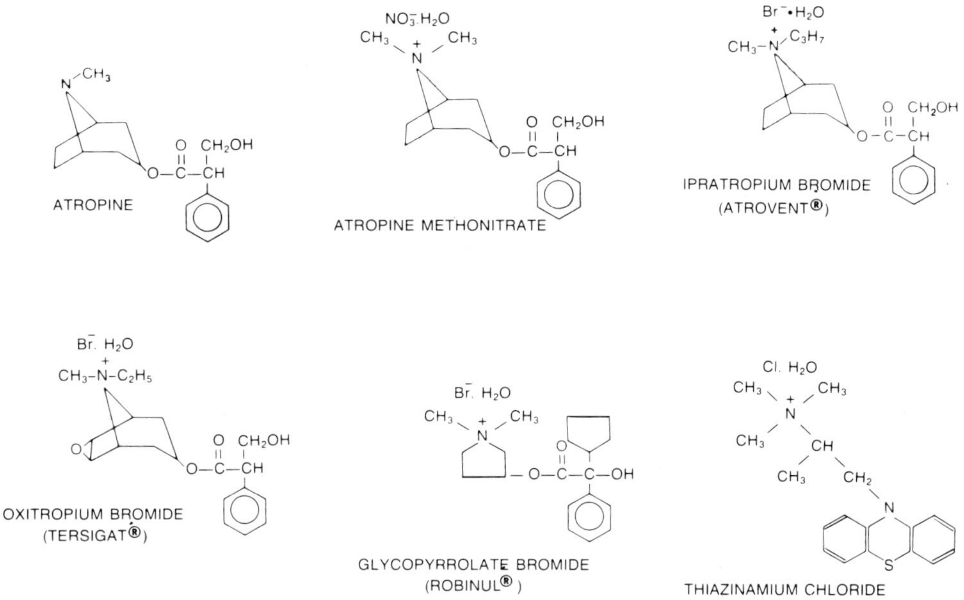

Figure 3 Structural formulas of atropine and some quaternary ammonium congeners. The ammonium group responsible for major differences between tertiary and quaternary compounds is in the upper left corner of each agent.

considered essential for binding to the receptor (Beers and Reich, 1970). Antagonists therefore probably compete with acetylcholine for the same binding site. The structure of atropine and its congeners (Fig. 3) typically consists of tropic acid esterified with an aromatic ring compound, tropine, nortropine, or scopine. Antimuscarinic agents with quite different structures exist (Weiner, 1980); these tend to be less specific than atropine.

One other important structural feature of anticholinergic agents is the valence of the nitrogen atom of the ammonium group; this determines the diffusibility of the molecule across membranes and, therefore, its distribution. Atropine and scopolamine are naturally occurring tertiary ammonium compounds, all of which are well absorbed from mucosal surfaces and cross membranes such as the blood-brain barrier. Quaternary ammonium compounds are synthetic congeners and carry a charge on the ammonium group. They therefore cross membrane barriers with difficulty (Levine, 1959).

B. Pharmacokinetics and Distribution

The parent compound is atropine, an alkaloid base. Atropine itself is almost insoluble but its salts (e.g., sulfate), are freely soluble in water, the solution being a little to the acid side of neutral. The pharmacology and pharmacokinetics of atropine are very well known and covered extensively in the standard texts. Atropine sulfate is well absorbed from the respiratory and alimentary mucosae (less well from the skin), and peak concentrations are reached within an hour. Following inhalation the blood level varies widely between subjects (an order of magnitude on either side of about 1 ng/ml) and corresponds poorly with the degree of bronchodilatation that results (Kradjan et al., 1981). After intramuscular administration in humans peak blood levels occur at 15-20 min (Kalser, 1971), the volume of distribution is about 10 times the blood volume, which suggests rapid equilibration between fluid compartments. Disappearance of atropine from the serum is variable, possibly due to genetic factors (Kalser, 1971); the serum half-life has been reported as approximately 3 hr in young adults and two to three times longer in children and the elderly (Virtanen et al., 1982). Atropine is largely excreted in the urine, mostly unchanged, within 24 hr. In lactating women, traces of atropine appear in breast milk. These properties are probably common to all tertiary ammonium congeners of atropine.

The pharmacologic properties of quaternary ammonium congener bronchodilators have been well studied only in the case of N-isopropyl-nortropine-tropic acid ester methyl bromide (ipratropium bromide, Atrovent) (Deckers, 1975; Wahl, 1975; Adlung et al., 1976; Rominger, 1979). It is freely soluble in water. Following oral administration peak blood levels, corresponding to only 0.2% of the administered dose, are reached in 2-3 hr, indicating poor absorption. Absorption may be higher in the case of other quaternary ammonium agents (Levine, 1959; Jonkman et al., 1977). Following inhalation of ipratropium, the peak level occurs at a similar time and corresponds to only 0.5% of the dose. The effective dosage for bronchodilatation is much lower following inhalation than other routes. The half-life in the blood is 1.5-4 hr, with a mean of about 3 hr. Its effect on the airways is longer and exceeds that of atropine. Over 90% of the orally administered dose is recovered in the feces. The remainder is converted to a number of inactive metabolites that appear in the urine (Deckers, 1975). Distribution studies show that ipratropium is largely excluded from the central nervous system. These properties are probably shared by other quaternary ammonium anticholinergic agents.

C. Specificity and Selectivity

Atropine is highly specific for muscarinic receptors. Related compounds in general have very similar actions; the search for receptor subtypes that has proved so fruitful in the field of adrenergic agents has been disappointing. Minor differences in specificity for gastrointestinal effects have been detected (Dotevall et al., 1982). In the respiratory field, among a range of atropine congeners ipratropium has been reported to have the most favorable ratio of bronchodilatation to inhibition of salivary secretion (Engelhardt and Klupp, 1975; Engelhardt, 1979), and almost no effect on respiratory mucociliary function at equivalent blood levels (Sackner et al., 1977a). At high blood levels quaternary ammonium congeners exhibit antinicotinic effects such as ganglion blockade and curariform neuromuscular blockade. Other, structurally distant agents, have less potent antimuscarinic effects and may have other actions. For example, thiazinamium chloride, a derivative of promethazine, has antiallergic as well as antimuscarinic properties (Lewis et al., 1982, 1984a,b; Chang et al., 1983). It inhibits platelet-activating-factor-induced platelet aggregation and the products of arachidonic acid metabolism, properties that are not related to its antimuscarinic action but that may prove to be useful in the treatment of asthma.

Of greater practical importance than the biochemical specificity of the agent is its absorbability from mucosae. Atropine and other tertiary ammonium compounds are so well absorbed and distributed in the body that widespread effects occur whether they are administered by mouth, by inhalation, or by injection. Quaternary ammonium compounds have similar effects only when given parenterally; even then they are excluded from the central nervous system by the blood-brain barrier. When inhaled they have negligible systemic effects but prolonged local effects presumably because they are not removed from the site of deposition by absorption. The sum of these properties gives inhaled quaternary ammonium agents a functional selectivity for the airways as well as a much wider therapeutic margin than atropine and other tertiary ammonium anticholinergic agents.

D. Effects and Tolerance

Detailed accounts of the pharmacologic actions of antimuscarinic agents on nonrespiratory systems are presented in recent reviews (Boushey and Gold, 1983; Weiner, 1980). Tolerance, subsensitivity, or tachyphylaxis to anticholinergic agents is minimal or absent, in keeping with the concept that tolerance to receptor antagonists does not occur (Shifrin and Klein, 1980; Nathanson, 1982).

However, chronic administration of an anticholinergic agent may result in up-regulation of the receptor so that withdrawal may leave the organ temporarily more sensitive to cholinergic stimuli (Wise et al., 1980; Newcomb et al., 1985). Thus, Newcomb et al. found that asthmatic subjects given ipratropium 60 μg four times daily for 3 weeks experienced no loss in its bronchodilator effect during this period; but their response to methacholine inhalation increased for 1-2 days after ipratropium withdrawal, that is, they were briefly more sensitive to a cholinergic stimulus than they had been before anticholinergic use. Whether this is clinically important is uncertain.

E. Toxicity and Side Effects

Atropine and Other Tertiary Ammonium Compounds

Toxic effects of atropine are dosage-related (Weiner, 1980). In adults a dose of 0.5 mg may cause dryness of the mouth and slight bradycardia. At 1 mg, there may be skin flushing, marked dryness of the mouth, and mild tachycardia. At 2-5 mg, tachycardia, palpitations, blurred vision due to pupillary dilatation, speech disturbances, urinary retention, and restlessness may occur. At doses of 10 mg or more, the above effects are more pronounced and ataxia, delirium, hallucinations, and coma may occur. Death is uncommon. Idiosyncrasy to atropine occurs but is uncommon.

Experience suggests that older patients with bronchitis and emphysema, who are often in poor general health and nutrition, are more liable to experience undesirable effects from atropine than the above account indicates; reversible psychotic reactions have been reported (Bergman et al., 1980).

Since the dosage of atropine that achieves useful bronchodilatation in adults is in the range of 0.5 to 2.5 mg, it is evident that the therapeutic margin of atropine is negligible. Its use in subjects with narrow-angle glaucoma and bladder neck obstruction is contraindicated.

When serious atropine-related side effects occur they can usually be readily reversed by administration of physostigmine (1.0-4.0 mg intravenously in an adult); it should be administered cautiously since it can exacerbate airways obstruction.

Quarternary Ammonium Compounds

In contrast, the quaternary ammonium compounds ipratropium and atropine methylnitrate have been taken in doses up to 30 mg and 3 mg, respectively, without untoward effects other than dryness of the mouth (Wahl, 1975; Gross and Skorodin, 1984a). Indeed, one patient accidentally received more than 32 mg atropine methylnitrate in a 60 min period. This was followed by headache but no serious consequences (Gross and Skorodin, 1985).

In experimental animals (Engelhardt and Klupp, 1975; Engelhardt, 1979) the LD_{50} of ipratropium was 10-20 mg/kg for intravenous administration, the cause of death being curariform respiratory paralysis due to ganglion blockade, a feature of parenteral administration of this class of agent in high dosage. The LD_{50} was 1-2 orders of magnitude higher with oral or inhalant administration, the cause of death being due to mucosal effects such as inhibition of secretions and gastric motility with consequent anorexia and weight loss.

Mucociliary Effects

In humans quaternary ammonium anticholinergic agents are almost exclusively administered by inhalation. A significant number of studies have focused on whether these agents have undesirable effects on respiratory secretions and mucosal transport, since most airway diseases are characterized by mucosal dysfunction (Wanner, 1977). Atropine reduces the secretory activity of human respiratory mucosae in vitro (Sturgess and Reid, 1972; Boat and Kleinerman, 1975). In animal experiments, atropine did not affect basal secretory activity but blocked vagally induced increases in mucus and electrolyte secretion (Marin et al., 1976; Ueki et al., 1980). The effect of this on mucus viscosity and transportability is small (Blanshard, 1960; Lopez-Vidriero et al., 1975; King et al., 1979). Results with ipratropium are similar (Krieger and Reitberger, 1975; Chervinsky, 1977). The beat frequency of respiratory tract cilia, which is markedly reduced by atropine and hyoscine (Corssen and Allen, 1959; Blair and Woods, 1969) was virtually unaffected by quaternary anticholinergic agents (Iravani and Melville, 1975).

Mucus transport in the respiratory tract (clearance rate) is markedly delayed by atropine or hyoscine in both humans (Pavia and Thomson, 1971; Yeates et al., 1975; Foster et al., 1976; Annis et al., 1976), the dog (Sackner et al., 1977a), and the donkey (Berger et al., 1978). However, ipratropium or methylscopolamine (a quaternary agent) either had no such effect (Pavia et al., 1979, 1980; Francis et al., 1977; Bell et al., 1984) or actually increased the clearance rate (Ruffin et al., 1978b). These latter studies included subjects with asthma or chronic bronchitis as well as normal subjects; many also included the administration of quite large dosages or ipratropium.

The volume of sputum production, a relatively insensitive indicator of mucosal function, was not materially altered by either atropine (Lopez-Vidriero et al., 1975) or ipratropium (Krieger and Reitberger, 1975; Chervinsky, 1977), even after prolonged use.

In normal humans, inhalation of ipratropium, 40 μg three times daily for up to 15 days, resulted in no histologic changes in biopsy specimens of the respiratory mucosae (Fasske et al., 1975).

The sum of all these data suggests that tertiary anticholinergics may interfere with certain aspects of mucociliary function, as was suspected half a century ago before the technology to prove it was available. However it is not certain that these effects are clinically deleterious. In contrast, no quaternary agents have been shown to have any such effects. The reason for the difference in mucociliary effects of the two classes of agents is a puzzle; the difference in absorption does not seem to be a plausible explanation because mucociliary effects are presumably local. Possibly there are differences in the selectivity of the receptors of the mucociliary apparatus for different agents (Hammer and Giachetti, 1983).

Effects on Hemodynamics

The cardiovascular effects of atropine are well known; small dosages (0.5 mg) produce mild bradycardia. Larger dosages produce tachycardia due in part to the release of vagal tone on the sinoatrial node, and modest increases in the cardiac output and pulse pressure due to peripheral vasodilatation. Vagally mediated cardiac reflexes may be blunted or abolished. The effects on the pulmonary circulation are complex; overall, there is a slight tendency for reduction in pulmonary and right ventricular pressures.

The cardiovascular effects of quaternary anticholinergics in humans have also been studied (Sackner et al., 1977; Ravez et al., 1979; Chapman et al., 1985). Administration of both conventional or large dosages (320 μg) by inhalation produced minimal changes. The heart rate decreased by a few beats/min and the stroke output increased correspondingly so that cardiac output was constant. Pulmonary artery, wedge, and systemic pressures and peripheral vascular resistance were unchanged, as were various parameters of left ventricular contractility. These findings contrasted markedly with the multiple hemodynamic effects of various β-adrenergic agonists with which ipratropium was compared in these studies.

Effects on Gas Exchange

Because all other bronchodilators, by any route of administration, can have an unfavorable effect on ventilation-perfusion ratios and arterial blood gas tensions, particularly in patients with bronchospasm, one is interested in knowing if anticholinergic bronchodilators have similar effects. Atropine itself has not been extensively or recently studied in this regard, but quaternary anticholinergic agents have been studied.

Field (1967) gave atropine methylnitrate by inhalation to normal subjects. He found a mean fall in the PaO2 of 2.4 mmHg and a mean increase in the alveolar-arterial PO_2 gradient of 3.0 mmHg, both changes being about one-third of those seen following isoproterenol inhalation. A number of studies on ipratropium also failed to find clinically significant effects on gas exchange or PaO_2, even when larger than usual dosages were given (Poppius et al., 1972; Hamm, 1975; Sackner et al., 1977; Thiessen and Pedersen, 1979; Minette and Marcq, 1979). Although these latter studies included patients with airways disease, none included patients with acute bronchospasm or serious hypoxemia, in whom the danger of an acute fall in PaO_2 is greatest. One such study in 12 patients with acute asthma and an initial mean PaO_2 of 63 mmHg (Leahy et al., 1983) found that whereas salbutamol administration by inhalation resulted in a mean decline in PaO_2 of 11 mmHg (measured first at 30 min), ipratropium inhalation resulted in a mean increase in PaO_2 of 3 mmHg, although the difference was not statistically different.

If we judge by available data, quaternary anticholinergics are probably safer in this respect than adrenergic agents, but further critical studies are called for.

Idiosyncrasy

Idiosyncrasy to anticholinergics is apparently very unusual. Paradoxical bronchoconstriction to ipratropium has been reported in a few patients (Connolly, 1982). This may be due to the bromide radical of ipratropium, since it also occurred with sodium bromide inhalation but not when atropine methonitrate was substituted (Patel and Tullett, 1983); or it might have been due to hypotonicity of the nebulization solution of ipratropium (Mann et al., 1984).

Other Effects

Many patients with airways obstruction who are candidates for bronchodilator therapy have concomitant diseases that may be unfavorably affected by anticholinergic therapy. Narrow-angle glaucoma and bladder neck obstruction in men are of particular concern. Atropine itself is contraindicated in these conditions because it dilates the pupil (potentially exacerbating glaucoma) and inhibits relaxation of the urinary sphincter during micturition (precipitating acute urinary retention). The latter has been a problem in some studies with atropine (Klock et al., 1975; Pak et al., 1982).

Studies with inhaled ipratropium that specifically examined the ocular effects showed that intraocular pressure, pupil size, and accommodation were unaffected even in patients with glaucoma and when larger than usual dosages were given (Scheufler, 1975; Thumm, 1975; Ruffin et al., 1978b). Ipratropium does affect the pupil when sprayed directly into the eye, however (Minette, 1975).

One detailed study of the effects of ipratropium on urinary flow (Molkenboer and Lardenoye, 1979) has been reported. In this double-blind controlled crossover study men aged 50-70 years received placebo or ipratropium 40 μg three times daily for 3 days. No effects on cytometrics were detected.

Tertiary ammonium congeners, when given to humans on a long-term basis, may impair the sleep pattern, short-term memory, learning, and mood (Drachman, 1977; Janowsky et al., 1972). These effects have not been seen with prolonged administration of quaternary ammonium agents.

Anticholinergic agents do not cause tremor, as is commonly observed after β-adrenergic administration, and no unfavorable interaction between anticholinergic agents and other bronchodilators has been reported.

In pregnancy and lactation, studies of the safety of anticholinergic agents in humans are incomplete. Extensive animal studies have not revealed any evidence of teratogenicity or toxicity to the embryo or fetus.

V. Available and Experimental Agents

A very large number of anticholinergics, antimuscarinic agents have been developed and used for a variety of therapeutic purposes (Weiner, 1980). Only a few

Table 1 Characteristics of Anticholinergic Agents

Agent	Proprietary name	Chemical type	Forms	Status in United States	Optimal dosage[a]	Approximate duration of action (hr)
Atropine sulfate		Tertiary		Available but not approved for respiratory use	2.5 mg nebulized solution	3-4
Atropine methonitrate		Quaternary		Investigational use only	1.5 mg nebulized solution	5-6
Ipratropium bromide	Atrovent	Quaternary	MDI 18 μg, solution	FDA approval pending, investigational use only	80 μg MDI 125 μg nebulized solution	5-6
Oxitropium	Tersigat	Quaternary		Investigational use only	500 μg MDI	8
Glycopyrrolate bromide	Robinul	Quaternary	solution: 0.2 mg/1 ml	Available but not approved for respiratory use	1.6 mg nebulized solution 0.32 μg/kg i.v.	6
Thiazinamium chloride		Quaternary		Investigational use only		6

[a]Approximately the smallest dosage that produces maximal bronchodilatation in an adult, see text for details.

of these have been studied and used for their respiratory effects. Some of the more commonly used ones are shown in Fig. 3. Their principal clinical properties are shown in Table 1. Virtually all studies in which "atropine" was used have actually used atropine sulfate although this is often not stated. Although many anticholinergic agents, especially atropine sulfate, have been given orally or parenterally, attention has been focused on the inhalational route, as this route provides the greatest ratio of airway to systemic effect and takes advantage of the poor absorption of quaternary ammonium congeners.

VI. Clinical Efficacy of Anticholinergic Agents

A. General Features

The bronchodilatory effects of anticholinergic agents in both normal subjects and subjects with airway obstruction have been reported in a large number of publications, some of which have been reviewed in detail (Pakes et al., 1980; Gross and Skorodin, 1984; Mann and George, 1985). The general features of their action that emerge from these studies are as follows. Their onset of action following inhalation occurs within seconds or minutes, but is slightly slower than that following adrenergic agents administered in the same way. Bronchodilatation develops somewhat slowly and reaches a peak between 30 min and 2 hr later than that after adrenergic agents. It persists longer at plateau and declines more slowly, however. The effects of quaternary ammonium compounds persist longer than tertiary ammonium compounds, usually 4-6 hr and often much longer.

Dose-Response

Dose-response data, which are available for a number of anticholinergic agents, need to be interpreted with the following considerations in mind. In general, nebulized agents are delivered to the site of effect, the lower respiratory tract, in lower proportional amounts than metered-dose cannister-delivered agents, due largely to differences in particle size. Nebulized medication tends to be deposited in the apparatus and the oropharynx. Thus equivalent effects of the same dosage of the same agent delivered by nebulization and metered dose inhaler were roughly 1:8 (Weber, 1979). However, the small volume nebulized, 1.0 ml, must have led to inefficient delivery. The use of spacers and other methodologic maneuvers, which must vary from study to study, also obviously affect deposition of the inhaled particles. Therefore the following dose-response data cannot be regarded as more than approximate.

Dose-response studies on nebulized atropine sulfate show optimal effect to be achieved by 0.05 mg/kg in children (Cavanaugh and Cooper, 1976), and 0.025-0.04 mg/kg in adults (Pak et al., 1982; Allen and Campbell, 1980a). For nebulized atropine methonitrate the optimal dosage is a little lower, or about 1.5 mg in an adult (Allen and Campbell, 1980a; Pierce et al., 1979). For nebulized ipratropium in stable airway disease, the optimal dosage in an adult has been reported as 54-78 μg (Gomm et al., 1983) and 125 μg (Jenkins et al., 1981), although higher dosages may be needed to reach maximal effect in acute severe bronchospasm (Ward et al., 1981). The optimal dosage in children is similar (Davis et al., 1984). Ipratropium delivered by metered dose inhaler achieves maximal effect in adults in a dosage between 40 and 82 μg (Storms et al., 1975; Gross, 1975; Yeager et al., 1976; Allen and Campbell, 1980b; Gomm et al., 1983; Hockley and Johnson, 1985). Higher dosages may be needed in patients with more severe disease. For oxitropium delivered by metered dose inhaler to adults the optimal dosage has been found to be approximately 500 μg (Peel and Anderson, 1984; Skorodin et al., 1986). For glycopyrrolate, the optimal dosage in healthy young volunteers was 3.2 μg/kg by intravenous injection (Gal and Suratt, 1981), or about 1.6 mg by inhalation of nebulized solution (Gal et al., 1984). For thiazinamium the optimal dosage has not been established; nebulized dosages of up to 4.5 mg have been used in clinical studies on adults (Wyeth Laboratories, personal communication).

For quaternary ammonium compounds the duration of effect seems to be more dosage-dependent than the peak airflow effect (see, for example, Ruffin and Newhouse [1978]), the highest dosage sometimes being still effective 10 hr after adminstration (Peel and Anderson, 1984).

B. Effects in Normal Subjects

Normal subjects who receive an anticholinergic agent experience significant increases in airflow and changes in static lung recoil and lung volumes. These effects are presumed to be due to the ablation of cholinergic tone in the airways and possibly in the parenchyma.

In these studies a variety of anticholinergic agents, atropine sulfate, scopolamine, ipratropium bromide, and glycopyrrolate, have been given by intravenous injection, by inhalation of nebulized solution, or by metered dose inhaler (Butler et al., 1960; Smith and DuBois, 1969; Kjellberg and Heinonen, 1974; De Troyer et al., 1979; Douglas et al., 1979b; Gal and Suratt, 1981; Gal et al., 1984; Islam and Ulmer, 1984). The results of these studies do not differ substantially from each other if one allows for differences in the site of effect due to the mode of administration.

Airflow parameters such as FEV_1 typically increased by up to about 10%, airway resistance decreased about 50%, and specific airway conductance increased about 100% at the time of peak effect of the agent. Flow rates at higher lung volumes increased consistently, but there was also some increase in flow rates at low lung volumes, particularly when the agent was given parenterally. Thus upstream resistance also fell, indicating some effect, albeit less, on small airways as well as large airways. Lung volumes changed very little, tending to fall in young subjects and rise in subjects over 47 years of age. Static lung recoil pressures fell about 20% when the agent was given parenterally, but not otherwise. The time course and duration of these effects did not differ substantially from those seen in patients with airways disease.

These results, which show a substantial bronchodilatory effect, provide an index of the amount of cholinergic tone in normal airways.

C. Efficacy Against Specific Stimuli

The effects of anticholinergic agents have been examined in terms of their ability to protect against the bronchoconstrictor effects of a wide variety of respiratory spasmogens. The clinical relevance of this type of experiment is based on the following implied logic: airway obstruction in subjects with airway disease is due to a number of factors, including the release of mediators. The extent to which the bronchospastic effects of a putative mediator can be blocked by anticholinergic agents indicates the role of the vagal parasympathetic system in bringing about the effects of that mediator. If it is blocked by the anticholinergic agent one can deduce that the mediator provokes bronchoconstriction by initiating a parasympathetic reflex. If not, the putative mediator may have a direct, local effect on airway effector cells, such as smooth muscle. One learns little about whether the mediator is relevant in the innate bronchospasm of that patient or whether the anticholinergic agent will be clinically beneficial.

Several caveats apply: one assumes that the mode of delivery of the stimuli imitates their natural release and does not initiate an artifactual parasympathetic reflex, and that the anticholinergic agent is delivered at the relevant site in sufficient dosage and is appropriately timed to inhibit a parasympathetic reflex. A problem in interpretation is also created by the fact that anticholinergic agents improve baseline airflow.

Since normal subjects respond only poorly, if at all, to possible respiratory stimuli, these experiments have mostly been performed on subjects with airway diseases. In the following sections details of the numerous studies (and literature citations) have been reviewed (Gross and Skorodin, 1984a).

Against Cholinergic-Induced Bronchoconstriction

Anticholinergic agents antagonize the effects of acetylcholine by competition for the cholinergic receptor. When given in sufficient dosage in advance of a cholinergic stimulus they block the effects of the cholinergic agent on airways. This is uniformly seen with all anticholinergic agents and against a variety of typical cholinergic spasmogens. It is seen in subjects of all ages, and with all varieties of airway diseases.

Against Histamine-Induced Bronchoconstriction

Protection against histamine-induced bronchoconstriction is less consistent. Atropine and ipratropium have been found to be at least partially protective in subjects with asthma or chronic bronchitis by some workers, but not by others. Most found that adrenergic agents provided more consistent protection against the effect of histamine. Possibly histamine causes bronchoconstriction both by direct action on H1 receptors on airway effector cells and by vagal reflexes, and only the latter are inhibited by anticholinergic agents.

Against Other Mediators

Inhaled prostaglandin F2α, leukotrienes, serotonin, and bradykinin produce bronchoconstriction in subjects with airway disease. Anticholinergic agents have been found to be at least partially protective against the effects of PGF2α, but not the remainder. Some questions hang over the interpretation of such experiments because these agents may be irritant to the airways.

Against β-Blockade

Administration of agents with any significant component of β-$_2$-blocking action can increase airway resistance in patients with airway obstruction (but not in subjects with normal airways). This effect is presumed to be due to removal of β-adrenergic opposition to cholinergic bronchomotor tone. Anticholinergic agents are effective not only in preventing β-blockade-induced bronchospasm but also in reversing it (MacDonald et al., 1967; Grieco and Pierson, 1971; DeVries, 1975; Germouty, 1975). Since β-blocking agents are occasionally given inadvertently to patients with obstructive airway disease, with results that can be catastrophic, and as adrenergic agents are ineffective in reversing the bronchospasm so induced, an anticholinergic bronchodilator is the treatment of choice.

Against Gases, Dusts, and Nonspecific Irritants

The small decrease in airway conductance that results from inhalation of sulfur dioxide by normal and atopic nonasthmatic subjects was prevented by prior administration of atropine (Nadel et al., 1965, Snashall and Baldwin, 1982) or ipratropium (Holzman et al., 1979). But asthmatic subjects, who are universally and innately more responsive to sulfur dioxide, were variably protected by anticholinergic agents, some not all, and others only partially at best (Snashall and Baldwin, 1982; Tan et al., 1982). In general, this pattern of response (normal subjects tending to be well protected and asthmatic subjects tending to be less well protected) was also found when other nonspecific stimuli were inhaled: carbon dust (Widdicombe et al., 1962; Simonsson et al., 1967; citric acid aerosol (Simonsson et al., 1967); ozone (Holzman et al., 1979); nebulized water (Fabbri et al., 1983); and cigarette smoke (Gayrard et al., 1975; Nolte, 1975).

One interpretation of these findings is that in normal subjects nonspecific irritants produce mild bronchoconstriction only through a vagal reflex. But in asthmatic subjects other, noncholinergic, bronchoconstricting mechanisms are also activated.

Against Antigen-Induced Bronchoconstriction

A considerable number of studies have been concerned with the question whether allergen-induced bronchospasm in extrinsic allergic subjects is mediated through a vagal reflex pathway. Animal experiments are inconclusive, on the one hand suggesting that it might be (Gold et al., 1972, Kessler et al., 1973); on the other suggesting that it is not (Justesen et al., 1970; Patterson and Harris, 1976; Krell et al., 1976; Abraham et al., 1981; Hirshman and Downes, 1981).

Studies in humans are similarly inconclusive. Several groups have found little evidence of protection against antigen-induced bronchospasm from prior and/or concomitant administration of a variety of anticholinergic agents (Fish et al., 1977; Ruffin et al., 1978a; Cockcroft et al., 1978; Rosenthal et al., 1977). Others, using essentially similar methodology, found at least partial protection in at least some of their experimental subjects (Itkin and Anand, 1970; Yu et al., 1972; Orehek et al., 1975; Vastag et al., 1976; Schultze-Werninghaus, 1981; Eiser and Guz, 1982).

If one assumes that each of these studies is methodologically sound, one can conclude that atopic asthmatic subjects vary considerably in the extent to which inhaled allergen produces bronchoconstriction through cholinergic mechanisms. In most subjects these mechanisms do not seem to be of great importance. Nevertheless, from a clinical standpoint, some subjects may obtain useful relief from symptoms due to allergen exposure by use of an anticholinergic agent, whatever the mechanism of that relief.

Exercise, Hyperventilation, and Cold Air-Induced Bronchospasm

Most workers now regard exercise, hyperventilation, and breathing cold air as more or less equivalent stimuli of bronchospasm in asthmatic subjects, their common factor being heat loss from the respiratory system (McFadden, 1981). A large number of studies have examined the use of anticholinergic agents either to throw light on the mechanism(s) of exercise-induced bronchospasm (EIB) as a model for naturally occurring bronchospasm, or to determine these agents' role in the management of EIB (Kiviloog, 1975, Tinkelman et al., 1976; Tashkin et al., 1977; Deal et al., 1978; Hartley and Davis, 1980; Neijens et al., 1981; Chen et al., 1981; Thomson et al., 1978; Borut et al., 1977; Griffin et al.,

1982; Wilson et al., 1982; Tullett et al., 1982; Sheppard et al., 1982; Wilson et al., 1984; Johnson et al., 1984).

As with allergen-induced bronchospasm, interpretation of experimental findings is complicated by the possibility of nonspecific bronchodilatation and, again, considerable variability in the degree of protection has been found between subjects, some experiencing good protection, others little. This variability does not appear to be explicable on the basis of the anticholinergic agent employed (most such agents have been studied), nor on the basis of the age of the patient population (both children and adults have been studied). The route by which the agent is delivered has been found to be a factor in its efficacy (Chen et al., 1981; Sheppard et al., 1983), and there may be a dosage effect: studies in which larger than usual dosages of anticholinergic agents have been used tended to provide better protection (Hartley, Davies, 1980; Sheppard et al., 1982). Nevertheless, large intersubject differences in protection remain. It is possible that those subjects whose EIB is due mainly to large airways constriction derive more protection from anticholinergic agents than other subjects (Thomson et al., 1978; McFadden et al., 1977) in keeping with the predominant site of action of these agents.

Almost certainly a large number of mechanisms other than vagally mediated reflexes can participate in the pathophysiology of EIB, and their relative importance differs among subjects. While anticholinergic agents usually afforded some protection, cromolyn was usually more effective and adrenergic agents were usually most effective in this regard.

Against Psychogenic Factors

In a guinea pig model of classic Pavlovian conditioned bronchospasm, atropine was found to be prophylactic against the bronchoconstrictive stimulus (Justesen et al., 1970).

Bronchospasm induced by suggestion in allergic human subjects was prevented by prior administration of atropine (McFadden et al., 1969). Subjects whose asthma was believed to be psychogenic in origin experienced greater and more prolonged bronchodilatation in response to ipratropium inhalation than a comparable group whose asthma was thought not to be psychogenic (Rebuck and Marcus, 1979). If one considers that psychogenic bronchospasm must be mediated through some connection between the cerebral cortex and the airways, it is reasonable that the pathway should involve the vagal efferents.

D. In "Stable Asthma"

Efficacy

An enormous number of studies have examined the efficacy of anticholinergic agents in "stable" asthma, a smaller number in acute severe asthma or "status asthmaticus," which is considered in the next section. Typically, the short-term effect has been studied in comparison to placebo and/or an adrenergic agent, spirometric or plethysmographic indices being used as the criteria of response. Maximum response, percent of achievable response, duration of response, or the time-integral (area under the curve) has been used to compare the response to the anticholinergic agent with that of other treatments. This comparison may or may not be clinically meaningful, but suffers scientifically from the fact that maximal therapeutic dosages of each agent are almost never used. Thus, when a given dosage of one agent is found to be more effective than a given dosage of a different class of agent it may be because of the dosages chosen rather than the intrinsic potency of the agents. The dosages chosen for such experiments are nearly always the choice of the pharmaceutical company sponsoring the study, and thus reflect their marketing intentions as much as any physiological interest. The results may nevertheless provide useful information, for example, about the relative responsiveness of different classes of patients to the given dosage, about responses within patients over time, subsensitivity, and some other aspects.

In stable asthmatic patients, a variety of anticholinergic agents given by mouth or, more commonly, by inhalation in usual clinical dosages produced bronchodilatation compared with placebo, but tended to be less potent in this regard than usual clinical dosages of a variety of β-2 adrenergic agents (reviewed in Pakes et al., 1980; Gross and Skorodin, 1984a), (Fig. 4). However, the degree of bronchodilatation resulting from anticholinergic agents varies considerably among patients, some respond as well to them as to adrenergic agents, others much less so. Also, some asthmatic subjects respond poorly to adrenergic agents but well to anticholinergic agents (Burge et al., 1980). Some of the factors that may account for these differences are considered below. Most studies show that the effect of anticholinergic agents is at least as prolonged as that of β-2 agents, and often more so. In some studies, such as those of Ullah et al. (1981) and Ruffin et al. (1977), administration of an adrenergic agent after the anticholinergic agent produced increases in the FEV_1 above the maximum achieved by the anticholinergic agent alone (Fig. 4), suggesting again that there are likely to be mechanisms of airflow obstruction in asthma which are independent of cholinergic activity.

Factors that Influence Response to Anticholinergic Agents

Extrinsic Atopic vs. Intrinsic Nonatopic Asthma

In most studies where comparisons were possible anticholinergic agents seemed to be about equally effective in both subtypes of asthma (although it was fairly clear that adrenergic agents were more effective in the atopic group) (Fig. 5) (Ruffin et al., 1982; Rebuck and Marcus, 1979; Ullah et al., 1981). However, in a series of reports on substantially larger numbers of subjects Jolobe (1983,

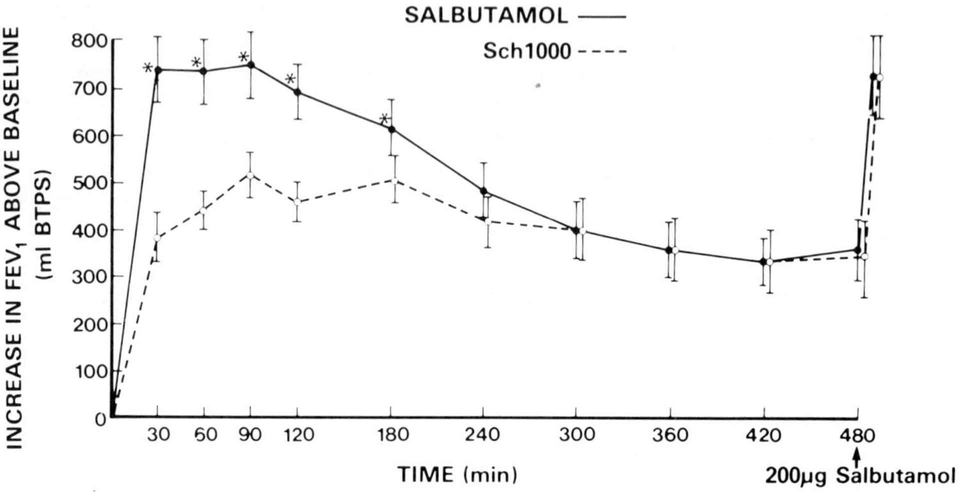

Figure 4 Responses of 25 asthmatic subjects to inhaled salbutamol (200 μg) and ipratropium (Sch 1000, 40 μg). Subjects received additional salbutamol at 8 hr. *, Significant difference between agents, $P < 0.05$ (from Ruffin et al., 1977, with permission).

Table 2 FEV1 Responses (% of Baseline) of Patients with Airway Diseases

Parameter	Atopic asthma	Intrinsic asthma	Chronic bronchitis
Number of patients	36	36	30
Age at onset (years)	27	43	48
Number with eosinophilia	19	36	0
Basal FEV1 (liters)	1.37 NS	1.28 NS	1.07 NS
Anticholinergic agent used	17[a]	28 NS	30[b]
Adrenergic agent used	19 NS	12 NS	6[b]

[a]Significant difference between adjacent values, $P<0.05$.
[b]Significant difference between atopic asthmatic and chronic bronchitic subjects, $P<0.01$.
NS, no significant difference between adjacent values.
Adapted from Jolobe (1984a), with permission.

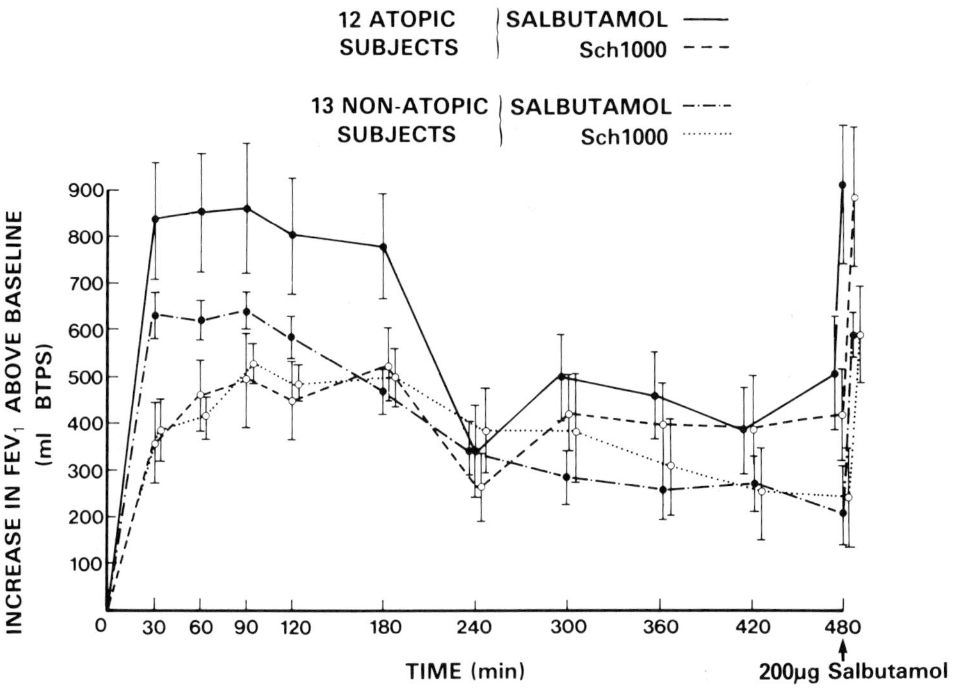

Figure 5 Responses of 12 atopic and 13 nonatopic asthmatic subjects to inhaled salbutamol (200 µg) and ipratropium (Sch 1000, 40 µg). Subjects received additional salbutamol at 8 hr (from Ruffin et al., 1977, with permission).

1984a,b,c) found that nonatopic subjects responded significantly better than atopic subjects to either atropine methonitrate or ipratropium (Table 2).

Age

Many authors have thought, and some have provided evidence (Partridge and Saunders, 1981; Ullah et al., 1981), that anticholinergic agents were more likely to be effective in patients over the age of 40, and with a longer history of asthma. But this is not borne out by others (Jolobe, 1984c).

Disease Status

In very few studies have the responses of patients to an agent been studied on more than one occasion, except in the context of the development of subsensitivity. Yet it was shown many years ago (Hume and Gandevia, 1957) and again more recently (Rebuck and Read, 1971) that a patient's response to an adrenergic agent is attenuated when he or she has an acute severe exacerbation of airways obstruction. In a retrospective study of patient records, Altounyan (1964) also found a decline in response to atropine methonitrate inhalation during periods of increased airflow obstruction. But in a similar retrospective survey, Jolobe (cited in Jolobe and Lane, 1981) was unable to confirm this. At present, there is not sufficient data to determine whether a patient's response to anticholinergic therapy is significantly altered during mild or severe exacerbations of asthma, seasonally, or from the influence of the many other factors that affect the patient's status. (The efficacy of anticholinergic therapy in acute severe asthma is discussed below.)

Concomitant Nonbronchodilator Therapy

Altounyan (1970) found that treatment of asthmatic subjects with cromolyn for 3 weeks increased their responsiveness to atropine methonitrate despite the absence of a change in baseline airflow. A course of prednisolone had a similar effect on atropine responsiveness, while improving baseline lung function. Similar findings have been reported by others (Lin et al., 1978; Lightbody et al., 1978; Jolobe and Lane, 1981). Thus, Jolobe and Lane found that administration of aerosol steroid for 4 weeks or more to asthmatic subjects (presumably stable) resulted not only in an improvement in their baseline FEV_1 but also in significant enhancement of their responsiveness to anticholinergic agents.

Combination with Other Agents in Asthma

Several studies have examined the question of whether an anticholinergic agent adds to the bronchodilatation achieved by an adrenergic agent or xanthine in subjects with asthma, and vice versa (Petrie and Palmer, 1975; Ruffin et al., 1977, 1982; Lightbody et al., 1978; Lin et al., 1978; Rebuck and Marcus, 1979; Marlin et al., 1979; Pierce et al., 1979; Kreisman et al., 1981; Ullah et al., 1981; Elwood and Abboud, 1982; Lefcoe et al., 1982; Bruderman et al., 1983; Rebuck et al., 1983). In most reports the combination of agents resulted in more bronchodilatation (higher peak and longer duration) than either alone, particularly if the anticholinergic agent was given first.

The manner in which these studies have generally been performed, namely using conventional, and possibly submaximal dosages of each agent, allows one only to conclude that better bronchodilatation was usually achieved by the combination. But this might well have been because more bronchodilator was given when the combination was used than with either agent alone. Nevertheless, this information might be of use in practice when a patient's condition is not optimally controlled by use of a single bronchodilator in conventional dosage, and one wishes to avoid the risks of giving larger dosages of that agent.

In Europe, where ipratropium has been in clinical use for a decade, fixed combinations of fenoterol and ipratropium have recently been introduced, either 50 μg plus 20 μg of the respective agents (Berodual) or 100 μg plus 40 μg (Duovent). The aim of the combination is to provide the rapid bronchodilatation of the β_2 adrenergic agent together with the prolonged effects of the anticholinergic agent, and the additive effects of the combination at intermediate times. Experience with one of these combinations, which reflects the previous literature cited above, has been reviewed (Hoffbrand and Phillips, 1984).

Analysis of a more physiological question, how much airflow obstruction is due to mechanisms reversible by adrenergic therapy and how much due to cholinergic mechanisms, can only be answered by giving optimal dosages of each class of agent. Ullah and associates (1981) gave cumulative dosages of salbutamol (total 600 μg) to asthmatic subjects; when maximal effect had been achieved they gave ipratropium bromide (80 μg) and found that the FEV_1 increased further (although only slightly). When they reversed the order of drug administration to ipratropium (120 μg) first, salbutamol was able to increase the FEV_1 futher (by a substantial amount). This result, which suggests that neither class of agent alone can bring about maximal bronchodilatation in asthmatic subjects, can be interpreted in at least two ways. Possibly airway obstruction in asthma is due to many factors, only some of which are reversed by each class of agent. Alternatively, the two agents have their effects at different anatomical sites in the airways, as was discussed above, and therefore have additive effects. But when both classes of agents are given by inhalation their site of effect is not distinguishable. The former explanation therefore seems more plausible. In asthma parasympathetic reflexes, and other noncholinergic mechanisms of airway obstruction operate to variable extents in individual subjects. Both classes of agents may therefore have a role in the therapy of individual subjects.

Long-Term Use in Asthma

Although atropine sulfate has been used on a long-term basis, there are few recent reports of this experience (Klock et al., 1975; Light and George, 1977). Ipratropium has been in general clinical use outside the United States for a decade and no major problems have been reported (Minette, 1975; Cockroft et al., 1982; Vakil et al., 1985). Nor has tolerance or subsensitivity been reported. In several reports it was mentioned, without documentation, that a reduction in other antiasthmatic therapy was achieved after the introduction of anticholinergic therapy into the patient's regimen.

E. In Acute Severe Asthma (Status Asthmaticus)

The place of an anticholinergic agent in the treatment of acute severe exacerbations of asthma (status asthmaticus) has been examined in several controlled studies. As initial therapy in adults, nebulized ipratropium solution (0.5-1.0 mg) was about as effective in improving airflow as 5-10 mg nebulized salbutamol (Ward et al., 1981; Leahy et al., 1983). But subsequent administration of salbutamol produced significantly more additional bronchodilatation over that achieved by initial ipratropium treatment than the reverse. Addition of ipratropium to an adrenergic agent, either simultaneously (Ward et al., 1981; Bryant, 1985) or in rapid sequence (Ward et al., 1985; Beck et al., 1985), consistently resulted in better airflow improvement than addition of placebo, or even addition of more adrenergic agent. One of these studies was on children (Beck et al., 1985) (Fig. 6). Even after the patient's initial response to treatment, atropine sulfate (Fairshter et al., 1981), or ipratropium (McGivern et al., 1984; Bryant, 1985), produced substantial further improvement in airflow and lung volumes.

Whether anticholinergic therapy can be regarded as an equally effective alternative to other conventional therapy in acute severe asthma cannot be deter-

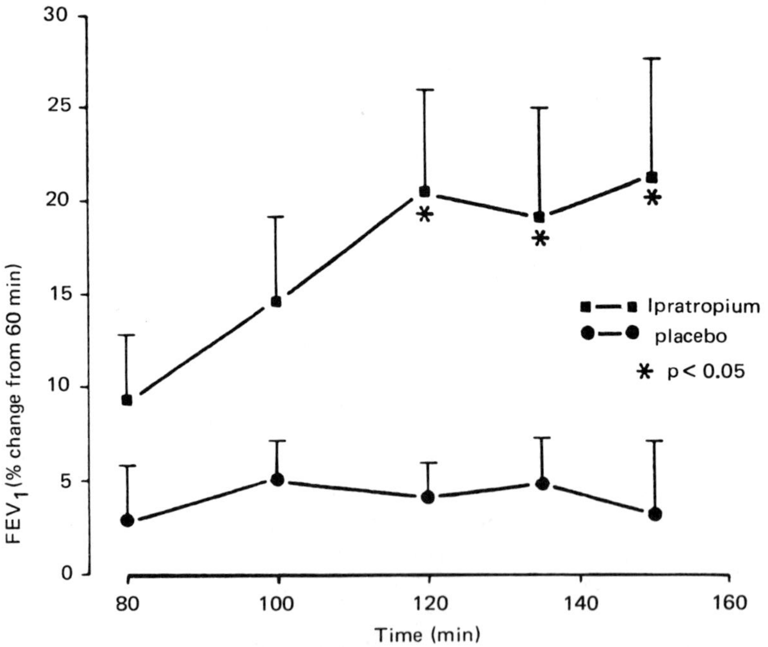

Figure 6 Responses of 25 children with acute severe asthma to nebulized ipratropium (250 μg) vs. placebo. All had received nebulized salbutamol at 20-min intervals for 1 hr previously and continued to receive it during the experimental period. *Significant difference between groups (from Beck et al., 1985, with permission).

mined on the basis of the above reports. However, one might be reluctant to rely solely on the anticholinergic agent without the confirmation of a larger experience. One must be concerned with at least two possible problems. They are slower to act than adrenergic agents, and status asthmaticus is one situation in which this is an important consideration. Second, the pathologic condition in status asthmaticus appears to be more marked in the small airways, and inhaled anticholinergic agents have less effect on the small airways than adrenergic agents, particularly when the latter are given parenterally.

However, the above reports strongly suggest that concomitant anticholinergic therapy, as an adjuvant to conventional therapy, would add significantly to the early management of acute severe bronchospasm without adding any hazard.

F. In "Stable" Chronic Bronchitis and Emphysema

Efficacy

Since the early studies of Crompton (1968), Astin (1972), and Poppius and Salorinne (1973), which showed that anticholinergic agents might be more potent bronchodilators than adrenergic agents in patients with chronic bronchitis, there has been a great deal of interest in this application of anticholinergic agents. As is well known, other conventional agents are not potent bronchodilators in chronic bronchitis and emphysema. Yet this large group of patients are highly symptomatic because of airway obstruction. Many publications have reported the effects of various anticholinergic agents in patients with predominant bronchitis and/or emphysema, although a component of asthma has not always been rigorously excluded.

These reports, only a few of which are cited here, show that in bronchitis/emphysema an anticholinergic agent was at least as effective as an adrenergic agent or a xanthine in improving airflow (Klock et al., 1975; Petrie and Palmer, 1975; Douglas et al., 1979; Minette and Marcq, 1979; Jenkins et al., 1981); or was more effective (Poppius and Salorinne, 1973; Baigelman and Chodosh, 1977; Chick and Jenne, 1977; Allen and Campbell, 1980; Marini and Lakshminarayan, 1980; Hughes et al., 1982; Passamonte and Martinez, 1984; Jolobe, 1984a). Moreover, the bronchodilator effect of an anticholinergic agent was apparent even when the subjects also received an adrenergic agent (Brown et al., 1984), or even an adrenergic agent plus therapeutic dosages of theophylline (Lefcoe et al., 1982; Passamonte and Martinez, 1984). Furthermore, some patients with bronchitis or emphysema who did not respond to all adrenergic agents responded to atropine (Klock et al., 1975; Marini and Lakshminarayan, 1980; Passamonte and Martinez, 1984).

In a multicenter study involving 261 patients, none of whom were atopic asthmatics, 40 μg ipratropium bromide was compared to 1.5 mg metaproterenol in parallel matched groups three times during a 90-day period (Tashkin et al., 1986). The group that received ipratropium inhalation consistently experienced more bronchodilatation throughout the 90-day study period than the group that received metaproterenol.

As was discussed in the preceding section, the use of agents in the dosages in which they are commercially supplied, as in most of the studied cited above, does not necessarily afford a valid comparison of the relative efficacy of each agent. More informative data are obtained on this point when maximal dosages are employed. Douglas et al. (1979) gave maximal dosages of salbutamol to patients with chronic bronchitis and found that ipratropium further increased the FEV_1. Likewise, Gross and Skorodin (1984b) found that atropine methonitrate inhalation improved the bronchodilatation achieved by maximal dosages of salbutamol in patients with emphysema, but that salbutamol did not improve the bronchodilatation achieved by atropine methonitrate. In fact, atropine methonitrate produced significantly more bronchodilatation and reduction in lung volumes than 760 μg salbutamol by metered dose inhaler. By itself it achieved as much bronchodilatation as was achievable with either agent, alone or in combination (Fig. 7). These results strongly support the view that anti-

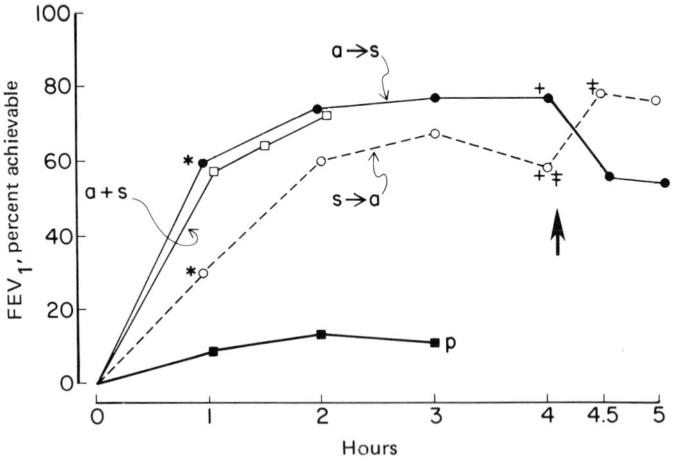

Figure 7 Responses of 10 patients with emphysema to atropine methonitrate (a) and salbutamol (s) in various sequences. a → s, atropine methonitrate hourly followed by salbutamol at the arrow; s → a, the same agents in reverse order; a + s, both agents simultaneously; p, placebo. Pairs of symbols indicate significant difference between values (from Gross and Skorodin, 1984b, with permission).

cholinergic agents are the most potent available bronchodilators in patients with chronic bronchitis and emphysema. Possible explanations why this is so are offered below.

The general features of bronchodilatation resulting from use of anticholinergics in bronchitis/emphysema are the same as in asthma. The onset of action, time to peak effect, duration of effect, and dose-response are the same as far as one can judge. The magnitude of response in terms of absolute increase in FEV_1 or decrease in specific resistance are similar too, being about 10-15% of predicted and about 50% of baseline, respectively. Due to a substantial decrease in residual volume of about 60% of the predicted value (Gross and Skorodin, 1984b) the vital capacity also increases, and usually by more than the FEV1 in absolute terms (Baigelman and Chodosh, 1977). More than in asthma, the bronchodilatory response, for example in terms of the increase in FEV_1, is fairly consistent between patients with all degrees of severity of airways disease. Minor day-to-day variation in the response to an anticholinergic agent within patients correlates inversely with the baseline FEV_1 on each day (Gross and Skorodin, 1984c), suggesting that the day-to-day fluctuations in baseline airflow are due to variations in baseline cholinergic tone.

As alluded to in the preceding paragraph, the amount of improvement in airflow is substantial. In absolute terms, the FEV_1 typically increased by 0.2-0.3 liters (Baigelman and Chodosh, 1977; Lefcoe et al., 1982), which is about the same as that achieved under the same conditions in asthmatic subjects although the baseline FEV1 differed substantially. The effects of anticholinergic agents are also reflected in other tests of airways function, such as specific conductance, and in the lung volume measurements where, for example, the residual volume fell by a mean of 1.1 liters (Table 3), (Gross and Skorodin, 1984b), a change that might contribute as much to symptomatic relief as the improvement in airflow.

The fairly impressive bronchodilatation seen in the studies cited above raises the question of whether the populations studied may have inadvertently included asthmatic subjects. The patient population was often not well enough characterized for one to be confident on this point and the distinction is often not easy to make (Fletcher and Pride, 1984). However, in several studies (for example, Jolobe, 1984a, b; Brown et al., 1984; Gross and Skorodin, 1984b), and one very large one (Tashkin et al., 1986), atopic asthma was specifically sought by all the usual criteria and excluded, and bronchitis/emphysema was positively identified in all subjects who were included. The amount of bronchodilatation achieved in these studies is comparable to that from other studies cited above where criteria for entry into the study were not as rigorous.

Table 3 Lung Volumes: Percent Predicted (±SD) in 10 Patients with Emphysema

	Base	Salbutamol	Atropine methonitrate	Base	Atropine methonitrate	Salbutamol	Base	Placebo	Both drugs
FRC	217	195[a]	187[a]	220	188[a]	197	211	207	189[a,b]
	(25)	(28)	(32)	(36)	(31)	(27)	(25)	(20)	(29)
RV	242	197[a]	182[a,b]	247	180[a]	190	238	237	181[a,b]
	(41)	(41)	(35)	(49)	(32)	(30)	(45)	(35)	(38)

Baseline value is followed by the value at plateau due to the first drug, and then the lowest value that occurred after administration of the second drug.
[a]Significantly different from corresponding baseline at P of 0.05 or less.
[b]Significant different from first drug on that day at P of 0.05 or less.
Reproduced from Gross and Skorodin (1984b), with permission.

Combination with Other Bronchodilators in Bronchitis/Emphysema

The combination of an anticholinergic agent with other bronchodilators invariably resulted in greater bronchodilatation than when other agents were used alone (Douglas et al., 1979; Lefcoe et al., 1982; Brown et al., 1984; Gross and Skorodin, 1984b). Whether other agents can add to the bronchodilatation achieved by an anticholinergic agent is doubtful. Thus Lefcoe and co-workers (1982) found no significant increase in airflow from the combination of ipratropium, fenoterol, and oxtriphylline than from ipratropium alone (Fig. 8). Jolobe (1984a,b) found only minimal augmentation in the FEV_1 by adrenergic agents after the patients had received an anticholinergic agent. And Gross and Skorodin (1984b) found that a large dosage of salbutamol failed to improve any index of airflow of lung volumes after a large dosage of atropine methonitrate. The conclusion one draws from these results is that all the available bronchodilatation in patients with bronchitis and emphysema can be achieved with an

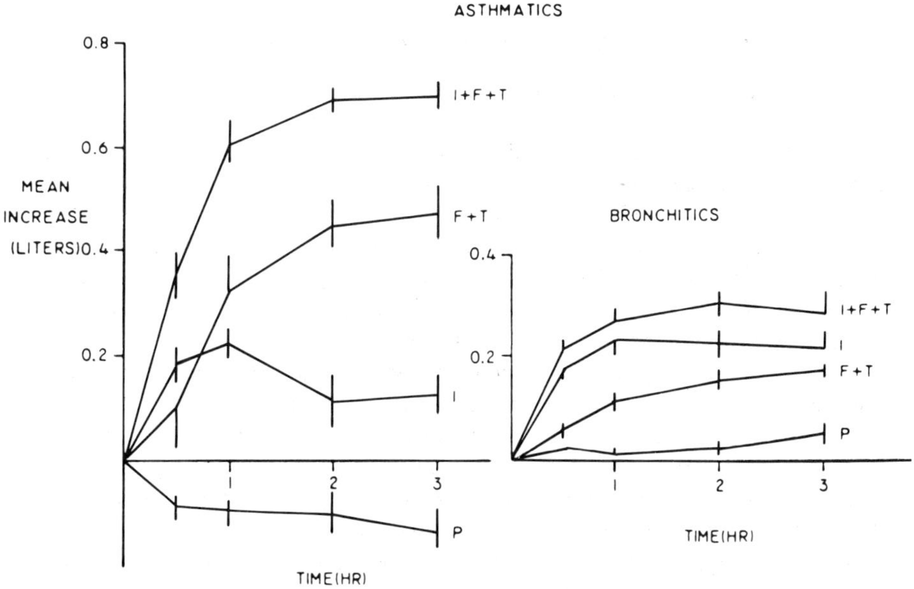

Figure 8 FEV1 responses of 15 patients with asthma and 15 with chronic bronchitis to agents indicated: I, ipratropium 40 μg aerosol; F, fenoterol 5 mg orally; T, oxtriphylline 400 mg orally; P, placebo (from Lefcoe et al., 1982, with permission).

anticholinergic agent alone and that the addition of an adrenergic or xanthine agent contributes little, if at all, to the bronchodilatation, although xanthines may ameliorate other aspects of respiratory mechanics in these patients.

Long-Term Use in Bronchitis and Emphysema

Long-term studies of the use of atropine sulfate are not documented in the literature. The regular, continuous use of ipratropium bromide for periods from 3 months to 4 years in dosages up to 400 μg daily has been reported for children (Mann and Hiller, 1982) and adults (Minette and Marcq, 1979; Cockcroft et al., 1982; Ulmer, 1975; Minette, 1975; Tashkin et al., 1986). There is also, of course, the considerable but unreported experience due to the clinical availability of ipratropium in the last decade outside the United States. No significant problems have emerged, nor have tolerance to the agent or unfavorable interactions with other agents been described. Some temporary loss of efficacy during acute exacerbations has been reported anecdotally but not documented (Minette, 1975). In one report, the initiation of long-term use of ipratropium permitted a reduction in the dosage of steroids in about half the patients (Ajewski and Popiak, 1979).

G. In Acute Exacerbations of Bronchitis and Emphysema

The use of nebulized atropine sulfate or glycopyrrolate in acute exacerbations of chronic bronchitis and emphysema is fairly widespread in the United States, but reports of this practice are lacking. Ipratropium solution has been used elsewhere for the same purpose. In a randomized double-blind study (Backman and Hellstrom, 1985), 40 patients with acute exacerbations received either fenoterol 0.5 mg or ipratropium 0.2 mg as nebulized aerosols three times daily for 1 week. They were studied twice, once on the day of admission to hospital because of the exacerbation, and again after 7 days of these treatments. Baseline airflow increased by the same amount over the 7-day course of the study in the two groups; the response over the first hour after ipratropium administration was greater than the response following fenoterol both on the 1st and the 7th day of hospitalization. Within groups the response to each agent remained constant, being the same on the 1st as on the 7th day of each treatment. Other parameters (pulse and blood pressure, arterial blood gases, and sputum production) did not differ between the groups during the study. But concomitant drug therapy, which included steroids, xanthines, and adrenergic agents in some patients, was not controlled for; however, concomitant adrenergic therapy was withheld for 8 hr before each testing period.

This report suggests that during acute exacerbations, as in stable bronchitis/emphysema, anticholinergic therapy is more effective than adrenergic therapy, and also that within patients, it is as effective during acute exacerbations as at other times. However, the reservations we expressed regarding the use of anticholinergic agents in acute severe asthma apply here as well. We assume that other reports on the same subject will appear shortly.

H. Efficacy in Asthma versus Bronchitis and Emphysema

A number of related questions can be considered: In which type of patient are anticholinergic agents most effective? How does their efficacy compare with other agents in each condition? What are the reasons for the differences? The answers to the first two questions have largely been dealt with in preceding sections.

The central fact seems to us to be that the increase in airflow brought about by an anticholinergic agent, expressed either as the absolute increase or, better, as a percent of the subject's predicted airflow, is about the same in all groups of patients. This emerges most clearly from studies that compare the different groups under similar conditions and report the results in comparable units (Chick and Jenne, 1977; Baigelman and Chodosh, 1977; Barber et al., 1977; Lefcoe et al., 1982; Jolobe, 1984a) (Fig. 8). Three points follow from this.

First, because the baseline airflow is usually higher in subjects with asthma the improvement *as a percent of baseline* appears to be less in asthmatics, and conversely more for subjects with bronchitis or emphysema. When the baselines were more or less comparable between groups, the improvement as a percent of baseline was also comparable (Chick and Jenne, 1977; Barber et al., 1977).

Second, patients with asthma generally respond well to adrenergic agents. Thus, if the amount of bronchodilatation is the sole consideration, adrenergic agents emerge as generally more potent than anticholinergic agents, particularly in atopic asthmatics.

Thirdly, patients with bronchitis and emphysema generally respond poorly to adrenergic agents. Thus by comparison, anticholinergic agents are more potent than adrenergic agents in this group.

The relative efficacy of the two major classes of bronchodilators is thus largely a function of the patient's response to the adrenergic agent. The difference in responsiveness to adrenergic agents between asthma and bronchitis/emphysema reflects the different pathophysiological mechanisms of airflow obstruction in these conditions. In asthma there are numerous mechanisms centering around the release of mediators and the inflammatory and allergic reaction, and these are at least partially amenable to adrenergic therapy. These mechanisms are minimal or absent in bronchitis/emphysema where much of the airflow obstruction is due to destructive changes in the lung parenchyma resulting in loss of recoil and instability of small airways, mechanisms which are not amenable to adrenergic therapy.

However, all patients and normal subjects have cholinergic bronchomotor tone amenable to anticholinergic drugs. The available evidence suggests that the reversal of normal physiological cholinergic tone accounts for the bronchodilatation that results from an anticholinergic agent. Some of the suggestive evidence, which derives from studies detailed in various parts of this chapter, is as follows. The amount of bronchodilatation achieved, in absolute terms, is fairly consistent among all groups of patients and normal subjects despite extreme differences in baseline airflow. Moreover, it is consistent at the same absolute level whether the patient is "stable" or in an acute phase of airway disease, such as status asthmaticus or acute exacerbation of bronchitis. When there are obstructive mechanisms over and above cholinergic tone, such as in asthma, the addition of agents active against these mechanisms (i.e., adrenergic agents), consistently produces more bronchodilatation than the anticholinergic agent alone. Challenge studies show that anticholinergic agents are not very effective against the bronchoconstriction due to mediators of asthma, and much of the effect they do have can be explained either by a change in the baseline (which is evident even before the mediator is administered) or by blocking an artefactual vagal reflex, which occurs when these irritant substances are inhaled. If intrinsic bronchoconstrictor mechanisms such as mediator effects are only minimally blocked by anticholinergic agents, then they cannot be contributing substantially to parasympathetic tone by the vagal reflex. Anticholinergic bronchodilatation in asthma must, therefore, be largely due to reversal of underlying cholinergic tone. As their effect in asthma is quantitatively similar to their effect in normal subjects, one can argue that cholinergic tone is normal in asthma.

When there are *not* additional obstructive factors, such as in emphysema, the anticholinergic agent alone produces all the available bronchodilatation. Again, since the amount of bronchodilatation produced is quantitatively similar to that in normal subjects, one deduces that the level of cholinergic tone is normal in emphysema.

The only pathway to bronchodilatation available for adrenergic agents in emphysema is by modulating cholinergic tone either at the peribronchial ganglia or at adrenergic receptors on airway smooth muscle cells. In either case their relaxant effect is dependent on a level of cholinergic tone which, if abolished, leaves no room for adrenergic bronchodilatation. By this reasoning it is more rational to use an anticholinergic than an adrenergic bronchodilator in emphysema, and this is confirmed in practice.

The clinical implications of this hypothesis are that anticholinergic agents are the logical first choice in chronic bronchitis and emphysema. In asthma they will usually produce some bronchodilatation, but not as much as an adrenergic agent or the combination of both types of agent.

References

Abraham, W. M., Olver, W., Jr., King, M. M., Yerger, L., and Wanner, A. (1981). Effects of pharmacologic agents on antigen-induced decreases in specific lung conductance in sheep. *Am. Rev. Respir. Dis. 124*: 554-558.

Adlung, J., Hohle, K. D., Zeren, S., and Wahl, D. (1976). Studies on pharmacokinetics and biotransformation of ipratropium bromide in man. *Arzneim. Forsch. 26*: 1005-1010.

Ajewski, Z., and Popiak, B. (1979). The relation between permanent administration of Atrovent and the dose of steroids in chronic bronchitis. Abstract. *Scand. J. Respir. Dis. 103* (Suppl): 205.

Allen, C. J., and Campbell, A. H. (1980a). Comparison of inhaled atropine sulfate and atropine methonitrate. *Thorax 35*: 932-935.

Allen, C. J., and Campbell, A. H. (1980b). Dose response of ipratropium bromide assessed by two methods. *Thorax 35*: 137-139.

Allison, D. G., Clay, T. P., Hughes, J. M. B., Jones, H. A., and Shevis, A. (1974). Effects of nasal stimulation on total respiratory resistance in the rabbit. *J. Physiol. (Lond.) 239*: 23-24.

Altounyan, R. E. C. (1964). Variation of drug action on airway obstruction in man. *Thorax 19*: 406-415.

Altounyan, R. E. C. (1970). Changes in histamine and atropine responsiveness as a guide to diagnosis and evaluation of therapy in obstructive airways disease. In *Disodium Cromoglycate in Allergic Airways Disease.* Edited by J. Pepys and A. W. Frankland. London, Buttersworths, pp. 47-53.

Annis, P., Landa, J., and Lichtiger, M. (1976). Effects of atropine on velocity of tracheal mucus in anesthetized patients. *Anesthesiology 44*: 74-77.

Ashutosh, K., Mead, G., Dickey, J. C. Jr., Berman, P., and Kuppinger, M. (1980). Density dependence of expiratory flow and bronchodilator response in asthma. *Chest 77*: 68-75.

Astin, T. W. (1972). Reversibility of airways obstruction in chronic bronchitis. *Clin. Sci. 42*: 725-733.

Backman, R., and Hellstrom, P-E. (1985). Fenoterol and ipratropium bromide in respiratory treatment of patients with chronic bronchitis. *Curr. Ther. Res. 38*: 135-140.

Baigelman, W., and Chodosh, S. (1977). Bronchodilator action of the anticholinergic drug, ipratropium bromide (Sch 1000), as an aerosol in chronic bronchitis and asthma. *Chest 71*: 324-328.

Barber, P. V., Chatterjee, S. S., and Scott, R. (1977). A comparison of ipratropium bromide, deptropine citrate and placebo in asthma and chronic bronchitis. *Br. J. Dis. Chest 71*: 101-104.

Barnes, P. J. (1984). The third nervous system in the lung: physiology and clinical perspectives. *Thorax 39*: 561-567.

Barnes, P. J., Dollery, C. T., and MacDermot, J. (1980a). Increased pulmonary alpha-adrenergic and reduced beta-adrenergic receptors in experimental asthma. *Nature 285*: 569-571.

Barnes, P. J., Karliner, J. S., and Dollery, C. T. (1980b). Human lung adrenoceptors studied by radioligand binding. *Clin. Sci. 58*: 457-461.

Barnes, P. J., Basbaum, C. B., and Nadel, J. A. (1983a). Autoradiographic localization of autonomic receptors in airway smooth muscle: marked differences between large and small airways. *Am. Rev. Respir. Dis. 127*: 758-762.

Barnes, P. J., Nadel, J. A., Roberts, J. M., and Basbaum, C. B. (1983b). Muscarinic receptors in lung and trachea. *Eur. J. Pharmacol. 86*: 103-106.

Beck, R., Robertson, C., Galdes, Sebaldt, M., and Levison, H. (1985). Combined salbutamol and ipratropium bromide by inhalation in the treatment of severe acute asthma. *J. Pediatr. 107*: 605-608.

Beers, W. H., and Reich, E. (1970). Structure and activity of acetyl choline. *Nature 228*: 917-922.

Bell, J. A., Bluestein, B. M., Danta, I., and Wanner, A. (1984). Effect of inhaled ipratropium bromide on tracheal mucociliary transport in bronchial asthma. *Mt. Sinai J. Med. 51*: 215-217.

Berger, J., Albert, R. E., Sanborn, K., and Lippman, M. (1978). Effects of atropine and methacholine on deposition and clearance of inhaled particles in the donkey. *J. Toxicol. Environ. Health. 4*: 587-604.

Bergman, K. R., Pearson, C., Waltz, G. W., and Evans, R. (1980). Atropine-induced psychosis: an unusual complication of therapy with inhaled atropine sulfate. *Chest 78*: 891-893.

Birdsall, N. J. M., Burgen, A. S. V., and Hulme, E. C. (1978). The binding of agonists to brian muscarinic receptors. *Mol. Pharmacol. 14*: 723-736.

Birdsall, N. J. M., Burgen, A. S. V., and Hulme, E. C. (1979). A study of the muscarinic receptors by gel electrophoresis. *Br. J. Pharmacol. 66*: 337-342.

Blair, A. M., and Woods, A. (1969). The effects of isoprenaline, atropine and disodium cromoglycate on ciliary motility and mucus flow measured in vivo in cats. *Br. J. Pharmacol. 35*: 379-380.

Blanshard, G. (1960). Sputum viscosity and postoperative pulmonary atelectasis. *Dis. Chest. 37*: 75-81.

Boat, T. F., and Kleinerman, J. L. (1975). Human respiratory tract secretions. 2. Effect of cholinergic and adrenergic agents on in vitro release of protein and mucous glycoprotein. *Chest 67* (Suppl): 32-34.

Borut, T. C., Tashkin, D. P., Fischer, T. J., Katz, R., Rachelefsky, G., Siegel, S. C., Lee, E., and Harper, C. (1977). Comparison of aerosolized atropine sulfate and Sch 1000 on exercise-induced bronchospasm in children. *J. Allergy Clin. Immunol. 60*: 127-133.

Boushey, H. A., and Gold, W. M. (1983). Anticholinergic drugs. In *Allergy: Principles and Practice,* 2nd ed. Edited by E. Middleton Jr., C. E. Reed, and E. F. Ellis. St. Louis, C. V. Mosby, pp. 633-651.

Boushey, H. A., Richardson, P. S., and Widdicombe, J. G. (1972). Reflex effects of laryngeal irritation on the pattern of breathing and total lung resistance. *J. Physiol. (Lond). 224*: 501-513.

Boushey, H. A., Richardson, P. S., Widdicombe, J. G., and Wise, J. C. M. (1974). The response of laryngeal afferent fibres to mechanical and chemical stimuli. *J. Physiol. (Lond.) 240*: 153-175.

Brown, I. G., Chan, C. S., Kelly, C. A., Dent, A. G., and Zimmerman, P. V. (1984). Assessment of the clinical usefulness of nebulized ipratropium bromide in patients with chronic airflow limitation. *Thorax 39*: 272-276.

Bruderman, I., Cohen-Aronovski, R., Smorzik, J. (1983). A comparative study of various combinations of ipratropium bromide and metaproterenol in allergic asthmatic patients. *Chest 83*: 206-210.

Bryant, D. H. (1985). Nebulized ipratropium bromide in the treatment of acute asthma. *Chest 88*: 24-29.

Burge, P. S., Harries, M. G., and I'Anson, E. (1980). Comparison of atropine with ipratropium bromide in patients with reversible airways obstruction unresponsive to salbutamol. *Br. J. Dis. Chest 74*: 259-262.

Butler, J., Caro, C. G., Alcala, R., and Dubois, A. B. (1960). Physiologic factors affecting airway resistance in normal subjects and in patients with obstructive respiratory disease. *J. Clin. Invest. 39*: 584-591.

Cabezas, G. A., Graf, P. D., and Nadel, J. A. (1971). Sympathetic versus parasympathetic nervous regulation of airways in dogs. *J. Appl. Physiol. 31*: 651-655.

Carlyle, R. F. (1963). The mode of action of neostigmine and physostigmine on guinea pig trachealis muscle. *Br. J. Pharmacol. 21*: 137-149.

Cavanaugh, M. J., and Cooper, D. M. (1976). Inhaled atropine sulfate: Dose response characteristics. *Am. Rev. Respir. Dis. 114*: 517-524.

Chang, J., Piperata, S., Skowronek, M., and Lewis, A. J. (1983). Effects of thiazinamium chloride, promezathine and chlorpromazine on thromboxane B2 synthesis, phagocytosis, and respiratory burst by rat alveolar macrophages. *Biochem. Pharmacol. 32*: 2671-2677.

Chapman, K. R., Smith, D. L., Rebuck, A. S., and Leenen, F. H. H. (1985). Hemodynamic effects of inhaled ipratripium bromide, alone and combined with an inhaled beta 2-agonist. *Am. Rev. Respir. Dis. 132*: 845-847.

Chen, W. Y., Brenner, A. M., Weiser, P. C., and Chai, H. (1981). Atropine and exercise-induced bronchoconstriction. *Chest 79*: 651-656.

Cheng, J. B., and Townley, R. G. (1982). Comparison of muscarinic and beta adrenergic receptors between bovine peripheral lung and tracheal smooth muscles: A striking difference in the receptor concentration. *Life Sci. 30*: 2079-2086.

Cheng, J. B., and Townley, R. G. (1983). Decreased sensitivity and response of isolated tracheal muscle to methacholine and histamine without changing the activity of pulmonary muscarinic receptors in the egg albumin-sensitized guinea pig. *Int. Arch. Allergy Appl. Immunol. 72*: 303-309.

Chervinsky, P. (1977). Double blind study of ipratropium bromide, a new anticholinergic bronchodilator. *J. Allergy Clin. Immunol. 59*: 22-30.

Chick, T. W., and Jenne, J. W. (1977). Comparative bronchodilator responses to atropine and terbutaline in asthma and chronic bronchitis. *Chest 72*: 719-723.

Cockcroft, D. W., Ruffin, R. E., and Hargreave, F. E. (1978). Effect of Sch 1000 on allergen-induced asthma. *Clin. Allergy 8*: 361-372.

Cockcroft, D. W., Cotton, D. J., and Berscheid, B. A. (1982). Long-term efficacy and safety of inhaled Sch 1000, an anticholinergic bronchodilator. *Curr. Ther. Res. 31*: 138-147.

Colebatch, H. J. H., and Halmagyi, D. F. J. (1963). Effect of vagotomy and vagal stimulation on lung mechanics and circulation. *J. Appl. Physiol. 18*: 881-887.

Connolly, C. K. (1982). Adverse reaction to ipratropium bromide. *Br. Med. J. 285*: 934-935.

Corssen, G., and Allen, C. R. (1959). Acetylcholine: its significance in controlling ciliary activity of human respiratory epithelium in vitro. *J. Appl. Physiol. 14*: 901-904.

Crompton, G. K. (1968). A comparison of responses to bronchodilator drugs in chronic bronchitis and chronic asthma. *Thorax 23*: 46-55.

Davis, A., Vickerson, F., Worsley, G., Mindorff, C., Kazim, F., and Levison, H. (1984). Determination of dose-response relationship for nebulized ipratropium in asthmatic children. *J. Pediatr. 105*: 1002-1005.

Deal, E. C. Jr., McFadden, E. R. Jr., Ingram, R. H. Jr., and Jaeger, J. J. (1978). Effects of atropine on potentiation of exercise-induced bronchospasm by cold air. *J. Appl. Physiol. 45*: 238-243.

Deckers, W. (1975). The chemistry of new derivatives of tropane alkaloids and the pharmacokinetics of a new quaternary compound. *Postgrad. Med. J. 51* (Suppl 7): 76-81.

DeKock, M. A. (1970). Mechanism of bronchial obstruction in man. In *International Bronchitis Symposium,* 3rd ed. Edited by N. G. M. Oriel and R. Vander Linde. New York, Thomas, pp. 300-315.

DeKock, M. A., Nadel, J. A., Zwi, S., Colebatch, H. J. H., and Olsen, C. R. (1966). New method for perfusing bronchial arteries: Histamine bronchoconstriction and apnea. *J. Appl. Physiol. 21*: 185-194.

De Troyer, A., Yernault, J-C., and Rodenstein, D. (1979). Effects of vagal blockade on lung mechanics in normal man. *J. Appl. Physiol. 46*: 217-226.

De Vries, K. (1975). The protective effect of inhaled Sch 1000 MDI on bronchoconstriction induced by serotonin, histamine, acetylcholine and propranolol (abstract). *Postgrad. Med. J. 51*: (Suppl 7): 106.

Dixon, W. E., and Ransom, F. (1912). Bronchodilator nerves. *J. Physiol. (Lond). 45*: 413-428.

Dotevall, G., Jaup, B. H., and Stochbrugger, R. W. (1982). Symposium on the selectivity of antimuscarinic compounds. *Scand. J. Gastroenterol. 17* (Suppl 72): 1-273.

Douglas, N. J., Davidson, I., Sudlow, M. F., and Flenley, D. C. (1979a). Bronchodilatation and the site of airway resistance in severe chronic bronchitis. *Thorax 34*: 51-56.

Douglas, N. J., Sudlow, M. F., and Flenley, D. C. (1979b). Effect of an inhaled atropinelike agent on normal airway function. *J. Appl. Physiol. 46*: 256-262.

Drachman, D. A. (1977). Memory and cognitive function in man: Does the cholinergic system have a specific role? *Neurology 27*: 783-790.

Eiser, N. M., and Guz, A. (1982). Effect of atropine on experimentally-induced airway obstruction in man. *Bull. Eur. Physiopathol. Respir. 18*: 449-460.

Ellis, J., and Lenox, R. H. (1985). Quaternary forms of classical muscarinic antagonists distinguish subpopulations of muscarinic receptors: correlation with gallamine-defined subpopulations. *Biochem. Biophys. Res. Commun. 126*: 1242-1250.

Elwood, R. K., and Abboud, R. T. (1982). The short-term bronchodilator effects of fenoterol and ipratropium in asthma. *J. Allergy Clin. Immunol. 69*: 467-473.

Engelhardt, A. (1979). Pharmacology and toxicology of Atrovent. *Scand. J. Respir. Dis. 103* (Suppl.): 110-115.

Engelhardt, A., and Klupp, H. (1975). The pharmacology and toxicology of a new tropane alkaloid derivative. *Postgrad. Med. J. 51* (Suppl 7): 82-85.

Fabbri, L. M., Hendrick, D. J., and Diem, J. E. (1983). Effect of atropine on the bronchial response of asthmatic subjects to the inhalation of ultrasonically nebulized distilled water. *J. Allergy Clin. Immunol. 71*: 468-472.

Fairshter, R. D., Habib, M. P., and Wilson, A. F. (1981). Inhaled atropine sulfate in acute asthma. *Respiration 42*: 263-272.

Fasske, E., Jungst, G., and Themann, H. (1975). Light and electron microscopic studies of human bronchial epithelium following treatment with Sch 1000 dose inhaler. (abstract). *Postgrad. Med. J. 51* (Suppl 7): 107.

Field, G. B. (1967). The effects of posture, oxygen, isoproterenol and atropine on ventilation-perfusion relationships in the lung in asthma. *Clin. Sci. 32*: 279-288.

Fish, J. E., Rosenthal, R. R., Summer, W. R., Menkes, H., Norman, P. S., and Permutt, S. (1977). The effect of atropine on acute antigen-mediated airway constriction in subjects with allergic asthma. *Am. Rev. Respir. Dis. 115*: 371-379.

Fletcher, C. M., and Pride, N. B. (1984). Definitions of emphysema, chronic bronchitis, asthma, and airflow obstruction: 25 years on from the Ciba Symposium. *Thorax 39*: 81-85.

Foster, W. M., Bergofsky, E. H., Bohning, D. E., Lippman, M., and Albert, R. E. (1976). Effects of adrenergic agents and their mode of action on mucociliary clearance in man. *J. Appl. Physiol. 41*: 146-152.

Francis, R. A., Thomson, M. L., Pavia, D., and Douglas, R. B. (1977). Ipratropium bromide: Mucociliary clearance rate and airway resistance in normal subjects. *Br. J. Dis. Chest 71*: 173-178.

Gal, T. J., and Suratt, P. M. (1981). Atropine and glycopyrrolate effects on lung mechanics in normal man. *Anesth. Analg. 60*: 85-90.

Gal, T. J., Suratt, P. M., and Lu, J-Y. (1984). Glycopyrrolate and atropine inhalation: comparative effects on normal airway function. *Am. Rev. Respir. Dis. 129*: 871-873.

Gandevia, B. (1975). Historical review of the use of parasympatholytic agents in the treatment of respiratory disorders. *Postgrad. Med. J. 51* (Suppl 7); 13-20.

Gayrard, P., Orehek, J., and Charpin, J. (1975). The prevention of the bronchoconstrictor effects of deep inspiration or of cigarette smoking in asthmatic patients by Sch 1000. (abstract). *Postgrad. Med. J. 51* (Suppl): 102.

Germouty, J. (1975). The possible antagonism between Sch 1000 and beta-blocking agents (abstract). *Postgrad. Med. J. 51* (Suppl 7): 103.

Gold, W. M. (1980). Role of cyclic nucleotides in airway smooth muscle. In *Physiology and Pharmacology of the Airways.* Edited by J. A. Nadel. New York, Marcel Dekker, pp. 123-190.

Gold, W. M., Kessler, G-F., and Yu, D. Y. C. (1972). Role of vagus nerves in experimental asthma in allergic dogs. *J. Appl. Physiol. 33*: 719-725.

Gomm, S. A., Keaney, N. P., Hunt, L. P., Allen, S. C., and Stretton, T. B. (1983). Dose response comparison of ipratropium bromide from a metered-dose inhaler and by jet nebulisation. *Thorax 38*: 297-301.

Grieco, M. H., and Pierson, R. N. Jr. (1971). Mechanism of bronchoconstriction due to beta-adrenergic blockade. *J. Allergy Clin. Immunol. 48*: 143-152.

Griffin, M. P., Fung, K. F., Ingram, R. H. Jr., and McFadden, E. R. Jr. (1982). Dose response effects of atropine on thermal stimulus-response relationships in asthma. *J. Appl. Physiol. 53*: 1576-1582.

Gross, N. J. (1975). Sch 1000: A new anticholinergic bronchodilator. *Am. Rev. Respir. Dis. 112*: 823-828.

Gross, N. J., and Skorodin, M. S. (1984a). Anticholinergic, antimuscarinic bronchodilators. *Am. Rev. Respir. Dis. 129*: 856-870.

Gross, N. J., and Skorodin, M. S. (1984b). Role of the parasympathetic system in airway obstruction due to emphysema. *N. Engl. J. Med. 311*: 421-425.

Gross, N. J., and Skorodin, M. S. (1984c). Role of the parasympathetic system in control of airways of patients with chronic obstructive airways disease (COPD). Abstract. *Am. Rev. Respir. Dis. 129*: A235.

Gross, N. J., and Skorodin, M. S. (1985). Massive overdose of atropine methonitrate with only slight untoward effects. *Lancet 2*: 386.

Haga, T. (1980). Molecular size of muscarinic acetylcholine receptors of rat brain. *FEBS Lett. 113*: 68-72.

Hamm, J. (1975). Hemodynamics and blood gas tensions. *Postgrad. Med. J. 51* (suppl 7): 149-150.

Hammer, K., and Giachetti, A. (1983). Muscarinic receptor subtypes M1 and M2: biochemical and functional characterization. *Life Sci. 31*: 2991-2998.

Hartley, J. P. R., and Davis, B. H. (1980). Cholinergic blockade in the prevention of exercise-induced asthma. *Thorax 35*: 680-685.

Heilbronn, E., and Bartfai, T. (1978). Muscarinic acetylcholine receptor. *Prog. Neurobiol. 11*: 171-188.

Hensley, M. J., O'Cain, C. F., McFadden, E. R. Jr., and Ingram, R. H. Jr. (1978). Distribution of bronchodilatation in normal subjects: beta agonists versus atropine. *J. Appl. Physiol. 45*: 778-782.

Hirshman, C. A., and Downes, H. (1981). Basenji-Breyhound dog model of asthma: influence of atropine on antigen-induced bronchoconstriction. *J. Appl. Physiol. 50*: 761-765.

Hockley, B., and Johnson, N. M. (1985). A comparison of three high doses of ipratropium bromide in chronic asthma. *Br. J. Dis. Chest 79*: 379-384.

Hoffbrand, B. I., and Phillips, V. J. (1984). Editors. The wheezy patient and Duovent. *Postgrad. Med. J. 60*: (Suppl 1): 1-42.

Holtzman, M. J., Cunningham, J. H., Sheller, J. R., Irsigler, G. B., Nadel, J. A., and Boushey, H. A. (1979). Effect of ozone on bronchial reactivity in atopic and nonatopic subjects. *Am. Rev. Respir. Dis. 120*: 1059-1067.

Holtzman, M. J., Sheller, J. R., DiMeo, M., Nadel, J. A., and Boushey, H. A. (1980). Effect of ganglion blockade on bronchial reactivity in atopic subjects. *Am. Rev. Respir. Dis. 122*: 17-25.

Holtzman, M. J., McNamara, M. P., Sheppard, D., Fabbri, L. M., Hahn, H. L. H., Graf, P. D., and Nadel, J. A. (1983). Intravenous versus inhaled atropine for inhibiting bronchoconstrictor responses in dogs. *J. Appl. Physiol. 54*: 134-139.

Hughes, J. A., Tobin, M. J., Bellamy, D., and Hutchison, D. C. S. (1982). Effects of ipratropium bromide and fenoterol in pulmonary emphysema. *Thorax 37*: 667-670.

Hume, K. M., and Gandevia, B. (1957). Forced expiratory volume before and after isoprenaline. *Thorax 12*: 276-278.

Ingram, R. H. Jr., Wellman, J. J., McFadden, E. R. Jr., and Mead, J. (1977). Relative contributions of large and small airways to flow limitation in normal subjects before and after atropine and isoproterenol. *J. Clin. Invest. 59*: 696-703.

Iravani, J., and Melville, G. N. (1975). Ciliary movement following various concentrations of different anticholinergic and adrenergic bronchodilator solutions in animals (abstract). *Postgrad. Med. J. 51* (Suppl 7): 108.

Islam, M. S., and Ulmer, W. T. (1984). Influence of the inhalative aerosol Atrovent on airway resistance and intrathoracic gas volume in healthy volunteers of different ages. *Respiration 45*: 225-231.

Itkin, I. H., and Anand, S. C. (1970). The role of atropine as a mediator blocker of induced bronchial obstruction. *J. Allergy Clin. Immunol. 45*: 178-186.

Janowsky, D. S., El-Yousef, M. K., Davis, J. M., and Sekerke, H. J. (1972). A cholinergic-adrenergic hypothesis of mania and depression. (1972). *Lancet 2*: 632-635.

Jeffery, P. K. (1981). The innervation of bronchial mucosa. In *Cellular Biology of the Lung.* Edited by G. Cumming and G. Bonsignore. New York and London, Plenum Press, pp. 1-25.

Jenkins, C. R., Chow, C. M., Fisher, B. L., and Marlin, G. E. (1981). Comparison of ipratropium bromide and salbutamol by aerosolized solution. *Aust. N.Z. J. Med. 11*: 513-516.

Johnson, B. E., Suratt, P. M., Gal, T. J., and Wilhoit, S. C. (1984). Effect of inhaled glycopyrrolate and atropine in asthma precipitated by exercise and cold air inhalation. *Chest 85*: 325-328.

Jolobe, O. M. P. (1983). Impaired atropine responsiveness in asthma: Role of atopy. *Respiration 44*: 97-102.

Jolobe, O. M. P. (1984a). Reversible airflow obstruction: Clinical spectrum and responsiveness to anticholinergic drugs. *Respiration 45*: 232-236.

Jolobe, O. M. P. (1984b). Asthma versus non-specific reversible airflow obstruction: clinical features and responsiveness to anticholinergic drugs. *Respiration 45*: 237-242.

Jolobe, O. M. P. (1984c). Atropine resistance in asthma: Definition and provisional hypothesis. *Respiration 46*: 174-179.

Jolobe, O. M. P., and Lane, D. J. (1981). Atropine responsiveness in asthma in relation to steroid aerosol therapy. *Br. J. Dis. Chest 75*: 413-416.

Jonkman, J. H. G., Van Bork, L. E., Wijsbeek, J., De Zeeuw, R. A., and Orie, N. G. M. (1977). Variations in the bioavailability of thiazinamium methylsulfate. *Clin. Pharmacol. Ther. 21*: 457-463.

Justesen, D. R., Braun, E. W., Garrison, R. G., and Pendleton, R. B. (1970). Pharmacologic differentiation of allergic and classically conditioned asthma in the guinea pig. *Science 170*: 864-866.

Kaiser, S. C. (1971). The fate of atropine in man. *Ann. N.Y. Acad. Sci. 179*: 667-683.

Karczewski, W., and Widdicombe, J. G. (1969). The effect of vagotomy, vagal cooling and efferent vagal stimulation on breathing and lung mechanics of rabbits. *J. Physiol. (Lond.) 201*: 259-270.

Kessler, G-F., Austin, J. H. M., Graf, p. D., Gamsu, G., and Gold, W. M. (1973). Airway constriction in experimental asthma in dogs: tantalum bronchographic studies. *J. Appl. Physiol. 35*: 703-708.

King, M., Cohen, C., and Viires, N. (1979). Influence of vagal tone on rheology and transportability of canine tracheal mucus. *Am. Rev. Respir. Dis. 120*: 1215-1219.

Kiviloog, J. (1975). The effect of pretreatment with atropine in exercise-induced bronchoconstriction. *Pediatrics 56* (Suppl): 940-941.

Kjellberg, M., and Heinonen, J. (1974). Atropine, neostigmine and airway resistance. *Acta Anaesthesiol. Scand. 18*: 209-214.

Klock, L. E., Miller, T. D., Morris, A. H., Watanabe, S., and Dickman, M. (1975). A comparative study of atropine sulfate and isoproterenol hydrochloride in chronic bronchitis. *Am. Rev. Respir. Dis. 112*: 371-376.

Kradjan, W. A., Lakshminarayan, S., Hayden, P. W., Larson, S. W., and Marini, J. J. (1981). Serum atropine concentrations after inhalation of atropine sulfate. *Am. Rev. Respir. Dis. 123*: 471-472.

Kreisman, H., Frank, H., Wolkove, N., and Gent, M. (1981). Synergism between ipratropium and theophylline in asthma. *Thorax 36*: 387-391.

Krell, R. D., Chakrin, L. W., and Wardell, J. R. Jr. (1976). The effect of cholinergic agents on a canine model of asthma. *J. Allergy Clin. Immunol. 58*: 19-30.

Krieger, E., and Reitberger, U. (1975). Sputum rheology following treatment with Sch 1000 MDI and orciprenaline MDI (abstract). *Postgrad. Med. J. 51* (Suppl 7): 108.

Langer, I. (1967). The bronchoconstrictor action of propranolol aerosol in asthmatic subjects (abstract). *J. Physiol. (Lond.) 190*: 41.

Leahy, B. C., Gomm, S. A., and Allen, S. C. (1983). Comparison of nebulized salbutamol with nebulized ipratropium bromide in acute asthma. *Br. J. Dis. Chest 77*: 159-163.

Lefcoe, N. M., Toogood, J. H., Blennerhassett, G., and Patterson, N. A. M. (1982). The addition of an aerosol anticholinergic to an oral beta agonist plus theophylline in asthma and bronchitis. *Chest 82*: 300-305.

Levine, R. M. (1959). The absorption of the quaternary derivatives of atropine and scopolamine. *Arch. Int. Pharmacodyn. Ther. 121*: 146-149.

Lewis, A. J., Dervinis, A., and Rosenthale, M. E. (1982). Bronchodilator and antiallergic effects of thiazinamium chloride in guinea pigs, rats, cats, and dogs. *Eur. J. Pharmacol. 80*: 171-184.

Lewis, A. J., Dervinis, A., and Chang, J. (1984a). The effects of antiallergic and bronchodilator drugs on platelet-activating factor induced bronchospasm and platelet aggregation. *Agents Actions 15*: 636-642.

Lewis, A. J., Dervinis, A., Rosenthale, M. E., Santilli, A. A., and Buzby, G. C. (1984b). The comparative bronchodilator properties of alkyl quaternary salts of promethazine. *Int. Arch. Allergy Appl. Immun. 75*: 282-283.

Lightboyd, I. M., Ingram, C. G., Legge, J. S., and Johnston, R. N. (1978). Ipratropium bromide, salbutamol and prednisolone in bronchial asthma and chronic bronchitis. *Br. J. Dis. Chest 72*: 181-186.

Lin, M. T., Lee-Hong, E., and Collins-Williams, C. (1978). A clinical trial of the bronchodilator effect of Sch 1000 aerosol in asthmatic children. *Ann. Allergy 40*: 326-332.

Lopez-Vidriero, M. T., Costello, J., Clark, T. J. H., Das, I., Keal, E. E., and Reid, L. (1975). Effect of atropine on sputum production. *Thorax 30*: 543-547.

Lundberg, J. M., Martling, C-R., and Saria, A. (1983). Substance P and capsaicin-induced contraction of human bronchi. *Acta Physiol. Scand. 119*: 49-53.

MacDonald, A. G., Ingram, C. G., and McNeill, R. S. (1967). The effect of propranolol on airway resistance. *Br. J. Anaesth. 39*: 919-926.

Mann, J. S., and George, C. F. (1985). Anticholinergic drugs in the treatment of airways disease. *Br. J. Dis. Chest 79*: 209-228.

Mann, J. S., Howarth, P. H., and Holgate, S. T. (1984). Bronchoconstriction induced by nebulised ipratropium bromide: relation to hypotonicity. *Br. Med. J. 289*: 469.

Mansfield, L. E., Hameister, H. H., Spaulding, H. S., Smith, N. J., and Glab, N. (1981). The role of the vagus nerve in airway narrowing caused by intraesophageal hydrochloric acid provocation and esophageal distention. *Ann. Allergy. 47*: 431-434.

Marin, M. G., Davis, B., and Nadel, J. A. (1976). Effect of acetylcholine on Cl- and Na+ fluxes across dog tracheal epithelium in vitro. *Am. J. Physiol. 231*: 1546-1549.

Marini, J. J., and Lakshminarayan, S. (1980). The effect of atropine inhalation in "irreversible" chronic bronchitis. *Chest 77*: 591-596.

Marlin, G. E., Berend, N., and Harrison, A. C. (1979). Combined cholinergic antagonist and beta-2 adreneceptor agonist bronchodilator therapy by inhalation. *Aust. N.Z. Med. J. 9*: 511-514.

Marquardt, D. L., Motulsky, H. J., and Wasserman, S. I. (1982). Rat lung cholinergic receptor: characterization and regulation by corticosteroids. *J. Appl. Physiol. 53*: 731-736.

Martinez, J., de Letona, J., Castro de la Mata, R., and Aviado, D. M. (1961). Local and reflex effects of bronchial artery injection of drugs. *J. Pharmacol. Exp. Ther. 133*: 295-303.

McFadden, E. R. Jr. (1981). An analysis of exercise as a stimulus for the production of airway obstruction. *Lung 159*: 3-11.

McFadden, E. R. Jr., Ingram, R. H. Jr., Haynes, R. L., and Wellman, J. J. (1977). Predominant site of flow limitation and mechanisms of postexertional asthma. *J. Appl. Physiol. 42*: 746-752.

McFadden, E. R. Jr., Luparello, T., Lyons, H. A., and Bleeker, E. (1969). The mechanism of action of suggestion in the induction of acute asthma attacks. *Psychosom. Med. 31*: 134-143.

McGivern, D. V., Fentem, P. H., MacFarlane, J. T., and Davies, D. (1984). Responses to the sequential administration of salbutamol and ipratropium bromide during recovery from acute severe asthma. *Thorax 39*: 227.

McNeill, R. S., and Ingram, C. G. (1966). Effect of propranolol on ventilatory function. *Am. J. Cardiol. 18*: 473-475.

Mills, J. E., Sellick, H., and Widdicombe, J. G. (1970). Epithelial irritant receptors in the lungs. In *Breathing: Hering-Breuer Centenary Symposium.* Edited by R. Porter. London, J. & A Churchill, pp. 77-92.

Minette, A. (1975). The effects of long-term treatment with Sch 1000 MDI. *Postgrad. Med. J. 51* (Suppl)7: 153-154.

Minette, A., and Marcq, M. (1979). Experience with Atrovent in coal miners. *Scand. J. Respir. Dis. 103* (Suppl): 192-199.

Mita, H., Yui, Y., Yasueda, H., Shida, T. (1983). Changes of alpha-1 and beta adrenergic and cholinergic muscarinic receptors in guinea pig lung sensitized with ovalbumin. *Int. Arch. Allergy Appl. Immunol. 70*: 225-230.

Molkenboer, J. F. W. M., and Lardenoye, J. G. (1979). The effect of Atrovent in micturition function, double blind cross-over study. *Scand. J. Respir. Dis. 103* (Suppl): 154-158.

Nadel, J. A. (1980). Autonomic regulation of airway smooth muscle. In *Physiology and Pharmacology of the Airways.* Edited by J. A. Nadel. New York, Marcel Dekker, pp. 217-257.

Nadel, J. A., and Widdicombe, J. G. (1962). Reflex effects of upper airway irritation on total lung resistance and blood pressure. *J. Appl. Physiol. 17*: 861-865.

Nadel, J. A., and Widdicombe, J. G. (1963). Reflex control of airway size. *Ann. N.Y. Acad. Sci. 108*: 712-722.

Nadel, J. A., Cabezas, G. A., and Austin, J. H. M. (1971). In vivo roentgenographic examination of parasympathetic innervation of small airways. Use of powdered tantalum and a fine focal spot x-ray tube. *Invest. Radiol. 6*: 9-17.

Nadel, J. A., Salem, H., Tamplin, B., and Yokiwa, Y. (1965). Mechanisms of bronchoconstriction during inhalation of sulfur dioxide. *J. Appl. Physiol. 20*: 164-167.

Nathanson, N. M. (1982). Regulation and development of muscarinic acetylcholine receptors. *TINS* Nov: 401-404.

Neijens, H. J., Wesselius, T., and Kerrebijn, K. (1981). Exercise-induced bronchoconstriction as an expression of bronchial hyperreactivity. A study of its mechanisms in children. *Thorax 36*: 517-522.

Newcomb, R., Tashkin, D. P., Hui, K. K., Conolly, M. E., Lee, M. E., and Dauphinee, B. (1985). Rebound hyperresponsiveness to muscarinic stimulation after chronic therapy with an inhaled muscarinic agent. *Am. Rev. Respir. Dis. 132*: 12-15.

Noble, M. D., Brown, T. H., and Peacock, J. H. (1978). Regulation of acetylcholine receptor levels by a cholinergic agonist in mouse cell cultures. *Proc. Natl. Acad. Sci. USA 75*: 3488-3492.

Nolte, D. (1975). The action of Sch 1000 on experimental bronchoconstriction induced by various types of non-specific and pharmacodynamic irritants in young asthmatics (abstract). *Postgrad. Med. J. 51* (Suppl 7): 103.

Olsen, C. R., Colebatch, H. J. H., Mebel, P. E., Nadel, J. A., and Staub, N. C. (1965). Motor control of pulmonary airways studied by nerve stimulation. *J. Appl. Physiol. 20*: 202-208.

Orehek, J., Gayrard, P., Grimaud, C. H., and Charpin, J. (1975). Bronchoconstriction provoquée par inhalation d'allegène dans l'asthme: Effet antagoniste d'un anticholinérgique de synthèse. *Bull. Eur. Physiopathol. Respir. 11*: 193-201.

Pak, C. C. F., Kradjan, W. A., Lashminarayan, S., and Marini, J. J. (1983). Inhaled atropine sulfate. Dose-response characteristics in adult patients with chronic airflow obstruction. *Am. Rev. Respir. Dis. 125*: 331-334.

Pakes, G. E., Brogden, R. N., Heel, R. C., Speight, T. M., and Avery, G. S. (1980). Ipratropium bromide: A review of its pharmacological properties and therapeutic efficacy in asthma and chronic bronchitis. *Drugs 20*: 237-266.

Partridge, M. R., and Saunders, K. B. (1981). Site of action of ipratropium bromide and clinical and physiological determinants of response in patients with asthma. *Thorax 36*: 530-533.

Passamonte, P. M., and Martinez, A. J. (1984). Effect of inhaled atropine or metaproterenol in patients with chronic airway obstruction and therapeutic serum theophylline levels. *Chest 85*: 610-615.

Patel, K. R., and Tullett, W. M. (1983). Bronchoconstriction in response to ipratropium bromide (Letter). *Br. Med. J. 286*: 1318.

Patterson, R., and Harris, K. E. (1976). The effect of cholinergic and anticholinergic agents on the primate models of allergic asthma. *J. Lab. Clin. Med. 87*: 65-72.

Pavia, D., and Thomson, M. L. (1971). Inhibition of mucociliary clearance from the human lung by hyoscine. *Lancet 1*: 449-450.

Pavia, D., Bateman, J. R. M., Sheahan, N. F., and Clarke, S. W. (1979). Effect of ipratropium bromide on mucociliary clearance and pulmonary function in reversible airways obstruction. *Thorax 34*: 501-507.

Pavia, D., Bateman, J. R. M., Sheahan, N. F., and Clarke, S. W. (1980). Clearance of lung secretions in patients with chronic bronchitis: effect of terbutaline and ipratropium bromide aerosols. *Eur. J. Respir. Dis. 61*: 245-253.

Peel, E. T., and Anderson, G. (1984). A dose response study of oxitropium bromide in chronic bronchitis. *Thorax 39*: 453-456.

Pernow, B. (1983). Substance P. *Pharmacol. Rev. 35*: 85-141.

Petrie, G. R., and Palmer, K. N. V. (1975). Comparison of aerosol ipratropium bromide and salbutamol in chronic bronchitis and asthma. *Br. J. Med. 1*: 430-432.

Pierce, R. J., Allen, C. J., and Campbell, A. H. (1979). A comparative study of atropine methonitrate, salbutamol, and their combination in airways obstruction. *Thorax 34*: 45-50.

Polak, J. M., and Bloom, S. R. (1982). Regulatory peptides in the respiratory tract of man and other animals. *Exp. Lung Res. 3*: 313-328.

Poppius, H., and Salorinne, Y. (1973). Comparative trial of a new anticholinergic bronchodilator, Sch 1000, and salbutamol in chronic bronchitis. *Br. Med. J. 4*: 134-136.

Poppius, H., Salorinne, Y., and Viljanen, A. A.(1972). Inhalation of a new anticholinergic drug, Sch 1000, in asthma and chronic bronchitis: Effect on airway resistance, thoracic gas volume, blood gases and exercise-induced asthma. *Bull. Eur. Physiopathol. Respir. 8*: 643-652.

Ravez, P., Riches, M., Halloy, J-L., and Robience, Y. (1979). Haemodynamic variables in chronic obstructive airways diseases. The influence of fenoterol and ipratropium bromide. *Clin. Trials 16*: 147-151.

Rebuck, A. S., Gent, M., and Chapman, K. R. (1983). Anticholinergic and sympathomimetic combination therapy of asthma. *J. Allergy Clin. Immunol. 71*: 317-323.

Rebuck, A. S., and Marcus, H. I. (1979). Sch 1000 in psychogenic asthma. *Scand. J. Respir. Dis. 103* (Suppl): 186-190.

Rebuck, A. S., and Read, J. (1971). Assessment and management of severe asthma. *Am. J. Med. 51*: 788-798.

Richardson, J. B., and Beland, J. (1976). Nonadrenergic inhibitory nervous system in human airways. *J. Appl. Physiol. 41*: 764-771.

Richardson, J. B., and Ferguson, C. C. (1979). Neuromuscular structure and function in the airways. *Fed. Proc. 38*: 202-208.

Richardson, P. S., and Sterling, G. M. (1969). Effects of beta-adrenergic receptor blockade on airway conductance and lung volume in normal and asthmatic subjects. *Br. Med. J. 3*: 143-145.

Rominger, K. L. (1979). Chemistry and pharmacokinetics of ipratropium bromide. *Scand. J. Respir. Dis. 103* (Suppl): 116-126.

Rosenthal, R. R., Norman, P. S., Summer, W. R., and Permutt, S. (1977). Role of the parasympathetic system in antigen-induced bronchospasm. *J. Appl. Physiol. 42*: 600-606.

Ruffin, R. E., and Newhouse, M. T. (1978). Ipratropium bromide (Sch 1000) monohydrate aerosol: bronchodilator effect of three dose levels in asthmatics. *Lung 155*: 141-146.

Ruffin, R. E., Fitzgerald, J. D., and Rebuck, A. S. (1977). A comparison of the bronchodilator activity of Sch 1000 and salbutamol. *J. Allergy Clin. Immunol. 59*: 136-141.

Ruffin, R. E., McIntyre, E., Crockett, A. J., Zeilonka, K., and Alpers, J. H. (1982). Combination bronchodilator therapy in asthma. *J. Allergy Clin. Immunol. 69*: 60-65.

Ruffin, R. E., Cockcroft, D. W., and Hargreave, F. E. (1978a). A comparison of the protective effect of fenoterol and Sch 1000 on allergen-induced asthma. *J. Allergy Clin. Immunol. 61*: 42-47.

Ruffin, R. E., Wolff, R. K., and Dolovich, M. B., Eng, P., Rossman, C. M., Fitzgerald, J. D., and Newhouse, M. T. (1978b). Aerosol therapy with Sch 1000: Short-term mucociliary clearance in normal and bronchitic subjects and toxicology in normal subjects. *Chest 73*: 501-506.

Sackner, M. A., Chapman, G. A., Dougherty, R. D. (1977a). Effects of nebulized ipratropium bromide and atropine sulfate on tracheal mucous velocity and lung mechanics in anesthetized dogs. *Respiration 34*: 181-185.

Sackner, M. A., Friedman, M., Silva, G., and Fernandez, R. (1977b). The pulmonary hemodynamic effects of aerosols of isoproterenol and ipratropium in normal subjects and patients with reversible airway obstruction. *Am. Rev. Respir. Dis. 116*: 1013-1022.

Salmon, D. M., and Honeyman, T. W. (1980). Proposed mechanism of cholinergic action in smooth muscle. *Nature 284*: 344-345.

Scheufler, G. (1975). Ophthalmotonometry, pupil diameter and visual accommodation following repeated administration of Sch 1000 MDI in patients with glaucoma (abstract). *Postgrad. Med. J. 51* (suppl y): 132.

Schultze-Werninghaus, G. (1981). Anticholinergic versus beta2-adrenergic therapy in allergic airways obstruction. *Respiration 41*: 239-247.

Sellick, H., and Widdicombe, J. G. (1971). Stimulation of lung irritant receptors by cigarette smoke, carbon dust and histamine. *J. Appl. Physiol. 31*: 15-19.

Sheppard, D., Epstein, J., Holtzman, M. J., Nadel, J. A., and Boushey, H. A. (1982). Dose-dependent inhibition of cold-air induced bronchoconstriction by atropine. *J. Appl. Physiol. 53*: 169-174.

Sheppard, D., Epstein, J., Holtzman, M. J., Nadel, J. A., and Boushey, H. A. (1983). Effect of route of atropine delivery on bronchospasm from cold air and methacholine. *J. Appl. Physiol. 54*: 130-133.

Shifrin, G. S., and Klein, W. L. (1980). Regulatin of muscarinic acetylcholine receptor concentration in cloned neuroblastoma cells. *J. Neurochem. 34*: 993-999.

Siman, R. G., and Klein, W. L. (1979). Cholinergic activity regulates muscarinic receptors in central nervous system cultures. *Proc. Natl. Acad. Sci. USA 76*: 4141-4145.

Simonsson, B. G., Jacobs, F. M., and Nadel, J. A. (1967). Role of autonomic nervous system and the cough reflex in the increased responsiveness of airways in patients with obstructive airway disease. *J. Clin. Invest. 46*: 1812-1818.

Skorodin, M. S., Gross, N. J., Moritz, T., King, F., Armstrong, W., Wells, D., Galowan, E., and Slutsky, L. (1986). Oxitropium bromide: a new anticholinergic bronchodilator. *Ann. Allergy* (in press).

Smith, T. C., and DuBois, A. B. (1969). Effects of scopolamine on the airways of man. *Anesthesiology 30*: 12-18.

Snashall, P. D., and Baldwin, C. (1982). Mechanisms of sulphur dioxide induced bronchoconstriction in normal and asthmatic man. *Thorax 37*: 118-123.

Storms, W. W., DoPico, G. A., and Reed, C. E. (1975). Aerosol Sch 1000: an anticholinergic bronchodilator. *Am. Rev. Respir. Dis. 111*: 419-422.

Sturgess, J., and Reid, L. (1972). An organ culture study of the effect of drugs on the secretory activity of the human bronchial submucosal gland. *Clin. Sci. 43*: 553-543.

Suzuki, R., Takagi, K., and Satake, T. (1985). Changes in muscarinic acetylcholine receptors in guinea-pig lung: Effects of aging, inhalation of an allergen, administration of drugs, and vagotomy. *Lung 163*: 173-182.

Tan, W. C., Cripps, E., Douglas, N., and Sudlow, M. F. (1982). Protective effect of drugs on bronchoconstriction induced by sulphur dioxide. *Thorax 37*: 671-676.

Tashkin, D. P., Katz, R. M., Kerschnar, H., Rachelefsky, G. S., and Siegel, S. C. (1977). Comparison of aerosolized atropine, isoproterenol, atropine plus isoproterenol, disodium cromoglycate and placebo in the prevention of exercise-induced asthma. *Ann. Allergy 39*: 311-318.

Tashkin, D. P., Ashutosh, K., Bleeker, E., Britt, J., Cugell, D., Cummiskey, J., DeLorenzo, L., Gilman, M., Gross, G., Gross, N., Kotch, A., Lakshminarayan, S., Maguire, G., Plummer, A., Renzetti, A., Sackner, M., Skorodin, M., and Wanner, A. (1986). Comparison of the anticholinergic ipratropium bromide with metaproterenol in chronic obstructive pulmonary disease: A 90-day multicenter study. *Am. J. Med.* in press.

Tattersfield, A. E., Leaver, D. G., and Pride, N. B. (1973). Effects of beta-adrenergic blockade and stimulation on normal human airways. *J. Appl. Physiol. 35*: 613-619.

Thiessen, B., and Pedersen, O. F. (1979). A double blind cross-over study of maximal expiratory flows and arterial blood gas tensions in normals, asthmathics, and bronchitics after salbutamol and ipratropin. *Scand. J. Respir. Dis. 103* (Suppl): 170-174.

Thomson, N. C., Patel, K. R., and Kerr, J. W. (1978). Sodium cromoglycate and ipratropium bromide in exercise-induced asthma. *Thorax 33*: 694-699.

Tinkelman, D. G., Cavanaugh, M. J., and Cooper, D. M. (1976). Inhibition of exercise-induced bronchospasm by atropine. *Am. Rev. Respir. Dis. 114*: 87-94.

Tomori, Z., and Widdicombe, J. G. (1969). Muscular, bronchomotor and cardiovascular reflexes elicited by mechanical stimulation of the respiratory tract. *J. Physiol. (Lond.) 200*: 25-49.

Tullett, W. M., Patel, K. R., Berlin, K. E., and Kerr, J. W. (1982). Effect of lignocaine, sodium cromoglycate, and ipratropium bromide in exercise-induced bronchospasm. *Thorax 37*: 737-740.

Ueki, I., German, V. F., and Nadel, J. A. (1980). Micropipette measurement of airway submucosal gland secretion. *Am. Rev. Respir. Dis. 121*: 351-357.

Ullah, M. I., Newman, G. B., and Saunders, K. B. (1981). Influence of age on response to ipratropium and salbutamol in asthma. *Thorax 36*: 523-529.

Ulmer, W. T. (1975). Repeated measurements of total airways obstruction, intrathoracic gas volume, PaO2, PaCO2, and clinical features in patients with chronic obstructive lung disease during long-term treatment with Sch 1000 inhalations (abstract). *Postgrad. Med. J. 51* (Suppl 7): 133.

Vakil, D. V., Ayiomamitis, A., and Nizami, R. M. (1985). Use of ipratropium aerosol in the long-term management of asthma. *J. Asthma 22*: 165-170.

Vastag, E., Vass, K., and Nagy, L. (1976). Bronchoconstriction reflex in bronchial asthma. *Pneumonologie* (Suppl): 259-265.

Vincent, N. J., Knudson, R., Leith, D. E., Macklem, P. T., and Mead, J. (1970). Factors influencing pulmonary resistance. *J. Appl. Physiol. 29*: 236-243.

Virtanen, R., Kanto, J., Iisalo, E., Iisalo, U. M., Salo, M., and Sjovall, S. (1982). Pharmacokinetic studies on atropine with special reference to age. *Acta Anaesthesiol. Scand. 26*: 297-300.

Wahl, D. (1975). Pharmacokinetics of C14-labelled Sch 1000 administered by inhalation, orally and intravenously. *Postgrad. Med. J. 51* (Suppl 7): 93-94.

Wanner, A. (1977). Clinical aspects of mucociliary transport. *Am. Rev. Respir. Dis. 116*: 73-125.

Ward, M. J., Fentem, P. H., Smith, W. H. R., and Davies, D. (1981). Ipratropium bromide in acute asthma. *Br. Med. J. 282*: 598-600.

Ward, M. J., MacFarlane, J. T., and Davies, D. (1985). A place for ipratropium bromide in the treatment of severe acute asthma. *Br. J. Dis. Chest 79*: 374-378.

Weber, R. W., Petty, W. E., and Nelson, H. S. (1979). Aerosolized terbutaline in asthmatics: Comparison of dosage strength, schedule, and methods of administration. *J. Allergy Clin. Immunol. 63*: 116-121.

Weiner, N. (1980). Atropine, scopolamine and related antimuscarinic drugs. In *The Pharmacologic Basis of Therapeutics,* 6th ed. Edited by A. G. Gilman, L. S. Goodman, and A. Gilman. New York, MacMillan, pp. 120-137.

Weiss, J. W., McFadden, E. R. Jr., and Ingram, R. H. Jr. (1982). Parenteral vs inhaled atropine: Density dependence of maximal expiratory flow. *J. Appl. Physiol. 53*: 392-396.

Widdicombe, J. G. (1954). Receptors on the trachea and bronchi of the cat. *J. Physiol. (Lond.) 123*: 71-104.

Widdicombe, J. G. (1977a). Some experimental models of acute asthma. *J. R. Coll. Physicians Lond. 11*: 141-155.

Widdicombe, J. G. (1977b). Reflex control of tracheobronchial smooth muscle in experimental and human asthma. In *Asthma: Physiology, Immunopharmacology, and Treatment.* Edited by L. M. Lichtenstein and K. F. Austen. New York, Academic Press, pp. 225-231.

Widdicombe, J. G. (1979). The parasympathetic nervous system in airways disease. *Scand. J. Respir. Dis. 103* (Suppl): 38-43.

Widdicombe, J. G., Kent, D. C., and Nadel, J. A. (1962). Mechanism of bronchoconstriction during inhalation of dust. *J. Appl. Physiol. 17*: 613-616.

Wilson, N. M., Barnes, P. J., Vickers, H., and Silverman, M. (1982). Hyperventilation induced asthma: evidence for two mechanisms. *Thorax 37*: 657-662.

Wilson, N., Dixon, C., and Silverman, M. (1984). Bronchial responsiveness to hyperventilation in children with asthma: inhibition by ipratropium bromide. *Thorax 39*: 588-593.

Wise, B. C., Shoji, M., and Kuo, J. F. (1980). Decrease or increase in cardiac muscarinic cholinergic receptor number in rats treated with methacholine or atropine. *Biochem. Biophys. Res. Commun. 92*: 1136-1142.

Woolcock, A. J., Macklem, P. T., Hogg, J. C., Wilson, N. J., Nadel, J. A., Frank, N. R., and Brain, J. (1969). Effect of vagal stimulation on central and peripheral airways in dogs. *J. Appl. Physiol. 26*: 806-813.

Yeager, H. Jr., Weinberg, R. M., Kaufman, L. V., and Katz, S. (1976). Asthma: Comparative bronchodilator effects of ipratropium bromide and isoproterenol. *J. Clin. Pharmacol. 16*: 198-204.

Yeats, D. B., Aspin, N., Levison, H., Jones, M. T., and Bryan, A. C. (1975). Mucociliary tracheal transport rates in man. *J. Appl. Physiol. 39*: 487-495.

Yu, D. Y. C., Galant, S. P., and Gold, W. M. (1972). Inhibition of antigen-induced bronchoconstriction by atropine in asthmatic patients. *J. Appl. Physiol. 32*: 823-828.

Zaid, G., and Beall, G. N. (1966). Bronchial response to beta-adrenergic blockade. *N. Engl. J. Med. 275*: 580-584.

Zuskin, E., Mitchell, C. A., and Bouhuys, A. (1974). Interaction between the effects of beta blockade and cigarette smoke on airways. *J. Appl. Physiol. 36*: 449-452.

17

Cromolyn Sodium

SHIRLEY MURPHY
University of New Mexico School of Medicine
Albuquerque, New Mexico

I. Introduction

Of the pharmacologic agents used to treat asthma, cromolyn sodium is unique in its serendipitous discovery, mode of action, and wide range of clinical applications. Although cromolyn sodium has been available for the treatment of asthma in the United States since 1973, continued investigation of this compound has led to new information about its mechanism of action and expanded clinical application.

Cromolyn sodium was discovered as a result of pharmaceutical research carried out in the United Kingdom in the mid-1950s with the naturally occurring antispasmodic, khellin (Cox, 1970). This furanochromone, derived from the Mediterranean plant *Ammi visnaga* (*Umbelliferae*), was investigated because its seeds had been used since ancient times as a smooth muscle relaxant and treatment for colic. Several derivatives were synthesized, but because of adverse side effects they were never investigated clinically. In 1956, Roger Altounyan, a physician, clinical pharmacologist, and an asthmatic himself, joined the research team. Because he doubted that animal testing was the best model for asthma pharmacology, he proceeded to evaluate new components with inhalation challenges on himself (Altounyan, 1967). With antigen challenge techniques, he made the observation that while khellin derivatives in which the 2-methyl group had been replaced by a carboxylic acid moiety had no bronchodilator properties, when taken prophylactically they inhibited the bronchoconstriction induced by antigen (Cox et al., 1970). On January 19, 1965, FPL 670 was synthesized. This unique bischromone offered the best protection for Dr. Altounyan's antigen-induced bronchospasm. These promising initial results were confirmed in clinical trials and this chrome-2-carboxylate, known as sodium cromoglycate or cromolyn sodium, subsequently became available for use in the treatment of asthma in the United Kingdom in 1968 and in the United States in 1973.

II. Basic Pharmacology

A. Chemistry

Cromolyn sodium is synthesized by linking two monochromone nuclei with a shared alkyl residue (Fig. 1) (Cox, 1970). It is a white hydrated powder that is a lipophobic, highly polar, acidic molecule with a pKa 2 and a molecular weight of just over 500 daltons (Brown et al., 1983). It is freely soluble in water up to 5% at 20°C, insoluble in alcohol, and sparingly soluble in common organic solvents such as dioxan, pyridine, ether, and chloroform. The OC=CC=P structure may produce the antiallergic activities of this compound (Pfister, 1972), while other structural sites determine absorptive properties. Cromolyn sodium is hygroscopic and its deliquescent point is around 93% relative humidity, which is much lower than the humidity of the airways.

B. Pharmacokinetics

Initial detailed studies in animals showed that following intravenous administration cromolyn sodium was cleared rapidly from plasma and excreted unchanged in both the urine and bile (Ashton et al., 1973). Inhalation studies in animals showed that the drug deposited in the lung was completely removed and only a small percentage of an oral dose was absorbed from the gastrointestinal tract. Regardless of the route of administration, metabolism of the drug has not been detected.

Early studies in human volunteers (Moss et al., 1971; Walker et al., 1972) indicated that following an intravenous dose, the majority of the drug was rapidly cleared from the plasma with about 50% of the total dose excreted in the urine and the rest in the biliary tract. In asthma patients and normal volunteers given oral doses of 20 mg and 500 mg, urinary excretion was only 0.5% of the administered dose, regardless of amount given. Because the extent of oral absorption is only 1%, the amount of drug that appears in plasma or urine after inhalation reflects the total dose to the lung.

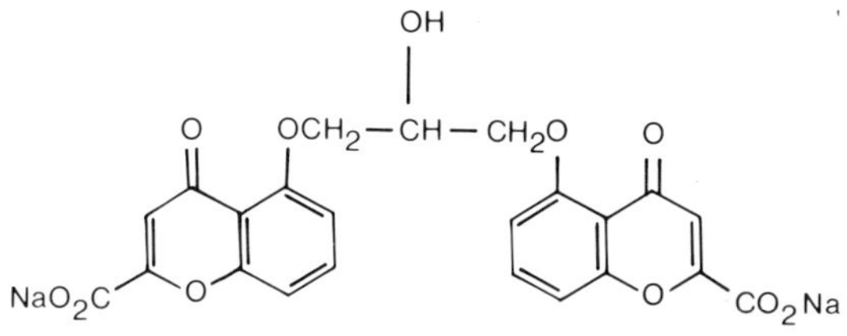

Figure 1 Chemical structure of cromolyn sodium (disodium cromoglycate).

Comparisons of relative bioavailability of drug delivered via the three formulations (Spincap, nebulizer solution, aerosol) of cromolyn sodium using the plasma concentration/time curves are difficult. Although these different formulations deliver different dosages, the same amount of drug can be deposited in the lung with the areas under the plasma concentration/time curves appearing identical. Thus, the pattern of distribution may be so varied that one formulation may be distributed in the large airways while another is mainly in the small airways. Until the exact location in the airways of the action of cromolyn sodium is determined, the relative bioavailability of these formulations may not be accurately reflected by comparing areas under the plasma concentration/time curves. Even with these limitations in interpreting the data, a sensitive radioimmunoassay (accurate to 0.5 ng/ml) has resulted in detailed pharmacokinetic information about cromolyn sodium (Brown et al., 1983).

The disposition of cromolyn sodium following intravenous administration fits a two-compartment open pharmacokinetic model. The values for the pharmacokinetic variables are listed in Table 1. The relative systemic bioavailability from the various inhalation formulations is very low. Fuller and Collier (1983), utilizing radioimmunoassay, demonstrated there was a greater variability with the Spinhaler than the nebulizer solution. The absorption rate constants (Ka) and relative bioavailability for the inhalational preparations are listed in Table 2. Due to the extremely poor absorption from the gastrointestinal tract, it is unlikely that the portion of drug swallowed contributed to the drug concentrations found following inhalation. Because of the relatively short terminal half-life of cromolyn sodium (11-20 min) and its low bioavailability, there should be no significant accumulation during continuous therapy.

The amount of cromolyn sodium absorbed after inhalation varies according to the delivery system and the dose. Twenty mg powder inhaled via Spincap using a peak inspiratory flow (PIF) of greater than 140 liters/min and breath-holding of 10 sec resulted in 1.30-3.96 mg actually reaching the plasma. When a solution of 10 mg/ml cromolyn sodium was inhaled for 5 min at 10 psi using a Minineb nebulizer, only 0.19-0.32 mg reached the plasma. However, increasing

Table 1 Pharmacokinetics of Intravenous Cromolyn Sodium

Alpha:	22.5 ± 10 hr^{-1}
Beta:	1.85 ± 0.13 $hour^{-1}$
T 1/2:	0.32 hr
Clp	0.35 ± 0.1 liters/kg hr^{-1}
Vd_{Beta}	0.2 ± 0.04 liters/kg

Adapted from Fuller and Collier, 1983.

the concentration of the solution to 30 mg/ml raised the plasma level to 0.33-0.45 mg (Fuller and Collier, 1983).

Brown and co-workers (1983) have demonstrated that a broad variation occurs in the plasma concentration versus time profiles generated by normal subjects compared to asthmatic patients following inhalation of cromolyn sodium (20 mg) via Spinhaler. Mean peak plasma concentration (44 ± 24 ng/ml in normals, 16 ± 15 ng/ml in asthmatics) and mean area under the curve (AUC 80 ± 39 in normals and 32 ± 30 ng/hr/ml in asthmatics) were higher in normal volunteers than in asthmatic patients (Fig. 2). Mean terminal plasma half-life was similar in the two groups (106 ± 64 min in normals, 96 ± 20 in asthmatics).

The percentage of Spincap dose deposited in the lungs was calculated using urine excretion data. Normals had 12 ± 5% deposited in the lungs, whereas asthmatic patients had only 5 ± 5% of the dose reach the lungs. The standard deviation was high in all these measurements reflecting marked intersubject variation. Peak plasma concentrations in the normal subjects ranged from 14 to 91 ng/ml while in the asthmatic patients it was 1 to 36 ng/ml (Brown et al., 1983).

This variation between normals and asthmatics may be explained on the basis of inspiratory flow rates and breath-holding time. The normal subjects

Table 2 Pharmacokinetics of Inhaled Cromolyn Sodium

	Ka $(hours)^{-1}$	Apparent bioavailability (%)
Capsule (20 mg via Spinhaler)	0.43 ± 0.21 (SD)	10
Nebulizer solution (10 mg/ml)	0.31 ± 0.16	2.3
Nebulizer solution (30 mg/ml)	1.12 ± 1.15	1.2

Adapted from Fuller and Collier, 1983.

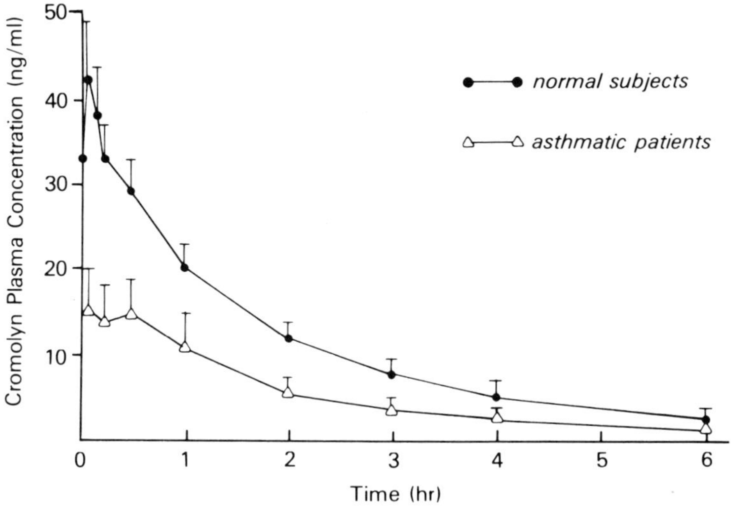

Figure 2 Comparison of plasma concentration (mean ± SEM) in 6 normal subjects and 10 asthmatic subjects after inhalation of cromolyn sodium 20 mg via Spinhaler (reproduced with permission from Brown et al., 1983).

generated peak inspiratory flow rates ranging from 67 to 161 liters/min while patients could only achieve 25-120 liters/min. Normal subjects utilized 10 sec of breath-holding whereas patients could only achieve 1-7 sec.

These findings concur with laboratory experimental observations. When the output of a Spinhaler containing a standard 20 mg Intal capsule is directed into a multistage liquid impinger and a flow rate of 30 liters/min is put through the system, only 3% of the drug is less than 10 μm aerodynamic diameter (Brown et al., 1983). However, if flow rates are increased to 90-120 liter/min, the respirable portion of the output increases dramatically to between 50 and 70% of the normal dose.

C. Mechanisms of Action

Mast Cell Stabilization

Despite intensive research, a precise mechanism to explain cromolyn sodium's clinical activity has not been completely delineated. The primary mode of action of cromolyn sodium is considered to be stabilization of mast cells, which prevents the subsequent release of mediators. Early laboratory studies using antigen challenge of tissues presensitized with reaginic (IgE) antibodies demonstrated that cromolyn sodium inhibited the release of biologically active chemi-

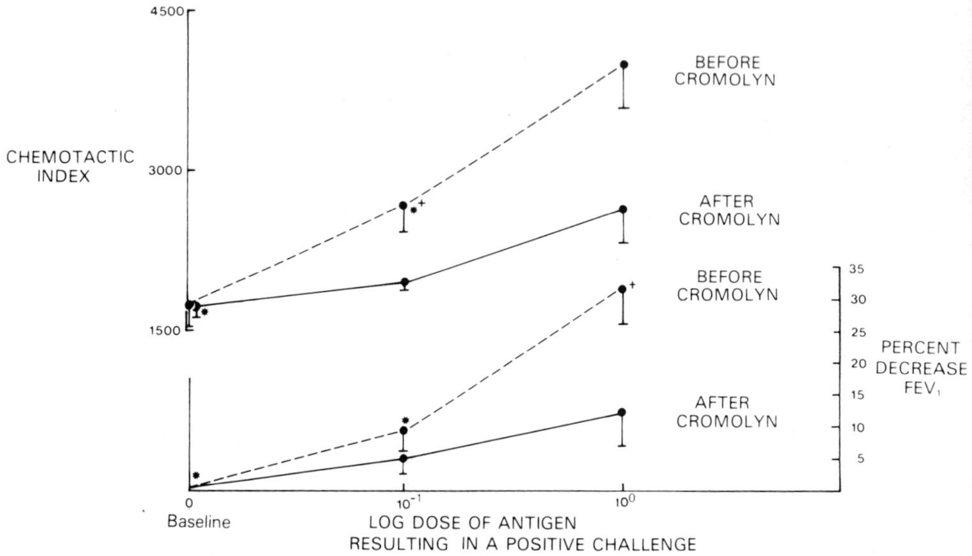

Figure 3 Serum neutrophil chemotactic activity and % decrease in FEV_1 after inhalation of increasing doses of ragweed in six subjects with positive challenges at 10° antigen dose, before (dashed line) and after (solid line) cromolyn sodium. *, $P < 0.05$, difference from 10° antigen dose. +, $P < 0.05$, difference between, before, and after cromolyn sodium (reproduced with permission from Atkins et al., 1978).

cal mediators (Cox, 1967). In rats sensitized with sera containing reaginic-like antibodies, cromolyn sodium inhibited passive cutaneous anaphylactic (PCA) reactions induced by antigen challenge (Goose and Blair, 1969). The local disruption of mast cells and the release of histamine induced by these antibodies were also inhibited by cromolyn sodium. However, the drug did not inhibit PCA reactions induced by serum containing nonreaginic antibodies. Thus, cromolyn sodium selectively inhibited reactions that involved reaginic (IgE) antibodies and mast cells (Cox, 1971). Further experiments established that cromolyn sodium also exerted an inhibitory effect on rat mast cells degranulated by nonimmunologic substances including phospholipase A (Orr and Cox, 1969), compound 48/80 (Orr et al., 1971), and the calcium ionophore A 23, 187 (Johnson and Bach, 1975).

In expanded studies, two experimental complications arose. First, cromolyn's protective effect against mast cell mediator release was found in some species including rats (Goose and Blair, 1969), primates, and humans (Assem and Mongar, 1970), but was absent in others. Secondly, cromolyn demonstrated

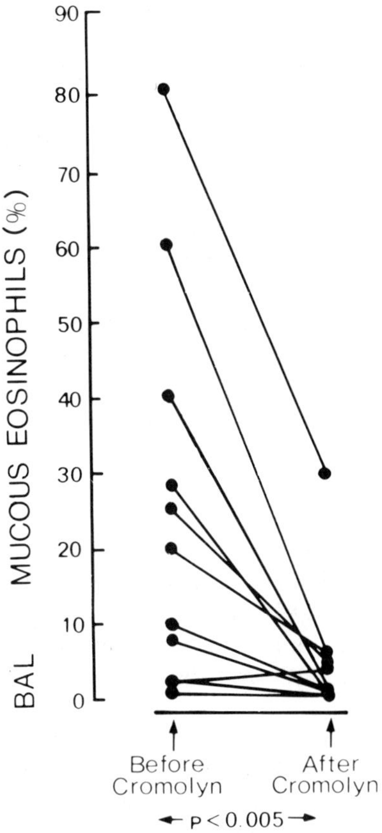

Figure 4 Reduction in mucous eosinophils obtained in bronchoalveolar lavage performed before and after 3 months of cromolyn sodium therapy (reproduced with permission from Diaz et al., 1984).

tissue specificity. It was active in preventing the release of mediators from mast cells derived from chopped lung (Sheard and Blair, 1970), but not in circulating basophils (Assem and Mongar, 1970) or skin (Patterson et al., 1971). Because of this variability in animal models and tissues, experimental evidence about the pharmacologic mechanisms of cromolyn sodium has been derived directly from human studies.

Recent studies have confirmed that cromolyn can block the release of both B-hexosaminidase and leukotrienes from mast cells. However, in some in vitro models coculturing mast cells with cromolyn for 5-7 days may be required to obtain the maximum inhibitory effect (Marquardt et al., 1985). This effect will persist if cells are washed free of cromolyn and returned to culture.

High concentrations of cromolyn sodium may be required for inhibition of IgE-dependent mast cell mediator release when human lung fragments or mast cells dispersed from human lungs are studied (Church and Young, 1983;

Church et al., 1983). The effect of cromolyn sodium has recently been examined in mast cells obtained by bronchoalveolar lavage. These cells may be more representative of mast cells in the lung lumen that come into contact with allergens (Flint et al., 1985). Cromolyn sodium is more effective in blocking mast cell mediator release in these cells than in chopped lung. Future research will delineate the exact population of human mast cells for which cromolyn is an effective inhibitor.

Antigen inhalation challenge in humans has further emphasized the role of cromolyn in stabilizing mast cells. Inhalation of ragweed in ragweed-sensitive asthmatics results in bronchospasm and the simultaneous release of quantifiable amounts of neutrophil chemotactic factor (NCF-A) into the sera of patients. Prior administration of cromolyn sodium blocks both the antigen-induced bronchospasm and the serum rise of chemotactic activity (Fig. 3) (Atkins et al., 1978). Neutrophil chemotactic factor (NCF-A) has a molecular weight of 500,000 daltons and is considered to be of mast cell origin (Nagy et al., 1982). This in vivo inhibition of NCF-A confirms the in vitro inhibition of mast cell mediator release by cromolyn sodium.

In a clinical study, 4 weeks of cromolyn sodium therapy in asthmatic patients resulted in a significant decrease in the number of eosinophils recovered in bronchoalveolar lavage fluid (Fig. 4) (Diaz et al., 1984). Thus, cromolyn sodium may block the release of other mast cell mediators such as eosinophil chemotactic factor (ECF-A) and leukotriene B_4 (LTB_4) that recruit eosinophils into tissue sites.

Further support is given to the mast cell stabilization theory by cromolyn sodium's therapeutic benefit in diseases involving type I immediate hypersensitivity reactions including allergic rhinitis (Handelman et al., 1977), allergic ocular disorders (Foster and Duncan, 1980), systemic mastocytosis (Frieri et al., 1985), and gastrointestinal allergy (Dahl, 1981).

Several theories as to the exact cellular mechanisms by which cromolyn sodium inhibits mast cell mediator release have been proposed and investigated, but none has been definitely established. Like many other secretory systems, the antigen-induced release of histamine and other mediators from mast cells requires extracellular calcium. The secretory process is initiated by aggregation of F_c receptors bound to mast cell membranes (Fewtrell and Metzger, 1980). After this trigger, a series of biochemical events occur resulting in the transient increase in permeability of the mast cell's plasma membrane for calcium ions. Although no direct evidence is available, this calcium influx may occur via membrane channels (Mazurek et al., 1980). Cross-linking of membrane-bound IgE by antigen results in opening the ion channels. Incubation of mast cells with cromolyn sodium abolishes or inhibits the channel conductance (Mazurek et al., 1984). Cromolyn sodium that has been covalently conjugated to fluorescent polyacrylamide or polyglutaraldehyde beads has been shown to bind to the mast cell membrane (Mazurek et al., 1980). Further studies on planar lipid bilayers containing membrane components of rat basophils have identified the calcium channel-forming membrane component as the cromolyn binding protein (CBP) (Mazurek et al., 1984). Cromolyn sodium has been shown to inhibit the uptake of radioactive calcium into rat purified mast cells following stimulation with either compound 48/80 (Spataro and Bosmann, 1976) or antigen (Forman and Garlano, 1976). Other observations have supported the hypothesis that the effect of cromolyn is at or near the mast cell surface (Spataro and Bosmann, 1976).

A biochemical basis by which cromolyn prevents mast cell mediator release may be through its ability to induce phosphorylation of a protein with a molecular weight of 78,000 daltons (Theoharides et al., 1980; Wells and Mann, 1983). Phosphorylation of this specific protein occurs 30-60 sec after stimulation of rat peritoneal mast cells, and coincides with the termination of the entire secretory process. These experiments suggest that cromolyn sodium activates a naturally occurring cell mechanism that is thought to represent an off switch to mast cell mediator release (Theoharides et al., 1980).

Effect on Other Inflammatory Cells

Although the key cell type affected by cromolyn has usually been considered to be the mast cell, cromolyn has been shown to inhibit the activation of other cell types (Kay and Barnes, 1985). Cromolyn sodium at a concentration of 10^{-7} moles/liter inhibits peripheral blood leukocyte activation as measured by formylmethionyl-leucyl-phenylalanine (FMLP)-induced enhancement of complement and IgG rosettes, as well as killing of target organisms (*Schistosomula* of *Schistosoma mansoni*) (Kay et al., 1985). Also, inhalation of cromolyn sodium prior to exercise challenge will inhibit the enhanced neutrophil and monocyte activation that occurs in asthmatic patients (Moqbel et al., 1985).

Andrij Holian (personal communication) examined the effects of cromolyn sodium on guinea pig alveolar macrophage activation. In a time- and concentration-dependent manner, cromolyn sodium inhibited macrophage stimulation by formyl peptide or leukotriene B_4, but had no effect on conconavalin A or phorbol-12, 13-dibutyrate stimulation. Cromolyn sodium also partially blocked formyl-peptide-stimulated phosphatidyl inositol turnover and elevated cAMP levels in alveolar macrophages. Cromolyn sodium slightly decreased the receptor binding affinity of 3H-FNLLP (tyr) to alveolar macrophages and decreased the number of receptor binding sites by 40%. These results suggest that cromolyn sodium inhibits FNLLP and LTB_4 stimulation at the receptor or coupling protein level, which Con A can bypass, prior to phospholipase C activation.

Cromolyn sodium has been shown to reduce significantly platelet-activating factor (PAF-acether)-induced immediate and delayed inflammatory responses in the skin of nonatopic volunteers (Basran et al., 1983). Pretreatment with intranasal cromolyn sodium will block the changes in nasal airway resistance induced by PAF (Karlsson and Pipkorn, 1984). However, intravenous administration of cromolyn failed to block PAF-acether-induced bronchoconstrictor responses in guinea pigs (Lewis et al., 1984). This lack of effect may be secondary to the species studied as cromolyn sodium has been previously shown to not be effective in guinea pigs (Cox et al., 1970b).

Cromolyn does not appear to antagonize the actions of type I immediate hypersensitivity mediators after they have been released from mast cells. It is not an antagonist of histamine, leukotrienes, bradykinin, or 5-hydroxytryptamine (Suschitzky and Sheard, 1984).

These new observations suggest that, besides acting on mast cells, cromolyn sodium may have a direct suppressive effect on other inflammatory cells, which could result in modulating inflammatory mechanisms in asthma.

Effect on Smooth Muscle

In animal pharmacologic experiments cromolyn sodium has not demonstrated smooth muscle relaxant properties (both in vitro and in vivo). However, cromolyn sodium administered by nebulization in stable asthmatic children was shown to be an effective bronchodilator, comparable in degree and duration of effect to salbutamol (Chung and Jones, 1979). However, when administered during an acute asthmatic attack cromolyn sodium showed little immediate bronchodilating effect (Hasham et al., 1981). Also, in a group of stable adult asthmatics no significant bronchodilation occurred following the administration of 60 mg cromolyn sodium delivered by nebulization (Thomson et al., 1981).

Hughes and co-workers (1982) compared the bronchodilator effects of cromolyn, salbutamol, and saline in 10 asthmatic children at rest. Cromolyn produced significant bronchodilation compared with saline as measured by PEFR only. The effect was not seen with FEV_1 or $FEF_{25-75\%}$. Salbutamol had a more immediate effect and produced a much greater degree of bronchodilation than cromolyn.

Most recently, Weiner and co-workers (1984) compared the effect of 20 mg nebulized cromolyn sodium and placebo in a double-blind crossover trial in 27 adult extrinsic asthmatics at rest and after exercise. PEFR measurements demonstrated that cromolyn produced significant bronchodilation at rest and could also reverse postexercise bronchoconstriction. Sixty mg cromolyn via Spinhaler or placebo were administered following exercise testing. FEV_1 and FEF_{20} measurements indicated that cromolyn increased the rate of recovery of the bronchoconstriction compared with placebo (Horn et al., 1984).

In isolated guinea pig tracheal strips, cromolyn attenuated the acetylcholine-induced contractile responses. Histamine, serotonin-bradykinin, and PGF2alpha-induced contractile responses were also attenuated dose-dependently (Kitamura et al., 1984). On the other hand, cromolyn potentiated the

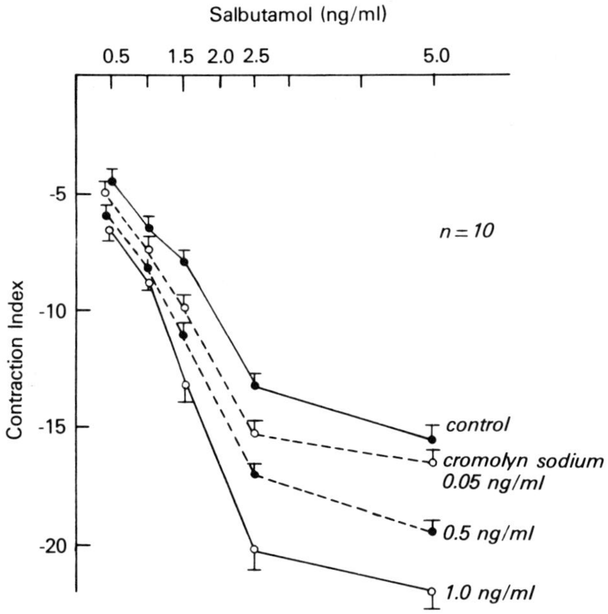

Figure 5 Effect of different dosages of cromolyn sodium on the dose-response curve of salbutamol in guinea pig tracheal strips. Cromolyn potentiated the salbutamol-induced relaxation responses and shifted the dose-response curve downward (reproduced with permission from Kitamura et al., 1984).

isoproterenol, epinephrine, PGE_2, and salbutamol-induced relaxation responses and shifted these dose-response curves downward (Fig. 5) (Kitamura et al., 1984). These experiments suggest that cromolyn may have a direct action on smooth muscle or may potentiate the relaxation induced by other pharmacologic agents.

Neuropharmacologic Effect

Cromolyn has been shown to inhibit bronchoconstriction induced in humans by a number of nonimmunologic triggers including exercise (Ben-Dov et al., 1983), inhalation of cold air (Fanta et al., 1981), sulfur dioxide (Sheppard et al., 1981a), and ultrasonically nebulized distilled water or fog (Fuller and Collier, 1984). Although mast cell mediator release has been shown to occur in both exercise (Lee et al., 1982) and fog challenge (Godden et al., 1983), other vagal reflex mechanisms may be involved.

Cromolyn sodium inhibits excitatory responses of "C" fiber sensory nerve endings in the dog lung (Dixon et al., 1980). These pulmonary nerve endings initiate reflex bronchoconstrictor responses in the dog (Harries, 1981).

Cromolyn sodium inhibits a component of the bronchoconstriction induced by leukotriene D_4, which is mediated by vagal reflex (Advenier et al., 1983). Based on these data, cromolyn may possess a neuropharmacologic effect that could explain its inhibitory effect on reflex-induced bronchospasm in humans.

D. Toxicity, Safety, and Adverse Reactions

Toxicity

Acute toxicity studies in a wide variety of species have demonstrated an extremely low order of toxicity for cromolyn sodium, whether administration was parenteral, oral or by inhalation. Parenteral administration in mice, rats, guinea pigs, hamsters, and rabbits demonstrated an LD_{50} of 4,000 mg/kg (Cox, 1970). In rhesus monkeys a single dose of cromolyn sodium produced no deaths at 6,000 mg/kg (Cox, 1970). The highest dosage administered by the oral route in rats and mice was 8,000 mg/kg and no deaths occurred (Cox et al., 1970b). By inhalation, even in long-term studies, it has proved impossible to achieve toxic dosage levels of cromolyn sodium in a range of mammalian species (Brogden et al., 1974).

During the course of toxicity studies on cromolyn sodium, focal proliferative arterial lesions affecting the medium-sized arteries of the kidneys of macaque monkeys were described. However, further histologic examinations of renal tissues from untreated monkeys as well as those which had received cromolyn sodium by various routes showed that the lesions were spontaneous and not related to the administration of the drug (Beach et al., 1981).

High-dosage parenterally administered cromolyn sodium has been shown to produce renal toxicity in rats given 200 mg/kg/day subcutaneously for 90 consecutive days. The primary lesion in rats was tubular degeneration in the proximal convoluted tubules. Dosages of 30 mg/kg/day in rats produced no lesions (Brogden et al., 1974).

Experimental studies in both conscious and anaesthetized animals from a wide variety of species have shown the drug to have no effect on the urinary, endocrine, or central nervous systems in dosages up to 10 mg/kg intravenously. It also has no effect on normal immunologic reactions, mucociliary activity, or lung surface active properties in animal studies. In most species the drug has no effect on the cardiovascular and respiratory systems. However, in marmosets and dogs there was an effect. In marmosets, dosages of 1 μg/kg intravenously produced an increase in blood pressure and heart rate while with higher dosages there was also transient apnea. In contrast, dosages of 10 μg/kg and above in dogs produced bradycardia and hypotension with apnea occurring in some cases. These effects were not observed in any other species. The pressor effect in the marmoset was due to sympathetic stimulation (via catecholamine release) and the reduction in blood pressure and heart rate in the dog was thought to be due to activation of baroreceptor reflex mechanisms originating in the pulmonary and coronary circulations (Cox, 1967, 1970; Cox et al., 1970b).

In mice, the LD_{50} of cromolyn sodium was not altered by the concurrent administration of isoproterenol, theophylline, ephedrine, triprolidine, mepyramine, prednisolone, and barbiturates (Cox et al., 1970b).

No evidence of chromosomal damage has been observed in mutagenesis studies and no evidence of impaired fertility was shown in laboratory reproduction studies. Six to eighteen-month studies in animals have shown no neoplastic effect (Cox et al., 1970b).

Pregnancy

Cromolyn sodium is listed as pregnancy category B (Intal package insert, revised 1985). Reproduction studies with cromolyn sodium administered parenterally to pregnant mice, rats, and rabbits in dosages up to 338 times the human clinical dosages produced no evidence of fetal malformations (Cox, 1970). Very low rates of placental and uterine transfer occur even with the injection of dosages of cromolyn sodium as high as 540 mg/kg into the caudal vein of the mouse. The maximal placental transfer seen was 0.08% of the intravenous dose. Cromolyn sodium was used to treat 296 asthmatic women throughout pregnancy in France. Malformations were observed in only four newborn infants (1.35%) which represents a frequency less than that reported for the whole population (2-3%) (Wilson, 1982).

In the lactating macaque monkey, excretion of cromolyn sodium into the milk after intravenous injection was less than 0.001% of the administered dosage, leading to the conclusion that the drug is not transferred into the milk to any appreciable extent (Fisons Corporation, personal communication, 1985).

Adverse Reactions

Long-term, worldwide clinical experience with the use of cromolyn sodium in various forms has shown that adverse reactions are rare. The most common side effects are transient cough and mild wheezing with use of the powder formulation which rarely require treatment or discontinuation of the drug.

According to American postmarketing experience accumulated since 1973, the following adverse reactions to cromolyn sodium has been reported in less than 1:10,000 patients: laryngeal edema, swollen parotic gland, angioedema, bronchospasm, joint swelling and pain, dizziness, dysuria and urinary frequency, nausea, cough, wheezing, headache, nasal congestion, rash, urticaria, and lacrimation.

Other adverse reactions have been reported in less than 1:100,000 patients, and it is unclear whether these were attributed to the drug: anaphylaxis, nephrosis, periarteritic vasculitis, pericarditis, peripheral neuritis, pulmonary infiltrates with eosinophilia, polymyositis, exfoliative dermatitis, hemoptysis, anemia, myalgia, hoarseness, photodermatitis, and vertigo.

Although most side effects are mild, there are a few case reports of more serious adverse experiences with cromolyn (Sheffer et al., 1975; Kus and Ciszek, 1978; Menon and Das, 1977). Anaphylaxis with inhaled cromolyn sodium was reported in a 7-year-old timothy-sensitive asthmatic girl after 1 week of inhalation. Sera were negative for IgG-anti-cromolyn sodium antibodies by the Farr technique, but passive transfer to the patient's mother was positive (Brown et al., 1981). In a prospective study of adverse reactions to cromolyn in 375 patients, the frequency of potential side effects of the drug was 2% (8/375) (Settipane et al., 1979). Dermatitis occurred in five patients, myositis in two and gastroenteritis in one. Immunologic evaluations including skin and serum tests for immediate and delayed reactivity all were negative, and all reactions were non-life-threatening and completely reversible.

III. Clinical Pharmacology

A. Acute Challenge

Antigen

Cromolyn sodium was developed through use of in vivo antigen challenge in asthmatic volunteers. Altounyan (1967, 1969) demonstrated that an inhalation of 20 mg cromolyn sodium given both 1 min and 1 hr before antigen challenge markedly inhibited the fall in FEV_1. However, the drug became progressively less effective when inhaled 1, 6, and 15 min after antigen challenge (Fig. 6).

Inhalation of various concentrations of cromolyn sodium 10 min before antigen challenge showed that the protective effect is present over a wide range of dosages. In fact, some protection occurs at a concentration of 5×10^{-7} which is equivalent to an inhaled dose of 150 ng cromolyn sodium (Altounyan, 1969). However, the degree of protection lessens when the time between drug inhalation and antigen challenge is lengthened to 2 hr or more (Fig. 7) (Cox and Altounyan, 1970a).

Early studies demonstrated the protective effect of cromolyn sodium in inhibiting bronchial reactions induced by a variety of antigens. Pepys and coworkers (1968) studied five patients with immediate bronchoconstrictive responses to grass pollen or mite antigen. The inhalation of 20 mg cromolyn sodium 10-12 min before antigen challenge completely inhibited the fall in FEV_1 in four patients. Booij-Noord et al. (1970) demonstrated that the inhalation of a 1% aerosol solution for 3 min (approximately 6 mg cromolyn sodium) 10

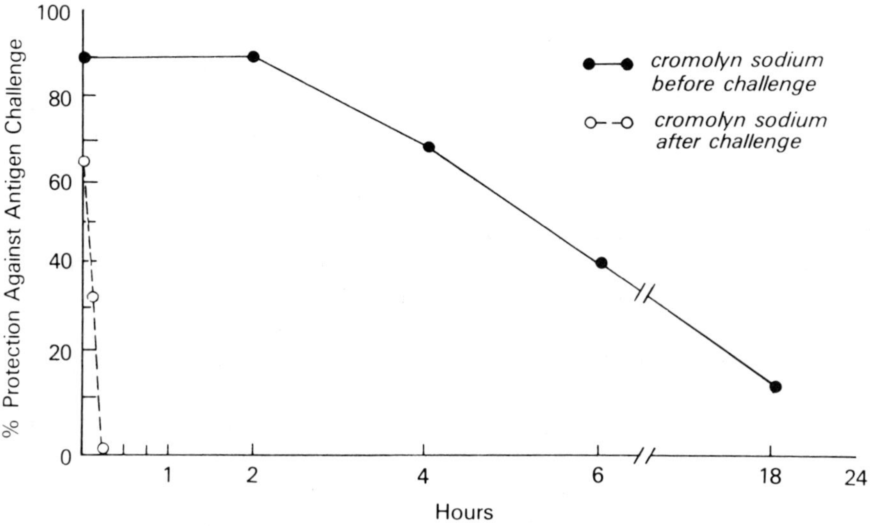

Figure 6 Protective effect of cromolyn sodium given before and after antigen aerosol challenge (protection expressed as percentage inhibition of antigen-induced fall in FEV_1 at intervals of 3 days between challenge). Cromolyn sodium 20 mg was administered at 0, 2, 4, 6, and 18 hr before challenge and at 1, 6, and 15 min after challenge (reproduced with permission from Altounyan, 1970).

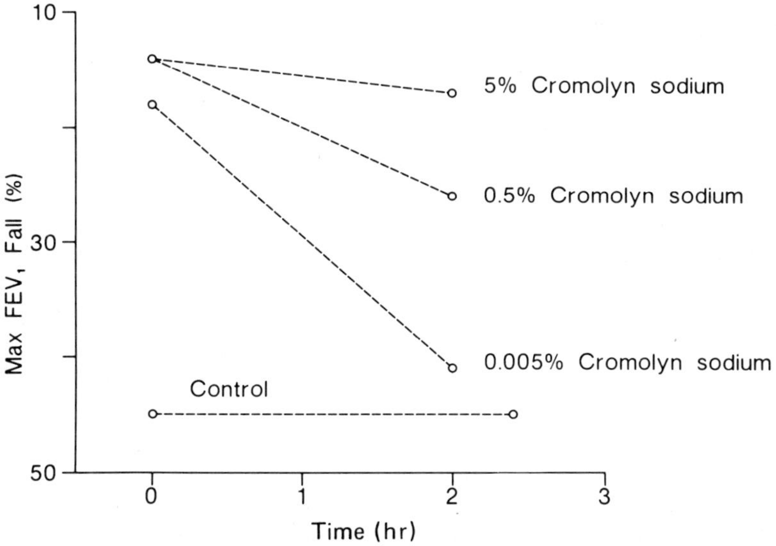

Figure 7 Maximum FEV_1 reduction after antigen alone (control line) and after antigen and varying concentrations of cromolyn sodium inhaled either 5 min or 2 hr before antigen challenge (reprinted with permission from Cox and Altounyan, 1970).

min prior to antigen challenge in 17 patients significantly inhibited the mean fall in FEV_1 and VC ($P < 0.005$). In a double-blind crossover comparison of cromolyn sodium and placebo in patients sensitive to grass pollen antigens, an inhalation of 20 mg cromolyn sodium 30 min prior to antigen challenge provided an average of 65.3 (± 3.4)% protection against the fall in FEV_1, which was significantly more protective than placebo (Grieco, 1972).

The duration of protection of cromolyn sodium against antigen challenge was examined by Kolotkin and co-workers (1973). A dose of 40 mg inhaled before challenge provided significant protection against antigen-induced bronchoconstriction at 30 min and 5 hr after inhalation but not at 24 hr. While protection was still present at 5 hr after inhalation of cromolyn when patients were challenged with the same antigen, it was lost when a different antigen was introduced.

From these studies and the numerous studies in the literature, it is apparent that cromolyn does not totally block every antigen challenge in every asthmatic person. The dosage of antigen relative to the amount of cromolyn inhaled and the patient's individual sensitivity to the challenging antigen may explain this variable response. Another explanation is offered by the work of Bryant and co-workers (1973), who showed that cromolyn sodium failed to protect against antigen challenge in patients whose immediate bronchoconstriction was due to IgG antibodies rather than IgE antibodies. Cromolyn sodium (20 mg) given 30 min before challenge was protective in 37 of 41 patients, but offered no protection in 12. In the protected patients, the serum IgE level was greater than 400 μg/ml (mean, 975 ± 75 μg/ml) and passive cutaneous anaphylaxis tests were positive in 13. In contrast, IgE levels in patients who were not protected were less than 400 μg/ml (mean 250 ± 53 μg/ml) and passive cutaneous anaphylaxis tests in eight patients suggested that the allergic reactions in this group were mediated by short-term anaphylactic IgG antibodies.

Mezey and co-workers (1978) measured tracheal mucous velocity (TMV) radiographically in asthmatics before and after the inhalation of ragweed antigen. Baseline TMV was significantly depressed in the asthmatics and the mean TMV was diminished to 72% of baseline immediately after bronchial provocation with a further reduction (47% of baseline) occurring 1 hr postchallenge. Inhalation of 20 mg cromolyn sodium increased the mean prechallenge TMV to 132% of baseline, which increased further to 162% of baseline after bronchial challenge. Thus, cromolyn sodium may have the potential of not only blocking the effect of acute antigen challenge on TMV but of also returning the impaired mucociliary function found in asymptomatic asthmatics to normal.

Cromolyn sodium is also protective against antigen challenge in animal models of asthma. Abraham and co-workers (1981) demonstrated that the nebulization of 1 mg/kg cromolyn sodium prevented the antigen-induced decrease in specific airway conductance (SG_L) induced by *Ascaris suum* in allergic sheep.

Many studies over the past 15 years have continued to demonstrate complete or partial inhibition of immediate bronchial reactions to antigen challenge, and controlled studies have documented the superiority of cromolyn sodium over placebo in this situation (Church and Warner, 1985).

Methacholine and/or Histamine Challenge

Conflicting results have been reported as to the immediate protective effect exerted by cromolyn sodium against the nonspecific constricting agents methacholine and histamine, that are not believed to induce their effect via mast cell mediator release (Patel, 1984).

Woenne and co-workers (1979) studied the inhalation of a 2% solution of cromolyn sodium compared with saline in inhibiting bronchoconstriction induced by methacholine and histamine in 30 asthmatic children. Seven of 17 children challenged with methacholine showed decreased sensitivity after pretreatment with cromolyn and in 4 of 13 children cromolyn inhalation attenuated the response to inhaled histamine.

Fabbri and co-workers (1982) found that 40 mg cromolyn sodium reduced the airway responsiveness to carbacol in both atopic and nonatopic subjects. Since the individual dose-response showed a parallel shift to the right without an obvious change in slope, they suggested that cromolyn may be a competitive antagonist of carbacol.

In a carefully controlled study in 16 adults, Lemire and co-workers (1984) demonstrated that 40 mg cromolyn sodium was no more protective than placebo lactose in altering the provocative concentration of histamine required to decrease FEV_1 by 20% (PC_{20}) to histamine. They also demonstrated that cromolyn had no acute bronchodilator effect.

As more standardized procedures for performing histamine and methacholine are developed, cromolyn will need to be reevaluated in these challenge situations. If cromolyn does prove to be protective against these challenges, it might have an action on cholinergic or irritant receptor sites.

Sulfur Dioxide Challenge

Cromolyn sodium was first shown to inhibit sulfur dioxide (SO_2)-induced bronchoconstriction in subjects with asthma by deVries and colleagues (1976) and confirmed by Snashall and Lewin (1976). Sheppard and co-workers (1981a) reported a randomized, double-blind study in six asthmatic subjects. Each subject inhaled 40 mg cromolyn or placebo 20 min before inhaling SO_2 for 10 min while exercising at a moderate rate (400 kpm/min) on a bicycle ergometer. In patients pretreated with cromolyn, SO_2 inhalation caused no increase in specific airway resistance (SR_{aw}) in four subjects and a small rise in two subjects (Fig. 8).

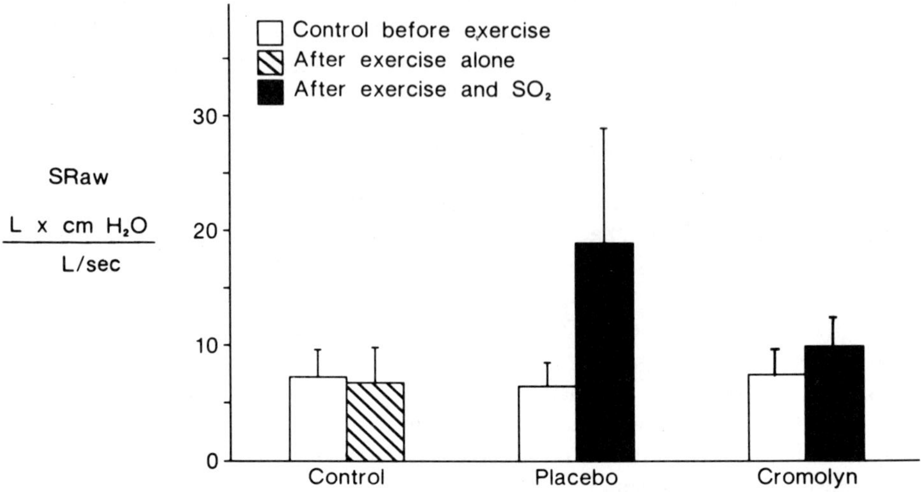

Figure 8 Effect of cromolyn sodium on the response to inhalation of SO_2 during exercise in six asthmatic subjects. All data represent mean ± SD. Exercise alone (left columns) did not increase SR_{aw}. Exercise and SO_2 after placebo (middle columns) increased SR_{aw} significantly ($P < 0.01$). Exercise and SO_2 after cromolyn (right columns) had a significantly smaller effect on SR_{aw} ($P < 0.025$) (reprinted with permission from Sheppard et al., 1981a).

A dosage-dependent protective effect of cromolyn sodium in reflex-mediated asthma induced by SO_2 has been demonstrated by independent investigators (Harries et al., 1981; Sheppard et al., 1981a). Sheppard and co-workers (1981a) demonstrated that the inhibitory dosage of cromolyn sodium against SO_2 is about twice that usually required for protection against antigen-induced bronchoconstriction. At this dosage the effect of cromolyn sodium is superior to that of atropine.

Myers and co-workers (1985) studied 10 asthmatic subjects who inhaled increasing concentrations of SO_2 following pretreatment with placebo, 20 mg cromolyn sodium, or 200 mg cromolyn sodium. The concentration of SO_2 needed to increase specific airway resistance was significantly greater after 200 mg cromolyn sodium than after 20 mg. In five of the patients methacholine responsiveness was tested and found to be unchanged by single doses of either 20 mg or 200 mg cromolyn sodium. These results indicated that cromolyn sodium inhibits SO_2-induced bronchoconstriction in a dosage-dependent manner and it does so without directly inhibiting smooth muscle responsiveness. Differences in dosages required to achieve comparable protection against SO_2-induced and antigen-induced bronchospasm may be additional evidence that the pharmaco-

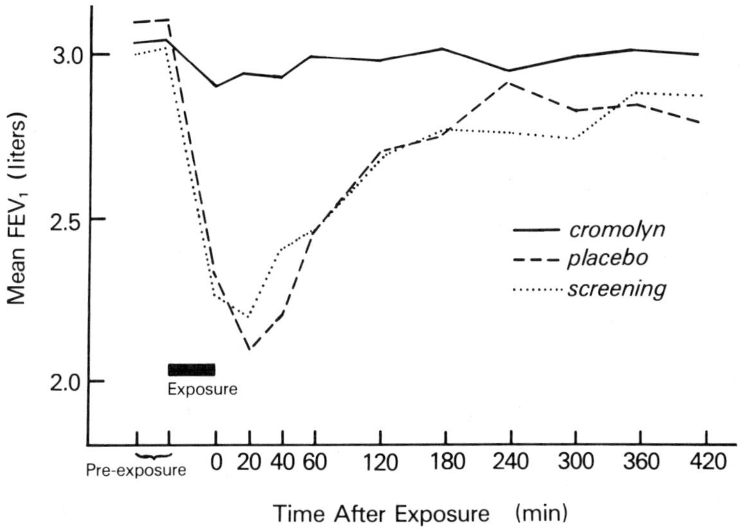

Figure 9 Mean FEV_1 before and after exposure to laboratory animals in 10 subjects with laboratory animal induced asthma on 3 exposure days. On screening day patient sat in animal room, placebo day they received lactose placebo, and on cromolyn day they were given 20 mg cromolyn powder via Spinhaler (reprinted with permission from Gross, 1980).

logic effects of cromolyn sodium may have different pathways. Since mast cell mediator release has not yet been demonstrated after SO_2-induced asthma, the effects of cromolyn may be acting through mechanisms other than mast cell stabilization.

Further evidence to support this concept comes from Allistone and coworkers (1985). They studied 10 healthy subjects in a double-blind crossover trial with intravenous infusions of saline or cromolyn sodium. After 20 min of infusion the sGAW of each subject was measured and the subject inhaled first a low and then a higher concentration of SO_2 while the infusions continued. During the infusion of cromolyn, the fall in sGAW was significantly less than with the saline solution. Plasma concentrations of cromolyn sodium at the end of the infusion were 100th of the lowest dosage required to stabilize mast cells in vitro indicating that cromolyn acted by a mechanism which did not involve mast cells.

Because of its effect in blocking both exercise-induced asthma and also that induced by SO_2, cromolyn sodium is a logical prophylactic approach in asthmatic patients whose exercise involves an environmental exposure to SO_2.

Occupational/Miscellaneous Challenges

Cromolyn sodium exerts a protective effect against exposure to several types of industrial agents including toluene diisocyanate, western red cedar and colophony (Pepys, 1981). In addition, cromolyn sodium has been shown to be effective in bakers' asthma. In a series of 17 long-term diseased bakers (duration of complaints between 1 and 20 years) a single dose of 20 mg of cromolyn sodium inhaled before specific challenge with wheat or rye flour suppressed the increase in airway resistance (R_{aw}) in 81 and 87%, respectively (Thiel and Ulmer, 1980). In addition, a clinical trial of cromolyn sodium in 36 bakers with flour-dependent asthma showed a 78% response and during a 3-year observation period only 6 persons had to change their occupation (Thiel and Ulmer, 1980).

Cromolyn sodium has also been studied in the control of allergy to laboratory animals. Gross (1980) reported a double-blind controlled challenge in 10 subjects with laboratory animal-induced bronchospasm. Cromolyn showed a significant protective effect in all subjects (Fig. 9).

Sulfiting agents, including bisulfites, sulfites, and metabisulfites, have been used for many years as preservatives/antioxidants. Many foods and drugs contain sulfites and severe asthmatic and anaphylactic episodes can be provoked by these agents (Schwartz, 1984). Nebulized cromolyn sodium and atropine demonstrate comparable blocking activities against metabisulfite reactions in sensitive patients (Simon et al., 1984). Also 200 mg oral cromolyn before challenge has been shown to block the reaction in a 58-year-old wine collector (Schwartz H, personal communication, 1985).

Pretreatment with cromolyn has also been reported to partially or completely block aspirin (ASA)-induced respiratory reactions (Delaney, 1976). Stevenson and co-workers showed that although pretreatment with 40 mg cromolyn solution by inhalation did not prevent reaction to ASA in 10 sensitive asthmatic patients, it did significantly prolong the elapsed times from ASA ingestion to onset of asthma (Stevenson et al., 1984).

Exercise/Cold Air

Cromolyn was first shown to inhibit exercise-induced asthma (EIA) by Davies (1968) and this observation has been confirmed by others (Silverman et al., 1973, 1972; Godfrey et al., 1974).

Several investigators have compared dose-response to different forms of cromolyn sodium. Schoeffel and co-workers (1983) investigated the effect of cromolyn sodium delivered as a pressurized aerosol, in a dosage of 2 or 4 mg in 15 patients known to have exercise-induced asthma. Overall, 87% of the patients had significant protection from EIA after 2 or 4 mg of cromolyn sodium. This value is slightly higher than 54% of 39 patients studied by Silverman and Turner-Warwick (1972). Corkey and co-workers (1982) compared the effect of cromolyn powder with and without lactose in inhibiting EIA. They found that cromolyn sodium only completely blocked EIA in 11% of studies, but was considered to be "clinically effective" in 59% of studies.

By contrast, using the pressurized metered-dose inhaler (MDI) delivery system for cromolyn sodium, Schoeffel and co-workers (1983) were able to show total inhibition of EIA in 66% and significant protection in 87% of patients. This apparent superiority of the MDI as a delivery system for cromolyn sodium may be due to several factors relating to particle size. Cromolyn sodium powder in a particle size of 2 μm has been shown to be more effective than particles of 11.7 μm in inhibiting EIA (Godfrey et al., 1974). These 2 μm particles are more likely to be deposited in the periphery of the lung than the 6-μm particles delivered via Spinhaler. This may be due to the hygroscopic properties of cromolyn sodium. As the powder is inhaled into the high humidity of the airways, water is absorbed by the cromolyn sodium and particles may increase up to 2.6 times their original size. This is supported by Smith and co-workers (1980) who demonstrated that only 0.99 mg of a 20-mg cromolyn sodium capsule was aerosolized into particles appropriate for pulmonary retention under conditions of 98% relative humidity. Because of this, a larger dose of cromolyn sodium may be deposited in the periphery of the lung when 2 mg is given by metered dose inhaler than with 20 mg via Spinhaler.

Patel and coinvestigators (1982) studied the protective effect of various concentrations of cromolyn sodium delivered in solution by nebulization in 10 patients with EIA. The inhibitory effect was significantly greater with 10, 20, and 40 mg/ml than at 2 mg/ml of cromolyn sodium with a concentration of 20 mg/ml giving the greatest protective effect. In an expanded study, Patel and Kerr (1984) investigated the protective effect of various concentrations of cromolyn compared at 20 min, 150 min, and 260 min after treatment. At the first two time periods all concentrations of cromolyn sodium (2 mg, 20 mg, 40 mg) showed statistically significant inhibition and the protection offered by the three concentrations were comparable. However, when the exercise challenge was performed 270 minutes after treatment, partial protection was observed with both the 20 mg and 40 mg, whereas 2 mg was no longer protective. In a further study (Tullett et al., 1985) the effects of 2, 10, and 20 mg cromolyn sodium delivered by metered dose inhaler, 12 mg delivered via Wright nebulization, and placebo were compared in EIA. Cromolyn sodium inhibited exercise at all doses with the protective effect of 20 mg cromolyn delivered by metered dose inhaler being similar to that observed with 12 mg of nebulized cromolyn (Fig. 10).

Cromolyn sodium in a dose of 40 mg delivered via Spinhaler has been shown to prevent bronchoconstriction stimulated by hyperventilation of cold air (Breslin et al., 1980; Fanta et al., 1981; Griffin et al., 1983). Latimer and colleagues (1984) expanded these earlier observations to examine the protective

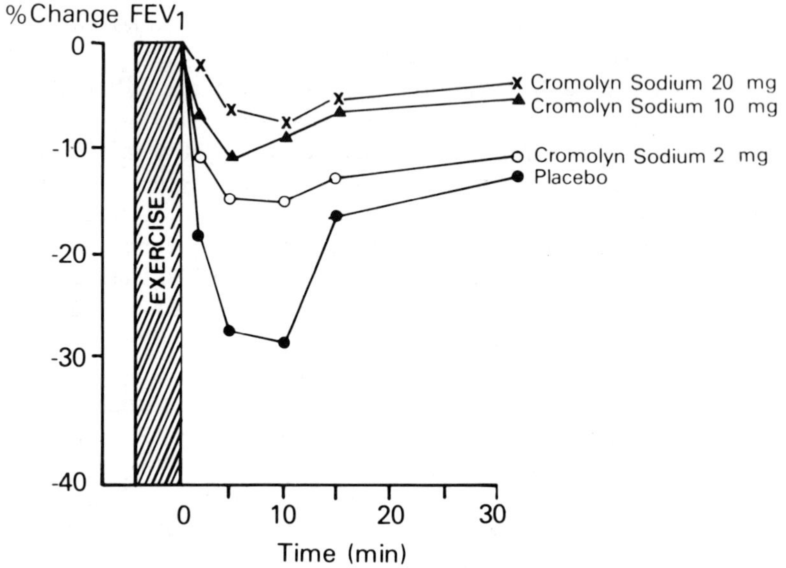

Figure 10 Mean percentage change in FEV_1 (from baseline after administration of drug) over 30 min after exercise following pretreatment with different dosages of cromolyn sodium aerosol (reproduced with permission from Tullet et al., 1985).

effect of three doses (2, 10, and 20 mg) of cromolyn sodium inhaled from a pressurized metered dose inhaler on the response to isocapnic hyperventilation of cold dry air in 10 asthmatic subjects. This was also compared to 20 mg cromolyn sodium powder inhaled from a spincap and placebo. All doses of cromolyn sodium significantly shifted the respiratory heat loss dose-response curve to the right of the placebo curve. There was no cromolyn sodium dose-response relationship between the three doses of aerosol or between the aerosol and the powder. The investigators concluded that 2 mg cromolyn sodium inhaled via a pressurized MDI gave the same magnitude of protection against bronchoconstriction stimulated by airway cooling as 20 mg cromolyn sodium delivered via Spinhaler or MDI.

B. Late Asthmatic Response

Inhalation challenge with antigen results in immediate bronchoconstriction in persons with allergic asthma. Many asthmatics will undergo a second bronchoconstrictive response 4-12 hr after the first which is known as the late or delayed asthmatic reaction (Booij-Noord et al., 1971). The early response can be rapidly reversed by $beta_2$-adrenergic agonists, whereas the late reaction responds poorly to these agents, is prolonged and more severe (Warner, 1976). Symptoms in patients with asthma more closely resemble the late rather than immediate response to antigen emphasizing the importance of the late asthmatic reaction (Larsen, 1985). Also, Warner (1976) reported a significant correlation between frequency of asthma attacks and the presence of late asthmatic response in children. Another important clinical observation was reported by Cockcroft and co-workers (1977c) who noted that allergen-induced late asthmatic responses provoked in the laboratory were associated with a prolonged increase in bronchial responsiveness to histamine and methacholine, whereas immediate asthmatic responses alone did not produce this increase in nonspecific hyperreactivity.

The exact pathogenesis of the late response is unknown although mast cells and IgE are thought to be important. Investigations in asthmatic patients utilizing the measurement of the mast-cell-derived mediator, neutrophil chemotactic factor, have found that it appears in two peaks in the sera of patients with both early and late asthmatic responses (Nagy et al., 1982). This mast cell etiology has been further confirmed using a unique rabbit model in which only a homocytotropic antibody analogous to human IgE is produced (Shampain et al., 1982).

Cromolyn sodium given before a variety of different antigen challenges has been shown to block the occurrence of both the immediate asthmatic bronchoconstrictive response and the more severe late onset or delayed response (Pepys et al., 1968; Booij-Noord et al., 1971; Hegardt et al., 1981). Late asthmatic reactions have also been reported following exercise-induced asthma. Feldman and associates demonstrated that cromolyn sodium had a greater protective effect in blocking exercise-induced acute asthmatic reactions than theophylline or metaproterenol (Feldman et al., 1982).

Two different animal models have been used to study the late asthmatic response. Abraham and co-workers (1983) have induced early and late asthmatic responses in sheep sensitive to *Ascaris suum.* In this model inhalation of cromolyn sodium (1 mg/kg) by nebulization prior to antigen challenge blocked both the early and late responses. The intravenous injection of methylprednisolone (15 mg/kg) 3 hr after antigen challenge blocked the late response to the same degree as the inhaled cromolyn given prior to challenge (Fig. 11). In asthmatic persons, corticosteroids have been shown to block the late response to antigen without affecting the early response (Booij-Noord et al., 1971). Larsen and colleagues (1984) in their IgE-mediated *Alternaria*-induced late asthmatic reaction in rabbits, have also shown that inhalation of cromolyn before challenge will block both the immediate and late asthmatic reactions. Corticosteroids will only prevent the development of the late response.

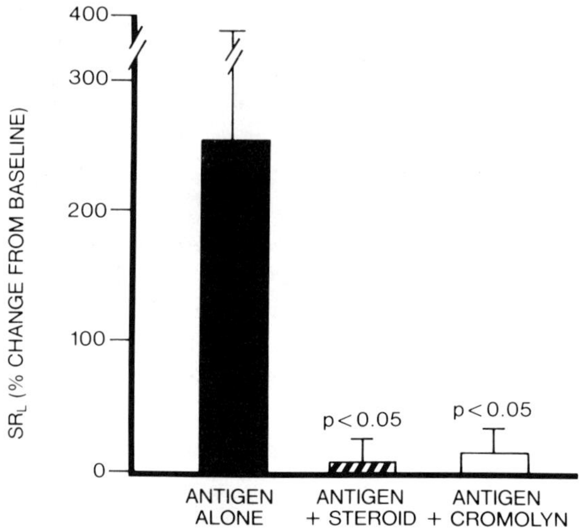

Figure 11 Effect of cromolyn sodium (1 mg/kg) by nebulization and intravenous methylprednisolone (15 mg/kg) in blocking the late response in sheep sensitive to *Ascaris suum.* Both treatments were equally effective (reproduced with permission from Abraham et al., 1983).

In experimental work in humans and animals, cromolyn consistently blocks both the immediate and delayed asthmatic response. Because of the association of the late response with severe asthma and also its correlation with increased bronchial hyperreactivity, the role of cromolyn in preventing the late response may be one of the keys to its ability to control and improve chronic clinical asthma.

C. Bronchial Hyperreactivity

One interesting aspect of the pharmacology of cromolyn sodium is its long-term effect on reducing bronchial hyperreactivity. Airways hyperreactivity is a characteristic feature of bronchial asthma, and the degree of bronchial responsiveness as measured by PC_{20} histamine has been shown to correlate with the occurrence and severity of asthma (Cockcroft et al., 1977b), with diurnal fluctuations in peak flow rate (Ryan et al., 1982), with the amount of medications needed to control symptoms (Juniper et al., 1981) and with airway responses to allergens (Cockcroft et al., 1977c).

The effect of cromolyn sodium on airway reactivity was first demonstrated by Roger Altounyan, M.D. (1970). Encouraged by the results he obtained in one asthmatic patient over a 5-year period, he proceeded to study 10

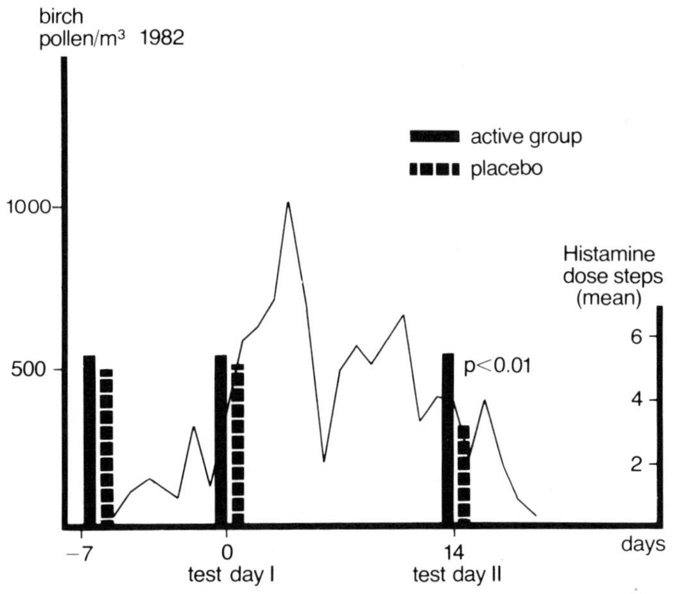

Figure 12 Cromolyn sodium (20 mg four times daily) blocked the seasonal increase in bronchial hyperreactivity occurring in birch pollen-sensitive asthmatics during the pollen season (reproduced with permission from Lowhagen and Rak, 1985b).

patients and found a reduction in their response to standardized histamine challenge following 6 weeks of cromolyn therapy. Dickson (1970) confirmed these results in a 1-year trial of cromolyn sodium in 24 severe extrinsic asthmatic children. However, Cockcroft and co-workers (1977b) and Ryo and associates (1976) were not able to demonstrate any effect of cromolyn on their patients' sensitivity to histamine. The most striking differences between their studies and those of Dickson and Altounyon was the duration of therapy with cromolyn. The negative studies used 1 week and 2 weeks, respectively, while in the two positive studies the duration of therapy was 6 weeks and 1 year.

Two recently published studies have examined the effect of cromolyn on histamine reactivity both in and out of pollen season. The first was a double-blind, randomized, crossover study in 14 atopic patients before, during, and after 4 weeks of treatment with cromolyn sodium or placebo (Lowhagen and Rak, 1985a). After cromolyn treatment the PC_{20} for histamine increased (less responsiveness) in 9 of 14 patients, however, the difference between placebo and active drug treatment was not statistically significant. The second study was randomized, double-blind group comparison in 22 birch pollen-sensitive asthmatics during the birch-pollen season (Lowhagen and Rak, 1985b). Patients received cromolyn sodium (20 mg four times daily) or placebo for 6 weeks. Responsiveness to histamine was significantly increased in the placebo group during the pollen season where the cromolyn-sodium-treated group, experienced no change in histamine responsiveness (Fig. 12). Thus, cromolyn sodium protected against pollen-induced increased bronchial hyperreactivity.

Change in responsiveness to methacholine challenge following cromolyn sodium therapy has produced conflicting results. Griffin and his colleagues (1983) found that after 2 weeks of cromolyn sodium therapy given during allergy season, there was a significant increase in challenge with eucapnic hyperventilation with frigid air. The $PD_{20}V_E$ rose significantly and remained elevated for the 4 weeks of the study. However, there was no change in the responsiveness to methacholine. Bleeker and co-workers (1982) also found that 4 weeks of cromolyn sodium therapy decreased their patients' sensitivity to inhaled antigen while the methacholine sensitivity remained unchanged. Cromolyn sodium therapy can attenuate the responsiveness to naturally occurring antigenic stimuli even when methacholine responsiveness is unchanged. In contrast to these results, Furukawa and his colleagues (1984) showed a significantly decreased sensitivity to methacholine in 23 children after a 3-month treatment period with cromolyn. These studies are summarized in Table 3.

Cromolyn will definitely block the seasonal rise in nonspecific airway reactivity to histamine, however, more information is required to determine its exact long-term effect with other challenge agents.

D. Clinical Trials

Although there are hundreds of published clinical trials with cromolyn sodium in the world-wide medical literature, the interpretation of many of the earlier studies is complicated by several factors (Shapiro and Konig, 1985). Many of the earlier studies did not include a placebo control group. Also, many of the original studies in the United Kingdom used cromolyn sodium in combination with 0.1 mg isoproterenol, which makes interpretation of the data difficult.

Another problem common to the study of all prophylactic, nonbronchodilating drugs for asthma is determining the best measurements of clinical response. Random spirometry or PEFR performed at infrequent intervals may have little relationship to the daily symptom scores. Also pulmonary function changes rapidly in bronchial asthma and the only reliable indicators of clinical asthma may be twice daily measurements (Chai et al., 1968).

Despite these problems, the majority of the results are very favorable with cromolyn sodium with the success rate ranging from 60 to 89% in numerous studies (Godfrey et al., 1975; Bernstein et al., 1972; Blumenthal et al., 1973; Brompton Hospital, 1972; Crisp et al., 1974; Chan-Yeung et al., 1971; and Friday et al., 1973).

Table 3 Effect of Cromolyn Sodium on Bronchial Reactivity

Reference	Duration of treatment	Challenge	Effect
Altounyan, 1970	6 weeks	Histamine	+
Dickson, 1970	1 year	Histamine	+
Ryo et al., 1976	2 weeks	Antigen Histamine Methacholine	+ - -
Cockcroft, 1976a	1 week	Histamine	-
Szmidt et al., 1979	3 weeks	Histamine	+
Dickson and Cole, 1979	10 years	Histamine Exercise	+ -
Griffin et al., 1983	4 weeks	Cold air Methacholine	+ -
Bleecker et al., 1982	4 weeks	Antigen Methacholine	+ -
Furukawa et al., 1984	3 months	Methacholine	+
Lowhagen and Rak, 1985a	4 weeks (out of season)	Hitamine	-
Lowhagen and Rak, 1985b	6 weeks (during season)	Histamine	+

Spincaps

In 1969 the Drug Committee of the American Academy of Allergy instituted a placebo-controlled trial of cromolyn sodium in 252 asthmatic patients (adults and children) in the United States (Bernstein et al., 1972). The objectives of the study were to determine the short-term therapeutic effectiveness and safety of cromolyn sodium (20 mg four times daily via Spinhaler) utilizing a 4-week double-blind placebo controlled study design. Cromolyn sodium was significantly better than placebo in patient symptom scoring, physician evaluation, and concomitant medication reduction, with 72% of the patients as evaluated by their physicians improved after active treatment. There was no significant side effects encountered in the study.

In 1972 the Brompton Hospital/Medical Research Council's long-term double-blind placebo controlled, parallel group study was published. It evaluated the efficacy and safety of cromolyn sodium in severe adult extrinsic and intrinsic asthmatics over a 1-year trial period and compared a standard 20 mg four times daily dosage with a reducing dosage.

At the end of 52 weeks there were 9/35 on cromolyn in whom treatment failed and 31/39 on either beta-agonists or placebo who dropped out of the study. Treatment with cromolyn sodium was statistically better from 4 weeks of treatment to the end of the study with patients on cromolyn sodium showing significant improvement in FEV_1 at both 24 and 52 weeks of treatment. Patients who received cromolyn sodium twice daily had the same control of their asthma as those who received four times daily dosage (Brompton Hospital, 1972).

No factors were predictive of response to cromolyn sodium including FEV_1, eosinophilia, allergy history, skin test results, and age. There were 3/20 (15%) treatment failures on cromolyn among 20 patients classified as extrinsic asthma and 4/9 (44%) failures in patients classified as intrinsic asthma. There was no evidence of any toxicity or adverse reactions during the study.

In a more recent study, lactose-free cromolyn sodium (20 mg four times daily via Spinhaler) was compared with placebo in a 12-week double-blind parallel group study of 30 adult asthmatic patients with mild to moderately severe asthma (Basran et al., 1984). The cromolyn-treated group demonstrated significantly better symptom scores, peak flow rates, and needed less additional inhaled bronchodilators.

Early placebo-controlled double-blind trials in childhood asthma included a 4-week crossover trial in 54 children with severe chronic asthma (McLean et al., 1973). Symptoms of wheezing, breathlessness, tightness, and coughing were significantly lower in the patients during the active drug period compared with the placebo period. Twenty percent of the subjects became essentially asymptomatic while on cromolyn sodium and 65% more were improved.

In another childhood study, 38 children with chronic asthma were given cromolyn sodium or placebo in a double-blind crossover of 8 weeks duration. A statistically significant difference ($P < 0.005$) in physicians ratings in favor of cromolyn therapy was found for both sequences (Hyde et al., 1973). Subsequently, 33 of these children received cromolyn sodium prophylactically for at least 12 months. Compared to the previous year, they experienced improved performance in physical exercise, lessened school absenteeism, reduced hospitalizations, and improved sleep patterns. Also a decreased frequency of attacks occurred in 26 of 33 with a reduced need for bronchodilators in 25 of 33 children, and improvement in peak expiratory flow rates measured during airborne pollen and mold seasons.

Tachyphylaxis to cromolyn sodium has been reported in rats (Thompson and Evans, 1973) but not confirmed in other animal species such as monkeys (El-Azab and Stewart, 1977). Long-term clinical trials in humans have not demonstrated any tachyphylaxis (Godfrey et al., 1975). Also, the dosage of cromolyn sodium can be decreased in many patients after 1 month of therapy to three times a day and further tapered to twice a day in some which does not point to tachyphylaxis as a phenomenon occurring in therapy (Furukawa et al., 1984).

Nebulizer Solution

Cromolyn sodium as a 1% solution has been studied in several clinical trials in very young asthmatic patients. Hiller and co-workers (1977) studied 17 asthmatic children under 5 years of age in a double-blind, placebo-controlled randomized 2-month crossover trial. Daily symptom scores kept by the parents showed improvement in 11 children during active treatment.

Mellon and colleagues (1982) studied 1% cromolyn sodium nebulizer solution in 19 young asthmatic children (mean, 5-9 years) who required daily oral bronchodilators but not corticosteroid maintenance. During the 8-week active treatment phase, significant reductions in asthmatic symptoms, physician assessment of asthma severity, and concomitant bronchodilator usage were observed in 16 of 19 children. These 16 patients continued to receive nebulizer cromolyn sodium treatment for at least 1 year after completion of the study. During the 6-month interval of cromolyn maintenance, there was a marked reduction in emergency visits ($P < 0.01$), corticosteroid courses, and hospitalizations.

In an open study, 50 children under 4 years of age with severe chronic asthma were treated with nebulized cromolyn sodium (20 mg inhaled for 10 min four times daily) for 6 months (Zareceansky et al., 1983). Thirty-three children showed marked improvement with no attacks occurring during the treatment period while 13 showed partial improvement. There was also a marked decrease in the use of other medications and in hospital admissions.

Pressurized Metered Dose Inhaler

Several well-controlled short-term trials evaluating cromolyn sodium delivered by pressurized metered dose inhaler (2 mg four times daily) have recently been conducted. Rubin and colleagues compared cromolyn sodium with matching placebo in a 12-week double-blind crossover trial in 31 adult asthmatics in Israel (Rubin et al., 1983). Patients who received cromolyn sodium showed improved breathlessness at rest ($P < 0.001$), breathlessness on exertion ($P < 0.05$), and morning peak expiratory flow rates ($P < 0.05$). Use of bronchodilators (theophylline and aerosol beta$_2$ agonists combined) significantly ($P < 0.001$) decreased during cromolyn sodium therapy.

A similar study was conducted in Belgium by Cordier (1984) who compared cromolyn sodium treatment with placebo in 29 adults with moderately severe or severe perennial asthma. Asthmatics who were treated with cromolyn sodium experienced reduced asthma symptoms as reported on patient daily diary cards ($P < 0.01$) and at clinic visits ($P < 0.01$). In the active drug group, monitoring peak expiratory flow rates (PEFR) significantly improved ($P < 0.05$) and $beta_2$-agonist usage decreased ($P < 0.001$).

Forty-six children (aged 4-13 years) with moderately severe or extrinsic asthma received either cromolyn sodium delivered by pressurized aerosol (2 mg four times daily) or placebo in a 12-week double-blind crossover trial (Geller-Bernstein and Levin, 1983). Asthma severity and pulmonary function tests after 3 and 6 weeks of treatment showed significant improvement in the cromolyn-sodium-treated group. Objective assessment using twice-daily peak expiratory flow rate also showed clear superiority of cromolyn sodium.

Cromolyn sodium (2 mg four times daily) via pressurized metered dose inhaler) was compared to placebo in a 1-week double-blind comparative group multicenter study with 83 adult and childhood asthmatic patients (Selcow et al., 1986). Subjects who received cromolyn sodium reported significant improvement ($P < 0.05$) in overall asthma scores, cough, physician assessment, FEV_1, and FVC. When data from the 35 adult asthmatics in the trial were analyzed separately, cromolyn sodium remained significantly better than placebo (Fig. 13).

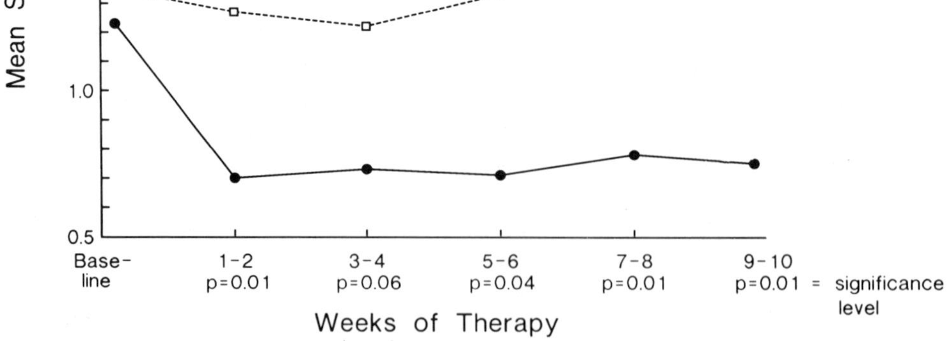

Figure 13 Changes in asthma severity in a placebo-controlled, multicenter study in 35 adult asthmatics receiving either cromolyn sodium or placebo (reproduced with permission from Selcow et al., 1986).

E. Comparison with Other Pharmacologic Agents

Theophylline

The first double-blind trial of cromolyn and theophylline was a collaborative 4-week study conducted in both London and Denver (Hambleton et al., 1977) involving moderate to severe asthmatics. Cromolyn and theophylline were equal, as there was no significant difference in therapy judged by peak expiratory flow rates, use of extra medications and, in 2 of the 3 patients', scoring criteria. Theophylline resulted in significantly fewer symptom-free days. These comparable results were surprising since cromolyn may take 4 weeks to be fully effective and the statistical analysis was based on the entire 4-week study period.

Newth and co-workers (1982) in an 8-week double-blind crossover study compared 1% nebulized cromolyn sodium (four times daily dosing) with liquid theophylline (every 6 hr dosing with serum levels 10-20 mg/liter) in controlling symptoms of chronic asthma in preschool children. Patients had an average of 61% symptom-free days while receiving cromolyn sodium compared with 46.5% when on theophylline ($P < 0.05$) (Fig. 14). Numerous adverse side effects were reported with theophylline therapy while none were reported for cromolyn sodium.

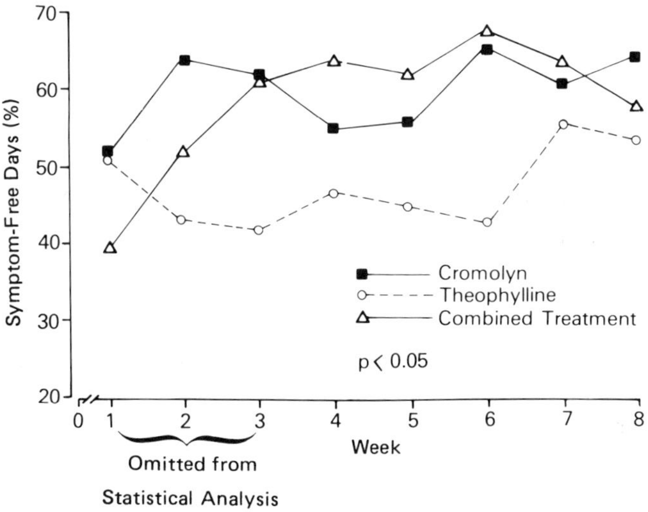

Figure 14 Comparison of nebulized cromolyn sodium, theophylline, and combined treatment in controlling asthma symptoms in preschool children. Patients receiving cromolyn sodium had an average of 61% symptom-free days as compared with 46.5% on theophylline ($P < 0.05$) (reproduced with permission from Newth et al., 1982).

Recently a 3 month double-blind placebo-controlled parallel group study in moderate childhood asthmatics compared cromolyn sodium (20 mg four times daily via Spinhaler) and sustained-release theophylline (Theo-Dur with serum levels adjusted to 15 μg/ml) in controlling asthma. Based on the degree of clinical improvement as reported on diary cards, by physician assessment of severity of asthma, and on the frequency of use of as-needed beta-adrenergic bronchodilators, theophylline and cromolyn were equally effective. This equal effectiveness of the two treatment regimens occurred despite the dosage of cromolyn sodium being tapered to three times daily in 100% of patients and twice daily in 77% of patients. The patients underwent methacholine challenge at the beginning and the end of the study to assess the degree of nonspecific bronchial hyperreactivity. Only the group who received active cromolyn sodium showed statistically significant reduction in their airway hyperreactivity. The patients in the group receiving active theophylline therapy experienced significantly more nausea and nervousness.

From these studies and others reported in the literature (Edmunds et al., 1980; Selcow et al., 1983) it appears that both drugs are equally effective and that cromolyn has fewer adverse effects and is considerably safer.

Corticosteroids

Cromolyn sodium was initially approved by the Food and Drug Administration for use in steroid-dependent asthmatics as a corticosteroid-sparing drug. This resulted from the observation in several early clinical studies that corticosteroid dosage could be reduced in some patients (Smith and Devey, 1968; Moran et al., 1968; Chai et al., 1971; Read and Rebuck, 1969).

In a double-blind crossover trial, Friday and co-workers (1973) gave 36 children with chronic intractable asthma, 23 of whom were corticosteroid-dependent, 20 mg inhaled cromolyn sodium or a placebo four times a day for two 4-week periods. Although in the very short treatment period cromolyn sodium was not statistically superior to the placebo in the severe patients, 36 patients noted subjective improvement from the cromolyn sodium and entered a 12-month open-ended clinical trial. Of the 18 steroid-dependent patients who completed 12 months of cromolyn sodium therapy, 7 discontinued corticosteroids, 10 decreased their dosage, and 1 patient increased his corticosteroid requirement.

It has been suggested that the combination of inhaled cromolyn sodium and inhaled corticosteroid may be more effective than either drug alone. Toogood and associates (1981) assessed the usefulness of adding cromolyn sodium to patients dependent on beclomethasone therapy. Thirty asthmatics who were well-controlled on high-dose beclomethasone (mean 1,040 μg) but with morning cortisol levels averaging 10 μg/dl were randomly allocated to placebo or cromolyn sodium (20 mg four times daily) used in addition to their beclomethasone and other regular asthma medications. After 4 weeks, the beclomethasone dose was halved and both groups were monitored subjectively and objectively for greater than 6 months. The distributions of good, fair, and poor risk-benefit responses were the same in both cromolyn sodium- and placebo-treated groups (P = 0.20). There was no discernible beclomethasone-sparing effect or other clinical advantage from adding cromolyn sodium to their established beclomethasone requirement.

In a recent double-blind 8-week study of bronchial hyperreactivity in non-atopic asthmatics, Lowhagen and Rak (1984) treated 40 adult intrinsic asthmatic patients with cromolyn sodium, budesonide, cromolyn sodium plus budesonide, or placebo. A mean decrease in sensitivity to histamine provocation was seen after both cromolyn sodium and budesonide but not after placebo. The combination of cromolyn sodium and budesonide gave no additional effect.

Two additional controlled trials have failed to show added benefit from combined and corticosteroid therapy (Dawood et al., 1977; Hiller and Milner, 1975). Patient selection bias could have yielded a cromolyn sodium unresponsive subset of asthmatics. Also, airway deposition of the drug in the formulation of cromolyn sodium utilized Spincaps and the dosage (20 mg four times daily) could have influenced these results. Despite these potential problems, it appears that the steroid-sparing effect of cromolyn sodium is not as marked as originally thought.

F. Clinical Applications and Practical Suggestions for Use

Three therapeutic forms of cromolyn sodium are available for use in the United States: 20 mg powdered capsule delivered via Spinhaler turbo inhaler, 1% solution containing 20 mg cromolyn sodium in 2 ml distilled water delivered by a compressor-driven nebulizer, and a pressurized metered-dose inhaler which delivers 1 mg per actuation.

Spinhaler

The Spinhaler was developed to overcome coordination problems in aerosol thrapy. It is a small open plastic tube containing a plastic propeller-like rotor that revolves at high speed when air is inhaled through the device. Twenty mg powdered cromolyn mixed with 20 mg lactose contained in a standard gelatin capsule is inserted into a cup in the propeller. Two perforations are made in the capsule by vertically sliding the sleeve down once, which activates a simple piercing mechanism. When air is inhaled through the mouthpiece, the turbo-vibratory action of the propeller causes the powdered drug to be dispersed into the inspired air through perforations in the capsule wall. The airstream inside the Spinhaler and the action of the propeller cause agglomerates of drug and lactose to break up with the resultant fine particles of cromolyn sodium passing with the inspired air into the respiratory tract. The remaining larger lactose particles are retained in the mouth and upper airway. Release of drug occurs early in the inhalation period and continues while adequate air flow into the lungs is maintained, providing distribution of cromolyn over the surface of the airways. The extent to which these clumps of powder are broken down to respirable particles is determined by the flow rate of air drawn through the device. When fast flow rates (29-120 liters/min) are achieved, the respirable portion of th output increases dramatically to between 50 and 70% of the normal dosage (Brown et al., 1983).

Although the Spinhaler eliminates patient coordination problems, careful attention should be paid when initially instructing patients. They should be encouraged to use high peak inspiratory flow rates with 10 sec of breath-holding.

The Spinhaler delivery system can be utilized by any patient older than about 4 years of age. Being a breath-activated system, it requires little coordination and no spacer devices are necessary. Also, there are no fluorocarbons to cause potential abuse. The starting dosage is usually one 20 mg capsule four times daily. When symptoms are in control, usually after 1-2 months of therapy the dosage can be decreased to three times a day and then twice daily.

Nebulizer Solution

Cromolyn sodium has been available in the United States as a 1% nebulizer solution since 1982. It contains 20 mg cromolyn sodium in 2 ml purified water with no preservatives and is packaged in 2-ml unit dose glass ampules. The clear, colorless solution has a pH of 4.0-7.0. It is delivered with a power-operated nebulizer via face mask or mouthpiece. The face mask has the potential of delivering the medication to the entire upper airway, which may be an advantage in patients who also have allergic rhinitis.

Cromolyn sodium nebulizer has been shown to be physically and chemically compatible for up to 60 min when mixed in vitro with metaproterenol sulfate solution, isoproterenol hydrochloride solution, isoetharine hydrochloride 0.25% inhalation solution, epinephrine hydrochloride solution, terbutaline sulfate sterile aqueous solution, and 20% acetyl-cysteine solution (Lesko and Miller, 1984). Similarly, cromolyn sodium did not adversely affect the stability of the individual bronchodilator/mucolytic drugs in the admixtures. Therefore it is possible to make a mixture of medications which can be simultaneously nebulized to the patient.

Cromolyn sodium has proven to be especially useful for children under 4, patients who are unable to tolerate the powder formulation because of extremely hyperreactive airways, patients with more severe disease who benefit from the bronchodilator/cromolyn sodium mixture, prevention of viral-induced wheezing in children and patients who have cough-variant asthma (Bernstein, 1985; Mellon et al., 1982). With the use of the nebulizer solution there is no

Table 4 Comparative Studies: Intal Capsules vs Intal Nebulizer Solution

Investigator	Type of study	Number and age range (yrs) of patients	Outcome
Matthew, 1977	EIB	10 (6-13)	Equal efficacy
Mellis and Levison, 1978	EIB	20 (11.8)	Equal efficacy
Marks, 1977	Bioavailability	6 (8-14)	Better absorption (urine assay) from capsules
Dahl and Hendriksen, 1979	EIB	10 (28)	Capsules marginally more effective than solution
Jones and Chung, 1979	EIB	51 (5-16)	Solution significantly better than powder 20 mg = 40 mg
MacDonald and Kennedy, 1980	Bioavailability and clinical efficacy	20 (45.4)	Better serum levels with capsules than solution. Equal efficacy
Frith et al., 1981	Bronchial provocation	10 (18-64)	Equal efficacy
Bungaard et al., 1981	EIB	4 (8-12)	Equal efficacy
Corkey et al., 1982	EIB	18 (14.1)	Equal efficacy

need to stop cromolyn when the patient is experiencing bronchospasm since a bronchodilator may be added directly to the solution.

A number of studies have compared cromolyn sodium nebulizer solution to cromolyn sodium capsules (Table 4). They have equal efficacy in the majority with nebulizer solution being superior in some clinical trials.

Metered Dose Inhaler

Cromolyn sodium became available in a pressurized metered dose aerosol unit in 1986. Each cannister contains micronized cromolyn sodium, sorbitan trioleate, with dichlorotetrafluoroethane and dichlorodifluoromethane as propellants. Each metered spray of 1 mg delivers approximately 800 μg cromolyn sodium to the patient with most of the individual particles of cromolyn sodium having a diameter not greater than 5 μm. The recommended dose is two inhalations or 1.6 mg four times daily at regular intervals. For the prevention of acute bronchospasms that follows exercise, exposure to cold dry air or environmental agents, the usual dose is two metered dose sprays 10-15 min before, but no more than 60 min before exposure to the precipitating factor.

Plasma levels obtained with 5 mg cromolyn sodium delivered via a metered dose inhaler are intermediate between those obtained with Intal capsules (20 mg) via the Spinhaler turboinhaler and Intal Nebulizer Solution (20 mg), delivered via a power-driven nebulizer and face mask (Cedric Grigg, Fisons Corporation, personal communication).

Several well-controlled studies have demonstrated that the pressurized aerosol (1.6 mg four times daily) is equivalent to 20 mg cromolyn sodium delivered via Spinhaler four times daily. It is also as effective in attenuating exercise-induced asthma as an inhalation of 20 mg powder.

Practical Suggestions for Use

Cromolyn sodium's unique prophylactic and safety properties have led to it being recommended as a first-line agent in the management of mild to moderately severe asthma (Bernstein, 1985; Shapiro and Konig, 1985).

As with all inhaled medications, it is important that patients learn proper inhalation techniques. The starting dosage of cromolyn is 20 mg via Spinhaler or nebulizer or 2 mg delivered by pressurized metered dose inhaler taken at regular intervals four times daily. When the patient is stabilized the Spincaps or nebulizer solution may be tapered to three times daily and then twice daily in some patients. If the results are equivocal after a 4-week trial, the clinical trial period should be extended from 8 to 12 weeks and the dosage should be doubled during the last 6 weeks of the trial (Bernstein, 1985).

Because there is a correlation between the degree of airway patency and the amount of cromolyn reaching the lungs (Benson et al., 1973), it is important that the airways are patent for maximal drug delivery. Depending on the degree of obstruction, this can be achieved with concomitant bronchodilator and/or corticosteroid therapy (Shapiro and Konig, 1985; Bernstein, 1985). It is important not to stop cromolyn if the patient is wheezing. Nebulizer solution may be used during wheezing episodes and the Spinhaler or MDI may be continued during an exacerbation of asthma by preceding it with a bronchodilator.

Taken acutely, cromolyn sodium is effective in blocking an encounter with a known allergen (animal or pollen exposure), exercise-induced asthma, cold air or fog-induced asthma, and reflex-induced bronchospasm (SO_2 exposure). Cromolyn sodium is most effective in blocking pollen-induced asthma if started 1 week before the anticipated exposure. However, it may be started at any time during the season.

Long-term use of cromolyn is appropriate for patients of any age with mild to moderately severe asthma requiring continuous medication, patients with dual or late asthmatic responses, and patients with excessive airways hyperreactivity.

References

Abraham, W. M., Oliver, W., King, M. M., Yerger, L., and Wanner, A. (1981). Effect of pharmacologic agents on antigen-induced decreases in specific lung conductance in sheep. *Am. Rev. Respir. Dis. 124*: 554-558.

Abraham, W. M., Delehunt, J. C., Yerger, L., and Marchette, B. (1983). Characterization of a late phase pulmonary response after antigen challenge in allergic sheep. *Am. Rev. Respir. Dis. 128*: 839-844.

Advenier, C., Cerrina, J., and Duroux, P. (1983). Sodium cromoglycate, verapamil, and nicardipine antagonism to leukotriene D_4 bronchoconstriction. *Br. J. Pharmacol. 78*: 301.

Advenier, C., Cerrina, J., and Duroux, P. (1983). *Br. J. Pharmacol. 78*: 301.

Allistone, A., Collier, J. G., Davidson, R. N., Fuller, R. W., and Richardson, P. S. (1985). The effect of intravenous sodium cromoglycate in the bronchoconstriction induced by sulphur dioxide inhalation in man. *Clin. Sci. 68*(2): 227-232.

Altounyan, R. E. C. (1967). Inhibition of experimental asthma by a new compound—disodium cromoglycate (Intal). *Acta Allergol. 22*: 487.

Altounyan, R. E. C. (1969). Disodium cromoglycate—development and clinical pharmacology. In *Progress in Bronchial Asthma. Proceedings of a Symposium on Disodium Cromoglycate.* Sydney, p. 15.

Altounyan, R. E. C. (1970). Changes in histamine and atropine responsiveness as a guide to diagnosis and evaluation of therapy in obstructive airways disease. In *Disodium Chromoglycate in Allergic Airways Disease.* Edited by J. Pepys and A. W. Frankland. London, Butterworths, pp. 47-54.

Ashton, M. J., Clark, B., Jones, K. M., Moss, G. F., Neale, M. G., and Ritchie, J.

T. (1973). The absorption metabolism and excretion of disodium cromoglycate in nine animal species. *Toxicol. Appl. Pharmacol. 26*: 319.

Assem, E. S. K., and Mongar, J. L. (1970). Inhibition of allergic reactions in man and other species by cromoglycate. *Int. Arch. Allergy Appl. Immunol. 38*: 68-77.

Atkins, P. C., Norman, M. E., and Zweiman, B. (1978). Antigen-induced neutrophil chemotactic activity in man. Correlation with bronchospasm and inhibition by disodium cromoglycate. *J. Allergy Clin. Immunol. 62*: 149-155.

Basran, G. S., Page, C. T., Paul, W., and Morley, J. (1983). Cromoglycate inhibits the responses to platelet-activating factor (PAF-acether) in man: An alternative mode of action for DSCG in asthma? *Eur. J. Pharmacol. 86*(1): 143-144.

Basran, G. S., Darbyshire, J. H., Nunn, A. J., and Turner-Warwick, M. (1984). Inhaled lactose-free sodium cromoglycate powder in the treatment of recurrent asthma. *Br. J. Dis. Chest 78*: 254-260.

Beach, J. E., Blair, A. M. J. N., and Clarke, A. J. (1981). Cromolyn sodium toxicity studies in primates. *Toxicol. Appl. Pharmacol. 57*: 367-400.

Ben-Dov, I., Bar-Yishay, E., and Godfrey, S. (1983). Heterogeneity in the response of asthmatic patients to pre-exercise treatment with cromolyn sodium. *Am. Rev. Respir. Dis. 127*: 113-116.

Benson, M. K., Curry, S. H., D'A Mills, G. G., and Hughs, D. T. D. (1973). Uptake of sodium cromoglycate in obstructive airway disease. *Clin. Allergy 3*: 389-394.

Bernstein, I. L. (1985). Cromolyn sodium in the treatment of asthma: Coming of age in the United States. *J. Allergy Clin. Immunol. 76*: 381-388.

Bernstein, I. L., Siegel, S. C., Brandon, M. L., Brown, E. G., Evans, R. R., Feinberg, A. R., Friedlander, S., Krumholz, R. A., Hadley, R. A., Handelman, N. I., Thurston, D., and Yamate, M. (1972). A controlled study of cromolyn sodium sponsored by the Drug Committee of the American Academy of Allergy. *J. Allergy Clin. Immunol. 50*: 235-245.

Bleecker, E. R., Britt, E. J., and Mason, P. L. (1982). The effect of cromolyn on antigen and methacholine airways reactivity during ragweed season in allergic asthma. *Chest 82*: 227.

Blumenthal, M. N., Schoenwetter, W. F., MacDonald, F. M., and McHugh, R. B. (1973). Cromolyn in extrinsic and intrinsic asthma. *J. Allergy Clin. Immunol. 52*: 105-113.

Booij-Noord, H., Orie, N. G. M., Berg, W. Chr., and deVries, K. (1970). Protection tests on bronchial allergen challenge with disodium cromoglycate and thiazinamium. *J. Allergy 46*: 1.

Booij-Noord, H., Orie, N. G. M., and deVries, K. (1971). Immediate and late bronchial obstructive reactions to inhalation of house dust and protective effects of disodium cromoglycate and prednisolone. *J. Allergy Clin. Immunol. 48*: 344-354.

Breslin, F. J., McFadden, E. R., and Ingram, R. H. (1980). The effects of cromolyn sodium on the airway response to hyperpnea and cold air in asthma. *Am. Rev. Respir. Dis. 122*: 11-16.

Brogden, R. N., Speight, T. M., and Avery, G. S. (1974). Sodium cromoglycate (cromolyn sodium): A review of its mode of action, pharmacology, therapeutic efficacy and use. *Drugs 7*: 164-282.

Brompton Hospital/Medical Research Council Collaborative Trial (1972). Long-term study of disodium cromoglycate in treatment of severe extrinsic or intrinsic bronchial asthma in adults. *Br. Med. J. 4*: 383-388.

Brown, L. A., Kaplan, R. A., Benjamin, P. A., Hoffman, L. S., and Shearer, W. T. (1981). Immunoglobulin E-mediated anaphylaxis with inhaled cromolyn sodium. *J. Allergy Clin. Immunol. 68*: 416-420, 1981.

Brown, L. A., Neale, K. M. G., Auty, R. M., Hodder, R. W., and Snashall, P. (1983). The pharmacokinetics of sodium cromoglycate. In *Proceedings of the Eleventh International Congress of Allergology and Clinical Immunology, London, October 1982.* Edited by G. W. Kerr and M. A. Ganderton. London, Macmillan, pp. 513-516.

Bryant, D. H., Burns, M. W., and Lazarus, L. (1973). New type of allergic asthma due to IgG "reaginic" antibody. *Br. Med. J. 4*: 589.

Bungaard, A., Pedersen, J. Z., Schmidt, A., and Bach-Mortensen, N. (1981). Should stable asthma be treated with nebulizer or/pressurized metered-dose spray? *Ugeskr Laeger 143*: 2878-2880 (in Danish, English summary).

Chai, H., Purcell, K., Brady, K., and Falliers, C. J. (1968). Therapeutic and investigational evaluation of asthmatic children. *J. Allergy 41*: 23-36.

Chai, H., Molk, L., Falliers, C. J., and Miklich, D. (1971). Steroid-sparing effects of disodium cromoglycate (DSC) in children with severe clinical asthma. In *New Concepts in Allergy and Clinical Immunology.* Edited by U. Serafini. Amsterdam, Excerpta Medica, pp. 385-91.

Chan-Yeung, M., Morton, J., and Grzybowski, S. (1971). A double-blind trial of disodium cromoglycate (Intal) in the treatment of bronchial asthma. *Can. Med. Assoc. J. 105*: 827-831.

Chung, J. T. N., and Jones, R. S. (1979). Bronchodilator effects of sodium cromoglycate and its clinical implications. *Br. Med. J. 11*: 1033.

Church, M. K., Holgate, S. T., and Pao, G. J-K. (1983). Histamine release from mechanically and enzymatically dispersed human lung mast cells: inhibition by salbutamol and cromoglycate. *Br. J. Pharmacol. 79*(Suppl.): 374.

Church, M. K., and Warner, J. O. (1985). Sodium cromoglycate and related drugs. *Clin. Allergy 15*: 311-320.

Church, M. K., and Young, K. O. (1983). The characteristics of inhibition of histamine release from human lung fragments by sodium cromoglycate, salbutamol, and chlorpromazine. *Br. J. Pharmacol. 78*: 671-679.

Cockcroft, D. W., Killian, D. N., Mellan, J. J. A., and Hargreave, F. E. (1977a).

Bronchial reactivity to inhaled histamine: a method and clinical survey. *Clin. Allergy* 7: 235-243.

Cockcroft, D. W., Killian, D. N., Mellan, J. J. A., and Hargreave, F. E. (1977b). Protective effect of drugs on histamine-induced asthma. *Thorax 32*: 429-437.

Cockcroft, D. W., Ruffin, R. E., Dolovich, J., and Hargreave, F. W. (1977c). Allergen-induced increase in non-allergic bronchial reactivity. *Clin. Allergy* 7: 503.

Cordier, R. (1984). Sodium cromoglycate delivered by pressurised aerosol in the treatment of adult asthma. *Clin. Trials J. 21*: 483-491.

Corkey, C., Mindorff, C., Levison, H., and Newth, C. (1982). Comparison of three different preparations of disodium cromoglycate in the prevention of exercise-induced bronchospasm. *Am. Rev. Respir. Dis. 125*: 623-626.

Cox, J. S. G. (1967). Disodium cromoglycate (FPL670) (Intal): A specific inhibitor of reaginic antibody/antigen mechanisms. *Nature 216*: 1328.

Cox, J. S. G. (1970). Review of chemistry, pharmacology, toxicity, metabolism, specific side-effects, antiallergic properties in vitro and in vivo of disodium cromoglycate. In *Disodium Cromoglycate in Allergic Airway Disease.* Edited by J. Pepys and A. W. Frankland. London, Butterworth, p. 13.

Cox, J. S. G. (1971). Disodium cromoglycate: mode of action and its possible relevance to the clinical use of the drug. *Br. J. Dis. Chest 65*: 189-204.

Cox, J. S. G. (1976). Disodium cromoglycate (cromolyn sodium) in bronchial asthma. In *Bronchial Asthma–Mechanisms and Therapeutics.* Edited by E. B. Weiss and M. S. Segal. Boston, Little, Brown and Co. pp. 805-836.

Cox, J. S. G., and Altounyan, R. E. C. (1970). Nature of modes of action of disodium cromoglycate (Lomudal). *Respiration 27*(Suppl.): 292.

Cox, J. S. G., Beach, J. E., and Blair, A. M. J. N. (1970). Disodium cromoglycate (Intal). *Adv. Drug Res. 5*: 115-196.

Crisp, J., Ostrander, C., Giannini, A., Stroup, C., and Diamer, W. C. (1974). Cromolyn sodium therapy for chronic perennial asthma. *JAMA 229*: 787-788.

Dahl, R. (1981). Oral and inhaled sodium cromoglycate in challenge test with fool allergies or acetylsalicylic acid. *Allergy 36*: 161.

Dahl, R., and Henriksen, J. M. (1979). Inhibition of exercise-induced bronchoconstriction by nebulised sodium cromoglycate in patients with bronchial asthma. *Scand. J. Respir. Dis. 60*: 51-55.

Davies, S. E. (1968). Effect of disodium cromoglycate on exercise-induced asthma. *Br. Med. J. 3*: 593-594.

Dawood, A. G., Hendry, A. T., and Walker, S. R. (1977). The combined use of betamethasone valerate and sodium cromoglycate in the treatment of asthma. *Clin. Allergy* 7: 161-165.

Delaney, J. C. (1976). The effect of sodium cromoglycate on analgesic induced asthmatic reactions. *Clin. Allergy 6*: 365.

deVries, K., Gokemerjer, J. D. M., Orie, N. G. M., Peset, R., and Sluiter, H. J. (1976). The response of the bronchial tree to allergic and non-allergic stimuli in patients with generalized obstructive lung disease. *Bull. Int. Union Tuberc. 51*: 617-619.

Diaz, P., Galleguillos, F. R., Gonzalez, M. C., Pantin, C. F. A., and Kay, A. B. (1984). Bronchoalveolar lavage in asthma: the effect of disodium cromoglycate (cromolyn) on leukocyte counts, immunoglobulins, and complement. *J. Allergy Clin. Immunol. 74*: 41-48.

Dickson, W. A. (1970). One-year's trial of Intal® compound in 24 children with severe asthma. In *Disodium Cromoglycate in Allergic Airways Disease.* Edited by J. Pepys and A. W. Frankland. London, Butterworth, pp. 105-120.

Dickson, W., and Cole, M. (1979). Severe asthma in children–a 10 year follow-up. In *The Mast Cell–Its Role in Health and Disease.* Edited by J. Pepys and A. M. Edwards. Tunbridge Wells, England, Pitman, p. 343.

Dixon, M., Jackson, D. M., and Richards, I. M. (1980). The action of sodium cromoglycate on "C" fibre endings in the dog lung. *Br. J. Pharmacol. 70*: 11-13.

Edmunds, A. T., Carswell, F., Robinson, P., and Hughes, A. O. (1980). Controlled trial of cromoglycate and slow-release aminophylline in perennial childhood asthma. *Br. Med. J. 281*: 842.

El-Azab, J., and Stewart, P. B. (1977). The difference in effect with predosing with antiallergic compounds between the rat PCA model and the monkey asthma model: Comparison of the effect of PR-D-92-EA and disodium cromoglycate. *Int. Arch. Allergy Appl. Immunol. 55*: 343.

Fabbri, L. M., Mapp, C. E., and Hendrick, D. J. (1982). Cromolyn reduces the airway response to carbacol. *Am. Rev. Respir. Dis. 125*(4, Part 2): 75A.

Fanta, C. H., McFadden, E. R., and Ingram, R. H. (1982). Effects of cromolyn sodium on the response to respiratory heat loss in normal subjects. *Am. Rev. Respir.Dis. 123*: 161-164.

Feldman, C. H., Fox, J., Kraut, E., Feldman, B. R., and Davies, W. J. (1982). Exercise induced asthma (EIA): Treatment for early and late responses. *Am. Rev. Respir. Dis. 125* (Part 2): 191.

Fewtrell, C., and Metzger, H. (1980). Larger oligomers of IgE are more effective than dimers in stimulating rat basophilic leukemic cells. *J. Immunol. 125*: 701-710.

Flint, K. C., Leung, K. B. P., Pearce, F. L., Hudspith, B. N., Brostoff, J., and Johnson, N. M. (1985). Human mast cells recovered by bronchoalveolar lavage: Their morphology, histamine release and the effects of sodium cromoglycate. *Clin. Sci. 68*: 427-432.

Forman, J. C., and Garlano, L. G. (1976). Cromoglycate and other antiallergic drugs: A possible mechanism of action. *Br. Med. J. 1*: 820.

Foster, C. S., and Duncan, J. (1980). Randomized clinical trial of topically administered cromolyn sodium for vernal keratoconjunctivitis. *Am. J. Ophthalmol. 90*: 175.

Friday, G. A., Facktor, M. A., Bernstein, R. A., and Fireman, P. (1973). Cromolyn therapy for severe asthma in children. *J. Pediatr. 83*: 299-304.

Frieri, M., Alling, D. W., and Methcalfe, D. D. (1985). Comparison of the therapeutic efficacy of cromolyn sodium with that of combined chlorpheniramine and cimetidine in systemic mastocytosis: results of a double-blind clinical trial. *Am. J. Med. 78*: 9-14.

Frith, P. A., Ruffin, R. E., Juniper, E. F., Dolovich, J., and Hargreave, P. E. (1981). Inhibition of allergen-induced asthma by three forms of sodium cromoglycate. *Clin. Allergy 11*(1): 67-77.

Fuller, R. W., and Collier, J. G. (1983). The pharmacokinetic assessment of sodium cromoglycate. *J. Pharm. Pharmacol. 35*: 289-292.

Fuller, R. W., and Collier, J. G. (1984). Sodium cromoglycate and atropine block the fall in FEV_1 but not the cough induced by hypotonic mist. *Thorax 39*: 766-70.

Furukawa, C. T., Shapiro, G. G., Kraemer, M. J., Pierson, W. E., and Bierman, C. W. (1984). A double-blind study comparing the effectiveness of cromolyn sodium and sustaine-release theophylline in childhood asthma. *Pediatrics 74*: 453-459.

Geller-Bernstein, C., and Levin, S. (1983). Sodium cromoglycate pressurised aerosol in childhood asthma. *Curr. Ther. Res. 34*: 345-349.

Godden, D., Jamieson, S., and Higenbottan, T. (1983). "Fog"-induced bronchoconstriction is inhibited by sodium cromoglycate but not lignocaine or ipratropium. *Thorax, 38*: 226.

Godfrey, S., Zeidifard, E., Brown, K., and Bell, J. H. (1974). The possible site of action of sodium cromoglycate assessed. *Clin. Sci. Mol. Med. 46*: 265-272.

Godfrey, S., Balfour-Lynn, L., and Konig, P. (1975). The place of cromolyn studies in the long-term management of childhood asthma based on a three- to five-year follow-up. *J. Pediatr. 87*: 465-473.

Goose, J., and Blair, A. M. J. N. (1969). Passive cutaneous anaphylaxis in the rat, induced with two homologous reagin-like antibodies sera and its specific inhibition with disodium cromoglycate. *Immunology 16*: 749.

Grieco, M. N. (1972). Crossover study of cromolyn sodium inhibition of aerosol antigen challenge. *Chest 61*: 432.

Griffin, M. P., MacDonald, N., McFadden, E. R. (1983). Short- and long-term effects of cromolyn sodium on the airway reactivity of asthmatics. *J. Allergy Clin. Immunol. 71*: 331-338.

Gross, N. J. (1980). Allergy to laboratory animals: epidemiologic, clinical, and physiologic aspects, and a trial of cromolyn in its management. *J. Allergy Clin. Immunol. 66*: 158-165.

Hambleton, G., Weinberger, M., Taylor, J., Cavanaugh, M., Ginchansky, E., Godfrey, S., Tooley, M., Bell, T., and Greenberg, S. (1977). Comparison of cromoglycate (cromolyn) and theophylline in controlling symptoms of chronic asthma. A collaborative study. *Lancet 1*: 381-385.

Handelman, N., Friday, G. A., and Schwartz, H. J. (1977). Cromolyn sodium nasal solution in the prophylactic treatment of pollen-induced seasonal allergic rhinitis: A tri-city study of efficacy and safety. *J. Allergy Clin. Immunol. 59*: 237.

Harries, M. G. (1981). Bronchial irritant receptors and a possible new action for cromolyn sodium. *Ann. Allergy 46*: 156-158.

Harries, M. G., Parkes, P. E. G., and Lessof, M. H. (1981). Roles of bronchial irritant receptors in asthma. *Lancet 1*: 5.

Hasham, F., Kennedy, J. D., and Jones, R. S. (1981). Actions of salbutamol, disodium cromoglycate and placebo administered as aerosols in acute asthma. *Arch. Dis. Child 56*: 722.

Hegardt, B., Pauwels, R., Van der Straaten, M. (1981). Inhibitory effect of KWO 2131, terbutaline and DSCG on the immediate and late allergin-induced bronchoconstriction. *Allergy 36*: 115-122.

Hiller, E. J., and Milner, A. D. (1975). Betamethasone 17 valerate aerosol and disodium cromoglycate in severe childhood asthma. *Br. J. Dis. Chest 69*: 103-106.

Hiller, E. J., Milner, A. D., and Lenney, W. (1977). Nebulized sodium cromoglycate in young asthmatic children. *Arch. Dis. Child. 52*: 875-876.

Horn, C. R., Jones, R. M., Lee, D., and Brennan, S. R. (1984). Bronchodilator effect of disodium cromoglycate administered as a dry powder in exercise-induced asthma. *Br. J. Pharmacol. 18*: 798-801.

Hughes, D., Mindorff, C., and Levison, H. (1982). The immediate effect of sodium cromoglycate on the airways. *Ann. Allergy 48*: 6-8.

Hyde, J. S., Isenberg, P. D., and Floro, L. D. (1973). Short- and long-term prophylaxis with cromolyn sodium in chronic asthma. *Chest 63*: 875-880.

Johnson, H. G., and Bach, N. K. (1975). Prevention of calcium ionophore-induced release of histamine in rat mast cells by disodium cromoglycate. *J. Immunol. 114*: 514.

Jones, R. S., and Chung, J. T. N. (1979). Comparison of action of disodium cromoglycate powder and solution on bronchoconstrictor mechanisms in asthmatic children. In *The Mast Cell: Its Role in Health and Disease.* Edited by J. Pepys and A. M. Edwards. Turnbridge Wells, pp. 287-292.

Juniper, E. F., Frith, P. A., and Hargreave, F. E. (1981). Airway responsiveness to histamine and methacholine: Relationship to minimum treatment to control symptoms of asthma. *Thorax 36*: 575-579.

Karlsson, G., and Pipkorn, U. (1984). Effect of disodium cromoglycate on changes in nasal airway resistance induced by platelet activating factor. *Eur. J. Clin. Pharmacol. 27*: 371-373.

Kay, A. B., and Barnes, P. J. (1985). Pharmacological modulation of the asthmatic response. In *Current Perspectives in the Immunology of Respiratory Diseases.* Edited by A. B. Kay and E. J. Goetzl. Edinburgh, Churchill Livingstone, pp. 30-31.

Kay, A. B., Papageorgiou, N., Lee, T. H., Carroll, M., and Durhan, S. R. (1983). Neutrophil and monocyte activation during exercise-induced asthma. *J. Allergy Clin. Immunol. 71*: 146.

Kitamura, S., Ishihara, Y., and Takaku, F. (1984). Effect of disodium cromoglycate on the action of bronchoactive agents in guinea pig tracheal strips. *Arzneim-Forsch./Drug Res. 34*(11): 1002-1004.

Kolotkin, B. M., Lee, C. K., and Townley, R. G. (1973). Duration and specificity of sodium cromolyn on allergen inhalation challenges in asthmatic patients. *J. Allergy Clin. Immunol. 51*: 87.

Kus, J., Ciszek, J. A., Kazimierczak, A. J., and Owczarek, J. (1978). Immediate allergic reaction to Intal in a patient with bronchial asthma. *Pneum. Pol. 46*: 745-749.

Lal, S., Malhotra, S. M., and Gribben, M. D. (1982). Comparison of sodium cromoglycate pressurized aerosol and powder in the treatment of asthma. *Clin. Allergy 12*: 197-201.

Larsen, G. L. (1985). Late-phase reactions: observations on pathogenesis and prevention. *J. Allergy Clin. Immunol. 76*: 665-669.

Larsen, G. L., Shampain, M. P., Marsh, W. R., and Behrens, B. L. (1948). Animal models of the late asthmatic response to antigen challenge. In *Asthma: Physiology, Immuno-pharmacology and Treatment.* Edited by A. B. Kay, K. F. Austen, and L. M. Lichtenstein. London, Academic Press, pp. 245-258.

Latimer, K. M., Roberts, R., Morris, M. M., and Hargreave, F. E. (1984). Inhibition by sodium cromoglycate of bronchoconstriction stimulated by respiratory heat loss: comparison of pressurised aerosol and powder. *Thorax 39*: 277-281.

Lee, T. H., Nagy, L., Nagakuru, T., Walport, M. J., and Kay, A. B. (1982). Identification and partial characterization of an exercise-induced neutrophil chemotactic factor in bronchial asthma. *J. Clin. Invest. 89*: 889-899.

Lemire, I., Cartier, A., Malo, J., Pineau, L., Ghezzo, H., and Martin, R. R. (1984). Effect of sodium cromoglycate on histamine inhalation tests. *J. Allergy Clin. Immunol. 73*: 234-239.

Lesko, L. J., and Miller, A. K. (1984). Physical-chemical compatibility of cromolyn sodium nebulizer solution-bronchodilator inhalant solution admixtures. *Ann. Allergy 53*(3): 236-238.

Lewis, A. J., Dervinis, A., and Chang, J. (1984). The effects of antiallergic and bronchodilator drugs on platelet-activating factor (PAF-acether) induced bronchospasm and platelet aggregation. *Agents Actions 15*: 636-642.

Lowhagen, O., and Rak, I. (1984). Effect of sodium cromoglycate and budesonide on bronchial hyperreactivity in non-atopic asthmatics. *Respiration 46*(Suppl. 1): 105.

Lowhagen, O., and Rak, I. (1985a). Bronchial hyperreactivity after treatment with sodium cromoglycate in atopic asthmatic patients not exposed to relevant allergens. *J. Allergy Clin. Immunol. 75*: 343-347.
Lowhagen, O., and Rak, I. (1985b). Modification of bronchial hyperreactivity after treatment with sodium cromoglycate during pollen season. *J. Allergy Clin. Immunol. 75*: 460-467.
Lozewicz, S., Robertson, C. F., Costello, J. F., and Price, J. F. (1984). Delivery of sodium cromoglycate by pressurized aerosol. *Clin. Allergy 14*: 187-191.
MacDonald, G. F., and Kennedy, D. J. (1980). Clinical trial–sodium cromoglycate (SCG) solution. *J. Can. Soc. Respir. Tech. 16*(2): 18-22.
Marks, M. B. (1977). Cromolyn sodium prophylaxis in asthmatic children under five. *Ann. Allergy 39*: 306-310.
Marquardt, D. L., Walker, L. L., and Wasserman, S. I. (1985). Cromolyn inhibition of mouse bone marrow-derived mast cell mediator release. *J. Allergy Clin. Immunol. 75*(2): 193.
Matthew, D. J. (1977). The use of nebulized sodium cromoglycate in children. *Acta Allergol. 32*(Suppl. 13): 34-43.
Mazurek, N., Berger, G., and Pecht, I. (1980). A binding site on mast cells and basophils for the antiallergic drug cromolyn. *Nature 286*: 722-723.
Mazurek, N., Schindler, H., Schurholz, T. H., and Pecht, I. (1984). The cromolyn binding protein constitutes the CA_2+ channel of basophils opening upon immunological stimulus. *Proc. Natl. Acad. Sci. 81*: 6841-6845.
McLean, W. L., Lozano, J., Hannaway, P., Sakowitz, S., and Mueller, H. L. (1973). Cromolyn treatment of asthmatic children. *Am. J. Dis. Child. 125*: 332-337.
Mellis, C. M., and Levison, H. (1978). Efficacy of sodium cromoglycate by nebulization. *Aust. Paediatr. J. 14*(3): 224.
Mellon, M. H., Harden, K., and Zeiger, R. S. (1982). The effectiveness and safety of nebulizer cromolyn solution in the young childhood asthmatic. *Immunol. Allergy Pract. 4*: 168-172.
Menon, M. P. S., and Das, A. K. (1977). Asthma and urticaria during disodium cromoglycate treatment. *Scand. J. Respir. Dis. 58*: 145-149.
Mezey, R. J., Cohn, M. A., Fernandez, R. J., Januszkiewicz, A. J., and Wanner, A. (1978). Mucociliary transport in allergic patients with antigen-induced bronchospasm. *Am. Rev. Respir. Dis. 118*: 677-684.
Moqbel, R., Durham, S. R., Carroll, M., McDonald, A. J., Walsh, G. M., McKay, J., Shaw, R. J., and Kay, A. B. (1985). Enhanced neutrophil and monocytotoxicty after exercise-induced asthma. *Thorax 40*: 218-219.
Moran, F., Bankier, J. D. H., and Boyd, G. (1968). Disodium cromoglycate in the treatment of allergic bronchial asthma. *Lancet 2*: 137.
Moss, G. F., Jones, K. M., Ritchie, J. T., and Cox, J. S. G. (1971). Plasma levels and urinary excretion of disodium cromoglycate after inhalation by human volunteers. *Toxicol. Appl. Pharmacol. 20*: 147.

Myers, D. J., Geffroy, B., and Boushey, H. (1985). The inhibition of sulfur dioxide induced bronchoconstriction in asthmatic subjects is dose dependent. *Clin. Res. 33*(1): 107A.

Nagy, L., Lee, T. H., and Kay, A. B. (1982). Neutrophil chemotactic activity in antigen-induced late asthmatic reactions. *N. Engl. J. Med. 306*: 497-501.

Newth, C. J. L., Newth, C. V., and Turner, J. A. P. (1982). Comparison of nebulised sodium cromoglycate and oral theophylline in controlling symptoms of chronic asthma in pre-school children: A double blind study. *Aust. NZ J. Med. 12*: 232.

Orr, T. S. C., and Cox, J. S. G. (1969). Disodium cromoglycate an inhibitor of mast cell degranulation and histamine release induced by phospholipase A. *Nature* (London) *223*: 197.

Orr, T. S. C., Hall, D. E., Gwilliam, J., and Cox, J. S. G. (1971). The effect of disodium cromoglycate on the release of histamine and degranulation of rat mast cells induced by compound 48/80. *Life Sci. 10*: 805.

Patel, K. R. (1984). Sodium cromoglycate in histamine and methacholine reactivity in asthma. *Clin. Allergy 14*: 143-145.

Patel, K. R., and Kerr, W. (1984). The dose-duration effect of sodium cromoglycate in exercise-induced asthma. *Clin. Allergy 14*: 87-91.

Patel, K. R., Berkin, K. E., and Kerr, J. W. (1982). Dose-response study of sodium cromoglycate in exercise-induced asthma. *Thorax 37*: 663-666.

Patterson, R., Talbot, C. H., and Broneonbrener, M. (1971). The use of IgE-mediated responses as a pharmacologic test system: The effect of disodium cromoglycate in respiratory and cutaneous reactions and on the electrocardiograms of rhesus monkeys. *Int. Arch. Allergy Appl. Immunol. 41*: 592-603.

Pepys, J. (1981). Basic mechanisms in acute and chronic allergic lung disease. *Immunol. Allergy Pract. 3*: 115-128.

Pepys, J., Hargreave, F. E., Chan, M., and McCarthy, D. S. (1968). Inhibitory effects of disodium cromoglycate on allergen-inhalation tests. *Lancet 2*: 134-137.

Pfister, J. R. (1972). Xanthone-2-carboxylic acids: a new series of antiallergic substances. *J. Med. Chem. 15*: 1032.

Prenner, B. M., Hyte, M. K., and Uryniak, T. J. (1982). The efficacy of 1% cromolyn sodium nebulizer solution in the treatment of young asthmatic children. *Ann. Allergy 48*: 254.

Read, J., and Rebuck, A. S. (1969). Steroid-sparing effect of disodium cromoglycate (Intal) in chronic asthma. *Med. J. Austral. 1*: 566-569.

Rubin, A. E., Alroy, G., and Spitzer, S. (1983). The treatment of asthma in adults using sodium cromoglycate pressurized aerosol: A double-blind controlled trial. *Curr. Med. Res. Opin. 8*: 553-558.

Ryan, G., Latimer, K. M., Dolovick, J., and Hargreave, F. E. (1982). Bronchial responsiveness to histamine: Relationship to diurnal variation of peak flow rate, improvement after bronchodilator in airway calibre. *Thorax 37*: 423-429.

Ryo, U. Y., Kang, B., and Townley, R. C. (1976). Cromolyn therapy in patients with bronchial asthma: Effect on inhalation challenge with allergen, histamine and methacholine. *JAMA 236*: 927-931.

Schoeffel, R. E., Anderson, S. D., and Lindsay, D. A. (1983). Sodium cromoglycate as a pressurised aerosol in exercise-induced asthma. *Aust. NZ J. Med. 13*: 157-161.

Schwartz, H. J. (1984). Observations on the uses of sulfiting agents in food and drugs. *Immunol. Allergy Pract. 6*: 302.

Schwartz, H. J. (1986). Observations on the use of oral sodium cromolyn in a sulfite sensitive asthmatic patient. Submitted for publication.

Selcow, J., Blumenthal, R., Spector, S., and Zeiger, R. (1986). A multicenter study to evaluate the clinical benefits of cromolyn sodium aerosol (1 mg) in the treatment of asthma. *J. Allergy Clin. Immunol. 77*(1): 149.

Selcow, J. E., Mendelson, L., and Rosen, J. P. (1983). A comparison of cromolyn and bronchodilators in patients with mild to moderately severe asthma in an office practice. *Ann. Allergy 50*: 13-18.

Settipane, G. A., Klein, D. E., Boyd, G. K., Sturam, J. H., Freye, H. B., and Weltman, J. K. (1979). Adverse reactions to cromolyn. *JAMA 23*: 811-813.

Shampain, M. P., Behrens, B. L., Larsen, G. L., and Henson, P. M. (1982). An animal model of late pulmonary responses to *Alternaria* challenge. *Am. Rev. Respir. Dis. 126*: 493-498.

Shapiro, G. G., and Konig, P. (1985). Cromolyn sodium: A review. *Pharmacotherapy 5*: 156-170.

Sheard, P., and Blair, A. M. J. N. (1970). Disodium cromoglycate: Activity in three in vitro models of the immediate hypersensitivity reaction in the lung. *Arch. Allergy Appl. Immunol. 38*: 217-244.

Sheffer, A. L., Rocklin, R. E., and Goetzel, E. J. (1975). Immunologic components of hypersensitivity reactions to cromolyn sodium. *N. Engl. J. Med. 293*: 1220-1224.

Sheppard, D., Nadel, J. A., and Boushey, H. A. (1981a). Inhibition of sulfur dioxide-induced bronchoconstriction by disodium cromoglycate in asthmatic subjects. *Am. Rev. Respir. Dis. 124*: 257-259.

Sheppard, D., Saisho, A., Nadel, J. A., and Boushey, H. A. (1981b). Exercise increases sulfur dioxide-induced bronchoconstriction in asthmatic subjects. *Am. Rev. Respir. Dis. 123*: 486-491.

Silverman, M., Konig, P., and Godfrey, S. (1973). The use of serial exercise tests to assess the efficacy and duration of drugs in asthma. *Thorax 28*: 574-578.

Silverman, M., and Turner-Warwick, M. (1972). Exercise-induced asthma: response to disodium cromoglycate in skin-test positive and skin-test negative subjects. *Clin. Allergy 2*: 137-142.

Simon, R., Goldfarb, G., and Jacobsen, D. (1984). Blocking studies in sulfite sensitive asthmatics. *J. Allergy Clin. Immunol. 73*: 136.

Smith, G., Hiller, C., Mazunder, M., and Bone, R. (1980). Aerodynamic size distribution of cromolyn sodium at ambient and airway humidity. *Am. Rev. Respir. Dis. 121*: 513-517.

Smith, J. M., and Devey, C. F. (1968). Clinical trial of disodium cromoglycate in the treatment of asthma in children. *Br. Med. J. 2*: 340.

Snashall, P. D., and Lewin, C. (1976). Mechanisms of sulfur dioxide induced bronchoconstriction in man. *Am. Rev. Respir. Dis. 113*(Suppl.): 87.

Spataro, A. C., and Bosman, H. B. (1976). Mechanisms of action of disodium cromoglycate-mast cell calcium ion influx after histamine releasing stimulus. *Biochem. Pharmacol. 25*: 505-510.

Stevenson, D. D., Simon, R. A., and Mathison, D. A. (1984). Cromolyn pretreatment delays onset of aspirin (ASA) induced asthmatic reactions. *J. Allergy Clin. Immunol. 73*(Part 2): 213.

Stokes, T. C., and Morley, J. (1981). Prospects for an oral Intal. *Br. J. Dis. Chest 75*: 1-14.

Suschitzky, J. L., and Sheard, P. (1984). The search for antiallergic drugs for the treatment of asthma—problems in finding a successor to sodium cromoglycate. *Progr. Med. Chem. 21*: 2-61.

Szmidt, M., Gorski, P., Rozniecki, J., and Rychlicka, I. (1979). Ocena zaleznosci miedzy wragliwoscia oskrzeli na wziewana histamine a histaminemia u chorych na astme atopwa podczas leczenia Intalem (DSCG). *Penumon. Pol. 47*: 517-522.

Theoharides, T. C., Sieghart, W., Greengard, P., and Douglas, W. W. (1980). Anti-allergic drug cromolyn may inhibit histamine secretion by regulating phosphorylation of a mast cell protein. *Science 207*: 80-82.

Thiel, H., and Ulmer, W. T. (1980). Bakers' asthma: Development and possibility for treatment. *Chest 78*(Suppl.): 400-405.

Thomson, D. S., and Evans, D. P. (1973). Inhibition of immediate hypersensitory reactions by disodium cromoglycate: Requirements for activity in two laboratory models. *Clin. Exp. Immunol. 13*: 537-544.

Thomson, N. C., Clark, C. J., Boyd, G., and Oran, F. (1981). Effect of sodium cromoglycate on bronchial smooth muscle. *Br. J. Clin. Pharm. 12*: 440.

Toogood, J. H., Jennings, B., and Lefcol, N.M. (1981). A clinical trial of combined cromolyn/beclomethasone treatment for chronic asthma. *J. Pediatr. 67*: 317-324.

Tullett, W. M., Tan, K. M., Wall, R. T., and Patel, K. R. (1985). Dose-response effect of sodium cromoglycate pressurised aerosol in exercise induced asthma. *Thorax 40*: 41-44.

Walker, S. R., Evans, M. E., Richards, A. J., and Paterson, J. W. (1972). The fate of [^{14}C] disodium cromoglycate in man. *J. Pharm. Pharmacol. 24*: 525.

Warner, J. O. (1976). Significance of late reactions after bronchial challenge with house dust mite. *Arch. Dis. Child. 51*: 905-911.

Weiner, P., Greif, J., Fireman, E. (1984). Bronchodilating effect of cromolyn sodium in asthmatic patients at rest and following exercise. *Ann. Allergy 53*: 186-188.

Wells, E., and Mann, J. (1983). Phosphorylation of a mast cell protein in response to treatment with anti-allergic compounds. (Implications for the mode of action of sodium cromoglycate.) *Biochem. Pharmacol. 32*: 837.

Wilson, J. (1982). Use of sodium cromoglycate during pregnancy (French). *J. Pharm. Med. 8*(2) (Suppl.): 45-51.

Woenne, R., Kattan, M., and Levison, H. (1979). Sodium cromoglycate-induced changes in the dose-response curve of inhaled methacholine and histamine in asthmatic children. *Am. Rev. Respir. Dis. 119*: 927-932.

Zareceansky, S., Nadel, G., Yahav, J., and Katznelson, D. (1983). Treatment of asthmatic patients under four years of age with sodium cromoglycate. *Harefuah 105*: 257-258.

18

Corticosteroids

JOHN H. TOOGOOD

University of Western Ontario
Victoria Hospital
London, Ontario, Canada

I. Mechanism of Action

Most of the effects of adrenocorticosteroid drugs that are useful in the treatment of asthma are expressed through interaction of the drug with a specific intracellular glucocorticoid receptor that is common to all steroid-responsive cells in the various body systems (Cupps and Fauci, 1982). During transport to a "target" tissue, the drug is metabolically inactive, bound mostly to transcortin, in the case of cortisol or prednisolone, or to albumin in the case of the other synthetic steroids. On reaching a "target" cell, the steroid dissociates from the carrier protein, diffuses into the cell, and binds there to the glucocorticoid receptor (Ballard, 1979). The steroid-receptor complex then translocates from the cytosol to the genome where it evokes production of a messenger ribonucleic acid, programmed for the synthesis of a regulatory protein. Many such proteins may be synthesized, each presumably responsible for a different facet of the broad spectrum of biological activities displayed by this class of drugs. Some of these proteins modulate the inflammatory process by blocking the synthesis and/or increasing the metabolic breakdown of inflammatory mediators (Hirata et al., 1980; Moore and Hoult, 1980). One such protein, lipomodulin (Moore and Hoult, 1980), or its partial degradation produce, macrocortin (Blackwell et al., 1980), inhibits the action of phospholipase A_2 on membrane phospholipids, thus blocking the synthesis of prostaglandins and leukotrienes. which are mediators known to be important in the pathogenesis of asthma (Kaliner, 1985; Lewis, 1985).

Because the multiple steps involved are rate-limiting, a significant time lapse is required for many of the effects of steroid treatment to be expressed. This is evident clinically in the delayed response of asthmatic subjects to treatment with systemic or inhaled steroids (IS) (Ellul-Micallef et al., 1980; Ellul-Micallef, 1982) and also in the steroid-induced shifting of blood leukocytes between marginated and circulating pools, and intravascular vs. extravascular compartments (Saavedra-Delgado et al., 1980; Cupps and Fauci, 1982; Slade and Hepburn, 1983). These changes are associated with evidence of a specific receptor-steroid interaction (Peterson et al., 1981). A pharmacologic dosage of prednisolone for example, causes the number of circulating neutrophils to increase temporarily, while eosinophils, monocytes, basophils, and lymphocytes decrease (Saavedra-Delgado et al., 1980; Chiang et al., 1980; Cupps and Fauci, 1982). The lymphocytopenia is primarily due to a drop in helper T cells (OKT4+), while the absolute numbers of B cells and suppressor T cells (OKT8+) remain relatively unchanged (Cupps and Fauci, 1982; Slade and Hepburn, 1983). These changes peak 4-6 hr after a bolus dose of prednisolone, then spontaneously reverse in 24-72 hr, and are followed by a transient "rebound" lymphocytosis, monocytosis, and neutrophilia (Toogood et al., 1985a). If the steroid treatment is continued, these short-term fluctuations remain fully and rapidly reversible: the steroid treatment has no cumulative effect on granulocyte or lymphocyte kinetics (Chiang et al., 1980). These intravascular changes are accompanied by reductions in chemotaxis and the influx of inflammatory cells to extravascular sites of tissue injury (Boggs et al., 1984), which is direct evidence of the anti-inflammatory actions of these drugs. The reduced chemotaxis reflects inhibition of both mediator release (Schleimer et al., 1984) and the capacity of inflammatory cells to respond to the mediators (Morris, 1985). The lymphocyte proliferative response to antigen and, to a lesser extent, to mitogens, is inhibited by steroids (Toogood et al., 1980b; Cupps and Fauci, 1982) as is the mixed leukocyte reaction (Katz and Fauci, 1979). In the rat, steroids (acting via lipomodulin) augment the formation by T cells of a lymphokine that inhibits both the production of IgE by B cells and the expression of IgE receptors (Uede et al., 1983). The IgE-dependent release of histamine from human basophils (but not from lung mast cells) is inhibited by steroid treatment, whereas nonspecific histamine release by calcium ionophore is not (Schleimer et al., 1984). The monocyte-macrophage-T helper lymphocyte interactions essential to the induction and regulation of the immune response are inhibited, since steroids block the release of interleukin 1 from macrophages. Type IV allergic phenomena, are especially steroid-sensitive (Cupps and Fauci, 1982). The bactericidal and fungicidal activities of monocytes or macrophages and the release of lysosomal enzymes from granulocytes are reduced (Rinehart et al., 1975). Steroids protect against the increased lysosomal release that ordinarily occurs with respiratory virus infections that exacerbate asthma (Busse et al., 1981). Steroids also constrict the microvasculature, reduce complement levels, and interfere with the passage of immune complexes across basement membranes (Cupps and Fauci, 1982). Thus these drugs can interfere with the inflammatory process at virtually every step in its evolution.

The overall impact of these events in the lung is well illustrated by the effect of steroid treatment on the late asthmatic response (LAR) to bronchial challenge with inhaled antigen (Booij-Noord et al., 1972). The LAR reflects the airways response to a chemotactic influx of neutrophils, basophils, monocytes, and eosinophils (Schleimer et al., 1984; Carroll et al., 1985; De Monchy et al., 1985), their activation to release mediators (Schleimer et al., 1984; Delehunt et al., 1984a; Durham et al., 1984; De Monchy et al., 1985), bronchospasm in response to some of the latter such as leukotrienes C, D, E, (Delehunt et al., 1984a), and local tissue damage produced by factors such as the major basic protein derived from eosinophil granules (De Monchy et al., 1985; Gleich et al., 1985). The LAR inflammatory response is triggered by an antigen-mediated mast cell activation occuring ~ 6 hr previously, and it can be blocked by pretreatment with steroid at or before the initial antigen challenge (Booij-Noord et al., 1972). The early asthmatic response to antigen can also be abrogated by steroid, provided the drug is administered long enough before the antigen challenge to allow time for production of the regulatory proteins responsible for the drug's effect. An interval of ~ 3 hr was found sufficient in sensitized sheep treated with systemic prednisolone (Delehunt et al., 1984b). In humans, daily treatment with IS for 1-4 weeks proved clinically effective; the degree of protection increased with the duration of treatment (Burge et al., 1982; Dahl and Johansson, 1982). This accumulative antianaphylactic action is in keeping with other evidence of the ability of steroids to inhibit the release of mediators from anaphylactic reactions in the skin, lymphocytes, or lung (Greaves and Plummer, 1974; Clissold and Heel, 1984).

Steroids can inhibit carbachol-induced bronchospasm (Israel et al., 1984), and also prevent or reverse the increase in nonspecific airway reactivity (NSAR) that occurs in association with seasonal exposure to inhaled antigens and activation of asthma symptoms (Sotomayor et al., 1984; Tyan et al., 1985). However steroid treatment does not necessarily normalize the heightened NSAR that may persist for years in some asthmatics despite symptom remission (Sotomayor et al., 1984; Israel et al., 1984). This suggests the mechanism of NSAR is heterogeneous and, as a corollary, that the responsiveness of NSAR to steroids may vary with the clinical circumstances.

Not all steroid effects show the above-mentioned time lag. Other pathways exist, independent of the cytosol receptor and the genome (Keller et al., 1982), and these may mediate the prompt drop in endogenous cortisol production that follows administration of an exogenous steroid (Saavedra-Delgado et al., 1980). This likely applies also to the capacity of steroids to prolong the action of endogenous catecholamines (but not albuterol or metaproterenol) by interfering with their extraneuronal uptake and inactivation (Jeffrey and Avner, 1980; Foster et al., 1983), since the effect is evident within minutes (Geddes et al., 1974). The reversal of β-adrenergic tachyphylaxis achieved by steroid treatment evolves more slowly (Ellul-Micallef and Fenech, 1975). This clinically valuable synergism between steroids and β-adrenergics reflects the capacity of the former to prevent (Davies and Lefkowitz, 1981) or reverse (Samuelson and Davies, 1984; Morris, 1985) the desensitizing effect of sustained adrenergic treatment upon cell responsiveness to the adrenergics. The desensitization is due to two distinct processes: down regulation (decrease in adrenergic receptor numbers) and functional uncoupling (inability of the agonist-bound receptor to initiate the usual physiological sequelae) (Samuelson and Davies, 1984). The steroid apparently acts to correct the impaired coupling, without affecting the down regulation (Samuelson and Davies, 1984). Steroids may also potentiate theophylline's smooth-muscle-relaxing effect (Kolbeck et al., 1979), possibly by altering calcium metabolism in the muscle (Morris, 1980).

Clinically advantageous steroid-bronchodilator interactions may also derive from the anti-inflammatory actions of theophylline and adrenergics per se (Sadoul et al., 1981). The latter inhibit mediator release from leukocytes (Kram et al., 1975; Martin et al., 1980) and reduce NSAR (McWilliams et al., 1984; Ahrens et al., 1984). Steroids, similarly to β-adrenergics, can accelerate mucociliary clearance in asthmatics (Santa Cruz et al., 1974; Bateman et al., 1980). Steroids also suppress the production of mucus in vivo (Moretti et al., 1984) and the in vitro response to mucus secretogogues such as leukotrienes and histamine (Maron et al., 1984; Morris, 1985). This is in keeping with the clinical benefits observed with steroid treatment in some patients with bronchial mucus hypersecretion.

This remarkably broad spectrum of biological activities accounts for the uniquely valuable role of corticosteroid drugs in the treatment of asthma. It is convenient to consider the latter in terms of their clinical use for acute and chronic asthma, respectively.

II. Systemic Steroids for Acute Asthma

The goals of treatment in severe acute asthma are to prevent death, accelerate recovery, and avoid recurrences. Corticosteroids are important in preventing death and recurrences, but they are less important than bronchodilators for accelerating recovery. If a patient with acute asthma is given an intravenous bolus of steroid, a significant ventilatory response may be detected after an hour or two, but the response does not peak until 5-9 hr later (Collins et al., 1975; Ellul-Micallef, Borthwick and McHardy, 1980; Fanta et al., 1983). Furthermore, it is overshadowed in most cases by the larger and more prompt response that can be achieved with subcutaneous epinephrine, inhaled or injected β-adrenergics, or intravenous theophylline, given alone or in combination (Pierson et al., 1974; McFadden et al., 1976; Britton et al., 1976; Kattan et al., 1980; Kemp et al., 1985). Thus, it is usually not possible to demonstrate a significant ventilatory response to steroid treatment, unless the patient is monitored for longer than 6 hr after the steroid was commenced and concomitant bronchodilator treatment is withheld during that time (Collins et al., 1975; Ellul-Micallef, 1982), or used in suboptimal dosage (Arnaud et al., 1979), or held stable while the steroid treatment is added to it (Loren et al., 1980; Fanta et al., 1983).

Therefore prompt and aggressive bronchodilator treatment is universally conceded to be mandatory for acute asthma, while the use of steroids remains more controversial (Pierson et al., 1974; McFadden et al., 1976; Britton et al., 1976; Kattan et al., 1980; Luksza, 1982). The arguments in favor of using a systemic steroid along with bronchodilators may be summarized as follows: (1) It is not possible to predict accurately which patient presenting with severe asthma may suddenly die (Speizer et al., 1968; MacDonald et al., 1976a; Wilson et al., 1981). (2) Failure to use steroids early and in adequate dosage has been cited as a frequent correlate of sudden death during severe asthma (Speizer et al., 1968; MacDonald et al., 1976a,b; Westerman et al., 1979; Wilson et al., 1981; Haskell et al., 1983). (3) The risks of such steroid treatment are negligible, when it is used in conventional dosage. (4) Steroids may exert an early normalizing effect on the arterial oxygen tension in acute asthma, beyond that obtainable with bronchodilators alone (Pierson et al., 1974; Ellul-Micallef et al., 1980). Since hypoxemia is an important determinant of asthmatic deaths (Kristoffersen et al., 1967), this effect may be clinically valuable, especially where oxygen therapy is not immediately accessible. (5) Steroids act rapidly to augment the bronchodilator action of β-adrenergic drugs (Ellul-Micallef and Fenech, 1975). This accelerates the recovery of asthmatic patients who have become refractory to β-adrenergic treatment (Fanta et al., 1983), and could be life-saving in some cases. (6) In some patients, iatrogenic adrenocortical insufficiency might contribute to their risk of death from severe asthma (Speizer et al., 1968). Steroid treatment could be critical in such patients. (7) The use of steroids (along with bronchodilators) in the emergency room has been shown to reduce significantly the incidence of subsequent asthma relapses in comparison with treatment by bronchodilators alone (Loren et al., 1980; Fiel et al., 1983; Fanta et al., 1983).

To initiate treatment, either IV hydrocortisone or methylprednisolone may be used (Collins et al., 1975; Fanta et al., 1983; Haskell et al., 1983). The penetrance of hydrocortisone from the blood into the lung is about twice that of methylprednisolone (Braude and Rebuck, 1982, 1983) although the latter is more potent on a weight for weight basis. However if given in sufficient dosage, either drug can be equally effective. In patients with established or incipient heart failure, the greater mineralocorticoid properties of hydrocortisone could be disadvantageous. However, in the absence of heart failure, any transient edema resulting from a few days' hydrocortisone treatment is clinically unimportant. The intravenous route is convenient but seldom essential since orally administered steroids are rapidly absorbed. The bioavailability of prednisolone is approximately the same, whether it is given intravenously or orally (McAllister et al., 1981). If the oral route is preferred, prednisone and prednisolone may be used interchangeably since they interconvert within an hour and the plasma level of therapeutically active prednisolone eventually achieved is determined more by the particular patient's conversion ratio than by which drug was given initially (Wilson et al., 1975; McAllister et al., 1981). Depot steroid injections cannot be relied upon to act quickly in acute asthma. An added disadvantage is that unexpected adverse effects cannot be terminated quickly by adjusting the dosage or stopping the drug. Adrenocorticotrophic hormone (ACTH) is effective for severe asthma, but its effect may be suboptimal in patients with adrenal hypofunction due to past steroid treatment. Furthermore, ACTH occasionally causes acute anaphylactic reactions.

The optimum dosage of steroid with which to start treatment has yet to be precisely defined (Fanta et al., 1983). However, 500 mg hydrocortisone given as an intravenous bolus and followed by 500 mg/24 hr by continuous drip, or 250 mg hydrocortisone given intravenously at 6-hr intervals, are known to be effective for acute asthma (Collins et al., 1975; Fanta et al., 1983). This dosage (14.3 mg/kg/24 hr) approximates or exceeds the maximally effective dosage (Pierson et al., 1974; Collins et al., 1975; Britton et al., 1976; Fanta et al., 1983; Haskell et al., 1983). By relating the blood to lung penetrance ratios of hydrocortisone and methylprednisolone (Braude and Rebuck 1982, 1983) to their respective anti-inflammatory potencies, it can be calculated that the clinical potency of 1000 mg hydrocortisone/day should approximate that of ~ 400 mg methylprednisolone/day. This is consistent with the results observed clinically, that is, both these dosages are able to achieve a maximal response in patients with status asthmaticus (Collins et al., 1975; Haskell et al., 1983) (see Fig. 1). There is no convincing evidence that very large dosages (2-3 g hydrocortisone per day or 1.0-2 g methylprednisolone) accomplish anything more. A better result can be achieved in a shorter time by ensuring prompt, aggressive bronchodilator treatment than by pushing the steroid dosage to heroic levels. Furthermore, sudden death may complicate intravenous high-dosage prednisolone "pulse" therapy, presumably due to cardiac arrhythmia triggered by acute electrolyte shifts (Bocanegra et al., 1981). This risk is likely to be enhanced if

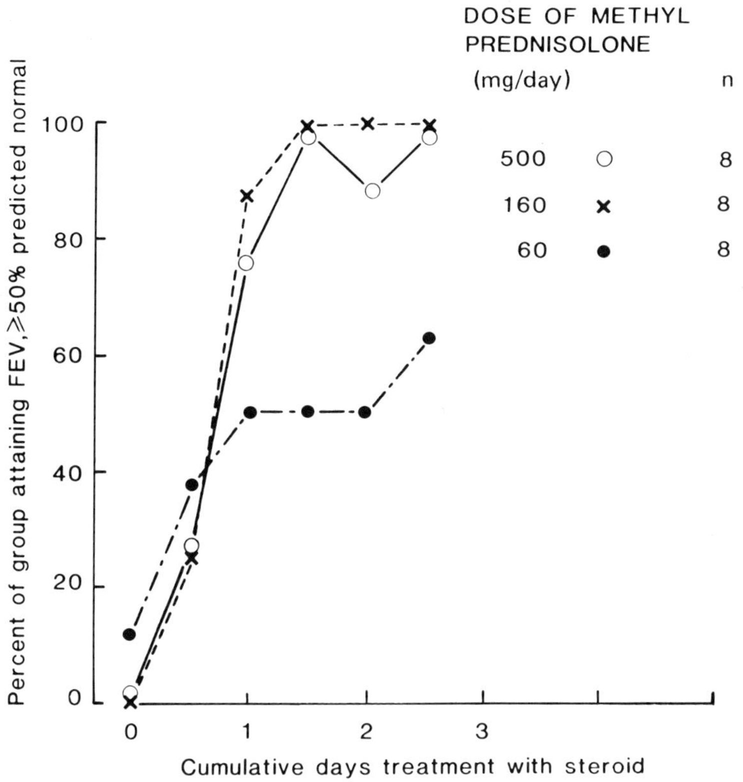

Figure 1 Response of severe acute asthma to intravenous steroid. Patients were randomized among three dosage regimens. A dosage of ~ 160 mg methylprednisolone/day achieved an optimal response in these adults with severe acute asthma (adapted from Haskell et al., 1983 *Arch Intern. Med. 143*: 1324, 1983).

intravenous β-adrenergics are used concurrently because they also produce significant hypokalemia (Elegbeleye et al., 1978; Nogrady et al., 1977). Hydrocortisone in dosages exceeding 1.0 g/day may induce a severe and protracted generalized myopathy (Marle and Woods, 1980), which is not seen with lower dosages.

As a general rule, after 24-48 hr, the intravenous hydrocortisone may be switched to oral prednisone in divided doses varying from 50 to ~150 mg per day, depending on the severity of the asthma and the patient's tolerance. We generally use 60-80 mg/day (0.85-1.2 mg/kg body weight), because CNS side effects are less of a problem if the prednisone dosage does not exceed 100 mg/day. The switch from hydrocortisone minimizes water retention but will not eliminate the continuing loss of potassium, so supplemental potassium should be given.

If diuretics are in use, a potassium-conserving formulation is preferred. This dosage of prednisone is continued until the patient is fully recovered. With high dosages, normalization of airflows may occur within 3 days (Haskell et al., 1983). However patients vary widely in their rate of recovery (Rebuck and Read, 1971). Our experience, using ~0.85 mg prednisone/kg/day, is that 10-14 days are generally required for improvement in the $FEF_{25-75\%}$ to plateau in the adult asthmatics with associated chronic obstructive pulmonary disease (COPD) who constitute the majority of our hospitalized asthmatic patients. This recovery period may appear shorter if a less sensitive index of the therapeutic response is used (e.g., symptoms, or the peak expiratory flow rate) and it may in fact be shorter in younger patients, or in those with less complicated obstructive airway pathologic conditions (Fanta et al., 1983). Whatever the initial dosage, cutting back too soon (before the response has plateaued) may adversely affect the patient's subsequent clinical course (Toogood, 1984c). Serial pulmonary function testing provides the most reliable guide to when to start reducing the steroid dosage (Rebuck and Read, 1971). The symptoms and signs of acute asthma consistently clear well before functional improvement reaches a plateau (Rebuck and Read, 1971; McFadden, 1975; Kelson et al., 1978) and it is difficult to estimate accurately the ventilatory reserve of a particular patient from the physical findings alone (Kelson et al., 1978). Furthermore, documentation of the patient's functional status after improvement has plateaued provides information that is valuable in drafting a plan for ambulatory management appropriate to the individual's needs. Patients with a lower ventilatory reserve due to a component of residual nonreversible COPD are at greater risk of asthma relapse (Toogood et al., 1981a; Toogood, 1984), so they merit closer surveillance. In particular, the 14 days after the patient leaves the hospital are known to be associated with a higher than usual risk of acute asthmatic relapse and death (MacDonald et al., 1976a; Kelson et al., 1978). Such relapses may relate to premature cutback of the initial high dosage of steroid while in hospital, to prescription of an inadequate steroid dosage at discharge, or to abrupt withdrawal from steroids after hospital discharge (MacDonald et al., 1976a; Haskell et al., 1983). In patients withdrawn from steroids, the acute relapse may evolve so quickly as to preclude effective emergency intervention (Haskell et al., 1983). In one review of 30 asthma fatalities, the interval from the onset of the terminal attack to death was less than 3 hr in 90% of cases (Speizer et al., 1968). Some patients die in 30 min (MacDonald et al., 1976a; Wilson et al., 1981; Haskell et al., 1983). It is reasonable to assume that the 2:1 preponderance of home over hospital deaths that has been noted in several independent reviews of asthma mortality (Speizer et al., 1968; MacDonald et al., 1976a,b; Wilson et al., 1981; Editorial, 1983; Haskell et al., 1983) relates at least in part to this accelerated course. Furthermore, hospital deaths from asthma also tend to occur soon after admission and unexpectedly (MacDonald et al., 1976b).

Given these considerations, it is clear that the key to dealing effectively with severe asthma is prevention.

The tactics of steroid withdrawal after the resolution of a severe attack can help achieve this aim. It is our usual practice to convert to morning dose, alternate-day prednisone within a week of discharge, subsequently taper the dose to about 10-20 mg on alternate mornings depending on the expected lability of the case, and then to follow the patient for 2-4 weeks to determine the degree of asthma lability on the reduced dosage. Bronchodilators, and IS where indicated, are used as well. By the latter weeks of follow-up, it has usually become apparent in whom the prednisone can safely be stopped and in whom a continuing preventative regimen is going to be required. Recurrence of symptoms on the "off-steroid" days indicates a need for more aggressive preventive tactics. At this point the therapist is faced with the choice between an inhaled or oral steroid formulation for continuing use. Inhaled steroids (IS) will be preferred for many patients.

III. Inhaled Steroids for Chronic Asthma

The topically active IS drugs currently used to treat asthma include beclomethasone diproprionate (BDP), betamethasone valerate (BV), budesonide (BUD), triamcinolone acetonide, and flunisolide. All are effective, (McAllen et al., 1974; Toogood et al., 1977b, 1982, Grieco et al., 1978; Ellul-Micallef, 1982; Orgel et al., 1983; Nyholm et al., 1984) and to date there is no convincing evidence that any one is clinically superior to another. Budesonide has the most advantageous ratio of topical anti-inflammatory potency to systemic glucocorticoid activity (Johansson et al., 1982). Both BV and BUD are not available at this time for clinical use in America.

When an IS drug is inhaled from a pressurized metered dose inhaler (MDI), the smallest aerosolized particles penetrate to the nonciliated peripheral airways and alveoli. From here, the drug is rapidly absorbed systemically and can exert systemic effects measurable in terms of eosinopenia or reduced hypothalamic-pituitary-adrenal (HPA) function (Mygind and Hansen, 1973; Toogood et al., 1977b, 1982; Wyatt et al., 1978). The systemic glucocorticoid activity of these drugs is weak relative to their topical potency (Harris, 1975; Johansson et al., 1982) but is materially greater than the same amount of prednisolone given by mouth (Johansson et al., 1982). Thus, if a sufficiently large dosage is given, systemic activity can easily be demonstrated with any IS drug. For BDP, 100 μg/day in four divided doses has been generally adopted as a "safe cut-off," to indicate the dosage above which systemic effects on endogenous HPA function or blood eosinophil counts are demonstrable in adults with statistically significant reliability.

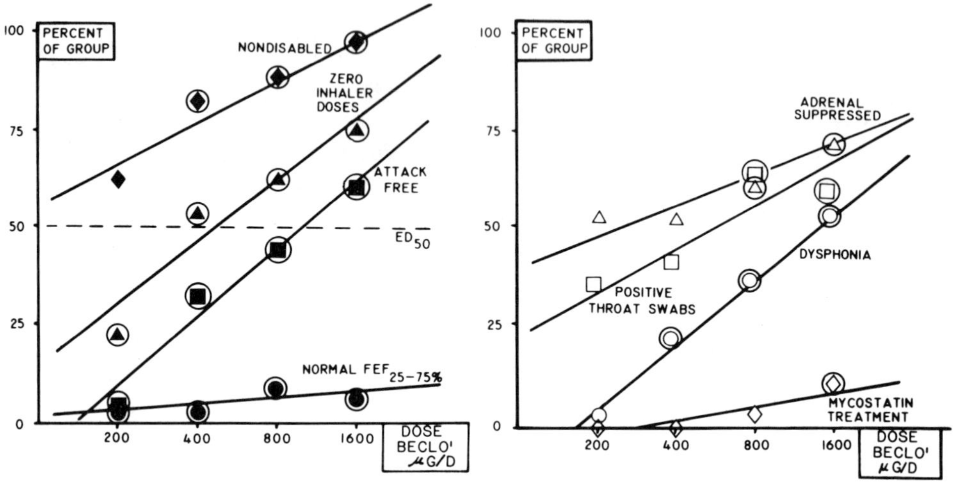

Figure 2 Response of 34 prednisone-dependent adult asthmatics to graded dosages of BDP. At each encircled point the mean change from the pre-BDP baseline value was significant ($p < 0.05$ or better). The effective BDP dose for 50% of the group (ED_{50}) may be determined by relating the intercepts of the dashed line with each regression line to the abscissa scale. The antiasthmatic effects, and the systemic and oropharyngeal complications of inhaled BDP, are all dose-dependent (adapted from J Allergy Clin Immunol 59: 298-308, 1977, Toogood et al., 1977b). The prednisone dosage was held stable in this study while the stepwise BDP increments were added as shown. Mean prednisone dosage = 11.0 mg/day. The high incidence of adrenal suppression in the group reflects their past systemic steroid therapy plus the effect of the combined oral and IS treatment.

However, the systemic activity of any particular dosage is quite variable from one patient to another because it depends on the fraction of the emitted dosage that actually reaches the lung periphery, which is the most important absorptive surface. This fraction is determined by variations in normal lung anatomy, by the presence or absence of associated chronic bronchitis and/or the severity of pulmonary functional impairment (each of which reduces peripheral delivery of the inhaled drug) (Ruffin et al., 1978; Messina and Smaldone, 1984), and especially by the inspiratory technique used (Newman et al., 1981b). Also, patients vary in their susceptibility to the systemic effects of steroid drugs because of intrinsic or acquired differences in their pharmacokinetics (Kozower et al., 1974; Gambertoglio et al., 1980). Finally, since IS and oral steroids bind to the same receptor, they exert additive glucocorticoid effects if used together (Toogood et al., 1977b; Wyatt et al., 1978).

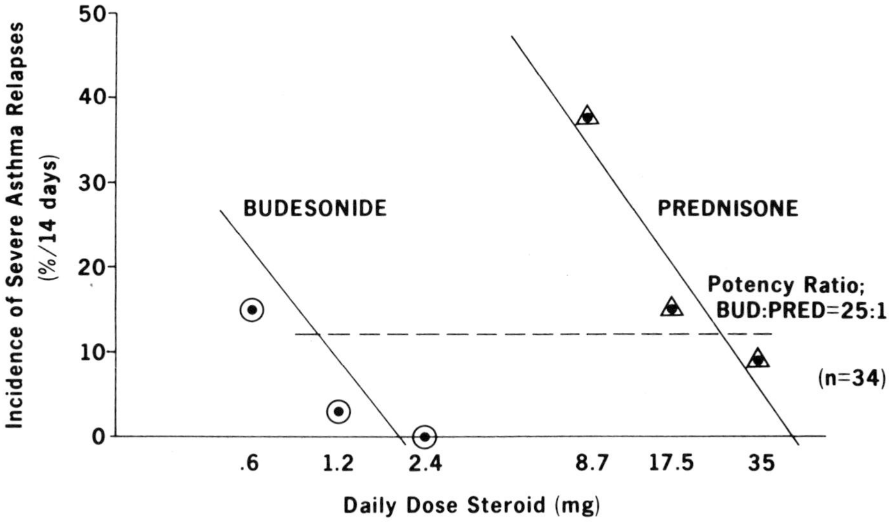

Figure 3 Incidence of disabling asthma relapses during a double-blind comparison of BUD (inhaled QID) or prednisone (single A.M. oral dose). All patients took three graduated doses of each drug, 2 weeks at each dosage level. The actual dosages prescribed varied with the patient's estimated asthma severity. The dosages shown are the group means. The data suggest that if a sufficiently large dosage is given, either oral or inhaled steroid may effectively control severe chronic asthma (Toogood et al., 1984c).

A. Effective Dosage

Both the benefits and adverse effects of IS treatment are dose-dependent, the relationship being approximately linear on log daily dose (Toogood et al., 1977b, 1982) (see Figs. 2-4). Patients vary not only in their initial responsiveness to a trial of IS (Toogood et al., 1977b) but also in their long-term dose requirements (Toogood et al., 1978). Certain patient and disease characteristics have been found to correlate significantly with the degree of responsiveness to IS treatment (Toogood et al., 1977a, 1981a, 1984b, 1985b). However, the usefulness of these variables as predictors of an individual patient's responsiveness in clinical practice is not clearly established. It seems better to rely on a trial of therapy than to restrict the use of the drug according to any particular constellation of patient or disease characteristics. For the purposes of such a trial, dosages higher than the conventionally recommended starting dosage of 400 μg BDP/day have been shown to be more efficient because (1) many patients who do not respond to a low dosage do so with a higher dosage (Toogood et al., 1977b;

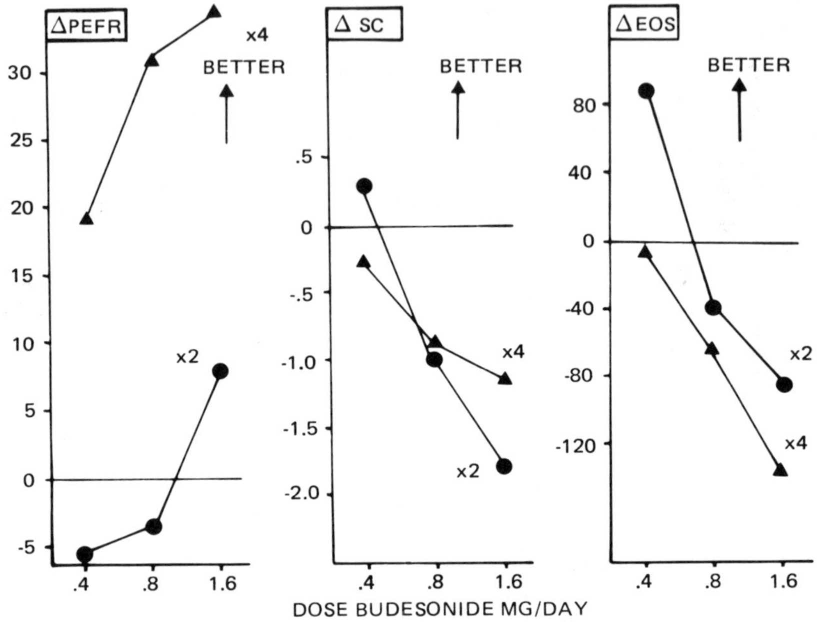

P FROM ANOVA	Δ PEFR	Δ SC	Δ EOS
DOSE	.001	.000	.000
FREQUENCY	.001	.94	.53
DOSE X FREQUENCY	.16	.40	.31

Figure 4 Influence of daily dosage and frequency on efficacy of inhaled BUD. All responses were dosage-dependent based on P values from ANOVA. Halving the dosage frequency (keeping to the same total dosage per day) had no statistically significant effect on the drug's systemic glucocorticoid potency as measured by changes in the blood eosinophils (Δ EOS) or the A.M. serum cortisol level (Δ SC), but reduced its antiasthmatic potency at least 10-fold (Δ PEFR) (P = 0.001). The difference in potency was entirely attributable to a comparison made when the asthma in these patients was clinically unstable. No difference was discernible when the same comparisons were repeated later when the asthma was stable (see Toogood et al., 1982).

Smith and Hodson, 1983); (2) high dosages give more accurately predictable results than low dosages in a trial of limited duration, such as 14 days (Toogood et al., 1977a); (3) a higher dosage is required to normalize pulmonary function than simply to control symptoms (Toogood et al., 1977b, 1983); and (4) normalization of pulmonary function is considered a more efficient goal of long-term asthma treatment than symptomatic treatment alone.

Where prednisone weaning is to be attempted under the aegis of IS therapy, clinical follow-up should continue for at least 6 months to avoid overestimating the effectiveness of the IS treatment. A review of the published experience of multiple investigators showed that after 6 months only about one-third of the prednisone-dependent asthmatics originally given IS treatment remained successfully controlled on IS treatment alone (Toogood et al., 1983). The remainder required either oral steroid alone or some combination of oral plus IS treatment. In less severe asthmatics, higher success rates with IS alone are noted.

The success rate obtainable with IS alone in severe asthmatics is determined to a large extent by the concentration of active drug in the formulations distributed commercially. The single-strength formulations now available are too weak to meet the needs of many severe asthmatics. When such patients are treated with more concentrated formulations (which makes it feasible to increase the daily dosage) the success rate with IS alone may, in fact, approximate that attainable with high-dosage oral steroid (Toogood et al., 1984c) (see Fig. 3). Concentrated formulations of BDP and Bud have recently been introduced for clinical use in Europe (Smith and Hodson, 1983; Toogood, 1983).

However, it is probably simplistic to view oral and inhaled steroids only as mutually interchangeable treatment modalities. They appear to supplement rather than substitute for each other (Toogood et al., 1984a) as evidenced by the fact that different factors determine the dosage requirements for each when they are given to the same patients in minimum effective dosages (Toogood et al., 1983, 1984a). Coexisting atopy has been found to be associated with a requirement for higher doses of BDP, but not of oral prednisone (Toogood et al., 1984a). The presence of nasal polyps and hyperplastic sinusitis is associated with a need for more BDP and more prednisone (Toogood et al., 1984a). Patients with associated chronic bronchitis also need more prednisone (but not more BDP), presumably to reduce or correct mucus plugging in the small airways and thereby ensure continuing accessibility of the inhaled drug (Toogood et al., 1984a). Among a large number of factors tested for their relative importance as determinants of the responsiveness of different patients to IS treatment. patient reliability proved to be of overriding importance (Toogood et al., 1984a). Its relationship to the long-term outcome of treatment was stronger than that of the severity of the pulmonary impairment, or the pathogenesis of the asthma (atopic vs. nonatopic). Patients with low reliability scores needed more prednisone, presumably because they comply as irregularly with the prescribed IS regimen as with other aspects of their treatment (Toogood et al., 1984a).

B. Risk vs. Benefit

The overall outcome of IS therapy in prednisone-dependent patients is generally favorable, both in patients who previously used daily prednisone and in those on alternate-morning treatment (Toogood, 1979; Toogood et al., 1978, 1984a). Both groups have been shown to experience similar degrees of symptom improvement without an increase in systemic steroid effect, but any actual improvement in HPA function may be confined to those previously dependent on daily prednisone (Toogood, 1979). Largely because of such evidence of persisting suppression of HPA function, it has been suggested that no clinically worthwhile advantage accrues from IS therapy in the more severely asthmatic patients, especially if the oral steroid cannot be completely withdrawn (Wyatt et al., 1978; Herxheimer, 1981; Vaz et al., 1982; Weinberger, 1982). However, it has been our experience that the addition of IS treatment conferred major reductions in symptom frequency and severity, in disability, and in iatrogenic risk (hypertension), and that these benefits accrued despite the fact that two-thirds of the group needed a combined oral/IS regimen to maintain optimal control of their asthma, and the overall prevalence of HPA axis functional suppression remained unchanged at about 50% of the group (Toogood et al., 1984a).

The practical importance of such persisting HPA dysfunction should not be exaggerated, since it is known that most steroid-dependent asthmatics can safely undergo severe stress, such as major surgery, even in the presence of demonstrably abnormal ACTH stimulation or insulin tolerance tests (Plumpton et al., 1969; Kehlet and Binder, 1973). Furthermore, deaths from Addisonian crisis appear remarkably rare in steroid-dependent patients, asthmatic or otherwise (Maunsell et al., 1968; Lieberman et al., 1972). Of greater concern are the risks of osteoporosis, cataract formation, and stunting of growth. Theoretically, there would appear to be no reason why any IS drug, if given in sufficient dosage, should not cause these untoward effects in a susceptible person. In practice, growth suppression has not been reported to occur in patients treated de novo with effective dosages of IS drugs (Godfrey et al., 1978; Graff-Lonnevig and Kraepelien, 1979). However existing growth suppression due to previous systemic steroid therapy may persist unchanged (Godfrey et al., 1978; Graff-Lonnevig and Kraepelien, 1979) despite an improvement in asthma severity that would have been expected to result in a spurt of "catch-up" growth. This is evident in up to 30% of some treated groups (Morris, 1985), which suggests that conventional doses of IS may act systemically to perpetuate established patterns of abnormal growth. More data are needed on the stature eventually attained at maturity by such patients. Posterior subcapsular cataracts have been reported in a few IS-treated patients, but their relationship to the IS treatment is uncertain (Rooklin et al., 1979; Kewley, 1980). The effects, if any, of IS drugs on bone, vitamin D and calcium metabolism have not been adequately studied to date.

C. Dosing Regimens

Conventionally, most IS drugs have been administered four times daily, and alternative regimens have received little study. If high dosages of BUD are used, scheduling the entire dosage for the morning has been shown to conserve HPA function (Toogood et al., 1982). However no similar sparing of the steroid-in-induced eosinopenia is evident, so it is not certain that a morning-dose schedule confers any clinically useful reduction in the risk of adverse systemic effects on extrapulmonary tissues. Also, morning dosing slightly reduces the drug's antiasthmatic potency (Toogood et al., 1982).

Opinions vary as to the ideal dosing frequency. From an overview of the published reports (Toogood, 1984), it is clear that for short periods of a few weeks to months, twice-daily treatment with IS (conserving the same daily dosage) can be equally as effective as four times daily, providing the asthma has been well stabilized beforehand by previous treatment (Toogood et al., 1982; Orgel et al., 1983; Nyholm et al., 1984; Meltzer et al., 1985). This probably applies to any of the IS drugs now in use. However, twice-daily dosing is significantly less effective than four times daily when the asthma is unstable (Toogood et al., 1982) (see Fig. 4). Thus, whenever chronic asthma enters an unstable phase, twice-daily dosing will become a major response-limiting factor that cannot be offset by large increments in daily dosage and/or by switching to a more concentrated formulation (Toogood et al., 1982; Toogood, 1983). In view of the characteristically variable course of chronic asthma, and the difficulty in accurately predicting its variations in the individual patient, it would therefore appear prudent to recommend four times daily dosing as the standard regimen. Benefit-to-cost and benefit-to-risk ratios also favor four times over three daily dosing: it has been shown that at any equivalent level of systemic glucocorticoid effect, the antiasthmatic efficacy of BUD is consistently greater if it is given four times rather than twice daily (Toogood et al., 1982). When a different approach was used in mild asthmatics, the 12-hr PEFR response to four divided doses of 100 μg of BUD was found to be equivalent to that of a single 1600 μg dose (Ellul-Micaleff and Johansson, 1983). Thus data from both short and long-term studies concur in indicating that an equivalent degree of asthma control can be achieved with lower per diem doses of BUD if more frequent dosing is used. This probably applies to the other IS drugs as well.

It has been suggested that reducing the frequency of IS treatment to twice daily may increase patient compliance and thus improve the long-term treatment outcome. Our own experience in studies during which we measured compliance objectively, has been that (1) the influence of symptom activity on IS usage overrides that of dosing frequency per se, (2) improved asthma control leads to dose omissions rather than vice versa, and (3) departures from the prescribed regimen inevitably occur, even in patients preselected for high reliability and monitored by frequent clinical follow-up (Toogood, 1985). From this we conclude that it is not necessary in ordinary clinical practice to advise patients to reduce the dose frequency of their IS drug; most will do that anyway, as symptoms remit. Instead one should inform each patient about the cost-benefit and risk-benefit advantages known to be associated with more frequent dosing of IS; counsel them to adhere to a four times daily regimen; and evaluate them to be sure that an optimal therapeutic response is sustained. If it is not, and lapses in dosing frequency are identified, the latter should be corrected.

D. Efficient Delivery

The antiasthmatic efficacy of any IS drug depends ultimately on how much gets into the lung. Under ideal conditions, about 10% of each dose emitted from the metered dose inhaler (MDI) enters the lung in well-trained, normal nonasthmatic test subjects, and about 3% may reach the distal airways (Newman et al., 1981a). Up to 80% inevitably deposits in the oropharynx where it commonly produces candidiasis or dysphonia.

Efficient intrapulmonary drug delivery requires discharge of the aerosol bolus from the MDI early in the inspiratory effort, and a slow inspiration (about 25 liters/min), followed by a 10-sec breath-holding pause (Newman et al., 1981b). A poorly coordinated inspiratory effort is common among asthmatic patients using inhaled drugs (Shim and Williams, 1980), and this can significantly reduce the effectiveness of IS treatment. Some of these problems can be corrected by attaching an extension tube (i.e., a "spacer") to the conventional MDI device. Spacers of different designs (Moren, 1978; Freigang, 1980; Corr et al., 1982) share the same operational principles. They reduce particle velocity, allow more of the propellant freons to evaporate by increasing the transit distance of the aerosol jet, and thus increase the proportion of small to large particles in the inspired bolus (Corr et al., 1982). Only the small particles of IS are wanted, since the larger particles preferentially deposit in the oropharynx or larger airways, with potentially counterproductive results.

The use of a tube or cone type spacer has been shown to reduce oropharyngeal candidiasis significantly during IS treatment (Toogood et al., 1984b), and to double the delivery of the drug to the lung in comparison to inhalation via the conventional MDI (Toogood et al., 1984b) (see Fig. 5). Efficacy increases commensurately. However, if the particular spacer device used is too small or inherently inefficient in design, excessive drug losses may occur within the device itself (Newman, 1983). The same may occur if the spacer is used incorrectly (Toogood et al., 1981b).

Patients often err by expelling more than one puff of drug at a time into the spacer, allowing more than 2 sec to elapse before starting their inspiration from the spacer, inspiring too rapidly (> 25 liters/min), or failing to hold their breath for 10 sec at the end of each deep inspiration. Together or singly these factors may lead to an unperceived reduction in the amount of drug actually reaching the lung, and insidious deterioration in asthma control (Toogood et al., 1981a).

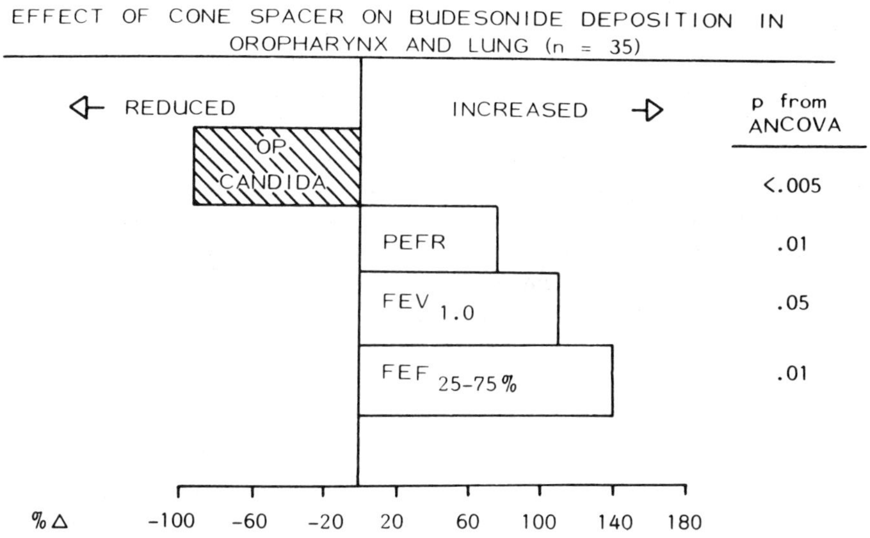

Figure 5 Effects of a spacer on BUD deposition. Inhaling BUD via a cone spacer instead of the conventional MDI reduced the oropharyngeal deposition of the drug by 94%, as reflected by change in the *Candida* colony counts, while doubling its delivery to the airways, as shown by the airflow indices (see Toogood et al., 1984b).

Patients who are reasonably adept at using the conventional MDI can improve its efficiency by using the "open mouth" technique (Dolovich et al., 1981). The MDI is held two fingerbreadths from the open mouth. As with the spacer, this lengthens the transit distance of the aerosol jet and reduces the size and velocity of the aerosolized drug particles. This diminishes particle impaction in the oropharynx and larynx and should, in theory, improve intrapulmonary delivery of the IS, as well as its penetrance to the distal airways. Unfortunately, many inept users of the MDI have difficulty mastering the open-mouth technique. For such patients, spacers often prove useful.

Spacers have been particularly recommended for use by children, but there are few data to substantiate their performance and safety in IS-treated children. In adult asthmatics, spacers slightly increase the amount of systemic absorption of IS from the lung (Toogood et al., 1984b). It is unlikely this implies a clinically important increase in the risk of adverse systemic effects (Toogood et al., 1984b), but until safety data are forthcoming from IS-treated children, it would seem prudent to reserve the use of spacers for cases in whom inefficient use of the MDI, or dysphonia, or candidiasis are compromising the effectiveness of the treatment.

Periodically, acute or subacute exacerbations of chronic asthma increase the degree of pulmonary impairment. This shifts the main site of deposition of any inhaled drug towards the larger, more central, airways. Clinically this is signalled by the advent of cough or bronchospasm triggered by each IS inhalation, in patients who had previously tolerated the drug well. The use of a spacer, and/or slowing the rate of inspiration, may improve these symptoms, but their full resolution generally requires more aggressive treatment aimed at reversing the functional impairment, such as a course of prednisone. After episodes of acute infective bronchitis, mucus plugging in small airways may persist for many weeks. Under these circumstances a course of prednisone can accelerate mucociliary clearance and restore the accessibility of the distal airways to the inhaled drug (Bateman et al., 1980).

E. Oropharyngeal and Other Local Complications

Candidiasis and dysphonia, especially the latter, are common during IS treatment (Toogood et al., 1980a). They often curtail effective dosage and lead some patients to abandon the treatment altogether. These complications are due to the active drug, rather than the freon propellants (Toogood et al., 1980a). The dysphonia is caused by a dyskinesia of the muscles that control phonation (Williams et al., 1983). Thus it is inappropriate to treat it with nystatin. It is alleviated by reducing the amount of IS deposition on and around the larynx, by reducing the daily dose, inhaling via a spacer, and /or reducing the speed of inspiration. A longer posttreatment breathhold may also help (Newman et al., 1982). Dysphonia is more common, severe, and persistent in patients with associated hypothyroidism (Toogood et al., 1980a); in those who habitually clear their throat (Toogood et al., 1980a); and in those who vocalize frequently in daily life, such as switchboard operators, sports coaches, singers, teachers, and preachers (Toogood et al., 1980a). Where such a codeterminant is present, dysphonia may persist despite all treatment measures (including complete cessation of IS treatment) until rigorous voice rest is imposed. Subsequently, the IS treatment can be resumed and is generally tolerated at the desired dosage, provided laryngeal abuse is avoided (Toogood et al., 1980a).

Oropharyngeal candidiasis, on the other hand, is due to a different set of pathogenetic determinants, including, in particular, concomitant prednisone and/or antibiotic use (Toogood et al., 1980a; Toogood et al., 1984d). The candidal overgrowth is due to inhibition by the IS drug of the normal host defense functions of T-lymphocytes, macrophages, and neutrophils at the oral mucosal surface. A 12-hr interval between doses appears long enough to allow temporary recovery of these functions, as evidenced by the fact that candidiasis is reduced and thrush virtually eliminated by giving the drug twice rather than four times daily (see Table 1). This applies to BUD and BDP (Smith and Hodson, 1983; Toogood et al., 1984d) and probably to the other IS drugs as well. Thus,

Table 1 Influence of Dose Frequency on the Incidence of Oropharyngeal Thrush During Budesonide Treatment

	Nystatin dosages/14 days (mean ± S.D.)			
	On BUD QID[a]	ON BUD BID[a]	P[b]	Patients developing clinical thrush
Prednisone-dependent (n = 19)	0.965 ± 4.58	0.07 ± 0.41	0.05	5/19
Not prednisone-dependent (n = 15)	0.166 ± 1.58	0		1/15

[a]Thirty-four asthmatics took the same daily doses of inhaled budesonide twice and four times daily, in a graded-dose crossover comparison. Eur J Resp Dis 65: 35-44, 1984; Toogood et al., 1984d.
[b]From paired t test.

a temporary switch to twice-daily dosing (keeping to the same total dosage per day) could be used preventively when the clinical circumstances are such as to increase the likelihood of thrush, for example, when antibiotics are prescribed for a patient who is already using high-dosage IS or a combined prednisone/IS regimen (Toogood et al., 1984d) (see Table 1). A better alternative in most cases however, would be a spacer, because this can accomplish the same thing without a potential reduction in antiasthmatic potency. Indeed, it usually enhances potency (Toogood et al., 1984b) (see Fig. 5).

Esophageal candidiasis is an unusual complication that also illustrates the interaction of multiple risk determinants (Stein et al., 1979): the topical immunosuppressive effect of the IS in the oropharynx and esophagus plus the additive effect of systemic steroids if these are used concomitantly; plus the candidogenic effect of frequent or prolonged antibiotic therapy; plus local damage to the integrity of the esophageal mucosa caused by acid reflux resulting from theophylline's effect on the cardiac sphincter. Hiatus hernia, when present, is an added risk factor. The problem may prove so persistent in some cases as to force the IS or theophylline or both to be discontinued. Some rare complications may occur, even with low dose IS therapy, such as the painful and protracted atrophic glossitis that sometimes complicates the prolonged use of broad-spectrum antibiotics along with topical steroid treatment (Toogood et al., 1980a); or esophagitis due to a combined *Candida*/herpes simplex infection (Hemstreet et al., 1980).

There has been no evidence by light or electron microscopy of histologic damage to the tracheobronchial epithelium or connective tissues after long-term IS use (Lundgren, 1977; Thiringer et al., 1977). The incidence of bacterial or viral respiratory infections is not increased by IS treatment (Tarlo et al., 1979;

Toogood et al., 1980a). Complicating pulmonary, bronchial, or systemic fungal infections have not been reported with long-term IS treatment, even with higher than usual dosages (Toogood et al., 1980a). Nevertheless any form of steroid therapy, oral or inhaled,ought to be avoided or used with great caution in the immunosuppressed or immunodeficient patient, because of the risks of opportunistic infection.

IV. Systemic Steroids for Chronic Asthma

Systemic steroids are preferred over IS for patients whose asthma can be satisfactorily controlled by infrequent short courses of prednisone, and for those whose asthma is already well stabilized on low-dosage alternate-day prednisone, without clinically important complications. Systemic steroids are also preferable for patients in whom poor compliance, drug costs, and/or inept use of the MDI compromise the usefulness of IS treatment; for severe asthmatics in whom a trial of IS at high dosage has proven clinically inadequate; and for patients who require continuing systemic steroid treatment for conditions other than asthma. Perhaps the most common example of the latter is nonatopic perennial hyperplastic rhinitis with recurrent nasal polyposis. Less common conditions include pulmonary infiltrates with eosinophilia (PIE syndrome), Churg-Strauss vasculitis, and allergic bronchopulmonary aspergillosis (ABPA).

In patients with ABPA, IS treatment can improve the asthma symptoms while leaving the recurrence rate of the segmental inflammatory lesions unchanged, or possibly even increased (Report 1979; Wang et al., 1979). Since it is the destructive effects of the latter, rather than the asthma, that lead to the bronchiectasis and widespread lung fibrosis characteristic of end-stage ABPA (Patterson et al., 1982), oral steroid should remain the mainstay of its long-term management (Fink, 1985). In patients with ABPA who require a prednisone dosage sufficiently large to cause significant adverse effects, supplemental bronchodilator and IS therapy should be used to facilitate reduction of the prednisone dosage and/or conversion to alternate-morning treatment. If that is achieved, subsequent assessment of the effectiveness of the new treatment regimen should be based on objective guidelines, rather than on symptoms alone. Useful data include serial chest x-rays, pulmonary function tests, sputum cultures, total serum IgE levels, specific IgG *Aspergillus* antibody titer, and blood eosinophil counts (Patterson et al., 1982). Monitoring is advisable because IS treatment may actually increase the *Aspergillus* content of the sputum in some cases (Turner-Warwick et al., 1975).

Intermittent short courses of systemic steroid are generally well tolerated: after 3 weeks' treatment with 20-mg prednisolone twice daily, endogenous cortisol production returns to normal within 3 days of stopping the drug (Webb and Clark, 1981). Furthermore, during the 3-day recovery period, the responsiveness of the HPA axis to stress remains prompt, albeit slightly reduced in magnitude (Streck and Lockwood, 1979). Growth retardation is negligible in patients who use systemic steroids infrequently (up to 3 weeks/year); slight to moderate if treatment is more frequent (4-12 weeks/year); and it only becomes significantly different from the growth of matched normal controls if steroids are used regularly (Chang et al., 1982).

If it is clinically necessary to use oral steroids regularly, endogenous HPA function is better conserved and hypercortisonism minimized if a rapidly metabolized drug such as prednisone or prednisolone is used and the entire daily dose is administered in the morning, (Myles et al., 1971; Huner and Allen, 1975) and the dosage is not too high (Huner and Allen, 1975). Conversion to alternate-morning prednisone treatment further decreases iatrogenic risks (Huner and Allen, 1975; Reimer et al., 1975; Weinberger, 1982). However, patients who need high doses daily may not be able to convert to alternate-morning treatment, because of its lesser efficacy (Huner and Allen, 1975). Even if they do, if the dosage remains high, established adverse effects such as impaired growth do not necessarily improve (Reimer et al., 1975). Indeed, there is conflicting evidence as to whether growth rates are faster or osteoporotic complications fewer on alternate-day than on daily prednisone, (Morris, 1975; Gluck et al., 1981; Chang et al., 1982; Adinoff and Hollister, 1983), despite the apparent advantages of the former regimen in terms of better intestinal calcium absorption (Klein et al., 1977) and less florid Cushingoid stigmata such as obesity and bruising (Huner and Allen, 1975; Weinberger, 1982). Adding IS treatment allows most patients on daily oral steroid to convert successfully to alternate day or intermittent usage (Toogood et al., 1978). Typically, this is followed by measurable improvement in HPA axis function, a reduction in the overt signs of hypercortisonism, and an accompanying improvement in asthma control (Toogood et al., 1978; Toogood, 1979).

Efforts to withdraw systemic steroids totally should not be unduly aggressive or persistent, since some asthmatic patients are at risk of sudden death if their oral steroid is stopped (Maunsell et al., 1968). We found the incidence of asthma relapse complicating attempted prednisone withdrawal during high dose BDP treatment to be higher in patients with associated nasal polyposis, ASA intolerance, chronic bronchitis, a previous need for more than one dose of prednisone per day, and a record of poor compliance with previous treatment (Toogood et al., 1984a). Tests of HPA function proved unreliable as predictors of the likelihood of asthma relapse in these patients (Toogood et al., 1984a). Nor have other investigators found such tests useful as predictors of the deaths that have occasionally complicated prednisone withdrawal under the aegis of IS treatment (Mellis and Phelan, 1977). Asthma relapse is the primary problem, and frequent follow-up is the only way to contain this risk. Follow-up should continue for an extended period of time because severe asthma relapse may occur as late as 4-8 months after withdrawal from regular oral steroid therapy (Maunsell et al., 1968; Mellis and Phelan, 1977).

Where close clinical surveillance is maintained, it is possible in some patients to prevent exacerbations of severe asthma because their occurrence is heralded by a gradual deterioration in pulmonary function progressing over days, weeks, or even months (Lal et al., 1972; Davis et al., 1980; Toogood, 1984). Intervention with a burst of systemic steroid can stem the decline and prevent or rapidly reverse the acute attack.

In patients whose asthma cannot be controlled on alternate-morning prednisone despite increasing the dosage and adding four-times-daily IS in high dosage, and in whom poor compliance with the treatment plan can be excluded, and who show no overt signs of hypercortisonism, a "fast metabolizer" state may reasonably be assumed. Differences in steroid pharmacokinetics are known to account for the low susceptibility of some subjects to the systemic effects of steroid treatment (Kozower et al., 1974; Gambertoglio et al., 1980). Faced with such a problem, a first step should be to discontinue, if possible, any concomitantly used drugs that accelerate steroid metabolism, such as phenobarbital or phenytoin (Brooks et al., 1972; Stjernholm and Katz, 1975). The options with regard to the steroid are: (1) Increase the daily dosage of prednisone and convert to a divided dose regimen to control the asthma; then gradually reduce the dosing frequency (maintaining the same dosage per day) to determine the lowest frequency needed to maintain satisfactory asthma control; or (1) substitute a more slowly metabolized steroid such as dexamethasone given once or twice daily; or (3) try the combination of daily methylprednisolone with troleandomycin (TAO). This macrolide antibiotic is ineffective for the treatment of asthma when used alone (Spector et al., 1974) and it has no effect on the glucocorticoid recepter per se (Engler et al., 1985), but it alters the pharmacokinetics of methylprednisolone to prolong its half life and mean residence time (Szefler et al., 1982). This increases both its antiasthmatic and systemic potencies (Zeiger et al., 1980; Harris and German, 1985). The interaction is specific for methylprednisolone: it does not occur with prednisone or prednisolone. TAO also impairs theophylline clearance (Weinberger et al., 1977) and as little as 250 mg daily may lead inadvertently to serious theophylline toxicity despite frequent monitoring of blood levels (J. H. Toogood, unpublished studies). TAO is also potentially hepatotoxic. This effect is dosage-related and reversible (Dasgupta and Marcoux, 1978). Recently, erythromycin base has been found to show the same potentiating activity on methylprednisolone as TAO (LaForce et al., 1982). Trials of the clinical value and safety of this less toxic combination are needed.

Some patients' conditions cannot be satisfactorily controlled despite daily prednisone treatment (single morning dose), plus IS therapy in moderate to high dosage, plus aggressive bronchodilator treatment. Some of these refractory patients improve if their treatment is shifted to divided dose daily prednisone. However, a few remain resistant to oral prednisone. This resistance cannot be explained on the basis of differences in steroid pharmacokinetics since prednisolone binding, distribution, and clearance have been found to be normal in such patients (Rose et al., 1980, 1981). The degree of resistance may fluctuate over time (Rose et al., 1980) so the process appears at least partly reversible. The mechanism(s) may relate to differences in the pathogenesis of the asthma (Rose et al., 1980), or in the numbers or functional integrity of steroid receptors (Rose et al., 1981). Down regulation of glucocorticoid receptors does occur in response to steroid treatment (Engler et al., 1985) but its clinical importance, if any, with respect to "steroid resistance" is unknown. Another theoretic possibility is the formation of auto- or anti-idiotypic antibodies with specificities directed against regulatory proteins such as lipomodulin (Hirata et al., 1981) or against the β-adrenergic receptor (Blecher et al., 1984). A particular subset of refractory asthmatics includes women whose asthma severity fluctuates with their menstrual cycle, becoming resistant to steroid and bronchodilator treatment during each premenstrual phase. The mechanism is obscure, but clinical benefit has been reported from inhibiting the endogenous production of pituitary gonadotropins (Pride and Yuen, 1984). Finally, behavioral factors must not be overlooked. These may bias the physician's assessment of some patients' responsiveness to treatment, and inflate the perceived need for steroid (Kinsman et al., 1977).

V. Therapeutic Options in Clinical Practice

In formulating a treatment plan for the individual patient, it is important to consider both the bronchospastic and inflammatory aspects of asthma. As a general rule, bronchodilators should be tried, with or without cromolyn, prior to long-term steroid therapy. Also an allergy assessment should be carried out. It is important that the latter not be overlooked because allergen avoidance alone can achieve clinically valuable reductions in symptom severity and in NSAR, as well as a major reduction in drug requirements (Murray and Ferguson, 1982, 1983).

For the stable moderate asthmatic who needs steroid treatment, IS is preferred over alternate-day systemic steroid, except for the special cases previously discussed above. If systemic steroids are needed, they should be used according to the following guideline: corticosteroids are the last drug to be added and the first to be discontinued. However, this caveat is less appropriate in the case of IS therapy. This is evidenced by an increasing trend toward administering IS as a "second-line" drug to patients with mild asthma (Crompton, 1983). In these circumstances, the IS is used not as an alternative to systemic steroid, but as an alternative to oral theophylline to supplement inhaled β-

Table 2 Prednisone-Budesonide Dose Equivalents: Equipotent Dosages of Prednisone Determined For Four Different Response Indices

Budesonide dosage/(mg/day)	FEV1[a]	Asthma severity[b]	Blood eosinophils[a]	Serum cortisol[a]
0.4	27.0	10.5	3.7	< 1.0
1.0	55.0	22.0	6.2	4.2
2.0	94.0	52.0	11.0	14.5

[a]Measured every 14 days at 8 A.M.
[b]A subjective symptom severity score recorded daily by patients using an analog scale (n = 17).

adrenergic therapy. The rationale is to achieve an improved level of asthma control, coupled with a reduced incidence of drug toxicity. The absence of any major adverse effects with low-dosage IS therapy (now documented by more than 8 million patient-years of clinical experience) contrasts with the morbidity and mortality known to be associated with theophylline (Woodcock et al., 1983), and the less serious adverse effects that limit the usefulness of oral β-adrenergics in some subjects (Gluckman, 1974; Committee on Drugs, 1985). There is a need for controlled studies to document the long-term efficiency of these competing treatment regimens in patients with mild asthma. It has also been suggested that the regular use of IS might diminish the likelihood of mild asthmatics progressing to develop nonreversible airflow limitation as a complication of chronic asthma (Bleecker, 1985). This hypothesis is based on (1) the observed association between increased NSAR and an accelerated rate of progression of chronic airflow limitation (Britt et al., 1980) and (2) the ability of steroid treatment, either oral or inhaled, to improve NSAR (Cockcroft et al., 1977; Israel et al., 1984; Bleecker, 1985). As yet, this hypothesis has not been subjected to critical evaluation, but it may lead to valuable new therapeutic insights.

At the other extreme of the clinical spectrum, it has been shown recently that some severe asthmatics who would appear to be permanently dependent on oral steroid to control their disease, can achieve a more favorable balance of symptom control vs. systemic steroid activity if switched to high-dosage IS therapy, using a concentrated formulation (Toogood et al., 1984c). This is illustrated by the data in Table 2.

These data derive from a double-blind, graded-dosage, crossover comparison of oral prednisone (single AM dose) vs. inhaled BUD (divided into four doses), which was designed to determine the exact dosage of each drug needed to achieve the same level of clinical response (Toogood et al., 1984c). In this particular group of adult asthmatics it was found that 2.0 mg BUD/day was needed to reduce the incidence of severe asthma relapses to zero (see also Fig. 3). Such a dosage was found to exert systemic effects equivalent to those produced by ~ 11-14 mg prednisone per day (Table 2). But a much higher dosage of prednisone was required to achieve an antiasthmatic response equal to that of 2.0 mg BUD/day (see Table 2). Indeed it is evident from the data in Table 2 that regardless of the dose of BUD used, and whether or not it exerts any "statistically significant" systemic glucocorticoid effect, its systemic activity is consistently less than that of oral prednisone if the two regimens are compared at equivalent levels of antiasthmatic efficacy. (Incidentally, it can also be seen from Table 2 that the relative potency of an inhaled IS vs. oral prednisone varies markedly depending on which index is used to measure the treatment response.)

Aside from the patient with frank asthma, a substantial number of patients who may be considered to have COPD on the basis of persisting symptoms and airflow limitation despite full bronchodilator therapy derive significant benefit from steroid treatment (Mandella et al., 1982; Blair and Light, 1984). A trial of therapy is the most reliable way to identify such patients since it is difficult to predict accurately their responsiveness from clinical data alone (Blair and Light, 1984). In particular, the failure of FEV_1 to improve with a bronchodilator, either inhaled or injected, does not preclude the possibility of a significant airflow improvement with steroid treatment (Blair and Light, 1984). This applies not only with oral, but also with inhaled steroids (see Fig. 6). In monitoring the response to such a therapeutic trial, it is useful to measure more than the airflow indices. Some patients report major improvement in symptoms and disability with high-dosage prednisone despite negligible changes in their airflow. This could be interpreted as nonspecific "steroid euphoria" if one were not aware of the concomitant improvements occurring in arterial oxygen tension, residual volume, and pulmonary diffusing capacity, changes that reflect improved small-airways function and lung mechanics, reduced hyperinflation, and symptomatic relief (Williams and McGavin, 1980; Blair and Light, 1984). Similarly, infantile bronchiolitis that is unresponsive to bronchodilators may respond well to nebulized BDP (Maayan et al., 1985).

The question of ambulant asthmatic patients "abusing" their bronchodilator inhalant merits special attention. The increasingly frequent use of the MDI signals in most cases a major deterioration in ventilatory function, due to β-adrenergic tachyphylaxis and/or an increasing inflammatory component to their diffuse airways obstruction. As the degree of ventilatory impairment increases, the efficiency of intrapulmonary delivery of the inhaled drug progressively falls, with the result that the patient has no alternative but to resort to more frequent use to try to compensate for the diminished effect of each dose. Warnings about the dangers of "inhaler abuse" are futile and inappropriate in

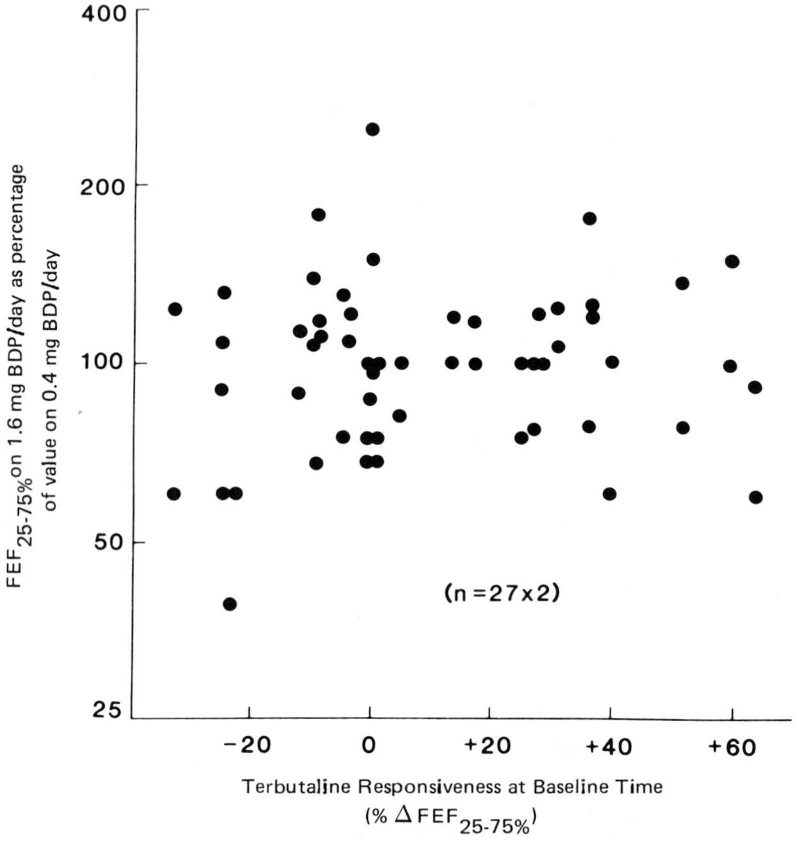

Figure 6 Responsiveness to inhaled steroid vs. bronchodilator "reversibility" of airflow limitation. $FEF_{25-75\%}$ doubled on the average, when the BDP dosage was increased from 0.4 to 1.6 mg/day. The degree of responsiveness of individual patients to the BDP was unpredictable from their response to 0.25 mg terbutaline subcutaneously. The latter was measured immediately prior to commencing the higher dosage of BDP (unpublished data from Toogood et al., 1981b).

these circumstances. What is urgently needed is an alternative form of treatment, namely systemic steroids. Restoration of the airways' responsiveness to adrenergics may begin within an hour of commencing the steroid (Ellul-Micallef and Fenech, 1975) although the widespread mucus plugging of small airways may take a week or more to fully resolve (Toogood, 1984). As control of the asthma is reestablished, the so-called "inhaler abuse" disappears spontaneously. Patients who have experienced such relapses should be put on a preventive steroid regimen and/or given a home supply of prednisone, along with written instructions outlining the indications for its use, and the details of dosage.

The advent of nocturnal asthma attacks in a previously well-controlled patient is another indication of deteriorating asthma control (Westerman et al., 1979; Editorial, 1983). These attacks may be viewed as an exaggeration of the normal circadian fluctuation in flow rates that may relate to variations in endogenous catecholamine output (Barnes et al., 1980) or in β-receptor functional activity (Reinhardt et al., 1980). They signal a need for more aggressive adrenergic treatment (Ayres et al., 1984) or supplemental treatment with oral or inhaled steroid (Horn et al., 1984) and/or sustained action theophylline (Barnes et al., 1982). If the nocturnal attacks fail to resolve fully, or recur repeatedly, adding cromolyn may prove helpful. In such severe and refractory cases, we generally administer the cromolyn as the nebulized solution.

Most patients whose chronic asthma is severe enough to require regular steroid treatment, are best treated with a combination of drugs. These are chosen to cover both the inflammatory and bronchospastic components of the disease, and to complement one another tactically. For example, one useful regimen would be daily theophylline and/or IS to provide a preventative first line of defense, plus an inhaled adrenergic as needed to deal with breakthrough symptoms, backed up by oral prednisone to be used in the event of a major symptom breakthrough. If high dosages of steroid are regularly required, either oral or inhaled, cotreatment with theophylline confers additive benefit that may permit optimal asthma control at a lower steroid dosage (Nassif et al., 1981). However, the adverse effects of theophylline sometimes offset any advantage from the combination (Appel, 1984). Adrenergic bronchodilators also give additive benefit (Clark and Anderson, 1978), but it is questionable whether routinely preceding each IS treatment with an inhalation of adrenergic bronchodilator materially improves intrapulmonary delivery of the IS drug. At least, the few studies that have examined the question have so far been unable to demonstrate any potentiation of the IS response (MacKay and Dyson, 1981; Muers and Dawkins, 1983; Toogood et al., 1984b). The available evidence suggests this objective can be better accomplished (at less cost to the patient) by using a spacer and training the patient to apply the principles of efficient inhalation technique (Toogood et al., 1984b).

Finally, it should be recognized that experienced physicians commonly use a "problem-solving" approach to decision making in practice. This expedites the clinical response, and is more versatile than step-by-step adherence to a hierarchic ranking of drug choices as "first-line, second-line," and so forth. The aim is to tailor a treatment plan appropriate to the different determinants of each individual patient, to their immediate and anticipated clinical needs and tolerances, lifestyle and age, and social and economic circumstances, and then to adapt the plan as needed to meet the changing exigencies of this characteristically variable disease.

Acknowledgments

The author is grateful for the expert assistance of J. Tasker in preparing the manuscript. Research support for clinical studies discussed in this chapter was provided by AB Draco, Sweden, Astra Pharmaceuticals Ltd., Canada, Fisons Corporation, Massachusetts, Medical Associates of Victoria Hospital Research Fund, Ontario Respiratory Diseases Foundation, Schering Corporation, Canada, and the Syntex Corporation, California.

The author is also grateful for the collaboration and support of Barbara Jennings, B.Sc., Jon Baskerville, Ph.D., N. M. Lefcoe, M.D., and the patients who voluntarily contributed many hours to these studies. Non sibi, sed omnibus.

References

Adinoff, A. D., and Hollister, J. R. (1983). Steroid-induced fracture and bone loss in patients with asthma. *N. Engl. J. Med. 309*: 265-268.

Ahrens, R. C., Bonham, A. C., Maxwell, G. A., and Weinberger, M. M. (1984). A method for comparing the peak intensity and duration of action of aerosolized bronchodilators using bronchoprovocation with methacholine. *Am. Rev. Respir. Dis. 129*: 903-906.

Appel, D. W. (1984). Effect of aminophylline when added to metaproterenol sulfate and beclomethasone dipropionate aerosol. *J. Allergy Clin. Immunol. 73(2)*: 291-297.

Arnaud, A., Vervloet, D., Dugue, P., Orehek, J., and Charpin, J. (1979). Treatment of acute asthma; effect of intravenous corticosteroids and beta-2 adrenergic agonists. *Lung 156*: 43-48.

Ayres, J., Fish, D. R., Wheller, D. C., Wiggins, J., Cochrane, G. M., and Skinner, C. (1984). Subcutaneous terbutaline and control of brittle asthma or appreciable morning dipping. *Br. Med. J. 288*: 1715-1716.

Ballard, P. L. (1979). Delivery and transport of glucocorticoids to target cells. *Monogr. Endocrinol. 12*: 25, 1979.

Barnes, P., Fitzgerald, G., Brown, M., and Dollery, C. (1980). Nocturnal asthma and changes in circulating epinephrine, histamine, and cortisol. *N. Engl. J. Med. 303*: 263-267.

Barnes, P. J., Greening, A. P., Neville, L., Timmers, J., and Poole, G. W. (1982). Single-dose slow-release aminophylline at night prevents nocturnal asthma. *Lancet 1*: 299-301.

Bateman, J. R. M., Agnew, J. E., Sheahan, N. F., Pavia, D., and Clarke, S. W. (1980). Tracheobronchial clearance and ventilatory function after medium dose oral corticosteroid therapy in stable asthmatics. *Progr. Respir. Res. 14*: 145-149.

Blackwell, G. J., Carnuccio, R., Di Rosa, M., Flower, R. J., Parente, L., and Persico, P. (1980). Macrocortin: A polypeptide causing the antiphospholipase effect of glucocorticoids. *Nature 287*: 147-149.

Blair, G. P., and Light, R. W. (1984). Treatment of chronic obstructive pulmonary disease with corticosteroids. Comparison of daily vs. alternate-day therapy. *Chest 86*: 524-528.

Blecher, M., Lewis, S., Hicks, J. M., and Josephs, S. (1984). Beta-blocking autoantibodies in pediatric bronchial asthma. *J. Allergy Clin. Immunol. 74*: 246-251.

Bleecker, E. R. (1985). Airways reactivity and asthma: significance and treatment. *J. Allergy Clin. Immunol. 75*: 21-24.

Bocanegra, T. S., Castaneda, M. O., Espinoza, L. R., Vasey, F. B., and Germain, B. F. (1981). Sudden death after methylprednisolone pulse therapy. *Ann. Intern. Med. 95*: 122.

Boggs, D. R., Athens, J. W., Cartwright, G. E., and Wintrobe, M. M. (1964). The effect of adrenal glucocorticosteroids upon the cellular composition of inflammatory exudates. *Am. J. Pathol. 44*: 763-773.

Booij-Noord, H., de Vries, K., Sluiter, H. J., and Orie, N. G. M. (1972). Late bronchial obstructive reaction to experimental inhalation of house dust extract. *Clin. Allergy 2*: 43-61.

Braude, A. C., and Rebuck, A. S. (1982). Pulmonary disposition of cortisol. *Ann. Intern. Med. 97*: 59-60.

Braude, A. C., and Rebuck, A. S. (1983). Prednisone and methylprednisolone disposition in the lung. *Lancet 2*: 995-997.

Britt, E. B., Cohen, B., Menkes, H., Bleecker, E., Permutt, S., Rosenthal, R., and Norman, P. (1980). Airways reactivity and functional deterioration in relatives of COPD patients. *Chest 77*: 260.

Britton, M. G., Collins, J. V., Brown, D., Fairhurst, N. P. A., and Lambert, R. G. (1976). High-dose corticosteroids in severe acute asthma. *Br. Med. J. 2*: 73-74.

Brooks, S. M., Werk, E. E., Ackerman, S. J., Sullivan, I., and Thrasher, K. (1972). Adverse effects of phenobarbital on corticosteroid metabolism in patients with bronchial asthma. *N. Engl. J. Med. 286*: 1125-1128.

Burge, P. S., Efthimiou, J., Turner-Warwick, M., and Nelmes, P. T. J. (1982). Double-blind trials of inhaled beclomethasone dipropionate and fluocortin butyl ester in allergen-induced immediate and late asthmatic reactions. *Clin. Allergy 12*: 523-531.

Busse, W. W., Anderson, C. L., and Cooper, W. (1981). Cortisol protection of the granulocyte response to isoproterenol during an in vitro influenza virus incubation. *J. Allergy Clin. Immunol. 67*: 78-84.

Carroll, M. P., Durham, S. R., Walsh, G., and Kay, A. B. (1985). Activation of neutrophils and monocytes after allergen and histamine-induced bronchoconstriction. *J. Allergy Clin. Immunol. 75*: 290-296.

Chang, K. C., Miklich, D. R., Barwise, G., Chai, H., and Miles-Lawrence, R. (1982). Linear growth of chronic asthmatic children: The effects of the disease and various forms of steroid therapy. *Clin. Allergy 12*: 369-378.

Chiang, J., Patterson, R., McGillen, J. J., Phair, J. P., Roberts, M., Harris, K. E., and Reising, K. S. (1980). Long-term corticosteroid effect on lymphocyte and polymorphonuclear cell function in asthmatics. *J. Allergy Clin. Immunol. 65*: 263-268.

Clark, R. A., and Anderson, P. B. (1978). Combined therapy with salbutamol and beclomethasone inhalers in chronic asthma. *Lancet 2*: 70-72.

Clissold, S. P., and Heel, R. C. (1984). Budesonide: A preliminary review of its pharmacodynamic properties and therapeutic efficacy in asthma and rhinitis. *Drugs 28*: 485-518.

Cockcroft, D. W., Ruffin, R. E., Dolovich, J., and Hargreave, F. E. (1977). Allergen-induced increase in non-allergic bronchial reactivity. *Clin. Allergy 7*: 503-513.

Collins, J. V., Clark, T. J. H., Brown, D., and Townsend, J. (1975). The use of corticosteroids in the treatment of acute asthma. *Q. J. Med. 44*: 259-273.

Committee on Drugs, The American Academy of Allergy and Immunology, Sly, R. M. (Chairman). (1985). Adverse effects and complications of treatment with beta-adrenergic agonist drugs. *J. Allergy Clin. Immunol. 75*: 443-449.

Corr, D., Dolovich, M., McCormack, D., Ruffin, R., Obminski, G., and Newhouse, M. (1982). Design and characteristics of a portable breath actuated, particle size selective medical aerosol inhaler. *J. Aerosol. Sci. 13*: 1-7.

Crompton, G. K. (1983). The use of inhaled steroids in the management of asthma. In *Steroids in Asthma.* Edited by T. J. H. Clark. Auckland, NZ, ADIS Press, pp. 166-192.

Cupps, T. R., and Fauci, A. S. (1982). Corticosteroid-mediated immunoregulation in man. *Immunol. Rev. 65*: 133-155.

Dahl, R., and Johansson, S-A. (1982). Importance of duration of treatment with inhaled budesonide on the immediate and late bronchial reaction. *Eur. J. Respir. Dis. 63*: Suppl. 122, 167-175.

Dasgupta, A., and Marcoux, J. P. (1978). Hepatic abnormalities associated with long-term use of troleandomycin in asthma: A case report. *Ann. Allergy 41*: 297.

Davies, A. O., and Lefkowitz, R. J. (1981). Agonist promoted high affinity state of the beta-adrenergic receptor in human neutrophils: Modulation by corticosteroids. *J. Clin. Endocrinol. Metab. 53*: 703-708.

Davis, B., Gett, P. M., and Sherwood Jones, E. (1980). A service for the adult asthmatic. *Thorax 35*: 111-113.

De Monchy, J. G. R., Kauffman, H. F., Venge, P., Koeter, G. H., Jansen, H. M., Sluiter, H. J., and De Vries, K. (1985). Bronchoalveolar eosinophilia during allergen-induced late asthmatic reactions. *Am. Rev. Respir. Dis. 131*: 373-376.

Delehunt, J. C., Perruchoud, A. P., Yerger, L., Marchette, B., Stevenson, J. S., and Abraham, W. M. (1984a). The role of slow-reacting substance of anaphylaxis in the late bronchial response after antigen challenge in allergic sheep. *Am. Rev. Respir. Dis. 130*: 748-754.

Delehunt, J. C., Yerger, L., Ahmen, T., and Abraham, W. M. (1984b). Inhibition of antigen-induced bronchoconstriction by methylprednisolone succinate. *J. Allergy Clin. Immunol. 73*: 479-483.

Dolovich, M., Ruffin, R. E., Roberts, R., and Newhouse, M. T. (1981). Optimal delivery of aerosols from metered dose inhalers. *Chest 80*: 911-915.

Durham, S. R., Lee, T. H., Cromwell, O., Shaw, R. J., Merrett, T. G., Merrett, J., Cooper, P., and Kay, A. B. (1984). Immunologic studies in allergen-induced late-phase asthmatic reactions. *J. Allergy Clin. Immunol. 74*: 49-60.

Editorial. (1983). Asthma at night. *Lancet 1*: 220-222.

Elegbeleye, O. O., Williams, K. O., and Femi-Pearse, D. (1978). Comparison of the metabolic effects of salbutamol administered in a one-minute bolus and a continuous infusion in patients with bronchial asthma. *Isr. J. Med. Sci. 14*: 455-458.

Ellul-Micallef, R. (1982). The acute effects of corticosteroids in bronchial asthma. *Eur. J. Respir. Dis. 63*: suppl. 122: 118-122.

Ellul-Micallef, R., and Fenech, F. F. (1975). Effect of intravenous prednisolone in asthmatics with diminished adrenergic responsiveness. *Lancet 2*: 1269-1270.

Ellul-Micallef, R., and Johansson, S-A. (1983). Dose frequency in chronic bronchial asthma with a new corticosteroid: budesonide. In *Evaluation of Budesonide–A New Glucocorticoid for Local Treatment of Bronchial Asthma.* S-A. Johansson. Doctoral thesis, Lund University, Lund, Sweden.

Ellul-Micallef, R., Borthwick, R. C., and McHardy, G. J. R. (1980). The effect of oral prednisolone on gas exchange in chronic bronchial asthma. *Br. J. Clin. Pharmacol. 9*: 479-482.

Engler, R. J. M., Chestnut, R. Y., Borst, G. C., and Eil, C. (1985). The effects of triacetyloleandomycin and oleandomycin phosphate on the glucocorticoid receptor in cultured skin fibroblasts. *J. Allergy Clin. Immunol. 75*: 395-400.

Fanta, C. H., Tossing, T. H., and McFadden, E. R., Jr. (1983). Glucocorticoids in acute asthma. A critical controlled trial. *Am. J. Med. 74*: 845-851.

Fiel, S. B., Swartz, M. A., Glanz, K., and Francis, M. E. (1983). Efficacy of short-term corticosteroid therapy in outpatient treatment of acute bronchial asthma. *Am. J. Med. 75*: 259-262.

Fink, J. N. (1985). Allergic bronchopulmonary aspergillosis. *Chest 87*: 81S-84S.

Foster, P. S., Goldie, R. G., and Peterson, J. W. (1983). Effect of steroids on beta-adrenoceptor-mediated relaxation of pig bronchus. *Br. J. Pharmacol. 78*: 441-445.

Freigang, B. (1980). Long-term follow-up of infants and children treated with beclomethasone aerosol by a special inhalation device. *Ann. Allergy 45*: 13-17.

Gambertoglio, J. G., Vincenti, F., Feduska, N. J., Birnbaum, I., Salvatierra, O., and Amend, W. J. C. (1980). Prednisolone disposition in Cushingoid and noncushingoid kidney transplant patients. *J. Clin. Endocrinol. Metab. 51*: 561-565.

Geddes, B. A., Jones, T. R., Dvorsky, R. J., and Lefcoe, N. M. (1974). Interactions of glucocorticoids and bronchodilators on isolated guinea pig tracheal and human bronchial smooth muscle. *Am. Rev. Respir. Dis. 110*: 420-427.

Gleich, G. J., Loegering, D. A., and Adolphson, C. R. (1985). Eosinophils and bronchial inflammation. *Chest 87*: 10S-13S.

Gluck, O. S., Murphy, W. A., Hahn, T. J., and Hahn, B. (1981). Bone loss in adults receiving alternate day glucocorticoid therapy. *Arthritis Rheum. 24*: 892-898.

Gluckman, L. (1974). Ventolin psychosis. *N.Z. Med. J. 80*: 411.

Godfrey, S., Balfour-Lynn, L., and Tooley, M. (1978). A three to five year follow-up of the use of the aerosol steroid beclomethasone dipropionate, in childhood asthma. *J. Allergy Clin. Immunol. 62*: 335-339.

Graff-Lonnevig, V., and Kraepelien, S. (1979). Long-term treatment with beclomethasone dipropionate aerosol in asthmatic children with special reference to growth. *Allergy 34*: 57.

Greaves, M. W., and Plummer, V. M. (1974). Glucocorticoid inhibition of antigen-evoked histamine release from human skin. *Immunology 27*: 359-364.

Grieco, M. H., Dwek, J., Larsen, K., and Rammohan, G. (1978). Clinical effect of aerosol triamcinolone acetonide in bronchial asthma. *Arch. Intern. Med. 138*: 1337-1341.

Harris, D. M. (1975). Some properties of beclomethasone dipropionate and related steroids in man. *Postgrad. Med. J. 51*: Supp. 4: 20-25.

Harris, R., and German, D. (1985). The incidence of corticosteroid side effects in chronic steroid dependent asthmatics on TAO (Troleandomycin) and methylprednisolone. *J. Allergy Clin. Immunol. 75*: 157.

Haskell, R. J., Wong, B. M., and Hansen, J. E. (1983). A double-blind randomized clinical trial of methylprednisolone in status asthmaticus. *Arch. Intern. Med. 143*: 1324-1327.

Hemstreet, M. P., Reynolds, D. W., and Meadows, J., Jr. (1980). Oesophagitis —a complication of inhaled steroid therapy. *Clin. Allergy 10*: 733-738.

Herxheimer, H. (1981). Should corticosteroid aerosols be used in severe chronic asthma? *Thorax 36*: 401-403.

Hirata, F., Schiffmann, E., Venkatasubramanian, K., Salomon, D., and Axelrod, J. (1980). A phospholipase A2 inhibitory protein in rabbit neutrophils induced by glucocorticoids. *Proc. Natl. Acad. Sci. USA, 77*: 2533-2536.

Hirata, F., del Carmine, R., Nelson, C. A., Axelrod, J., Schiffmann, E., Warabi, A., DeBlas, A. L., Nirenberg, M., Manganiello, V., Vaughan, M., Kumagai, S., Green, I., and Decker, J. L. (1981). Presence of autoantibody for phospholipase inhibitory protein, lipomodulin, in patients with rheumatic diseases. *Proc. Natl. Acad. Sci. USA 78*: 3190-3194.

Horn, C. R., Clark, T. J. H., and Cochrane, C. M. (1984). Inhaled therapy reduces morning dips in asthma. *Lancet 1*: 1143-1145.

Huner, G. G., and Allen, G. L. (1975). Daily and alternate day corticosteroid regimens in treatment of giant cell arteritis. *Ann. Intern. Med. 82*: 613-618.

Israel, R. H., Poe, R. H., Wicks, C. M., Greenblatt, D. W., and Kallay, M. C. (1984). The protective effect of methylprednisolone on carbachol-induced bronchospasm. *Am. Rev. Respir. Dis. 130*: 1019-1022.

Jeffrey, J. L., and Avner, B. P. (1980). Blockade of uptake 2: The mechanism of rapid corticosteroid induced potentiation of bronchodilator drugs in tracheal smooth muscle. *Proc. West. Pharmacol. Soc. 23*: 355.

Johansson, S-A., Anderson, K. E., Brattsand, R., Gruvstad, E., Hedner, P. (1982). Topical and systemic glucocorticoid potencies of budesonide and beclomethasone dipropionate in man. *Eur. J. Respir. Dis. 63*: suppl. 122: 74-82.

Kaliner, M. (1985). Mast cell mediators and asthma. *Chest 87*: 2S-5S.

Kattan, M., Gurwitz, D., and Levison, H. (1980). Corticosteroids in status asthmaticus. *J. Pediatr. 96*: 596-599.

Katz, P., and Fauci, A. S. (1979). Autologous and allogenic intercellular interactions: modulation by adherent cells, irradiation, and in vitro and in vivo corticosteroids. *J. Immunol. 123*: 2270.

Kehlet, H., and Binder, C. (1973). Adrenocortical function and clinical course during and after surgery in unsupplemented glucocorticoid treated patients. *Br. J. Anaesth. 45*: 1043-1048.

Keller, B. T., Landes, G. M., and Kitos, P. A. (1982). Evidence for more than one mechanism of action of the glucocorticoid hormones. *Biochim. Biophys. Acta 717*: 228-235.

Kelson, S. G., Kelson, D. P., Fleegler, B. F., Jones, R. C., and Rodman, T. (1978). Emergency room assessment and treatment of patients with acute asthma. *Am. J. Med. 64*: 622-628.

Kemp, J. P., Orgel, H. A., Meltzer, E. O., and Welch, M. J. (1985). Comparison of subcutaneous albuterol (ALB), terbutaline (TER), and epinephrine (EPI) in acute asthma. *J. Allergy Clin. Immunol. 75*: 162.

Kewley, G. D. (1980). Possible association between beclomethasone dipropionate aerosol and cataracts. *Aust. Paediatr. J. 16*: 117-118.

Kinsman, R. A., Wray Dahlem, N., Spector, S., and Staudenmayer, H. (1977). Observations on subjective symptomatology, coping behavior and medical decisions in asthma. *Psychosom. Med. 39*: 102-119.

Klein, R. G., Arnaud, S. B., Gallagher, J. C., DeLuca, H. F., and Riggs, B. L. (1977). Intestinal calcium absorption in exogenous hypercortisonism. Role of 25-Hydroxyvitamin D and corticosteroid dose. *J. Clin. Invest. 60*: 253-259.

Kolbeck, R. C., Downing, D. L., Harrison, G. N., Chaudhary, B. A., and Speir, W. A. (1979). Potentiation of the bronchodilator response to theophylline and isoproterenol: In vitro studies with hydrocortisone. *Am. Rev. Respir. Dis. 119*: 137.

Kozower, M., Veatch, L., and Kaplan, M. M. (1974). Decreased clearance of prednisolone, a factor in the development of corticosteroid side effects. *J. Clin. Endocrinol. Metab. 38*: 407-412.

Kram, J., Bourne, H., Maibach, H., and Melmon, K. (1975). Cutaneous immediate hypersensitivity in man: effects of systemically administered adrenergic drugs. *J. Allergy Clin. Immunol. 56*: 387.

Kristoffersen, M. G., Rattenborg, C. C., and Holaday, D. A. (1967). Asphyxial death: The roles of acute anoxia, hypercarbia and acidosis. *Anethesiologia 28*: 488-497.

LaForce, C. F., Szefler, S. J., Miller, M. F., Ebling, W., and Brenner, M. (1982). Inhibition of methylprednisolone elimination in the presence of erythromycin therapy. *J. Allergy Clin. Immunol. 72*: 34-39.

Lal, S., Harris, D. M., Bhalla, K. K., Singhal, S. N., and Butler, A. G. (1972). Comparison of beclomethasone dipropionate aerosol and prednisone in reversible airways obstruction. *Br. Med. J. 3*: 314-317.

Lewis, R. A. (1985). Leukotrienes and other lipid mediators of asthma. *Chest 87*: 5S-10S.

Lieberman, P., Patterson, R., and Kunske, R. (1972). Complications of long-term steroid therapy for asthma. *J. Allergy Clin. Immunol. 49*: 329-336.

Loren, M. L., Chai, H., Leung, P., Rohr, C., and Brenner, A. M. (1980). Corticosteroids in the treatment of acute exacerbations of asthma. *Ann. Allergy 45*: 67-71.

Luksza, A. R. (1982). A new look at adult asthma. *Br. J. Dis. Chest 76*: 11-14.

Lundgren, R. (1977). Scanning electron microscope studies of bronchial mucosa before and during treatment with beclomethasone dipropionate inhalation. *Scand. J. Respir. Dis. 57*: Suppl. 101, 179.

Maayan, C., Yitzhaki, T., and Bar-Yishay, E. (1985). Response of lung function to treatment in infants with bronchiolitis. *J. Allergy Clin. Immunol. 75*: 172.

MacDonald, J. B., Seaton, A., and Williams, D. A. (1976a). Asthma deaths in Cardiff 1963-74: 90 deaths outside hospital. *Br. Med. J. 1*: 1493-1495.

MacDonald, J. B., MacDonald, E. T., Seaton, A., and Williams, D. A. (1976b). Asthma deaths in Cardiff 1963: 74: 53 deaths in hospital. *Br. Med. J. 2*: 721-723.

MacKay, A. D., and Dyson, A. J. (1981). How important is the sequence of administration of inhaled beclomethasone dipropionate and salbutamol in asthma. *Br. J. Dis. Chest 75*: 273-276.

Mandella, L. A., Manfreda, J., Warren, C. P. W., and Anthonisen, N. R. (1982). Steroid response in stable chronic obstructive pulmonary disease. *Ann. Intern. Med. 96*: 17-21.

Marle, W. V., and Woods, K. L. (1980). Acute hydrocortisone myopathy. *Br. Med. J. 281*: 271.

Maron, Z., Shelhamer, J., Alling, D., and Kaliner, M. (1984). The effects of corticosteroids on mucous glycoprotein secretion from human airways in vitro. *Am. Rev. Respir. Dis. 129*: 62-65.

Martin, G. L., Atkins, P. C., Dunsky, E. H., and Zweiman, B. (1980). Effects of theophylline, terbutaline, and prednisone on antigen-induced bronchospasm and mediator release. *J. Allergy Clin. Immunol. 66*: 204-212.

Maunsell, K., Pearson, R. S. B., and Livingstone, J. L. (1968). Long-term corticosteroid treatment of asthma. *Br. Med. J. 1*: 661-665.

McAllen, M. K., Kochanowski, S. J., and Shaw, K. M. (1974). Steroid aerosols in asthma: An assessment of betamethasone valerate and a 12-month study of patients on maintenance treatment. *Br. Med. J. 1*: 171-175.

McAllister, W. A. C., Winfield, C. R., and Collins, J. V. (1981). Pharmacokinetics of prednisolone in normal and asthmatic subjects in relation to dose. *Eur. J. Clin. Pharmacol. 20*: 141-145.

McFadden, E. R., Jr. (1975). The chronicity of acute attacks of asthma—mechanical and therapeutic implications. *J. Allergy Clin. Immunol. 56*: 18-26.

McFadden, E. R., Kiser, R., deGroot, W. J., Holmes, B., Kiker, R., and Viser, G. (1976). A controlled study of the effects of single doses of hydrocortisone on the resolution of acute attacks of asthma. *Am. J. Med. 60*: 52-59.

McWilliams, B. C., Menendex, R., Kelly, H. W., and Howick, J. (1984). Effects of theophylline on inhaled methacholine and histamine in asthmatic children. *Am. Rev. Respir. Dis. 130*: 193-197.

Mellis, C. M., and Phelan, P. D. (1977). Asthma deaths in children—a continuing problem. *Thorax 32*: 29-34.

Meltzer, E. O., Kemp, J. P., and Welch, J. M. (1985). Effect of dosing schedule on efficacy of beclomethasone dipropionate aerosol in chronic asthma. *Am. Rev. Respir. Dis. 131*: 732-736.

Messina, M. S., and Smaldone, G. C. (1984). Evaluation of quantitative aerosol techniques for use in bronchoprovocation studies. *J. Allergy Clin. Immunol. 75*: 252-257.

Moore, P. D., and Hoult, J. R. S. (1980). Anti-inflammatory steroids reduce tissue PG synthetase activity and enhance PG breakdown. *Nature 288*: 269-270.

Moren, F. (1978). Drug deposition of pressurized inhalation aerosols. I. Influence of actuator tube design. *Int. J. Pharm. 1*: 205-212.

Moretti, M., Giannico, G., Marchioni, C. F., and Bisetti, A. (1984). Effects of methylprednisolone on sputum biochemical components in asthmatic bronchitis. *Eur. J. Respir. Dis. 65*: 365-370.

Morris, H. G. (1975). Growth and skeletal maturation in asthmatic children: Effect of corticosteroid treatment. *Pediatr. Res. 9*: 579-583.

Morris, H. G. (1980). Factors that influence clinical responses to administered corticosteroids. *J. Allergy Clin. Immunol. 66*: 343-346.

Morris, H. G. (1985). Mechanisms of action and therapeutic role of corticosteroids in asthma. *J. Allergy Clin. Immunol. 75*: 1-14.

Muers, M., and Dawkins, K. (1983). Effect of a timed interval between inhalation of beta-agonist and corticosteroid aerosol on the control of chronic asthma. *Thorax 38*: 378-382.

Murray, A. B., and Ferguson, A. C. (1982). Reduction of bronchial hyperreactivity during prolonged allergen avoidance. *Lancet 2*: 1212.

Murray, A. B., and Ferguson, A. C. (1983). Dust-free bedrooms in the treatment of asthmatic children with house dust or house dust mite allergy: A controlled trial. *Pediatrics 71*: 418-422.

Mygind, N., and Hansen, I. (1973). Beclomethasone dipropionate aerosol effect on the adrenals in normal persons. *Acta Allergol. 28*: 211-218.

Myles, A. B., Bacon, P. A., and Daly, J. R. (1971). Single daily dose corticosteroid treatment. *Annu. Rheum. Dis. 30*: 149-153.

Nassif, E. G., Weinberger, M., Thompson, R., and Huntley, W. (1981). The value of maintenance theophylline in steroid-dependent asthma. *N. Engl. J. Med. 304*: 71-75.

Newman, S. P. (1983). Pressurized aerosols inhaled through extension devices. *J. Aerosol. Sci. 14*: 69.

Newman, S. P., Pavia, D., Moren, F., Sheahan, N. F., and Clarke, S. W. (1981a). Deposition of pressurized aerosols in the human respiratory tract. *Thorax 36*: 52-55.

Newman, S. P., Pavia, D., and Clarke, S. W. (1981b). How should a pressurized beta-adrenergic bronchodilator be inhaled? *Eur. J.Respir. Dis. 62*: 3-21.

Newman, S. P., Pavia, D., and Garland, N. (1982). Effects of various inhalation modes on the deposition of radioactive pressurized aerosols. *Eur. J. Respir. Dis. 63*: Suppl. 199, 57.

Nogrady, S. G., Hartley, J. P. R., and Seaton, A. (1977). Metabolic effects of intravenous salbutamol in the course of acute severe asthma. *Thorax 32*: 559-562.

Nyholm, E., Frame, M. H., and Cayton, R. M. (1984). Therapeutic advantages of twice-daily over four-times daily inhalation budesonide in the treatment of chronic asthma. *Eur. J. Respir. Dis. 65*: 339-345.

Orgel, H. A., Meltzer, E. O., and Kemp, J. P. (1983). Flunisolide aerosol in treatment of steroid-dependent asthma in children. *Ann. Allergy 51(1)*: 21-25.

Patterson, R., Greenberger, P. A., Radin, R. C., and Roberts, M. (1982). Allergic bronchopulmonary aspergillosis: Staging as an aid to management. *Ann. Intern. Med. 96*: 286-291.

Peterson, A. P., Altman, L. C., Hill, J. S., Gosney, K., and Kadin, M. E. (1981). Glucocorticoid receptors in normal human eosinophils: comparison with neutrophils. *J. Allergy Clin. Immunol. 68*: 212-217.

Pierson, W. E., Bierman, C. W., and Kelley, V. C. (1974). A double-blind trial of corticosteroid therapy in status asthmaticus. *Pediatrics 54*: 282-288.

Plumpton, F. S., Besser, G. M., and Cole, P. V. (1969). Corticosteroid treatment and surgery. *Anaesthesia 24*: 3-11.

Pride, S. M., and Yuen, B. H. (1984). Relief of asthma in two patients receiving danazol for endometriosis. *Can. Med. Assoc. J. 131*: 763-764.

Rebuck, A. S., and Read, R. (1971). Assessment and management of severe asthma. *Am. J. Med. 51*: 788-798.

Reimer, L. G., Morris, H. G., and Ellis, E. F. (1975). Growth of asthmatic children during treatment with alternate day steroids. *J. Allergy Clin. Immunol. 55*: 224-231.

Reinhardt, D., Schuhmacher, P., Fox, A., Stemman, E. A., and Wegner, F. (1980). Comparison of the effects of theophylline, prednisolone and sleep withdrawal on airway obstruction and urinary cyclic AMP/cyclic GMP excretion of asthmatic children with and without nocturnal asthma. *Int. J. Clin. Pharmacol. 18*: 399-404.

Report to the Research Committee of the British Thoracic Association. (1979). Inhaled beclomethasone dipropionate in allergic bronchopulmonary aspergillosis. *Br. J. Dis. Chest 73*: 349-356.

Rinehart, J. J., Sagone, A. L., Balcerzak, S. P., Ackerman, G. A., and LoBuglio, A. F. (1975). Effects of corticosteroid therapy on human monocyte function. *N. Engl. J. Med. 292*: 236-241.

Rooklin, A. R., Lampert, S. I., Jaeger, E. A., McGeady, S. J., and Mansmann, H. C., Jr. (1979). Posterior subcapsular cataracts in steroid-requiring asthmatic children. *J. Allergy Clin. Immunol. 63*: 383-386.

Rose, J. Q., Nickelsen, J. A., Middleton, E., Yurchak, A. M., Park, B. H., and Jusko, W. J. (1980). Prednisolone disposition in steroid-dependent asthmatics. *J. Allergy Clin. Immunol. 66*: 366-373.

Rose, J. Q., Nickelsen, J. A., Ellis, E. F., Middleton, E., Jr., and Jusko, W. J. (1981). Prednisolone disposition in steroid-dependent asthmatic children. *J. Allergy Clin. Immunol. 67*: 188-193.

Ruffin, R. E., Wolff, R. K., Dolovich, M. B., Rossman, C. M., Fitzgerald, J. D., and Newhouse, M. T. (1978). Aerosol therapy with Sch 1000. Short-term mucociliary clearance in normal and bronchitic subjects and toxicology in normal subjects. *Chest 73*: 501-506.

Saavedra-Delgado, A. P., Mathews, K. P., Pan, P. M., Kay, D. R., and Muilenberg, M. L. (1980). Dose-response studies of the suppression of whole blood histamine and basophil counts by prednisone. *J. Allergy Clin. Immunol. 66*: 464-471.

Sadoul, P., Puchelle, E., Zehm, J., Jacquot, J., Aug, F., and Polu, J. (1981). Effect of terbutaline on mucociliary transport and sputum properties in chronic bronchitis. *Chest 80*: 885-889.

Samuelson, W. M., and Davies, A. O. (1984). Hydrocortisone-induced reversal of beta-adrenergic receptor uncoupling. *Am. Rev. Respir. Dis. 130*: 1023-1026.

Santa Curz, R., Landa, J., Hirsch, J., and Sackner, M. A. (1974). Tracheal mucous velocity in normal man and patients with obstructive lung disease: effects of terbutaline. *Am. Rev. Respir. Dis. 109*: 458-463.

Schleimer, R. P., MacGlashan, D. W., Peters, S. P., Naclerio, R., Pround, D., Adkinson, N. R., and Lichtenstein, L. M. (1984). Inflammatory mediators and mechanisms of release from purified human basophils and mast cells. *J. Allergy Clin. Immunol. 74*: 473-481.

Shim, C., and Williams, M. H., Jr. (1980). The adequacy of inhalation of aerosol from canister nebulizers. *Am. J. Med. 69*: 891-894.

Slade, J. D., and Hepburn, B. (1983). Prednisone-induced alterations of circulating human lymphocyte subsets. *J. Lab. Clin. Med. 101*: 479-487.

Smith, M. J., and Hodson, M. E. (1983). High-dose beclomethasone inhaler in the treatment of asthma. *Lancet 1*: 265-269.

Sotomayor, H., Badier, M., Vervloet, D., and Orehek, J. (1984). Seasonal increase of carbachol airway responsiveness in patients allergic to grass pollen. *Am. Rev. Respir. Dis. 130*: 56-58.

Spector, S. L., Katz, F. H., and Farr, R. S. (1974). Troleandomycin: Effectiveness in steroid-dependent asthma and bronchitis. *J. Allergy Clin. Immunol. 54*: 367-368.

Speizer, F. E., Doll, R., Heaf, P., and Strang, L. B. (1968). Investigation into use of drugs preceding death from asthma. *Br. Med. J. 1*: 399-343.

Stein, M. R., Shay, S. S., and Jacobson, K. (1979). Monilial eosphagitis in asthmatic patients treated with beclomethasone. *J. Allergy Clin. Immunol. 63*: 172.

Stjernholm, M. R., and Katz, F. H. (1975). Effects of diphenylhydantoin, phenobarbital, and diazepam on the metabolism of methylprednisolone and its sodium succinate. *Clin. Endocr. Metabl. 41*: 887-893.

Streck, W. F., and Lockwood, D. H. (1979). Pituitary adrenal recovery following short-term suppression with corticosteroids. *Am. J. Med. 66*:910-914.

Szefler, S. J., Brenner, M., Jusko, W. J., Spector, S. L., Flesher, K. A., and Ellis, E. F. (1982). Dose and time-related effect of troleandomycin on methylprednisolone elimination. *Clin. Pharmacol. Ther. 32*: 166-171.

Tarlo, S., Broder, I., Spence, L. (1979). A prospective study of respiratory infection in adult asthmatics and their normal spouses. *Clin. Allergy 9*: 293-301.

Thiringer, G., Eriksson, N., Malmberg, R., Svedmyr, N., and Zettergren, L. (1977). Bronchoscopic biopsies of bronchial mucosa before and after beclomethasone dipropionate therapy. *Scand. J. Respir. Dis. Suppl 101*: 173-177.

Toogood, J. H. (1979). Steroids in asthma. *Lancet 2*: 1185-1186. Ibid 1:54, 1980.

Toogood, J. H. (1983). Concentrated aerosol formulations in asthma. *Lancet 2*: 790-791.

Toogood, J. H. (1984). Guidelines to steroid therapy in asthma and rhinitis. *J. Respir. Dis. 5(5)*: 41-55.

Toogood, J. H. (1985). An appraisal of the influence of dose frequency on the antiasthmatic activity of inhaled corticosteroids. *Ann. Allergy 55*: 2-4.

Toogood, J. H., Baskerville, J., Errington, N., Jennings, B., Chuang, L., and Lefcoe, N. (1977a). Determinants of the response to beclomethasone aerosol at various dosage levels: A multiple regression analysis to identify clinically useful predictors. *J. Allergy Clin. Immunol. 60*: 367-376.

Toogood, J. H., Lefcoe, N. M., Haines, D. S. M., Jennings, B., Errington, N., Baksh, L., and Chuang, L. (1977b). A graded dose assessment of the efficacy of beclomethasone dipropionate aerosol for severe chronic asthma. *J. Allergy Clin. Immunol. 59*: 298-308.

Toogood, J. H., Lefcoe, N. M., Haines, D. S. M., Chuang, L., Jennings, B., Errington, N., Baksh, L., and Cauchi, M. (1978). Minimum dose requirements of steroid-dependent asthmatic patients for aerosol beclomethasone and oral prednisone. *J. Allergy Clin. Immunol. 61*: 355-364.

Toogood, J. H., Jennings, B., Greenway, R. W., and Chuang, L. (1980a). Candidiasis and dysphonia complicating beclomethasone treatment of asthma. *J. Allergy Clin. Immunol. 65*: 145-153.

Toogood, J. H., Khan, R. H., Baskerville, J. C., and Jennings, B. H. (1980b). Effect of corticosteroid on lymphocyte responsiveness in pigeon breeder's lung. *Clin. Allergy 10*: 547-553.

Toogood, J. H., Jennings, B., Lefcoe, N., and Simmons, M. (1981a). Therapeutic implications of small airways dysfunction in chronic asthma. *Am. Rev. Respir. Dis. 123*: 113.

Toogood, J. H., Jennings, B., Baskerville, J., Lefcoe, N., and Newhouse, M. (1981b). Assessment of a device for reducing oropharyngeal complications during beclomethasone treatment of asthma. *Am. Rev. Respir. Dis. 123*: 113.

Toogood, J. H., Baskerville, J. C., Jennings, B., Lefcoe, N. M., and Johanson, S-A. (1982). Influence of dosing frequency and schedule on the response of chronic asthmatics to the aerosol steroid, budesonide. *J. Allergy Clin. Immunol. 70*: 288-298.

Toogood, J. H., Jennings, B., and Baskerville, J. (1983). Tactics for clinical trials of therapy in patients with chronic asthma. *J. Asthma 20(S-1)*: 51-60.

Toogood, J. H., Jennings, B., Baskerville, N. M. (1984a). Personal observations on the use of inhaled corticosteroid drugs for chronic asthma. *Eur. J. Respir. Dis. 65*: 321-338.

Toogood, J. H., Baskerville, J., Jennings, B., Lefcoe, N. M., and Johansson, S-A. (1984b). Use of spacers to facilitate inhaled corticosteroid treatment of asthma. *Am. Rev. Respir. Dis. 129*: 723-729.

Toogood, J. H., Baskerville, J., Jennings, B., and Johansson, S-A. (1984c). A role for more concentrated formulations of inhaled steroid in the treatment of chronic asthma. *Ann Roy Coll Phys Surg Cda 17*(4): 297.

Toogood , J. H., Jennings, B., Baskerville, J., Anderson, J., and Johansson, S-A. (1984d). Dosing regimen of budesonide and occurrence of oropharyngeal complications. *Eur. J. Respir. Dis. 65*: 35-44.

Toogood, J. H., Baskerville, J., and Johansson, S-A. (1985a). Anomalous effects of steroid treatment on circulating leukocytes. *J. Allergy Clin. Immunol. 75*: 158.

Toogood, J. H., Baskerville, J., and Johansson, S-A. (1985b). Factors accounting for steroid resistance in chronic asthma. *Chest 88(1)*: 52S.

Turner-Warwick, M., Citron, K. M., Carroll, K. B., Heard, B. E., Mitchell, D. N., and Pepys, J. (1975). Immunologic lung disease due to aspergillosis. *Chest 68*: 346-355.

Tyan, G., Latimer, K. M., Juniper, E. F., Roberts, R. S., and Hargreave, F. E. (1985). Effect of beclomethasone diproprionate on bronchial responsiveness to histamine in controlled nonsteroid-dependent asthma. *J. Allergy Clin. Immunol. 75*: 25-30.

Uede, T., Hirata, F., Hirashima, M., and Ishizaka, K. (1983). Modulation of the biologic activities of IgE binding factors. *J. Immunol. 130*: 878-879.

Vaz, R., Senior, B., Morris, M., and Binkiewicz, A. (1982). Adrenal effects of beclomethasone inhalation therapy in asthmatic children. *J. Pediatr. 100*: 660-662.

Wang, J. L. F., Patterson, R., Roberts, M., and Ghory, A. C. (1979). The management of allergic bronchopulmonary aspergillosis. *Am. Rev. Respir. Dis. 120*: 87-92.

Webb, J., and Clark, T. J. H. (1981). Recovery of plasma corticotrophin and cortisol levels after a three-week course of prednisolone. *Thorax 36*: 22-24.

Weinberger, M., Hudgel, D., Spector, S., and Chidsey, C. (1977). Inhibition of theophylline clearance by troleandomycin. *J. Allergy Clin. Immunol. 59*: 228-231.

Weinberger, M. (1982). Safety of oral corticosteroids. *Eur. J. Respir. Dis. 63*: Suppl. 122:243-251.

Westerman, D. E., Benatar, S. R., Potgieter, P. D., and Ferguson, A. D. (1979). Identification of the high-risk asthmatic patient. Experience with 39 patients undergoing ventilation for status asthmaticus. *Am. J. Med. 66*: 565-572.

Williams, A. J., Baghat, M. S., Stableforth, D. E., Cayton, R. M., Shenoi, P. M., and Skinner, C. (1983). Dysphonia caused by inhaled steroids: Recognition of a characteristic laryngeal abnormality. *Thorax 38*: 813-821.

Williams, I. P., and McGavin, C. R. (1980). Corticosteroids in chronic airways obstructions: can the patient's assessment be ignored? *Br. J. Dis. Chest 74*: 142-148.

Wilson, C. G., Ssendagire, R., May, C. S., and Paterson, J. W. (1975). Measurement of plasma prednisolone in man. *Br. J. Clin. Pharmacol. 2*: 321-325.

Wilson, J. D., Sutherland, D. C., and Thomas, A. C. (1981). Has the change to beta-agonists combined with oral theophylline increased cases of fatal asthma? *Lancet 1*: 1235-1237.

Woodcock, A. A., Johnson, M. A., and Geddes, D. M. (1983). Theophylline prescribing, serum concentrations and toxicity. *Lancet 2*: 610-612.

Wyatt, R., Washek, J., Weinberger, M., and Sherman, B. (1978). Effects of inhaled beclomethasone dipropionate and alternate-day prednisone on pituitary-adrenal function in children with chronic asthma. *N. Engl. J. Med. 299*: 1387-1392.

Zeiger, R. S., Schatz, M., Sperling, W., Simon, R. A., and Stevenson, D. D. (1980). Efficacy of troleandomycin in outpatients with severe corticosteroid-dependent asthma. *J. Allergy Clin. Immunol. 66*: 438-446.

19

Bronchodilator Management of the Adult in the United States

CHARLES E. REED

Mayo Medical School and Mayo Clinic
Rochester, Minnesota

I. Historical Introduction

The aim of this chapter will be to discuss treatment with bronchodilators from the perspective of opinions and attitudes that have been prevalent in the United States, to express my personal point of view on various somewhat controversial issues, and finally, to present guidelines for their use. Details of treatment with the individual agents are discussed in other chapters.

Current practice in the United States is best understood as a process that is still evolving. Not long after aerosol epinephrine became available and was found to be an effective bronchodilator, Benson and Perlman cautioned that some patients become worse after using it, and they reported fatal asthma associated with frequent heavy inhalation (Benson and Perlman, 1948). They suggested that the desquamation of the ciliated bronchial epithelium observed in their fatal cases was due to intense vasoconstriction from epinephrine and concluded that aerosol bronchodilators should not be used for asthma. Although we now consider that the epithelial desquamation is part of the disease and not its treatment, their concern was sufficiently persuasive that many allergists avoided aerosol treatment of ambulatory patients, preferring oral bronchodilators, usually ephedrine, theophylline, or their combination. Meanwhile thoracic

Table 1 Commonly Available Theophylline Preparations

Generic name	Trade name	% Theophylline	Available Theophylline (mg)[a]	Form
Theophylline (anhydrous)	Aerolate	100	160/15 ml	Elixir (20% alcohol)
			III 65; Jr 125; Sr 260[b]	Bead-filled capsule
			80/15 ml	
	Constant-T		200, 300[b]	Slow-release tablet
	Duraphyl		200, 300[b]	Slow-release tablet
	Elixicon		100/5 ml	Suspension
	Elixophyllin		80/15 ml	Elixir (20% alcohol)
			100, 200	Tablet
	Elixophyllin SR		125, 250[b]	Bead-filled capsule
	La-BID		250 (scored)[b]	Slow-release tablet
	Physpan		130, 260[b]	Bead-filled capsule
	Quibron		150/15 ml plus 90 mg guaifenesin	Elixir (15% alcohol)
			150 plus 90 mg guaifenesin	Capsule
	Quibron-300		300 plus 180 mg guaifenesin	Capsule
	Quibron Plus		150/15 ml plus 25 mg ephedrine, 100 mg guaifenesin, 20 mg butabarbital	Elixir (15% alcohol)

	150 plus 25 mg ephedrine. 100 mg guaifenesin, 20 mg butabarbital	Capsule
Quibron-T-Dividose	300	Tablet
Quibron-T-SR Dividose	300[b]	Slow-release tablet
Respbid	250,500	Slow-release tablet
Slobid	50, 100, 200, 300[b]	Bead filled capsules
Slo-Phyllin	80/15 ml	Syrup
	100, 200	Tablet
Slo-Phyllin Gyrocap	60, 125, 250[b]	Bead-filled capsule
Somophyllin-T	100, 200	Capsule
Somophyllin-CRT	50, 100, 250[b]	Bead-filled capsule
Sustaire	100, 300 (scored)[b]	Slow-release tablet
Theobid Curacap	130, 260[b]	Bead-filled capsule
Theoclear 80	80/15 ml	Syrup
Theo-Dur	100, 200, 300 (scored)[b]	Slow-release tablet
Theo-Dur sprinkle	50, 75, 125, 200[b]	Bead-filled capsule
Theo-24	100, 300[b]	Bead-filled capsule
Theolair	150-250	Tablet
Theolair SR	250, 500 (scored)[b]	Slow-release tablet
Theon	50/5 ml	Elixir (10% alcohol)
Theon 300	130, 260[b]	Bead-filled capsule
Theophyl	225/30 ml	Elixir
	225	Tablet
Theophyl Chewable	100 (scored)	Chewable tablet
Theophyl-SR	125, 250[b]	Bead-filled capsule

Table 1 (Continued)

Generic name	Trade name	% Theophylline	Available Theophylline (mg)[a]	Form
Theophylline (anhydrous) (continued)	Theospan SR		65, 130, 250[b]	Bead-filled capsule
	Theostat		80/25 ml	Syrup (1% alcohol)
			100, 200	Tablet
	Uniphil		200, 400[b]	Slow-release tablet
Aminophylline (theophylline ethylenediamine)	(Various brands)	86	100, 200	Tablet
			250/10 ml	Injectable
	Phyllocontin		225[b]	Slow-release tablet
	Somophyllin		105/5 ml	Syrup
	Somophyllin-DF		105/5 ml	Dye-free solution
	Somophyllin Rectal Solution		300/5 ml	Rectal solution
	Aminodur		300 mg[b]	Slow-release tablet
Oxtriphylline (choline theophyllinate)	Choledyl	64	100/5 ml	Elixir (20% alcohol)
			50/5 ml	Syrup
			100, 200	Enteric-coated tablet
	Choledyl-SA		400, 600[b]	Slow-release tablet
	Brondecon		100/5 ml plus 50 mg guaifenesin	Elixir (20% alcohol)
			200 plus 100 mg guaifenesin	Tablet

Theophylline sodium glycinate	Asbron-G	51	300/15 ml plus 100 mg guaifenesin	Elixir (15% alcohol)
			300	Tablet
	Synophylate		330/15 ml	Elixir (20% alcohol)
			330	Tablet
Theophylline (calcium salicylate)	Theokin	51	448/15 ml	Elixir (9.5% alcohol)
			448 plus 450 KI	Tablet
Dyphylline[c]	Airet	0	100/15 ml	Elixir
			200, 400	Tablet
	Airet L.A.		400 (scored)[b]	Slow-release tablet
	Lufyllin		100/115 ml	Elixir (20% alcohol)
			250 ml	Injectable
			200, 400	Tablet

[a]Available theophylline/total volume or theophylline salt.
[b]Sustained.
[c]Dyphylline is a xanthine bronchodilator but not a true theophylline; it does not yield theophylline in solution or in vivo; its bronchodilator activity is substantially less than that of theophylline.
Modified from Siegel, S. C., Katz, R. M., and Rachelfsky, G. S. (1983). In *Allergy Principles and Practice,* ed. 2. Edited by E. Middleton, E. F. Ellis and C. E. Reed. St. Louis, C. V. Mosby, pp. 889-890.

physicians accumulated convincing evidence of efficacy of adrenergic aerosols, particularly among hospitalized patients. Thus, a divergence of practice developed, and inpatients were often treated with aerosol epinephrine, usually with an intermittent positive-pressure breathing apparatus. The introduction of aerosol isoproterenol was welcomed as an advance because isoproterenol lacked the vasoconstrictive effect of epinephrine and was perceived as safer. Also about this same time, newly developed metered-dose inhalers provided a delivery system with advantages of convenience and reproducible dosing. But before long isoproterenol was also indicted for causing death in asthma patients. Speizer et al. reported an association between an increase in mortality from asthma in the United Kingdom and sales of aerosol isoproterenol (Speizer et al., 1968). Van Metre, after reviewing 58 patients who died between 1952 and 1966 stated, "Nine of 17 patients, whose deaths were caused primarily by asthma, used these preparations excessively and apparently more and more to accomplish less and less" (Van Metre, 1969). About this same time Ouellette and I cared for six middle-aged women who, after admission to the hospital for treatment of status asthmaticus, were discovered to have extensive subendocardial myocardial infarction though they had no prior history of coronary artery disease. In a futile attempt to relieve the asthma, all of them had emptied a canister of isoproterenol. We concluded that the isoproterenol, probably coupled with hypoxemia from asthma, had caused the subendocardial damage similar to the damage it can cause in experimental animals. Although we assumed that these adverse reactions occurred from abuse of isoproterenol rather than its proper use, a widespread opinion developed that any aerosol adrenergic bronchodilator therapy was dangerous.

The next important development was the study of Weinberger and Bronsky that showed that addition of ephedrine to an optimal dose of theophylline did not increase bronchodilatation but only added toxicity (Weinberger and Bronsky, 1974). The fact that theophylline fitted simple mathematical models of pharmacokinetics made it feasible to use the drug at optimal therapeutic doses even though it has a low therapeutic index. By monitoring blood levels and by taking into account factors that alter theophylline metabolism, it was possible to achieve reasonable bronchodilatation without serious toxicity. Therefore theophylline became popular in the United States as the first choice bronchodilator (Table 1).

Meanwhile pharmaceutical chemists were developing selective adrenergic agonists which in animals have predominantly β-2-adrenergic activity and cause myocardial damage only in very high concentrations. After introduction of albuterol aerosol in the United States, the tide of opinion turned and is now running rather strongly in favor of selective β-2 adrenergic aerosols as the initial therapy. These bronchodilators have the advantages over isoproterenol not only of causing less myocardial toxicity in animals and having a duration of action several hours longer but also of being less likely to be abused. Minor adverse effects of theophylline such as nervousness, insomnia, headaches, and indigestion are common at therapeutic doses, occurring in as many as half of the patients who take them. Not uncommonly they are unpleasant enough to require changing the medication regimen. There also has been concern about the possible long-term result of the central nervous system stimulation on school-aged children's behavior and learning. Selective β-2 adrenergic agonists aerosols offer more effective bronchodilatation with fewer side effects.

However, introduction of sustained release tablets of theophylline made once or twice a day dosing practical and smoothed out the fluctuation of blood levels associated with rapidly absorbed theophylline preparations. The result was increased compliance and fewer of the minor side effects mentioned above. Furthermore, because of simplicity and familiarity oral medication remains popular with patients and physicians alike. It has also become apparent that the blood level found to be necessary for full bronchodilatation in severely ill hospitalized patients is not necessary for milder cases. Lower levels, 5-10 μg/ml rather than 15-20 μg/ml, suffice (Katz et al., 1983; Klein et al., 1983). Although ephedrine is rarely prescribed now, the orally active β-2 selective adrenergic agonists have found a place as effective and practical bronchodilators for patients who cannot inhale aerosols efficiently, particularly infants and the elderly. Theophylline increases the myocardial damage of β-2 adrenergic agonists in experimental animals. Therefore, concern about the potential for added toxicity of the combinations leads many clinicians to prefer the aerosol route for the β agonists for patients being treated with theophylline.

What of the future? The theoretical arguments in favor of the specificity and selectivity of the aerosol route of administration seem persuasive, but there two practical difficulties remain to be completely solved. First, proper technique for inhaling therapeutic aerosols is difficult for many patients to learn. Full bronchodilatation requires careful instruction and repeated personal coaching. Second, the adrenergic aerosols presently available have a duration of action in most patients with chronic airway obstruction of only 3-4 hr. A duration of 8-12 hr is desirable so that patients can sleep through the night. A longer duration of action also provides a more convenient dosing schedule, thereby improving compliance. Several new β-2 adrenergic aerosols will soon be released that maintain bronchodilatation for 6 hr, but at this time it seems unlikely that the goal of a 12-hr aerosol will be achieved. Another pharmaceutical development coming soon is sustained-release information for twice a day, or perhaps once a day dosing with selective β-2 adrenergic agonist tablets. Anticholinergic aerosols may turn out to have an advantage over adrenergic agonists in duration of action, but this point has not yet been investigated thoroughly.

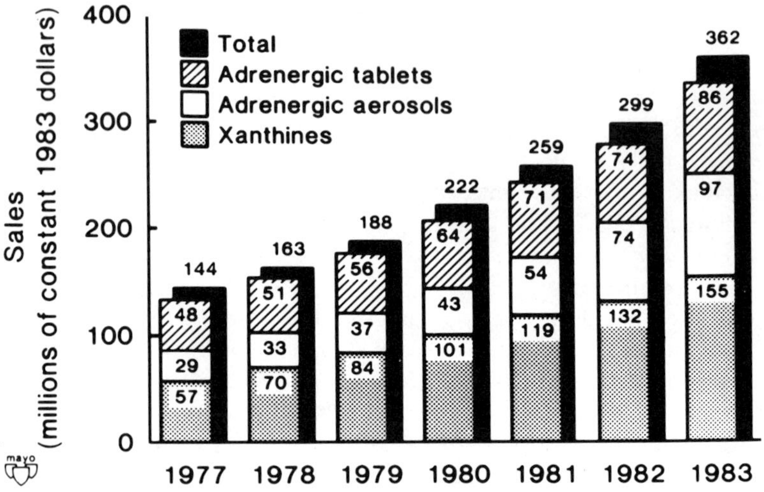

Figure 1 Sales of medications for obstructive lung diseases from 1977 to 1983, sales corrected for inflation and expressed as constant 1983 dollars. Numbers of prescriptions have increased similarly (data not shown). Sales have increased in all categories of drugs, though the ratio of increase has been greater in 1982 and 1983 for adrenergic aerosols than the other categories. The difference between the gain of the bronchodilator and the total is made up of glucocorticoids, both tablets and aerosols and by cromolyn and expectorants (data courtesy of Dr. Sidney Regnier, Warner Lambert Corporation, New York, New York). (Reprinted by permission from C. E. Reed.)

II. Bronchodilator Sales and Hospitalization for Asthma

Between 1960 and 1983 sales of drugs for bronchial therapy increased from about $20,000,000 to about $362,000,000 (Figs. 1 and 2). (Values corrected for inflation and expressed as constant 1983 dollars.) Sales have increased in all categories of drugs but in the past 2 years the rate has slowed for theophylline while it has increased for adrenergic aerosols. From their experience with their own patients, allergists and chest physicians generally believe that vigorous outpatient treatment of asthma with bronchodilators and glucocorticoids will prevent the need for hospital treatment, a belief we share with our colleagues in the United Kingdom (Arnold et al., 1983). Therefore it is surprising that this very substantial increase in prescriptions for bronchial therapy has not been reflected in a reciprocal decline in hospital treatment for asthma. In fact, the numbers of patients treated in the hospital has increased at about the same rate as sales of drugs (Fig. 2). There has been a decline in the length of stay in the hospital,

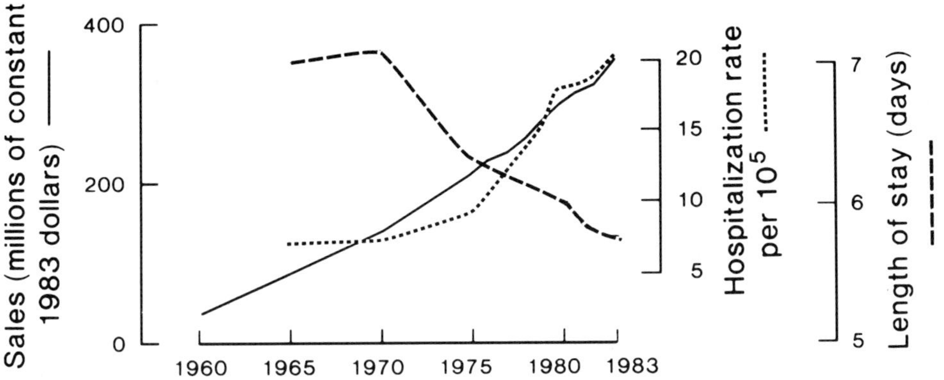

Figure 2 Sales of medications for obstructive lung disease and hospitalization for asthma, 1960-1983, corrected for inflation and expressed in constant 1983 dollars. Hospitalization rates expressed as patient discharges per 100,000 population (data courtesy of Dr. Sidney Regnier, Warner Lambert Corporation, New York, New York; and Dr. Fred T. Nobrega, Health Care Studies Unit, Mayo Clinic, Rochester, Minnesota, and the National Center for Health Care Statistics). (Reprinted by permission from C. E. Reed.)

however. Both hospitalization rate and length of stay have changed in a parallel fashion in all age groups. The reasons for this striking change in treatment of asthma and chronic obstructive pulmonary (COPD) in the past 20 years are unknown but a number of factors can be mentioned. One is that new bronchodilators have been vigorously promoted by the pharmaceutical industry with the result that physicians' prescribing patterns have changed. Since these agents are safe and effective for asthma, the change is for the better. Furthermore, physicians have been recognizing COPD earlier and treating it more vigorously with bronchodilators. In the early part of the period most of the bronchodilator treatment was for asthma; now it includes COPD. But this change in prescribing patterns does not explain the rise in hospitalization for asthma. The criteria for hospitalization may have changed, but there is no evidence for this explanation and it seems unlikely, especially since the change has occurred for all age groups and is nationwide. The increased rate may be due to change in the nomenclature or methods of coding. Also some physicians may be more likely now than in the past to diagnose asthma rather than bronchitis. The fact that the same parallel increase in drug sales and asthma hospitalization rate has occurred in New Zealand implies that it is not the result of changes in the organization of the system of medical care. In my opinion the most likely explanation is that asthma has increased in frequency, severity, or both, though I know of no data that support this (Jackson et al., 1983). The question needs research.

III. Aerosol Inhalation

Specificity is the main advantage of the aerosol route. Inhaled drugs are concentrated in the airways. The dose reaching other organs is much reduced and the dose required for bronchodilation is substantially less (Louridas et al., 1983). The main disadvantage is that effective inhalation requires learning a complex muscular skill. Infants and the elderly or arthritic cannot use metered dose inhalers and many others have difficulty in learning the proper technique. Considerable attention has been devoted to devising equipment and techniques for improving compliance and efficacy, but oral medication will always remain important. In acute asthmatic attacks aerosol β-adrenergic agonists from a compressed-air-driven jet nebulizer are as effective as an epinephrine injection and more effective than a bolus of intravenous aminophylline, even in patients who have failed to respond to aerosol sympathomimetics before coming to the emergency room (Rossing et al., 1983). In patients with stable airway obstruction, aerosol albuterol was more effective than a combination of theophylline and an oral β agonist (Rossing et al., 1980, 1981, 1982; Becker et al., 1983; Tinkelman et al., 1983). Other studies have demonstrated that β-adrenergic agonists from a metered dose inhaler are as effective as compressed-air-driven nebulizer; in fact, the dose required is considerably less (Shim and Williams, 1984). Intermittent positive pressure devices provide no benefit over simple aerosols (Intermittent Positive Pressure Breathing Trial Group, 1983).

Most of the particles from a nebulizer deposit in the mouth and pharynx and ultimately are swallowed. For drugs that are well absorbed from the gastrointestinal tract the swallowed medication contributes to side effects more than to efficacy. For the others the fraction deposited in the mouth is simply wasted. The fraction deposited in the mouth can be decreased by decreasing the particle momentum by reducing both its size and velocity. Particle size of powders is determined in the manufacturing process for metered dose inhalers and the size of droplets by the design of wet nebulizers. Particle velocity is determined both by the velocity of the jet from the nebulizer and by the inspiratory flow rate. Velocity can be reduced by introducing a spacer between the inhaler and the mouth and by having patients inhale slowly. Such a spacer may also reduce particle size by allowing time for the freon propellent to evaporate. Despite these compelling theoretical advantages, using a spacer does not seem to improve bronchodilatation if patients activate a metered dose inhaler at the start of inspiration. Spacers and expansion chambers seem to be most helpful for patients who have trouble coordinating inspiration with activation. It is also likely that spacers are helpful for the administration of aerosol glucocorticoids.

IV. Anticholinergic Aerosols

The anatomical fact that cholinergic innervation is the pathway for reflex bronchoconstriction lends appeal to the concept that anticholinergic drugs would be effective bronchodilators, as indeed they are. The belief, widely held 40 years ago, that they would aggravate the airway obstruction by drying mucus has proved to be unfounded (Bell et al., 1984). The primary reason for mucus plugs is structural damage of the ciliated epithelium, not change in secretion of mucus glands. But at the present writing no metered dose inhaler preparations of anticholinergic drugs are approved in the United States. The only agent available is atropine which has been invaluable as a research tool, but has limited therapeutic application and is less effective than adrenergic aerosols (Peerless et al., 1983). The effective dose from a compressed-air powered nebulizer is of the order of 1-2 mg, and is associated with systemic anticholinergic effects. These systemic effects usually make it unacceptable in comparison with adrenergic agonists. Quaternary amine anticholinergic aerosols such as atropine methyl nitrate or ipratropium are available in other countries. They have the important advantage over atropine of being poorly absorbed from the gut and therefore being relatively free of systemic anticholinergic effects. When they become available it seems likely that American physicians will find a place for them, particularly in the treatment of patients who tolerate adrenergic aerosols poorly. Considerably more experience will be needed to define their role in comparison to other bronchodilators. It is possible that the next major new development in bronchodilator drugs will come in this category. As mentioned above, an important potential advantage for anticholinergics is prolonged duration of action (Anderson, 1983). In general antagonists can be found that have greater affinity for receptors than agonists do and therefore have a more prolonged effect.

V. Bronchodilator Regimens

Despite the effort expended on comparing bronchodilator regimens, no final conclusion emerges, except perhaps that the choice of a bronchodilator must be individualized to meet the particular patient's needs. These needs change with changing activity of the disease. For treatment of acute attacks an aerosol adrenergic agonist is most effective. The dose may need to be repeated at short intervals to achieve maximal effect, presumably because partial dilatation from the first dose allows deeper penetration of the next. Emergency room treatment with aerosol adrenergic agonist was effective even in patients who reported that using metered dose inhalers at home had not controlled the attack (Rossing et al., 1983). Microgram for microgram, metered dose inhalers are more effective than wet aerosols, but during severe attacks the more passive inhalation at tidal volume over several minutes achieves better delivery to the airway and a better response. In either case, the usually recommended dose does not provide maximal bronchodilatation and may need to be increased fourfold for optimal results (Nelson et al., 1983).

It is not at all certain that intravenous theophylline adds to the bronchodilatation that can be achieved with aerosol β-adrenergic agonists, although every patient admitted to a hospital in the United States for treatment of severe asthma has probably received this treatment as a matter of course. Such practice is not necessarily futile because theophylline has other beneficial actions, increasing respiratory drive and relieving diaphragmatic fatigue. The practice may also be valuable in achieving a smoother, more consistent, bronchodilatation than aerosols can. Because of their short duration isoproterenol and isoetharine have been largely supplanted by the longer-acting agents metaproterenol and terbutaline, but even these begin to fade after an hour.

Aerosol atropine is often added to the treatment regimen of severe asthma in the hospital, though there is no convincing evidence that it adds substantially to bronchodilatation. In general, atropine is less effective than adrenergic agonists. Its chief merit may be somewhat longer action and less direct effect on ventricular myocardium, though these possibilities have not been adequately investigated. Some clinicians suspect that there is a subset of patients with moderately severe chronic asthma who respond better to anticholinergics than to adrenergic agonists. This hypothesis is difficult to test rigorously. Cough and copius thin mucus are characteristics that are said to predict an especially good response to anticholinergic aerosols. This question of whether subsets of asthmatic patients exist who selectively respond better to one category of bronchodilator than another is an important subject of future research. Lacking guidance from controlled trials, the clinician falls back on the art of medical practice and matches the patient with the regimen by trial and error. Differences in the factors that provoke attacks such as exercise, allergy, or infection, differences in personality and socioeconomic status; differences in response to unwanted side effects as well as the therapeutic benefit all affect the final choice.

VI. Combination Treatments

Combining bronchodilators with the aim of improving results with fewer side effects has been traditional for generations. This goal is as reasonable now as it was in our grandparents' day. Recently there have appeared reports of increasing bronchodilatation by combining adrenergic agonists and theophylline in various doses and routes of administration (Shim and Williams, 1983; Busse and Smith,

1983; Sahay and Chatterjee, 1983). When both drugs are given orally the increased benefit is usually accompanied by increased side effects, since both can cause insomnia, nervousness, tremor, and tachycardia. Theophylline and adrenergic agonists have opposite effects on gastric acid secretion, so the combination may be better tolerated by patients who are especially prone to the gastric effects of theophylline. For most patients, however, side effects can be minimized by combining aerosol adrenergic agonist with oral theophylline.

Similarly, combinations of submaximal doses of anticholinergic and adrenergic aerosols are more effective than either one alone, but it remains to be proved that the combination has a practical advantage over larger doses of the adrenergic agonist (Ruffin et al., 1982; Elwood and Abboud, 1982; Rebuck et al., 1983). My opinion is that there is an advantage in combining the speed of onset of the adrenergic agonist with the longer action of the cholinergic antagonist, and that dispensing the two together in the same metered dose inhaler would improve compliance because it is cheaper and more convenient.

VII. Limitations of Bronchodilators in the Treatment of Chronic Airway Obstruction

It seems to me that one of the generalizations from the Weinberger and Bronsky study has not received sufficient emphasis: *Once maximum bronchodilatation has been achieved, adding additional bronchodilators can only increase toxicity; increased benefit is impossible.*

Airway obstruction in asthma has two components: bronchospasm and inflammation of the bronchial wall. There is mucosal and submucosal edema and desquamation of the ciliated epithelium. Without cilia the mucociliary escalator fails and plugs of mucus mixed with inflammatory exudate and bits of desquamated epithelium (Creola bodies) fill the lumen. In treating asthma we should pay more attention than we commonly do to controlling bronchial inflammation. Perhaps this change in emphasis would come easier if we renamed asthma "chronic desquamating eosinophilic bronchitis," which is a concise description of its histopathologic appearance. How can inflammation be recognized? Clues are eosinophils and desquamated epithelial cells in the sputum, persistent nocturnal asthma disturbing sleep, and wide diurnal swings in peak flow rates. The diagnostic criterion is obstruction that does not respond to bronchodilators but does respond to glucocorticoids.

The fixed airway obstruction in COPD has a complex histopathologic basis including emphysema and other irreversible changes. Here too, increasing the dose of bronchodilators, or pyramiding additional classes of bronchodilators, is often counterproductive.

VIII. Summary Recommendations

The cardinal rule in bronchodilator therapy is to individualize the program for each patient, and to modify it to meet changing circumstances. Patients vary greatly in their response to and tolerance of specific drugs. It is very important to monitor the effect of treatment with pulmonary function tests because subjective reports of symptom severity or the physical examination are frequently misleading. Simple spirometry to determine FEV_1 is the most reliable measurement, but peak flow meters offer an economical alternative. They are especially useful for home recording of peak flow rates twice daily to help in management of patients wtith severe asthma. Early recognition of changes in flow, or loss of response to bronchodilators allows adjustment of the program to meet changing circumstances. If an asthmatic patient's flow no longer responds well to bronchodilators, a brief course of prednisone can be started or maintenance treatment with aerosol glucocorticoids added before the obstruction has become so severe that hospital care will be needed.

The following statements are offered as guidelines of bronchodilator therapy. Doses are indicated in Appendix II of this volume.

A. Treatment of Mild Intermittent Asthma

Noncatecholamine β-adrenergic agonists delivered with a metered dose inhaler are simplest, safest, and most effective. Careful instruction in proper inhalation technique is essential, and it is wise to watch each patient inhale the aerosol at each visit and correct errors. Improper inhalation technique is the most common reason for poor response. The method that I recommend is to hold the aerosol 2 or 3 cm in front of the open mouth, and discharge the puff just after starting a slow steady inhalation from functional residual volume. Slow inhalation continues to total lung capacity and the breath held for at least 10 sec. In some patients, inhalation to total lung capacity causes rather severe cough and reflex bronchoconstriction, and a shallower breath is better. Several good β-agonists are available; metaproterenol albuterol, terbutaline, and bitolterol are licensed in the United States at the date of this writing. Fenoterol and procaterol may be licensed in the near future. The usual dose is two puffs, but if the obstruction is not relieved promptly two more puffs can be inhaled 15 min later. Other good alternatives to metered dose inhalers for the infant, the arthritic, or the occasional adult who cannot master the psychomotor skills needed for effective inhalation, are an oral β-2 agonist syrup or tablet or a rapidly absorbed theophylline preparation.

B. Treatment of Mild to Moderate Chronic Asthma or COPD

Because of the simplicity of dosing and better patient compliance, slow-release long-acting theophylline tablets or capsules are ordinarily the best first choice.

It is rarely desirable to attempt to achieve peak blood levels over 15 μg/ml; levels of 8-10 μg/ml are usually effective. Higher levels are often associated with frequent unpleasant side effects that render the treatment more uncomfortable than the disease. My preference is to schedule the dose to achieve the peak blood level between 4 and 8 AM, when the obstruction is at the worst of its diurnal swing. The timing of administration depends on the pharmacokinetic properties of the specific preparation. For example Theo-Dur reaches peak level at about 6-7 hr and should be taken at bedtime. Uniphyl reaches peak level at about 11 hr and should be taken with supper. If this low dose of theophylline once or twice a day does not provide sufficient bronchodilatation, add aerosol β-agonist, either occasionally as needed for symptoms, or on a regular schedule four times a day. In asthma if this combination does not control the obstruction, the next step is to add aerosol glucocorticoid or cromolyn. In COPD the next step is not so obvious. Alternatives include increasing theophylline, increasing β-agonists, and adding aerosol or oral glucocorticoids. It is not established, however, that adding additional bronchodilators improves the COPD patient's well-being. Distinction between asthma and COPD is by no means easy, and many patients have elements of both. Serial spirometry is the best objective way to assess the results of treatment and to determine the amount of reversal of the obstruction that can be obtained. It is important not to give medication that does not provide objective benefit and may do harm. Occasional patients who cannot use metered dose inhalers can use wet aerosols generated with a small electric pump and a jet nebulizer. For equal efficacy the dose of a wet adrenergic aerosol needs to be considerably greater than with a metered dose inhaler. Cromolyn can also be given by wet aerosol 20 mg four times a day. There is no evidence however that wet aerosol glucorticoids have any less systemic effect than equivalent oral dose of prednisone and are not recommended. In my experience aerosol atropine adds little bronchodilatation to adequate amounts of β-agonists and can be recommended only in exceptional circumstances.

C. Treatment of Acute Asthma Attacks

It is now quite clear that large doses of adrenergic aerosols are as effective as epinephrine injections, and more effective than intravenous aminophylline even in patients who appear at the emergency room having failed to respond to the adrenergic aerosol at home. In managing the patient in the emergency room objective spirometric evaluation of the response to treatment is essential. In acute asthma the aerosol should be delivered by jet nebulizer and inhaled at tidal volume for 5-15 min. It is important to remember that the dose of aerosol may need to be larger and repeated more often than recommended by the manufacturer. My own choice is metaproterenol 5-15 mg or terbutaline 0.5-1 mg repeated every 15 min until the FEV_1 does not increase further and then repeated every 3 hr as needed. If the obstruction is not substantially reversed within 1 hr a course of prednisone is indicated. Admission to the hospital is indicated if the FEV_1 changes little or not at all within 1 hr.

D. Treatment of Severe Chronic Asthma

Most experts in the United States have recommended increasing the dose of theophylline to achieve peak blood levels of about 20 μg/ml at 6 AM and a trough of 15 μg/ml during the day. Adrenergic aerosols are inhaled every 3 or 4 hr (unless the patient is asleep) and as large a dose of aerosol glucocorticoid as is feasible prescribed (up to five inhalations four times a day). Our colleagues from the United Kingdom would reverse this sequence, adding the aerosol glucorticoids before increasing theophylline. I must say I am persuaded by their arguments and also by my own experience that long-term treatment of patients over 60 years of age with these higher doses of theophylline is associated with a high frequency of toxicity, particularly upper gastrointestinal bleeding and cardiac arrhythmias. I have not found addition of aerosol atropine sulfate to be useful. The place of quaternary amine anticholinergics remains to be defined. if this regimen does not control symptoms well enough for the patient to lead a normal life, maintenance oral prednisone should be added.

E. Treatment of Severe COPD

Management is much the same as for asthma, but three additional points deserve mention. The response to glucocorticoids is often more subjective than objective. In my opinion the long-term side effects of prednisone outweigh its benefits unless objective changes are demonstrated. The effects of theophylline on skeletal muscles of respiration and on the respiratory centers in the CNS may justify increasing the dose to the maximum tolerated aiming, to maintain blood levels of 15-20 μg/ml. Beta adrenergic agonists similarly improve diaphragmatic function. To capitalize on this effect the oral route is preferred and the attendant muscle tremor must be accepted. Patients with severe COPD often have heart disease, so the cardiac effects of bronchodilators require careful individual consideration.

F. Management of the Hospital Patient

This topic is discussed in other chapters.

References

Anderson, G. (1983). Anticholinergic drugs in airways obstruction. *Postgrad. Med. J. 59*: 64-65.

Arnold, A. G., Lane, D. J., and Zapata, E. (1983). Current therapeutic practice in the management of acute severe asthma. *Br. J. Dis. Chest 77*: 123-135.

Becker, A. B., Nelson, N. A., and Simons, F. E. R. (1983). Inhaled salbutamol (albuterol) vs injected epinephrine in the treatment of acute asthma in children. *J. Pediatrics 102*: 465-469.

Bell, J. A., Bluestein, B. M., Danta, I., and Wanner, A. (1984). Effect of inhaled ipratropium bromide on tracheal mucociliary transport in bronchial asthma. *Mt. Sinai J. Med. 51*: 215-217.

Benson, R. L., and Perlman, F. (1948). Clinical effects of epenephrine by inhalation. *J. Allergy 19*: 129.

Busse, W. W., and Smith, A. (1983). Combination low-dose metaproterenol-theophylline therapy in asthma. *J. Asthma 20*: 85-91.

Elwood, R. K., and Abboud, R. T. (1982). The short-term bronchodilator effects of fenoterol and ipratropium in asthma. *J. Allergy Clin. Immunol. 69*; 467-473.

Fanta, C. H., Rossing, T. H., and McFadden, E. R., Jr. (1982). Emergency room treatment of asthma. Relationships among therapeutic combinations, severity of obstructions, and time course of response. *Am. J. Med. 72*: 416-422.

Intermittent Positive Pressure Breathing Trial Group (1983). Intermittent positive pressure breathing therapy of chronic obstructive pulmonary disease. *Ann. Intern. Med. 99*: 612-620.

Jackson, R. T., and Mitchell, E. A. (1983). Trends in hospital admission rate and drug treatment of asthma in New Zealand. *N. Z. Med. J. 96*: 728-730.

Katz, R. M., Rachelefsky, G. S., Siegel, S. C., and Mickey, R. (1983). Theophylline administration in children with asthma: Optimal pulmonary function and possible tolerance to chronic administration. *Ann. Allergy 50*: 23-26.

Klein, J. J., Lefkowitz, M. S., Spector, S. L., and Cherniack, R. M. (1983). Relationship between serum theophylline levels and pulmonary function before and after inhaled beta-agonist in "stable" asthmatics." *Am. Rev. Respir. Dis. 127*: 413-416.

Louridas, T., Kakoura, M., Galanis, N., Patakas, D., and Kastritsi, K. (1983). Bronchodilatory effect of inhaled versus oral salbutamol in bronchial asthma. *Respiration 44*: 439-443.

Nelson, H. S., Spector, S. L., Whitsett, T. L., George, R. B., and Dwek, J. H. (1983). The bronchodilator response to inhalation of increasing doses of aerosolized albuterol. *J. Allergy Clin. Immunol. 72*: 371-375.

Peerless, A. G., Rachelefsky, G. S., Mickey, M. R., Katz, R. M., and Siegel, S. C. (1983). Bronchodilator characteristics of nebulized metaproterenol sulfate, isoetharine, and atropine in chronic asthma. *J. Allergy Clin. Immunol. 72*: 702-708.

Rebuck, A. S., Gent, M., and Chapman, K. R. (1983). Anticholinergic and sympathomimetic combination therapy of asthma. *J. Allergy Clin. Immunol. 71*: 317-323.

Rossing, T. H., Fanta, C. H., Goldstein, D. H., Snapper, J. R., and McFadden, E. R., Jr. (1980). Emergency therapy of asthma: Comparison of the acute effects of parenteral and inhaled sympathomimetics and infused aminophylline. *Am. Rev. Respir. Dis. 122*: 365-371.

Rossing, T. H., Fanta, C. H., and McFadden, E. R., Jr. (1981). A controlled trial of the use of single versus combined drug therapy in the treatment of acute episodes of asthma. *Am. Rev. Respir. Dis. 123:* 190-194.

Rossing, T. H., Fanta, C. H., and McFadden, E. R., Jr. (1983). Effect of outpatient treatment of asthma with beta agonists on the response to sympathomimetics in an emergency room. *Am. J. Med. 75*: 781-784.

Ruffin, R. E., McIntyre, E., Crockett, A. J., Zielonka, K., and Alpers, J. H. (1982). *J. Allergy Clin. Immunol. 69*: 60-65.

Sahay, J. N., and Chatterjee, S. S. (1983). A 21-day double-blind study of the effect of adding sustained-release theophylline (Nuelin sa) to inhaled salbutamol in patients with asthma. *Br. J. Dis. Chest 77*: 66-70.

Shim, C. S. and Williams, M. H., Jr. (1983). Bronchodilator response to oral aminophylline and terbutaline versus aerosol albuterol in patients with chronic obstructive pulmonary disease. *Am. J. Med. 75*: 697-701.

Shim, C. S., and Williams, M. H., Jr. (1984). Effect of bronchodilator therapy administered by canister versus jet nebulizer. *J. Allergy Clin. Immunol. 73*: 387-390.

Speizer, F. E., Doll, R., Heaf, P., and Shang, L. B. (1968). Investigation into use of drugs preceding death from asthma. *Br. Med. J. 1*: 339.

Tinkelman, D. G., Vanderpool, G. E., Carroll, M. S., Lotner, G. Z., and Spangler, D. L. Comparison of nebulized terbutaline and subcutaneous epinephrine (EPI) in the treatment of acute asthma. *Ann. Allergy 50*: 398-401.

Van Metre, T. E. (1969). Adverse effects of inhalation of excessive amounts of nebulized isoproterenol in status asthmaticus. *J. Allergy 43*: 101-113.

Weinberger, M. M., and Bronsky, E. A. (1974). Evaluation of oral bronchodilator therapy in asthmatic children. *J. Pediatr. 84*: 421.

20

Bronchodilator Management of the Adult in the United Kingdom

CHRISTOPHER HARDY* and STEPHEN T. HOLGATE

Southampton General Hospital
University of Southampton
Southampton, England

I. Introduction

Asthma has a reported prevalence in the United Kingdom of 2-4% of the population. However 11% of 2700 7-year-old school children studied in northeast England (Lee et al., 1983) and 27% of 2000 adults studied in Hampshire (Mortagy, 1982) had experienced recurrent intermittent wheezing during the preceding 2 years. The apparent discrepancy between the prevalence of wheeze and the clinical diagnosis of asthma may largely be explained by the fact that asthma in the general population is underdiagnosed and consequently undertreated. Even if a diagnosis of asthma is established treatment may be suboptimal. A study of the adequacy of treatment taken by 120 asthmatic subjects treated by two general practitioners in the London area reported a positive correlation between asthma severity and number of antiasthma therapies being taken. Patients with a forced expiratory volume in 1 sec (FEV_1) within normal limits received an average of 1.2 therapies compared with 2.4 therapies when the FEV_1 was less than 50% predicted (Horn and Cochrane, 1984). However, in this study only 50% of the subjects who had an FEV_1 of less than 50% of their predicted value were taking one or both regular β-adrenoreceptor agonists and

* *Present affiliation:* Wythenshawe Hospital, Manchester, England

corticosteroids by any route of administration. This and similar studies illustrate that for optimal treatment of asthma symptoms, the use of drugs must be accompanied by improved education both of patients and their medical practitioners. With the assumption that asthma is underdiagnosed and undertreated, this chapter presents current trends in the management of air flow limitation in the United Kingdom with particular reference to bronchodilator therapy.

Data on the sales of bronchodilator drugs in the United Kingdom during the years 1977-1981 showed a striking increase in prescriptions for sympathomimetic aerosols (42%) and inhaled corticosteroid therapy (69%) with lesser increases in preparations of theophylline (30%) and sodium cromoglycate (20%) (Keating et al., 1984). These changes in prescribing habits may reflect an increase in the number of patients being treated for asthma or an increase in the number of treatments each patient receives, a combination of the two, or increased use of bronchodilators by patients with obstructive airways diseases other than classic asthma. This chapter will concentrate on the clinical applications of β-adrenoreceptor agonists, steroids, methylxanthines, anticholinergic agents, H_1-antagonists, and cromolyn sodium as applied to the treatment of asthma and chronic bronchitis. The increased use of nebulizers as a form of inhalation therapy in the United Kingdom will also be appraised.

The ideal bronchodilator should fulfill certain criteria, particularly if it is to be used on a long-term, regular basis (Tattersfield, 1984).

1. It should be effective in producing its therapeutic effect with a satisfactory onset and duration of action.
2. It should be convenient to take.
3. It should have a low toxicity.
4. It should have an additive or interactive effect with other bronchodilators.
5. Drug tolerance should not develop.

II. Beta-Adrenoceptor Agonists

Beta adrenoreceptor agonists are the mainstay of treatment of asthma in the United Kingdom. On the basis of the pharmacology of these drugs, the selective β_2-adrenoreceptor agonists confer obvious advantages over the older nonselective agents such as epinephrine, isoprenaline, and ephedrine (Tattersfield and McNichol, 1969) (Tables 1 and 2). There are now many selective β_2-adrenoreceptor agonists to choose from which differ little in their speed of onset, duration of action, and capacity to bronchodilate. However, individual responses to the different agents vary, so it may be worth trying different preparations (Madsen et al., 1979). Many β_2-adrenoreceptor agonists are available in intravenous, oral, pressurized aerosol, and nebulizer solution preparations. Physicians should familiarize themselves with the efficacy and limitations of one or two of these preparations rather than practice polypharmacy.

A. Oral vs. Inhaled Therapy

Inhaled β-adrenoreceptor agonist therapy has many advantages over oral therapy. Thus in Europe a considerable body of opinion favors aerosol administration to the virtual exclusion of oral therapy, except for use by the very young and the elderly. Administration of drugs by the inhaled route results in targeting of high concentrations of drug locally to the airways, thereby minimizing unwanted systemic effects. In addition, the inhaled route of administration results in rapid bronchodilatation reaching maximum 15 min after inhalation and lasting between 4 and 6 hr. The major objection to inhaled therapy observed particularly at the two age extremes is difficulty in synchronizing inhalation with actuation of the inhaler. Poor inhalation technique may be circumvented by using a breath-actuated device such as the dry powder inhaler (Rotahaler) or by the insertion of a spacer device between the aerosol and the patient, such as a Volumatic (Allen & Hanbury's) or the pear or nebuhaler spacer (Astra) (Fig. 1). Alternatively, β-adrenoreceptor agonists may be delivered by nebulizer.

B. Correct Use of Inhalers

Up to 30% of patients with asthma fail to obtain maximum benefit from their inhalers because of an inability to use them correctly (Orehek, 1976; Paterson and Crompton, 1976). For example, it is reported that about 2% of patients do not remove the cap from the inhaler before use. Thus the technique of inhalation needs to be carefully taught and checked by the physician or assistant regularly. Allen & Hanbury's devised the following instructions in agreement with the Asthma Society and Friends of the Asthma Research Council of the United Kingdom, circulated to all practicing physicians in the United Kingdom in January 1985 (Figs. 2 and 3).

1. The cover should be removed from the mouthpiece and the inhaler shaken vigorously.
2. Holding the inhaler, breathe out gently but not fully and then immediately place the mouthpiece in the mouth and close lips around it. After starting to breathe in slowly and deeply through your mouth, press the inhaler firmly as shown to release the contents and continue to breathe in. Hold your breath for 10 sec or as long as is comfortable before breathing out slowly. If you are to take a second inhalation you should wait at least 1 min before repeating step 2. After use replace the cover on the mouthpiece.

Table 1 Selective β_2-Adrenoceptor Agonists Available in the United Kingdom

Drug	Selectivity β_2	β_1	α	Type	Route(s)	Advantages/disadvantages
Salbutamol (Albuterol) (Ventolin)	+++	+	–	Saligenin	p.o.s.r., p.o., mdi, rhlr, neb. soln, sc, im, iv.	Duration of action 4 hr, Volumatic spacer device, 200 doses per canister
Terbutaline sulfate (Bricanyl)	+++	+	–	Resorcinol	p.o.s.r., p.o., mdi, neb. soln. sc, im, iv.	Long duration of action: 16 hr Nebuhaler spacer device 400 doses per canister
Fenoterol hydrobromide (Berotec)	+++	+	–	Resorcinol	mdi neb. soln.	Long duration of action: 6-8 hr 200 doses per cannister
Pirbuterol (Exirel)	++++	+	–	Synthetic heterocyclic catecholamine analog	po, mdi.	Highly selective: 7 times as β_2-specific as salbutamol: Long duration of action: 5-6 hr 200 doses per cannister

Reproterol hydrochloride (Bronchodil)	+++	+	–	Resorcinol/theophylline derivative	po, mdi, neb. soln.	Rapid onset of bronchodilatation Long duration of action = 8 hr 400 doses per cannister
Rimiterol hydrochloride (Pulmadil)	+++	+	–	Catecholamine	mdi. neb. soln.	Short duration of action: 2-3 hr
Combined preparations						
Fenoterol hydrobromide and ipratropium bromide (Duovent)					mdi	β_2-agonist combined with an anticholinergic agent
Salbutamol and beclomethasone dipropionate (Ventide)					mdi	β_2-agonist combined with a corticosteroid

p.o., oral; p.o.s.r., oral slow release preparation; mdi, metered dose inhaler; rhlr, Rotahaler; neb. soln., nebulizer solution; sc, subcutaneous; iv, intravenous; im, intramuscular.

Table 2 Nonselective β-Adrenoceptor Agonists Available in the United Kingdom

Drug	Selectivity			Type	Route(s)	Advantages/disadvantages
	β_2	β_1	α			
Isoetharine hydrochloride (Numotac)	+++	++	–	Catecholamine	p.o.	
Epinephrine	+++	+++	+++	Catecholamine	mdi, sc, im.	Cardiovascular effects limit use
Ephedrine hydrochloride	+	+	+++	Catecholamine	p.o.	Urinary retention Cardiovascular effects limit use
Isoprenaline sulfate	+++	+++	–	Catecholamine	p.o., mdi.	Short duration of action: 2 hr
Orciprenaline sulfate (Alupent)	+++	++	–	Resorcinol	p.o., mdi, im.	
Methoxyphenamine hydrochloride				Catecholamine	p.o.	

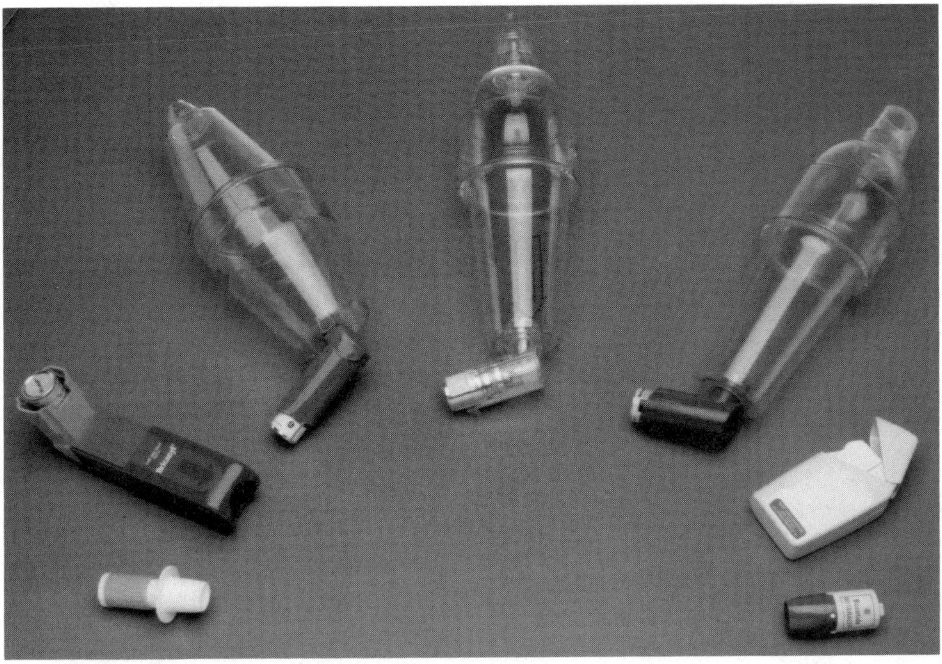

Figure 1 Devices for maximizing delivery of bronchodilator agents to the airways. Clockwise left to right: (1) Spinhaler (salbutamol, cromoglycate), (2) spacer (terbutaline, budesonide), (3) Volumatic (salbutamol, beclomethasone), (4) + (5) Nebuhaler (terbutaline, budesonide), (6) breath-actuated inhaler (rimiterol), (7) Rotohaler (salbutamol, beclomethasone).

In addition to these instructions the patient may also be advised:

1. To hold the chin up during inhalation as this makes a relatively straight passage between the inhaler and the lungs;
2. That only one actuation inhalation should be used;
3. Before using a new aerosol and on every occasion when the aerosol has not been used for a week or more, it is a wise precaution to test-fire it into the air.

C. Advanced Inhalation Techniques

For those patients who have mastered the standard technique there is evidence that two other methods of inhalation can increase the proportion of inhaled drug reaching the lungs (Dolovitch et al., 1981). These two methods involve either

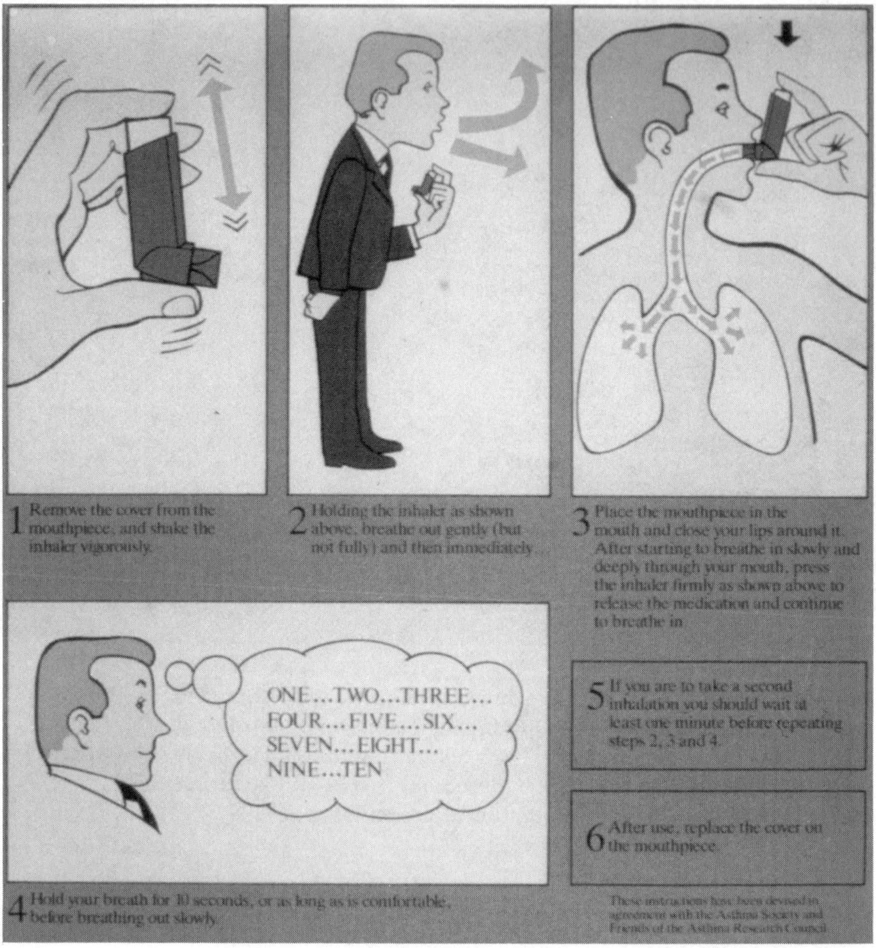

Figure 2 Instructions on the correct use of a simple pressurized aerosol (M.D.I.). (Printed with kind permission of Allen and Hanburys, Greenford, England.)

(1) holding the mouth wide open and placing the inhaler between the lips thus enlarging the oral cavity, or (2) holding the inhaler a few centimeters away from the open mouth and triggering inhalation.

D. Regular or On-Demand Therapy

Traditionally β-adrenoreceptor agonists have been used on an on-demand basis for the immediate relief of symptoms. Many patients with mild asthma prefer

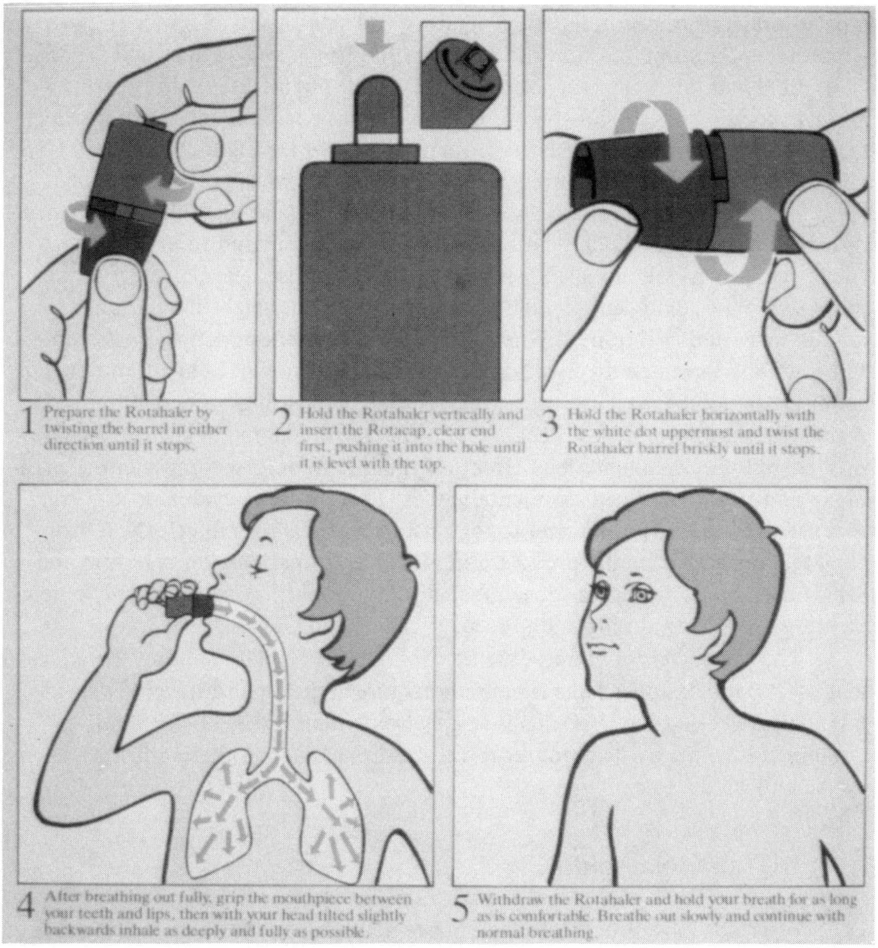

Figure 3 Instructions on the correct use of a Rotahaler (printed with kind permission of Allen and Hanburys, Greenford, England).

this regimen to taking regular treatment, although they often do so without obtaining maximum benefit from the drugs as assessed by objective measurements such as FEV_1. Many such asthmatics who have few symptoms prefer not to take regular therapy, fearing that a drug tolerance may develop. This point has also been of concern to medical practitioners, particularly following the reported rise in deaths of asthmatic patients associated with increased sales of isoproterenol in the late 1960s. There have now been over 40 studies conducted in which patients given maximum recommended dosages of oral or inhaled preparations have failed to demonstrate significant tolerance to β_2-adrenoreceptor stimulation in the airways (Stainforth and Tattersfield, 1983).

Beta$_2$-adrenoreceptor agonists possess a prophylactic role in protecting against specific bronchoconstrictor stimuli such as exercise, and when taken regularly they produce more even bronchodilatation throughout the 24-hr period. Therefore, any patient experiencing frequent wheezing or occasional episodes of more severe asthma should be advised to take these drugs regularly rather than on demand. The published data sheets circulated to practitioners advise patients to take inhaled β-adrenoreceptor agonist treatment of two puffs four times daily, supplemented by up to a further eight inhalations in any 24-hr period as required. Whether regular treatment with β-agonists confers any long-term benefit in chronic asthma is not known. Beta-adrenoreceptor agonists are potent mast cell stabilizers, acutely decreasing bronchial hyperreactivity in subdilator doses (Peel and Gibson, 1980; Salome et al., 1983) and may therefore have a beneficial effect on the inflammatory component of asthma in addition to acting as bronchodilators. There is some evidence, however, that regular use of β_2-adrenoceptor agonists have little overall effect on bronchial reactivity. Histamine provocation in eight asthmatic patients before and after treatment with regular dose inhaled salbutamol for 4 weeks failed to demonstrate any change in histamine recovery (Peel and Gibson, 1980).

The pressurized metered-dose aerosols conventionally contain the equivalent of 200 inhalations. Thus if patients require additional refill cannisters at less than 2-weekly intervals, this is suggestive of their asthma being inadequately controlled by β-adrenoreceptor agonists alone and that additional therapy is indicated.

III. Corticosteroids

Corticosteroids have proven efficacy in the management of chronic and deteriorating asthma (MRC, 1956a; Ellul-Micallef, 1981). Yet the evidence for corticosteroid therapy being of benefit once acute severe asthma has supervened is difficult to find (Grant, 1982). Difficulty in defining what acute severe asthma is may be responsible in part for the differing opinions on the efficacy of corticosteroid therapy. Clark defined acute severe asthma as an increase in severity of symptoms not mitigated by an increase in treatment (Clark, 1983). However, Luksza proposes that acute severe asthma is a completely distinct entity from deteriorating asthma, characterized by severe cardiovascular changes including tachycardia and pulsus paradoxus (Luksza, 1982a). Luscka studied 60 patients with acute severe asthma admitted to a general hospital in Liverpool. He found no additional benefit of corticosteroid therapy over that achieved with nebulized bronchodilators and intravenous theophylline (Luksza, 1982b).

All the asthmatic patients recruited into this study were of grade II-III disability according to the clinical assessment of severity of asthma of Sherwood Jones (1971). This, taken together with a high rate of assisted ventilation and over 50% of the subjects having received no corticosteroids prior to admission, suggests that the patients studied were highly selected and were neither typical nor perhaps relevant to patients with acute asthma seen in everyday clinical practice.

However, there are at least two studies suggesting that corticosteroids may be of benefit in acute severe asthma. In children, one prominent study demonstrated significant improvement in arterial hypoxemia compared with a control group not receiving corticosteroid therapy (Pierson et al., 1974). In a Medical Research Council Study (MRC, 1956b) 32 patients with "status asthmaticus" who had not responded to usual bronchodilator therapy (including subcutaneous epinephrine, inhaled isoprenaline, and intravenous aminophylline) 24 hr post-admission were allocated to one of two groups: placebo and bronchodilator therapy or a course of cortisone acetate commencing at 350 mg daily, tailored by 25 mg daily for a total of 2 weeks and similar bronchodilator therapy. Clinical improvement was monitored by chest auscultation and measurements of temperature, heart rate, and respiratory rate with no formal test of the airway caliber. After 4 days of treatment 10 of 15 patients allocated to the cortisone treatment group had significant improvement of the measured indices compared to only 4 of 12 on placebo. However, at 3 months postadmission there was no significant difference in the presence or severity of symptoms between the two treatment groups, nor was the occurrence of further attacks of bronchoconstriction influenced. In a randomized placebo controlled study, acutely ill asthmatics responding poorly to 8 hr of conventional bronchodilator therapy showed significantly more rapid resolution of airway obstruction on intravenous hydrocortisone, although blood gas values did not differ from the control group (Fanta et al., 1983). It may be concluded from these studies that corticosteroids are most effective in deteriorating asthma to prevent the onset of acute severe asthma, but probably also in the management of acute severe asthma itself.

The indications for corticosteroid therapy in asthma can thus be summarized as follows:

1. In chronic asthma where symptoms are not adequately controlled by regular β_2-adrenoreceptor agonist therapy, when corticosteroid therapy may potentiate the bronchodilatation achieved by beta adrenoceptor agonists in some patients (Shenfield et al., 1975).
2. In the management of deteriorating asthma, defined by an increasing severity of symptoms not responding to the patient's usual or increased bronchodilator therapy.
3. In the management of acute severe asthma.

4. Many authorities would also suggest a trial of corticosteroid therapy in any patient with severe airflow obstruction reflected by an FEV_1 of 1.5 liters/sec or less.

Turner-Warwick (1977) identified the following three types, based on the day-to-day patterns of airflow obstruction with peak expiratory flow measurements:

1. The brittle asthmatic exhibiting frequent and pronounced fluctuations in peak expiratory flow readings,
2. The early morning "dipper" characterized by nocturnal or early morning wheeze.
3. A subgroup of "irreversible asthmatics" who show little or no diurnal variation in airflow obstruction, and yet respond to corticosteroid therapy in the absence of response to other bronchodilator drugs.

This subgroup of asthmatic patients are in danger of being mislabeled as having chronic bronchitis, particularly if they smoke. Thus, a trial of corticosteroid therapy in patients with severe airflow obstruction is indicated even when the patient presents with a clinical pattern that is not "typical" of asthma. Ideally, confirmation of clinical improvement with corticosteroid treatment is best supplied by an objective measurement of airflow limitation such as peak expiratory flow rate (PEFR), since subjective improvement is not uncommon and may be related purely to an increase in well being attributable to systemic corticosteroid therapy. However, one point worthy of note is that patients may undergo considerable relief of symptoms by a reduction in lung volume that may accompany corticosteroid treatment without a major change in airflow measurement.

The advent of inhaled corticosteroid therapy, with the targeting of high concentrations of drugs locally to the airways, has reduced the need for oral corticosteroids with all their concomitant complications (B.T.T.A., 1976; Cameron et al., 1983; Hodson et al., 1974).

In the 1974 MRC Brompton Hospital trial 28 weeks of treatment of asthmatic patients already receiving oral prednisone with inhaled beclomethasone dipropionate (400 μg daily) resulted in a considerable reduction in oral steroid requirements (Hodson et al., 1974). This steroid-sparing effect was particularly marked in subjects originally receiving 5-9 mg prednisone daily, in whom beclomethasone enabled 50% of the subjects to stop oral steroid therapy altogether. In the remaining subjects who required more than 9 mg prednisone, inhaled corticosteroid therapy enabled a reduction in therapy to be achieved in 50%, but cessation of treatment was unusual. In a similar study of 138 patients being maintained on prednisolone (8-9 mg daily), inhaled beclomethasone dipropionate enabled 80% of patients to discontinue their oral therapy, and at 6 months

60% still required inhaled steroid therapy only. The mean daily reduction in oral prednisolone was 8 mg in those patients taking inhaled steroid, and 5 mg in those patients allocated to inhaled placebo (B.T.T.A., 1976). Thus, in moderately severe asthma not adequately controlled by β_2-adrenoreceptor agonist therapy alone, inhaled corticosteroids provide effective control in up to 75% of patients. Those subjects with the lowest FEV_1/FVC ratio often show the greatest response to corticosteroid therapy (Imbeau and Geller, 1978). The beneficial effect of inhaled corticosteroids is largely maintained even after 10 years of treatment (Kennedy et al., 1981).

A variety of inhaled corticosteroid preparations are available to medical practitioners in the United Kingdom (see Table 3), with little to choose between them. Recently, a combination inhaler, Ventide, containing salbutamol (100 mg) and beclomethasone (50 μg) has been marketed. Though patient compliance overall is more likely with such a preparation than prescribing the individual inhaled drugs, combined preparations represent an inflexible regimen. Inhaled corticosteroids are prescribed as a regular regime, usually two puffs three or four times daily. However, two studies have shown adequate control of most asthmatic patients with 4 puffs taken twice daily (Munch et al., 1982; Willey et al., 1982). Since oral corticosteroids are usually prescribed only once daily McGivern has compared the efficacy of a single inhalation of beclomethasone with the usual multiple inhalation regimen (McGivern et al., 1984). In all the subjects studied the dosages were designed so that the single dose exceeded the sum total of the multiple dose regimen. For the group as a whole, while taking the single large inhalation, asthma symptoms deteriorated and were accompanied by objective deterioration in peak expiratory flow rate measurements. The condition of two of the 12 patients studied deteriorated to such an extent while taking the large single inhalation that they had to be withdrawn from the study. Further studies are required to ascertain whether a larger single inhaled dose of corticosteroid than that used in this study is capable of controlling the symptoms of asthma.

Patients are frequently advised to inhale their β_2-adrenoreceptor agonist first, wait 5 min, and then inhale the corticosteroid to ensure penetration of the steroid aerosol to the peripheral airways. Several studies, however, have failed to show that this method of taking inhaled corticosteroids is any more efficacious than taking the two treatments in random order (Muers and Dawkins, 1983). Nevertheless, this sequence of administering the two drugs is logical and theoretically instructive to the asthmatic patients in helping them to understand the different modes of action of the two inhaled drugs and is therefore likely to increase compliance.

Inhaled corticosteroids, administered in larger than conventional dosages to patients who have not adequately responded to a standard dosage regimen, often results in further improvement in symptoms and lung function (Costello

Table 3 Inhaled Corticosteroid Preparations Available in the United Kingdom

Drug	Inhaler type	Metered inhalation/ actuation	Advised dosage regime (adult)
Beclomethasone dipropionate	1. pressurized aerosol	1. Becotide = 50 μg	1. 100 μg, 3-4 times daily
(Becotide, Becloforte)	2. dry powder rotahaler 3. Neb. soln.	1. Becloforte = 250 μg 2. Rotahaler = 100, 200 μg	1. 250/500 μg 3-4 times daily 2. 200 μg, 3-4 times daily 3. 100 μg, twice daily to a maximum 1 mg
Betamethasone valerate (Bextasol)	pressurized aerosol	100 μg	200 μg, 3-4 times daily
Budesonide (Pulmicort)	pressurized aerosol ± nebuhaler spacer device	200 μg	200 μg, twice daily to a maximum 1.2 mg daily
Combined preparation			
Beclomethasone dipropionate and salbutamol (Ventide)	pressurized aerosol	50 μg with 100 μg salbutamol	100 μg, 3-4 times daily

and Clark, 1974; Smith and Hodson, 1983b). However, in administering inhaled doses of 400-1,000 μg/day from a standard beclomethasone dipropionate inhaler (50 μg/actuation), Costello and Clark (1974) noted a threefold increase in the incidence of oral candidiasis.

In 1982 a high-dosage beclomethasone inhaler (Becloforte, 200 μg/actuation) was introduced in the United Kingdom. The effect of high-dosage beclomethasone (1,000-2,000 μg/daily) was investigated using this inhaler in 293 asthmatic patients not adequately controlled by either inhaled beclomethasone dipropionate 400 μg/daily (131 patients), or by inhaled beclomethasone 400 μg/daily in addition to oral corticosteroids (162 patients) (Smith and Hodson, 1983b). Control of the asthma improved in 62% of patients and was accompanied by significant increases in peak expiratory flow rates, and a reduction in the number of acute severe asthmatic attacks. Of those patients who were also receiving oral corticosteroids, 27% were able to discontinue their oral therapy, and a further 39% were able to decrease the dosage. Thus in those patients receiving 1-5 mg prednisolone at the start of the study, 35% were able to stop oral steroid therapy compared to 7% of those patients who were taking 15 mg or more of prednisolone. However, although 80% of patient who were able to discontinue oral steroid therapy had been taking 2-10 mg/day, the greatest mean daily reduction was achieved in those patients taking more than 16 mg/day. Overall, high dose inhaled beclomethasone achieved a mean 5.5-mg reduction in oral dosage, in addition to the steroid-sparing effect expected with beclomethasone dipproprionate in conventional dosage (Hodson et al., 1974). No increased incidence of oropharyngeal candidiasis was noted with high dose inhaled therapy compared to the use of standard doses (12% vs. 9%). It is important to note that although high dose inhaled corticosteroids are efficacious in chronic asthmatic patients whose condition does not respond to conventional doses of inhaled beclomethasone or those requiring large doses of oral corticosteroids, they are not advocated in the management of deteriorating and acute severe asthma when corticosteroids administered orally are still the treatment of choice.

Complications of inhaled corticosteroid therapy are few. They include stomatitis and hoarse voice, usually secondary to infection with *Candida albicans,* although with high doses dysphonia may be caused by a local steroid myopathy. Oral *Candida* infection is related to the frequency of administration rather than dose of inhaled corticosteroid (Costello and Clark, 1974; Smith and Hodson, 1983b) and infection rate is markedly decreased if patients rinse their mouths after inhalation. An occasional minimal suppression of the hypothalamic pituitary adrenal axis may occur, but even with doses as high as 2000 μg/day of beclomethasone this is not clinically significant (Smith and Hodson, 1983a). Fears that inhaled steroids would increase the incidence of chest infection in asthmatic subjects have not been substantiated in several clinical trials that examined the sputa of subjects for pathogens. Furthermore the prescription rate of antibiotics before and after institution of corticosteroid inhalers is no different (Toogood et al., 1977). Histologic and electron microscopic studies of lung biopsies from patients treated for up to 3 years with high dose inhaled corticosteroids have revealed no permanent pathologic changes (Andersson et al., 1977; Thiringer et al., 1975).

Oral corticosteroids are usually prescribed as a single dose in the morning, if possible on an alternate day basis, since this causes less hypothalamic-pituitary-adrenal suppression. In deteriorating asthma and asthma characterized by severe airflow limitation ($FEV_1 < 1.5$ liters), it is customary to administer a trial short course of oral corticosteroid in the form of 30-60 mg prednisolone daily for 1-2 weeks or until symptoms are controlled. The dose is thereafter rapidly reduced over a 2-week period, followed by reversion to the original baseline therapy. In severe airflow obstruction not responding to bronchodilator therapy, oral steroids are continued for up to 4 weeks and a decision based on symptoms and objective measurements is made as to whether or not to continue or terminate treatment. If a clinical response is achieved, then attempts should be made to decrease oral therapy rapidly and institute inhaled steroids, either in the standard or high dose form.

One of the main indications for corticosteroids in the United Kingdom is severe asthma refractory to β-adrenoceptor agonist therapy alone. Under these conditions corticosteroids have an additive rather than a synergistic effect. Inhaled corticosteroids control symptoms in up to 75% of asthmatic subjects, reducing the need for oral corticosteroid therapy with all its attending complications. Since asthma is an inflammatory disease of the airways (Laitinen et al., 1985), with acquired bronchial hyperreactivity being its attendant physiological consequence, some authorities are now advocating inhaled corticosteroids as a first line therapy for symptomatic asthma, any additional symptoms being controlled by β-adrenoceptor agonist inhalation as required. Corticosteroids for oral and parenteral administration available in the United Kingdom are outlined in Table 4.

IV. Methylxanthines

Only with the development of slow release preparations have methylxanthines been more widely prescribed in the treatment of airflow limitation in the United Kingdom. At present, the major indication for methylxanthine therapy is the presence of troublesome nocturnal symptoms (Barnes et al., 1982a). Outside of this indication, many physicians believe that there is little place for aminophylline and theophylline in the routine management of adult asthma and they should be considered only as adjuncts to therapy with β-adrenoceptor agonists and corticosteroids. This clearly represents a major difference in clinical practice compared to the United States. Methylxanthines administered by the oral route

Table 4 Oral and Parenteral Corticosteroid Preparations Available in the United Kingdom

Drug	Route of administration	Dosage	Relative potency ratio
Hydrocortisone	p.o.		
	iv: hydrocortisone sodium succinate hydrocortisone sodium phosphate	100-500 mg 3-4 times daily	5
Methylprednisolone	p.o.	up to 40 mg daily	
	iv: methylprednisolone sodium succinate	up to 120 mg daily for 3 days as infusion or slow iv bolus	1
Prednisolone	p.o. plain enteric coated	acute severe, deteriorating asthma: initially 40 mg daily until improvement, then a reducing regimen maintenance: 2.5-20 mg daily	1.25
	iv: prednisolone sodium phosphate	4-60 mg in divided doses	
	im: prednisolone acetate	25-100 mg once/twice daily	
Prednisone	p.o.	see prednisolone	1.25
Triamcinolone	p.o.	up to 24 mg daily in divided doses	
	im: triamcinolone acetonide	depot: 40-100 mg	1

Table 5 Xanthine Preparations Available in the United Kingdom

Product name	Xanthine	Other active ingredients	Sustained release
Amesec Capsules	Aminophylline 130 mg	Ephedrine Hcl 25 mg	No
Aminophylline Injection 250 mg/10 ml, 500 mg/2 ml	Aminophylline	–	N/A
Aminophylline Suppositories 50, 100, 150, 180, 360 mg	Aminophylline	–	N/A
Aminophylline Tablets 100 mg	Aminophylline	–	No
Anestan Tablets	Theophylline hydrate 60 mg	Ephedrine Hcl 15 mg Salicylamide 130 mg	No
Asmapax Tablets	Theophylline hydrate 65 mg	Ephedrine Hcl (as resinate) 50 mg	No
Bronchipax Tablets	Theophylline hydrate 40 mg	Ephedrine Hcl 30 mg Salicylamide 250 mg	No
Choledyl Tablets	Choline theophyllinate 100 mg, 200 mg	–	No
Choledyl Syrup	Choledyl theophyllinate 62.5 mg/ml	–	N/A
Do-Do Tablets	Theophylline sodium glycinate 50 mg/anhydrous caffeine 30 mg	Ephedrine Hcl 22 mg	No
Etophyllate Tablets	Acepifylline 250 mg	–	No

Etophyllate Tablets forte	Acepifylline 500 mg	–	No
Etophyllate Syrup	Acepifylline 125 mg/5 ml	–	N/A
Etophyllate Syrup forte	Acepifylline 500 mg/5 ml	–	N/A
Etophyllate Suppositories	Acepifylline 500 mg	–	N/A
Etophyllate Suppositories pediatric	Acepifylline 100 mg	–	N/A
Franol Expectorant	Theophylline (as monohydrate) 60 mg	Phenobarbitone 4 mg ephedrine 4.75 mg guaiphenesin 25 mg/5 ml	N/A
Franol Plus Tablets	Theophylline 120 mg	Ephedrine sulph. 15 mg, phenobarbitone 8 mg, thenyldiamine 10 mg	No
Franol Tablets	Theophylline 120 mg	Ephedrine Hcl 11 mg phenobarbitone 8 mg	No
Franolyn Expectorant	Theophylline 60 mg	Guaiphenesin 25 mg Ephedrine 4.75 mg/5 ml	N/A
Franolyn Tablets	Theophylline 120 mg	Ephedrine Hcl 11 mg	No
Labophylline Tablets	Theophylline 100 mg	Lysine 74 mg	No
Lasma Tablets	Theophylline 300 mg	–	Yes
Millophylline Tablets	Etamiphylline camsylate 100 mg	–	No
Millophylline Injection	Etamiphylline camsylate 700 mg/5 ml	–	N/A

Table 5 (continued)

Product name	Xanthine	Other active ingredient	Sustained release
Millophylline suppositories	Etamiphylline Camsylate 200 mg	–	N/A
Nethaprin Dospan Tablets	Bufylline 180 mg	Etafedrine Hcl 50 mg, doxylamine succ. 25 mg, phenylephrine Hcl 25 mg	No
Nethaprin Expectorant	Bufylline 60 mg	Etafedrine Hcl 20 mg, doxylamine Succ. 6 mg, guaiphenesin 100 mg/5 ml	N/A
Noradran Syrup	Diprophylline 50 mg	Guaiphenesin 25 mg, diphenhydramine Hcl 5 mg, ephedrine Hcl 7.5 mg/5 ml	N/A
Nuelin SA Tablets	Theophylline 175 mg	–	Yes
Nuelin SA 250 Tablets	Theophylline 250 mg	–	Yes
Nuelin Tablets	Theophylline 125 mg	–	No
Nuelin Liquid	Theophylline 60 mg/5 ml (as sodium glycinate)	–	N/A
Phyldrox Tablets (and tablets e/c)	Theophylline 128 mg	Ephedrine Hcl 12 mg phenobarbitone 8 mg	No
Phyllocontin Tablets	Aminophylline 225 mg	–	Yes
Phyllocontin Forte Tablets	Aminophylline 350 mg	–	Yes

Phyllocontin Paedriatic Tablets	Aminophylline 100 mg	–	Yes
Pro-Vent Capsules	Theophylline 300 mg	–	Yes
Sabidal Retention Enema	Choline theophyllinate 78.5 mg/3 ml, 157 mg/3 ml	–	N/A
Sabidal SR 90 Tablets	Choline theophyllinate 142 mg (= 90 mg theophylline)	–	Yes
Sabidal SR 270 Tablets	Choline theophyllinate 424 mg	–	Yes
Silbephylline Tablets	Diprophylline 200 mg	–	No
Sibephylline Syrup	Diprophylline 100 mg/5 ml	–	No
Silbephylline Injection	Diprophylline 500 mg/2 ml	–	N/A
Silbephylline Suppositories	Diprophylline 400 mg	–	N/A
Slophylline Capsules 60 mg 125 mg, 250 mg	Theophylline	–	Yes
Tancolin Childrens Linctus	Theophylline 15 mg	Dextromethorphan hbr 2.62 mg, Ascorbic acid 12.35 mg/5 ml	N/A
Taumasthman Tablets	Theophylline 100 mg Caffeine 50 mg	Phenazone 100 mg Ephedrine hcl 10 mg atropine sulf. 0.3 mg	No
Tedral Tablets	Theophylline 120 mg	Ephedrine hcl 24 mg	No
Tedral Elixir	Theophylline 30 mg	Ephedrine hcl 6 mg/5 ml	N/A
Tedral SA Tablets	Theophylline 180 mg	Ephedrine hcl 48 mg	Yes
Thean Tablets	Proxyphylline 300 mg	–	No
Theodrox Tablets	Aminophylline 195 mg	Dried aluminum hydroxide gel 260 mg	No

Table 5 (Continued)

Product name	Xanthine	Other active ingredients	Sustained release
Theo-Dur Tablets 200 mg 300 mg	Theophylline	–	Yes
Theograd Tablets	Theophylline 350 mg	–	Yes
Uniphyllin Tablets	Theophylline 400 mg	–	Yes
Uniphyllin Paediatric Tablets	Theophylline 200 mg	–	Yes

Products containing acepifylline, aminophylline, choline theophyllinate, bufylline, diprophylline, etamiphylline, proxyphylline and theophylline are included. Caffeine is also a xanthine but is included only when another xanthine is also present.
N/A = not applicable.

have been shown to possess a similar bronchodilator capacity to β-adrenoceptor agonists administered orally (Wolfe et al., 1978) or by inhalation (Marlin et al., 1978). These authors studied the comparative acute effects on airway caliber of inhaled rimiterol (500 μg), oral theophylline (375 mg), and similar doses of inhaled rimiterol 2 hr after administration of oral theophylline in eight patients with chronic asthma (mean baseline FEV_1 = 39%) predicted). The mean increase in FEV_1 of 30% was similar for rimiterol and theophylline when administered alone, whereas in combination an additive effect was apparent, achieving a mean increase in FEV_1 of 50% (Marlin et al., 1978). Thus oral methylxanthines produce significant subjective and objective improvement in up to 50% of asthmatic patients whose condition is not adequately controlled with β-adrenoceptor agonist and corticosteroid therapy (Greening et al., 1981). The reticence in prescribing theophyllines in the United Kingdom is related to their narrow therapeutic index (peak plasma levels > 20, troughs < 10 mg/ml) and the lack of the facility in monitoring blood levels. Achieving therapeutic plasma levels of theophylline is made difficult by the wide individual variations of absorption and pharmacokinetics after recommended standard dosages. The rate of elimination of theophylline is determined by various exogenous and endogenous factors, including the presence of other disease states, such as cardiac failure and hepatic impairment, interactions with other drugs including cimetidine (Reitberg et al., 1981) and erythromycin (Kozak et al., 1977) possibly as a consequence of altered hepatic P450, P448 synthesis, and smoking (Powell et al., 1977). Monitoring plasma levels is therefore desirable if not mandatory if theophylline and aminophylline are used. The necessity for monitoring serum drug levels has been emphasized in a study at the Brompton Hospital, where 130 consecutive outpatients on stable conventional oral dosages of theophylline were studied (Woodcock et al., 1983). Toxic levels of theophylline were found in 8% of these patients, whereas 49% had subtherapeutic plasma levels. It is interesting that a report of a toxic level always prompted a reduction in dosage, whereas a report of a subtherapeutic level resulted in an increase in therapy in only a third of patients. Similar variations in plasma theophylline levels were reported in 44 consecutive cases of deteriorating asthma admitted to the hospital in Malmo, Sweden (Toennesen, 1982). Five of the 44 had toxic levels with 30 in the subtherapeutic range, which emphasizes that although toxicity does occur in occasional patients undertreatment is more common. To facilitate the measurement of theophylline levels in a domiciliary setting there are now available blood spot tests (Gamlen et al., 1984) and assays in saliva (Koysooko et al., 1974; Ebden et al., 1984) both of which have been shown to correlate well with plasma levels.

Methylxanthines are particularly indicated in the more hyperreactive asthmatic subjects with nocturnal and early morning symptoms, for which there are a wide range of theophylline preparations available (see Table 5). Most physicians in the United Kingdom use slow release theophylline such as Uniphyllin, Nuelin SA or Aminophylline, either as a single nocturnal dosage or in a twice daily dose regimen. It has been suggested that twice daily treatment is unnecessary for the management of nocturnal asthma and that if the agent is only given at night, side effects are better tolerated by the sleeping patient. In the study reported by Barnes et al. (1982a), the nocturnal dose of slow release aminophylline was titrated to that giving a plasma theophylline concentration of approximately 10 μg/ml 10 hr after treatment. The mean variation between morning and evening peak expiratory flow rate was reduced from 22 to 5%, accompanied by subjective improvement with decreased night-time bronchodilator therapy. The doses given ranged from 550 to 775 mg, which are considerably higher than the manufacturer's standard recommended dose. However, these patients did not have severe nocturnal asthma, as evidenced by mean morning peak expiratory flow rates of 283 liters/min before treatment and 332 liters/min after aminophylline treatment. Several studies have shown that the pharmacokinetics of theophylline differ at night compared to the day, with prolongation of the half-life at night. These altered nocturnal pharmacokinetics may improve control of nocturnal asthma, yet also increase the risk of toxicity (Jonkman and Van der Boom, 1983; Primrose, 1983; Thompson et al., 1981). Thus an incremental dosage regimen starting from low doses such as 200 mg twice daily is recommended with plasma monitoring of levels in an attempt to avoid toxicity. The rapid release preparations of aminophylline and theophylline are rarely used because of the high incidence of side effects such as gastric irritation, headache, and CNS stimulation that coincide with the rapid high peaks of plasma theophylline. Various modifications such as choline theophyllinate are available which are reported to be better tolerated. Acepifylline (Etophylate), diprophylline (Silbephylline), and etamphylline (Millophyline) are better-tolerated theophylline derivatives, but their efficacy in relation to theophylline is doubtful and consequently they are not widely used (Table 5).

Methylxanthines are also indicated in the treatment of acute, severe asthma when they are given intravenously as aminophylline or, in subjects with ethylenediamine sensitivity, as lysine theophylline. They are usually given after nebulized beta-adrenoceptor agonist therapy if this drug alone has not produced useful reversal of symptoms. It is standard to achieve therapeutic plasma levels with an initial intravenous loading dose of 5.6 mg/kg aminophylline given over 15 min (Mitenko and Ogilvie, 1973) followed by maintenance therapy of 0.5 mg/kg/hr not exceeding 1/g in the first 24 hr. Plasma levels of theophylline should be measured as soon as steady state is achieved. When altered pharmacokinetics are anticipated, for example, in the elderly and patients with cardiac failure, these doses should be halved. Since an increasing number of chronic asthmatics are prescribed regular oral theophylline therapy, a potential problem in acute severe asthma is the inadvertant administration of standard doses of parenteral aminophylline with the potential of precipitating theophylline toxicity (Stewart et al., 1984). A thorough drug history should be taken in all cases of acute, severe asthma. If the subjects are taking regular oral methylxanthine therapy or have had intravenous aminophylline administered by their physician prior to referral to hospital, extreme care should be taken when considering the further administration of intravenous aminophylline. Such patients should be given nebulized β-adrenoceptor agonist alone and only if their response to this is not adequate should parenteral aminophylline be considered. Under these conditions the loading dose should be omitted and the maintenance regimen modified to give half the dose employed in the standard regimen.

Several commerical preparations of methylxanthines combined with a wide variety of other drugs are still available in the United Kingdom (Table 5). Most require a medical practitioner's prescription, but some may be purchased over the counter without a prescription. There is little to commend these preparations and certainly those containing sedative components should be avoided. The dangers of such medications was apparent in the Brompton Hospital study already referred to (Woodcock et al., 1983). Duplicate prescribing of two theophylline-containing preparations was responsible for the toxic levels seen in six of the asthmatic subjects, who represented 33% of patients who had toxic levels while taking oral theophylline. In these six cases a slow release theophylline preparation had been prescribed by the hospital and a combined preparation containing theophylline by the patient's physician. This may have been the result of poor communication between the hospital and the physician or, more likely, lack of awareness of the exact constituents of commercial preparations containing several components. The use of approved drug name prescribing, rather than proprietary preparation prescribing, a restricted use of compound preparations, and improved education of medical practitioner's might reduce the risk of duplicate prescribing.

V. Anticholinergics

Anticholinergic agents, acting as competitive antagonists at muscarinic cholinergic receptors, induce bronchodilatation by reducing vagal tone to bronchial smooth muscle. Atropine sulfate and atropine methylnitrate have been available in the United Kingdom for intravenous use and inhalation for many years but their systemic side effects, including urinary retention and glaucoma, have limited their use. However, the introduction of ipratropium bromide (a quaternary ammonium derivative) has stimulated a resurgence in the use of anticholinergic agents for the treatment of airflow limitation. Ipratropium bromide, administered by inhalation either from a pressurized aerosol or nebulizer, has provided an anticholinergic agent that exhibits bronchial selectivity because of its poor absorption into the circulation (Engelhardt and Klupp, 1975). It is surprising that this muscarinic antagonist has little inhibitory effect on mucociliary clearance or on increasing mucus viscosity, effects that have been attributed to its anticholinergic forerunners (Pavia et al., 1979). In the majority of subjects with classic asthma, bronchodilatation induced by ipratropium bromide is generally less than that achieved with β_2-adrenoreceptor agonists (Ruffin et al., 1977). There are, however, a small subgroup of asthmatic subjects who seem to respond better to ipratropium bromide than to β-adrenoreceptor agonists, presumably because their asthma is largely dependent on increased vagal tone. However, generally ipratropium bromide is only used in asthmatic subjects who are symptomatic despite regular use of a β-adrenoreceptor agonist or other prophylactic therapy. Some studies have suggested that there may be a small additive bronchodilator effects of ipratropium with β_2-adrenoreceptor agonists, but, if true, this is of questionable clinical significance. There is some evidence that older patients with asthma are more likely to respond to ipratropium bromide therapy than β-adrenoreceptor agonist therapy (Ullah et al., 1981). This may reflect a functional decrease in numbers of β_2-adrenoreceptors in this age group (Hume and Rhys-Jones, 1961).

Anticholinergic agents have also been advocated in the management of acute severe asthma (Fairshter et al., 1981; Altounyan, 1964). However, it has been shown that during periods of greatly increased airways resistance, as occurs in acute severe asthma, there is a progressive decline in the response of the airways to anticholinergic agents (Altounyan, 1964). Altounyan studied 96 patients with airflow obstruction. In these patients it was difficult to differentiate between chronic bronchitis and intrinsic and extrinsic asthma on the basis of a history and examination alone. He treated them all with 2 weeks of corticosteroids and divided them into two groups: corticosteroid-responsive (60 patients) and corticosteroid-nonresponsive (36 patients) based on measurements of FEV_1. The effect of nebulized isoprenaline and nebulized atropine methylnitrate was then compared in the two groups. He found that in corticosteroid-nonresponsive patients, atropine afforded significant reversal of airways limitation, the response being at least equal to, and in some cases greater, than that achieved with nebulized isoprenaline. This was a uniform effect and there was no correlation between the previous degree of airways obstruction and the relative efficacy of the atropine. Corticosteroid-responsive subjects also showed benefit from atropine of at least equal efficacy to nebulized isoprenaline, but only during phases of relative remission. Thus during periods of increased airways obstruction there was a progressive decline of atropine responsiveness when compared to the bronchodilator effect of isoprenaline. He extrapolated his findings to patients with corticosteroid-responsive airflow limitation (who might now be defined as asthmatic patients) and suggested that in patients already receiving corticosteroids a good atropine response implied adequate corticosteroid control, whereas a poor response indicated inadequate control. Similar findings of the decreased bronchodilator response to anticholinergic agents during an acute attack compared to a period of remission have been confirmed (Ullah et al., 1981).

In practice, ipratropium bromide is seldom used in the treatment of acute severe asthma, although two recent studies demonstrated that combined nebulization of ipratropium bromide 0.5-1.0 mg/ml with salbutamol 5-10 mg/ml produced a greater benefit than either drug when given alone (Ward et al., 1981; Leahy et al., 1983). Although ipratropium bromide has a longer duration of action than $beta_2$-adrenoceptor agonists its speed of onset is slower, with peak effects not occurring until 1-2 hr after administration. In addition, ipratropium bromide in nebulized form and possibly by metered dose inhaler may cause paradoxical bronchoconstriction. This initially was suggested to be due to the bromide moiety (Patel and Tullett, 1983) though the bronchoconstriction induced by ipratropium bromide nebulizer solution may be caused by the hypotonic vehicle in which it was initially marketed (Mann et al., 1984). As a consequence ipratropium bromide has now been reformulated as an isotonic solution.

In the United Kingdom there is now available a combined β_2-adrenoreceptor agonist, fenoterol (90 μg) and ipratropium bromide (36 μg) inhaler marketed under the name of Duovent. The use of ipratropium bromide in chronic bronchitis and emphysema, where it may have a greater therapeutic potential than in asthma, will be discussed in a later section.

VI. Sodium Cromoglycate

Sodium cromoglycate was synthesized in 1965 and shortly afterwards shown to inhibit exercise-induced asthma and antigen-induced early and late asthmatic reactions. The clinical efficacy of inhaled cromoglycate in chronic asthma has been demonstrated in several studies (Howell and Altounyan, 1967; Brompton-MRC, 1972). Comparison of cromoglycate with isoprenaline and placebo demonstrated that cromoglycate had a small variable effect upon simple objective parameters of lung function (FEV_1/FVC). However, cromoglycate did appear to be more efficacious than isoprenaline or placebo therapies, as evidenced by significant subjective improvement accompanied by decreased use of other bronchodilators and a lesser need to institute oral corticosteroids. Howell demonstrated significant clinical improvement in 10 corticosteroid-dependent asthmatic patients with decreased early morning tightness, decreased shortness of breath and wheeze on exercise, and reduced bronchodilator usage in all subjects, yet only 4 of the 10 showed spirometric improvement. He concluded that reliance on simple spirometry alone would have led to a failure to recognize the therapeutic value of cromoglycate. When asthmatic patients responsive to cromoglycate received either cromoglycate or placebo over 12 months, 50% continued to do well with placebo substitution, in comparison to 87% taking cromoglycate (Northern General Hospital et al., 1976). Hambleton found cromoglycate to be of similar efficacy to regular theophylline in chronic asthma (Hambleton et al., 1977). In view of the apparent efficacy and high margin of clinical safety, cromoglycate initially appeared an attractive candidate for the prophylactic treatment of chronic asthma. Although it is proven to be of use in children, its prophylactic use in adults is somewhat disappointing. Cromoglycate appears to be efficacious in up to 20% of adult asthmatic patients but there appears to be no way of predicting this small number of cromoglycate responders. There is no selective response in either extrinsic or intrinsic asthma although cromoglycate is often given to young adults with extrinsic asthma on an empirical basis and in the belief that its action is mediated. as a mast-cell-stabilizing agent. Cromoglycate may be administered as an inhaled dry powder from a Spinhaler, as a pressurized metered dose aerosol, or more recently by nebulizer solution, which enables larger doses to be administered (Hiller et al., 1977). Although therapeutic effect in asthma has been largely ascribed to stabilization of bronchial mast cells, antagonism of bronchoconstriction evoked by sulfur dioxide, inhaled adenosine, isocapnic hyperventilation, exercise, and propranolol suggests that cromolyn sodium has other actions in addition to mast cell stabilization. Its antagonism of exercise-induced bronchoconstriction may be due to the prevention of airway cooling (Cox, et al., 1971; Pichurko et al., 1984).

The therapeutic effect of sodium cromoglycate may not be apparent until 1 month of regular use and therefore any potential therapeutic effect should not be assessed until this period of treatment has been completed. Original studies suggested that sodium cromoglycate may have a steroid-sparing effect but this has now been disputed in controlled studies. Many of the early studies on the efficacy and safety of cromoglycate were carried out when the only alternative therapies were isoprenaline sulfate or oral corticosteroids. The recognition that inhaled selective β-adrenoreceptor agonists and inhaled corticosteroids constitute more effective bronchodilator therapy in the majority of asthmatic subjects has diminished the early popularity of sodium cromoglycate. A preliminary study of a new inhaled cromone sodium nedocromil, a paranoquinaline dicarboxylic acid, in a double-blind trial in patients with chronic asthma has shown this to be a potentially promising drug (Lal et al., 1984).

VII. Antihistamines

In 1946 histamine was shown to be a bronchoconstrictor agent in humans (Curry, 1946). Inhaled and intravenous histamine decreased vital capacity in asthmatic subjects with no effect in nonasthmatic subjects. Bronchial hyperreactivity to inhaled histamine is now a well recognized feature of asthma and is widely used as a diagnostic test (Cockcroft et al., 1977).

With its release from human lung mast cells, endogenous histamine is a putative inflammatory mediator in the pathogenesis of bronchial asthma. However, in asthma there have been conflicting reports of plasma histamine levels which may be related in part to unreliable assay techniques. The development of more sensitive radioenzymatic assays has shown that in stable asthmatic subjects there is an increased plasma histamine level (Barnes et al., 1982b), which exhibits a diurnal variation with increased levels apparent at night (Barnes et al., 1980). Taken together with the finding that asthmatic airways exhibit an increased sensitivity to histamine at night (DeVries et al., 1962), this observation implies a causal role for this mast cell mediator in the pathogenesis of nocturnal symptoms.

The development of the early H_1-antihistamines in the 1940s brought effective treatment to such allergic conditions as hay fever, rhinitis, and urticaria, but their place in the management of asthma is less certain. Little evidence to support their efficacy together with central nervous system side effects limited their use (Levy and Seabury, 1947). There was a revival of interest in antihistamines in asthma in the 1970s when the newer antihistamines were shown to be bronchodilators when administered parenterally (Popa, 1977). In contrast, when delivered by the inhaled route antihistamines invariably caused bronchoconstriction, with the notable exception of clemastine which was a bronchodilator (Nogrady et al., 1978). The bronchodilator effect of inhaled clemastine is variable, occurring in only 50 percent of asthmatic subjects with lower starting values of FEV_1 (Thomson and Kerr, 1980). In addition to their bronchodilator properties, antihistamines protect against a variety of nonspecific bronchial provocants such as antigen and exercise (Eiser et al., 1980; Hartley and Nogrady, 1980).

Further interest in antihistamines came with the discovery of H_2 receptors. H_2 receptors are reported to be present in the airways and cause bronchodilatation when stimulated. Cimetidine, a competitive H_2-antagonist when administered orally or by inhalation, has been shown to protect against exercise and histamine-induced bronchoconstriction (Eiser et al., 1981).

Recently there has also been renewed interest in H_1-receptor antagonists in asthma with the development of two new potent compounds, astemizole and terfenadine, which are free of anticholinergic and sedative side effects. In addition to a small bronchodilator effect, pretreatment with terfenadine attenuates the bronchoconstrictor response to exercise (Patel, 1984), with little or no effect on allergen- (Chan et al., 1985) and methacholine-induced bronchoconstriction (Patel and Kerr, 1985). Astemizole 10 mg daily for 2 weeks, administered to allergic asthmatic subjects, protects against histamine-induced bronchoconstriction and inhibits the immediate airways response to antigen, without significant effect on mast cell mediator release as assessed by the increment in plasma histamine levels postchallenge (Howarth and Holgate, 1985). In 58 grass-pollen-sensitive patients, astemizole 10 mg daily initiated before the onset of the grass pollen season, significantly reduced the subjective severity of wheezing during the hay fever season. However, more detailed clinical studies are required before these new H_1-antagonists can be recommended in the management of asthmatic patients.

VIII. Practical Applications

A. Chronic Asthma

In mild asthma, in which subjects may experience symptoms only after exercise or accompanying severe chest infections, it is common practice to prescribe an inhaled β-adrenoreceptor agonist such as salbutamol (Albuterol) only when symptoms are present (as required therapy) rather than regularly. The β-adrenoreceptor agonist may be inhaled either to reverse bronchoconstriction or prophylactically 5-10 min before exercise is undertaken. However, when symptoms become more persistent a regular prophylactic regimen of three to four times daily is preferred. Failure of this regimen to produce adequate symptomatic control requires a check of the patient's inhaler technique. If this is acceptable, a regular inhaled corticosteroid is advocated initially four times daily, then reduced if possible to a twice-daily regime. The majority of inhaled corticosteroids administered by pressurized aerosol involve the administration of 400 to a maximum 800 μg beclomethasone, 600-800 μg betamethasone, or 400-1200 μg budesonide daily. There is now available a high-dose inhaled beclomethasone aerosol with each actuation delivering 250 μg drug, with an advised maximum daily dose of between 1 and 2 mg. Inhaled corticosteroids control symptoms in up to 75% of asthmatic patients irrespective of whether their asthma is extrinsic (allergic) or intrinsic (nonallergic) in nature, and, in chronic asthmatics, reduce the need to prescribe oral corticosteroids. If symptoms are not controlled on a low-dose inhaled corticosteroid regimen, then transfer to a high-dose inhaled corticosteroid regime may prevent progression to oral corticosteroid therapy. When adequate improvement is maintained with inhaled corticosteroids, their regular use supplemented by β-adrenoreceptor agonist therapy when symptoms develop is favored over than using both agents regularly.

If response to inhaled corticosteroids is inadequate, then oral corticosteroids, such as prednisolone 30-40 mg initially, are instituted assuming that there are no contraindications to their use. If systemic contraindications are present, then any risks of corticosteroid therapy should be carefully evaluated. Oral corticosteroids, when administered in large doses (prednisolone 30-60 mg daily, dependent upon the size of the patient) enable the degree of reversibility of airways obstruction to be assessed. If a useful clinical effect is achieved the dose is then tailored to a maintenance dose and supplemented with inhaled steroids for their oral steroid-sparing effect.

The role of methylxanthines, sodium cromoglycate, and anticholinergics in the management of chronic asthma has not been fully evaluated and currently they form third-line therapy. As discussed earlier, the most common indication for theophylline therapy is in asthmatic subjects who experience severe nocturnal and early morning symptoms. Depending on the half-life of the theophylline preparation being used, theophyllines may be prescribed either as a single dose at night or as a twice-daily 12-hourly dosage. It is desirable that plasma levels be assayed 10-12 hr after administration to ensure that adequate therapeutic levels are achieved. If slow-release theophyllines are to be used effectively in treating nocturnal asthma, the dose must be progressively titrated until the therapeutic range is achieved or until side effects prohibit a further increase. Theophylline side effects may occur even with therapeutic blood levels. In the survey by Woodcock et al. (1983) side effects were most common with plasma levels in excess of 20 mg/ml (62% of their cases). However, in this study side effects were almost equally seen in 24% of patient with levels in the therapeutic range and in those with subtherapeutic blood levels of less than 10 mg/ml (6%). It is therefore theoretically possible to induce side effects while giving a dose unlikely to provide much clinical benefit. Slow-release oral methylxanthine preparations at night may be insufficient in controlling nocturnal asthma. Patients with severe nocturnal symptoms may need multiple drugs to diminish their nocturnal symptoms, including a slow-release oral β_2-adrenoceptor agonist (Fairfax et al., 1980), a high dose of β_2-adrenoceptor agonist by metered dose inhaler, and serious consideration for inhaled and/or oral corticosteroids. The response of nocturnal asthma to bronchodilator therapy is variable. At one extreme, treatment with a single drug may be very effective yet other asthmatics may be refractory to all available treatments. The reasons for these widely differing responses reflects the severity of bronchial hyperreactivity and the overall heterogeneity of asthma (Turner-Warwick, 1977).

The role of sodium cromoglycate and anticholinergic agents in the day-to-day management of adult chronic asthma is less clearly defined. Since most patients with chronic asthma respond to inhaled β_2-adrenoreceptor agonists and corticosteroids, the introduction of sodium cromoglycate, which is effective only in up to 20% of asthmatic subjects, has largely been superseded by these other more efficacious agents. There is a tendency for physicians to try their young, highly atopic (extrinsic, allergic) asthmatic subjects on sodium cromoglycate in the belief that they are more responsive to the drug than older patients, though objective evidence for this is lacking. As described earlier, Altounyan has shown that anticholinergic agents have a varying bronchodilator effect in asthmatic subjects and seem to lose their bronchodilator effect in more severe asthma. Anticholinergics tend to be used only when they can be demonstrated

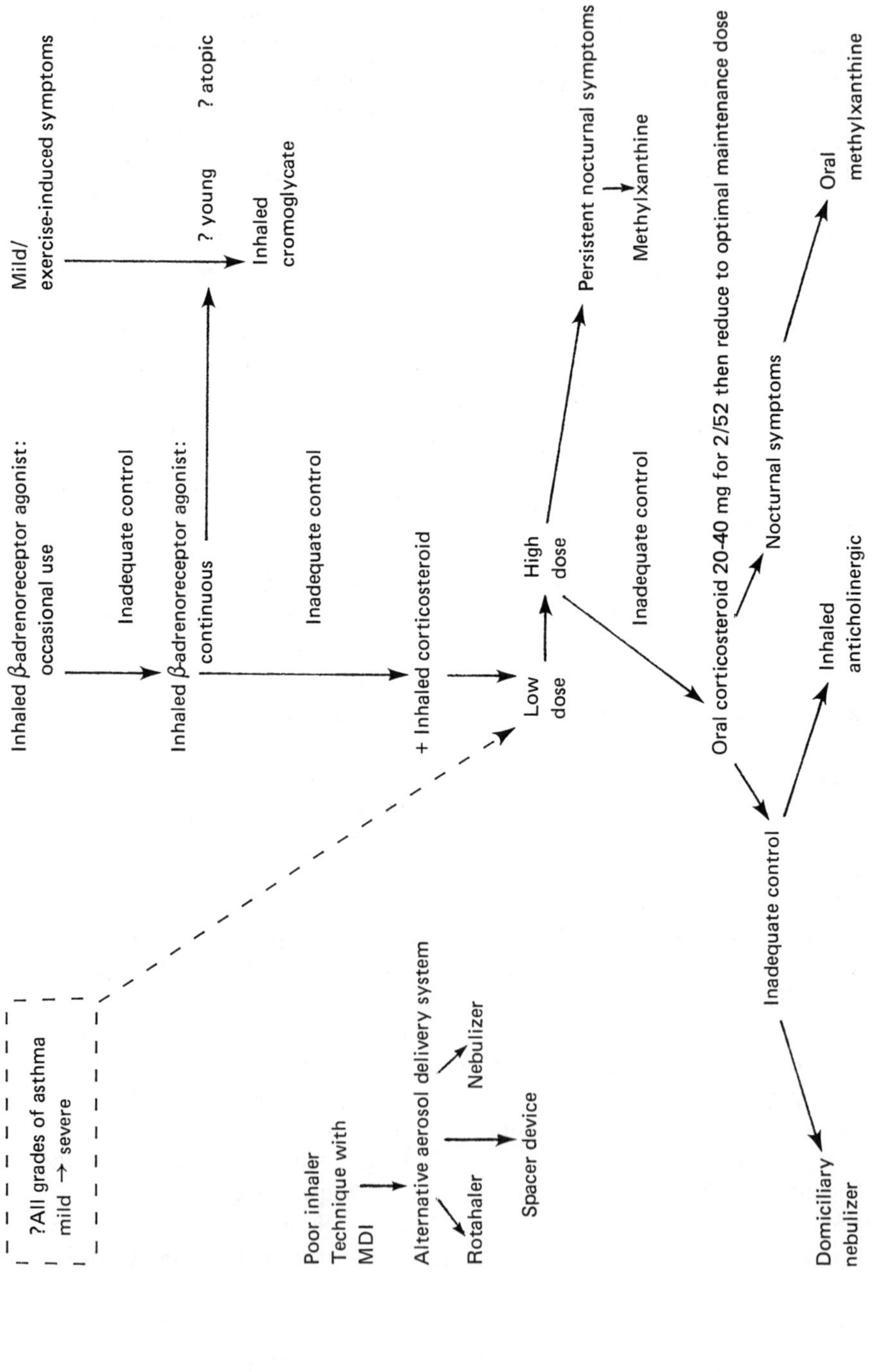

Figure 4 Management of chronic asthma in the United Kingdom.

to produce objective improvement in airflow obstruction over and above that produced by β_2-adrenoceptor agonists.

The management of chronic asthma in the United Kingdom is summarized in the algorithm in Figure 4. Suboptimal response to β_2-adrenoceptor agonist therapy may be due either to poor inhaler technique or the presence of severe resistant asthma. In such patients additional aids to facilitate the delivery and inhalation of the drugs such as breath-activated inhalers, spacer devices, or the use of domiciliary nebulizers may prove more effective than metered dose inhaler therapy (Fig. 1).

B. Deteriorating and Acute Severe Asthma

Theory

The difficulty in defining deteriorating asthma as distinct from acute severe asthma has already been alluded to and indeed many patients with acute severe asthma admitted to hospital have a condition superimposed upon a background of deteriorating asthma although occasionally these attacks occur more abruptly after a relatively trouble-free period. Despite the introduction of a wide variety of new and selective bronchodilators and the more widespread use of inhaled and oral steroids, it is worrying to observe that the annual death rates associated with asthma have shown no significant improvement in the United Kingdom since the introduction of epinephrine in 1890. Approximately 1,500 patients die from asthma in the United Kingdom each year.

Bronchodilator Therapy

Beta-Adrenoreceptor Agonists

Response to bronchodilator aerosols in patients with bronchial asthma declines with increasing severity of airflow obstruction, thereby increasing the need for larger and more frequent doses to produce a therapeutic effect (Hume and Rhys-Jones, 1961). This decreased bronchodilator responsiveness cannot be accounted for by failure of aerosol penetration to peripheral airways in the more constricted subject since, in these patients oral or intravenous β_2-adrenoreceptor agonists are no more effective than inhaled and nebulized salbutamol (Hetzel and Clark, 1976; Nogrady et al., 1977). The first-line treatment for acute severe and deteriorating asthma is nebulized β_2 adrenoceptor agonists such as salbutamol (2.5-5 mg/ml) delivered either by passive inhalation or with an attachment enabling intermittent positive pressure breathing (IPPB). However, Fergusson has shown no additional advantage of IPPB over passive inhalation (Fergusson et al., 1983). Alternative β_2-agonists available for nebulization are shown in Tables 1 and 2. Although nebulized bronchodilators are preferable in acute severe asthma, dry powder inhalers (e.g., Rotohaler) have been shown to be effective in 60% of subjects with peak expiratory flow rates less than 100 1/min (Webber et al.,

1982). Terbutaline, when delivered by a spacer mechanism, is as effective as administration by nebulizer (Morgan et al., 1982).

There are potential problems in delivering high concentrations of β_2-adrenoceptor agonists to the airways sufficient to achieve bronchodilatation in patients with greatly increased airways resistance. These include muscle cramps, tremor, and in susceptible subjects with ischemic heart disease, angina (Neville et al., 1982). It has also been shown that β_2-adrenoceptor drugs administered intravenously or by inhalation in acute severe asthma may increase the degree of arterial hypoxemia (Alliot, 1972). The mechanism of this drug-related increase in hypoxemia is considered to result from increased ventilation perfusion inequality in areas of lung where bronchodilators increase ventilation to underperfused alveoli. However, two controlled studies have failed to confirm increased hypoxemia in patients with acute severe asthma treated with high dose nebulized salbutamol (Gunawardena et al., 1984; Douglas, 1985). Douglas studied 32 patients admitted to hospital with a mean FEV_1 40% predicted and mean PaO_2 of 63 mmHg. In a double-blind study they were randomized to three doses of salbutamol (1.25, 2.5, and 5 mg) administered by air-driven nebulizers and observed for 2 hr, during which time they did not receive any extra treatment with corticosteroids or oxygen. At both 15 and 60 min postnebulization no significant change in PaO_2 could be demonstrated. In this study, however, nebulized salbutamol alone produced only a slight improvement in the degree of airflow obstruction with mean FEV_1 rising from 0.8 to 1.1 liters, and FVC from 1.3 to 1.8 liters. They also noted that maximum bronchodilatation was achieved 10 min postnebulization with no further significant bronchodilation occurring after that time. However, only one inhalation of salbutamol was given and the risk of aggravating hypoxemia could be greater with multiple dosing. In a hospital setting nebulizers for aerosolizing salbutamol are driven by oxygen and therefore the risk of hypoxemia is limited. At home, however, where asthmatic subjects self-administer their nebulized bronchodilators, which are driven by air compressors, the risk of drug-induced hypoxemia may be significantly increased.

Anticholinergic Agents

Ipratropium bromide is effective in acute severe asthma (Ward et al., 1981). Equivalent bronchodilatation to that produced by 5 mg nebulized salbutamol occurs with 0.5-1 mg nebulized ipratropium bromide. There is evidence that the combination of ipratropium bromide with a β_2-adrenoreceptor agonist may produce increased bronchodilatation over that produced by either agent alone. Salbutamol appears to further the bronchodilatation when given 1 hr after nebulized ipratropium bromide. However, when these bronchodilators are given in reverse order there appears to be no enhancement of bronchodilatation with ipratropium bromide over and above that of salbutamol (Ward et al., 1982).

Practice

Deteriorating Asthma

There is no simple formula for the management of the asthmatic with worsening symptoms. The physician must monitor carefully the response to therapy and modify treatment accordingly. Deteriorating asthma is characterized by worsening symptoms, fall in peak expiratory flow rate measurements, and increased bronchodilator aerosol usage. Any obvious precipitating cause of the deterioration should be identified and treated accordingly. For example, excessive purulent sputum should be treated with antibiotics. In all cases of deteriorating asthma, bronchodilator therapy should be increased in association with a course of corticosteroid therapy. Some general practitioners loan home nebulizers during acute exacerbations in an attempt to abort the attack, in the hope of preventing the need to hospitalize the patient with acute severe asthma.

Corticosteroids in deteriorating asthma are usually given orally either as a 7-day course of 40 mg prednisolone daily or as a decreasing course, starting at 40 mg daily for 2 days followed by a progressive reduction in the dose by 5 mg on alternate days. At review by the physician, the response to this treatment can be monitored and a decision made to continue with the corticosteroid therapy using the present regimen or to intensify or stop treatment depending upon the response. Some practitioners prefer to give a single intravenous steroid injection as symptoms begin to deteriorate. In a general practice in Oxfordshire it has been shown that hydrocortisone given intravenously (200 mg) to patients with deteriorating asthma diminishes the need for hospital admission (Arnold et al., 1983).

Acute Severe Asthma at Home

With the circadian rhythm of airway caliber many asthmatic subjects experience a severe exacerbation of their symptoms during the night, often after a more prolonged period of deterioration. Nowadays many general practitioners possess portable ultrasonic or jet nebulizers, making it possible to administer nebulized β_2-adrenoreceptor agonists as the first line of emergency treatment of severe and persistent attacks of asthma. Nebulized salbutamol 2.5-5 mg or terbutaline 2-5 mg in 4 ml normal saline are the most commonly used drugs. Ampoules of prediluted drug are also available. Since portable domiciliary nebulizers are invariably driven by air rather than oxygen, with concern about increasing arterial hypoxemia, caution should be taken about administering repeated doses or larger doses than those already mentioned (Douglas, 1985). If the practitioner does not possess a nebulizer than a spacer device such as the Pear or Nebuhaler for use with terbutaline, the Volumatic for use with salbutamol, or a dry powder inhaler (Rotahaler) for salbutamol convey advantages over the metered dose inhaler by increasing drug penetration into the lungs. If a nebulizer or the alternative facilities for aerosolizing beta$_2$-agonists are not available or if there is no significant improvement in symptoms 10 min after administration of the beta$_2$-agonist, intravenous aminophylline or β_2-agonist is usually helpful. Many regimens have been suggested, often depending upon evaluation of body weight. However, in practical terms for a general practitioner seeing the patient in the home, 250 mg aminophylline given by the intravenous route slowly (over 15 min) provides effective bronchodilatation with a relatively large safety margin. If the patient is already taking regular oral theophyllines, intravenous aminophylline should preferably be avoided or given with great care. Under these circumstances it is generally advisable to give a parenteral β_2-adrenoceptor agonist. The most commonly used are terbutaline 0.5 mg (subcutaneous) or salbutamol either 5 mg (intramuscular) or 250 μg (intravenous). In the United Kingdom these parenteral therapies have superseded the use of subcutaneous epinephrine, because of the latter's undesired systemic effects, particularly tachycardia. Parenteral β_2-adrenoreceptor agonists are occasionally self-administered by asthmatic patients who develop a sudden onset of severe life-threatening asthma, in an attempt to abort attacks. In addition to β_2-agonist or aminophylline therapy, patients with acute severe asthma at home should be given hydrocortisone 200 mg intravenously followed by a short course of oral corticosteroid therapy. A thorough assessment of the patient's previous maintenance therapy should be made and any necessary adjustments made. If available, the loan to the patient of a peak flow meter for readings three times a day will give a good objective measurement of the response to treatment.

It is unfortunate that many patients with deteriorating asthma are treated initially with antibiotics when there is often no evidence of a bacterial infection and corticosteroids are unwittingly omitted (Cochrane and Clark, 1975; MacDonald et al., 1976). In Luksza series (Luksza, 1982b), 48 of 90 asthmatic subjects admitted with acute severe asthma had received no corticosteroid therapy at all prior to their hospital admission. Similarly, only 2 of 16 young asthmatics in Auckland, New Zealand, dying from asthma had received corticosteroid therapy (Wilson et al., 1981). It therefore remains possible that the absence of impact of drug therapy on asthma mortality indicates that patients are either not receiving corticosteroids at all or soon enough when they deteriorate.

Acute Severe Asthma in the Hospital

Patients with acute severe asthma at home who do not respond promptly to treatment administered by the general practitioner are usually referred to hospital where management is easier, including facilities for continuing assessments. However, treatment of acute severe asthma in hospital is very similar to that in the home. Again, nebulized selective β_2-adrenoceptor agonists are the mainstay of treatment. These are usually administered at 4-hr intervals, though some physicians prefer to alternate a β-adrenoceptor agonist and the anticholinergic ipratropium bromide at 2-hr intervals. If the patient is unable to tolerate a mask or nasal prongs, or requires assisted ventilation, then the β_2-agonist may be administered by the intravenous route. It is common hospital practice to administer aminophylline intravenously and to provide simultaneously β_2-adrenoceptor agonists by the nebulized route. However, with the potential danger that many asthmatics may have already received preparations of oral theophylline and the published evidence that intravenous aminophylline may add little to nebulized β-adrenoceptor agonist therapy alone (Ward et al., 1982), the administration of aminophylline in acute asthma is undergoing review. Nevertheless, aminophylline administered by the intravenous route is highly effective in aborting severe attacks of asthma. Providing it is administered with care and the precautions about previous treatment taken, its use should not be dismissed.

Some physicians prefer to administer β_2-adrenoceptor agonists intravenously rather than by the nebulized route, although there is no evidence that this route confers any benefit over nebulization. Lawford et al. have compared, in 16 patients with acute severe asthma, nebulized salbutamol (10 mg in 10 ml saline), and intravenous salbutamol (20 μg/min) both delivered for 45 min (Lawford et al., 1978). Increases in FEV_1 of 40% were similar with both routes, as were changes in peak flow and arterial blood gas tensions. However, undesirable side effects including tachycardia and dizziness were apparent in five of the nine receiving intravenous therapy, of sufficient severity that it had to be stopped in two. Similar findings were observed by Hetzel in controlled chronic asthmatic subjects. Aerosolized salbutamol was equipotent to intravenous salbutamol, with less side effects and a longer duration of action (Hetzel and Clark, 1976).

The advised regimen for intravenous therapy with salbutamol is 250 μg by slow intravenous injection followed by an infusion of 5 μg/min, though infusion rates of 3-20 μg may be individually tailored to the patients response. Similarly, terbutaline may be given intravenously with a loading dose of 250-500 μg given slowly followed by a maintenance regimen of 1.5-5 μg/min.

It is usual practice to administer corticosteroids to patients with acute, severe asthma. Suggested regimens include bolus injections of intravenous hydrocortisone sodium succinate or hydrocortisone sodium phosphate 200 mg every 4 hr. In addition prednisolone is given usually in a starting dose of 30-40 mg daily. When the patient has responded, this is decreased by 5 mg on alternate days, until the corticosteroid is withdrawn altogether or a maintenance dose achieved. Prednisolone is available in an enteric-coated preparation which is suggested to be less ulcerogenic, although clinical pharmacologists believe that the ulcer-producing and exacerbating properties of corticosteroids are a systemic rather than local effect (Duprez and Simons, 1963). In addition, the degree of absorption of enteric-coated corticosteroid preparations is less reliable than the uncoated preparations (Mant, 1979), although the absorption and bioavailability of the newly developed cellulose acetate pthalate (CAP) preparation is more uniform and predictable than its shellac-based forerunners (Lee et al., 1979).

Some physicians prefer to administer parenteral corticosteroids by continuous infusion rather than as an individual injection. Intravenous hydrocortisone may be given in normal saline as 200 mg every 6 hr or prednisolone sodium phosphate may be given, up to 60 mg daily in sodium chloride.

In addition to treating the attack of acute severe asthma intensely, hospital admission also enables a thorough assessment of the patient's asthma, facilitating appropriate changes in baseline asthma treatment where required. Nocturnal asthma and early morning "dipping" may follow an attack of acute severe asthma (Shenfield et al., 1975) and require intensification of treatment.

A closer liaison between hospital practitioner and patient may be of benefit in asthmatic subjects who experience frequent severe attacks of asthma and in whom there is an increased risk of death (MacDonald et al., 1976). There are several centers in the United Kingdom, such as Edinburgh, where a hospital self-referral system is operative (Crompton et al., 1979). Lowry in Belfast has selected his high-risk asthmatic patients and carefully educated them in the correct use of their treatment, particularly with regard to instituting or increasing corticosteroid treatment in deteriorating asthma (Lowry, 1981). He also has arranged a 24-hr telephone link with the hospital so that patient can easily seek advice on adjustments in treatment and, if it is felt appropriate, may arrange their own admission to hospital. Such liaison with physicians may decrease the number of asthmatic patients requiring admission and may ensure prompt effective treatment of any acute severe attack. High-risk patients who may benefit from a closer liaison may be identified as those with a history of sudden or severe attacks, with severe nocturnal or early morning symptoms, or frequent attendance by a medical practitioner either in the home or with hospitalization (Research Committee of the British Thoracic Association, 1982).

C. Chronic Bronchitis and Emphysema

The role of bronchodilator therapy in the management of chronic obstructive bronchitis and emphysema is less clearly defined than in clinical asthma. Clinically many patients with chronic obstructive lung disease experience symptomatic improvement and increased exercise tolerance when a trial of bronchodilator therapy is instituted, yet often in these patients conventional dosages of β_2-adrenoceptor agonists reveal no obvious objective improvement with a tendency for bronchodilator therapy to be withheld. There are various explanations for this disparity between patient's and practitioner's observations. When airway dose-response curves to inhaled β_2-adrenoceptor agonists are performed in chronic obstructive bronchitis there is often no measurable response to conventional bronchodilator doses and yet with higher doses a response may be obtained (Connellan and Wilson, 1978; Prior and Cochrane, 1982; Corris et al., 1983). The dose at which maximum bronchodilatation is produced in chronic obstructive bronchitis is more variable when compared to asthma. Secondly the test of pulmonary function most appropriate to these patients may not be the forced expiratory volume in 1 sec (FEV_1) or peak expiratory flow rate (PEFR). Measurements of thoracic gas volume measured before and after bronchodilator therapy may be more appropriate than a measure of airway caliber (Jennings and Cochrane, 1984). Several studies have also demonstrated improvements in 6- and 12-min exercise testing in the absence of significant changes in spirometric values (McGavin et al., 1976), implying that the work of breathing is greatly reduced.

Theory of Chronic Obstructive Lung Disease: Which Bronchodilator?

Beta-Adrenoreceptor Agonist Therapy

Beta-adrenoreceptor agonists are effective bronchodilators in most patients with chronic obstructive lung disease so long as they are given in high enough doses (Connellan and Wilson, 1979). An additional potential beneficial effect of selective β_2-adrenoceptor agonists in chronic obstructive lung disease is that they increase mucociliary clearance (Santa Cruz et al., 1974), although there is little evidence to suggest that reducing the volume of sputum within the airways decreases airways resistance (Cochrane et al., 1977). Selective β_2-adrenoceptor agonists may also reduce the pulmonary atrial pressure in this group of patients in whom pulmonary hypertension is frequently present. Intravenous salbutamol causes small falls in pulmonary vascular resistance (Iodice et al., 1970) and similar changes have also been reported with oral salbutamol (Winter et al., 1984). Since in chronic obstructive lung disease there is a correlation between survival and the magnitude of the pulmonary artery pressure (Wietzenblum et al., 1981), fall in pulmonary artery pressure may be of long-term benefit. However, all of these have been short-term and long-term studies of systemic β_2-adrenoceptor agonists on pulmonary artery pressure are urgently required to determine whether their short-term effects on the pulmonary circulation are sustained. Generally most physicians still use inhaled therapy for its effects on lung volume and the airways, though by this route β-adrenoreceptor agonists do not affect the pulmonary artery pressure because of their deposition in the airways. Beta$_2$-adrenoceptor agonists may also increase cardiac output in patients with chronic obstructive airways disease. This may contribute to the increasing arterial hypoxemia observed in one study, probably resulting from increased ventilation perfusion mismatch (Peacock et al., 1983).

Anticholinergic Agents

There is evidence that the vagal component of bronchoconstriction is more prominent with increase in age and airways obstruction (Ullah et al., 1981).

Anticholinergic agents have been shown to be as efficacious as β_2-adrenoreceptor agonists in patients with non-corticosteroid-responsive chronic obstructive disease (Altounyan, 1964). Inhaled ipratropium bromide is an effective bronchodilator in chronic obstructive airways disease (Douglas et al., 1979). However, as is the case for β_2-adrenoreceptor agonists, larger doses of ipratropium bromide than used in asthma may be necessary. The standard inhaled dose of 40 μg four times daily may need to be increased to 120 μg four times daily to achieve adequate bronchodilatation (Gomm et al., 1983). There is also evidence to suggest that in some patients β_2-adrenoreceptor agonists and ipratropium bromide have an additive effect in producing bronchodilatation (Howarth et al., 1982). In a study of 12 patients with severe chronic airways limitation not responsive to conventional doses of inhaled β_2-agonists from a metered dose inhaler, whose mean FEV_1 and transfer factor were 35 and 45% of predicted values, respectively, a combination of ipratropium bromide (1 mg) and salbutamol (5 mg) delivered by nebulizer produced greater bronchodilatation than either agent administered alone (Howarth et al., 1982). Such observation has lead to the development of a combined aerosol inhaler containing fenoterol hydrobromide 90 μg, ipratropium bromide 36 μg by metered Duovent inhalation (Table 1).

Methylxanthines

The benefits of theophylline for chronic bronchitis have to be balanced against possible hazards, which may be greater in patients with chronic airflow obstruction than in those with asthma. Clearance of theophylline may be affected by age, smoking, the presence of cor pulmonale, concurrent respiratory viral infections, impaired liver function, and intercurrent antibiotic therapy. The efficacy of methylxanthines is controversial with many of the studies based on single-dose administration rather than on long-term maintenance treatment. In a study of 24 patients fulfilling the British Medical Research Council's criteria for chronic bronchitis and with a mean FEV_1 of 0.8 liters, oral salbutamol 4 mg, and slow-release aminophylline 450 mg as single doses produced similar, significant increases in FEV_1 of 8 and 6%, respectively, with no significant change in FVC. (Leitch et al., 1981). However, when both drugs were administered together greater increases in FEV_1 and FVC were observed of 22 and 13%, respectively. Improved spirometric performance on the combination of salbutamol and aminophylline was not matched by a significantly increased 12-min walk test over the study days on aminophylline alone and salbutamol alone. However, on each of the 3 study days there was a mean 6% increased walked distance. They also observed that the 12-min walked distance, although very reproducible for any individual, did not correlate with the subject's FEV_1. Eaton et al. (1982) studied 14 men with chronic obstructive lung disease with placebo or two doses of theophylline to achieve plasma concentrations in the low and high therapeutic range for 1 week. They found that although theophylline increased forced expiratory volume (7% low-dose, 12% high-dose) and increased heart rate (8% low-dose, 20% high-dose) there was no significant difference in exercise performance on treadmill testing or bicycle ergometry and no subjective symptomatic improvement.

A recent study investigated the response to slow-release theophylline in 20 patients with chronic obstructive bronchitis who had a mean FEV_1 of 0.8 liters and showed no significant bronchodilatation with inhaled β_2-selective agonists (Evans, 1984). Fourteen were considered to have emphysema based on low transfer factors (carbon monoxide transfer coefficient $< 68\%$ predicted). The doses of theophylline ranged from 200 to 800 mg to maintain "therapeutic" plasma levels. Changes in spirometry, subjective breathlessness scores using visual analog scales, and 6-min walk tests were assessed 12 hr after administration of oral theophylline and the results correlated with plasma theophylline levels. There was good intrasubject correlation between theophylline dosage and plasma theophylline levels, though there was a three to fourfold intersubject variation. In contrast to the earlier studies, theophylline, even at the highest dose given, produced no overall improvement in FEV_1, FVC, and PEFR though this was not totally unexpected since patients showing no bronchodilator response to a β_2-adrenoceptor agonist are also unlikely to respond to theophylline. There was no correlation between theophylline dose, plasma theophylline concentration, and 6 min walking distance, nor was any subjective improvement in the degree of breathlessness observed. The incidence of side effects was unacceptably high with theophylline doses of 600 mg or more. A study of patients with chronic obstructive bronchitis already stabilized on high maintenance doses of theophylline showed that theophylline alone failed to provide maximal bronchodilatation and an increased spirometric response could be gained by either inhaled β_2-agonists or atropine sulfate (Passamonte and Martinez, 1984). Niewoehner and Leatherman commented that this study did not investigate whether theophylline was necessary to achieve maximal bronchodilatation produced by these other agents (Niewoehner and Leatherman, 1984). However, theophylline may produce a bronchodilator response in addition to that produced by a β_2-agonist (Barclay et al., 1981).

It is also suggested that methylxanthines improve the mechanical performance of the diaphragm though this is of questionable clinical relevance (Moxham, 1984). In normal volunteers, intravenous aminophylline has been shown to have an enhancing action on diaphragm contractility observed during voluntary contractions of nonfatigued diaphragm. This effect is even more pronounced when the diaphragm is fatigued, both in reversing fatigue and to delay its onset (Aubier et al., 1981). Respiratory muscle fatigue is a contributing factor to dyspnea and respiratory failure in patients with chronic obstructive lung disease (Grassino, 1979). It is possible that pharmacologic activity of theophylline and related drugs may be of some benefit and result in improved subjective findings without spirometric change. In addition methylxanthines have a stimulant effect on the medullary respiratory centers (Dowell et al., 1965) and have also been shown to increase hypoxic ventilatory drive in normal subjects (Sanders et al., 1980). However in this study increased respiratory drive was based on the finding of a theophylline-induced increase in minute volume and some of the presumed central stimulatory effect of theophyllines may in fact have been due to increased efficiency of the respiratory muscles including the diaphragm (Roussos and Macklem, 1977). In general, the indiscriminate use of oral methylxanthines for treating chronic bronchitis seems difficult to justify, with their apparent small advantages and increased risks of theophylline intoxication when compared to their use in asthma (Mountain and Neff, 1984).

Corticosteroids

In most patients with chronic airflow obstruction, airflow is limited mainly by emphysema with distortion and diminished support to the airways. In a few patients with severe airflow limitation, the predominant pathologic features are inflammatory, accompanied by hyperplasia of goblet cells and enlargement of the mucus glands in the small and large airways (Mitchell et al., 1976) and smooth muscle hypertrophy reminiscent of asthma (Hossain and Heard, 1970). Corticosteroids might be expected to influence the airflow limitation in these patients where inflammation accompanies bronchoconstriction but would not be expected to influence the effects of emphysema. During acute exacerbations in both groups of patients, airflow may be temporarily increased by inflammation and bronchoconstriction (Fletcher and Peto, 1977) and in theory would be amenable to corticosteroid therapy.

Placebo-controlled studies in patients with stable airflow limitation have reported response rates to a 2-week course of oral corticosteroids of 17 and 23%, respectively (Mandella et al., 1982; Stokes et al., 1982). The responders did not readily identify themselves from the nonresponders but an increase in FEV_1 after a bronchodilator, spontaneous variability of the FEV_1, and blood eosinophilia were more common among responders, whereas a low carbon monoxide transfer factor and appreciable pressure-dependent collapse of the airways on an expiratory flow-volume curve indicated that a response to corticosteroids was less likely (Harding and Freedman, 1978). However, it might be argued that patients responding to bronchodilators or with a spontaneous variability in FEV_1 might be better classified as suffering from chronic asthma rather than chronic bronchitis and therefore, not surprisingly, respond to corticosteroid therapy. Since FEV_1 usually declines at a constant rate in heavy smokers of around 80 ml each year, a more rapid rate of decline is suggestive of an additional cause of their airways obstruction which may be relieved by corticosteroids (Fletcher and Peto, 1977). In a study of patients with chronic bronchitis during an acute exacerbation treated with both bronchodilators and antibiotics, FEV_1 increased by 40% after 3 days in only 3 of 21 patients, whereas when intravenous methylprednisolone 0.5 mg/kg every 6 hr was added to the regimen, 40% increases in FEV_1 occurred in 12 of 22 patients (Albert et al., 1980). This observation suggests that corticosteroids are efficacious in the management of chronic bronchitis with acute exacerbations, presumably through their anti-inflammatory activity.

A frequently used regimen of a "trial of corticosteroids" in chronic airflow obstruction is oral prednisolone, 30-40 mg daily for 2-4 weeks (Rudd, 1984). Inhaled corticosteroids may identify most corticosteroid responders, though addition or replacement with oral prednisolone may often result in further improvement (Harding and Freedman, 1978). A response to corticosteroids in most studies is taken as an increase of 20% in measures of airflow. However, a response in one airflow measurement is not necessarily accompanied by a similar change in another. The FVC may increase without change in FEV_1 (Stokes et al., 1982; Williams and McGavin, 1980) and occasionally home recording of PEFR indicates improvement whereas clinic spirometric measurements do not (Rudd et al., 1982). Changes in 12-min walking distances do not necessarily reflect changes in airflow measurements (McGavin et al., 1976). If the patient does not respond to corticosteroids when given as a trial of prednisolone 40 mg daily for 3 weeks, then these agents may be stopped abruptly with a return of pituitary and adrenal function to normal within 3 days of stopping treatment (Webb and Clark, 1981). Patients who respond symptomatically to a trial of steroids may subsequently be started on an inhaled corticosteroid preparation with gradual withdrawal of the oral steroid. At the time of writing there is no evidence to indicate whether long-term corticosteroid therapy of patients with chronic obstructive lung disease conveys a maintained bronchodilator response or has a favorable effect on long-term prognosis. It should be noted that chronic asthma may masquerade as chronic bronchitis; these patients often respond to a prolonged course of corticosteroids (Webb et al., 1981).

Practice

A trial of bronchodilator therapy is offered to all patients with chronic obstructive lung disease. Frequently symptoms may be inappropriately ascribed as being totally due to previous smoking habits. Bronchodilator therapy may not only identify a small proportion of patients with chronic bronchitis and emphysema who respond to drug therapy but may also differentiate those subjects labeled as having chronic irreversible airways disease from those with chronic severe asthma. Treatment is initiated with inhaled $beta_2$-adrenoreceptor agonists, although large doses are often required. The high-dose requirement, particularly when accompanied by poor inhaler technique, favors the addition of an inhaler aid for drug administration. Spacer devices such as the Volumatic or Nebuhaler are frequently helpful, though if they fail a trial of nebulized β_2-agonists is worthwhile. An objective assessment of response to long-term therapy is advisable using such measurements as symptom scores, spirometry, residual volume and exercise tolerance. Ipratropium bromide, in large doses (80-120 μg four times daily) may confer additional symptomatic relief on some patients (Gomm et al., 1983). If patients are unable to use any of the inhaler devices, oral β-adrenoceptor agonists or methylxanthines are worthy of trial.

A trial of corticosteroids is reasonable in patients with chronic limitation of airflow who, despite treatment with maximum doses of bronchodilators, remain symptomatic. Up to 20% of patient with chronic obstructive lung disease respond well to corticosteroids that may be accompanied by revelation of β_2-adrenoceptor agonist reversibility. A trial of corticosteroids will also reveal patients with chronic severe asthma masquerading as chronic irreversible lung disease (Turner-Warwick, 1977). The advised regimen of oral corticosteroids is prednisolone 30-40 mg daily for 2-4 weeks. By using such a short trial of oral prednisolone, inappropriate long-term therapy and its potential side effects are avoided. A study in 19 patients with chronic airflow limitation reported that in the majority of patients most responses were complete by the 8th day and all by the 11th day of such a course (Webb et al., 1981). Inhaled corticosteroids may identify most responders but later treatment with oral prednisolone further improves the condition of some patients. Assessment of response should include symptom scoring, regular spirometry together with measurement of residual volume and exercise testing. If there is a good response to oral corticosteroids it is advisable to substitute inhaled corticosteroid therapy. Very rarely does a patient who benefits from systemic treatment fail to respond to inhaled corticosteroid therapy. If the trial of corticosteroids has no effect then it may be stopped abruptly with minimal disturbance in adrenal function (Webb and Clark, 1981).

The treatment of chronic bronchitis and emphysema is not limited solely to bronchodilator drugs and corticosteroid therapy. Other supportive measures include health education and advice on stopping smoking, diuretics and digoxin where appropriate in cor pulmonale, domiciliary oxygen therapy (Nocturnal Oxygen Trial Group; 1980; MRC Working Party, 1981) venesection (Harrison and Stokes, 1982) and occasionally the addition of dihydrocodeine to reduce breathlessness and increase exercise tolerance in patients incapacitated with emphysema (Johnson et al., 1983). Patients with acute exacerbations of chronic airflow limitation benefit from intensive management including bronchodilators, antibiotics, and corticosteroid therapy (Albert et al., 1980), suggesting that the limitation of airflow has been increased by inflammation and bronchoconstriction (Fletcher and Peto, 1977).

Nebulizer Therapy at Home

In the last 2 years there has been a nebulizer "epidemic" in the United Kingdom (Editorial, 1984). Beta_2-adrenoreceptor agonists are the predominant agents nebulized, though ipratropium bromide, corticosteroids and sodium cromoglycate are also available for administration by nebulizer. In 1983, 17,000 nebulizer compressor units were sold. Most of these units were sold for use at home for the treatment of asthma and chronic airways obstruction, often without specific medical evaluation of the patients and adequate follow-up (Laroche et al., 1985). Nebulizers are of proven efficacy in the treatment of deteriorating and acute severe asthma (Grant, 1983), but their value in long-term domiciliary use has not been adequately tested either in asthma or in chronic obstructive bronchitis. Uncontrolled studies of long-term use of nebulized β_2-adrenoreceptor agonists in domiciliary practice have revealed symptomatic relief in bronchitis, emphysema (Conellan and Wilson, 1979), and some patients with asthma as reflected by a reduction in adjuvant bronchodilator therapy, though there has been no apparent improvement in resting lung function, nor frequency of hospital admissions (Higgs et al., 1984). Long-term nebulized β_2-adrenoceptor agonist therapy does not appear to induce tolerance (Higgs et al., 1984; Stainforth and Tattersfield, 1983).

When one compares the efficiency of drug delivery to the lungs by both metered dose inhalers and nebulizers (Newman et al., 1985; Lewis et al., 1981), 10-15% of the dose administered reaches the lungs by both routes of delivery. Similar bronchodilatation is achieved with a given dose by either delivery system, but dose for dose higher blood levels are apparent with a metered dose inhaler than a nebulizer (Cushley et al., 1983). This is possibly due to the period over which the dose is inhaled or secondary to increased alveolar absorption with a metered dose inhaler, since subjects inhale to total lung capacity rather than breathe tidally as with a nebulizer. Such high blood levels are attended by increased side effects such as tremor, tachycardia, and even angina (Neville et al., 1982). Nebulizers therefore provide a convenient way of delivering large doses of bronchodilator agents to the lung, which may be necessary in acute severe asthma to relieve bronchoconstriction, whereas in chronic asthma maximum bronchodilatation can be achieved just as efficiently with recommended doses from metered dose inhalers with and without spacer devices (O'Reilly et al., 1983). Thus, in chronic asthma the nebulizer may serve only to increase the risk of side effects rather than improve therapeutic efficacy. With increased doses, benefit decreases and side effects increase exponentially. Therefore unless there is clear evidence of patients benefiting from larger doses of β_2-adrenoreceptor agonists, low doses such as 2.5-5.0 mg are advisable. A recent questionnaire survey of hospital practice in Britain showed a five-fold variation in the dose of salbutamol used in nebulizers and a 20-fold variation in the diluent volume, with a resultant overall estimated 11-fold difference in the dose delivered to the airways (Stainforth et al., 1983b).

Two small groups of patients may benefit from nebulized aerosol therapy rather than metered dose inhalers. Coordination necessary to activate metered dose inhalers is often a problem in the very young and very old and when either hand weakness or deformity is apparent. In a small number of patients with very reactive airways the act of inspiration to total lung capacity using a metered dose inhaler may produce bronchoconstriction. In patients whose lack of coordination reduces the efficacy of a metered dose inhaler or who require large doses of bronchodilators to achieve their therapeutic effect such as in chronic obstructive bronchitis, spacer devices such as Nebuhaler or Volumatic or dry powder inhalations (Rotahalers) have often proven equally efficacious to nebulized aerosols (Cushley et al., 1983). They are also simpler to use and cheaper devices. Two types of nebulizer are available in the United Kingdom: the ultrasonic nebulizer and the air-compressor-driven jet nebulizer, such as an Inspiron nebulizer. Ultrasonic nebulizers do have the advantages of being silent in operation and may be more effective than jet nebulizers when delivering bronchodilators (Stainforth et al., 1983a), but appear to induce more cough and bronchoconstriction when administering hypotonic solutions (Lewis et al., 1984). This adverse effect of ultrasonic nebulizers has been ascribed to particle size and particle charge (Lewis et al., 1985).

Although nebulizers are useful in the management of acute, severe, and deteriorating asthma it is not clear whether nebulizers benefit patients with chronic symptoms as compared to other forms of treatment. It is the practitioners prerogative to identify patients in whom nebulizer therapy may appear the most appropriate. Thereafter, long-term prospective studies are required in the domiciliary setting to assess the efficacy of nebulizer treatment, with regular review of these patients. Other patients, many of whom nowadays request domiciliary nebulizer therapy after proper assessment using other inhaler devices, may be best advised to continue with simple inhalers or use a spacer mechanism rather than to purchase a nebulizer. Nebulizers for use at home are not available from the National Health Service, but some hospitals operate a short-term loan system.

IX. Summary

Bronchodilator therapy is of symptomatic benefit to patients with asthma and some patients with chronic bronchitis and emphysema. The effects of bronchodilators on longer-term outcome are not clear. In all forms of obstructive airways disease inhaled β-adrenoreceptor agonist therapy forms the mainstay of treatment, with much larger doses necessary to achieve a response in chronic bronchitic than in asthmatic patients. Where response is inadequate, corticosteroids, preferably by the inhaled route, may be beneficial in up to 75% of patients with asthma, and 20% of those with other chronic obstructive lung disease. With the exception of their use in nocturnal asthma, the role of methylxanthines and likewise anticholinergic agents in the treatment of obstructive airways disease is considered contentious in the United Kingdom. Since sodium cromoglycate is efficacious in only up to 20% of cases of adult asthma it has largely been superseded by β_2-adrenoceptor agonists and inhaled corticosteroids. The role of antihistamines in the management of asthma is less clearly defined and they are very rarely prescribed.

It is surprising that despite improved bronchodilator therapy, including the introduction of prophylactic agents in the past 30 years, there is still a considerable, possibly unacceptable, morbidity and mortality from asthma in the United Kingdom. Mortality statistics obtained from the Office of Population Censuses and Surveys show that 1500 people die from asthma per year in England and Wales. There is no evidence that the true prevalence of asthma has changed over this period of time, though this cannot be excluded. If the morbidity and mortality of asthma are to be reduced the detection, assessment, and management of patients with acute and chronic asthma in the community needs to be improved. In a retrospective analysis of 90 deaths from asthma the British Thoracic Association identified avoidable factors in 82% of cases. These included a failure to diagnose asthma (10%), a lack of appreciation of the severity of the attack of asthma by some patients (so-called "poor perceivers") (Rubinfield and Pain, 1976), their relatives, and their medical practitioners (Shim and Williams, 1980) with a resultant delay initially in seeking medical attention, but also in referral to hospital, and undertreatment, particularly with regard to corticosteroid therapy (60%).

Improved education of patients by both the medical profession and the British and Regional Asthma Associations, membership in which should be encouraged, may circumvent some of these shortcomings. Patients need to be taught how to recognize a deterioration in their asthma, particularly a failure to respond to their usual bronchodilator therapy, and the onset of nocturnal and early morning wheeze. Instruction is important in the appropriate manipulation of their bronchodilator therapy, including the institution of a short course of high-dose oral corticosteroids, and possibly the self-administration of parenteral β-agonists in sudden severe asthma. Finally, an explanation of when and how to seek emergency help when self-treatment fails is essential, and self-admission policies such as those in use in Edinburgh and Belfast are to be encouraged.

Acknowledgments

The authors thank the Drug Information Centre at Southampton General Hospital for helping in the compilation of comprehensive tables and Mrs. M. Dowling and Mrs. S. Foulkes for preparation of the manuscript.

References

Albert, R. K., Martin, T. R., and Lewis, S. W. (1980). Controlled clinical trial of methylprednisolone in patients with chronic bronchitis and acute respiratory insufficiency. *Ann. Intern. Med. 92*: 753-758.

Alliot, R. J. (1972). Effects of salbutamol and isoprenaline/phenylephrine in reversible airways obstruction. *Br. Med. J. 1*: 539-542.

Altounyan, R. E. C. (1964). Variation of drug action on airway obstruction in man. *Thorax 19*: 406-415.

Andersson, E., Smidt, C. M., Sikjaer, B., Hinge, G., and Poynter, D. (1977). Bronchial biopsies after beclomethasone dipropionate aerosol. *Br. J. Dis. Chest 77*: 35-43.

Arnold, A. G., Lane, D. J., and Zapata, E. (1983). Acute severe asthma: Factors that influence hospital referral by the general practitioner and self referral by the patient. *Br. J. Dis. Chest 77*: 51-59.

Aubier, M. A., De Troyer, A., Sampson, M., Macklem, P. T., and Roussos, L. (1981). Aminophylline improves diaphragm contractility. *N. Engl. J. Med. 305*: 249-2.

Barclay, J., Whiting, B., Meredith, P. A., and Addis, J. G. (1981). Theophylline-salbutamol interaction: Bronchodilator response to salbutamol at maximally effective plasma theophylline concentrations. *Br. J. Clin. Pharmacol. 11*: 203-208.

Barnes, P., Fitzgerald, G., Brown, M., and Dollery, C. (1980). Nocturnal asthma and changes in circulating epinephrine, histamine and cortisol. *N. Engl. J. Med. 303*: 263-267.

Barnes, P. J., Greening, A. P., Neville, L., Timmers, J., and Poole, G. W. (1982a). Single dose slow release aminophylline at night prevents nocturnal asthma. *Lancet 2*: 299-301.

Barnes, P. J., Ind, P. W., and Brown, M. J. (1982b). Plasma histamine and catecholamines in stable asthmatic subjects. *Clin. Sci. 62*: 661-665.

British Thoracic and Tuberculosis Association (1976). A controlled trial of inhaled corticosteroids in patients receiving prednisone tablets for asthma. *Br. J. Dis. Chest 70*: 95-103.

Brompton Hospital/Medical Research Council Collaborative Trial (1972). Long term study of disodium cromoglycate in treatment of severe extrinsic or intrinsic bronchial asthma in adults. *Br. Med. J. 4*: 383-388.

Cameron, S. J., Cooper, E. J., Crompton, G. K., Hoare, M. V., and Grant, I. W. B. (1983). Substitution of beclomethasone aerosol for oral prednisolone in the treatment of chronic asthma. *Br. Med. J. 4*: 205-207.

Chan, T. B., Shelton, D., and Eiser, N. (1985). Effects of an oral "antihistamine" on antigen-induced asthma. *J. Allergy Clin. Immunol. 75*: 141-146.

Clark, T. J. H. (1983). Acute severe asthma. In *Asthma,* 2nd Ed. Edited by T. J. H. Clark and S. Godfrey. London, Chapman and Hall, 1983, pp. 393-414.

Cochrane, G. M., and Clark, T. J. H. (1975). A survey of asthma mortality in patients between ages 35 and 64 in the Greater London Hospitals in 1971. *Thorax 30*: 300-305.

Cochrane, G. M., Webber, B. A., and Clarke, S. W. (1977). Effects of sputum on pulmonary function. *Br. Med. J. 2*: 1181-1183.

Cockcroft, D. W., Killian, D. N., Mellon, J. J. A., and Hargreave, F. E. (1977). Bronchial reactivity to inhaled histamine: A method and clinical survey. *Clin. Allergy 7*: 235-243.

Connellan, S. J. B., and Wilson, R. S. E. (1978). Nebulised salbutamol in adult asthma. *Lancet 1*: 662-663.

Connellan, S. J., and Wilson, R. S. E. (1979). The use of domiciliary nebulised salbutamol in the treatment of severe emphysema. *Br. J. Clin. Pract. 33*: 135-136.

Corris, P. A., Neville, E., Nariman, S., and Gibson, G. J. (1983). Dose-response relationship of inhaled salbutamol powder in chronic airflow obstruction. *Thorax 38*: 292-296.

Costello, J. F., and Clark, T. J. H. (1974). Response of patients receiving high dose beclomethasone dipropionate. *Thorax 29*: 571-573.

Cox, J. S. J., Woodward, G. D., and McGore, W. C. (1971). Solid state chemistry of cromolyn sodium. *J. Pharm. Sci. 60*: 1458-65.

Crompton, G. K., Grant, I. W. B., and Bloomfield, P. (1979). Edinburgh emergency asthma admission service: Report on 10 years experience. *Br. Med. J. 2*: 1199-1201.

Curry, J. J. (1946). The action of histamine on the respiratory tract in normal and asthmatic subjects. *J. Clin. Invest. 25*: 785-791.

Cushley, M. J., Lewis, R. A., and Tattersfield, A. E. (1983). Comparison of three techniques of inhalation on the airway response to terbutaline. *Thorax 38*: 908-913.

DeVries, K., Goeij, T., Booij-Nord, H., and Orie, N. E. M. (1962). Changes during 24 hours of the lung function and histamine hyperreactivity of the bronchial tree in asthmatic and bronchitic patients. *Int. Arch. Allergy 20*: 93-101.

Dolovitch, M., Ruffin, R. E., Roberts, R., and Newhouse, M. J. (1981). Optimal delivery of aerosols from metered dose inhalers. *Chest 80*: 911.

Douglas, J. C. (1985). Nebulised salbutamol without oxygen in severe acute asthma: How effective and how safe? *Thorax 40*: 180-183.

Douglas, N. J., Davidson, I., Sudlow, M. F., and Flenley, D. C. (1979). Bronchodilation and the site of airway resistance in severe chronic bronchitis. *Thorax 34*: 51-56.

Dowell, A. R., Heyman, A., Sieker, H. O., and Tripathy, K. (1965). Effect of aminophylline on respiratory-center sensitivity in Cheyne-Stokes respiration and in pulmonary emphysema. *N. Engl. J. Med. 273*: 1447-1453.

Duprez, A., and Simons, M. (1963). A propos de quelques drames abdominaux au cours de traitements à la cortisone. *Acta Gastroenterol. Belg. 26*: 609-620.

Eaton, M. L., MacDonald, F. M., Church, T. R., and Niewoehner D. G. (1982). Effects of theophylline on breathlessness and exercise tolerance in patients with chronic airflow obstruction. *Chest 82*: 538-42.

Ebden, P., Leopold, D., Buss, D., Smith, A. P., and Routledge, P. A. (1984). Saliva theophylline concentrations as a guide to total (and free) plasma concentrations. *Thorax 39*(3): 228.

Editorial (1984). The nebuliser epidemic. *Lancet* 789-790.

Eiser, N. M., Mills, J., McKrae, K. D., Snashall, P. D., and Guz, A. (1980). Histamine receptors in normal human bronchi. *Clin. Sci. 58*: 537-544.

Eiser, N. M., Mills, J., Snashall, P. D., and Guz, A. (1981). The role of histamine receptors in asthma. *Clin. Sci. 60*: 363-370.

Ellul-Micallef, R. (1981). Acute effects of corticosteroids in bronchial asthma. *Eur. J. Respir. Dis. 122*: 118-125.

Engelhardt, A., and Klupp, H. (1975). The pharmacology and toxicity of a new tropane alkaloid derivative. *Postgrad. Med. J. 51*(suppl 17): 82-85.

Evans, W. V. (1984). Plasma theophylline concentrations, six minute walking distances, and breathlessness in patients with chronic airflow obstruction. *Br. Med. J. 289*: 1649-1651.

Fairfax, A. J., McNabb, W. R., Davies, H. J., and Spiro, S. G. (1980). Slow releast oral salbutamol and aminophylline in nocturnal asthma. *Thorax 35*: 526-530.

Fairshter, R. D., Habib, M. P., and Wilson, A. F. (1981). Inhaled atropine sulfate in acute asthma. *Respiration 42*: 263-272.

Fanta, C. H., Rossing, T. H., and McFadden, E. R. Jr. (1983). Glucocorticoids in acute asthma. A critical controlled trial. *Am. J. Med. 74*: 845.

Fergusson, R. J., Carmichael, J., Rafferty, P., Willey, R. F., Crompton, G. K., and Grant, I. W. B. (1983). Nebulised salbutamol in life-threatening asthma, is IPPB necessary? *Br. J. Dis. Chest 77*: 255-261.

Fletcher, C., and Peto, R. (1977). The natural history of chronic airflow obstruction. *Br. Med. J. 1*: 1645-1648.

Gamlen, T. R., Coombes, E. J., Batstone, G. F., Cushley, M. J., and Holgate, S. T. (1984). Monitoring theophylline therapy using dried blood spot samples. *Thorax 39*(3): 228.

Gomm, S. A., Keaney, N. P., Hunt, L. P., Allen, S. C., and Stretton, T. J. (1983). Dose-response comparison of ipratropium bromide from a metered dose inhaler and by jet nebulisation. *Thorax 38*: 297-301.

Grant, I. W. B. (1982). Are corticosteroids necessary in the treatment of severe acute asthma? *Br. J. Dis. Chest 76*: 125-129.

Grant, I. W. B. (1983). Asthma in New Zealand. *Br. Med. J. 286*: 374-377.

Grassino, A. (1979). Inspiratory muscle fatigue as a factor limiting exercise. *Bull. Eur. Physiopathol. Respir. 15*: 105-111.

Greening, A. P., Baillie, E., Gribbin, H. R., and Pride, N. B. (1981). Sustained release oral aminophylline in patients with airflow obstruction. *Thorax 36*: 303-307.

Gunawardena, K. A., Patel, B., Campbell, I. A., MacDonald, J. B., and Smith, A. P. (1984). Oxygen as a driving gas for nebulisers. Safe or dangerous? *Br. Med. J. 288*: 272-274.

Hambleton, G., Weinberger, M., Taylor, J., Cavanaugh, M., Ginchansky, E., Godfrey, S., Tooley, M., Bell, T., and Greenberg, S. (1977). Comparison of cromoglycate (cromolyn) and theophylline in controlling symptoms of chronic asthma. A collaborative study. *Lancet 1*: 381-385.

Harding, S. M., and Freedman, S. (1978). A comparison of oral and inhaled steroids in patients with chronic airways obstruction: Features determining response. *Thorax 33*: 214-218.

Harrison, B. D. W., and Stokes, T. C. (1982). Secondary polycythaemia, its causes effects and treatment. *Br. J. Dis. Chest 76*: 313-340.

Hartley, J. P. R., and Nogrady, S. G. (1980). Effect of an inhaled antihistamine on exercise-induced asthma. *Thorax 35*: 675-679.

Hetzel, M. R., and Clark, T. J. (1976). Comparison of intravenous and aerosol salbutamol. *Br. Med. J. 2*: 919.

Higgs, C. M. B., Harvey, J. E., Jones, P., and Tanser, A. R. (1984). Effects of long-term domiciliary nebuliser treatment. *Thorax 39*: 689.

Hiller, E. J., Milner, A. D., Lenney, W. (1977). Nebulised sodium cromoglycate in young asthmatic children. *Arch. Dis. Child. 52*: 875-876.

Hodson, M. E., Batten, J. C., Clarke, S. W., and Gregg, I. (1974). Beclomethasone dipropionate aerosol in asthma. *Am. Rev. Respir. Dis. 110*: 403-408.

Horn, C. R., and Cochrane, G. M. (1984). Undertreatment of asthma in general practice. *Thorax 39*: 687.

Hossain, S., and Heard, B. E. (1970). Hyperplasia of bronchial muscle in chronic bronchitis. *J. Pathol. 101*: 171-184.

Howarth, P. H., and Holgate, S. T. (1985). Astemizole, a H_1-antagonist in allergic asthma. *J. Allergy Clin. Immunol. 75*: 166: 248.

Howarth, P. H., Stainforth, J. N., and Holgate, S. T. (1982). Bronchodilator efficacy of nebulised salbutamol and ipratropium bromide in chronic airflow obstruction. *Thorax 37*: 789.

Howell, J. B. L., and Altounyan, R. E. C. (1967). A double blind trial of disodium cromoglycate in the treatment of allergic bronchial asthma. *Lancet 2*: 539-542.

Hume, K. M., and Rhys-Jones, E. (1961). The response to bronchodilators in intrinsic asthma. *Q. J. Med. 30*: 189-199.
Imbeau, S. A., and Geller, M. (1978). Aerosol beclomethasone treatment of chronic severe asthma. *JAMA 240*: 1260-1262.
Iodice, F., Rufolo, L., Piscione, F., and De Michele, G. (1980). Haemodynamic and ventilatory effects of intravenous salbutamol in patients affected by COLD. *Respiration 40*: 272-277.
Jennings, S., and Cochrane, G. M. (1984). Complex pulmonary function data. *Chest 85*: 712.
Johnson, M. A., Woodcock, A. A., and Geddes, D. M. (1983). Dihydrocodeine for breathlessness in pink puffers. *Br. Med. J. 286*: 675.
Jonkman, J. H. G., and Vander Boom, W. J. V. (1983). Nocturnal theophylline plasma concentration. *Lancet 1*: 1278-1279.
Keating, G., Mitchell, E. A., Jackson, R., Beaglehole, R., and Rea, H. (1984). Trends in sales of drugs for asthma in New Zealand, Australia and the United Kingdom, 1975-81. *Br. Med. J. 289*: 348-351.
Kennedy, M. C. S., Haslock, M. R., and Thursby-Pelham, D. C. (1981). Aerosol therapy for asthma: a 10 year follow-up of treatment with beclomethasone dipropionate in 100 asthmatic patients. *Pharmatherapeutica 2*:648-657.
Koysooko, R., Ellis, E. F., and Levy, G. (1974). Relationship between theophylline concentration in plasma and saliva of man. *Clin. Pharmacol. Ther. 15*: 454-60.
Kozak, P. P., Cummins, L. H., and Gillman, S. A. (1977). Administration of erythromycin to patients on theophylline. *J. Allergy Clin. Immunol. 60*: 149-151.
Laitinen, L. A., Neino, M., Laitinen, A., Kava, T., Haahtela, T., (1985). Damage of the airway epithelium and bronchial reactivity in patients with asthma. *Am. Rev. Respir. Dis. 131*: 599-606.
Lal, S., Malhotra, S., Gribben, D., and Hodder, O. (1984). Nedocromil sodium: A new drug for the management of bronchial asthma. *Thorax 39*: 809-812.
Laroche, C. M., Harris, A. V. K., Newton, R. C. F., and Britton, M. G. (1985). Domiciliary nebulisers in asthma: A district survey. *Br. Med. J. 290*: 1611-1613.
Lawford, P., Jones, B. J. M., and Milledge, J. S. (1978). Comparison of intravenous and nebulised salbutamol in initial treatment of severe asthma. *Br. Med. J. 1* (6105) 84.
Leahy, B. C., Gomm, S. A., and Allen, S. C. (1983). Comparison of nebulised salbutamol with nebulised ipratropium bromide in acute asthma. *Br. J. Dis. Chest 77*: 159-163.
Lee, D. A. H., Taylor, G. M., Walker, J. G., and James, V. H. T. (1979). The effect of food and tablet formulation on plasma prednisolone levels following administration of enteric-coated tablets. *Br. J. Clin. Pharmacol. 7*:523-528.

Lee, D. A., Winslow, N. R., Speight, A. W. P., and Hay, E. W. (1983). Prevalence and spectrum of asthma in childhood. *Br. Med. J. 286*: 1256-1258.

Leitch, A. C., Morgan, A., Ellis, D. A., Bell, G., Haslett, C., and McHardy, G. J. R. (1981). Effect of oral salbutamol and slow release aminophylline on exercise tolerance in chronic bronchitis. *Thorax 36*: 787-789.

Levy, L., and Seabury, J. H. (1947). Spirometric evaluation of benadryl in asthma. *J. Allergy 18*: 244-250.

Lewis, R. A., Fleming, J. S., Balachandran, W., and Tattersfield, A. E. (1981). Particle size distribution and deposition from a jet nebuliser: Influence of humidity and temperature. *Clin. Sci. 62*: 5P.

Lewis, R. A., Ellis, C. J., Fleming, J. S., and Balachandran, V. W. (1984). Ultrasonic and jet nebulisers: Differences in their physical properties and fractional deposition and in the airway response to nebulised water and saline solutions. *Thorax 39*: 712.

Lewis, R. A., Ellis, C. J., Bailey, A., Hashish, A., and Balachandran, W. (1985). Cough induced by ultrasonically nebulised water is related to aerosol particle charge. *Thorax 40*: 718-719.

Lowry, R. (1981). Oral theophylline and fatal asthma. *Lancet 2*: 200.

Luksza, Q. (1982a). A new look at adult asthma. *Br. J. Dis. Chest 76*:1-14.

Luksza, A. R. (1982b). Acute severe asthma treated without steroids. *Br. J. Dis. Chest 76*: 15-19.

MacDonald, J. B., Seaton, A., and Williams, D. A. (1976). Asthma deaths in Cardiff, 1963-1974: 90 deaths outside hospital. *Br. Med. J. 1*: 1493-95.

Madsen, B. W., Tandon, M. K., and Paterson, J. W. (1979). Cross-over study of the efficacy of four B_2-sympathomimetic bronchodilator aerosols. *Br. J. Clin. Pharmacol. 8*(1): 75-82.

Mann, J. S., Howarth, P. H., and Holgate, S. T. (1984). Bronchoconstriction induced by nebulised ipratropium bromide: Relation to hypotonicity. *Br. Med. J. 289*: 469.

Mant, T. G. K. (1979). Investigation of a case of prednisolone malabsorption. *Postgrad. Med. J. 55*: 421-422.

Marlin, G. E., Hartnett, B. J. S., and Hacket, N. B. (1978). Assessment of combined oral theophylline and inhaled B-adrenoreceptor agonist bronchodilator therapy. *Br. J. Clin. Pharmacol. 5*: 45-50.

Marlin, G. G., Berend, N., and Harrison, A. C. (1979). Combined cholinergic antagonist and B_2-adrenoceptor agonist bronchodilator therapy by inhalation. *Aust. N.Z. J. Med. 9*: 511.

McGavin, C. R., Gupta, S. P., and McHardy, G. J. R. (1976). Twelve minute walking test for assessing disability in chronic bronchitis. *Br. Med. J. 1*: 822-3.

McGivern, D. V., Ward, M., MacFarlane, J. T., and Roderick Smith, W. H. (1984). Failure of once daily inhaled corticosteroid treatment to control chronic asthma. *Thorax 39*: 933-934.

Medical Research Council Working Party (1981). Long term domiciliary oxygen therapy in chronic hypoxic cor pulmonale complicating chronic bronchitis and emphysema. A clinical trial. *Lancet 1*: 681-685.

Mendella, L. A., Manfreda, J., Warren, C. P. W., and Anthonisen, N. R. (1982). Steroid response in stable chronic obstructive pulmonary disease. *Ann. Intern. Med. 96*: 17-21.

Mitchell, R. S., Standford, R. E., Johnson, J. M., Silvers, G. W., Dart, G., and George, M. S. (1976). The morphologic features of the bronchi, bronchioles and alveoli in chronic airway obstruction: A clinicopathologic study. *Am. Rev. Respir. Dis. 114*: 137-145.

Mitenko, P. A., and Ogilvie, R. I. (1973). Rational intravenous doses of theophylline. *N. Engl. J. Med. 289*: 600-603.

Morgan, M. D. L., Singh, B. V., Frame, M. H., and Williams, S. J. (1982). Terbutaline aerosol given through pear spacer in acute severe asthma. *Br. Med. J. 285*: 849-850.

Mortagy, A. (1982). The Epidemiology of Asthma. Southampton University Ph.D. Thesis.

Mountain, R. D., and Neff, T. A. (1984). Oral theophylline intoxications: A serious error of patient and physician understanding. *Arch. Intern. Med. 144*: 724-727.

Moxham, J. (1984). Respiratory muscle fatigue—aspects of detection and treatment. *Bull. Eur. Physiopathol. Respir. 20*: 437-44.

MRC (1956a). Cortisone acetate in chronic asthma. *Lancet 2*: 798-803.

MRC (1956b). Cortisone acetate in status asthmaticus. *Lancet 2*: 803-806.

Muers, M., and Dawkins, K. (1983). Effect of a timed interval between inhalation of beta-agonist and corticosteroid aerosols on the control of chronic asthma. *Thorax 38*: 378-382.

Munch, E. P., Taudorf, E., and Wecke, B. (1982). Dose frequency in the treatment of asthmatics with inhaled topical steroids. *Eur. J. Respir. Dis. 63*: 143-153.

Neville, E., Corris, P. A., Vivian, J., Nariman, S., and Gibson, G. J. (1982). Nebulised salbutamol and angina. *Br. Med. J. 285*: 849-850.

Newman, S. P., Pavia, D., Moren, F., Sheahan, N. F., and Clarke, S. W. (1981). Deposition of pressurised aerosols in the human respiratory tract. *Thorax 36*: 52-55.

Niewoehner, D. G., and Leatherman, J. W. (1984). Bronchodilator therapy in chronic airflow obstruction. *Chest 86*: 161-162.

Nocturnal Oxygen Therapy Trial Group (1980). Continuous or nocturnal oxygen therapy in hypoxaemic chronic obstructive lung disease. A clinical trial. *Ann. Intern. Med. 93*: 391-398.

Nogrady, S. O., Hartley, J. P. R., and Seaton, A. (1977). Metabolic effects of intravenous salbutamol in the course of acute severe asthma. *Thorax 32*: 559.

Nogrady, S. G., Hartley, J. P. R., Handslip, P. D. J., and Hurst, N. P. (1978). Bronchodilatation after inhalation of the antihistamine clemastine. *Thorax 33*: 479-482.

Northern General Hospital, Brompton Hospital and Medical Research Council Collaborative Trial (1976). Sodium cromoglycate in chronic asthma. *Br. Med. J. 1*: 361-364.

Orehek, J. (1976). Patient error in use of bronchodilator metered aerosols. *Br. Med. J. 1*: 76.

O'Reilly, J. F., Buchanan, D. R., and Sudlow, M. J. (1983). Pressurised aerosol with conical spacer is an effective alternative to nebuliser in chronic stable asthma. *Br. Med. J. 286*: 1548.

Passamonte, P. M., and Martinez, A. J. (1984). Effect of inhaled atropine or metaproterenol in patients with chronic airway obstruction and therapeutic serum theophylline levels. *Chest 85*: 610-615.

Patel, K. R. (1984). Terfenadine in exercise-induced asthma. *Br. Med. J. 288*: 1496-1497.

Patel, K. R., and Tullett, W. M. (1983). Bronchoconstriction in response to ipratropium bromide. *Br. Med. J. 286*: 1318.

Patel, K. R., and Kerr, J. W. (1985). Effect of terfenadine on methacholine-induced bronchoconstriction in asthma. *J. Allergy Clin. Immunol. 75*: no. 1, Pt 2, 168: 253.

Paterson, I. C., and Crompton, G. K. (1976). Use of pressurised aerosols by asthmatic patients. *Br. Med. J. 1*: 76-77.

Pavia, D., Bateman, J. R. M., Sheahan, N. F., and Clarke, S. W. (1979). Effect of ipratropium bromide on mucociliary clearance and pulmonary function in reversible airways obstruction. *Thorax 34*: 501-507.

Peacock, A., Busst, C., Dawkins, K., and Denison, D. M. (1983). Response of pulmonary circulation to oral pirbuterol in chronic airflow obstruction. *Br. Med. J. 287*: 1178-1180.

Peel, E. T., and Gibson, G. J. (1980). Effects of long-term inhaled salbutamol therapy on the provocation of asthma by histamine. *Am. Rev. Respir. Dis. 121* (6): 973-979.

Pierson, W. E., Bierwan, C. W., and Kelley, V. C. (1974). A double blind trial of corticosteroid therapy in status asthmaticus. *Pediatrics 54*: 282-288.

Pichurko, B. M., McFadden, J. E. R., Bowman, F., Solway, J., Burns, S., and Daring, N. (1984). Influence of cromolyn sodium on airway temperature in normal subjects. *Am. Rev. Respir. Dis. 130*: 1002-1005.

Popa, V. T. (1977). Bronchodilating activity of an H_1-blocker, chlorpheniramine. *J. Allergy Clin. Immunol. 59*: 54-63.

Powell, J. R., Thiercelin, J. F., Vozen, S., Sansom, L., and Riegelmen, S. (1977). The influence of cigarette smoking and sex on theophylline disposition. *Am. Rev. Respir. Dis. 116*: 17-23.

Primrose, W. R. (1983). Asthma at night. *Lancet 1*: 927.

Prior, J. G., and Cochrane, G. M. (1982). Assessment of optimum dose of inhaled terbutaline in patients with chronic asthma. The use of simple cumulative dose-response curves. *Br. J. Dis. Chest 76*: 266-268.

Reitberg, D. P., Bernhard, H., and Schentag, J. J. (1981). Alteration of theophylline clearance and half-life by cimetidine in normal volunteers. *Ann. Intern. Med. 95*: 582-585.

Research Committee of the British Thoracic Association (1982). Death from asthma in two regions of England. *Br. Med. J. 285*: 1251-1255.

Roussos, C. S., and Macklem, P. T. (1977). Diaphragmatic fatigue in man. *J. Appl. Physiol. 43*: 189-197.

Rubinfield, A. R., and Pain, M. C. F. (1976). The perception of asthma. *Lancet 1*: 882-884.

Rudd, R. (1984). Corticosteroids in chronic bronchitis (Editorial). *Br. Med. J. 288*: 1553-1554.

Rudd, R., Gellert, A., and Empey, D. (1982). Steroid responsiveness and chronic airflow obstruction. *Lancet 2*: 820.

Ruffin, R. E., Fitzgerald, J. D., and Rebuck, A. J. (1977). A comparison of the bronchodilator activity of SCH 1000 and salbutamol. *J. Allergy Clin. Immunol. 59*: 136-141.

Salome, C. M., Schoeffel, R. E., Yan, K., and Woolcock, A. J. (1983). Effect of aerosol fenoterol on the severity of bronchial hyperreactivity in patients with asthma. *Thorax 38*: 854-858.

Sanders, J. S., Berman, T. M., Bartlett, M. M., and Kronenberg, R. S. (1980). Increased hypoxic ventilatory drive due to administration of aminophylline in normal man. *Chest 78*: 279-282.

Santa Cruz, R., Landa, J., Hirsch, J., and Sackner, M. A. (1974). Tracheal mucous velocity in normal man and patients with obstructive lung disease; effects of terbutaline. *Am. Rev. Respir. Dis. 109*: 458-463.

Shenfield, G. M., Hodson, M. E., Clarke, S. W., and Paterson, J. W. (1975). Interaction of corticosteroids and catecholamines in the treatment of asthma. *Thorax 30*: 430-435.

Sherwood Jones, E. (1971). The intensive therapy of asthma. *Proc. R. Soc. Med. 64*: 1151-1152.

Shim, C. S., and Williams, M. H. (1980). Evaluation of the severity of asthma: patient versus physician. *Am. J. Med. 68*: 11-13.

Smith, M. J., and Hodson, M. E. (1983a). Effects of long term high dose beclomethasone dipropionate on adrenal function. *Thorax 38*(9): 676-681.

Smith, M. J., and Hodson, M. E. (1983b). High dose beclomethasone inhaler in the treatment of asthma. *Lancet 1*: 265-269.

Stainforth, J. N., and Tattersfield, A. E. (1983). Airway responsiveness to high dose nebulised salbutamol in chronic asthma. *Clin. Sci. 64*: 13P.

Stainforth, J. N., Sturgiss, P. J., and Tattersfield, A. E. (1983a). Effect of salbutamol delivered by metered dose inhaler and jet nebuliser on FEV_1 and heart rate in patients with chronic asthma. *Thorax 38*: 707-708.

Stainforth, J. N., Lewis, R. A., and Tattersfield, A. E. (1983b). Dosage and delivery of nebulised beta-agonists in hospital. *Thorax 38*: 751-754.

Stewart, M. F., Barclay, J., and Warburton, R. (1984). Risk of giving intravenous aminophylline to acutely ill patients receiving maintenance treatment with theophylline. *Br. Med. J. 288*: 450.

Stokes, T. C., Shaylor, J. M., O'Reilly, J. F., and Harrison, B. D. W. (1982). Assessment of steroid responsiveness in patients with chronic airflow obstruction. *Lancet 2*: 345-348.

Tattersfield, A. E. (1984). Bronchodilators in the prevention of asthma. In *Bronchodilator Therapy, the Basis of Asthma and Chronic Obstructive Lung Disease Management,* 1st Ed. Edited by T. J. H. Clarke, Auckland, N.Z., Adis, 1984, p. 76.

Tattersfield, A. E., and McNichol, M. W. (1969). Salbutamol and isoprenaline. A double-blind trial to compare bronchodilator and cardiovascular activity. *N. Engl. J. Med. 281*: 1323-1326.

Thiringer, G., Eriksson, N., Malmberg, N., Svedmyr, N., and Zettergren, L. (1975). Bronchoscopic biopsies of bronchial mucosa before and after beclomethasone dipropionate therapy. *Postgrad. Med. J. 51*(suppl 4): 30-31.

Thompson, P. J., Butcher, M. A., Frazer, L. A., and Marlin, G. F. (1981). Pharmacokinetics of a single evening dose of slow release theophylline in patients with chronic lung disease. *Br. J. Clin. Pharmacol. 12*: 443-444.

Thomson, N. C., and Kerr, J. W. (1980). Effect of inhaled H_1- and H_2-receptor antagonists in normal and asthmatic subjects. *Thorax 35*: 428-434.

Toennesen, J. (1982). Oral theophylline and fatal asthma. *Lancet 2*: 200.

Toogood, J. H., Lefcoe, N. M., Haines, D. S. M., Jennings, B., Errington, N., Baksh, L., and Chuang, L. (1977). A graded dose assessment of the efficacy of beclomethasone dipropionate aerosol for severe chronic asthma. *J. Allergy Clin. Immunol. 59*: 298-308.

Turner-Warwick, M. (1977). On observing patterns of airflow obstruction in chronic asthma. *Br. J. Dis. Chest 71*: 73-86.

Ullah, M., Newman, G. B., and Saunders, K. B. (1981). Influence of age on response to ipratropium and salbutamol in asthma. *Thorax 36*: 523-529.

Ward, M. J., Fentem, P. H., Roderick Smith, W. H., and Davies, D. (1981). Ipratropium bromide in acute asthma. *Br. Med. J. 282*: 598-600.

Ward, M. J., Macfarlane, J. T., and Davies, D. (1982). Treatment of acute severe asthma with intravenous aminophylline and nebulised ipratropium after salbutamol. *Thorax 37*: 785.

Webb, J., and Clark, T. J. H. (1981). Recovery of plasma corticotrophin and cortisol levels after a three-week course of prednisolone. *Thorax 36*: 22-24.

Webb, J., Clark, T. J. H., and Chilvers, C. (1981). Time course of response to prednisolone in chronic airflow obstruction. *Thorax 36*: 18-21.

Webber, B. A., Collins, J. V., and Braithwaite, M. A. (1982). Severe acute asthma: A comparison of three methods of inhaling salbutamol. *Br. J. Dis. Chest 76*: 69-74.

Wietzenblum, E., Hirth, C., Duculone, A., Mirham, R., Rasaholinjarsahany, J., and Ehrhart, M. (1981). Prognostic value of pulmonary artery pressure in chronic obstructive pulmonary disease. *Thorax 36*: 752-758.

Willey, R. F., Godden, D. J., Carmichael, J., Preston, P., Frame, M., and Crompton, G. K. (1982). Comparison of twice daily administration of a new corticosteroid budesonide with beclomethasone dipropionate four times daily in the treatment of chronic asthma. *Br. J. Dis. Chest 76*: 61-68.

Williams, I. P., and McGavin, C. R. (1980). Corticosteroids in chronic airways obstruction: can the patient's assessment be ignored? *Br. J. Dis. Chest 74*: 142-148.

Wilson, J. D., Sutherland, D. C., and Thomas, A. C. (1981). Has the change to beta-agonists combined with oral theophylline increased cases of fatal asthma? *Lancet 1*: 1235-1237.

Winter, R. J. D., Langford, J. A., and Rudd, R. M. (1984). Effects of oral and inhaled salbutamol and oral pirbuterol on right and left ventricular function in chronic bronchitis. *Br. Med. J. 288*: 824.

Wolfe, J. D., Tashkin, D. P., Calverese, B., and Simmons, M. (1978). Bronchodilator effects of terbutaline and aminophylline alone and in combination in asthmatic subjects. *N. Engl. J. Med. 298*: 363-367.

Woodcock, A. A., Johnson, M. A., and Geddes, D. M. (1983). Theophylline prescribing, serum concentrations and toxicity. *Lancet 2*: 610-612.

21

Bronchodilator Treatment of Children

ELLIOT F. ELLIS

Children's Hospital of Buffalo
State University of New York at Buffalo
Buffalo, New York

The goal of the treatment of asthma in children is to provide a degree of symptom control that will permit normal school attendance, full participation in recreational activities, including competitive sports, uninterrupted sleep at night, minimal use of hospital facilities, and reasonably normal pulmonary function. Under optimal circumstances, these objectives should be accomplished without significant adverse effects from the therapeutic agents prescribed. Normalization of pulmonary function, as desirable as it may be, is often difficult to achieve in those children who have asthma of severe degree. Experienced clinicians who routinely monitor pulmonary function by spirometry recognize children who, by thorough questioning and all clinical criteria, appear to have satisfactory control of asthma yet will be found to have significant impairment of expiratory air flow, particularly when measured at low lung volumes, presumably indicating peripheral airway obstruction (Hill et al., 1972; Cooper et al., 1977). The question frequently arises: does one treat the patient, or the pulmonary function test? The issue is particularly important since systemic corticosteroids, often in daily dosage, may be required to restore pulmonary function measurements to normal, and for this one pays a price in terms of adverse drug effect. The aggressiveness with which pharmacologic therapy is applied to asthmatic children depends upon the tolerance of the physician, the parents, and the child for asthma symptoms. Some physicians appear to have an enormous degree of tolerance for patient symptoms as do some parents who believe it has to be that way. Physicians (most of the good ones) who have low asthma symptom tolerance are more liberal in their use of drugs, to the great benefit of their patients. Despite lack of proof that optimal pharmacologic therapy alters the natural history of asthma, there is little question that the availability of many new drugs and new information about old drugs (theophylline is the best example) has substantially improved the quality of life for asthmatic children and their families. Unfortunately, there is still a good deal of what may be described as "throwing of drugs" at patients without apparent rhyme or reason. The challenge to the physician is to match treatment with severity of the disease. Towards this end, it is useful to have a scheme for classifying asthma according to severity on the basis of history, physical findings, radiographic, and pulmonary function criteria. While no classification scheme has been validated, one can devise an asthma severity index based upon frequency of exacerbations, utilization of physician or hospital resources, exercise tolerance, sleep interruption due to asthma, school attendance, hyperinflation on physical examination and by x-ray, and degree of airflow limitation and air trapping (Ellis, 1983). Therapy may then be applied in a rational way by a stepwise increase according to the patient's needs.

As a general rule, children with mild asthma require therapy as needed only with adrenergics (preferably by the inhalational route) and/or theophylline. Treatment is only required for 4-5 days and may then be discontinued. Children with a moderate degree of asthma do better in terms of symptom control when treated with a regular around-the-clock medication program with adrenergics and/or theophylline and/or cromolyn. While corticosteroids may be required during an acute exacerbation, they are not used on a regular basis. Children with severe asthma need polypharmacy treatment including some combination of adrenergic agents, theophylline, cromolyn, and the regular use of corticosteroids either in a systemic alternate-day regimen or with an inhaled surface-active drug.

Several drugs under investigation or presently available for treatment of asthma in Europe and Canada are not yet marketed in the United States. Ipratropium bromide, a congener of atropine, has good bronchodilator effect in many subjects. In children, ipratropium, when used on a regular basis, increases peak expiratory flow rate and reduces nocturnal asthma symptoms (Mann and Hiller, 1982). Its role (and that of atropine) in treatment of the acute attack of asthma or its day-to-day management has yet to be defined.

Lodoxamide, a drug with cromolyn-like actions, has been investigated in both oral and inhaled formulations. In a recent study of adults with perennial asthma, the inhaled drug could not be distinguished from placebo (Mann et al., 1985). Ketotifen, an orally administered drug with antihistaminic properties, has been received favorably in Europe for treatment of asthma. It does not alter bronchial hyperreactivity in children and (Graff-Lonnevig and Hedlin, 1985) has received mixed reviews. Groggins and co-workers (1981), in a double-blind crossover study, failed to show any effect on asthma in children. On the other hand, a multicenter trial in asthmatic subjects 12 years of age and older in the United States, in which ketotifen was compared with theophylline and placebo, was interpreted to show a favorable effect of the drug (Tinkelman et al., 1985). Sedation and weight gain may limit the usefulness of this drug, which may be indicated in children with mild disease (Mann and Hiller, 1982).

The specific details of the pharmacologic treatment of asthma are best approached by considering the treatment of acute asthma, in a physician's office or in the hospital emergency room, and the day-to-day ambulatory management of the disease.

I. Acute Asthma

Adrenergics are the drugs of choice for the acute attack of asthma. Epinephrine, in a dose of 0.01 mg/kg, is still the most commonly used adrenergic agent in the emergency room or office setting for treatment of the acute symptoms of asthma in a child. Recently there have been a number of head-to-head comparisons of epinephrine and aerosolized β_2 agents for relieving acute symptoms of asthma (Ben-Zvi et al., 1982). The aerosolized drugs have been shown to be as effective as epinephrine in terms of speed of onset (more so in fact), extent of improvement, and duration of activity (Dulfano and Glass, 1976). However, in a busy hospital emergency room or physician's office it is often more expeditious to give an epinephrine injection than it is to deliver the inhaled drug in the form of a "wet" aerosol. In emergency rooms, where a source of compressed air, nebulizer, mask, and accessories are readily available, aerosolized adrenergic agents are the drugs of choice for treatment of acute asthma systems. We use a Maxi-Myst compressor with nebulizer or mask to aerosolize 0.5 cc isoetharine (Bronkosol) or 0.5 cc metaproterenol (Alupent) in 2 cc saline over a few minutes with the patient continuously inhaling the drug. If one treatment does not suffice, another is given in 20 min. Should the child not obtain the satisfactory response to the inhaled drug, then an injection of epinephrine is given. Conversely, in the face of an inadequate response to an epinephrine injection, treatment with an aerosolized drug is tried. While the alternating use of injectible and aerosolized adrenergic agents for treatment of the acute attack of asthma has not been studied, this procedure has proven efficacious in some children who, for reasons that are unclear, are relatively resistant at the time to the inhaled or aerosolized agent. In terms of choice of specific drugs for inhalation in the United States, isoetharine (Bronkosol) and metaproterenol (Alupent) are the most widely used solutions for "wet" aerosols. It is useful to remember that isoproterenol is the most potent of the inhaled β-adrenergic agonists, and it is not unusual to see a child with a poor response to Bronkosol or Alupent who improves substantially following inhalation of isoproterenol 1:200, 0.25 cc in 2 cc saline. Terbutaline has promoted as an alternative to epinephrine as an injectible agent for acute asthma. In children at least, terbutaline has no substantial advantage over epinephrine if the latter is given in modest, but therapeutic, dosages (Simons and Gillies, 1981).

If the child fails to respond to two treatments with adrenergic agents, either injected or inhaled over the course of 1 hr, little is gained by trying a third treatment (Ben-Zvi, 1983). Aminophylline 6 mg/kg (equivalent to approximately 5 mg/kg theophylline) should be infused intravenously over 20 minutes diluted with 5% D/W in 1/2 normal saline other suitable fluid. While one would anticipate that children already receiving theophylline, especially in a sustained-release formulation, might have a preexisting serum theophylline concentration that would dictate reducing the intravenous dose, experience has shown that regardless of the history, the serum theophylline concentration is almost always 5 mg/liter or less (Canavan et al., 1980). Furthermore, because of the relationship between theophylline volume of distribution, dose, and serum concentration, each mg/kg of theophylline infused will increase the serum concentration by no more than 2 mg/liter at the peak (Weinberger et al., 1981). Thus, a dose of 5 mg/kg will boost a preexisting serum concentration by 10 mg/liter at the most, and this should not be a cause for concern. Nonetheless, if there is reason to believe that the child's serum concentration may already be in the therapeutic range, one may wish to reduce the intravenous dose by 50%. Should the child fail to respond to intravenous aminophylline, admission to the hospital is indicated. With a satisfactory response, the patient may be sent home with instructions for oral medications and arrangements for follow-up. Children who are corticosteroid-dependent, those who have been treated with steroids in the past 6 months, or who are borderline in terms of the decision to admit to the hospital or send home, should be given a dose of corticosteroids and treatment should be continued over the next 5-7 days. We find it convenient to give the initial steroids as methylprednisolone 1-2 mg/kg, using the intravenous line put in place for the aminophylline. Oral steroids in divided doses are prescribed on a twice-daily regimen (1-2 mg/kg) for 3-4 days and then at a daily dosing interval either as a constant dose or in decreasing fashion, over the 5-7-day course of treatment. Neither the constant or decreasing dosage regimen has been shown to be superior to the other.

Physicians should recognize that frequent acute episodes of asthma requiring emergency room visits represent (excluding the most severely affected subjects) failure of ambulatory treatment. Anticipatory management of the acute exacerbation often aborts the episode and prevents its progression. The idea that the best time to treat a severe attack of asthma is 2 days "before it gets there" is a sound one.

II. Day-to-Day Management of Asthma

The drugs used for treatment of the acute attack of asthma (the adrenergics, theophylline, and systemic corticosteroids) also have a major role in the ambulatory management of the disease. In addition to these agents, cromolyn sodium (Intal) and the new generation of inhaled corticosteroids are used in the day-to-day treatment program.

The previously noted principle of matching treatment with severity of disease, guides the physician in drug selection. Children who have mild intermittent symptoms are most effectively and safely treated with an inhaled adrenergic bronchodilator administered on an as-required basis. For children 6 years or older, two inhalations of albuterol, metaproterenol, terbutaline, bitolterol, or procaterol, three to four times a day from a metered dose inhaler for a few days, is frequently all that is needed during an exacerbation of symptoms. Similarly, the child with asthma who notes symptoms only following exercise may be prophylactically treated with two inhalations of an adrenergic agent from a metered dose inhaler immediately prior to exercise and postexercise if needed. Cromolyn and, to some extent, theophylline, which are both effective in modulating the exercise-induced asthma response, are substantially less active than the adrenergic aerosols (Godfrey and Konig, 1975). Adrenergic drugs, by the oral route, have little to recommend them in comparison to the aerosolized formulations. Many studies have established that the aerosol route of administration gives better bronchodilator effect and is more effective in preventing exercise-induced asthma than the orally administered drug (Anderson et al., 1976). Furthermore, the dose by the aerosol route is 10-15 times less than that required when the drug is given by mouth. Since adverse effects of the adrenergic drugs are dose-related, their frequency is greatly diminished when the drugs are inhaled. All of the foregoing assumes that the metered dose inhaler is being used properly (Harper and Strunk, 1981). Unfortunately, studies have shown that not only do substantial numbers of patients use the metered dose inhalers incorrectly (Epstein et al., 1979; MacFarlane and Lane, 1980), but also that their instructors (physicians and other personnel) are often deficient in their knowledge of the correct technique for effective use of the metered dose inhaler (Table 1). A variety of so-called spacers or holding chambers have been developed for use by subjects (children under 6 and some adults) who do not possess the necessary coordination of hand and respiration to use a metered dose inhaler effectively. These devices, which vary in size and design, provide a reservoir into which drug is delivered from the metered dose inhaler (Rivlin et al., 1984). The aerosol remains suspended in the chamber for up to 5 sec, permitting the patient to inhale at will. One such device, the Inhal-Aid, has a 700 cc reservoir, sells for $18 in drug stores, and has been widely accepted by children (Huntley and Weinberger, 1984). Children

Table 1 Optimal Use of Metered Dose Inhaler (MDI)

Hold MDI 4 cm from wide open mouth
Actuate MDI at end expiration (FRC)
Inspire slowly (over 5-6 sec)
Breath-hold for 10 sec
Space inhalations a few minutes apart

as young as 4 years and even some 3-year-olds have been able to use the Inhal-Aid successfully. For even younger children, the delivery of bronchodilator aerosols with the use of an air compressor, tubing, nebulizer, and mask has been extremely useful for both the regular three to four times per day administration of adrenergic drugs and for more frequent use during an exacerbation of disease. We have used the Maxi-Myst (Mead Johnson, $300), Pulmon-Aid (DeVilbiss, $159) or Schuco-Myst (Schuco Co., $159) in children as young as 18 months of age, to deliver aerosolized medication successfully. Isoetharine, in a dose of 0.5 cc in 2 cc saline, or metaproterenol, 0.5 cc in 2 cc saline, appears to be both safe and effective in young children. With the use of a mask, it is possible to reduce the drug concentration since more drug is delivered to the patient than from the hand-held nebulizer. If the frequency of symptoms in a young child or economic considerations do not justify providing a compressor-driven nebulization device, the use of a liquid formulation of an adrenergic agent is an acceptable, although less effective, alternative to aerosol treatment. Metaproterenol syrup (Alupent, Metaprel) or albuterol (ventolin) syrup in a dose of 1.0-1.5 mg/kg/day in three to four divided doses is recommended for children under 9 years of age.

Generally, the short-lived exacerbations of asthma experienced intermittently by children with a mild degree of disease are easily handled by the use of adrenergic drug treatment as prescribed above. However, if less than optimal symptom control is achieved theophylline, which has an additive bronchodilator effect when combined with adrenergic agents (Vermeire, 1982; Marlin et al., 1978; Wolfe et al., 1978), may be added to the treatment regimen. For the few days of treatment required, it is generally not necessary to prescribe a sustained-release theophylline product; a rapidly absorbed formulation may be used. The increased dosing frequency required by the use of a rapidly absorbed theophylline product is not a problem since the adrenergic aerosol will require frequent dosing (every 3-4 hr or less) during a flare of symptoms.

To summarize, exacerbation of symptoms in a child with mild asthma on the basis of a history of infrequent cough and wheezing, good exercise tolerance, uninterrupted sleep at night, and good school attendance is managed very nicely with adrenergic drugs alone, preferably by aerosol, or in combination with a rapidly absorbed theophylline product. Treatment lasts no longer than 5-7 days and then may be discontinued.

Those children who suffer from more frequent symptoms and signs of increased airway reactivity, whose exercise tolerance is less than optimal, who may have some interruption of nighttime sleep and miss school from time to time due to asthma, benefit from a regular program of asthma drug therapy, so-called around-the-clock therapy. According to the physician's estimate of the degree of symptoms in the very heterogeneous population of children with asthma, an adrenergic aerosol alone, such as albuterol, metaproterenol, terbutaline, procaterol, or bitolterol, two inhalations four times a day may be all that is necessary. More often than not, and particularly to control nighttime or early morning symptoms, the addition of a sustained-release theophylline product will be required. Adrenergic aerosols, which at best exert bronchodilator effect for not much longer than 6 hr, present a problem in symptom control for children who sleep 8-10 hr or more at night. This assumes that one does not wish to awaken the child in the middle of the night for an aerosol treatment, which is an inconvenience not only for the child but also for the parent. Theophylline in a sustained-release formulation is the only agent that will provide nighttime and early morning control of asthma symptoms (cromolyn also has diminishing efficacy after 6 hr) (Kolotkin et al., 1973).

A considerable degree of knowledge concerning the clinical pharmacology of theophylline is required to use it safely and effectively (Hendeles and Weinberger, 1983). To accomplish this, the physician must be aware of the following: (1) both efficacy as a bronchodilator (Mitenko and Ogilvie, 1973; Levy and Koysooko, 1975; Simons et al., 1982) and toxicity (Zwillich et al., 1975; Jacobs et al., 1976; Hendeles et al., 1977) are related to serum concentrations; (2) the therapeutic index is low, that is, the range of serum concentration between that optimal for bronchodilator activity and that which is toxic is narrow; (3) theophylline is eliminated principally by biotransformation in the liver and, therefore, drug concentration in the body is subject to developmental (age), environmental (diet, other drugs given concurrently, cigarette smoking), and disease (cirrhosis, congestive heart failure, viral illnesses) factors that may influence theophylline-metabolizing enzymes (Miller et al., 1983; Jonkman and Upton, 1984) (Table 2); (4) substantial intersubject variation in elimination rate occurs both in children and adults, indicating the need for individualization of therapy (Ellis et al., 1976); (5) sustained-release formulations are indicated to minimize fluctuations of serum concentration over a dosing interval, particularly in patients with serum half-lives of less than 6 hr (the majority of the pediatric population) (Hendeles et al., 1984; Riegelman and Jenne, 1980). Unfortunately, in some children sustained release products are not absorbed as regularly and to the

Table 2 Factors Influencing Theophylline Clearance

Factors	Decreased clearance	Increased clearance
Age	Prematures Neonates ? Age > 50 years	Age 1-16 years
Weight	Obesity (in relation to total body weight)	
Diet	Dietary methylxanthines High carbohydrate	Low carbohydrate High protein Charcoal-broiled meats
Habits		Cigarette smoking (tobacco or marijuana)
Drugs	Troleandomycin Erythromycin Cimetidine Influenza vaccine	Phenytoin Phenobarbital Isoproterenol (intravenous) Terbutaline
Disease	Cirrhosis Congestive heart failure Chronic obstructive pulmonary disease Acute pulmonary edema Acute viral illnesses	

same extent as rapidly absorbed liquids or uncoated tablets; this leads to unpredictable fluctuations in serum concentration that are difficult to interpret on the basis of single serum theophylline determinations (Rogers et al., 1985). Furthermore, with certain products and not others administration with food has a substantial effect on the rate of drug absorption (Pedersen and Moller-Petersen, 1984; Hendeles et al., 1985). It is safest to start therapy with a modest dose of theophylline, using ideal body weight should the patient be obese. If the bronchodilator response is inadequate, the dose may be increased by 25% at 3-4-day intervals (Hendeles et al., 1978). Under ideal circumstances, all children who are treated with theophylline on a chronic basis should have a serum concentration measured initially and at approximately 6-month intervals thereafter, but this rarely occurs in routine ambulatory practice. Many experienced physicians find it satisfactory to reserve monitoring of serum theophylline concentration for those children who either have an unsatisfactory response to the usual dose given at the usual dosing interval or develop adverse effects on this dose. When a decision is made to obtain a specimen for measurement of serum theophylline concentration, certain information is required to interpret the result properly. For example, one needs to know which product the patient is receiving (rapidly absorbed or slow-release), dosage, duration of therapy at a given dose (to ensure steady state), dosing interval timing of last dose, timing of blood sample collection, concurrent drug therapy, and presence of other disease states. Unfortunately, often this information is not provided, the laboratory report therefore cannot be meaningfully interpreted, and a good deal of money is wasted. Many reliable laboratory methods for theophylline analysis (TDX and EMIT are the most widely used) are available that are specific, sensitive, rapid, and require only a small serum sample. Recently several methods that require only fingerprick blood have been introduced. AccuLevel is a noninstrumental method for assay of theophylline on a fingerprick whole blood sample (Vaughan et al., 1986). The test takes only 15 min, has a high degree of correlation with standard laboratory methods, and is particularly suitable for office or night and weekend monitoring in hospital emergency rooms. Even more recently, we have developed a filter paper spot test that requires only a fingerprick blood sample and the Abbott TDX System (a fluorescence polarization immunoassay) for analysis (Li, 1986). The assay takes about 15 min to run and it is particularly suited for monitoring patients who live in remote areas, who can simply mail the filter paper specimen to the laboratory. There are at least 26 sustained release formulations on the market, including a generic formulation sold under various labels and this creates a problem for the physician, who is well advised to learn to use two or three products and forget the rest. The choice of one slow-release product over another is often based on the strength of the dosage form available relative to the patient's needs, for example, 250 mg every 8 hr vs. 200 mg every 8 hr. The physician should select the dosage form that most closely approximates the dose desired. The selection may be based on the dosage form itself, for example, tablets vs. bead-filled capsules. The latter are particularly useful in children since the contents of the capsule may be mixed with liquids or moist foods. Even with sustained release formulations, many children with particularly rapid theophylline clearance require dosing every 8 hr to prevent peaks and troughs of serum theophylline concentration. Older children, particularly adolescents, eliminate the drug more slowly and may be effectively treated with 12-hr dosing regimens. There is a spectrum of theophylline release rates even among the slow release products. For example, some are slow (Slophyllin), others slower (Theo-Dur, Slo-Bid), and a few very slow (Theo-24 and Uniphyl). The latter two products are probably not suitable for children because their bioavailability has been shown to be significantly reduced in this age group. This is probably due to the fact that the short gastro-

Table 3 Theophylline Dosing Recommendations

Age	Dosage (mg/kg/24 hr)
Initial dose	
2-6 mos	8
6-8 mos	12
8-12 mos	14
1-16 yrs	16
Adjusted dose (increase at 3-4-day intervals)	
1-9 yrs	24
9-12 yrs	20
12-16 yrs	18
Adults	12

intestinal transit time of children virtually ensures that the drug will be out of the tract before it is completely absorbed. A theophylline drug regimen based upon age is shown in Table 3.

The serum theophylline concentration required for optimal bronchodilator effect is a subject of some controversy and varies according to the severity of the patient's asthma. It is clear that some children obtain very satisfactory control of symptoms of asthma at serum concentrations between 5 and 10 μg/ml (Rachelefsky et al., 1978). It is important to treat the patient and not the theophylline "level." We prefer not to exceed steady-state serum concentrations of 15 μg/ml in most children because various factors including temporary disease states might reduce theophylline clearance and permit the drug to accumulate in the body to toxic levels. The physician must be aware of the adverse effects of theophylline and its treatment (Ellis, 1985). It is essential that parents be instructed that nausea, vomiting, headache, and jitteriness are signs and symptoms of theophylline toxicity and, in their presence, the next dose or two should be omitted and medical advice sought. Children are particularly vulnerable to theophylline intoxication because they have little control over theophylline drug administration, which is most often in the hands of their parents. Rectal suppositories containing theophylline should not be used in children because of the well-documented evidence of erratic absorption (Bolme et al., 1979). On the other hand, rectal solutions (Somophyllin-Fisons) may be very effectively used if the parents are given specific instructions concerning the dose and frequency of administration (Mason et al., 1980).

Table 4 Measures to Reduce Local and Systemic Effects of Aerosolized Steroids

Actuate inhaler 2.5 cm from mouth
Use before meals
Use a spacer or holding chamber into which aerosol is delivered
Rinse mouth and throat after inhalation

Recently there has been renewed interest in cromolyn sodium as an alternative to theophylline in children who need combination therapy for asthma control (Berman, 1983; Bernstein, 1981). When first introduced in the United States for treatment of asthma in 1972, cromolyn was recommended for use in patients with moderate to severe degrees who failed to respond to theophylline and were often corticosteroid-dependent. Experience quickly showed that the response to cromolyn in this population was unimpressive and the drug was never widely used. Subsequently, it has been shown that cromolyn is most effective in children with mild degrees of asthma. The outstanding advantage of cromolyn is that for all practical purposes it is virtually free of both short- and long-term adverse effects. Inhalation of cromolyn powder requires the use of a special inhaler device (Spinhaler) and requires a good deal of patient compliance. Unfortunately, the inhalation technique differs from that which provides optimal bronchodilator aerosol to the lungs (see Table 1). When using the Spinhaler, the child is instructed to exhale fully and then take a forceful, rapid, and deep inspiration to deliver the powder to the airways. At about $50 per month the drug is costly, which presents a problem for some families. Generally, cromolyn is begun in a dose of one capsule (20 mg) given four times a day. While favorable results often appear within 7-10 days of the institution of treatment, one ought to continue the agent for at least a month before concluding that it is ineffective. If the child responds favorably to four-times-a-day dosing, after several months three-times-a-day administration may be tried. The frequency of cromolyn dosing in some children may be further reduced to a twice-a-day schedule. Whether a child who can get by on twice-a-day dosing needs the drug at all has been debated by clinicians. In addition to its well-publicized "mast-cell-membrane-stabilizing" effects, the fact that cromolyn is one of the few drugs (corticosteroids may be another) that appears to exert a dampening effect on airway hyperreactivity with prolonged usage makes it particularly attractive (Breslin et al., 1980). The availability of cromolyn solution for nebulization permits it to be given to children who are too young to use the Spinhaler device successfully (Newth et al., 1982). We find cromolyn solution, alone or in combination with Bronkosol or Alupent (0.5 cc in 2 cc cromolyn) nebulized using a source of compressed air as described above to be very useful in young asthmatic children who are subject to frequent exacerbations of asthma precipitated by viral respiratory infections during the cold weather months. The regular use of cromolyn solution in this manner on a four-times-a-day basis appears to be successful (well-controlled studies have not been done) in reducing the frequency and severity of exacerbations of asthma.

A minority of children with asthma, perhaps 10-15% of the affected population, will have a degree of asthma incompatible with a normal life style despite a trial of optimal drug therapy, thorough investigation of the role that allergic factors play in the disease, and attention to possible psychosocial problems. These children are candidates for the regular administration of corticosteroids. Children who require a "burst" of daily corticosteroids more than once every 6 weeks are also candidates for a continuous corticosteroid treatment program. The reluctance of some physicians to use corticosteroids in children with moderate to severe asthma is appalling and shows lack of recognition of the fact that the asthma represents a far greater threat to the child's well-being than do the possible adverse effects of the corticoids, the great majority of which can be avoided. Because of the increasing recognition of the role of inflammation of the airways as a major contributor to the hyperreactive state (Nadel and Holtzman, 1984), there is an even greater rationale for the use of corticosteroids in asthma treatment programs. Once the physician concludes that oral corticosteroids are required on a regular basis for satisfactory asthma control, the child should first be given a 7-10-day course of prednisone or prednisolone, in the same way much as if one were treating an acute exacerbation.

At the end of this period, a change to alternate-day therapy is initiated by doubling the last daily dose which is then given as a single early morning dose every 48 hr. If the patient continues to do well after 10-14 days, the dose is first reduced by 5-mg increments and then by 2.5 mg increments as the dosage approaches 15 mg every other day. Many children receive very satisfactory control of asthma on an alternate-day regimen of 5-20 mg prednisone given as a single dose early in the morning every 48 hr. Since alternate-day corticosteroid therapy regimens were introduced by Harter and co-workers in 1963, it has become evident that many patients with corticosteroid-responsive diseases can be managed satisfactorily with minimal adverse effects. A very small segment of the steroid-dependent childhood asthmatic population will be unable to tolerate an alternate-day regimen. These children become symptomatic on the night of the second day (the off day) at which time the tissue effect of the dose given 36 hr earlier will have dissipated. Such patients will require daily therapy, preferably given as a single early-morning dose.

Of the long list of adverse effects associated with corticosteroid treatment regimens, all of which are dose- and dosing-interval related, the great majority may be avoided by the use of an alternate-day regimen. A single exception appears to be the development of posterior subcapsular cataracts which, while more common in patients who have received steroids in high daily doses or in intermittent (3 days on, 4 days off) regimens, have also been observed in children treated principally with alternate-day dosing. Asthma in children can be a life-threatening condition and is capable of causing chronic invalidism. The judicious use of alternate-day steroid therapy in selected cases should override the physician's reluctance to use these important anti-inflammatory drugs in the treatment of asthma in children. On the other hand, corticosteroids should not be used as a substitute for a plan of comprehensive disease management.

With the development of the new generation of surface-active aerosol corticosteroids, the relative merits of these agents compared to the alternate-day systemic steroid regimen has been a subject of interest (Weinberger, 1982; Ellis, 1984). Although beclomethasone, the most widely used of the aerosolized steroids, is well absorbed from mucosal surfaces, it is rapidly inactivated in the liver into metabolites devoid of glucocorticoid activity. At the usual dosage of two inhalations (84 μg four times a day) systemic effects are minimal, if any. As with other inhaled drugs, considerable patient compliance, which is not often attained in children under 6-7 years of age, is required for optimal aerosol delivery to the airways. When introducing aerosolized corticosteroids, it is important to "clear the airways" by giving the patient a 7-10 day course of systemic steroids. The aerosols are then introduced in a dose of two inhalations four times a day. As the patient begins to improve, the dose is gradually reduced to whatever extent possible as dictated by the degree of asthma control. Some children will do well on two inhalations twice a day. It is important that the child and his or her parents understand that during an exacerbation of asthma, introduction of systemic steroids is required.

In terms of adverse effects oropharyngeal candidiasis has not been a significant problem in children. Studies in which bronchial biopsies were obtained following up to 18 months of inhaled corticosteroid treatment have not shown evidence of epithelial atrophy or thinning of underlying connective tissue (Thiringer et al., 1977). Nonetheless, the possible long-term adverse effects of these potent surface active steroids on the pharynx and airways are unknown and of concern to physicians who treat children. Methods used to minimize adverse effects of the aerosol agents are shown in the Table 4.

The relative benefits of inhalational corticosteroids compared to alternate-day prednisone regimens are yet to be determined. The use of either alternate-day prednisone or inhalation corticosteroids in children does not commit them to a life of steroid therapy. The prognosis of asthma in childhood is excellent, with the majority of patients having remission of the disease with continued growth. In a disease with the potential for causing chronic disability, and even death, the physician must do whatever is necessary to provide the child with an opportunity to grow, develop, and lead a normal life. It is important for physicians to appreciate that death and severe disability from asthma occur more often from lack of appropriate drug treatment than from use of it (Stewart et al., 1981).

References

Anderson, S., Seale, J. P., Rozea, P., Bandler, L., Theobald, G., and Lindsay, D. A. (1976). Inhaled and oral salbutamol in exercise-induced asthma. *Am. Rev. Respir. Dis. 114*: 493-500.

Ben-Zvi, Z., Lam, C., Hoffman, J., Teets-Grimm, K. C., and Kattan, M. (1982). An evaluation of the initial treatment of acute asthma. *Pediatrics 70*: 348-353.

Ben-Zvi, Z., Lam, C., Spohn, W. A., Gribetz, I., Mulvihill, M. N., and Kattan, M. (1983). An evaluation of repeated injections of epinephrine for the initial treatment of acute asthma. *Am. Rev. Respir. Dis. 127*: 101-105.

Berman, B. A. (1983). Cromolyn: Past, present and future. *Pediatr. Clin. North Am. 30*: 915-930.

Bernstein, I. L. (1981). Cromolyn sodium in the treatment of asthma: Changing concepts. *J. Allergy Clin. Immunol. 68*: 247-253.

Bolme, P., Edlund, P. O., Eriksson, M., Paalzow, L., and Windbladh, B. (1979). Pharmacokinetics of theophylline in young children with asthma: Comparison of rectal enema and suppositories. *Eur. J. Clin. Pharmacol. 16*: 133-139.

Breslin, F. J., McFadden, E. R. Jr., and Ingram, R. H. Jr. (1980). The effects of cromolyn sodium on the airway response to hypernea and cold air in asthma. *Am. Rev. Respir. Dis. 122*: 11.

Canavan, J. W., Ellerstein, N. S., and Sullivan, T. D. (1980). Intravenous administration of aminophylline in asthmatic children taking theophylline orally. *J. Pediatr. 97*: 301-303.

Cooper, D. M., Cutz, E., and Levison, H. (1977). Occult pulmonary abnormalities in asymptomatic asthmatic children. *Chest 7*: 361-365.

Dulfano, M. J., and Glass, P. (1976). The bronchodilator effects of terbutaline: Route of administration and patterns of response. *Ann. Allergy 37*: 357-366.

Ellis, E. F. (1983). Asthma in childhood. *J. Allergy Clin. Immunol. 72*: 526-539.

Ellis, E. F. (1984). Corticosteroid regimens in pediatric practice. *Hosp. Pract. 19*: 143-151.

Ellis, E. F. (1983). Theophylline toxicity. *J. Allergy Clin. Immunol. 76*: 297-301.

Ellis, E. F., Koysooko, R., and Levy, G. (1976). Pharmacokinetics of theophylline in children with asthma. *Pediatrics 58*: 542-547.

Epstein, S. W., Manning, C. P. R., Ashley, M. J., and Corey, P. N. (1979). Survey of the clinical use of pressurized aerosol inhalers. *Can. Med. Assoc. J. 120*: 813-816.

Godfrey, S., and Konig, P. (1975). Suppression of exercise-induced asthma by salbutamol, theophylline, atropine, cromolyn and placebo in a group of asthmatic children. *Pediatrics 56*: 930, 1975.

Graff-Lonnevig, V., and Hedlin, G. (1985). The effect of ketotifin on bronchial hyperreactivity in childhood asthma. *J. Allergy Clin. Immunol. 76*: 59-63.

Groggins, R. C., Hiller, E. J., Milner, A. D., and Stokes, G. M. (1981). Ketotifin in the prophylaxis of childhood asthma. *Arch. Dis. Child. 56*: 304-305.

Harper, T. B., and Strunk, R. C. (1981). Techniques of administration of metered-dose aerosolized drugs in asthmatic children. *Am. J. Dis. Child. 135*: 218-221.

Harter, J. G., Reddy, W. J., and Thorn, G. W. (1963). Studies on an intermittent corticosteroid dosage regimen. *N. Engl. J. Med. 209*: 591-596.

Hendeles, L., Weinberger, M., Milavetz, G., Hill, M., and Vaughan, L. (1985). Food-induced dose dumping from a "once-a-day" theophylline product as a cause of theophylline toxicity. *Chest 87*: 758-765.

Hendeles, L., Bighley, L., Richardson, R. H., Hepler, C. D., and Carmichael, J. (1977). Frequent toxicity from IV aminophylline infusions in critically ill patients. *Drug Intell. Clin. Pharmacol. 11*: 12-18.

Hendeles, R., Iafrate, R., and Weinberger, M. (1984). A clinical and pharmacokinetic basis for the selections and use of slow release theophylline products. *Clin. Pharmacokinet. 9*: 95-135.

Hendeles, L., and Weinberger, M. (1983). Theophylline: A "state of the art" review. *Pharmacotherapy 3*: 2-44.

Hendeles, L., Weinberger, M., and Wyatt, R. (1978). A guide to oral theophylline therapy for the treatment of chronic asthma. *Am. J. Dis. Child. 132*: 876-880.

Hill, D. J., Landau, L. I., and Phelan, P. D. (1972). Small airway disease in asymptomatic asthmatic adolescents. *Am. Rev. Respir. Dis. 106*: 873-880.

Huntley, W., and Weinberger, M. (1984). Evaluation of bronchodilation from aerosol beta 2 agonists delivered by the Inhal-Aid device to young children. *J. Asthma 21*: 265-270.

Jacobs, M. H., Senior, R. M., and Kessler, G. (1976). Clinical experience with theophylline: Relationships between dosage, serum concentration and toxicity. *JAMA 235*: 1983-1986.

Jonkman, J. H. G., and Upton, R. A. (1984). Pharmacokinetic drug interactions with theophylline. *Clin. Pharmacokinet. 9*: 309-334.

Kolotkin, B. M., Lee, C. K., and Townley, R. G. (1973). Sodium cromolyn in antigen inhalation challenges in asthmatic patients. *J. Allergy Clin. Immunol. 51*: 87-88.

Levy, G., and Koysooko, R. (1975). Pharmacokinetic analysis of the effect of theophylline on pulmonary function in asthmatic children. *J. Pediatr. 86*: 789-793.

Li, P. K., Lee, J. T., Conboy, K. A., and Ellis, E. F. (1986). Fluorescence-polarization-immunoassay for the theophylline modified for use with dried blood spots on filter paper. *Clin. Chem. 32*: 552-555.

MacFarlane, J. T., and Lane, D. J. (1980). Irregularities in the use of regular aerosol inhalers. *Thorax 35*: 477-478.

Mann, N. P., and Hiller, E. S. (1982). Ipratropium bromide in children with asthma. *Thorax 37*: 72-74.

Mann, J. S., Clement, P., Sheridan, A. Q., Soryal, I., Fairfax, A. J., and Holgate, S. T. (1985). Inhaled lodoxamide tromethamine in the treatment of perennial asthma: A double-blind placebo-controlled study. *J. Allergy Clin. Immunol. 76*: 83-90.

Marlin, G. E., Hartnett, B. J. S., Berend, N., and Hacket, N. B. (1978). Assessment of combined oral theophylline and inhaled beta-adrenoceptor agonist bronchodilator therapy. *Br. J. Clin. Pharmacol. 5*: 45-50.

Mason, W. D., Lanman, R. C., Amick, E. N., Arnold, J., and March, L. (1980). Bioavailability of theophylline following a rectally administered concentrated aminophylline solution. *J. Allergy Clin. Immunol. 66*: 119-122.

Miller, J. L., Baciewicz, A. M., Bauman, J. H., and Self, T. H. (1983). Factors modifying serum theophylline concentrations. *Immunol. Allergy Pract. 5*: 130-151.

Mitenko, P. A., and Ogilvie, R. I. (1973). Rational intravenous doses of theophylline. *N. Engl. J. Med. 289*: 600-603.

Nadel, J. A., and Holtzman, M. S. (1984). Regulation of airway responsiveness and secretion: Role of inflammation. In *Asthma: Physiology, Immunopharmacology and Treatment.* Edited by A. B. Kay, K. F. Austin, and L. M. Lichenstein. London, Academic Press, pp. 129-155.

Newth, C. J. L., Newth, C. V., and Turner, J. A. P. (1982). Comparison of nebulized sodium cromoglycate and oral theophylline in controlling symptoms of chronic asthma in preschool children: A double blind study. *Aust. NZ J. Med. 12*: 232.

Pedersen, S., and Moller-Petersen, J. (1984). Erratic absorption of a slow-release theophylline sprinkle product. *Pediatrics 74*: 534-538.

Rachelefsky, G., Katz, R., and Siegel, S. (1978). A sustained release theophylline preparation: Efficacy in childhood asthma with low serum theophylline level. *Ann. Allergy 40*: 252-261.

Riegelman, S., and Jenne, J. (1980). Controlled release theophylline. *Chest 78*: 250-251.

Rivlin, J., Mindorff, C., Reilly, P., and Levison, H. (1984). Pulmonary response to a bronchodilator delivered from three inhalation devices. *J. Pediatr.* *104*: 470-473.

Rogers, R., Kalisker, A., Wiener, M., and Szefler, S. (1985). Inconsistent absorption from a sustained-release theophylline preparation during continuous therapy in asthmatic children. *J. Pediatr.* *106*: 496-501.

Simons, F. E., and Gillies, J. D. (1984). Dose response of subcutaneous terbutaline and epinephrine in children with acute asthma. *Am. J. Dis. Child.* *135*: 214-217.

Simons, F. E. R., Luciuk, G. H., and Simons, K. S. (1982). Sustained-release theophylline for treatment of asthma in preschool children. *Am. J. Dis. Child.* *136*: 790-793.

Stewart, C. J., Nunn, A. J., Stableforth, D., and Somner, A. R. (1981). Deaths in asthma: Disease or treatment? (Letter) *Lancet* *2*: 747.

Thiringer, G., Ericksson, N., Malmberg, N., Svedmyr, N., and Zettergren, L. (1977). Broncoscopic biopsies of bronchial mucosa before and after beclomethasone diproprionate therapy. *Scand. J. Respir. Dis.* *101*: 173-177.

Tinkelman, D. G., Moss, B. A., Bukantz, S. C., et al. (1985). A multicenter trial of the prophylactic effect of ketotifen, theophylline, and placebo in atopic asthma. *J. Allergy Clin. Immunol.* *76*: 487-497.

Vaughan, L. M., Weinberger, M. M., Milavetz, G., Tillson, S., Ellis, E., Jenne, J., Szefler, S., Wiener, M., Conboy, C., Shaughnessy, T., and Carrico, J. (1986). Multicentre evaluation of disposable visual measuring device to assay theophylline from capillary blood sample. *Lancet* *1*: 184-186.

Vermeire, P. (1982). Combined use of theophylline and beta-2-agonists. (editorial) *Eur. J. Respir. Dis.* *63*: 372-375.

Weinberger, M. (1982). Safety of oral corticosteroids. *Eur. J. Respir. Dis.* *63*: 243-251.

Weinberger, M., Hendeles, L., and Ahrens, R. (1981). Clinical pharmacology of drugs used for asthma. *Pediatr. Clin. North Am.* *28*: 47-75.

Wolfe, J. D., Tashkin, D. P., Calvarese, B., and Simmons, M. (1978). Bronchodilator effects of terbutaline and aminophylline alone and in combination in asthmatic patients. *N. Engl. J. Med.* *298*: 363-367.

Zwillich, C. W., Sutton, F. D., Neff, T. A., Cohn, W. M., Matthay, R. A., and Weinberger, M. M. (1975). Theophylline-induced seizures in adults: correlation with serum concentrations. *Ann. Intern. Med.* *82*: 784-787.

22

Acute Life-Threatening Asthma

CHARLES SCOGGIN

University of Colorado Health Sciences Center
Denver, Colorado

I. Introduction

Part of the broad clinical spectrum of asthma in adults is the acute, life-threatening episode. This is characterized by increasing airway obstruction, and if unabated, progressive hypoxemia, carbon dioxide retention, and respiratory acidosis (McFadden et al., 1973). Fortunately, improved techniques of treatment, probably due in large part to effective use of bronchodilators, has led to a progressive decrease in the mortality rate of asthma. At present, less than 1% of all asthmatic attacks result in death (Scoggin et al., 1977). This chapter will focus on the pathophysiology, assessment, and, most of all, treatment of acute life-threatening asthma in the adult patient.

II. Pathophysiology

What's wrong in asthma? A number of circumstances can precipitate acute asthma (Bousher et al., 1980). Some factors known to cause acute episodes of asthma, such as exercise, rarely result in life-threatening asthma. Others, such as upper respiratory tract infections, are common precipitants of acute episodes.

Regardless of what triggers asthma, the common pathophysiological finding is airflow obstruction. Airflow obstruction is due to three factors: smooth muscle constriction, mucosal edema, and excessive production of mucus. Thus the term "bronchospasm," which is commonly used to explain air flow obstruction in asthma, really involves two other factors beyond smooth muscle constriction. As acute asthma develops, progressive abnormalities are seen in arterial blood gases (McFadden and Lyons, 1968). Obstruction of airways leads to hypoxemia. As asthma worsens further, alveolar hypoventilation occurs and carbon dioxide retention and respiratory acidosis result. Increased airway resistance causes increased work of breathing, which may lead to metabolic acidosis as well. Development of severe metabolic lactic acidosis indicates a particularly severe episode of acute asthma (Appel et al., 1983).

III. Assessment

All the factors involved in the pathogenesis of asthma act in concert to explain the abnormalities of arterial blood gases seen in life-threatening asthma; decreased PO_2, increased PCO_2, and reduced arterial pH. They also provide parameters by which to assess severity and response to treatment: determination of air flow by spirometry or peak flow meter and arterial blood gas measurements. It is difficult to quantitate precisely the severity of asthma based on measurements of air flow alone. In general, patients who present with a forced expiratory volume in the first second of less than 1 liter or a peak flow rate of less than 80 liters/min have severe air flow obstruction (Kelsen et al., 1978; Franklin, 1981). Because of the difficulty in precisely predicting severity of asthma based upon any single parameter, other parameters have been assessed for usefulness in determining severity of asthma. Acute asthma may cause an increase in variation of systolic blood pressure with respiration (pulsus paradoxus) (Shim and Williams, 1978). Pulsus paradoxus greater than 20 mmHg is an indication of a severe episode. Pulse rate, respiratory rate, accessory respiratory muscle use, and subjective appreciation of dyspnea are other parameters that have been proposed. In fact, one study found that all these factors could be combined to generate a scoring system by which to assess asthma (Fischl et al., 1981). Recently, such an approach has been shown to not be universally effective (Rose et al., 1984; Centor et al., 1984). One investigation found that the position of the patient when he or she presented with asthma was also a useful indicator of severity of the episode (Brenner et al., 1983). Patients who could not lie flat, but had to sit or even stand, had the most severe asthma. Routine chest x-ray is not cost effective and should be performed only if one suspects a condition such as pneumonia or pneumothorax (Gershel et al., 1983). Our center does not utilize blood or sputum eosinophilia as a routine factor in assessing asthma. While sputum eosinophilia declines in the face of treatment with such medications as cortico-

Table 1 Historical Factors Suggesting a Life-Threatening Episode of Asthma

Previous history of severe asthma requiring corticosteroids
Previous history of asthma requiring intubation and mechanical ventilation
Pulmonary or cardiac condition coexisting with asthma
Failure of bronchodilators usually effective for control
Asthma induced by β-adrenergic blocking agents
Repeated visits to emergency room
Increasing use of inhaler without relief
Breakthrough of acute asthma despite steroid therapy

steroids, it has been shown that, contrary to previous reports, sputum eosinophilia may not disappear even though acute asthma has resolved (Baigelman et al., 1983).

Historical information should be focused. What factors may have precipitated an acute episode should be determined, such as viral infection. It is also important to ascertain whether other conditions that complicate the management of patients with acute asthma, such as coronary artery disease, may be present. It is also helpful if the patient can relate what has been effective in controlling previous acute episodes. A more detailed history can be obtained once the crisis has passed. Physical examination should center on characterizing breath sounds and determining if heart failure is coexisting with respiratory failure. Remember that breath sounds are usually decreased, and may be absent due to severe air flow obstruction. Likewise heart tones may be difficult to hear. Table 1 lists historical factors that suggest a life-threatening situation. Such patients are also most likely to require corticosteroids for control of their acute asthma.

In summary, other than history and physical examination, we recommend quantifying air flow obstruction by either peak flow meter or spirometry. This establishes a baseline value by which to gauge response to subsequent treatment. Arterial blood gas measurement need not be performed on all patients with acute asthma. Arterial blood gas levels should be obtained in those with clinically suspected severe respiratory failure or in whom there is clinical deterioration in the face of therapy in this circumstance. These levels are helpful in determining if oxygenation is adequate and whether or not carbon dioxide and systemic acidosis are present.

IV. Treatment

Certain therapeutic modalities should be avoided in acute asthma. Because of the sensitive nature of asthmatic airways, irritants such as acetycystine (Mucomyst) should be avoided. Likewise, cool mist and moisture generated from ultrasonic nebulizers may be poorly tolerated. Cromolyn and beclomethasone are excellent medications for the prevention of asthma, but because of their particular nature, they also can irritate the inflamed airway which occurs in acute asthma. Finally, sedative-hypnotic medications should be used rarely if at all in acute asthma. Patients with acute asthma are often agitated; however, this is a reflection of their physiological distress. Because sedative agents depress respiration, they may turn a patient who cannot breathe into one who will not breathe.

A. Oxygen

Because a universal finding in acute life-threatening asthma is hypoxemia, oxygen should be administered in sufficient amounts to assure an oxygen saturation

Table 2 Bronchodilator Treatment of Acute Asthma

Begin with β-adrenergic medications:
Epinephrine 1:1000 subcutaneously
60 kg body weight = 0.3 ml
60-80 body weight = 0.4 ml
80 kg body weight = 0.5 ml
or
Terbutaline sulfate subcutaneously, 0.25 ml
or
Inhaled isoetharine mesylate, 0.5 ml, via nebulizer diluted 1:3 with saline solution or water
or
Inhaled metaproterenol sulfate, 0.3 ml, via nebulizer diluted 1:3 with saline solution or water.
If no response in 30 min and patient's condition is not deteriorating, repeat β-adrenergic medication
If patient's condition still does not improve, or deteriorates, begin theophylline 3-5 mg/kg (Aminophylline, 4-6 mg/kg) as loading dosage. Use lower dosage if patient has been taking theophylline preparation.
If patient still does not improve, begin corticosteroids. Hydrocortisone 200 mg (or equivalent in alternative preparation) every 4 hr.

of at least 90%. This may be done using either a nasal cannula or a face mask. Some patients find face masks to be particularly uncomfortable during acute episodes and for this reason we favor using nasal prongs. In contrast to the observation of high-flow oxygen inducing hypoventilation in patients with acute episodes of respiratory failure due to chronic obstructive pulmonary disease, administration of high-flow oxygen does not appear to have the effect of increasing hypoventilation in acute asthma.

B. Beta-Adrenergic Amines

Beta-adrenergic sympathomimetic amines are the first agents of choice in the treatment of acute episodes of asthma (Rossing et al., 1980). These medications and their dosages in adults are listed in Table 2. The route of administration may be either subcutaneous or by inhalation. Inhalation is preferred since it has the potential advantage of decreasing systemic side effects. Intermittent positive pressure devices should not be used (Karetsky, 1975). Because their airways may be very irritable, some patients may be unable to tolerate inhaled drugs. In this case, subcutaneous injection is a reasonable alternative (Ben-Ziv et al., 1983). Sequential inhalation using a metered dose device and spacer or a liquid nebulizer is probably the preferred method of delivery of inhaled β-adrenergic sympathomimetic amines (Shim and Williams, 1980). The patient can take one or two puffs and wait a few minutes to allow onset of bronchial dilatation. A second and third administration are then given at divided intervals. The advantage of this approach is that the airways are progressively dilated to allow deeper breaths and further penetration of the medications into the airways of the lung with each subsequent treatment.

Whether or not patients who present with acute episodes of asthma who have been previously treating themselves with β-adrenergic medications receive further benefit from administration of these medications in the emergent setting has been questioned. A recent study has provided evidence that drug resistance does not appear to occur in these patients and that further administration of β-adrenergic medications may be effective in improving airflow (Rossing et al., 1983). A word of caution, however. It has been shown that excessive use of β-adrenergic medications can lead to serious hypokalemia (Kung et al., 1984).

C. Theophylline

Patients who do not respond to β-adrenergic sympathomimetic amine treatment with resolution of symptoms and improvement in airflow should also be treated with intravenous theophylline. It has been demonstrated that adult patients who present with severe airflow obstruction (forced expiratory volume in the first second less than 1 liter) respond best to a combination of intravenous theophylline and β-adrenergic sympathomimetic amines (Rossing et al., 1978). The usual

$$\text{Adjusted theophylline influsion rate} = \text{initial theophylline infusion rate} \times \frac{\text{target theophylline level}}{\text{measured theophylline level}}$$

Example:

Initial theophylline infusion rate	0.5 mg/kg/hr
Measured theophylline level	5 μg/ml
Target theophylline level	15 μg/ml

$$\text{Adjusted theophylline infusion rate} = 0.5 \text{ mg/kg/hr} \times \frac{15\ \mu\text{g/ml}}{5\ \mu\text{g/ml}}$$

$$= 1.5 \text{ mg/kg/hr}$$

Figure 1 Formula for adjustment of theophylline infusion based on blood theophylline level, assuming steady-state levels. For dosage of aminophylline, multiply theophylline infusion rate by 1.25. *Editors' note*: Please refer to Appendix for details of dosage regimens.

loading dosage of theophylline in adults is 3-6 mg/kg administered in dextrose and water over 15-20 min (Zwillich et al., 1975). This is equivalent to 4-6 mg/kg aminophylline. Patients with liver disease or congestive heart failure should be approached with great caution. They may receive the usual loading dose, but the maintenance dose requirements may be drastically reduced.

Patients with theophylline levels in the range of 5-20 mg/ml should be started on a maintenance infusion of theophylline and not necessarily receive a further loading dosage. The initial maintenance dosage of theophylline in stable nonsmokers and critically ill adults is 0.5 mg/kg/hr (0.5 mg aminophylline) if the target concentration is 10 μg/ml (Powell et al., 1978; Westerfield et al., 1981) (see Appendix). Theophylline levels in the blood should be monitored to determine whether or not adequate theophylline is being given. Such monitoring should also be used to gauge whether levels associated with toxicity are present. The so-called "therapeutic range" has been defined as 10-20 μg/ml. Levels above 20 μg/ml, while leading to increased bronchodilatation, also increased the likelihood of serious complications, particularly seizure (Zwillich et al., 1975). Increasing the theophylline dosage within the therapeutic range may speed the resolution of acute asthma (Vozeh et al., 1982). Patients given theophylline in dosages that result in high levels (15-20 μg/ml) appear to respond better as judged by such factors as total time on intravenous therapy than those patients whose dosages result in lower blood levels. A formula for adjusting theophylline infusion based on blood level is shown in Figure 1. It must be reemphasized that theophylline must be regarded as a potentially lethal drug. Controlled infusion devices should be utilized to protect the patient from inadvertent overinfusion. Should it become necessary to lower serum levels of theophylline in a patient, oral-activated charcoal should be administered in a dosage of 30 g every 2 hr (Mahutte et al., 1983). This will not only result in binding theophylline that may be present within the intestine, but will also actively lower serum theophylline levels (see chapter on theophylline toxicity).

D. Corticosteroids

If acute asthma is not controlled by β-adrenergic and intravenous theophylline treatment or if features of a life-threatening attack are present (Table 1), therapy with intravenous corticosteroids should be begun. A recent controlled clinical trial has demonstrated the efficacy of corticosteroids in acute asthma (Fanta et al., 1983). Appropriate dosages have stirred a minor controversy (Haskell et al., 1983); however, 200 mg hydrocortisone or its equivalent intravenously every 4 hr as initial therapy is a reasonable starting point. In patients who do not respond, progressive increase of dosage is justified. Since the onset of action corticosteroids may take up to 6 hr, they should be started early in the course of treatment of acute asthma. Thus, if a patient's condition has not "broken" in 1-2 hr after starting β-adrenergic and theophylline treatment, or if they show progressive deterioration in spite of such treatment as defined by deteriorating air flow and worsening arterial blood gases, corticosteroids should be given. One should not be timid in the management of acute asthma. After the acute episode is resolved, the patient can be placed on oral steroids and administration adjusted based on the clinical circumstances. Some patients will require long-term steroids, while some patients will be able to be rapidly tapered off corticosteroids. Use of corticosteroids in these situations is discussed in other chapters of this book. The principles of treatment of acute asthma are summarized in Table 3.

E. Anticholinergics

Certain patients with acute asthma may favorably respond to inhaled anticholinergic treatment (Nadel, 1984). This may be in the form of inhaled atropine or a similar agent, iprotropium bromide. The latter compound is presently not available in the United States. Atropine is delivered as a nebulized solution in the dosage of 1-3 mg per treatment. Obtaining an atropine formulation may be difficult. Concentrated atropine solutions are available; however, they have been

Table 3 Principles of Management

Maintain adequate oxygenation
Begin with inhaled or subcutaneous β-adrenergic therapy
Add intravenous theophylline if FEV_1 less than 1 liter or no response to β-adrenergic
Use corticosteroids early if patient is not responding to β-adrenergic and theophylline therapy

concocted for other than respiratory treatment purposes. For this reason, they should be checked to make certain they do not contain preservatives such as formaldehyde, which is highly irritating when inhaled. Atropine may be particularly effective in patients who have cough as a major manifestation of their acute episode. When these agents are given by inhalation, systemic side effects are rare. While some patient may note dryness of the mouth, drying of respiratory secretions does not appear to present a clinical problem (Chopra, 1978). Caution should be exerted in administration of atropine to prevent inadvertent spray into the eye. Atropine may be coadministered with β-adrenergic sympathomimetic solutions (Brady and Easton, 1979). This is easily accomplished by mixing the two solutions together in their usual dosages.

F. Other Measures

Other pharmacologic modalities described as being effective in the treatment of acute severe asthma include rectal ether, general anesthesia, and intravenous β-adrenergic sympathomimetic amines (Scoggin, 1981). Because of the severe toxicity associated with ether and intravenous β-adrenergic medications such as isoproterenol, these approaches have not been adopted as customary treatment (Kurland et al., 1979). Their use is discouraged except in desperation, when all else has failed. The use of α-receptor blockers (Utting, 1979) and calcium channel blockers (Williams et al., 1981) remains experimental.

Chest physiotherapy and inhaled moisture may aid patients with particularly thick mucus secretion (Menkes and Britt, 1980; Brain, 1980). Bronchial lavage has been used in the treatment of both acute and chronic asthma. The rationale for its use is that it may serve to irrigate the lung of obstructing mucus impactions. Like the modalities mentioned above, its use is reserved for desperate situations. Prewarmed irrigating fluid, 30-60 ml, is injected down in the tracheal tube and then aspirated back. A more formal approach is to use a wedged bronchoscope to lavage particular segments of the lung selectively.

While antibiotics are often given empirically to patients with acute asthma, the majority of organisms that infect patients with asthma are nonbacterial (Hudgel et al., 1979). For this reason, we discourage the routine use of broad-spectrum antibiotics in the treatment of asthma.

Because of their high respiratory rates and poor fluid intake due to symptoms of shortness of breath, patients with asthma may present with dehydration. It is important to rehydrate them, but vigorous hydration in excess of that physiologically required to correct dehydration is not necessary (Straub et al., 1968). In fact, overhydration may result in acute pulmonary edema.

Some attacks of acute asthma may either present or progress to the point that intubation and mechanical ventilation are necessary. It should be stressed that an elevated arterial PCO_2 level should not be the sole criteria for mechanical ventilation (Mountain and Sahn, 1983). In fact, intubation and mechanical ventilation are to be avoided (Scoggin et al., 1977). With appropriate treatment, the hypercapnia seen with acute asthma usually resolves quickly (Mountain and Sahn, 1983). Criteria for mechanical ventilation are cardiopulmonary arrest or progressive clinical deterioration with tiring of the patient and resultant carbon dioxide retention as defined by serial blood gas analysis. When intubating adult patients, the orotracheal route should be used and a large-diameter endotracheal tube with a low-pressure prestretched cuff employed. Volume-cycled ventilators capable of delivering high pressures should be used because patients with acute life-threatening asthma require high inspiratory pressures to deliver adequate tidal volumes. These high pressures lead to a major complication of barotrauma which can result in pneumothorax and pneumomediastinum. It has been suggested that this can be avoided by ventilating patients wtih low pressures, although this leads to hypoventilation, hypercarbia, and respiratory acidosis (Davioli and Perret, 1984). Serum pH can be controlled by bicarbonate infusion (Menitove and Gadring, 1983).

Finally, some special patients may present with acute, life-threatening asthma: elderly patients, particularly those with heart disease; pregnant patients; and patients with acute asthma provoked by β adrenergic blockade therapy.

V. Elderly Patients with Heart Disease

The medications used to treat acute asthma, such as the β-adrenergic sympathomimetic amines, have very definable effects on the heart. Not only do they increase heart rate, but they also increase myocardial oxygen consumption by stimulating myocardial contraction. Such effects could potentially have an adverse consequence in patients with such conditions as coronary artery disease. It must also be remembered that acute asthma and hypoxemia may be deleterious (Josephson et al., 1980). Age or heart disease is not a contraindication to the use of any of the agents appropriate for the treatment of asthma; however, all must be used with caution. Monitoring of heart rate and rhythm is appropriate in such circumstances. By using theophylline and β-adrenergic medications in combination, it may be possible to reproduce therapeutic effects with fewer side effects than if either class of medications were used alone and in higher amounts. Furthermore, since uncontrolled asthma itself places a burden on the cardiovascular system, oxygenation should be monitored with arterial blood gas determination or ear oximetry. Corticosteroids should be utilized early in the course of treatment of these patients.

VI. Pregnant Patients

The only factor that has been conclusively associated with adverse outcome for mother or child in acute asthma is uncontrolled asthma (Turner et al., 1980; Weinstein et al., 1979). The same medications used to treat life-threatening asthma in the nonpregnant patient should be used in the pregnant patient. Some agents, particularly the β-adrenergic sympathomimetic amines, may interrupt active labor (Ingemarsson, 1976; Coutinhok, 1971). Corticosteroids are given as in the nonpregnant patient (Snyder and Snyder, 1978). Arterial blood gas measurement or ear oximetry should be used to ensure that the mother, and consequently the fetus, is receiving adequate oxygen.

VII. The Surgical Patient

Acute asthma may occasionally complicate either the preoperative patient or the postoperative patient. A rare but potentially disastrous surgical complication of acute asthma is the problems created for the management of the acute abdomen by corticosteroid treatment for asthma. Acute asthma in the postoperative period is treated exactly the same way as in acute asthma alone. Corticosteroids should be employed even though they may have the theoretic possibility of decreasing wound healing and increasing the likelihood of infection.

VIII. Patients with Acute Asthma Induced by Beta-Adrenergic Blocking Agents

Beta-adrenergic blocking agents continue to have a wider and wider application in clinical medicine. All agents have the potential for inducing acute asthma. Even topical administration, such as into the eye for glaucoma, can trigger acute asthma. Beta blockade affect may persist for days. Some agents that are more selective for the β_1 receptors of the cardiovascular system may be less likely to cause bronchospasm and their effects more easily overcome by bronchodilator treatment (Johnsson et al., 1975). Treatment of bronchospasm induced by β-

adrenergic blockade therapy is similar to that for acute asthma in general (Johnson et al., 1975). Beta-adrenergic sympathomimetic amines are the agents of first choice.

References

Appel, D., Rubenstein, R., Schrager, K., and Williams, M. H. (1983). Lactic acidosis in severe asthma. *Am. Med. J. 75*: 580-585.

Baigelman, W., Chodosh, S., Pizzuto, D., and Cupples, L. A. (1983). Sputum and blood eosinophils during corticosteroid treatment of acute exacerbations of asthma. *Am. J. Med. 75*: 929-936.

Ben-Zvi, Z., Lam, Carin, Spohn, W. A., Gribetz, I., Mulvihill, M. N., and Kattan, M. (1983). An evaluation of repeated injections of epinephrine for the initial treatment of acute asthma. *Am. Rev. Respir. Dis. 127*: 101-105.

Bousher, H. A., Holtzman, M. J., Sheller, J. R., and Nadel, J. A. (1980). State of the art—bronchial hyperreactivity. *Am. Rev. Respir. Dis. 121*: 389-413.

Brady, R., and Easton, J. (1979). The value of atropine in the documentation of reversible airways obstruction. *Ann. Allergy 42*: 211-217.

Brain, J. (1980). Aerosol and humidity therapy. *Am. Rev. Respir. Dis. 122*: 17-21.

Brenner, B. E., Abraham, E., and Simon, R. R. (1983). Position and diaphoresis in acute asthma. *Am. J. Med. 74*: 1005-1009.

Centor, R. M., Yarbrough, B., and Wood, J. P. (1984). Inability to predict relapse in acute asthma. *N. Engl. J. Med. 310*: 577-580.

Chopra, S. K. (1978). Effects of atropine on mucociliary transport velocity in anesthetized dogs. *Am. Rev. Respir. Dis. 118*: 367-371.

Coutinhok, E. M., and Vieira Lopes, A. C. (1971). Inhibition of uterine motility by aminophylline. *Am. J. Obstet. Gynecol. 110*: 726-729.

Darioli, R., and Perret, C. (1984). Mechanical controlled hypoventilation in status asthmaticus. *Am. Rev. Respir. Dis. 129*: 385-387.

Fanta, C. H., Rossing, T. H., and McFadden, E. R. (1983). Glucocorticoids in acute asthma: A critical controlled trial. *Am. J. Med. 74*: 845-851.

Fischl, M. A., Pitchenik, A., and Gardner, L. B. (1981). An index predicting relapse and need for hospitalization in patients with acute bronchial asthma. *N. Engl. J. Med. 305*: 783-789.

Franklin, W. (1981). Asthma in the emergency room: Assessment and treatment. *N. Engl. J. Med. 305*: 826-828.

Gershel, J. C., Goldman, H. S., Stein, R. E. K., Shelov, S. P., and Ziprkowski, M. (1983). The usefulness of chest radiographs in first asthma attacks. *N. Engl. J. Med. 309*: 336-339.

Haskell, R. J., Wong, B. M., and Hansen, J. E. (1983). A double-blind, randomized clinical trial of methylprednisolone in status asthmaticus. *Arch. Intern. Med. 143*: 1324-1327.

Hudgel, D. W., Langston, L., Selner, C., and McIntosh, K. (1979). Viral and bacterial infections in adults with chronic asthma. *Am. Rev. Respir. Dis. 120*: 393-397.

Ingemarsson, I. (1976). Effect of terbutaline on premature labor. *Am. J. Obstet. Gynecol. 125*: 520-524.

Johnsson, G., Svedmyr, N., and Thiringer, G. (1975). Effects of intravenous propranolol and metoprolol and their interaction with isoprenaline on pulmonary function, heart rate and blood pressure in asthmatics. *Eur. J. Clin. Pharmacol. 8*: 175-180.

Josephson, G. W., Kennedy, H. L., MacKenzie, E. J., and Gibson, G. (1980). Cardiac dysrhythmias during the treatment of acute asthma. *Chest 78*: 429-435.

Karetsky, M. S. (1975). Asthma mortality associated with pneumothorax and intermittent positive-pressure breathing. *Lancet 1*: 828-829.

Kelsen, S. G., Kelsen, D. P., Fleegler, B. F., Jones, R. C., and Rodman, T. (1978). Emergency room assessment and treatment of patients with acute asthma: adequacy of the conventional approach. *Am. J. Med. 64*: 622-628.

Kung, M., White, J. R., and Burki, N. K. (1984). The effect of subcutaneously administered Terbutaline on serum potassium in asymptomatic adult asthmatics. *Am. Rev. Respir. Dis. 129*: 329-332.

Kurland, G., Williams, J., and Lewiston, N. (1979). Fatal myocardial toxicity during continuous infusion of intravenous isoproterenol therapy of asthma. *J. Allergy Clin. Immunol. 63*: 407-411.

Mahutte, C. K., True, R. J., Michiels, T. M., Berman, J. M., and Light, R. W. (1983). Increased serum theophylline clearance with orally administered activated charcoal. *Am. Rev. Respir. Dis. 128*: 820-822.

McFadden, E. R. Jr., Lyons, H. A. (1968). Arterial-blood gas tension in asthma. *N. Engl. J. Med. 278*: 1027-1032.

McFadden, E. R., Kiser, R., and deGroot, W. J. (1973). Acute bronchial asthma: Relations between clinical and physiologic manifestations. *N. Engl. J. Med. 288*: 221-225.

Menitove, S. M., and Godring, R. M. (1983). Combined ventilator and bicarbonate strategy in the management of status asthmaticus. *Am. J. Med. 74*: 898-901.

Menkes, H., and Britt, J. (1980). Rationale for physical therapy. *Am. Rev. Respir. Dis. 122*: 127-131.

Mountain, R. D., and Sahn, S. A. (1983). Hypercapnia in acute asthma resolves rapidly without mechanical ventilation. *Clin. Res. 32*: 37A.

Nadel, J. A. (1984). Adoration of the vagi. *N. Engl. J. Med. 311*: 463-464.
Powell, J. R., Vozeh, S., Hopewill, P., Costello, J., Sheiner, L. B., and Riegelman, S. (1978). Theophylline deposition in acutely ill hospitalized patients. The effect of smoking, heart failure, severe airway obstruction and pneumonia. *Am. Rev. Respir. Dis. 118*: 229-238.
Rose, C. C., Murphy, J. G., and Schwartz, J. S. (1984). Performance of an index predicting the response of patients with acute bronchial asthma to intensive emergency department treatment. *N. Engl. J. Med. 310*: 573-577.
Rossing, T. H., Fanta, C. H., Goldstein, D. H., Snapper, J. R., and McFadden, E. R. Jr. (1980). Emergency therapy of asthma: Comparison of the acute effects of parenteral and inhaled sympathomimetics and infused aminophylline. *Am. Rev. Respir. Dis. 122*: 365-371.
Rossing, T. H., Fanta, C. H., and McFadden, E. R. Jr. (1981). A controlled trial of the use of single vs. combined-drug therapy in the treatment of acute episodes of asthma. *Am. Rev. Respir. Dis. 123*: 190-194.
Rossing, T. H., Fanta, C. H., and McFadden, E. R. (1983). Effect of outpatient treatment of asthma with beta agonists on the response to sympathomimetics in an emergency room. *Am. J. Med. 75*: 781-784.
Scoggin, C. H. (1981). Acute and status asthma. In *Clinical Strategies in Adult Asthma.* Edited by C. H. Scoggin and T. L. Petty. Lea and Febiger, Philadelphia, p. 53.
Scoggin, C. H., Sahn, S. A., and Petty, T. L. (1977). Status asthmaticus: A nine year experience. *JAMA 238*: 1158-1162.
Shim, C., and Williams, M. H. (1978). Pulsus paradoxus in asthma. *Lancet 1*: 530-531.
Shim. C., and Williams, M. H. (1980). Bronchial response to oral versus aerosol metaproterenol in asthma. *Ann. Intern. Med. 93*: 428-431.
Snyder, R. D., and Synder, D. (1978). Corticosteroids for asthma during pregnancy. *Ann. Allergy 41*: 340-341.
Straub, P. W., Buhlmann, A. A., and Rossier, P. H. (1968). Hypovolemia in status asthmaticus. *Lancet* 1923.
Turner, E. S., Greenberger, P. A., and Patterson, R. (1980). Management of the pregnant asthmatic patient. *Ann. Intern. Med. 93*: 905-918.
Utting, J. A. (1979). Alpha-adrenergic blockade in severe asthma. *Br. J. Dis. Chest 73*: 317.
Vozeh, S., Kewitz, G., Perruchoud, A., Tschan, M., Kipp, C., Eitz, M., and Follath, F. (1982). Theophylline serum concentration and therapeutic effect in severe acute bronchial obstruction: The optimal use of intravenously administered aminophylline. *Am. Rev. Respir. Dis. 125*: 181-184.
Weinstein, A. M., Dubin, B. D., Podleski, W. K., et al. (1979). Asthma and pregnancy. *JAMA 241*: 1161-1165.
Westerfield, B. T., Carder, A. J., and Light, R. W. (1981). The relationship be-

tween arterial blood gases and serum theophylline clearance in critically ill patients. *Am. Rev. Respir. Dis. 124*: 17-20.

Williams, D. D., Barnes, P. J., Vickers, H. P., and Rudolph, M. (1981). Effect of nifedipine on bronchomotor tone and histamine reactivity in asthma. *Br. Med. J. 283*: 348.

Zwillich, C. W., Sutton, F. D. Jr., Tan, TA, et al. (1975). Theophylline-induced seizure in adults: correlation with serum concentrations. *Ann. Intern. Med. 82*: 784-787.

23

Treatment of the Life-Threatening Asthma Attack in Children

HOWARD EIGEN

Indiana University School of Medicine
James Whitcomb Riley Hospital for Children
Indianapolis, Indiana

BENNIE McWILLIAMS

University of New Mexico School of Medicine
Albuquerque, New Mexico

I. Introduction

Treatment of the life-threatening asthma episode in children is based on therapy of the three major components: bronchospasm, excessive secretions, and edema of the airways. Mechanical obstruction may be more important in children than in adults owing to the small size of the child's airway. Furthermore, the young child or infant operates at a mechanical disadvantage to breathing. The chest wall structures are soft, giving less leverage to the accessory inspiratory muscles and the diaphragm contains fewer slow fibers in infants than in adults, thus reducing stamina.

Although some clinicians are still unwilling to diagnose asthma in patients under the age of 2 years, this failure to recognize the reversibility of disease in infants may lead to a delay in instituting appropriate therapy. While it may be true that for a given degree of obstruction bronchiolar muscle spasm plays a less important role than edema and mucus because of the relatively poor muscular development until age 2-3 years (Matsuba and Thurlbeck, 1972), status asthmaticus can occur at any age and reversible airway obstruction has been demonstrated in young infants. In children, there is an increase in the density of bronchial mucous glands and, as in adults, the secretions of these glands are thick and tenacious (Field, 1968; Matsuba and Thurlbeck, 1971). This excess production of mucus in an airway with a small diameter leads to profound physical obstruction that is not responsive to bronchodilator drugs. In young children the precipitating factor for the severe asthma attacks is most often viral (Minor et al., 1974) and young children suffer a high number (estimated at six to eight a year) of viral respiratory infections in the first 2 years of life. Because upper respiratory infections can increase airway reactivity for 6 weeks, the airways of some children are in a constant state of hyperreactivity and increased obstruction for many weeks or months at a time.

II. Evaluation

Evaluation of a child with acute wheezing should start with a brief physical examination. After one is certain that the patient is not obviously hypoxemic and that air movement is adequate, a brief history can be obtained from patient and parents. Each child has a characteristic pattern to his or her wheezing attacks, so a description of the child's previous episodes and how he or she responded to drug therapy is very helpful. The relative severity of the present episode can be assessed at this time. One needs to determine the doses of *all* medications taken regularly and as extra therapy for the present wheezing attack.

Specific methods of evaluation are available that allow assessment of the severity of an attack and the likelihood of admission to the hospital. Commey and Levison (1976) evaluated 62 children by comparing subjective symptoms, physical signs, with pulmonary function studies including lung volumes. They found that dyspnea, subjective wheezing, and auscultatory findings had no discriminant value. However, supraclavicular retraction and sternocleidomastoid contraction were invariably associated with pulmonary function values indicative of severe disease. All patients with FVC, FEV_1, and MEFR values below 50% predicted had sternocleidomastoid contraction with inspiration. Pulsus paradoxus is also a sign of severely impaired lung function and is valuable in assessing children with status asthmaticus. In a study of children ages 13 months to 15 years, Galant et al. (1978b) found that increasing pulsus paradoxus correlated with worsening clinical score. Pulsus paradoxus was significantly greater (mean 22 mmHg) in children with PCO_2 above 40 mmHg than in those with PCO_2 below 40 (mean pressure change, 12 mmHg). The measurement of pulsus paradoxus is difficult in the tachypneic child but, using the special techniques described by Gallant, it provides a useful window into the pathophysiology of the severely ill asthmatic child.

Examination of the chest for wheezes, air entry, and crackles may be helpful in gauging severity but these signs can be misleading, especially in a quiet chest. A child who is severely obstructed will have a quiet, nearly wheeze-free chest because air flow is not sufficient to create a wheeze. Perhaps the best use of the chest exam is in assessing the presence of loud wheezing, indicating that the child is not likely to be severely obstructed. The percussion note is hyper-resonant under these circumstances and offers little help in assessing severity.

Arterial blood gas analysis is an essential part of the evaluation of children with status asthmaticus. Nearly one-quarter of children with asthma will be hypoxemic even when well clinically (Cooper et al., 1977). When symptomatic, essentially all children suffer hypoxemia, the degree being correlated with the degree of airway obstruction (Weng et al., 1970), FEV_1 having the strongest correlation ($r = 0.69$) with the degree of hypoxemia. Thus during an acute exacerbation we treat all acutely wheezing patients as if they were hypoxemic. Oxygen is given by mask at a known inspired concentration. An arterial blood sample is analyzed for PO_2 PCO_2, and pH in any child admitted to hospital or as clinical judgment dictates. One expects acutely wheezing adults to be hyperventilating, with PCO_2 in the low 30s (mmHg), but this is seen less frequently in children. With clinical wheezing, an arterial PO_2 of 50–70 mmHg ($FIO_2 = 0.21$) can be expected (Weng et al., 1970). Deviation from this pattern, especially if PCO_2 is 45 mmHg or higher, indicates severe obstruction and usually requires placement of an indwelling arterial catheter and observation in an intensive care unit.

Extensive pulmonary function testing during an acute episode is generally not feasible, but measurement of peak expiratory flow rate can help assess the initial severity and is useful in making judgment in the emergency room about the patient's responsiveness to bronchodilators. Repeated peak flow attempts may worsen obstruction and so testing should be used judiciously. If a child is essentially unresponsive to the first or second aerosol treatment, admission to the hospital is almost certain to be necessary. A Wright peak flow meter that has a low range of 60 liters/min or less is needed to measure peak flow and can generally be used successfully even by preschool children.

A. Chest Radiograph

The chest radiograph has taken its place as one of the routine examinations in the evaluation of the seriously ill asthmatic child, presumably to identify free air (pneumothorax or pneumomediastinum), infiltrate, or atelectasis. The chest radiograph typically shows air trapping, usually bilateral and symmetrical, which varies in degree with the severity of the episode. Patches of atelectasis may accompany the overinflation. Varying in size from subsegmental to lobar, these areas of atelectasis may change in location as bronchi open and close and are often misconstrued as being of infectious cause. Signs of pulmonary artery hypertension may be seen as well (Levison et al., 1974). Although the incidence of abnormal chest roentgenograms in asthmatic children is reported as 43-75% (Eggleston et al., 1974; Dubretzky and Philson, 1968; Gillies et al., 1978) of those children hospitalized for asthma, the rate is more on the order of 25% if the obvious diagnosis of hyperaeration is excluded. Brooks and colleagues (1982) evaluated the significance of radiographic abnormalities in the management of 128 children admitted for asthma by comparing x-ray findings with clinical assessment. Seven patients had abnormal radiographs of which three had been expected to be abnormal by clinical evaluation. Fourteen patients clinically predicted to have pneumonia or pneumothorax had, in fact, normal chest roentgenograms. No significant alterations in the plan of treatment were required as the result of chest radiographic findings.

The incidence of pneumomediastinum and infiltrates has been found to be age-dependent, with infiltrates occurring primarily in younger (less than 6 years old) and pneumomediastinum in older (more than 10 years old) children (Eggleston et al., 1974). Rarely is free air clinically significant either by causing obvious symptoms or by requiring evacuation. Although some authors (Jorgenson et al., 1963) suggest removal of any amount of free air, we would opt for nonintervention unless the patient shows signs of marked restriction, tension pneumothorax, or cardiac compromise.

III. Treatment

A. Oxygen

Delivery of an oxygen-enriched gas is a paramount concern since all patients with severe wheezing must be considered to be hypoxemic. The gas should be humidified using water vapor. Distilled water or saline aerosol should be avoided since particulate water can stimulate bronchospasm, bronchoconstriction, and cough (Sheppard et al., 1983). This is true whether the child uses a mask or is placed in a mist tent for oxygen delivery. Aerosol tents have the added disadvantage of chilling small children. There is no evidence that large amounts of water delivered to the respiratory tract hasten the clearance of mucous plugs, but dry oxygen may stimulate bronchospasm.

Asthmatic children are not at risk for developing hypercarbia as a result of breathing oxygen-enriched gas. We initially provide 30-40% oxygen and then adjust the mixture as needed once measurements of oxygen saturation or PaO_2 are made.

B. Hydration

Reestablishing adequate hydration is an important part of treating children. Children are generally 5-10% dehydrated when admitted to the hospital and this deficit should be repaired. Data in laboratory animals (Stalcup and Mellins, 1977) indicates that free lung water will increase as pleural pressure becomes more negative, as is the case in severely obstructed patients. This leads to clinically apparent interstitial pulmonary edema if the child is rehydrated too vigorously. Interstitial edema will decrease compliance and increase the work of breathing, which increases oxygen requirements. Florid pulmonary edema has been reported in severely obstructed asthmatic children (Levison et al., 1974).

C. Sympathomimetic Drugs

Sympathomimetic therapy is the mainstay of treatment in life-threatening pediatric asthma (Fanta et al., 1982). Sympathomimetic agents have β-2 receptor agonist properties that directly cause bronchial smooth muscle relaxation (McFadden, 1981). Beta agonists may also improve pulmonary function by other mechanisms, such as by increasing the strength of diaphragmatic contractions (Aubier et al., 1984; Howell and Roussos, 1984) and by increasing mucociliary clearance (Wanner, 1977). Pure β_2 receptor stimulation causes bronchodilatation as well as vasodilatation, but the side effects of sympathomimetics result from α- and β_1-receptor stimulation.

Beta-2-agonist agents may be classified according to their base structure: catecholamine, resorcinol, and saligenin. Catecholamines (epinephrine, isoproterenol, and isoetharine) are quickly taken up into cells by the uptake-2 process for catecholamines and inactivated by catechol-O-methyl transferase (COMT). Because of this inactivation, they are not effective when given orally and have a relatively short duration of action. Resorcinols (metaproterenol, terbutaline, and fenoterol) and saligenins (albuterol, salbutamol) are not degraded by COMT and thus are effective when given orally and have a longer duration of action than catecholamines.

Catecholamine Base

Epinephrine

Epinephrine is very commonly used in episodes of acute asthma and is considered by some to be the treatment of choice in acute asthma in children (Lulla and Newcoms, 1980). Epinephrine stimulates α, β_1, and β_2 receptors. It is routinely administered in a dosage of 0.01 cc/kg body weight (1:1,000 solution) to a maximum of 0.3 cc subcutaneously every 15 min. It is a very potent bronchodilator, but its α and β_1 properties as well as its short duration of action (Nelson, 1982) limit its usefulness in life-threatening asthmatic episodes. Epinephrine may also be given as an aerosol but again its short duration of action as well as β_1 and α-agonist effects limit its usefulness.

Isoproterenol

Isoproterenol (Isuprel) is a selective β-agonist, but stimulates both β_1 and β_2 receptors. When given intravenously it causes bronchodilatation and vasodilatation as well as positive cardiac inotropic and chronotropic effects. Isoproterenol may be given by the inhaled route at a dosage of 0.1-0.5 mg by metered dose inhaler (MDI) or 2.5 mg by pressure-driven nebulizer. Isoproterenol is very seldom used by this route because other more selective β_2 agonists are available. Isoproterenol has been recommended as a continuous infusion beginning at a dosage of 0.05-0.1 μg/kg per min and increasing by 0.1-μg/kg per min until a clinical response is obtained or side effects occur. Side effects include tachycardia greater than 180-200 beats/min, ST-T wave changes and CPK-MB enzyme elevations (Matson et al., 1978; Kurland et al., 1979, Maguire et al., 1986). Intravenous isoproterenol causes pulmonary vasodilatation before its bronchodilatory effects are noted. This may produce acute hypoxemia by inhibiting hypoxic vasoconstriction in the pulmonary bed (McFadden, 1981) and so worsening ventilation/perfusion matching. Thus, a severe asthmatic may have an acute decrease in PaO_2 at the beginning of an isoproterenol infusion. This effect, however, is usually short-lived (McFadden, 1981).

Isoetharine

Isoetharine (Bronkosol) is produced by the introduction of a β-ethyl group on the side chain, which decreases β_2 effects by 10 but reduces β_1 activity by 300. Thus, it is a relatively more selective β_2 agent than is isoproterenol. Because of its catecholamine base structure, it is degraded by COMT, and has a relatively short duration of action (2 hr). It is administered in a dosage of 0.3-0.5 cc of a 1% solution diluted with normal saline.

Resorcinol Base

Metaproterenol

Metaproterenol (Alupent, Metaprel) is not inactivated by COMT, giving it both oral activity and a longer duration of action. Its selectivity is similar to that of isoetharine but its duration of action is approximately 4 hr in pediatric patients (Lee, 1981). As an aerosol it is administered at a dosage of 0.1-0.3 cc of a 5% solution diluted with normal saline to a total volume of 2-3 ml and given every 4 hr. This interval may be decreased in severe asthma episodes to every 30 min.

Terbutaline

Terbutaline (Brethine, Bricanyl) is a tertiary butyl derivative of metaproterenol. It produces powerful β_2 activity with very little β_1 activity, especially when given by inhalation. It is used subcutaneously in a dose of 0.01 mg/kg (Amory et al., 1975), by continual intravenous infusion (See Appendix), or by aerosol. For aerosol administration, a dosage of 0.1-0.3 mg/kg (a 1 mg/ml solution is used in the United States) is diluted with normal saline (Isles and Levison, 1985), and given every 4 hr. In a severe life-threatening attack, the interval may be decreased to every 15-30 min. Terbutaline has a 4-6 hr duration of action when given by inhalation (Formgren, 1970).

Fenoterol

Fenoterol (Berotec) is another long-acting β_2-specific agonist with a resorcinol base. Ben-Zvi and co-workers (1982) found that fenoterol produced better bronchodilatation in children than epinephrine and fewer side effects. Its specificity and duration of action are similar to those of terbutaline, although Gray et al. (1982), by administering increasing doses of terbutaline and fenoterol to adults, found fenoterol to produce more systemic side effects than terbutaline. Fenoterol may be used orally, parenterally, or by aerosol. It is currently not available in the United States but is scheduled for release in a metered dose inhaler in the near future.

Saligenin Base: Albuterol

Albuterol (salbutamol, Ventolin, Proventil) was the first highly selective β_2-agonist available. Outside the United States it is used for the treatment of severe asthma by intravenous and aerosol administration. The intravenous dosage of albuterol is 10 μg/kg over 10 min followed by a continuous infusion of 0.2 μg/kg/min up to a maximum of 2 μg/kg/min (Isles and Levison, 1985). In the United States it is available only as an oral tablet or by metered dose inhaler (MDI). It has a duration of action of 4-6 hr.

D. Other Sympathomimetics

Newer β_2-selective sympathomimetics (rimiterol, carbuterol, salmefamol, soterenol, tretoquinol, and quinterenol) have recently been developed and clinical studies with these medications are currently underway.

As mentioned previously, sympathomimetics may be administered orally, parenterally, or topically (aerosol). In life-threatening episodes, the parenteral and aerosol routes are used exclusively (Fanta et al., 1982). Traditional therapy of acute asthmatic episodes consists of subcutaneous epinephrine and, in the more severe cases, intravenous isoproterenol. The development of more selective and longer-acting β_2 agonists, along with their use by inhalation, has changed the approach to pediatric patients with severe asthma.

Epinephrine was the first sympathomimetic to be given by the topical or aerosol route in asthmatics over 40 years ago (Barger and Dale, 1910; Graeser and Rome, 1935). Nebulized sympathomimetics, however, were used little until 1969 (Pierson and Grieco, 1969). Since that time the aerosol route has been used with increasing frequency in the treatment of children. The site of deposition of aerosolized particles depends on the size of the particles, although the factors affecting deposition are complex (Raabe, 1982). During a severe wheezing attack generalized airway narrowing causes an increase in air velocity leading to increased deposition of inhaled particles in the central airways by impaction (Raabe, 1982; Crompton et al., 1982). In addition, a large amount of an inhaled beta agonist, may be swallowed, especially in children. Thus, part of the effectiveness of β-agonists may be a result of absorption from the gastrointestinal tract. In studies utilizing oral activated charcoal to prevent absorption from the gastrointestinal tract, the therapeutic effects of inhaled isoproterenol (Davies, 1982) and terbutaline (Davies, 1984) have been shown to be an effect of local action and not systemic absorption. Because there is a decreased tidal volume and preferential deposition in central airways during an asthma attack, one might suppose the systemic route to be preferable in severe asthma episodes. This finding has been reported (Editorial, 1978) but no difference in clinical efficacy between aerosolized and systemically administered beta-agonists was found in pediatric patients in two studies (Edmunds and Godfrey, 1981; Schwartz et al., 1980). Similar results have been reported in studies of adults (Tinkleman et al., 1983; Lawford et al., 1978; Pliss and Gallagher, 1981). Rossing et al. (1980) found no evidence that the deposition of aerosols in the large airways impairs the clinical actions of beta agonists. In fact, the aerosol administration of β agonists was shown in children to have pharmacologic activity in both large and small airways (Bentar and Konig, 1974; Posey and Tinkleman 1979) as has been shown in adults (Hetzel and Clark, 1976; Larsson and Svedmyr, 1977; Wagner et al., 1978; Antic and Macklem, 1976; Mosberg, 1984) even in the presence of severe airways obstruction (Becker et al., 1983). Numerous reports have compared subcutaneous epinephrine to inhaled sympathomimetics in pediatric asthmatic patients.

Uden et al. (1985) compared the effects of aerosolized terbutaline and subcutaneous epinephrine in 19 pediatric patients. Their mean initial FEV_1 was 30% predicted and FEF 25-75 was 20% predicted. The FEV_1 and FEF_{25-75} improved to approximately 50 and 40% predicted, respectively, 1 hr following either mode of therapy. Becker et al. (1983) compared inhaled salbutamol (albuterol) and subcutaneous epinephrine in 40 children with acute asthmatic attaks. Initial FEV_1 and FEF_{25-75} values were 45% predicted and 15% predicted and increased to 65% predicted and 30% predicted, respectively, with either mode of therapy. There were no significant differences in other pulmonary function parameters or vital signs between the groups receiving aerosolized salbutamol (albuterol) and subcutaneous epinephrine. Side effects of nausea, vomiting, tremor, headache, palpitations, excitement, and pallor were documented more often in the epinephrine-tested patients. Similar findings in a comparison using aerosolized fenoterol and subcutaneous epinephrine have been reported by Ben-Zvi et al. (1982). Garra et al. (1977) found aerosolized metaproterenol and isoproterenol to improve pulmonary status in asthmatic children, with few side effects.

Studies comparing oral and aerosol administration of sympathomimetics have also been enlightening. Lee (1981) examined the effects of oral, aerosol, and combined oral/aerosol administration of metaproterenol in 17 asthmatic children. There was a greater improvement in FEV1 following its aerosol administration. Combined oral/aerosol administration produced no significantly greater clinical improvement than aerosol alone. The side effects of either oral or combined oral/aerosol administration were much greater than either placebo or aerosol administration alone. Similar studies in adults comparing oral and aerosolized administration of metaproterenol (Shim and Williams, 1980), terbutaline (Pierce et al., 1981) and albuterol (Hetzel and Clark, 1976) have found equal or greater clinical effectiveness of the aerosol route in moderate to severe asthmatics, while causing little or no systemic side effects.

A number of comparisons of sympathomimetics in children and adults give us information for making a rational choice of the drug to be used. In comparing isoetharine to metaproterenol using a single dose from a metered dose inhaler in a double-blind comparison in adults (Emirgil et al., 1976), the duration of response to metaproterenol was found to be 4 hr and that of isoetharine (as Bronkosol; isoetharine 680 μg + phenylephrine 140 μg) to be 2 hr (Emirgil et al., 1976). No significant side effects were observed with either drug. This short duration of action makes isoetharine a relatively poor choice in the seriously ill child. Aerosolized terbutaline and isoproterenol have been compared (Huhti, 1972) and terbutaline produced equal improvement in pulmonary function tests, without the sytemic side effects seen with isoproterenol administration (Formgren, 1970). In addition, the duration of action of terbutaline was increased over that of isoproterenol. Thus, aerosolized isoproterenol is also a poor choice as a bronchodilator in the seriously ill child. Similar studies comparing aerosolized terbutaline with aerosolized metaproterenol (Formgren, 1970; Roth et al., 1977; Chester et al., 1978) have been performed showing terbutaline to have both earlier and higher peak activities as well as more prolonged effects than metaproterenol. Albuterol (salbutamol) is widely used by nebulizer (Editorial, 1978) and has been advocated as the drug of choice in studies of selective β_2-agonists in the treatment of pediatric asthma (Konig, 1978). When compared with other sympathomimetics, terbutaline, albuterol, and fenoterol are relatively equipotent and all have greater bronchodilatory effects than metaproterenol while causing fewer side effects (Geumei and Miller, 1977). Albuterol was found to have slightly better bronchodilatory effects than terbutaline in some children (Francis et al., 1983). Conversely, terbutaline was found to have slightly less systemic effects than fenoterol when given in equipotent doses (Gray et al., 1982). Similar differences, but not quite as pronounced, between inhaled terbutaline and albuterol have been demonstrated (Freedman, 1972; Simonsson et al., 1972). In addition to these advantages, terbutaline in adult studies does not appear to have the same adverse effects on ventilation/perfusion relationships as seen with albuterol (Harris, 1973) and isoproterenol (McFadden, 1981). Giving repeated doses of nebulized terbutaline has been demonstrated to produce progressive improvement in pulmonary function (Pancorbo et al., 1983; Heimer et al., 1980; Williams, 1973; Riley et al., 1979).

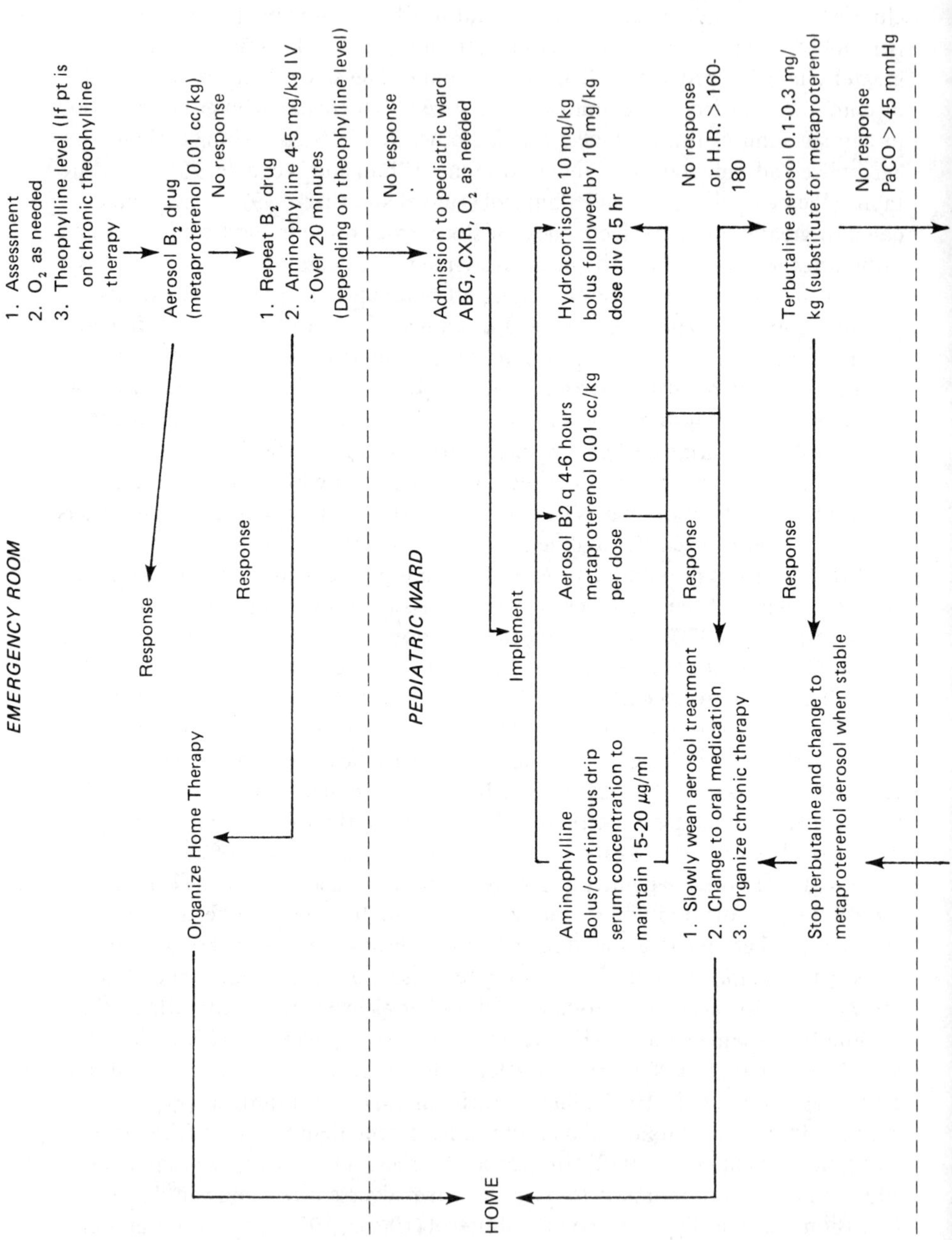
EMERGENCY ROOM
1. Assessment
2. O_2 as needed
3. Theophylline level (If pt is on chronic theophylline therapy
Aerosol B_2 drug (metaproterenol 0.01 cc/kg)
No response
Response
1. Repeat B_2 drug
2. Aminophylline 4-5 mg/kg IV Over 20 minutes (Depending on theophylline level)
Response
Organize Home Therapy
No response
PEDIATRIC WARD
Admission to pediatric ward ABG, CXR, O_2 as needed
Implement
Aminophylline Bolus/continuous drip serum concentration to maintain 15-20 μg/ml
Aerosol B2 q 4-6 hours metaproterenol 0.01 cc/kg per dose
Hydrocortisone 10 mg/kg bolus followed by 10 mg/kg dose div q 5 hr
No response or H.R. > 160-180
Response
1. Slowly wean aerosol treatment
2. Change to oral medication
3. Organize chronic therapy
Terbutaline aerosol 0.1-0.3 mg/kg (substitute for metaproterenol
Response
Stop terbutaline and change to metaproterenol aerosol when stable
No response $PaCO_2$ > 45 mmHg
HOME

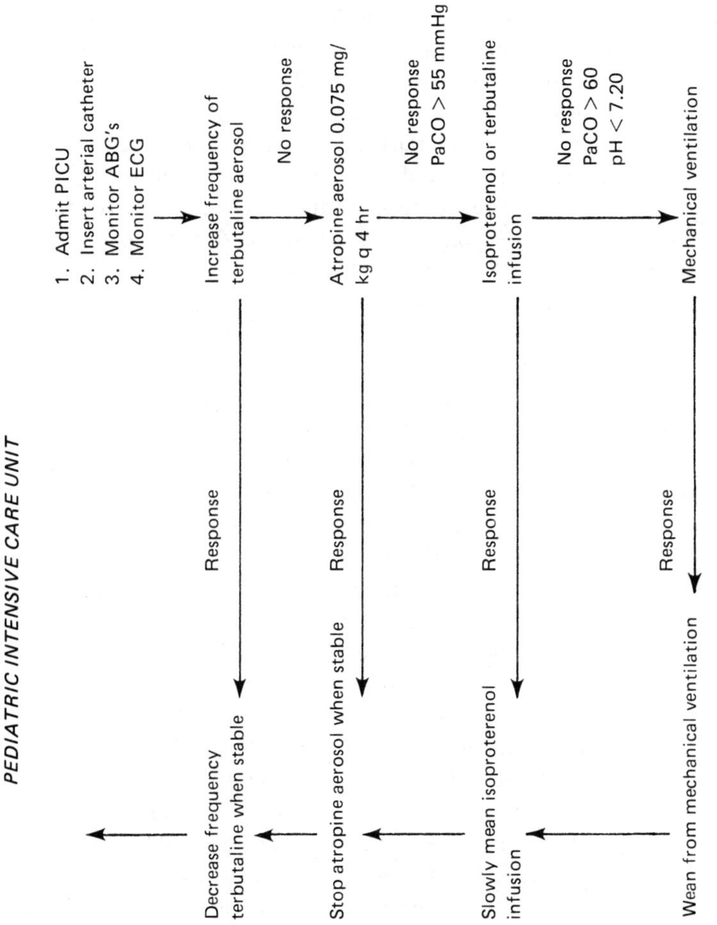

Figure 1 Steps in treating acute asthma.

In life-threatening pediatric asthmatic attacks with impending respiratory failure, the greatly decreased vital capacity as well as preferential deposition in the less obstructed airways may prevent optimal bronchodilatation by inhaled sympathomimetics. Intravenous sympathomimetics may, in these relatively rare instances, prevent the need for mechanical ventilation. In one study, 37 pediatric patients were studied whose previous therapy included aminophylline at therapeutic blood concentrations, corticosteroids, and isoetharine nebulized at a dosage of 0.01 ml/kg of the nebulizer solution diluted 1:10 or 1:20 given up to every hour. Thirty-four patients responded to the addition of intravenous isoproterenol at a mean dosage of 0.2 μg/kg/min. Two patients required mechanical ventilation and one patient, who was subsequently found to have Wolfe-Parkinson-White syndrome, required discontinuation of isoproterenol therapy secondary to arrhythmias (Herman et al., 1983).

The superiority of sympathomimetics over aminophylline in acute asthma has been well documented (Fanta et al., 1982; Rossing et al., 1980). The efficacy of combination therapy with methylxanthines and sympathomimetics in acute asthma is well known. Galant et al. (1978), for instance, demonstrated an additive effect between sympathomimetics and aminophylline in children similar to that seen in studies in adults (Rossing et al., 1981; Wolfe et al., 1978). However, recent work in adults found no additive therapeutic effect when aminophylline was added to metaproterenol aerosol. The aminophylline-treated patients patients had a significantly more side effects (Siegel et al., 1985).

The treatment of a serious asthma episode starts in the emergency room (Fig. 1). Traditionally, the treatment for asthmatic children in the emergency room has been the use of subcutaneous epinephrine (Table 1) in repeated doses, generally two or three, given 20-30 min apart. Failure to respond to this regimen had been defined as status asthmaticus. If a response was obtained, a long-acting epinephrine preparation (Sus-Phrine) was given and the child sent home.

Ben Zvi and colleagues (1983) evaluated this therapeutic regimen comparing single- and multiple-dose regimens in four groups of patients (total of 88 children and young adults aged 6-20 years). Patients received (1) epinephrine-epinephrine-Sus-Phrine (group EES); (2) Sus-Phrine only (group S); (3) Sus-Phrine-placebo-placebo (group SPP); or (4) epinephrine only (group E). At 5 min those receiving epinephrine had a greater FEV_1 than those treated with Sus-Phrine (groups SSP and S). This difference was not sustained at 25 min up to 2 hr. Side effects (tremor, palpitation, and nausea) were significantly greater in those patients receiving epinephrine than in those treated with Sus-Phrine. The failure rate (inadequate response or relapse) was 17.8% for groups EES, S, and SPP combined, with no difference in failure rate among them. Among those receiving only epinephrine there was a 46% failure rate. Thus, there was little therapeutic advantage of giving multiple epinephrine injections over a single injection of Sus-Phrine for the initial treatment of acute asthma.

Table 1 Treatment Regimens for Asthma

	Systemic administration			Inhaled administration	
	Oral	Subcutaneous	IV	Metered dose	Nebulizer[a]
Catecholamine base					
Epinephrine (Adrenaline)	–	0.01 ml/kg (1:1,000)	–	–	–
Epinephrine suspension (Sus-Phrine)	–	0.005 ml/kg	–	–	–
Isoproterenol (Isuprel)	–	–	(see Appendix)	2 puffs 4 times daily	0.1 ml (1% soln)
Isoetharine (Bronkosol)	–	–	–	2 puffs 4 times daily	0.24 ml (1% soln)
Resorcinol base					
Metaproterenol (Alupent, Metaprel)	0.5 mg/kg/dose 3-4 times daily	–	–	2 puffs 4 times daily	0.01-0.02 ml/kg
Terbutaline (Brethine, Bricanyl)	0.035 mg/kg/dose 3-4 times daily	0.005 mg/kg (0.1% soln)	(see Appendix)	2 puffs 4 times daily	0.1-0.3 ml/kg (0.1% soln or 1 mg/ml)
Fenoterol (Berotec)	0.1 mg/kg/dose 3-4 times daily	–	–	2 puffs 4 times daily	0.03 ml/kg (0.5% soln)[b]
Salinigen base					
Albuterol (Ventolin, Proventil)	0.15 mg/kg/dose 3-4 times daily	–	0.2-2.0 μg/kg/min	2 puffs 4 times daily	0.1 cc (5% soln)[b]

[a]All doses are diluted with saline to 2-3 cc total volume recommended nebulized doses are given every 4-6 hr, but the frequency of the more selective β-agonists (e.g., Terbutaline) may be increased up to every 30 min in a very severe attack.
[b]Not available in the United States.

In assessing 269 patients, ages 5-21 years, presenting with acute asthma, Schwartz et al. (1980) reported a cumulative effect for single doses of epinephrine. Based on clinical assessment, 25% of patients could be discharged home after each of the three epinephrine doses (0.01 mg/kg) given 5 min apart. Although this appears to demonstrate a cumulative effect of epinephrine, no patients were given a single dose of epinephrine and followed for the same period of time, so these results may represent the bronchodilator effect of the first dose and of the subsequent time lag during which the patient improved slowly. Since pulmonary function was not tested serially there may have been residual obstruction that went undetected by clinical examination.

Terbutaline by injection has been suggested for use in acute asthma, presumably because it has greater β_2 specificity and fewer side effects. Based on clinical outcome, Schwartz et al. (1980) did not find terbutaline given by subcutaneous injection more effective than epinephrine and, contrary to its supposed β_2 specificity, terbutaline caused the highest frequency of adverse side effects, with patients noting most often, tremor, vomiting, and tachycardia. A higher incidence of side effects was also reported by Davis et al. (1977). The subcutaneous administration of terbutaline in asthmatic children was found to cause cardiac side effects similar to those of epinephrine (Sly et al., 1977), but in another comparison tremor was its only major side effect, while subcutaneous epinephrine caused excitement, agitation, tremor, and headache (Simons and Gillies, 1981).

From the available data, if one wishes to use injectable medication in the emergency room, it seems best to give Sus-Phrine as a single subcutaneous injection. However, the worldwide experience with inhaled bronchodilators indicates that they are both safer and more effective than injectable sympathomimetics. We should examine these drugs, find the most effective one, and identify the technical and pharmacologic factors that contribute to efficacy. The objective is to find the most specific β_2 agent and the one having the longest duration of action by the route of administration to be used. In the emergency room, inhalation is helpful. The drugs available for use are listed in Table 1. Not all are available in the United States at the time of writing but are in various preapproval stages. Epinephrine can be used by inhalation but is a weak bronchodilator and has a duration of action of only 20-30 min. Isoproterenol has been used and recommended in a dosage of 0.25-0.5 ml of a 1:200 solution because it is free of α-adrenergic effects and has a longer duration of action than epinephrine. Compared to the newer β_2 agonists, isoproterenol is relatively short-acting, being effective for 60 min, and causes tachycardia and arrhythmias. A report of chest pain in a child being treated with inhaled isoproterenol followed by electrocardiographic changes indicating myocardial ischemia (ST segment and depression and T wave inversion) during infusion (Matson et al., 1978) indicates the potential dangers of its use.

In the United States availability of the highly selective β-agonists (terbutaline, albuterol, and fenoterol) in a nebulizer formulation is limited and thus, the first-line sympathomimetic in severe asthma is metaproterenol by nebulizer. In the more severe patients we recommend administering terbutaline by nebulizer, which is available as a 1 mg/1 cc parenteral preparation. This is usually administered at a dosage of 0.1-0.3 mg/kg every 4 hr but the interval may be decreased to every 15-30 min in severe cases.

Theophylline

Theophylline has been used as a bronchodilator for over 50 years and is still considered a mainstay of drug treatment for status asthmaticus. Its mechanism of action has often been postulated to be inhibition of phosphodiesterase, which increases intracellular cyclic AMP causing bronchial smooth muscle relaxation. However, other phosphodiesterase inhibitors such as dipyridamole do not produce bronchodilation. Theophylline also blocks adenosine receptors, which may explain its cardiac, central nervous system, and diuretic effect, but does not completely explain its activity as a bronchodilator.

Maselli and co-workers (1970) demonstrated the effectiveness of intravenous aminophylline (theophylline ethylenediamine) in a group of mild to moderately ill children. In these children FEV_1 improved in proportion to the serum theophylline concentration. A rapid infusion or intravenous injection of aminophylline at 4 mg/kg achieved a rapid increase in mean theophylline concentration to a level of 8 μg/ml accompanied by an improvement in FEV_1 to 65% above baseline value at 15 min and 78% above baseline by 2 hr. Despite a rapid fall in serum theophylline concentration, FEV_1 remained stable until the end of an 8 hr period, then declined markedly. Mitenko and Ogilvie (1973) later demonstrated, in a small group of adults, that the improvement in FEV_1 varies directly with the logarithm of the plasma concentration between theophylline serum concentrations of 5 and 20 mg/liter.

Because of its narrow therapeutic range, the dosing of theophylline in any form is difficult. Add to this the wide variability among children in plasma half-life for theophylline and absorption in the case of oral dosing, and it is evident that one must spend considerable time and energy calculating and adjusting theophylline dosages for children with status asthmaticus. The half-life of theophylline in children from 1 to 16 years of age has been shown to average between 3.0 and 3.69 hr (Ellis et al., 1976; Loughnan et al., 1976; Levy and Koysooko, 1975) which is approximately half that seen in the nonsmoking adult.

To avoid a sawtooth plasma theophylline concentration curve, which would occur with a short half-life if the doses were given every 6 or 8 hr, Mitenko and Ogilvie (1972) devised a method for intravenous administration that combines a loading dose with a constant infusion. This approach increases theophylline serum concentration rapidly and avoids the 4 to 5 half-life delay in achieving steady-state serum concentrations that would occur if a constant infusion were started without a loading dose.

In practice, however, the pharmacokinetic data required for this method are rarely known and, even if they had been calculated on a previous admission, theophylline pharmacokinetics are affected by a variety of drugs (including cimetidine and erythromycin) and clinical states (diet, smoking), making each new admission an experiment in clinical pharmacology. Theophylline clearance is increased by isoproterenol infusion by a mechanism unrelated to acidemia or increased renal clearance (Hemstreet et al., 1982). Whether a similar phenomenon exists in children with inhaled isoproterenol or with other sympathomimetics given either systemically or by inhalation is not known. Furthermore, the apparent volume of distribution (V_D) varies among patients and within the same patient.

Loading Dose

A bolus, calculated to achieve a serum concentration of between 15 and 20 mg/liter, assuming an average V_D, is administered. Ideally, this is done after a serum theophylline concentration, measured from blood drawn immediately upon the patient's arrival in the emergency room, is returned by the laboratory so that the physician knows the starting serum concentration. However, it is rare for this measurement to be back from the laboratory quickly enough to make the calculation and an empirical calculation must be done. We, therefore, give a loading dose calculated on the assumption that 1 mg/kg raises the serum concentration 2 mg/liter in the average patient. Our goal is to raise the serum level by 10-12 mg/liter.

The loading dose is given over 20 min to avoid excessively high theophylline blood concentrations. If the patient has taken a theophylline preparation within 6 hr the loading dose should be adjusted downward. The loading dose is then followed by a constant infusion of aminophylline calculated to maintain the desired serum concentration at steady state.

Maintenance Dose

The constant infusion rate can present similar problems because the clearance (Cl) varies widely among children and will change within the same child from time to time. The clearance is the product of the elimination rate constant and the distribution volume ($Cl = Kel \times V_D$). The constant infusion rate is the product of the clearance and the desired plasma concentration.

As a starting point in patients who have documented theophylline serum concentrations in the therapeutic range, we convert the total daily oral dose of theophylline to aminophylline. For example, a child with an adequate theophylline concentration (e.g., 16 mg/liter) while receiving 150 mg of a slow release oral preparation every 8 hr would have a total dose of 450 mg anhydrous theophylline or 530 mg aminophylline. This converts to an hourly dose of 22 mg aminophylline (530 mg per day/24 hr = 22 mg/hr). A short cut calculation is to multiply the total daily *theophylline* dose by 0.05, which results in the hourly dose of *aminophylline* (450 mg/24 hr × 0.05 = 22.5 mg/hr aminophylline).

If the infusion is to be started when the last oral dose is expected to peak, it is safer to withhold the bolus dose until the serum theophylline concentration is reported from the laboratory. Subsequently, small bolus doses and adjustments in the infusion rate will be required to maintain the serum concentration high in the therapeutic range. The same assumptions are used for these incremental changes as for the loading dose.

Oral theophylline medications should not be substituted for intravenous drugs to treat a seriously ill child. If intravenous access is impossible we would recommend the use of inhaled sympathomimetics until the problem is remedied or the child is transferred to another facility. A rectal solution is available (Somophyllin Rectal Solution, Fisons) for use if intravenous access is not available, but it suffers from some of the same problems as oral dosing in that absorption may be delayed or the dose expelled. This should not be confused with rectal suppositories, which have no place in the treatment of childhood asthma.

The management of seriously ill asthmatic children is predicated on having available a laboratory that can perform accurate and reproducible theophylline serum concentration determinations 24 hr a day. Unfortunately, there is wide variability in the results reported from different clinical laboratories (Bonham et al., 1980).

The question of whether to use a continuous infusion of aminophylline or bolus dosing every 4-6 hr has been a long-standing topic of discussion. In a study of 11 asthmatic children requiring bronchodilators but who were not in status asthmaticus Goldberg and co-workers (1980) found pulmonary function was significantly better in children receiving continuous infusion than those treated with boluses of aminophylline at 4-hr intervals. Intermittent administration may be useful in settings in which constant infusion cannot be maintained reliably. In practice, a 2-hr dose of aminophylline is put in the pediatric drip chamber when giving a constant infusion as compared to 4-6 hr dose when using the intermittent method, making the continuous regimen safer in case a large amount of fluid is administered quickly in error.

Corticosteroids

The role of corticosteroids in the treatment of children with asthma has always been problematic. Steroids have been advocated as a last resort and the use of this class of drugs is seen as committing the patient to their use during all future admissions for acute wheezing. On the other hand, it was stated that to be effective steroids had to be given early in the course because they took 6-8 hr to "kick in." Thus, the paradox existed of wishing to use corticosteroids early enough for maximum effect but not so as to commit a patient to their use until one is certain they were absolutely necessary. Fortunately, these impressions were not built on a foundation of scientific data.

The literature on the use of steroids in the acute wheezing attack in children remains confusing. Parenteral corticosteroid therapy was evaluated in 45 children hospitalized in status (Pierson et al., 1974). Measurements at 3 and 24 hr postadmission showed no difference in FEV_1, FVC, and clinical score between the steroid and placebo groups. There was an improvement in PaO_2 in both groups but the steroid group had a significantly higher PaO_2 after 24 hr than did the placebo patients. The steroid group had an initial PaO_2 of 58.5 mmHg which improved to 78.1 mmHg at 24 hr while the placebo group increased from 57.9 to 64.4 mmHg over 24 hr ($P < 0.005$). This study included children who were already steroid dependent.

Kattan and colleagues (1980) studied a similar group of children hospitalized for status asthmaticus, but excluded children who were already steroid dependent. The rest were treated with aminophylline and salbutamol in addition to either hydrocortisone or placebo. These workers monitored PEFR and clinical score over 36 and 48 hr, respectively. Both groups' condition was moderately severe on admission and in both groups clinical score and flows improved with time. However, there was no difference demonstrated between steroid and controls.

Since Pierson et al. had included children already on steroids and had used isoproterenol, a less effective sympathomimetic, the studies are not directly comparable. It may be that steroids potentiate a relatively less effective bronchodilator, isoproterenol, but have their effect masked by a more potent agent, salbutamol. Kattan failed to monitor blood gas tensions and so may have lost the crucial difference claimed for steroids: an early improvement in arterial hypoxemia, presumably through an improvement in small airways functioning.

Shapiro et al. (1983), in evaluating the effect of oral methylprednisolone on asthmatic children with acute wheezing not requiring hospitalization, found that steroids accelerated the recovery of $FEF_{25\text{-}75\%}$ to normal, indicating an effect on small airway function. Both Pierson and Shapiro found short-term steroid therapy to be safe and Shapiro found no difference in the adrenal response to cosyntropin between steroid- and placebo-treated patients.

These data do not provide much assistance in making a rational decision about the use of steroids in a child with status asthmaticus. Given the apparent safety of the drug used short term and the evidence of effectiveness in some patients, we continue to recommend their use in the standard dosages of 10-20 mg/kg of hydrocortisone (or equivalent) per 24 hr. There does not appear to be a definite benefit of one steroid preparation over another.

E. Intravenous Sympathomimetics

In an effort to avoid the use of mechanical ventilation in the severely obstructed asthmatic, Downes et al. (1973) proposed the use of a constant intravenous infusion of isoproterenol to promote bronchodilation.

Their criterion for its use was a PCO_2 greater than 55 mmHg despite conventional therapy. In 18 episodes studied there was a prompt and sustained reduction in PCO_2 obviating mechanical ventilation but without improving oxygenation. With this therapy a pediatric patient in impending respiratory failure, despite vigorous conventional therapy (sympathomimetics, aminophylline, anticholinergics, and corticosteroids), is given intravenous isoproterenol in a dosage of 0.05-0.1 μg/kg/min and the dosage is increased, if necessary, as previously described. The ability of isoproterenol to prevent the need for mechanical ventilation has been documented (Cotton and Parry, 1975; Woods et al., 1972). Again, care must be used when administering isoproterenol because of its effects of worsening ventilation/perfusion matching (McFadden, 1981). Acute hypoxemia may occur secondary to vasodilation in areas with reflex vasoconstriction. Other common side effects of isoproterenol include its cardiac effects, antidiuretic effects (Tinkelman et al., 1983), and increased theophylline clearance (Levi et al., 1976). Others (Parry et al., 1976) have reported difficulties with cardiac arrhythmias and have noted rebound bronchospasm during administration when decreasing the dose.

Studies of the newer β-agonists such as terbutaline and albuterol indicate that they are more effective by the inhaled route than when given intravenously. In stable asthmatic adults, albuterol (salbutamol) given by aerosol produced longer-lasting bronchodilation than intravenous drugs (Hetzel and Clark, 1976). The peak increase in flows was similar but the intravenous dose produced an increase in heart rates whereas the aerosol did not. Terbutaline produces a greater peak effect on FEV_1 and less tremor when given by inhalation than intravenously (Thiringer and Svedmyr, 1976). There appears to be no selective response of the small airways to intravenous terbutaline (Pierce et al., 1981). In our institutions, when a patient is not responding to conventional therapy we begin terbutaline by inhalation repeated as frequently as every half hour. This is done in the pediatric intensive care unit with constant cardiac monitoring after placement of an indwelling arterial catheter for frequent monitoring of PCO_2 and PO_2. In our clinical experience inhaled terbutaline does not result in a tachycardia and usually causes a decrease in the heart rate toward normal levels. On the rare occasion when this therapy fails intravenous terbutaline is preferable to isoproterenol since it results in fewer side effects. No intravenous albuterol preparation is available in the United States at this time.

IV. Respiratory Failure

Respiratory failure from acute asthma is reported in 5-6% of patients, but is less frequent in our experience, usually occurring at the onset of therapy in children who did not arrive at the hospital early enough in the course of their attack. Simons et al. (1977) assessed 13 asthmatic children who had 19 episodes of respiratory failure. They could discern no difference in pharmacologic treatment of these children prior to the need for ventilation, but found that delayed or inappropriate therapy was a contributing factor in most instances.

The ventilatory management of asthmatic patients may be difficult, but the mortality rate for asthmatics requiring mechanical ventilation is low (Richards et al., 1979).

The intubation of an asthmatic child may pose considerable risks. These patients are hypoxemic and acidotic, both of which may be aggravated during intubation. In addition, vagal stimulation may potentiate bronchospasm and worsen hypoxemia and acidosis. Many different intubation regimens are acceptable, but intubation of an asthmatic with respiratory failure should be performed by a physician skilled and experienced in intubation. We routinely premedicate with sodium pentothal (3-5 mg/kg IV), atropine (0.01-0.02 mg/kg IV), and succinylcholine (1-2 mg/kg IV). Because of the danger involved in paralyzing patients with severe respiratory compromise, other institutions recommend sedating with Valium and intubating patients without paralysis. The decision of whether or not to paralyze patients for intubation depends largely on the experience of the individual institution. Intubation must be done quickly to prevent the patient from becoming more acidotic and hypoxic. A nasal endotracheal tube is preferable because of its increased stability and patient comfort.

A volume-cycled ventilator should be used to maintain a constant tidal volume despite changing airway resistance. Since an asthmatic has a long time constant for exhalation, we use relatively high flow rates and choose tidal volumes that will maximize expiratory time. We prefer a combination of settings that allow audible exhalation to stop before the next breath begins, which generally results in low ventilator rates (8-12 breaths/min). Recent reports (Darioli and Perret, 1984; Menitone and Goldring, 1983) have advocated a "controlled hypoventilation." This approach corrects hypoxemia but not hypercarbia, while acidosis is controlled by using sodium bicarbonate. Darioli and Perret (1984) reported 26 adult asthmatic patients with 34 episodes of acute respiratory acidosis requiring intubation and mechanical ventilation. Sedation and muscle relaxants were used as necessary for ventilator synchronization. Controlled hypoventilation was used until the patient's ventilation and oxygenation improved. No deaths and no pneumothoraces were reported. Although there were no studies using this approach in pediatric patients, we have successfully used this approach in our most severely ill asthmatic patients. It is not always needed, however.

Because exhaled airflow obstruction is the main pathologic finding in severe asthma, positive end expiratory pressure (PEEP) has been thought to be contraindicated in mechanically ventilated asthmatics (Qvist et al., 1982). (Pierce et al., 1981) recently reported the use of PEEP in adult asthmatics, reasoning that PEEP may decrease airways closure and facilitate emptying of gas from the lungs. They presented two cases, an adult and a 9-year-old girl, who received 25 cmH_2O PEEP, respectively, with clinical improvement. Other reports (Martin et al., 1982; Tenaillon et al., 1983) have advocated a similar approach to patients who are unable to be ventilated and oxygenated with little or no PEEP. This approach, however, is controversial and should only be considered as an alternative when other standard methods have failed.

Sedation and paralysis are very important in the ventilatory management of asthmatics, especially if controlled hypoventilation is being utilized. Although opioids such as morphine and meperidine cause histamine release, Simons et al. (1977) did not find any worsening in bronchospasm. We use morphine 0.2 mg/kg IV and/or Valium 0.1-0.3 mg/kg IV for sedation and pancuronium 0.1 mg/kg IV for continued paralysis.

Medical management prior to mechanical ventilation should be continued as before and the patient weaned from mechanical ventilation as the first step in withdrawing support. Once the patient is extubated, other medical management may be weaned as indicated.

References

Amory, S. W., Brunham, S. C., and Chenz, F. W. (1975). Comparison of the cardiopulmonary effects of the subcutaneously administered epinephrine and terbutaline in patients with reversible airway obstruction. *Chest 67*: 279-286.

Antic, R., and Macklem, P. T. (1976). The influence of clinical factors on site of airways obstruction in asthma. *Am. Rev. Respir. Dis. 114*: 851-859.

Aubier, M., Viires, N., Murciano, D., Medrano, G., Lecocguic, Y., and Pariente, R. (1984). Effects and mechanism of action of terbutaline on diaphragmatic contractility and fatigue. *J. Appl. Physiol. 56*: 922-929.

Barger, G., and Dale, H. H.(1910). Chemical structure and sympathomimetic action of amines. *J. Physiol. 4*: 19-59.

Becker, A. B., Nelson, N. A., and Simons, F. E. R. (1983). Inhaled salbutamol (albuterol) versus injected epinephrine in the treatment of acute asthma. *J. Pediatr. 102*: 465-469.

Bentar, S. R., and Konig, P. (1974). Maximal expiratory flow and lung volume changes associated with exercise induced asthma in children and the effect of breathing a low density gas mixture. *Clin. Sci. Mol. Med. 46*: 317-329.

Ben-Zvi, Z., Lam, C., Hoffman, J., et al. (1982). An evaluation of the initial treatment of acute asthma. *Pediatrics 70*: 348.

Ben-Zvi, Z., Lam, C., Spohn, W. A., Gribetz, I., Mulvihill, M. N., and Kattan, M. (1983). An evaluation of repeated injections of epinephrine for the initial treatment of acute asthma. *Am. Rev. Respir. Dis. 127*: 101-105.

Bonham, A., Hendeles, L., Weinberger, M., and Vaughan, L. (1980). The reliability of serum theophylline determinations from clinical laboratories. *Am. Rev. Respir. Dis. 122*: 829.

Brooks, L. J., Cloutier, M. M., and Afshani, E. (1982). Significance of roentgenographic abnormalities in children hospitalized for asthma. *Chest 82*: 315-318.

Chester, E. H., Euggett, W. E., Montenegro, H. D., et al. (1978). Bronchodilating effect of terbutaline aerosol. *Clin. Pharmacol. Ther. 23*: 630-634.

Commey, J. O. O., and Levison, H. (1976). Physical signs in childhood asthma. *Pediatrics 58*: 537-541.

Cooper, D. M., Cutz, E., and Levison, H. (1977). Occult pulmonary abnormalities in asymptomatic children. *Chest 71*: 361-365.

Cotton, E. K., and Parry, W. (1975). Treatment of status asthmaticus and respiratory failure. *Pediatr. Clin. North Am. 22*: 163.

Crompton, G., Moren, F., Simonnson, B. G. (eds.). (1982). Inhalation therapy in the management of airway obstruction. *Eur. J. Respir. Dis.* Suppl. 119:1-125.

Darioli, R., and Perret, C. (1984). Mechanical controlled hypoventilation in status asthmaticus. *Am. Rev. Respir. Dis. 129*: 385-387.

Davies, D. S. (1982). Pharmacokinetic studies with inhaled drugs. *Eur. J. Respir. Dis. 63*(Suppl 119): 67-72.

Davies, D. S. (1984). The fate of inhaled terbutaline. *Eur. J. Respir. Dis. 65* (suppl 134): 141-147.

Davis, W. J., Pang, L. M., Cherniack, W. J., and Mellins, R. B. (1977). Terbutaline in the treatment of acute asthma in childhood. *Chest 72*: 614-617.

Downes, J. J., Wood, D. W., Harwood, I., Sheinkopf, H. N., and Raphaely, R. C. (1973). Intravenous isoproterenol infusion in children with severe hypercapnia due to status asthmaticus. *Crit. Care Med. 1*: 63-68.

Dworetzky, M., and Philson, A. D. (1968). Review of asthmatic patients hospitalized in the pavilion service of the New York Hospital from 1948 to 1963. *J. Allergy 41*: 181.

Editorial. (1978). Management of severe acute asthma. *Br. Med. J. 1*: 873.

Edmunds, A. T., and Godfrey, S. (1981). Cardiovascular response during severe acute asthma and its treatment in children. *Thorax 36*: 534.

Eggleston, P. A., Ward, B. H., Pierson, W. E., Bierman, C. W. (1974). Radiographic abnormalities in acute asthma in children. *Pediatrics 54*: 442-449.

Ellis, E. F., Koysooko, R., and Levy, G. (1976). Pharmacokinetics of theophylline in children with asthma. *Pediatrics 58*: 542.

Emirgil, C., Dwyer, K., and Sobol, B. J. (1976). A comparison of the duration of action and the cardiovascular effects of metaproterenol and an isoetharine-phenylephrine combination. *Curr. Ther. Res. 19*: 317-378.

Fanta, C. H., Rossing, T. H., McFadden, E. R., Jr. (1982). Emergency room treatment of asthma. *Am. J. Med. 72*: 416.

Field, W. E. (1968). Mucous gland hypertrophy in babies and children 15 years or less. *Br. J. Dis. Chest 62*: 11.

Formgren, H. (1970). Clinical comparison of inhaled terbutaline and orciprenaline in asthmatic patients. *Scand. J. Respir. Dis. 51*: 203-211.

Francis, P. W., Kelly, C. A., and Zimmerman, P. V. (1983). Comparison of salbutamol powder with terbutaline aerosol administered with a tube spacer in asthmatic children. *Aust. Pediatr. J. 19*: 245-247.

Freedman, B. J. (1972). Trial of a terbutaline aerosol in the treatment of asthma and a comparison of its effects with those of a salbutamol aerosol. *Br. J. Dis. Chest 66*: 222-229.

Galant, S. P., Groncy, C. E., Duriseti, S., et al. (1978a). Effect of metaproterenol in chronic asthmatic children receiving therapeutic doses of theophylline. *J. Allergy Clin. Immunol. 61*: 73.

Galant, S. T., Groncy, C. E., and Shaw, K. C. (1978b). The value of pulsus paradoxus in assessing the child with status asthmaticus. *Pediatrics 61*: 46-51.

Garra, B., Shapiro, G. G., Dorsett, C., et al. (1977). A double-blind evaluation of the use of nebulized metaproterenol and isoproterenol in hospitalized asthmatic children and adolescents. *J. Allergy Clin. Immunol. 60*: 63.

Geumei, A. M., and Miller, W. F. (1977). New oral bronchodilator drug with relative selective stimulation of beta-2-adrenergic receptors. *Chest 72*: 267.

Gillies, J. D., Reed, M. H., and Simons, F. E. R. (1978). Radiographic findings in acute childhood asthma. *J. Can. Assoc. Radiol. 29*: 28.

Goldberg, P., Leffert, F., Gonzalez, M., Gogenola, L., and Zerbe, G. (1980). Intravenous aminophylline therapy for asthma. *Am. J. Dis. Child. 134*: 596-599.

Graeser, J. B., and Rome, A. H. (1935). Inhalation of epinephrine for the relief of asthmatic symptoms. *J. Allergy 6*: 415-416.

Gray, B. J., Frame, M. H., and Costello, J. F. (1982). A comparative double-blind study of the bronchodilator effects and side effects of inhaled fenoterol and terbutaline administered in equipotent doses. *Br. J. Dis. Chest 76*: 341.

Harris, L. (1973). Comparison of cardiorespiratory effects of terbutaline and salbutamol aerosols in patients with reversible airways obstruction. *Thorax 28*: 592-595.

Heimer, D., Shim, C., and Williams, M. H. (1980). Bronchodilator response to metaproterenol aerosol. *J. Allergy Clin. Immunol.* 75-77.

Hemstreet, M. P., Miles, M. V., and Rutland, R. O. (1982). Effect of intravenous isoproterenol on theophylline kinetics. *J. Allergy Clin. Immunol. 69*: 360-364.

Herman, J. J., Noah, Z. L., and Moody, R. R. (1983). Use of intravenous isoproterenol for status asthmaticus in children. *Crit. Care Med. 11*: 716-720.

Hetzel, M. R., and Clark, T. J. H. (1976). Comparison of intravenous and aerosol salbutamol. *Br. Med. J. 2*: 16 October: 919.

Howell, S., and Roussos, C. (1984). Isoproterenol and aminophylline improve contractility of fatigued canine diaphragm. *Am. Rev. Respir. Dis. 129*: 118-124.

Huhti, E. (1972). Clinical comparison of terbutaline and isoprenaline administered by inhalation: A double-blind study. *Ann. Clin. Res. 4*: 152-157.

Isles, A. F., and Levison, H. (1985). Pediatric asthma. In *Bronchial Asthma.* Boston/Toronto, Little, Brown and Company, pp. 857-871.

Jorgenson, J. R., Falliers, C. J., and Bukantz, S. C. (1963). Pneumothorax and mediastinal and subcutaneous emphysema in children with bronchial asthma. *Pediatrics 31*: 824-832.

Kattan, M., Gurwitz, D., and Levison, H. (1980). Corticosteroids in status asthmaticus. *J. Pediatr. 96*: 596-599.

Konig, P., (1978). Treatment of severe attacks of asthma in children with nebulized beta-2-adrenergic agents. *Ann. Allergy 40*: 185.

Kurland, G., Williams, J., and Lewiston, N. J. (1979). Fatal myocardial toxicity during continuous infusion intravenous isoproterenol therapy of asthma. *J. Allergy Clin. Immunol. 63*: 407.

Larsson, S., and Svedmyr, N. (1977). Bronchodilating effect and side effects of beta-2-adrenoceptor stimulants by different modes of administration (tablets, metered aerosols and combinations thereof). A study of salbutamol in asthmatics. *Am. Rev. Respir. Dis. 116*: 961-969.

Lawford, P., Jones, B. J. M., and Milledge, J. S. (1978). Comparison of intravenous and nebulized salbutamol in the initial treatment of severe asthma. *Br. Med. J. 1*: 84.

Lee, H. S. (1981). Comparison of oral and aerosol adrenergic bronchodilators in asthma. *J. Pediatr. 99*: 805-807.

Levi, J., Coburn, J., and Kleeman, C. R. (1976). Mechanism of the antidiuretic effect of beta adrenergic stimulation in man. *Arch. Intern. Med. 136*: 25.

Levison, H., Collins-Williams, C., Bryan, A. C., et al. (1974). Asthma: current concepts. *Pediatr. Clin. North Am. 21*: 951.

Levy, G., and Koysooko, R. (1975). Pharmacokinetic analysis of the effect of theophylline on pulmonary function in asthmatic children. *J. Pediatr. 86*: 789.

Loughnan, P. M., Sitar, D. S., Ogilvie, R. J., et al. (1976). Pharmacokinetics analysis of the disposition of intravenous theophylline in young children. *J. Pediatr. 88*: 874.

Lulla, S., and Newcoms, R. W. (1980). Emergency management of asthma in children. *J. Pediatr. 97*: 346.

Maguire, J. F., Geha, R. S., and Umetso, D. T. (1986). Myocardial specific creatinine phosphokinase isoenzyme elevation in children with asthma treated with intravenous isoproterenol. *J. Allergy Clin. Immunol. 78*: 631-636.

Martin, J. G., Shore, S., and Engel, L. A. (1982). Effect of continuous positive airway pressure on respiratory mechanics and pattern of breathing in induced asthma. *Am. Rev. Respir. Dis. 126*: 812-817.

Maselli, R., Casal, G., and Ellis, E. F. (1970). Pharmacologic effects of intravenously administered aminophylline in asthmatic children. *J. Pediatr. 76*: 777-782.

Matson, J. R., Laughlin, G. M., and Strunk, R. C. (1978). Myocardial ischemia complicating the use of isoproterenol in asthmatic children. *J. Pediatr. 92*: 776.

Matsuba, K., and Thurlbeck, W. M. (1971). The number and dimensions of small airways in nonemphysematous lungs. *Am. Rev. Respir. Dis. 104*: 516.

Matsuba, K., and Thurlbeck, W. M. (1972). A morphometric study of bronchial and bronchiolar walls in children. *Am. Rev. Respir. Dis. 105*: 908.

McFadden, E. R., Jr. (1981). Beta-2-receptor agonists: Metabolism and pharmacology. *J. Allergy Clin. Immunol. 68*: 91.

Menitone, S. M., and Goldring, R. M. (1983). Combined ventilator and bicarbonate strategy in the management of status asthmaticus. *Am. J. Med. 74*: 898-901.

Minor, T. E., Dick, E. C., DeMeo, A. N., Ouellette, J. J., Cohen, M., and Reed, C. E. (1974). Viruses as precipitants of asthmatic attacks in children. *JAMA 227*: 292-298.

Mitenko, P. A., and Ogilvie, R. I. (1972). Rapidly achieved plasma concentrations plateaus with observations on theophylline kinetics. *Clin. Pharmacol. Ther. 13*: 329.

Mitenko, P. A., and Ogilvie, R. I. (1973). Rational intravenous doses of theophylline. *N. Engl. J. Med. 289*: 600.

Mosberg, B. (1984). Asthma—site of airway obstruction and aerosol deposition. *Eur. J. Respir. Dis. 65* (Suppl 136): 49-53.

Nelson, H. S. (1982). Beta receptor agonists. *Chest* (Suppl.) *82*: 335.

Pancorbo, S., Fifield, G., Davies, S., Fraser, G., Helmink, R., and Heissler, J. (1983). Subcutaneous epinephrine versus nebulized terbutaline in the emergency treatment of asthma. *Clin. Pharm. 2*: 45-48.

Pang, L. M., Rodriguez-Martinez, F., Davis, W. J., et al. (1977). Terbutaline in the treatment of status asthmaticus. *Chest 72*: 469-473.

Parry, W. H., Martorano, F., and Cotton, E. K. (1976). Management of life-threatening asthma with intravenous isoproterenol infusions. *Am. J. Dis. Child. 130*: 39-42.

Pierce, R. J., Payne, C. R., Williams, S. J., Denison, D. M., and Clark, T. J. H. (1981). Comparison of intravenous and inhaled terbutaline in the treatment of asthma. *Chest 79*: 506-511.

Pierson, R. N., and Grieco, M. H. (1969). Isoproterenol aerosols in normal and asthmatic subjects. *Am. Rev. Respir. Dis. 100*: 533-541.

Pierson, W. E., Bierman, C. W., and Kelley, V. C. (1974). A double-blind trial of corticosteroid therapy in status asthmaticus. *Pediatrics 54*: 282-288.

Pliss, L. B., and Gallagher, E. J. (1981). Aerosol versus injected epinephrine in acute asthma. *Ann. Emerg. Med. 10*: 353.

Posey, W. C., and Tinkleman, D. G. (1979). Dose-response characteristics of nebulized isoproterenol in asthmatic children. *J. Allergy Clin. Immunol. 63*: 258-266.

Qvist, J., Anderson, J. B., Pemberton, M., et al. (1982). High-level PEEP in severe asthma. *N. Engl. J. Med. 307*: 1347-1348.

Raabe, O. G. (1982). Deposition and clearance of inhaled aerosols. In *Mechanisms in Respiratory Toxicology,* Volume I. Edited by H. Witschi and P. Nettesheim. Boca Raton, CRC Press.

Richards, W., Lew, C., Carney, J., Platzker, A., and Church, J. A. (1979). Review of intensive care unit admission for asthma. *Clin. Pediatr. 18*: 345-352.

Riley, G. J., Liu, R. T., and Edelman, N. H. (1979). Enhanced responses to aerosolized bronchodilator therapy in asthma using respiratory maneuvers. *Chest 76*: 501-507.

Rossing, T. H., Fanta, C. H., Goldstein, D. H., Snapper, J. R., and McFadden, E. R. Jr. (1980). Emergency therapy of asthma. Comparison of the acute effects of parenteral and inhaled sympathomimetics and infused aminophylline. *Am. Rev. Respir. Dis. 122*: 365-371.

Rossing, T. H., Fanta, C. H., and McFadden, E. R. Jr. (1981). A controlled trial of the use of simple versus combined drug therapy in the treatment of acute episodes of asthma. *Am. Rev. Respir. Dis. 123*: 190.

Roth, M. J., Wilson, A. F., and Novey, H. S. (1977). A comparative study of the aerosolized bronchodilators, isoproterenol, metaproterenol, and terbutaline in asthma. *Ann. Allergy 38*: 16-21.

Schwartz, A. L., Lipton, J. M., Warburton, D., Johnson, L. B., and Twarog, F. J. (1980). Management of acute asthma in childhood: A randomized evaluation of beta-adrenergic agents. *Am. J. Dis. Child. 134*: 474.

Shapiro, G. G., Furukawa, C. T., Pierson, W. E., Gardinier, R., and Bierman, C. W. (1983). Double-blind evaluation of methylprednisolone versus placebo for acute asthma episodes. *Pediatrics 71*: 510-514.

Sheppard, D., Rizk, N. W., Boushey, H. A., and Bethel, R. A. (1983). Mechanism of cough and bronchoconstriction induced by distilled water aerosol. *Am. Rev. Respir. Dis. 127*: 691-694.

Shim, C., and Williams, M. H. (1980). Bronchial response to oral versus aerosol metaproterenol in asthma. *Ann. Intern. Med. 93*: 428-431.

Siegel, D., Sheppard, D., Gelb, A., and Weinberg, P. F. (1985). Aminophylline increases the toxicity but not the efficacy of an inhaled beta-adrenergic agonist in the treatment of acute exacerbations of asthma. *Am. Rev. Respir. Dis. 132*: 283-286.

Simons, F. E. R., Pierson, W. E., and Bierman, C. W. (1977). Respiratory failure in childhood status asthmaticus. *Am. J. Dis. Child. 131*: 1097-1101.

Simons, F. E. R., and Gillies, J. D. (1981). Dose response of subcutaneous terbutaline and epinephrine in children with acute asthma. *Am. J. Dis. Child. 135*: 214-217.

Simonsson, B. G., Stiksa, J., and Strom, B. (1972). Double-blind trial with increasing doses of salbutamol and terbutaline aerosols in patients with reversible airways obstruction. *Acta Med. Scand. 192*: 371-376.

Sly, R. M., Badier, B., and Faciani, J. (1977). Comparison of subcutaneous terbutaline with epinephrine in the treatment of asthma in children. *J. Allergy Clin. Immunol. 59*: 128.

Stalcup, S. A., and Mellins, R. B. (1977). Mechanical forces producing pulmonary edema in acute asthma. *N. Engl. J. Med. 297*: 592-596.

Tenaillon, A., Salmona, J. P., and Burdin, M. (1983). Continuous positive airway pressure in asthma. *Am. Rev. Respir. Dis. 127*: 658.

Thiringer, G., and Svedmyr, N. (1976). Comparison of infused and inhaled terbutaline in patients with asthma. *Scand. J. Respir. Dis. 57*: 17-24.

Tinkelman, D. G., Vanderpool, G. E., Carroll, M. S., Lotner, G. Z., and Spangler, D. L. (1983). Comparison of nebulized terbutaline (Terb) and subcutaneous epinephrine (Epi) in the treatment of acute asthma. *Ann. Allergy 50*: 398-401.

Uden, D. L., Goetz, D. R., Kohen, D. P., and Fifield, G. C. (1985). Comparison of nebulized terbutaline and subcutaneous epinephrine in the treatment of acute asthma. *Ann. Emerg. Med. 14*: 229-232.

Wagner, P. D., Dantzker, D. R., Zacovani, V. E., et al. (1978). Ventilation-perfusion inequality in asymptomatic asthma. *Am. Rev. Respir. Dis. 118*: 511-524.

Wanner, A. (1977). Clinical aspects of mucociliary transport. *Am. Rev. Respir. Dis.* (State of the art) *116*: 73.

Weng, T. R., Langer, H. M., Featherby, E. A., and Levison, H. (1970). Arterial blood gas tensions and acid-base balance in symptomatic and asymptomatic asthma in childhood. *Am. Rev. Respir. Dis. 101*: 274-282.

Williams, M. H. (1973). Pathophysiology and treatment of severe asthma. *NY State J. Med. 73*: 2446-2451.

Wolfe, J. D., Tashkin, D. P., Calorese, B., et al. (1978). Bronchodilator effects of terbutaline and aminophylline alone and in combination in asthmatic patients. *N. Engl. J. Med. 298*: 363.

Wood, D. W., Downes, J. J., Scheinkopf, H., et al. (1972). Intravenous isoproterenol in the management of respiratory failure in childhood status asthmaticus. *J. Allergy Clin. Immunol.* *50*: 75.

24

The Office Approach to Unusual Causes of Asthma

SHELDON L. SPECTOR

UCLA School of Medicine
and Allergy Medical Clinic
Los Angeles, California

I. Assessment of the Asthmatic State

Before bronchodilator therapy can be initiated in an asthmatic patient who is difficult to manage, it is important to assess properly those factors that might be contributing to the intractability.

A. Home Monitoring

It is remarkable how patients differ in their subjective experience of obstructive symptoms. Some patients are very much aware of small changes in pulmonary functions while others can have rather big changes in pulmonary function parameters without even knowing the direction, that is toward bronchoconstriction or bronchodilatation. This lack of awareness could be due to a variety of factors, such as the site of obstruction or the psychological make-up of that individual. Therefore we need to use objective means of monitoring flow.

The peak flow meter is presently the most frequently used home monitoring device. Peak expiratory flow rate (PEFR) requires a brief maximum exhalation from total lung capacity. The Wright peak flow meter has made PEFR measurements popular due to its simplicity and low price. Even more inexpensive are smaller versions of the Wright peak flow meter such as the Armstrong Mini-Wright peak flow meter, Vitalography pulmonary monitor, and Health-Scan peak flow meter. These instruments have been difficult to calibrate. Moreover, PEFR depends on effort and probably also on the size of the trachea and largest bronchi rather than smaller airways. In fact, certain patients with airway obstruction may be able to reach relatively high peak flow rates, yet have decreased flow rates at lower lung volumes. Thus PEFR may underestimate the severity of lower airway obstruction.

The three most commonly used portable flow meters were recently assessed (Eichenhorn et al., 1982). The Armstrong Mini-Wright peak flow meter met the flow range criteria established by the American Thoracic Society and the American College of Chest Physicians for flow devices, while the Health-Scan-Organon peak flow meter met the criteria for accuracy and reproducibility. We have studied the standard Wright peak flow meter with the Mini-Wright peak flow meter over 6 months and found them both to be stable (Morrill et al., 1981).

Home monitoring of peak expiratory flow rates might improve understanding and compliance on the part of patients. Parents are often surprised to see that bronchial obstruction exists in their children whom they thought were basically asymptomatic. It also gives information as to how long a given bronchodilator lasts, or if exposure to a particular allergen is actually causing symptoms.

B. Patterns of Asthma

Around-the-clock measurements of peak expiratory flow rates done at 3-4 hr intervals with a portable Wright peak flow meter were performed in children at a Denver residential center for severe asthma. There was a statistically significant elevation of PEFR in the early afternoon (Halberg and Falliers, 1966). Measurements of airway resistance confirmed variability of pulmonary function measurements at the Swiss Alpine Center for Asthma (Zuidema and van Essel, 1965). Airway resistance also varied significantly over 24 hr. Best values were recorded around noon, while between 4 and 6 AM the patients were at their worst. Spirometry and Wright PEFR were not as sensitive in the detection of circadian pattern differences as the airway resistance.

Asthmatic subjects typically have greater daily fluctuations of pulmonary functions than subjects without asthma. In fact, comparative study of monozygotic twins showed that the asymptomatic adult with a past history of asthma had greater amplitudes of peak expiratory flow fluctuations than the control twin with no background of asthma.

Nocturnal Asthma

Certain subgroups of asthmatic subjects experience an exaggerated nocturnal diminution in pulmonary function with resulting asthmatic symptoms. Even some healthy individuals show periodicity in airway conductance which can be reduced or abolished after inhalation of isoproterenol (Graham et al., 1967). Thus, asthma itself may only exacerbate a normal circadian rhythm in airway caliber seen in many individuals.

The postulated reasons for exacerbation of symptoms of asthma at night have been manifold. Some investigators found the most marked bronchoconstriction among patients with intrinsic asthma, especially between the hours of noon and midnight (Todisco et al., 1980). They reported extrinsic asthmatics to be less consistent in their daily cycle, although generally worse around 3 AM at the time when the urinary catechols were found to be at their lowest levels. Other investigators report that nocturnal asthma is equally common in intrinsic and extrinsic asthmatics (Clark and Hetzel, 1977). One theory links nocturnal asthma to allergic sensitivity from house dust mite or feathers in bedding. Although allergens can cause increased bronchial reactivity at night often manifesting as recurrent nocturnal attacks, one group did not find that the decrement in peak flow was affected by living in an allergen-free chamber (Reinberg et al., 1974).

Bronchial reactivity to allergens, histamine, and cholinergic agents such as methacholine also varies depending on the time of day.

In one study the reactivity to histamine correlated with the amplitude of diurnal variability in PEFR before and after inhalations of 200 μg albuterol (Ryan et al., 1981). Large morning and evening PEFR differences were associated with higher sensitivity to inhaled histamine and with the greatest bronchodilator responses to albuterol. Bronchial sensitivity to acetylcholine changes in accordance with the circadian cycle and has been found to be highest in the early afternoon in phase with the noted peak in expiratory flow rates (Reinberg et al., 1974). Although the peak flow rhythm does not seem to correlate with plasma cortisol changes (Soutar et al., 1975), the rhythm in circulating catecholamines may be partly responsible (Barnes et al., 1980; Soutar et al., 1977). On the other hand, sympathomimetic drugs do not always abolish the peak flow rhythm. Perhaps the best explanation for nocturnal asthma is that it is due to a multiplicity of factors or different factors in different individuals. Thus, one has to consider a combined or isolated effect of rhythms of catecholamines, vagal tone, β-2 receptor responsiveness, mucociliary clearance, immunologic response and gastrointestinal reflux (Hetzel, 1981). In addition, theophylline blood levels are lower on a twice-daily theophylline preparation given at night compared to the same preparation given during the day (Scott et al., 1981). It has even been suggested that the nocturnal fall in body temperature alone might cause nocturnal asthma (Chen and Chai, 1982).

Is it important to recognize nocturnal asthma as an entity? Amplitudes in peak flow rate over 50% of the average daily reading have been associated with an increased risk of ventilatory arrest and sudden death during recovery from asthma attacks in or out of the hospital (Hetzel et al., 1977; Bateman and Clarke, 1979). It is my personal opinion, however, that nocturnal symptoms occur most often in a subgroup of patients who are usually not well controlled during the day as well. As such, the *total* asthma treatment program is revamped rather than the nocturnal treatment by itself. One approach to accomplish this goal is to use β-agonist bronchodilator aerosols and/or theophylline throughout the day and night to raise the threshold rather than treating symptoms as they occur. Vigorous treatment with aerosolized bronchodilators at bedtime may be almost as effective as oral theophylline preparations, yet the latter has the advantage of a more prolonged duration of action. Other attempts at treatment should correspond to the primary causative mechanism such as the use of an antacid for gastroesophageal reflux, sleeping in a warm environment to overcome the effect of cold air, and minimization of allergenic contact if immunologic factors are suspected.

II. Identification and Treatment of Specific Triggers

A. Thyroid Status in Asthma

The hyperthyroid state has been associated with severe intractable asthma (Feinberg, 1944; Settipane et al., 1972). Striking improvement of asthma follows treatment of the hyperthyroidism. Although the latter authors suggested that the relationship between thyroid disease and asthma might be due to an overall decrease in cyclic AMP, an elevation of cyclic AMP levels in plasma, adipose tissue and skeletal muscle in patients with hyperthyroidism has been found (Karlberg et al., 1974). Hyperthyroidism can affect corticosteroid metabolism (Dazord et al., 1972; Hellman et al., 1961; Kenney et al., 1967; Martin et al., 1963; Ruder et al., 1972) so that the conversion of hydrocortisone to its inactive 11-ketonic derivative and also the rate of steroid reduction in the liver are increased (Ruder et al., 1972). This in turn increases urinary excretion of conjugated cortisol catabolites and diminishes the level of active circulating hormone (i.e., unbound cortisol).

Although the previous theories are interesting, the mechanism responsible for the increased severity of asthma with thyrotoxicosis is still unclear. From a clinical point of view, however, adrenergic drugs should be used with caution in patients with hyperthyroidism. Intravenous aminophylline may also provoke an increased susceptibility to tachycardias and arrhythmias due to an increased release of adrenal catecholamines. When both hyperthyroidism and asthma are present simultaneously, the treatment of thyroid crisis with propranolol is contraindicated. Propranolol should also be avoided in the treatment of other clinical conditions such as hypertension and angina pectoris in patients with asthma.

B. Beta-Adrenergic Receptor Blockers

Propranolol and the so-called "selective" β-blocking analogs are being used more and more frequently in the treatment of conditions such as hypertension, cardiac arrhythmias, and even migraine headaches. Beta-adrenoceptor-blockers have been associated with exacerbations of wheezing in asthmatic patients, and induction of bronchoconstriction in patients with mild hyperreactive airways disease such as allergic rhinitis patients and chronic bronchitis (Ouillette and Reed, 1967). Even ocular preparations containing β-blockers such as pindolol can cause bronchoconstriction through absorption into the systemic circulation from the ocular surface. Substitutions can often be made for the β-blockers, (e.g., a calcium channel blocker to treat hypertension in asthmatics). In the unusual circumstance when a selective β-blocking agent might be necessary, agents such as metoprolol can be tried (Formgren, 1976) and the patient observed for bronchoconstriction. One technique to minimize bronchoconstriction is to titrate the β-blocker down to the smallest dose that will produce the desired effect, and then add a β-agonist to counteract residual bronchial obstruction.

C. Compliance

Compliance is a major problem in health care. In many chronic diseases, failure of compliance with medication is a major cause of treatment failure. For example, a study of men on antihypertensive treatment showed a compliance rate of only 53% and poor compliance correlated closely with failure to achieve the target blood pressure (Sackett et al., 1975; Haynes et al., 1976). In other studies, only 55% of patients complied with antituberculosis chemotherapy as outpatients (Allen et al., 1964) and only 36% of children were compliant with oral penicillin prophylaxis against rheumatic fever (Gordis et al., 1969).

Compliance is an especially important concern for the successful treatment of asthma. Studies in asthmatic patients have revealed various levels of compliance. One study reported that 75% of patients taking a regularly scheduled short-acting preparation of theophylline achieved therapeutic serum levels (Beer et al., 1982); however, another study reported that only 11% of patients taking a short-acting theophylline preparation achieved therapeutic levels (Enley and Goldstein, 1976). Compliance may be improved by decreasing the number of doses required per day. Children taking a twice-a-day corticosteroid preparation were found to be 75% more compliant than when taking an aerosol formulation every 6 hr (Mecoy and Lab, 1980). Furthermore, only a 7% failure rate in patient compliance was found to occur with a once a day dosing regimen whereas a 60% compliance failure rate occurred with a divided dose taken several times during the day (Ayd, 1974). Thus, a 24-hr controlled-release theophylline product should produce greater patient compliance and, consequently, better management of asthma.

An accurate assessment of patient compliance is difficult to achieve because the methods used have many sources of error. For example, many methods often involve patient reporting, which is subject to as much as 50% error (Kinsman et al., 1981). Also, problems are encountered when either the number of unused tablets vs. prescribed tablets are compared, drug or metabolite levels are measured in the serum, urine, or saliva, or when compliance is derived from observing the expected response to treatment.

We attempted to overcome many problems inherent in these methods using a "nebulizer chronolog" for the administration of medication. This device enabled us to document accurately the date and time of pill or aerosol dispensation as an objective measure of patient compliance. Patients were instructed to take one puff four times daily of a cromolyn-like compound or an identical-appearing placebo nebulizer placed in the nebulizer chronolog. Aerosol treatments were spaced at approximately 4-hr intervals between waking hours of the 12-week study. The chronolog was adapted to hold any standard bronchodilator bottle and fit nicely into a pocket or purse. Each act of squeezing triggered a microswitch. The time within 4 min of its use was then stored in the memory inside the chronolog. Up to 256 uses over a 2-month period could be stored at one time. The information was printed out in a translator at the site of patient follow-up. Concomitant with the nebulization patients recorded the number of times they used the nebulizer each day on a diary sheet. They also were asked to fill out a "battery of asthma illness behavior," the so-called BAIB, developed to study the psychological characteristics of asthmatic patients (Kinsmen et al., 1982).

We found that eight subjects showed compliance for 12 days, two subjects for 24 days, three subjects for 36 days, one subject for 48 days, and five subjects for 60 days. Mean compliance rate was 47.4%, that is, medications were taken by the 19 subjects four times a day an average of 47.4% of the time. The mean rate of overusage was 5.3%. One would expect a greater rate of overusage than underusage for an asthma drug, but the mean rate of underusage was 48%, and all patients underused medications on occasion. Nine of 19 underused medications at least half of the time. The highest rate of underusage was *95.6%*. The lowest rate of underusage was 5.2%.

The diary did not correspond to the chronolog. According to the diary, 1 patient complied on 24 days, 3 patients complied on 36 days, 2 patients complied on 60 days, and 13 patients complied on 72 days. None recorded overuse; yet 13 subjects reported underuse on 8 days, 3 subjects reported underuse on 16 days, 2 subjects reported underuse on 24 days, and 2 subjects reported underuse on 24 days; 2 subjects reported underuse on 40 days. Often patients reported that they had used the nebulizer, yet it was not confirmed by the chronolog. Additionally, compliance fell as the study progressed. The two best compliers (assessed by the chronolog) completed all three tests of the BAIB appropriately with rates of compliance of 83.5 and 82.5%. The two worse compliers failed to complete the BAIB appropriately, and their rates of compliance were only 4.3 and 11.6%, which suggests that subjects who dislike filling out forms are the worst compliers. Other psychological profiles may emerge from the BAIB as more patients are analyzed to identify noncompliers.

Presently serum theophylline levels remain the most readily available means to assess compliance. In view of our data with the nebulizer chronolog it would not be surprising to find that compliance is a major issue in the treatment of asthma, especially if a medication must be administered at frequent intervals throughout the day.

D. Gastroesophageal Reflux

There appears to be an association between asthma and gastroesophageal reflux in adults and children (Berquist et al., 1981; Mays, 1976). In an attempt to demonstrate the existence of microaspiration from the gastrointestinal tract into the lungs we gave a radioisotope to asthmatic patients with a history suspicious for aspiration. The isotope was swallowed at bedtime. We demonstrated it in the lungs the following morning in two of seven patients (Reich et al., 1977). Reflex mechanisms may be playing an important role in the observed bronchospasm (Mansfield and Stein, 1978).

In some patients medical or surgical correction of reflux results in a marked dimunition or even disappearance of the asthmatic state. Oral bronchodilators commonly used in asthma relax the gastroesophageal junction and actually contribute to the reflux. If possible, they should be discontinued in favor of cromolyn sodium or aerosolized bronchodilators.

E. Sinus Disease

The precise role of sinus infections in the initiation and perpetuation of asthma has not been clearly elucidated. Wheezing and respiratory distress appear to be prominent features during and following infections of the sinuses and respiratory tract in some patients. In patients with asthma in whom infection appears to play an important role ("intrinsic" or "infective" asthma), sinus infections may spread to the tracheobronchial trees (Quinn and Meyer, 1929; McCaurin, 1935). If this is true, eradication of severe sinus disease should improve the patient's pulmonary status. There is also some evidence to suggest that spread of infection may be from the tracheobronchial tree to the paranasal sinuses (Hogg, 1950).

Chronic sinusitis may or may not be associated with tenderness after percussion or applied pressure over the sinuses. Although transillumination of the sinuses might have some value in the diagnosis of sinusitis, it is certainly not as accurate as radiographs.

In an unpublished study of sinus disease, sinus tissue from asthmatic subjects showed evidence of fairly intense immunologic activity, but data are lacking to support the notion that an allergic reaction is responsible for initiating the sinusitis. It is possible that the immunologic changes occur after the disease process has been established by a different mechanism.

In our experience sinus infections should be treated vigorously. Moisturizing with such agents as saline or propylene and polyethylene glycol may be useful and is not associated with side effects (Spector et al., 1982). Moisture provided by a facial sauna is another modality that may help certain patients. Oral decongestants and antihistamines provide adequate control of sinusitis in some patients, and antibiotics should be given if signs of an active infection are present. Oral corticosteroids for a short period of time are sometimes beneficial but should be used only in the most severe and persistent situations. Intranasal corticosteroids have met with some success; dexamethasone may be tried for a short period of time but can produce pituitary-adrenal suppression with prolonged or persistent use. Beclomethasone or flunisolide probably does not suppress the pituitary-adrenal axis when given in recommended doses. Surgical procedures such as antrostomies or the Caldwell-Luc procedure are the last resort.

III. Triggers that Involve Standardized Provocative Challenges

A. Exercise-Induced Asthma

It has been estimated that exercise produces bronchial obstruction in 75-80% of children with asthma (Jones, 1966). The incidence is still not well appreciated since standardized techniques to measure exercise-induced asthma (EIA) have not customarily been utilized. The free running test and treadmill exercise test are probably the most asthmogenic forms of exercise.

The latter has been most extensively standardized since the load, time, and speed can be prearranged, allowing for more reproducibility. The equipment is expensive but usually allows for adequate cardiac monitoring. This is an important asset for adults, and even advisable for children if a significant stress is anticipated. The main disadvantage is the expense of the equipment. Although the bicycle ergometer has also been standardized, it probably does not produce the same real-life situation. Both the free run and modifications such as stair climbing can be nicely adapted to an office procedure. The exercise may involve running on a flat surface or up and down a stairway for 2-6 min so that the heart rate is raised to at least 80% of maximum for a valid test. In the office lung function measurements can be taken immediately and at 5, 10, 15, and 30 min thereafter. The usual endpoint is a 20% drop in FEV_1 or peak expiratory flow rate.

Once these tests have been standardized to the office setting, preventive or blocking types of drugs or medication can be used in a particular asthmatic subject. Examples include cromolyn sodium, sympathomimetics, inhaled atropine, oral sympathomimetics, or theophylline. Even a face mask has been shown to block exercise-induced bronchospasm with the rebreathing of warm air. Various authors have reviewed those agents found most useful in blocking exercise-induced asthma (Anderson et al., 1979; Bierman and Pierson, 1984). Most studies support the contention that β-adreno receptor-stimulating agents administered as aerosols before exercise are the most effective in ameliorating or preventing EIA in both adults and children. Cromolyn sodium runs a close second since it inhibits EIA in the majority of patients. In certain individuals methylxanthines, α-adrenergic antagonists, and anticholinergic drugs prevent EIA. The variable effectiveness of different bronchodilators can be due to the heterogeneity of mechanism for EIA or the lack of standardization of the procedure itself.

B. Sensitivity to Aspirin and Nonsteroidal Anti-Inflammatory Agents

Aspirin idiosyncrasy has been a well recognized problem in a subpopulation of asthmatics for many years. The term "aspirin idiosyncrasy" best describes the pulmonary symptoms associated with relatively small doses of aspirin (as well as tartrazine and certain nonsteroidal anti-inflammatory substances) and is preferred over "aspirin allergy." The characteristic findings in patients with idiosyncrasy include rhinorrhea, nasal polyps, or sinusitis in an adult or child with asthma. The term "triad asthma" has been used in the past but is inappropriate since we now know that a given individual may lack some of the "triad" such as nasal polyps, yet have the typical adverse reaction. The incidence of idiosyncrasy varies considerably depending on the population surveyed and the methods used to diagnose this entity. In general, oral challenge studies reveal a significantly higher incidence that those studies that look at historical data alone.

For many years, we have used the following protocol to safely challenge our asthmatic population to tartrazine, and other agents. Based on their history, patients are classified into four groups: group I: patients with no history of idiosyncrasy who had ingested aspirin within a month before admission; group II: patients with no history of idiosyncrasy who had ingested no aspirin for at least a month before admission; group III: patients who, according to their history, are uncertain of the relationship of their asthma attacks and aspirin ingestion; and group IV: patients who, according to their history, had had asthma attacks within 24 hr of ingesting aspirin.

For the purpose of the oral challenges, groups I and II are treated similarly and groups III and IV are treated similarly. All medications except corticosteroids are withheld for 6-12 hr prior to testing. Occasional patients are unable to maintain a stable baseline FEV_1 and medications are not withheld for those patients. Groups I and II are screened in a double-blind manner and are successively given placebo and 75, 325, and 650 mg aspirin on different days. A positive challenge is a 20% or greater fall in the FEV_1 within 4 hr after ingestion of aspirin. If a test dose is borderline or questionable, it is repeated on a double-blind basis with a placebo.

Patients with a suggestive history of tartrazine idiosyncrasy are tested with placebo and 1, 5, 15, 25, and 50 mg tartrazine in a double-blind study. If a patient believes he or she can tolerate colored food, such as Tang, yellow Jello, or other foods, the test is performed on a double-blind basis with both placebo and 50 mg tartrazine.

When we used these procedures, a recent compilation of our results indicates that 44, or 19%, of 230 patients tested with aspirin had positive responses; 11, or 4%, of 277 tested with tartrazine had a positive response; 2, or 2.2%, of 92 tested to sodium salicylate had a positive response. All 11 of our tartrazine responders were also aspirin idiosyncratic.

The procedure as described has proved to be safe and the bronchial obstruction easily reversible with bronchodilators. Patients should also be observed for rhinorrhea and symptoms of sinusitis following the challenge.

Our current attitudes regarding the performance of aspirin and tartrazine challenge on asthmatics follow. We do not recommend routine challenge, since we advise all persons with or without asthma and/or rhinitis to use acetaminophen as an analgesic or an antipyretic. Aspirin forms covalent bonds with body constituents and has the potential for as yet unrecognized adverse effects. We do recommend aspirin challenges for asthmatics who *need* aspirin or other nonsteroidal anti-inflammatory medications for the treatment of a concomitant disease such as rheumatoid arthritis. This is necessary because many patients do not recognize a relationship between aspirin ingestion and asthmatic symptoms, which furthermore, can develop after a latent period. People with a history suggestive of asthma following ingestion of either aspirin or yellow-colored food should be tested for tartrazine-induced asthma. Perhaps difficult-to-control asthmatics should also be tested for tartrazine-induced asthma. It should be recognized that acetaminophen or sodium salicylate can also induce bronchospasm in some asthmatics.

Before the bronchodilator therapy of aspirin idiosyncrasy can be discussed, other therapeutic aspects should be considered involving all manifestations of aspirin idiosyncrasy. Sinus infections should be treated vigorously, as has been described. Although nasal polyps occasionally respond to the previously mentioned medical management program for sinusitis, this is uncommon. Polyps are sometimes injected with steroids such as dexamethasone with varying degrees of success. However, if they are numerous and cause marked discomfort and anosmia, a polypectomy should be done (Brown, et al., 1979; Holopainen et al., 1979; Moloney, 1980). Some European investigators advocate the treatment of nasal polyps with intranasal corticosteroids such as beclomethasone dipropionate (Mygind et al., 1975). Aerosol nasal steroids may play an even more impressive role in delaying or preventing recurrence of nasal polyps *after* polypectomy.

Treatment of asthma should follow good general principles, as outlined in reviews of the subject (Spector, 1979, 1985). Although the usual medications prescribed for asthmatic patients should be employed in idiosyncratic patients as well, certain agents have been used specifically in an attempt to block an aspirin challenge. For example, the H_1 receptor-blocking antihistamine clemastine given to 10 asthmatic patients with known aspirin idiosyncrasy provided complete protection in 3 patients, partial protection in 4 patients, and no protection in the remaining 3 patients against aspirin-induced bronchospasm and other symptoms (Szczelik and Serwonska, 1979). Cromolyn sodium (20-40 mg) blocked the bronchoconstrictive effect of aspirin both when inhaled and after the challenge when a progressive decrease in FEV_1 was occurring (Martelli and Usandivaras, 1977). The favorable influence of cromolyn as well as aminophylline in protecting against aspirin-induced bronchospasm has also been noted (Pasargiklian et al., 1977).

In 1922 a patient was described who originally reacted to 100 mg of aspirin but underwent desensitization with increasing doses of aspirin and after 7 days of treatment could tolerate 600 mg of aspirin (Widal et al., 1922). A specially prepared solution of lysine acetylsalicylic (LASA 18% w/v) has been administered by inhalation (Bianco et al., 1977) to two patients who received the solution on 4 consecutive days. The bronchial response progressively faded and by the fourth day had disappeared. If the "desensitized" patient stopped taking aspirin for more than 1-2 days, the bronchial response reappeared. After 6 or 7 days, the "desensitized" state was lost and a full response to a second challenge occurred.

Two asthmatic patients with aspirin idiosyncrasy have been described who became refractory to the adverse effects of aspirin with daily aspirin administration (Stevenson et al., 1980). Although both parents were taking small doses of alternate-day corticosteroids, their clinical courses improved while they continued to take daily aspirin. These initial observations were extended to a double-blind placebo cross-over study on the effects of daily aspirin given to aspirin-sensitive patients. It was found that aspirin-sensitive patients can be "desensitized" by repeated cautious challenges so that they tolerate a 640 mg dose. As long as aspirin is taken daily, the state of desensitization persists. When aspirin is discontinued, the sensitivity gradually returns over several days. Following desensitization, treatment with usual therapeutic doses of aspirin in some aspirin-sensitive patients (approximately 10-25%) reduces the ongoing inflammation in the respiratory tract; however, in approximately 10% of patients such treatment seems to intensify the ongoing pulmonary process.

Aspirin desensitization does not influence cholinergic sensitivity. There is no change in methacholine reactivity. Until the efficacy of aspirin desensitization is determined, the most practical subgroup for this treatment is those aspirin-sensitive asthmatic individuals who also suffer from arthritis, chronic headache, and/or arterial thromboembolism, that is, conditions that are logically treated with aspirin.

C. Tartrazine

Tartrazine (FD&C No. 5) is a yellow azobenzene dye that is a common food and drug additive. As with aspirin sensitivity, urticaria and angioedema have been described with its use as well as symptoms of bronchial obstruction. In 1969, three patients were described who developed urticaria after ingestion of pills containing yellow dye (Lockey, 1959). Other investigators have confirmed this association (Douglas, 1975; Michaelsson and Juhlin, 1973; Neuman et al., 1978). The incidence of wheezing in association with tartrazine differs widely according to the dose of tartrazine used and the population surveyed. In one series, 1 out of 13 aspirin-intolerant patients could not tolerate tartrazine (Samter and Beers, 1968). Another found positive reactions in 2 of 35 patients tested (Delaney, 1976). In another, no pediatric patient had an adverse reaction to tartrazine (Vedanthan et al., 1977). In one very interesting report bronchospasm occurred in 7 of 44 asthmatic patients in an open study (Weber et al., 1979). Yet in the same patients after double-blind challenge, not a single case of tartrazine idiosyncrasy could be confirmed among the 44 aspirin-idiosyncratic asthmatic patients. The Scripps investigators found 2 of 30 aspirin-sensitive asthmatic individuals to be tartrazine-sensitive by oral challenge (Mathison et al., 1983).

Although a positive reaction is undoubtedly dose-related, most investigators have used relatively small doses to elicit a positive response. One group using only 0.22-0.44 mg found that 3 of 40 patients had bronchospasm and another 3 had urticaria (Settipane and Pudopakkam, 1975). Another using 1-2 mg had a very high incidence of positive reactions, (7 of 8 patients) (Juhlin et al., 1972). In tests on patients with a suspicious or strong history of aspirin idiosyncrasy, we found that approximately 33% of 50 patients at the National Jewish Hospital in Denver developed wheezing after tartrazine (Spector et al., 1979). When almost all asthma patients were challenged in a double-blind fashion with doses of tartrazine up to 50 mg; we found 11 of 277 patients with a positive response. More such double-blind studies using a range of doses are needed to assess the importance of tartrazine-induced asthma.

Tartrazine is present in a great variety of foods and medications. Beginning in June, 1980, all manufacturers were required to list yellow dye No. 5 on the label. This ruling should make the need for extensive lists of drugs containing tartrazine (Smith and Slavin, 1976) somewhat less important in the future and, we hope, make the consumer more aware of possible adverse reactions.

In our hands, tartrazine challenges are performed initially with increasing doses in a manner similar to aspirin challenges. Presently the challenge dose is guided by a detailed history with specific questions regarding tolerance or intolerance to certain foods known to contain tartrazine. Patients with negative findings on aspirin challenge and no history of aspirin or tartrazine sensitivity receive 50 mg of tartrazine. Patients with a positive aspirin challenge who give a positive or questionable history of tartrazine sensitivity receive in a double-blind manner 1, 5, 15, 25, and 50 mg of tartrazine randomized with placebo on separate days.

The doses of sodium salicylate and acetaminophen used for challenge are 600 and 650 mg, respectively. In patients with a positive aspirin challenge and a suspicious history, these medications are tested incrementally as with aspirin, beginning with the dose in milligrams that provokes a positive aspirin challenge.

For all compounds tested, challenges are monitored with half-hourly pulmonary function studies including forced vital capacity (FVC) and FEV_1. Peak expiratory flow rates are observed, and the occurrence of rhinorrhea, which often precedes a drop in pulmonary function, is monitored. A positive test is considered to be a fall in FEV_1 to 20% or greater within 4 hr. Others prefer to use a 30% fall in FEV_1 (Mathison and Stevenson, 1979). The best of two consistent forced expiratory efforts is recorded on each occasion. Patients are tested only when their FEV_1 is equal to or exceeds 80% of their best known function. Questionable results are repeated with placebos in a double-blind fashion. Ideally, challenges should be performed with at least a 3-day interval between doses. It is difficult to make definite recommendations regarding proper timing until refractory or insensitivity periods are better understood. As a general rule, there is a corresponding sensitivity to aspirin and other drugs, which inhibit cyclooxygenase; that is, if low doses of aspirin provoke symptoms, so will low doses of prostaglandin synthetase inhibitors such as fenoprofen or indomethacin (Mathison and Stevenson, 1979; Szczeklik and Gryglewski, 1972).

We have challenged 230 asthmatic patients and correlated response with group (I–IV). The fact that 15 of 171, or 8.8%, of the group I or II patients with no history or suspicion of aspirin idiosyncrasy nevertheless had a positive aspirin challenge implies that the entity is not suspected by many susceptible individuals. During the challenge with aspirin, 14 had rhinorrhea and 10 had nasal stuffiness, and these symptoms helped convince us that a true reaction was occurring. Since about 35% of the patients who were quite certain they had aspirin idiosyncrasy had a negative challenge, overdiagnosis from the history in others is possible. However, other explanations for the negative test in the group IV patients are also possible. These include changes in thresholds, temporary refractoriness, or even loss of aspirin idiosyncrasy. We have carefully documented one circumstance in which a patient with a known strongly positive oral challenge and abnormal collagen-induced platelet aggregation subsequently showed negative findings after administration of 600 mg aspirin. The rechallenge was prompted by the fact that her platelet aggregation study had reverted to normal.

The response of asthmatic patients challenged with tartrazine had a mean duration of 2.3 hr, which emphasizes that a delayed reaction may occur with tartrazine as well as with aspirin. Approximately half of the patients who had a positive response to tartrazine also had nasal symptoms. Treatment should consist of avoiding tartrazine-containing foods and beverages. The usual bronchodilators, cromolyn-like derivatives, and corticosteroids appear to "block" or counteract the unusual adverse reactions to tartrazine.

D. Sulfite (Metabisulfite) Sensitivity

Sulfites have been used for hundreds of years as food preservatives or fresheners due to their known properties as sanitizing agents, inhibitors of microorganisms, and antioxidants. Life-threatening reactions have occurred in a number of patients after ingestion, inhalation, or parenteral administration. The greatest exposure to sulfites occurs with restaurant meals, especially in salad bars. For example, it has been estimated that sausages contain 40-45 mg per serving, dehydrated fruits 45-90 mg per serving, and wine 15-30 mg per serving. Various medications such as epinephrine and most local anesthetics also contain sulfites. Many life-threatening reactions have been documented after ingestion, inhalation, or parenteral administration of sulfites (Allen and Kollet, 1981; Koepke et al., 1983; Mathison et al., 1983; Stevenson and Simon, 1981; Werth, 1982). In the experience of investigators at the Scripps Clinic, the amounts of sulfite in the usual doses of subcutaneous medications (i.e., epinephrine or local anesthetics) do not usually provoke asthma in sulfite-sensitive individuals, but the amounts present in bronchodilator solutions such as Bronkosol and Isuprel do when these bronchodilators are administered by nebulization. While the usual Alupent solution contains metabisulfite, unit doses of Alupent and terbutaline solution packaged for subcutaneous administration do not contain metabisulfites and can be utilized for aerosol administration. What may not be appreciated is the *lack* of significant bronchodilator response in patients with metabisulfite sensitivity, rather than a decrement in pulmonary function subsequent to metabisulfite use as is typically described in susceptible individuals.

Suggested protocols for potassium metabisulfite ($K_2S_2O_5$) oral challenge based on the original Scripps experience with five asthmatic subjects consisted of challenges with gelatin capsules containing 1, 5, 10, 25, 50, and 100 mg of $K_2S_2O_5$ administered sequentially at 30-min intervals with a positive endpoint of 20-25% fall in FEV_1 (Mathison et al., 1983). It has been observed that certain individuals respond to an epilingual solution even though they may not have responded to the oral gelatin-filled capsule. Therefore, 1 ml epilingual metabisulfite at 1 mg/ml is squirted over the tongue with a syringe, followed by the same quantity of a 10 mg/ml solution if the previous reaction is negative. Typical symptoms after $K_2S_2O_5$ ingestion are sudden onset of flushing, weakness, chest tightness, and severe wheezing and dyspnea, within minutes after the ingestion. Patients with asthma can normally take their usual medications such as theophylline and corticosteroids, but cromolyn, anticholinergics, antihistamines, and vitamin B 12 should not be given soon after or before the challenge. One source of $K_2S_2O_5$ is Mallickrodt Laboratories. (USP grade $K_2S_2O_5$). To mitigate against a potential false-positive reactions, suspected positives should be reproduced using a double-blind protocol. In the Scripps experience none of the sulfite-sensitive patients had aspirin idiosyncrasy or tartrazine sensitivity. Those patients who have asthma or anaphylaxis during a restaurant meal usually have a positive challenge after small doses of 5-25 mg $K_2S_2O_5$. However, these patients are not as common as the group of asthmatics who respond to 50-200 mg $K_2S_2O_5$ and tend to have mild wheezing but not anaphylaxis. An occasional patient will wheeze only after the oral mucosal surface exposure. Although the mechanism of sulfite sensitivity is unknown, it has been postulated that the irritant receptors are stimulated by free sulfite radicles or SO_2.

The mechanism does not appear to be an immediate hypersensitivity reaction since skin tests for immediate hypersensitivity, peripheral blood leukocyte, and histamine release upon challenges are negative. It also has been postulated that a subgroup of these patients do not degrade sulfites appropriately, that is, they lack a sufficient quantity of sulfite oxidase. Treatment of these reactions primarily involves avoidance of foods containing sulfites. Although aqueous epinephrine and injectable dexamethasone contain metabisulfites, the quantity is usually insufficient to produce an asthmatic attack. It is also unclear whether β-adrenergic bronchodilators containing sulfites can generate enough SO_2 during aerosolization to produce clinically relevant asthma. Treatment of these severe attacks involves some of the usual medications used to treat any asthmatic situation. However, cromolyn, ipratropium, antihistamines, and aerosolized bronchodilators containing no metabisulfite have been successfully used to block these reactions. A subgroup of sensitive patients respond to vitamin B 12, an enzyme important in the sulfite oxidase pathway. Further investigation is underway to allow better understanding of the mechanism behind metabisulfite sensitivity and thereby improve on present therapy.

E. Monosodium Glutamate

Although monosodium glutamate (MSG) occurs in our diet as an artificially added enhancer of flavors in our foods, MSG is also a sodium salt of glutamic acid, a nonessential amino acid that forms 20% of dietary protein. Apparently two groups of patients have been described who experience asthma, in particular after a Chinese meal. The first group experiences symptoms 1 or 2 hr after this meal, and the second has a more delayed reaction, with asthma appearing 6-12 hr after MSG ingestion (Allen and Baker, 1981). In later study six asthmatics experienced wheezing attacks after ingestion of various doses of MSG, as encountered in Chinese restaurants (Allen, personal communication, 1983). Monosodium glutamate is found particularly in tomatoes, mushrooms, soy sauce, yeast extracts, meat extracts, wine, Parmesan cheese, Camembert cheese, and blue-veined cheese. Hydrolized vegetables contain around 20% MSG. It is also found in stock cubes. It may be added to various Chinese, Japanese, and Asian meals. For example, won ton soup can contain 2 or 3 g.

A protocol for MSG challenges used by Allen suggests that the patient receive an additive-free diet for 5 days prior to challenge, and that the challenge be performed in a hospital due to the potential severity of the asthmatic attack and delayed-onset reactions. After an overnight fast single-blind, placebo-controlled challenges are performed, randomized so that the sequence of challenges involved the smallest dose of MSG given first. Only one MSG dose or placebo is given per day. The dosage sequence is 0.5-, 1.5-, 2.5-, and 5-g capsules given on separate days, mixed with placebo. The mechanism behind MSG-stimulated asthma is not clear. Monosodium glutamate is reported to be neuroexcitatory, both centrally and peripherally. The early reaction and associated "Chinese restaurant syndrome" might be due to stimulation of peripheral sensory receptors leading to reflex bronchoconstriction, while the late reaction could be due to alteration in central control of reflex bronchoconstriction (Allen and Baker, 1981).

Avoidance of MSG is obviously an important aspect of treatment but difficult to accomplish in practice. Presently there are no restrictions on the use of this flavor enhancer in either manufactured or restaurant foods. Presumably the usual bronchodilators can reverse a severe reaction. The existence and incidence of these reactions must be further clarified in other centers.

IV. Unusual Treatment Modalities: What to Do When Standard Treatment Fails

Since this volume is dedicated to bronchodilator therapy, a point of clarification is in order. Some of the agents described here act as true bronchodilators in a subgroup of patients. Others may act more like "stabilizers," with a net effect of more bronchodilatation than previously if the patient is evaluated over 24 hr.

A. Iodides

Iodides are often listed under the category of "expectorants." Just as this inclusive category is controversial, so are iodides themselves as prescribed for expectoration or any other purpose in the treatment of asthma. Currently available forms include saturated solution of potassium iodide, potassium iodide solution (Pima), iodinated glycerol (Organidin), or sodium iodide solution (for intravenous use, 500 mg/500 ml fluid).

The exact mode of action of iodides is unknown. It has been postulated that they act by stimulating the production of a watery mucus as well as proteolytic liquefaction (Boyd, 1954), or even improved mucociliary clearance. However, iodides seem to be effective in only a relatively small subgroup of asthmatic subjects, leading to less than an enthusiastic response to their use. It has been suggested that it is "time to abandon the use of iodides in the management of pulmonary diseases" (Hendeles and Weinberger, 1980). These investigators have taken this position since they believe there are more effective pharmacologic agents available and do not find that iodides have expectorant action. They list a multitude of side reactions such as goiter (hypothyroidism); metallic taste; rare sensitivity reactions including erythema nodosa, ioderma, urticaria, bullous eruptions, drug fever, hypersensitivity angiitis, parotid swelling, increased salivation, serum sickness, and rhinitis. In children, hypothyroidism, goiter, and even thyrotoxicosis (with preexisting goiter) have been reported. The American Academy of Pediatrics has recommended that the use of iodides be limited to those children with chronic disease who have a reproducible, clear amelioration with its use (Committee on Drugs for the American Academy of Pediatrics, 1976). The dosage should be as low as possible and used for the shortest time. There is no doubt that iodides, especially in association with prolonged use, can cause goiter in children and should not be used in pregnant or breastfeeding women due to the thyroid effect and hypothyroidism, and in adolescents due to acneiform lesions. On the other hand, should we abandon their use completely if there is evidence that at least some patients respond to them in a beneficial way? In one study, 10 of 200 asthmatics showed an exceptionally favorable response to potassium iodide, 300-600 mg, four times a day (Siegal, 1964) and confirmatory statements were published by the reviewers with the article. Another group reported that 18% of 52 children ages 8-16 who received potassium iodide randomly in doses of 300 mg or 900 mg daily compared to placebo had significant improvement (Falliers et al., 1966). The study continued for a 12-week course and was conducted double blind. An additional 46% reported moderate improvement. Although side effects such as thyroid enlargement and acneiform lesions did occur, there were a surprisingly large number of responders in this age group. A more recent report summarized the results of a double-blind randomized study carried out in 11 centers (Repsher et al., 1983). Eighty patients were treated for 28 days with iodopropylidene glycerol, two tablets four times a day (Organidin) or placebo. After assessing 41 response parameters it was found that 78% had significant improvement as measured predominantly by improved breath sounds and sputum production, decreased cough severity and frequency, and decreased bronchodilator aerosol use. In this study 3 of 51 patients had a rash. In my experience, some patients respond on a short-term basis to iodine therapy, usually adults with sputum production as a common characteristic of their symptoms. On the other hand, many characteristics of responders do not fit within this category, and if the usual treatment fails, iodides are a suggested approach for a limited time in a subgroup of asthmatic patients.

B. Alpha-Adrenergic Blockers

Evidence has accumulated to show that there are α-receptors in the tracheobronchial smooth muscle of humans and other mammals (Beil and de Kock, 1978; Maguire and Nair, 1978; Mathe et al., 1971; Seale et al., 1976; Szentivanyi et al., 1979). Previous difficulty in demonstrating their presence may be associated with the fact that the density of α-receptors may change after allergic or pharmacologic manipulation and may be more prevalent with disease than in the normal state (Kneussl and Richardson, 1978). Alpha adrenergic responsiveness has been compared in patients with allergic rhinitis, normal controls, and asthmatic subjects by the capacity of phenylephrine to constrict the cutaneous vascular bed and dilate the pupillary sphincter muscle (Henderson et al., 1979). Compared to normal patients and those with allergic rhinitis, asthmatic subjects require much less phenylephrine to reduce cutaneous blood flow. In those asthmatics with the greatest susceptibility to changes in pupillary diameter, α-blockers have been used as a potential treatment for asthma since as early as the 1950s. It has been reported that oral or intravenous dibenamine produced relief in 8-14 hr in 20 severely asthmatic subjects (Klotz and Bernstein, 1950). The drug was administered orally in 18 and intravenously in 2 of the subjects. Improvement was assessed by increased vital capacity and clinical judgment. Many investigators have reported that α-adrenergic agents can prevent exercise-induced asthma. Aerosolized thymoxamine prevented EIA in 12 of 13 patients (Patel et al., 1976). Other preparations include aerosolized phentolamine 5 mg, oral indoramin, and recently inhaled prazosin (2 mg) (Beil and de Kock, 1978; Bianco et al., 1965; Seale et al., 1976; Kamburoff, 1980).

In one report, phentolamine controlled a severe incapacitating EIA in a 45-year-old woman with asthma who did not respond to the usual medications (Gross et al., 1974). She demonstrated an improvement in her exercise-induced bronchospasm after aerosolized phentolamine 5 mg, on long-term oral treatment with 300 mg in 24 hr. She was the same person who demonstrated an idiosyncratic response to isoproterenol. This was subsequently confirmed in another patient. This patient was one of a series of patients subsequently tested at National Jewish Hospital in an attempt to categorize subgroups of asthmatic patients by the use of 5 mg/ml phentolamine aerosol. Of 68 patients, only 16% demonstrated bronchodilatation, 72% had no response, and 12% had actual bronchoconstriction (Spector, 1979). Others have reported bronchoconstriction in certain individuals (Shiner and Molho, 1981). In three relatively long-term investigations of the effect of oral indoramin in asthma, one investigator reported no pulmonary function improvements (Uttling, 1979), another group found small increases in 8 of 30 patients with a tendency for unresponsiveness to salbutamol but improvement on indoramin (Campbell and Dyson, 1977), and a third group in a 3-month trial of indoramin found three of eight asthmatics, had marked increase daily flow rates (Black et al., 1978). The α-antagonist, thymoxamine, was found to restore the bronchodilator effect of metaproterenol in a group of steroid-dependent asthmatic subjects (Griffen et al., 1972), and the combination of isoproterenol and either thymoxamine or phentolamine produced marked improvement in airway conductance, significantly greater than that produced by isoproterenol by itself (Patel and Kerr, 1975). Similar results were obtained in a subsequent study of thymoxamine (Patel, 1976). Thus, it would appear that a subset of asthmatic subjects may respond to α-antagonists with bronchodilatation or with improved responsiveness to beta stimulation when unresponsiveness to the latter developed. A further clue to the responder group may be an idiosyncratic response to isoproterenol.

C. Troleandomycin

Troleandomycin (TAO), a macrolide antibiotic, was studied in a double-blind crossover design of 74 corticosteroid-dependent asthmatic and bronchitic subjects at the National Jewish Hospital in Denver (Spector et al., 1974). We found that 50 were marked responders, 13 probable responders, an 11 nonresponders. Some severely asthmatic patients could be changed from daily steroids to an alternate-day program or from a high alternate-day dosage to a much lower one. The favorable interaction occurs exclusively with methylprednisolone. The initial 0.75-1 g troleandomycin can be reduced to a daily maintenance level of 0.25-0.5 g after the desired effect is established, given with 8-12 mg every other day of methylprednisolone. Although troleandomycin commonly induces abnormal findings on liver chemistry tests, especially in the higher doses, this is not a prerequisite for troleandomycin responsiveness. Responding patients often stop producing sputum if this had been a component of their asthmatic state.

Although the mechanism of action of TAO is not understood, its antibiotic effect does not explain its beneficial effect. For example, TAO has been found to augment the suppressive effect of glucocorticosteroids on mitogen-induced blast transformation (Ong et al., 1978). It has been found to lower plasma triglyceride, an effect not found with high doses of steroids. It also seems to interact with other medications usually present in asthmatic subjects.

We first studied the inhibition of theophylline clearance by TAO. This can even lead to theophylline toxicity. Subsequent studies have shown that this is not responsible for its beneficial effect (Weinberger et al., 1977). Troleandomycin was also shown to reduce methylprednisolone elimination. In the presence of TAO, the pattern of elimination changes from a linear to a nonlinear one (Szefler et al., 1980). There is no such effect on prednisolone elimination, indicating that the effect of TAO on corticosteroid disposition is steroid-specific (Szefler et al., 1982). Troleandomycin is also found to increase the threshold response to methacholine (Spector et al., 1974).

In practice we have used TAO only in our most severe asthmatic subjects who have not responded to the usual therapy. In one study, 15 of 16 severe corticosteroid-dependent outpatients became well controlled on TAO and methylprednisolone (Zeiger et al., 1980). Since we are still unsure of TAO's mode of action or its ability to improve the overall long-term risk-benefit ratio of corticosteroid treatment, we are hesitant to recommend it for other than the most intractable case of asthma. Although we still give a "loading dose" of 500-750 mg TAO, we will rapidly decrease the dose of TAO and methylprednisolone once the responder state has been established. This usually takes 7 to 10 days. A maintenance dose of 250 mg TAO given daily, or on alternate days, with 4-12 mg methylprednisolone is usually possible in a few weeks, once the responder state has been established. Troleandomycin still serves as the last treatment modality to be added to a program.

References

Allen, D. H., and Baker, G. J. (1981). Chinese restaurant asthma. *N. Engl. J. Med. 305*: 1114-1115.

Allen, D. H., and Kollet, P. (1981). Life threatening asthmatic reactions to the food and drug preservative sodium metabisulfite. (abstract 284) American Academy of Allergy, San Francisco.

Allen, E. A., Stewart, M., and Jeney, P. (1964). The efficacy of post-sanatorium management of tuberculosis. *Can. J. Public Health 55*: 323.

Anderson, S., Seola, J. P., Ferris, L., Shaeffel, R., and Lendsay, D. A. (1979). An evaluation of pharmacology for exercise-induced asthma. *J. Allergy Clin. Immunol. 64*: 612.

Ayd, F. J., Jr. (1974). Single daily dose of antidepressants (editorial). *JAMA 230*: 263-264.

Barnes, P., Fitzgerald, G., Brown, M., and Dollery, C. (1980). Nocturnal asthma and change circulating epinephrine, histamine and cortisol. *N. Engl. J. Med. 303*: 263.

Bateman, J. R. M., and Clarke, S. W. (1979). Sudden deaths in asthma. *Thorax 34*: 40.

Beer, S., Laver, J., and Benson, L. (1982). Comparison of serum theophylline levels in asthmatic children receiving sustained-release and rapid-release theophylline tablets. *Isr. J. Med. Sci. 18*: 25.

Beil, M., and deKock, M. A. (1978). Role of alpha adrenergic receptors in exercise-induced bronchoconstriction. *Respiration 35*: 78.

Berquist, W. E., Rachelefsky, G. S., and Kadden, M. (1981). Gastroesophageal reflux-associated recurrent pneumonia and chronic asthma in children. *Pediatrics 68*: 29-35.

Bianco, S., Griffin, J. P., Kamburoff, A. C., and Prime, F. J. (1965). Prevention of exercise-induced asthma by indoramin. *J. Pharm. Pharmacol. 17*: 449.

Bianco, S., Robuschi, M., and Petrigni, G. (1977). Aspirin-induced tolerance to aspirin-asthma detected by a new challenge test. *J. Med. Sci. 5*: 129.

Bierman, C. W., Pierson, W. E. (eds.) (1984). International Symposium on Special Problems and Management of Allergic Athletes. *J. Allergy Clin. Immunol. 73*: No. 5, Part 2.

Black, J. L., Temple, D. M., and Anderson, S. D. (1978). Long-term trial of an alpha adrenoreceptor blocking drug (indoramin) in asthma. *Scand. J. Respir. Dis. 59*: 307.

Boyd, E. M. (1954). Respiratory tract fluid and expectorants. *Pharmacol. Rev. 6*: 521.

Brown, B. L., Harner, S. G., and Van Dellen, R. G. (1979). Nasal polypectomy in patients with asthma sensitivity to aspirin. *Arch. Otolaryngol. 105*: 413.

Campbell, I. A., and Dyson, A. J. (1977). Indoramin: An alpha adrenoreceptor antagonist for airway obstruction. *Br. J. Dis. Chest 71*: 105.

Chen, W. Y., and Chai, H. (1982). Airway cooling and nocturnal asthma. *Chest 81*: 675.

Clark, T. J. H., and Hetzel, M. R. (1977). Diurnal variation of asthma. *Br. J. Dis. Chest 71*: 87.

Committee on Drugs for the American Academy of Pediatrics (1976). Evidence of efficacy of iodides as an expectorant. *Pediatrics 57*: 272.

Dazord, A., Saez, J., and Bertrand, J. (1972). Metabolic clearance rates and interconversion of cortisol and cortisone. *J. Clin. Endocrinol. Metab. 35*: 24.

Delaney, J. C. (1976). Response of patients with asthma and aspirin idiosyncrasy to tartrazine (a dye commonly used in the food and drug industries). *Practitioner 217*: 285.

Douglas, H. M. G. (1975). Reactions to aspirin and food additives in patients with chronic urticaria, including the physical urticarias. *Br. J. Dermatol. 93*: 135.

Eichenhorn, M. S., Beauchamp, R. K., Harper, P. A., and Ward, J. C. (1982). An assessment of three portable peak flow meters. *Chest 82*: 306-309.

Eney, R. D., and Goldstein, E. O. (1976). Compliance of chronic asthmatics with oral administration of theophylline as measured by serum and salivary levels. *Pediatrics 57*: 513.

Falliers, C. J., McCann, W. P., Ellis, E. F., and Yazdi, N. (1966). Controlled study of iodotherapy for childhood asthma. *J. Allergy 38*: 183-192.

Falliers, C. J., Cardoso, RdeA, Bane, H., et al. (1971). Discordant allergic manifestations in monozygotic twins: Genetic identity vs. clinical, physiologic and biochemical differences. *J. Allergy 47*: 207.

Feinberg, S. M. (1944). *Allergy in Practice.* Chicago, Year Book.

Formgren, H. (1976). The effect of metoprolol and practolol on lung function and blood pressure in hypertensive asthmatics. *Br. J. Clin. Pharmacol. 3*: 1007.

Gordis, L., Markowitz, M., and Lilienfeld, A. M. (1969). Why patients don't follow medical advice: A study of children on long term anti-streptococcal prophylaxis. *J. Pediatr. 75*: 856.

Graham, W. G. B., Heim, E., and Constantine, H. P. (1967). Measurement of airway variation and bronchial reactivity in normal and asthmatic subjects. *Am. Rev. Respir. Dis. 96*: 266.

Griffin, J. P., Kamburoff, P. L., Prime, F. J., and Arab, A. G. (1972). Thymoxamine and airways obstruction. *Lancet 1*: 1288.

Gross, G. N., Souhrada, J. F., and Farr, R. S. (1974). The long term treatment of an asthmatic patient using phentolamine. *Chest 66*: 397.

Halberg, F., and Falliers, C. J. (1966). Variability of physiologic circadian crests in groups of children studied "transversely." *J. Pediatr. 68*: 741.

Haynes, R. B., Sackett, D. L., Gibson, E. S., et al. (1976). Improvement of medication compliance in uncontrolled hypertension. *Lancet 1*: 1265.

Hellman, L., Bradlow, H. L., Zumoff, B., and Gallagher, T. F. (1961). The influence of thyroid hormone on hydrocortisone production and metabolism. *J. Clin. Endocrinol. Metab. 21*: 1231.

Hendeles, L., and Weinberger, M. (1980). A time to abandon the use of iodides in the management of pulmonary diseases. *J. Allergy Clin. Immunol. 66*: 177-178.

Henderson, W. R., Shelhame, J. H., Reingold, D. B., et al. (1979). Alpha-adrenergic, hyperresponsiveness in asthma: Analysis of vascular and pupillary responses. *N. Engl. J. Med. 300*: 642.

Hetzel, M. R. (1981). The pulmonary clock. *Thorax 36*: 481.

Hetzel, M. R., Clark, T. J. H., and Branthwaite, M. A. (1977). Asthma: An analysis of sudden deaths and ventilatory arrests in hospital. *Br. Med. J. 1*: 808.

Hogg, J. C. (1950). Discussion on the role of sinusitis in bronchiectasis. *Proc. R. Soc. Med. 43*: 1089.

Holopainen, J., Makinen, J., Paavolainen, M., et al. (1979). Nasal polyposis: Relatinship to allergy and acetylsalicylic acid intolerance. *Acta Otolaryngol. 87*: 330.

Jones, R. S. (1966). Assessment of respiratory function in the asthmatic child. *Br. Med. J. 2*: 972.

Juhlin, L., Michaellsson, G., and Zetterstrom, O. (1972). Urticaria and asthma induced by food and drug additives in patients with aspirin hypersensitivity. *J. Allergy Clin. Immunol. 50*: 92.

Kamburoff, P. L. (1980). Effects of different drugs on exercise-induced asthma (EIA). *Eur. J. Respir. Dis. Suppl. 106*: 65.

Karlberg, B. E., Henriksson, K. G., and Andersson, R. G. G. (1974). Cyclic-adenosine 3′5′ monophosphate concentration in plasma, adipose tissue, and skeletal muscle in normal subjects and in patients with hyper- and hypothyroidism. *J. Clin. Endocrinol. Metab. 39*: 96.

Kenney, F. M., Iturzaeta, N., Preeyasombat, C., et al. (1967). Cortisol production rate. VII. Hypothyroidism and hyperthyroidism in infants and children. *J. Clin. Endocrinol. Metab. 27*: 1616.

Kinsman, R. A., Chai, H., Dickey, D. W., Jones, R., Morrill, C. G., Perry, G. B., Spector, S. L., and Weiser, P. C. (1981). U.S. Environmental Protection Agency, Contract No. 68-02-3208.

Kinsman, R. A., Dirks, J. F., and Jones, N. F. (1982). In *Handbook of Clinical Health Psychology*. Edited by Millon, Green, and Meagher. New York, Plenum Press.

Klotz, S. D., and Bernstein, C. (1950). The use of Dibenamine in the severe asthmatic state and related chronic pulmonary conditions. *Ann. Allergy 8*: 767.

Kneussl, M. P., and Richardson, J. B. (1978). Alpha-adrenergic receptors in human and canine tracheal and bronchial smooth muscle. *J. Appl. Physiol. 45*(2): 307.

Koepke, J. W., Selner, J. C., and Dunhill, A. L. (1983). Presence of sulfur dioxide in commonly used bronchodilator solutions. *J. Allergy Clin. Immunol. 72*: 504-508.

Lockey, S. D. (1959). Allergy reactions due to FDC & yellow No. 5 tartrazine, an analine dye used as a coloring and identifying agent in various steroids. *Ann. Allergy 17*: 719.

Maguire, W. C., and Nair, S. (1978). Ventilation and perfusion effects of inhaled alpha and beta agonists in asthma patients. *Chest 73* (Supp): 983.

Mansfield, L. E., and Stein, M. R. (1978). Gastroesophageal reflux and asthma: A possible reflex mechanism. *Ann. Allergy 41*: 224-226.

Martelli, N. A., and Usandivaras, G. (1977). Inhibition of aspirin induced bronchoconstriction by sodium cromoglycate inhalation. *Thorax 32*: 683.

Martin, M. M., Mintz, D. H., and Tamagaki, H. (1963). Effect of altered thyroid function upon steroid circadian rhythm in man. *J. Clin. Endocrinol. Metab. 23*: 242.

Mathe, A. A., Astrom, A., and Persson, N. A. (1971). Some bronchoconstricting and bronchodilating responses of human isolated bronchi: Evidence for the existence of a-adrenoreceptors. *J. Pharm. Pharmacol. 23*: 905.

Mathison, D. A., Pleskow, W. W., Simon, R. A., and Stevenson, D. D. (1983). Aspirin and chemical sensitivities and challenges in asthmatic patients. In *Provocative Challenge Procedures: Bronchial, Oral, Nasal, and Exercise,* vol. II. Edited by S. L. Spector. CRC Press, Boca Raton, pp. 103-114.

Mathison, D. A., and Stevenson, D. D. (1979). Hypersensitivity to nonsteroidal anti-inflammatory drugs: Indications and methods for oral challenges. *J. Allergy Clin. Immunol. 64*: 669-674.

Mays, E. E. (1976). Intrinsic asthma in adults, association with gastroesophageal reflux. *JAMA 236*: 2626.

McCaurin, J. G. (1935). A review of the interrelationship of paranasal sinus disease and certain chest conditions, with especial consideration of bronchiectasis and asthma. *Ann. Otol. Rhinol. Laryngol. 44*: 344.

Mecoy, R. J., and Lab, B. (1980). Beclomethasone dipropionate in twice daily treatment of asthma. *Aust. Fam. Physician 9*: 721.

Michaelsson, G., and Juhlin, L. (1973). Urticaria induced by preservatives and dye additives in food and drugs. *Br. J. Dermatol. 88*: 525.

Moloney, J. R. (1980). Nasal polyps, nasal polypectomy, asthma, and aspirin sensitivity. *J. Laryngol. Otol. 5*; 183-189.

Morrill, C. G., Dickey, D. W., Weiser, P. C., Kinsman, R. A., Chai, H., and Spector, S. L. (1981). Calibration and stability of standard MiniWright peak flow meters. *Ann. Allergy 46*: 70-73.

Mygind, N., Brake-Pedersen, C., Przty, S., and Sorensen, H. (1975). Treatment of nasal polyps with intranasal beclomethasone dipropionate aerosol. *Clin. Allergy 5*: 159.

Neuman, I., Elian, R., Nahum, et al. (1978). The danger of "yellow dyes" (tartrazine) to allergic subjects. *Clin. Allergy 8*: 65.

Ong, K., Grieco, M. H., and Rosner, W. (1978). Enhancement by oleandomycin of the inhibitory effect of methylprednisolone on phytohemagglutinin-stimulated lymphocytes. *J. Allergy Clin. Immunol. 62*: 115.

Ouellette, J. J., and Reed, C. E. (1967). The effect of partial beta adrenergic blockade on the bronchial response of hay fever subjects to ragweed aerosol. *J. Allergy 39*: 160.

Pasargiklian, M., Bianco, S., Allegra, L., et al. (1977). Aspects of bronchial reactivity to prostaglandins and aspirin in asthmatic patients. *Respiration 34*: 79.

Patel, K. R. (1976). Alpha-adrenoceptor blocking drugs in asthma. *Br. J. Clin. Pharmacol. 3*: 601.

Patel, K. R., and Kerr, J. W. (1975). Alpha-receptor blocking drugs in bronchial asthma. *Lancet 1*: 348.

Patel, K. R., Kerr, J. W., MacDonald, E. B., and McKenzie, A. M. (1976). The effect of thymoxamine and cromolyn sodium on post-exercise bronchoconstriction in asthma. *J. Allergy Clin. Immunol. 57*: 285.

Quinn, L. H., and Meyer, P. P. (1929). The relationship of sinusitis and bronchiectasis and asthma. *Arch. Otolaryngol. 10*: 152.

Reich, S., Early, W., Raven, T., Goodman, M., and Spector, S. (1977). Evaluation of gastropulmonary aspiration by a radioactive technique. *J. Nucl. Med. 18*: 1079-1081.

Reinberg, A., Gervais, P., Frambourg, J. C., Halberg, F., Abulker, C., Vignaud, C., and Dupont, J. (1970). Rhythmes circadiens de fonctions respiratoires et de la témperature d'asthmatiques sejournant en milieu hypoallergenique. *Presse Med. 78*: 1817.

Reinberg, A., Gervais, P., Morin, M., and Abulker, C. (1974). Circadian rhythms in the threshold of bronchial response to acetylcholine in healthy and asthmatic subjects. In *Chronobiology*. Edited by L. E. Scheving, F. Halberg, and J. E. Pauly. Tokyo, Igaku Shoin Ltd., pp. 174-177.

Repsher, L. H., Glassman, J. M., and Soyka, J. P. (1983). Evaluation of iodoprophylidene glycerol as adjunctive therapy in stable, chronic asthmatic patients on theophylline maintenance. *Todays Ther. Trends 1*: 77-89.

Ruder, H., Corvol, P., Mahoudeau, J. A., et al. (1972). Effects of induced hyperthyroidism on steroid metabolism in man. *J. Clin. Endocrinol. Metab. 33*: 382.

Ryan, G., Latimer, K., and Hargreave, F. E. (1981). Relationship between bronchial reactivity to histamine and daily variation of peak flow rate (abstract 167). American Academy of Allergy, San Francisco.

Sackett, D. L., Haynes, R. B., Gibson, E. S., et al. (1975). Randomised clinical trial of strategies for improving medication compliance in primary hypertension. *Lancet 1*: 1205.

Samter, M., and Beers, R. F. (1968). Intolerance to aspirin: clinical studies and consideration to pathogenesis. *Ann. Intern. Med. 68*: 975.

Scott, P. H., Tabachnik, E., MacLeod, S., Correia, J., Newth, C., and Levison, H. (1981). Sustained-release theophylline for childhood asthma: Evidence for circadian variation of theophylline pharmacokinetics. *J. Pediatr. 99*: 476-479.

Seale, J. P., Anderson, S. D., and Lindsay, D. A. (1976). A trial of an alpha-adrenoceptor blocking drug (indoramin) in exercise-induced bronchoconstriction. *Scand. J. Respir. Dis. 57*: 261.

Settipane, G. A., and Pudupakkam, R. (1975). Aspirin tolerance. III. Subtypes, familial occurrence and crossreactivity with tartrazine. *J. Allergy Clin. Immunol. 56*: 215.

Settipane, G. A., Schoenfeld, E., and Hamolsky, M. W. (1972). Asthma and hyperthyroidism. *J. Allergy Clin. Immunol. 49*: 348.

Shiner, R. J., and Molho, M. J. (1981). A comparative study between an alpha adrenergic antagonist and a beta adrenergic agonist agent in bronchial asthma. *Am. Rev. Respir. Dis. 123*: 39.

Siegal, S. (1964). The asthma-suppressive action of potassium iodide. *J. Allergy 35*: 252-270.

Simonsson, B. G., and Svedmyr, N. (1977). Bronchoconstrictor drugs. *Pharmacol. Ther. 3*: 329.

Smith, L. J., and Slavin, R. G. (1976). Drugs containing tartrazine dye. *J. Allergy Clin. Immunol. 58*: 456.

Soutar, C., Costello, J., Ijaduola, O., and Turner-Warwick, M. (1975). Nocturnal and morning asthma: Relationship to plasma corticosteroids and response to cortisol infusion. *Thorax 30*: 436.

Soutar, C. A., Carruthers, M., and Pickering, C. A. C. (1977). Nocturnal asthma and urinary adrenaline and noradrenaline excretion. *Thorax 32*: 677.

Spector, S. H. (1985). Asthma in adults. In *Advances in the Treatment of Bronchial Asthma.* Philadelphia, W. B. Saunders.

Spector, S. L. (1979a). Management of chronic symptoms in the asthmatic patient. *Hosp. Med. 15*: 16.

Spector, S. L. (1979b). Precautions on the use of alpha-adrenergic antagonists on asthmatic patients. Letter to the Editor. *N. Engl. J. Med. 301*: 388-389.

Spector, S. L., Katz, F. H., and Farr, R. S. (1974). Troleandomycin: Effectiveness in steroid dependent asthma and bronchitis. *J. Allergy Clin. Immunol. 54*: 367-369.

Spector, S. L., Wangaard, C. H., and Farr, R. S. (1979). Aspirin and concomitant idiosyncrasies in adult asthmatic patients. *J. Allergy Clin. Immunol. 64*: 500.

Spector, S. L., Toshener, D., Gay, I., and Rosenmann, E. (1982). Beneficial effects of propylene and polyethylene glycol and saline in the treatment of perennial rhinitis. *Clin. Allergy 12*: 187.

Stevenson, D. D., and Simon, R. A. (1981). Sensitivity to metabisulfites in asthmatic subjects. *J. Allergy Clin. Immunol. 68*: 26.

Stevenson, D. D., Simon, R. A., and Mathison, D. A. (1980). Aspirin-sensitive asthma: Tolerance to aspirin after positive oral aspirin challenges. *J. Allergy Clin. Immunol. 66*: 82.

Szczeklik, A., Gryglewski, R. J., Czerniawska-Mysic, G., and Zmuda, A. (1972). Aspirin-induced asthma: Hypersensitivity to fenoprofen and ibuprofen in relation to their inhibitory action of prostaglandin generation by different microsomal enzyme preparation. *J. Allergy Clin. Immunol. 58*: 10.

Szczeklik, A., and Serwonska, M. (1979). Inhibition of idiosyncratic reactions to aspirin in asthmatic patients by clemastine. *Thorax 34*: 654.

Szefler, S. J., Rose, J. Q., Ellis, E. F., Spector, S. L., Green, A. W., and Jusko, W. J. (1980). The effect of troleandomycin on methylprednisolone elimination. *J. Allergy Clin. Immunol. 66*: 447-451.

Szefler, S. J., Ellis, E. F., Brenner, M., Rose, J. Q., Spector, S. L., Yurcahk, A. M., Andrews, F., and Jusko, W. J. (1982). Steroid-specific and anticonvulsant interaction aspects of troleandomycin-steroid therapy. *J. Allergy Clin. Immunol. 69*: 445-460.

Szentivanyi, A., Heim, O., and Schultze, P. (1979). Changes in adrenoceptor densities in membranes of lung tissue and lymphocytes from patients with atopic disease. *Ann. N.Y. Acad. Sci. 322*: 295.

Todisco, T., Grassi, V., Sorbini, C. A., et al. (1980). Circadian rhythms of respiratory function in asthmatics. *Respiration 40*: 128.

Utting, J. A. (1979). Alpha adrenergic blockade in severe asthma. *Br. J. Dis. Chest 73*: 117.

Vedanthan, P. K., Menon, M. M., Bell, T. D., and Bergin, D. (1977). Aspirin and tartrazine oral challenge: Incidence of adverse response in chronic childhood asthma. *J. Allergy Clin. Immunol. 60*: 8.

Weber, R. W., Hoffman, M., Raine, D. A., and Nelson, H. S. (1979). Incidence of bronchoconstriction due to aspirin, azo dyes and preservatives in a population of prerennial asthmatics. *J. Allergy Clin. Immunol. 64*: 32.

Weinberger, M., Hudgel, D., Spector, S., and Chidsey, C. (1977). Inhibition of theophylline clearance by troleandomycin. *J. Allergy Clin. Immunol. 59*: 228.

Werth, G. R. (1982). Inhaled metabisulfite sensitivity (correspondence). *J. Allergy Clin. Immunol. 70*: 143.

Widal, M. F., Abramin, P., and Lemoyez, J. (1922). Anaphylaxis et idiosyncrase. *Presse Med. 30*: 189.

Zeiger, R. S., Schatz, M., Sperling, W., Simon, R. A., and Stevenson, D. D. (1980). Efficacy of troleandomycin in outpatients with severe, corticosteroid-dependent asthma. *J. Allergy Clin. Immunol. 66*: 438-446.

Zuidema, P., and van Essel, A. D. (1965). Messung von Tagesschwankungen des bronchialen Stsromungswiderstandes bei Asthmatikern—Vergleichende Untersuchung versciedener Methoden. *Schweiz Med Wocheschr 95*: 805.

25

Theophylline Toxicity

H. WILLIAM KELLY

University of New Mexico School of Medicine
Albuquerque, New Mexico

I. Introduction

Theophylline is often defined as a drug with a narrow therapeutic index, that is, significant toxicity occurs at serum theophylline concentrations just above those that produce the optimal therapeutic effect. In actuality, the toxicity of theophylline defines the upper limit of its therapeutic range. The first reports of serious toxicity including death from intravenous aminophylline (Merrill, 1943; Bresnick et al., 1948) appeared in the 1940s. A series of reports in the 1950s (Soifer, 1957), however, clearly delineated the wide range of symptoms produced by theophylline intoxication. The many pharmacologic actions of theophylline (Rall, 1980) undoubtedly account for the diversity of toxicological symptoms.

Unfortunately, most of the literature on theophylline toxicity is in the form of case reports or small series. Therefore it is difficult to define a completely accurate serum theophylline concentration to toxic effect relationship. Figure 1 summarizes the relationship of toxicity to theophylline concentration and was compiled from 13 studies in the literature that attempted to correlate serum theophylline concentration with effect. The total population of 329 cases consists of ambulatory patients as well as inpatients. As can be seen, the

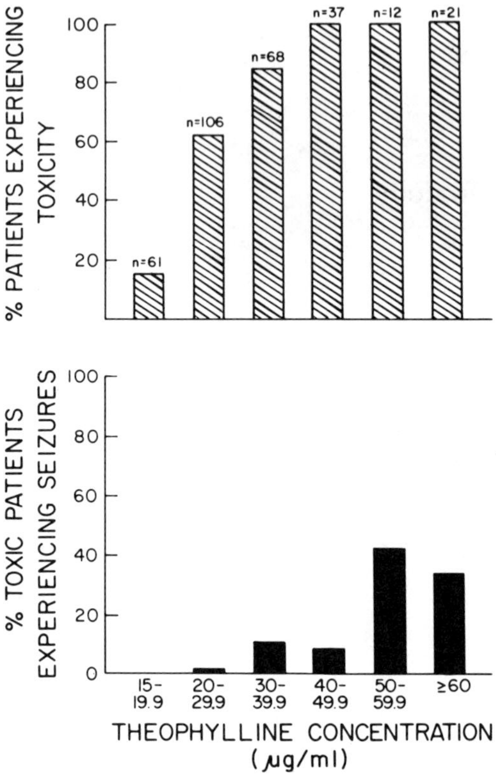

Figure 1 (Top) Prevalence of symptomatic toxicity at various ranges of theophylline concentrations. n, total number of patients at the concentration range. (Bottom) Prevalence of seizures in the toxic patients. Data from Burkle and Gwizdala, 1981; Greenberg et al., 1984; Helliwell and Berry, 1979; Hendeles et al., 1977; Jacobs et al., 1976; Jenne et al., 1972; Kordash et al., 1977; Kraemer et al., 1982; Mountain and Neff, 1984; Park et al., 1983a,b.

prevalence of toxicity increases dramatically at theophylline concentrations greater than 20 μg/ml. There exists, however, a significant interpatient variability in response particularly within the theophylline concentration range of 15-30 μg/ml. While the reasons for this variability are not obvious, age and underlying disease states are significant factors.

In a recent review of 28 cases of acute theophylline intoxication in children (Gaudreault et al., 1983), severe manifestations (cardiac arrhythmias and/or seizures) occurred only at theophylline concentrations greater than 60 μg/ml with the majority occurring at concentrations greater than 100 μg/ml. On

Table 1 Signs and Symptoms of Theophylline Toxicity

Sinus tachycardia	Anxiety
Anorexia	Seizure
Nausea	Supraventricular tachycardia
Tremulousness	Ventricular and atrial ectopic beats
Vomiting	Obtundation
Nervousness	Diarrhea
Irritability	Hypotension
Headache	Hyperglycemia
Hematemesis	Cardiopulmonary arrest
Agitation	Urinary retention
Disorientation	Hypokalemia

the other hand, Hendeles and co-workers (1977) found that a mean theophylline concentration of 46.5 μg/ml was associated with severe toxicity in acutely ill older patients. Three elderly patients (aged 75, 92, and 95 years) with chronic obstructive pulmonary disease exhibited severe toxicity at theophylline concentrations of 17, 24, and 20.5 μg/ml, respectively (Nakada et al., 1983).

Population differences cannot explain all the variability. Mountain and Neff (1984) found a significant variability in signs and symptoms in 21 outpatients with chronic obstructive pulmonary disease requiring hospitalization for theophylline intoxication. Theophylline concentrations ranged from 22.4 to 104.8 μg/ml. Anorexia, nausea, and vomiting were the most common clinical signs and symptoms but were not universally present. Two of the patients with the highest concentrations (78.5 and 104.8 μg/ml) exhibited only gastrointestinal symptoms, while 13 patients with a mean concentration of 35 μg/ml exhibited cardiac arrhythmias or seizures. This study aptly illustrates the highly variable susceptibility to specific adverse effects. It is extremely important for the clinician to realize that life-threatening toxicities may not be preceded by the more common minor toxic reactions. Therefore, routine serum concentration monitoring is essential for the safe use of theophylline.

In a two-year study of elevated serum theophylline concentrations in 87 patients Burkle and Gwizdala (1981) failed to demonstrate a single toxic symptom present in 100% of the outpatients. They classified their patients into three groups according to serum theophylline concentration: group 1 (20-29.9 μg/ml), group 2 (30-39.9 μg/ml), group 3 ($>$40 μg/ml). The most frequent toxicities were tachycardia (group 1, 57%; group 2, 88%; group 3, 84%) and nausea (group 1, 33%; group 2, 54%; group 3, 63%). Other studies have demonstrated similar results (Jacobs et al., 1976; Mountain and Neff, 1984). Table 1 lists the signs and symptoms of theophylline toxicity in order of decreasing frequency.

II. Neurotoxicity

A. Theophylline-Induced Seizures

The methylxanthines are potent central nervous system stimulants (Rall, 1980). Theophylline administration can produce headache, nervousness, hyperactivity, anxiety, and insomnia at concentrations within the therapeutic range of 10-20 μg/ml. At higher theophylline concentrations irritability, agitation, encephalopathy, and seizures become more frequent (Burkle and Gwizdala, 1981; Greenberg et al., 1984; Zwillich et al., 1975). Seizures are the most serious neurotoxicity of theophylline, having been associated with a 50% mortality rate in some small series (Park et al., 1983b; Helliwell and Berry, 1979; Zwillich et al., 1975). Although well over 100 cases of theophylline-induced seizures have been reported in the literature over the past 30 years, little is known of their incidence, relationship to serum concentration, pathophysiology, predisposing factors, response to anticonvulsants, or associated mortality. This is largely due to the fact that most reports are in the form of single cases or small series. This creates a significant selection bias, since often only the more severe or unusual cases are reported. Despite this problem, 100 cases of theophylline-associated seizures from 52 references were analyzed in an attempt to shed light on some of these questions.

Morbidity and Mortality

Of the 100 cases reviewed there was an overall mortality rate, directly associated with the seizure, of 29%. The combined rate of mortality plus significant neurologic sequelae was 34%. Table 2 summarizes the relationship of age and theophylline concentration to mortality in patients with seizures. Age was determined in 84 cases and serum theophylline concentrations were determined in 65 instances. When more than one serum theophylline determination was made, the peak concentration was utilized. Seventeen of the patients were treated with a method of removing theophylline (see below). The combined mortality and severe morbidity in these patients was 29.4%.

The overall mortality rate of 29% is lower than the 50% previously reported (Helliwell and Berry, 1979; Zwillich et al., 1975). This may be due to the inclusion of pediatric patients (Table 2), who appear to have a better outcome than adults. There also appears to be less of a disparity between the theophylline concentrations in elderly patients dying and surviving (Table 2). This may

Table 2 Relationship of Age and Theophylline Concentration to Mortality with Theophylline-Induced Seizures

				Theophylline concentrations (μg/ml)		
Age (yr)	Number	Deaths	No.	Total	Died	Survived
< 2 (3 days-18 months)	18[a]	2 (11%)	13	109 (36-300)	150 (150)	101 (36-300)
2-15	11[b]	4 (36%)	7	110 (33-224)	–	110 (33-224)
16-49	10[c]	3 (30%)	7	135 (21.3-290)	187 (85-290)	115 (21.3-190)
50-69	24	8 (33%)	19	75.2 (30-260)	87 (30-260)	66 (37-203)
> 70	21	9 (43%)	19	45.6 (21.5-86)	48.4 (25-80)	44 (21.5-86)
Total			65	80.1 (21.3-300)	89.5 (25-290)	71.1 (21.3-300)

[a]Two patients survived with severe neurologic sequelae.
[b]One patient survived with severe neurologic sequelae.
[c]Two patients survived with severe neurologic sequelae.
Source: Data derived from Reinhardt et al., 1982; Winek et al., 1980; McDonald et al., 1978; Jacobs and Senior, 1974; Simons et al., 1980; Kordash et al., 1977; Nicholson and Chick, 1973; Jenne et al., 1972; Weinberger and Ginchansky, 1977; Woodcock et al., 1983; Mattay et al., 1976; Vincent et al., 1978; Vaucher et al., 1977; Parfrey and Davies, 1970; Dean and Brown, 1982; Anderson et al., 1983a,b; Kadlec et al., 1978; Gotz et al., 1979; Haddad and Sakai, 1982; Wells and Ferlauto, 1979; Gal et al., 1980; Buchanan et al., 1979; Schwartz, 1974; Gaudrault et al., 1983; Greenberg et al., 1984; Miceli et al., 1979, 1980; Fleetham, 1979; Sahney et al., 1983; Russo, 1979; Ehlers et al., 1978; Lawyer et al., 1978; Yarnell and Chu, 1975; Nakada et al., 1983; Faden, 1976; Burgan et al., 1982; Helliwell and Berry, 1979; Kraemer et al., 1982; Lambert et al., 1981; Jacobs et al., 1976; Burkle and Gwidzala, 1981; Mountain and Neff, 1984; White and Daeschner, 1956; Soiffer, 1957; Rounds, 1954; Nolke, 1956; McKee and Haggerty, 1957; Zwillich et al., 1975; Veum and Schwartz, 1956; Mahutte et al., 1983; Jefferys et al., 1980; Park et al., 1983a,b.

be due to the more complicated nature of the illness in elderly patients or to the inability of their cardiovascular or CNS systems to withstand the insult.

Predisposing Factors

Age appears to be a significant factor when one is analyzing the frequency of seizures for a given theophylline concentration. In a review of 43 pediatric patients, Gaudreault and co-workers (1983) found that all patients with seizures had serum theophylline concentrations greater than 60 μg/ml, with two-thirds greater than 100 μg/ml, suggesting a relative resistance to seizures in pediatric patients. Kraemer and colleagues (1982) reported two cases of theophylline-induced seizures in children with peak concentrations of 33 μg/ml and 48 μg/ml, again emphasizing the significant variability within an age group.

Figure 1 gives the prevalence of seizures at increasing theophylline concentrations. The overall prevalence of 21% for theophylline concentrations greater than 40 μg/ml is in agreement with the study of Burkle and Gwizdala (1981). A significant increase in seizure frequency occurs at theophylline concentrations greater than 50 μg/ml. To evaluate this relationship further, the data from eight studies of theophylline intoxication were combined and the concentrations of theophylline in patients with and without seizures were compared (Table 3). This would appear to confirm that theophylline concentrations greater than 50 μg/ml are more likely to induce seizures. The wide range of concentrations in both groups also confirms a significant interpatient variability.

There appears to be a number of predisposing factors other than age. Decreased serum protein binding of theophylline may increase the entry into the central nervous system (Letarte and duSouich, 1984). Theophylline binding to protein ranges from 30 to 80%, with a mean of 60% (Lesko et al., 1981). Protein binding is reduced in elderly patients (Antal et al., 1981; Lesko et al., 1981), and

Table 3 Theophylline Concentrations in Toxic Patients With and Without Seizures

	Without seizures	Seizures	Deaths
Number of patients	65	25	12
Mean theophylline concentration (μg/ml)	40.8	56.9	52.7
Range	15.8-104.8	25-180	25-120

Data from Greenberg et al., 1984; Helliwell and Berry, 1979; Jacobs et al., 1976; Kraemer et al., 1982; Mountain and Neff, 1984; Park et al., 1983a,b; Woodcock et al., 1983; Zwillich et al., 1975.

in those with hepatic cirrhosis (Mangione et al., 1978), acidosis (Vallner et al., 1984), hypoxemia and hypercarbia (Letarte and duSouich, 1984), and in neonate (Aranda et al., 1976). In the study by Zwillich and associates (1975), the one patient with seizures associated with a theophylline concentration less than 30 μg/ml demonstrated evidence of significant hepatic dysfunction (elevated bilirubin level and prothrombin time). The three elderly patients reported by Nakada and associates (1983) who had seizures with theophylline concentrations of 17, 24, and 20.5 μg/ml had markedly depressed serum albumin levels of 2.2, 2.0, and 2.2 g/dl, respectively. If one corrects for a normal serum albumin of 4 g/dl, the patients would have free theophylline concentrations representative of total concentrations of 25, 35.6, and 30.3 μg/ml, respectively (Winter, 1980). These patients also had severe chronic obstructive pulmonary disease with hypercarbic acidosis. Unfortunately, most of the reports of theophylline-induced seizures do not document the serum albumin level.

In a patient with hepatic failure, theophylline-induced seizures, and a serum albumin of 2.6 mg/dl (Lawyer et al., 1978) a plasma theophylline concentration of 40 μg/ml was accompanied by a corresponding cerebrospinal fluid (CSF) concentration of 37.4 μg/ml (93.5%). In contrast, an infant who received an accidental overdose of theophylline (Simons et al., 1980) had a theophylline CSF-to-plasma ratio of 60% with normal serum albumin levels and protein binding studies. One of the two children who had seizures in association with theophylline concentrations less than 40 μg/ml had a low serum albumin dose to the nephrotic syndrome (Miceli et al., 1979).

Although the changes in plasma protein binding induced by acidosis, hypoxemia, and hypercarbia are slight in relation to differences produced by hypoalbuminemia, they have been shown to produce an elevated CNS-to-serum ratio of theophylline in the animal model (Letarte and du Souich, 1984). While we are still unable to predict with certainty the impact of any given abnormality, it has become increasingly obvious that the serum theophylline concentration must be interpreted in light of the clinical situation. In other words, a serum theophylline concentration of 20 μg/ml may be required to produce optimal results in an otherwise healthy young adult asthmatic and be exceedingly hazardous in the elderly cirrhotic with severe obstructive pulmonary disease.

Other predisposing factors appear to be respiratory failure and mechanical ventilation (Yarnell and Chu, 1975; Fleetham et al., 1979; Faden, 1976), underlying neurologic disorders (Covelli et al., 1983), and duration of the elevated theophylline concentration (Simons et al., 1980; Soiffer, 1957; Sahney et al., 1983).

Most patients who develop seizures from theophylline will exhibit prodromal signs and symptoms of theophylline toxicity including tachycardia, persistent nausea and vomiting, irritability, tremor, and agitation (Burkle and Gwizdala, 1981; Gaudreault et al., 1983; Mountain and Neff, 1984). However, a number of reports have presented patients without other apparent signs or symptoms of theophylline toxicity prior to the seizure (Yarnell and Chu, 1975; Zwillich et al., 1975). These reports were of older patients with severe chronic obstructive pulmonary disease (COPD) and other complicating illnesses that could produce clinical signs and symptoms (tachycardia and agitation) similar to those due to theophylline toxicity. This emphasizes the need for routine monitoring of theophylline concentrations along with careful clinical monitoring of the patient to detect early signs of theophylline toxicity particularly in the complicated elderly patients. Pediatric patients usually present with intractable vomiting or irritability, and agitation.

Clinical and Electroencephalographic Characteristics

Theophylline-induced seizures are focal in onset but rapidly progress to become generalized, tonic-clonic in nature (Soifer, 1957; Schwartz and Scott, 1974; Nakada et al., 1983). However, the seizures may remain focal in nature (Yarnell and Chu, 1975), or they may take on an encephalopathic picture with obtundation and periodic seizures (Faden, 1976; Schwartz and Scott, 1974). In severe overdoses, or if theophylline is not discontinued, the patient will progress to status epilepticus (Jacobs and Senior, 1974; Lawyer et al., 1978). Patients usually die of cardiorespiratory arrest or unresponsive hypotension (Helliwell and Berry, 1979; Anderson et al., 1983; Burgan et al., 1982). The electroencephalogram characteristically shows periodic lateralized epileptiform discharges or related activity (Nakada et al., 1983; Yarnell and Chu, 1975). This type of activity is characteristic of metabolic or anoxic insults superimposed on preexisting subclinical brain lesions (Chu, 1980).

Mechanisms

The mechanism of theophylline-induced seizure is currently unknown although theophylline is epileptogenic when applied directly to the cerebral cortex (Chu, 1981). At high concentrations theophylline may increase cyclic guanosine monophosphate levels; this agent is involved in producing epileptic discharges (Phillis, 1977). It is more likely due to theophylline antagonism of adenosine (Rall, 1980). Adenosine inhibits both spontaneous firing of central neurons and generation of postsynaptic potentials (Daly et al., 1981). Theophylline-induced cerebral vasoconstriction reduces blood flow and may produce a relative hypoxia, which could initiate the epileptic discharges (Yarnell and Chu, 1975; Schwartz and Scott, 1974). This may explain the increased susceptibility in patients with hypoxia and in elderly patients.

Brain scans taken to document structural abnormalities (Nakada et al., 1983) and cerebral spinal fluid studies (Simons et al., 1980) are unremarkable. However, an abnormal neurologic history or brain scan may predispose patients to developing a seizure at lower theophylline concentrations (Covelli et al., 1983). Autopsies from patients who did not die immediately following the seizures variably show no abnormalities or mild cortical hemorrhagic infarcts (Yarnell and Chu, 1975; Nakada et al., 1983). Autopsies of patients who died of the theophylline intoxication show diffuse cerebral edema (Soiffer, 1957).

Anticonvulsant Therapy

Theophylline-induced seizures are relatively resistant to anticonvulsant therapy (Zwillich et al., 1975). Fifty-four of the initial 100 cases (Table 2) were documented to receive anticonvulsants. A positive therapeutic response was documented in 16 cases (30%). Three cases responded to phenobarbital and 13 responded to diazepam or diazepam plus phenobarbital. Twenty-one patients received phenytoin, and in no case was it documented to be effective except in one patient who received the combination of diazepam and phenytoin (Jacobs and Senior, 1974). Three patients receiving intravenous diazepam suffered cardiorespiratory arrests requiring intubation and mechanical ventilation. Pediatric patients appear to be more responsive than adults to anticonvulsant therapy (Gaudreault et al., 1983). Some authorities have suggested that phenobarbital be administered prophylactically in patients with extremely high theophylline serum concentrations (>60 μg/ml) or are exhibiting signs of significant agitation. Prophylactic phenobarbital, but not phenytoin, prevented seizures and improved survival when administered to rabbits following toxic doses of theophylline (Goldberg et al., 1986).

B. Behavioral Neurotoxicity

Hyperactivity and insomnia are frequent complaints noted by parents in small children receiving theophylline in therapeutic "nontoxic" concentrations. Recent interest and concern has been expressed in a possible link between theophylline and learning and behavioral disorders in school-aged children (Furukawa et al., 1984). Theophylline alters the normal human sleep rhythm (Nobuyuki et al., 1984). Theophylline intoxication in elderly patients presenting with agitation, confusion, and bizarre behavior has occasionally been confused with psychosis or dementia (Wasser et al., 1981; Drummond, 1982). The diverse symptoms of neurotoxicity require the physician to have a high index of suspicion and to monitor elderly patients who are taking theophylline carefully.

III. Gastrointestinal Toxicity

Gastrointestinal symptoms are some of the most frequent clinical manifestations of theophylline toxicity. Anorexia, nausea, and vomiting are not uncommon in patients with theophylline concentrations in the high therapeutic range of 15-20 μg/ml (Jacobs et al., 1976; Jenne et al., 1972), but are rare at concentrations less than 15 μg/ml (Kordash et al., 1977). Persistent vomiting with hematemesis, often described as "coffee grounds," occurs frequently in pediatric intoxication (McKee and Haggerty, 1957).

A. Hemorrhage

Gastric hemorrhage may contribute to the hypotension seen in theophylline intoxication. At least one death associated with theophylline intoxication was believed to be the direct result of a massive gastrointestinal hemorrhage (McDonald et al., 1978). The mechanism of gastrointestinal hemorrhage is most likely multifactorial. Autopsy findings have revealed esophageal, gastric, and duodenal ulcers (Soifer, 1957). Theophylline, even in therapeutic concentrations, increases gastric acid secretion (Foster et al., 1979). The ulcers may be a result of the combination of stress and theophylline. Esophageal ulcerations with perforations may result from the persistent vomiting. The emetic effect of theophylline is primarily due to the stimulation of the vomiting center in the medulla oblongata (Borison and Wang, 1953). Theophylline is a weak base and direct irritation of the gastric mucosa may also play a role in the discomfort and nausea resulting from oral theophylline therapy.

B. Gastroesophageal Reflux

At therapeutic concentrations, theophylline decreases lower esophageal sphincter pressure (Stein et al., 1980). This effect was associated with a positive intraesophageal acid reflux test and symptoms of heartburn in a group of normal adults (Berquist et al., 1981). Gastroesophageal reflux is associated with chronic asthma and recurrent obstructive bronchitis (Danus et al., 1979). Although the precise cause-and-effect relationship between chronic lung disease and gastroesophageal reflux is still speculative, theophylline will aggravate the reflux.

IV. Cardiovascular Toxicity

A. Mechanisms

Theophylline exerts its effects on cardiovascular system through complex and incompletely understood mechanisms. The first deaths following rapid intravenous administration of aminophylline (Merrill, 1943; Bresnick et al., 1948) were characterized by severe hypotension and cardiac arrest. High concentrations of theophylline at the myocardium were also thought to be responsible for cardiac arrest and sudden death in critically ill patients receiving aminophylline through central venous catheters (Camarata et al., 1971). The exact mechanism of this phenomenon is unknown, but is thought to be a result of central vagal stimulation producing bradycardia in conjunction with peripheral vasodilation (Andersson and Persson, 1980).

Theophylline has both positive inotropic and chronotropic effects due to direct effects on the myocardium and pacemaker regions as well as the release of epinephrine from the adrenal gland and norepinephrine locally in the myocardium (Rall, 1980; Andersson and Persson, 1980). A reflex tachycardia from peripheral vasodilation also occurs (Ogilvie et al., 1977). The result of these combined effects is that sinus tachycardia is the most frequent adverse reaction seen with theophylline intoxication. It is not unusual for patients to have a modest increase of 3-16 beats/min in heart rate with theophylline concentrations in the therapeutic range (Ogilvie et al., 1977). Burkle and Gwizdala (1981) found tachycardia (heart rate $>$ 100 beats/min) to be the most prevalent sign of toxicity, occurring in over 80% of the patients with theophylline concentrations greater than 30 μg/ml. Unfortunately, many of the patients treated with theophylline have conditions that also produce tachycardia, such as hypoxia or heart failure. This decreases the reliability of tachycardia as a sign of theophylline toxicity in these patients. In patients taking theophylline, persistent sinus tachycardia without another obvious cause should be considered a sign of theophylline toxicity and should alert the physician to measure the theophylline level.

A variety of cardiac arrhythmias have been associated with theophylline intoxication. Premature atrial and or ventricular contractions have been the most frequently reported (Mountain and Neff, 1984; Greenberg et al., 1984). Supraventricular tachycardia, multifocal atrial tachycardia, and atrial fibrillation also occur, though less commonly (Levine et al., 1985; Greenberg et al., 1984; Pfeifer and Greenblatt, 1978; Mountain and Neff, 1984).

The cause of cardiac arrhythmias in theophylline intoxication is multivariate. Elderly patients with chronic obstructive pulmonary disease have a high incidence of ectopic activity and tachyarrhythmias (Klieger and Senior, 1974; Flick and Block, 1979). Horowitz and associates (1975) demonstrated that intravenous aminophylline lowered the ventricular fibrillation threshold in dogs and this effect was more pronounced with hypoxemia. Theophylline in therapeutic concentrations has been shown to exacerbate cardiac arrhythmias in patients with chronic obstructive pulmonary disease and preexisting arrhythmias (Shim et al., 1976; Patel et al., 1981).

B. Response to Therapy

The cardiac arrhythmias are generally responsive to therapy. The supraventricular tachycardias respond to intravenous verapamil (Burgan et al., 1982; Greenberg et al., 1984), while ventricular tachycardia and ectopic activity have responded to propranolol, procainamide, or lidocaine (Pfeifer and Greenblatt, 1978; McDonald et al., 1978). However, a number of cases have been reported in which lidocaine failed to control the ectopic activity until the theophylline concentration fell below toxic levels (Greenberg et al., 1984; Ehlers et al., 1978; Dean and Brown, 1982; True et al., 1984).

V. Miscellaneous Toxicity

A. Metabolic

Theophylline produces a marked diuresis (Rall, 1980) which could aggravate the hypotension in acute overdoses. Patients receiving the drug chronically develop a tolerance to the diuretic effect (Andersson and Persson, 1980), therefore this effect is of little consequence to patients who have been receiving the drug chronically. The metabolic effects of theophylline are varied. Many of the patients with theophylline intoxication demonstrate hyperglycemia, hypokalemia, and metabolic acidosis (Soiffer, 1957; Ellis, 1984). The hyperglycemia and hypokalemia may both be secondary to excess catecholamine release (Rall, 1980).

The hyperglycemia is generally not severe but may aggravate the hypotension by producing an osmotic diuresis. The persistent vomiting may contribute to the hypokalemia. Combined with a metabolic acidosis and diuresis, the patients may develop a significant total body potassium loss with attendant electrocardiographic changes (Ellis, 1984). This further emphasizes the need for appropriate cardiographic monitoring for theophylline intoxication.

B. Urinary Retention

A few reports of urinary retention from theophylline have appeared (Owens and Tannenbaum, 1981; Mountain and Neff, 1984). Theophylline inhibits ureteral peristalsis, decreases the resting tone of the bladder (Wein et al., 1972), and inhibits the contractile response of the detrusor muscle (Leoni et al., 1973). These effects may result in urinary retention, particularly in elderly men whose urinary outflow tract may already be compromised.

VI. Treatment

The initial treatment of theophylline intoxication includes immediate discontinuation of the drug or attempts to decontaminate the gastrointestinal tract with oral agents. The use of systemic removal techniques is still somewhat controversial (Greenberg et al., 1984; Park et al., 1983b). The controversy is due to the variable outcome of severe overdoses. Patients treated conservatively with only supportive therapy often have excellent outcomes (Dean and Brown, 1982; Gaudreault et al., 1983). As stated previously, the combined morbidity and mortality rate of patients with seizures was not markedly improved in those treated

Table 4 Comparison of Outcomes in Patients Manifesting Severe Theophylline Toxicity Treated with Hemoperfusion

	Survived without sequelae		Died or survived with sequelae
Number of patients	8		4
Mean age (yrs) (range)	27 (1-66)		25 (7 mo-50)
Peak theophylline concentration (μg/ml) (range)	89 (40.5-170)	NS	93 (46-190)
Time from symptom[a] onset and treatment (hr) (range)	6.1 (3-12)	$p = 0.01$[b]	18.8 99-36)

[a]Serious toxicity, such as seizure or significant arrhythmia.
[b]Mann-Whitney U test for nonparametric data.
Data from Chang, 1980; Connell et al., 1982; Ehlers et al., 1978; Fleetham, 1979; Greenberg et al., 1984; Jefferys et al., 1980; Lawyer et al., 1978; Park et al., 1983a,b; Russo, 1979; Sahney et al., 1983.

with removal techniques. However, all the patients with poor outcome had their treatment delayed for at least 9 hr after the onset of severe toxicity (Table 4). Patients in whom therapy was initiated within 2-7 hr of ingestion or onset of severe toxicity (including seizures, coma, arrhythmias, and cardiopulmonary arrests) recovered without sequelae (Table 4).

Evidence that duration of exposure to toxic concentrations may be a more important determinant of outcome than the absolute peak concentration would support the need for aggressive systemic removal of theophylline. Support for this concept comes from the inconsistent relation of peak theophylline concentration to severity of toxicity and the rapid improvement in patients corresponding to the rapid removal of theophylline (Table 5) (Sahney et al., 1983; Connell et al., 1982). Kadlec and co-workers (1978) presented the case of a child who developed seizures 15 hr after ingestion of theophylline at a concentration of 55 μg/ml, after presenting with only lethargy and vomiting with a theophylline concentration of 102 μg/ml. This patient exhibited saturation kinetics with a prolonged elimination half-life of 12.6 hr at high theophylline concentrations. Jacobs and Senior (1974) reported an adult

Table 5 Theophylline Removal Techniques

Reference Patient's age (years) Sex	Removal method	Theophylline conc. (μg/ml) start/end	Duration of removal (hr)	Endogenous clearance (ml/min)	Clearance of removal technique (ml/min)	Half-life (hr) endogenous/removal	Comments
Ehlers et al., 1978 48 F	HP FBC	170/20	6	38.5	61-163	8.1/2	Hemoperfusion begun following onset of seizures and two cardiorespiratory arrests 9 hr after admission. Patient survived with neurologic sequelae. Hemoperfusion decreased platelets and serum calcium
Greenberg et al., 1984 35 F	HP FBC	170/40	8.5	16.1	ND	16/4.7	Hemoperfusion started 4 hr following onset of seizures, arrhythmias, and refractory hypotension. Coagulopathy during hemoperfusion. *Enterobacter* sepsis and aspiration pneumonia. Recovered without sequelae
Park et al., 1983 11 mo F	HP FBC	70/16	3.5	ND	4.9/kg	12/0.7	Hemoperfusion started after seizures developed. 14 hr after ingestion. Patient died.
14 M	HP FBC	71/NR	5.5	ND	2.3/kg	9/1.5	No severe toxicity. Recovered
16 F	HP FBC	75/NR	5.5	ND	2.3/kg	12/2.1	No severe toxicity. Recovered
18 M	HP FBC	80/NR	3.5	ND	ND	7/1.5	No severe toxicity. Recovered
24 F	HP FBC	84/NR	4.5	ND	ND	6/1.0	No severe toxicity. Recovered
77 F	HP FBC	55/NR	3	ND	ND	30/1.2	Multifocal atrial tachycardia. Recovered

							Adverse effects of hemoperfusion were: hypotension in 2 patients; all patients developed thrombocytopenia and hypocalcemia
Jefferys et al., 1980 15 F	HP FBC	120/31	3	ND	97	ND/ND	Hemoperfusion started over 6 hr after cardiorespiratory symptoms and onset of arrhythmias; 16 hr after ingestion. No rebound seizures prior to hemoperfusion. Complications included aspiration pneumonia and acute renal failure requiring hemodialysis. Recovered
Lawyer et al., 1978 50 F	HP Resin	30/15.4	4	ND	225	54.5/3.9	Hemoperfusion started after 36 hr of status epilepticus. Patient was a chronic alcoholic; died 2 weeks following hemoperfusion from pneumonia. Rebound
Fleetham 1979 63 M	HP Resin	36.6/14.1	2.5	ND	ND	13.3/1.8	Hemoperfusion started 5 hr after status epilepticus and cardiac arrhythmias. No adverse effects from hemoperfusion. Patient recovered
Russo 1979 66 F	HP FBC	37/15	4	20	25-113	ND/ND	Hemoperfusion started 12-18 hr after onset of seizures and arrhythmias following a cardiac arrest. Hematocrit, platelet, and white blood cell count decreased during hemoperfusion. Rebound seen at 2 hr. Patient recovered
Connell et al., 1982 26 F	HP FBC	60/33	3	62	75	ND/ND	Hemoperfusion 4 hr after admission. Secondary rise 10 hr following hemoperfusion due to sustained-release tablets ingested.
	HP FBC	51/15	3	62	233	ND/ND	
Chang et al., 1980 3 F	HP ACAC	74/14.4	3	ND	3.8-5.8	ND/ND	Hemoperfusion started 8 hr following accidental intravenous overdose. Patient had hematemesis and tachycardia. Recovered without sequelae. Platelet level dropped during hemoperfusion

Table 5 (Continued)

Reference Patient's age (years) Sex	Removal method	Theophylline conc. (μg/ml) start/end	Duration of removal (hr)	Endogenous clearance (ml/min)	Clearance of removal technique (ml/min)	Half-life (hr) endogenous/removal	Comments
Sahney et al., 1983 4 F	HP FBC	46/6	1.75	ND	ND	ND/ND	Hemoperfusion started 7 hr after seizures. Patient incoherent at beginning became alert after hemoperfusion. Recovered without sequelae
7 mo F	HP FBC	48.6/2	2.5	ND	ND	ND/ND	Hemoperfusion started 16 hr following onset of seizures. Progressed to coma and cardiac arrest prior to starting. Seizures stopped 2 hr after hemoperfusion; patient survived with severe neurologic sequelae
1 F	HP FBC	56/12.5	2	ND	137/ $1.73m^2$	ND/ND	Hemoperfusion started 18 hr after ingestion and 3 hr after onset of seizures. Comatose at start; became alert 1.5 hr into hemoperfusion. Recovered without sequelae
1 F	PD	70/N	2	ND	16/ $1.73m^2$	ND/ND	Peritoneal dialysis started prior to hemoperfusion; no clinical improvement on peritoneal dialysis. Concentration dropped from 70-56 μg/ml 1 hr
Miceli et al., 1979 2.5 M	PD	37.2/6.2	33	ND	1.3	ND/9.5	Peritoneal dialysis started after seizure. Patient recovered without sequelae
Miceli et al., 1980	PD	110/4	27	ND	5.1	ND/9.5-5.4	Peritoneal dialysis started after seizures and coma. Patient survived with severe neurologic sequelae
Levy et al., 1977 47 F	HD	NR/NR	3	ND	32.8	ND/ND	Patient surgically anephric receiving aminophylline for wheezing during hemodialysis with coil dialyzer

Lee et al., 1979 69 M	HD	11/4	3	ND	88.1	ND/3.1	Uremic patients requiring dialysis received 250 mg aminophylline intravenously
52 F	HD	8.16/2.9	3	ND	88.1	ND/2.0	Cardis-Dow hollow fiber dialyzer. Blood flow was 180-250 ml/min. Patients not studied off dialysis
31 F	HD	5/2.3	3	ND	88.1	ND/2.7	
Kradjan et al., 1982 8 pts: 52	HD		4	48.7	52.3	7.3/2.7	Mean values for 8 patients with chronic renal failure. Blood flow through dialyzer: 200 ml/min
Anderson et al., 1983 11 pts: 42/45	HD	6.3/NR	3.3	ND	83.0	5.0/2.3	Mean values for 11 patients with chronic renal failure. Dialyzer blood flow was 300 ml/min
Snodgrass et al., 1980 29 F	HD	70/28.5	5.25	27.8	74.8	13.1/4.3	Patient exhibited hypotension and PACs recovered without sequelae
Mahutte et al., 1983 72 M	GID	28.6/12	8	ND	ND	34.4/5.7	Oral charcoal 30 g every 2 hr for 4 doses was started 4 hr after onset seizures and PVCs. Initial prolonged half-life may have been due to continued absorption from sustained-release product. Patient recovered without sequelae
8 pts: 25-38	GID		8	35.6	37	10.2/4.6	Oral activated charcoal, 30 g every 2 hr 4 times after 8 mg/kg aminophylline given intravenously
Gal et al., 1984 23 F	GID	54/1.6	30	ND	ND	17.2/5.9	Oral activated charcoal 50 g every 6 hr started 18 hr after peak concentration of 111 μg/ml. Initial prolonged half-life may have been due to continued absorption of sustained-release product

Table 5 (Continued)

Reference Patient's age (years) Sex	Removal method	Theophylline conc. ($\mu g/ml$) start/end	Duration of removal (hr)	Endogenous clearance (ml/min)	Clearance of removal technique (ml/min)	Half-life (hr) endogenous/removal	Comments
True et al., 1984 72 M	GID	26.8/10.3	8	ND	ND	16.2/5.9	Oral activated charcoal 30 g every 2 hr for 4 doses was started 7.5 hr after admission with arrhythmias. Patient ingested sustained-release theophylline. Recovered without sequelae
66 M	GID	50/ND	12	ND	ND	23/13.9	Oral activated charcoal 30 g every 4 hr for four doses was started 5 hr after admission for arrhythmia and nausea with a theophylline level of 58 $\mu g/ml$
Berlinger et al., 1983 6 pts: 20-30 M	GID	NR/NR	12	ND	ND	6.4/3.3	Following 6 mg/kg intravenous aminophylline, 6 subjects received activated charcoal in 300 ml water; 40 g at time 0 and 20 g at 2, 4, 6, 9, and 12 hr or just water in a randomized crossover study
Radomski et al., 1984 6 pts: 56-67	GID	NR/NR	12	ND	ND	12.7/4.0	Patients with hepatic cirrhosis received 6 mg/kg aminophylline intravenously; activated charcoal 40 g at time 0 and 20 g at 2, 4, 6, 9, and 12 hr or an equal volume of water
5 pts:	GID	NR/NR	12	ND	ND	6.4/3.2	Healthy young volunteers received same as above

HP, hemoperfusion; FBC, fixed-charcoal; ACAC, albumin-collodion-activated charcoal; PD, peritoneal dialysis; HD, hemodialysis; GID, gastrointestinal dialysis with activated charcoal; NR, not recorded; ND, not determined.

patient who developed seizures after 2 days of theophylline concentrations greater than 60 μg/ml. Patients on continuous intravenous administration appear to have seizures and poorer outcomes at lower theophylline concentrations (Zwillich et al., 1975) than patients with more acute intoxications (Greenberg et al., 1984; Park et al., 1983b). Olson and co=workers (1985) recently confirmed that patients chronically overdosed exhibit severe symptoms at lower serum theophylline concentrations (40-70 μg/ml) than patients presenting with acute single ingestions (>100 μg/ml).

A. Hemoperfusion

Data on the available methods for removal of systemic theophylline are included in Table 5. Exchange transfusions in neonates and small infants are ineffective for removing substantial amounts of theophylline (Assael et al., 1977; Wells and Ferlauto, 1979) and these are not included in the table. Hemoperfusion through fixed bed charcoal or resin is the most efficient means of removing theophylline. Hemoperfusion can increase the clearance of theophylline by four or five times (see Table 5). The efficiency of hemoperfusion appears to be limited only by the achievable blood flow through the system (Ehlers et al., 1978). Extraction efficiencies are decreased with higher theophylline concentrations (Park et al., 1983b) and after 1-2 hr with the same cartridge, due to saturation (Russo, 1979; Ehlers et al., 1978). Thrombocytopenia and hypocalcemia are the most common adverse effects from hemoperfusion but generally do not cause significant problems. However, hemoperfusion requires a high level of skill that may not be available at all institutions, thus delaying treatment and leading to a poor outcome (Sahney et al., 1983; Park et al., 1983b).

B. Hemodialysis and Peritoneal Dialysis

Hemodialysis is less efficient than hemoperfusion but appears to be an effective means for the removal of theophylline (Table 5). One case report of successful avoidance of severe toxicity in a massive overdose due to removal by hemodialysis has appeared in the literature (Snodgrass et al., 1980). Like hemoperfusion, hemodialysis requires a high level of expertise, which may not be readily available. Peritoneal dialysis is more readily available, however, it has limited efficiency in clearing theophylline (Brown et al., 1981) and has not proven to be satisfactory in the treatment of theophylline intoxication (Sahney et al., 1983).

C. Gastrointestinal Dialysis

Continuous administration of oral activated charcoal to produce a "gastrointestinal dialysis" has been proposed by Levy (1982) and used successfully in cases of theophylline intoxication (see Table 5). The gastric juice concentrations of theophylline parallel the plasma theophylline concentration (Lawyer et al.,

1978; Miceli et al., 1980). The activated charcoal adsorbs the theophylline producing a gradient and thereby increasing theophylline clearance across the mucosa (Berlinger et al., 1983; Radomski et al., 1984). The most efficacious method of administering the charcoal has yet to be established but larger dosages, up to 40 g every 4 hr, resulted in incremental increases in clearance. Administering the same total dosage in smaller doses at more frequent intervals (20 mg every 2 hr) may produce further slight increases in clearance (Park et al., 1983a). The obvious advantages of oral activated charcoal include ease of administration, availability, decreased cost, and lack of significant adverse effects. It would be the method of choice for treating oral intoxication because it would also prevent continued absorption. This may be particularly advantageous now with the increasing use, and therefore misuse, of sustained-release theophylline preparations (True et al., 1984; Connell et al., 1982; Gal et al., 1984).

Oral activated charcoal should be started in all patients following attempts to decontaminate the stomach with lavage. The charcoal should be given as a slurry at a dosage of 20-40 g every 2-4 hr. An oral cathartic such as sodium sulfate or magnesium citrate may be used to prevent constipation. Serum theophylline concentrations should be measured immediately and frequently enough (every 4 hr) to evaluate therapy. Preparations for hemoperfusion should be started for patients with theophylline concentrations greater than 60 μg/ml or less than 60 μg/ml who present with seizures, arrhythmias, hypotension, coma, or cardiac arrest. Hemoperfusion should be started based on the clinical picture: in any patient with symptoms unresponsive to supportive care or deteriorating after 4-6 hr of oral charcoal therapy.

VII. Causes

The causes of theophylline intoxication are multivariate but fall into two general categories: intentional ingestions, which are generally unpreventable; and unintentional overdoses by patients and clinicians. Two recent publications (Woodcock et al., 1983; Mountain and Neff, 1984) have addressed the multiplicity of factors involved in unintentional overdoses and emphasized the need for better education of patients and physicians in the safe and effective use of theophylline. Duplicate prescribing by different physicians, unrecognized drug interactions, excessive dosage prescribed, and patients exceeding the prescribed dosage were the primary causes of theophylline intoxication. In the 2-year study by Burkle and Gwizdala (1981), 89% of inpatients with toxic theophylline concentrations received theophylline dosages that exceeded recommended guidelines that took pathophysiological factors into consideration. Patients with limited physiological reserve, such as those with congestive heart failure, liver cirrhosis, or cor pulmonale, and those receiving multiple drugs are at particularly high risk for theophylline intoxication and may tolerate the toxicity less well. An evaluation of the numerous case reports of severe theophylline intoxication validates these findings. Physicians should weigh carefully the risk-to-benefit ratio before prescribing theophylline in potentially high-risk patients. Dosage should be guided by theophylline concentration measurements and patients and their caretakers should be carefully educated in the appropriate use of the drug. All parties involved—the physician, patient, nurse, and pharmacist—should communicate actively to improve the safety of theophylline therapy.

References

Anderson, J. R., Poklis, A., McQueen, R. C., Purtell, J. N., and Slavin, R. G. (1983). Effects of hemodialysis on theophylline kinetics. *J. Clin. Pharmacol. 23*: 428-432.

Anderson, J. R., Poklis, A., and Slavin, R. G. (1983). A fatal case of theophylline intoxication. *Arch. Intern. Med. 143*: 559-560.

Andersson, K. E., and Persson, C. G. A. (1980). Extrapulmonary effects of theophylline. *Eur. J. Respir. Dis. 61* (Suppl) *109*: 17-28.

Antal, E. J., Kramer, P. A., Mercik, S. A., Chapron, D. J., and Lawson, I. R. (1981). Theophylline pharmacokinetics in advanced age. *Br. J. Clin. Pharmacol. 12*: 637-645.

Aranda, J. V., Sitar, D. S., Parsons, W. D., Loughnan, P. M., and Neims, A. H. (1976). Pharmacokinetic aspects of theophylline in premature newborns. *N. Engl. J. Med. 295*: 413-416.

Assael, B. M., Caccamo, M. L., Gerna, M., Latini, R., Mandelli, M., Marini, A., Sereni, F., and Tognoni, G. (1977). Effect of exchange transfusion on elimination of theophylline in premature neonates. *J. Pediatr. 91*: 331-332.

Berlinger, W. G., Spector, R., Goldberg, M. J., Johnson, G. F., Quee, C. K., and Berg, M. J. (1983). Enhancement of theophylline clearance by oral activated charcoal. *Clin. Pharmacol. Ther. 33*: 351-354.

Berquist, W. E., Rachelefsky, G. S., Kadden, M., Siegel, S. C., Katz, R. M., Mickey, M. R., and Ament, M. G. (1981). Effect of theophylline on gastroesophageal reflux in normal adults. *J. Allergy Clin. Immunol. 67*: 407-411.

Borison, H. L., and Wang, S. C. (1953). Physiology and pharmacology of vomiting. *Pharmacol. Rev. 5*: 193-230.

Bresnick, E., Woodward, W. K., and Sageman, C. B. (1948). Fatal reactions to the intravenous administration of aminophylline. *JAMA 136*: 397-398.

Brown, G. S., Lohr, T. O., Mayor, G. H., Freitag, J. J., Sanchez, T. V., and Prasad, J. M. (1981). Peritoneal clearance of theophylline. *Am. J. Kidney Dis. 1*: 24-26.

Buchanan, N., Wainwright, L., and De Villiers, F. (1979). Theophylline poisoning in an infant: A case report. *S. Afr. Med. J. 56*: 811-812.

Burgan, T. H. S., Gupta, I., and Bate, C. M. (1982). Fatal overdose of theophylline simulating acute pancreatitis. *Br. Med. J. 284*: 939-940.

Burkle, W. S., and Gwizdala, C. J. (1981). Evaluation of "toxic" serum theophylline concentrations. *Am. J. Hosp. Pharm. 38*: 1164-1166.

Camarata, S. J., Weil, M. H., Hanashiro, P. K., and Shubin, H. (1971). Cardiac arrest in the critically ill: I. A study of the predisposing causes in 132 patients. *Circulation 44*: 688-695.

Chang, T. M. S., Espinosa-Melendez, E., Francoeur, T. E., and Eade, N. R. (1980). Albumin-collodion activated charcoal hemoperfusion in the treatment of severe theophylline intoxication in a 3-year-old patient. *Pediatrics 65*: 811-814.

Chu, N. S. (1980). Periodic lateralized epileptiform discharges with preexisting focal brain lesions–role of alcohol withdrawal and anoxic encephalopathy. *Arch. Neurol. 37*: 551-554.

Chu, N. S. (1981). Caffeine- and aminophylline-induced seizures. *Epilepsia 22*: 85-94.

Connell, J. M. C., McGeachie, J. F., Knepil, J., Thomson, A., and Junor, B. (1982). Self-poisoning with sustained-release aminophylline: Secondary rise in serum theophylline concentration after charcoal haemoperfusion. *Br. Med. J. 284*: 943.

Covelli, H. D., Knodel, A., and Heppner, B. (1983). The changing characteristics of theophylline-induced seizures. *Chest* (abstract) *84*: 332.

Daly, J. W., Bruns, R. F., and Snyder, S. H. (1981). Adenosine receptors in the central nervous system: Relationship to the central actions of methylxanthines. *Life Sci. 28*: 2083-2097.

Danus, O., Cesar, C., Larrain, A., and Pope, C. G. (1976). Esophageal reflux–an unrecognized cause of obstructive bronchitis in children. *J. Pediatr. 89*: 220-224.

Dean, L. S., and Brown, J. W. (1982). Massive theophylline overdose: Survival without hemoperfusion. *JAMA 248*: 1742.

Drummond, I. (1982). Aminophylline toxicity in the elderly. *Br. Med. J. 285*: 779-780.

Ehlers, S. M., Zaske, D. E., and Sawchuk, R. J. (1978). Massive theophylline overdose: Rapid elimination by charcoal hemoperfusion. *JAMA 240*: 474-475.

Faden, A. (1976). Encephalopathy following treatment of chronic pulmonary failure. *Neurology 26*: 337-339.

Fleetham, J. A., Ginsburg, J. C., Nakatsu, K., Wigle, R. D., and Munt, P. W. (1979). Resin hemoperfusion as treatment for theophylline-induced seizures. *Chest 75*: 741-742.

Flick, M. R., and Block, A. J. (1979). Nocturnal vs diurnal cardiac arrhythmias in patients with chronic obstructive pulmonary disease. *Chest 75*: 8-11.

Foster, L. J., Turdeau, W. L., and Goldman, A. L. (1979). Bronchodilator effects on gastric acid secretion. *JAMA 241*: 2613-2615.

Furukawa, C. T., Shapiro, G. G., Du Hamel, T., Weimer, L., Pierson, W. E., and Bierman, C. W. (1984). Learning and behavior problems associated with theophylline therapy. *Lancet 1*: 621 (letter).

Gal, P., Miller, A., and McCue, J. D. (1984). Oral activated charcoal to enhance theophylline elimination in an acute overdose. *JAMA 251*: 3130-3131.

Gal, P., Roop, C., Robinson, H., and Erkan, N. V. (1980). Theophylline-induced seizures in accidentally overdosed neonates. *Pediatrics 65*: 547-549.

Gaudreault, P., Wason, S., and Lovejoy, F. H. (1983). Acute pediatric theophylline overdose: A summary of 28 cases. *J. Pediatr. 102*: 474-476.

Goldberg, M. J., Spector, R., and Miller, G. (1986). Phenobarbital improves survival in theophylline-intoxicated rabbits. *Clin. Toxicol. 24*(3): 203-211.

Gotz, V. P., Drayer, D. E., Schned, E. S., and Reidenberg, M. M. (1979). Unusual cause of theophylline toxicity. *N. Y. State J. Med. 79*: 1232-1234.

Greenberg, A., Piraino, B. H., Kroboth, P. D., and Weiss, J. (1984). Severe theophylline toxicity: Role of conservative measures, antiarrhythmic agents, and charcoal hemoperfusion. *Am. J. Med. 76*: 854-860.

Haddad, Z. H., and Sakai, R. (1982). Massive accidental theophylline ingestion: Linear first order elimination kinetics in an infant. *Ann. Allergy 48*: 178-179.

Helliwell, M., and Berry, D. (1979). Theophylline poisoning in adults. *Br. Med. J. 2*: 1114-1115.

Hendeles, L., Bighley, L., Richardson, R. H., Hepler, C. D., and Carmichael, J. (1977). Frequent toxicity from iv aminophylline infusions in critically ill patients. *Drug Intell. Clin. Pharm. 11*: 12-18.

Jacobs, M. H., and Senior, R. M. (1974). Theophylline toxicity due to impaired theophylline degradation. *Am. Rev. Respir. Dis. 110*: 342-345.

Jacobs, M. H., Senior, R. M., and Kessler, G. (1976). Clinical experience with theophylline: Relationships between dosage, serum concentration, and toxicity. *JAMA 235*: 1983-1986.

Jefferys, D. B., Raper, S. M., Helliwell, M., Berry, D. J., and Crome, P. (1980). Haemoperfusion for theophylline overdose. *Br. Med. J. 1*: 1167.

Jenne, J. W., Wyze, E., Rood, F. S., and MacDonald, F. M. (1972). Pharmacokinetics of theophylline: Application to adjustment of the clinical dose of aminophylline. *Clin. Pharmacol. Ther. 13*: 349-360.

Jonkman, J. H. S., Jenne, J. W., and Simon, F. E. R. (Eds.). *Theophylline in the Treatment of CRAO.* Amsterdam, Excerpta Medica, pp. 33-38.

Kadlec, G. J., Jarboe, C. H., Pollard, S. J., and Sublett, J. L. (1978). Acute theophylline intoxication. Biphasic first order elimination kinetics in a child. *Ann. Allergy 41*: 337-339.

Kleiger, R. G., and Senior, R. M. (1974). Long term electrocardiographic monitoring of ambulatory patients with chronic airway obstruction. *Chest 65*: 483-487.

Kordash, T. R., Van Dellen, R. G., and McCall, J. T. (1977). Theophylline concentrations in asthmatic patients after administration of aminophylline. *JAMA 238*: 139-141.

Kradjan, W. A., Martin, T. R., Delaney, C. J., Blair, A. D., and Cutler, R. E. (1982). Effect of hemodialysis on the pharmacokinetics of theophylline in chronic renal failure. *Nephron 32*: 40-44.

Kraemer, M. J., Furukawa, C. T., Koup, J. R., Shapiro, G. G., Pierson, W. E., amd Bierman, C. W. (1982). Altered theophylline clearance during an influenza B outbreak. *Pediatrics 69*: 476-480.

Lambert, M., Mahieu, P., Hassoun, A., and Jacqmin, P. (1981). About three cases of acute theophylline intoxication: Clinical, toxicological and pharmacokinetic studies. *Acta Clin. Belg. 36*: 30-36.

Lawyer, C., Aitchison, J., Sutton, J., and Bennett, W. (1978). Treatment of theophylline neurotoxicity with resin hemoperfusion. *Ann. Intern. Med. 88*: 516-517.

Lee, C. S., Marbury, T. C., Perrin, J. H., and Fuller, T. J. (1979). Hemodialysis of theophylline in uremic patients. *J. Clin. Pharmacol. 19*: 219-226.

Leoni, J., Wein, A., and Schoenberg, H. (1973). The effects of isoproterenol and aminophylline on detrusor muscle contractility in an organ bath apparatus. *Invest. Urol. 10*: 458-463.

Lesko, L. J., Tabor, K. J., and Johnson, B. F. (1981). Theophylline serum protein binding in obstructive airways disease. *Clin. Pharmacol. Ther. 29*: 776-781.

Letarte, L., and duSouich, P. (1984). Influence of hypercapnia and/or hypoxemia and metabolic acidosis on theophylline kinetics in the conscious rabbit. *Am. Rev. Respir. Dis. 129*: 762-766.

Levine, J. H., Michael, J. R., and Guarnieri, T. (1985). Multifocal atrial tachycardia: A toxic effect of theophylline. *Lancet 1*: 12-14.

Levy, G. (1982). Gastrointestinal clearance of drugs with activated charcoal. *N. Engl. J. Med. 307*: 676-678.

Levy, G., Gibson, T. P., Whitman, W., and Proknal, J. (1977). Hemodialysis clearance of theophylline. *JAMA 237*: 1466-1467.

Mahutte, C. K., True, R. J., Michiels, T. M., Berman, J. M., and Light, R. W. (1983). Increased serum theophylline clearance with orally administered activated charcoal. *Am. Rev. Respir. Dis. 128*: 820-822.

Matthay, R. A., Matthay, M. A., and Weinberger, M. M. (1976). Grand mal seizure induced by oral theophylline. *Thorax 31*: 470-471.

McDonald, J. M., Ladenson, J. H., Turk, J., Dietzler, D. N., and Weidner, N. (1978). Theophylline toxicity. *Clin. Chem. 24*: 1603-1608.

McKee, M., and Haggerty, R. J. (1957). Toxic hazards: Aminophylline poisoning. *N. Engl. J. Med. 256*: 956-957.

Merrill, G. A. (1943). Aminophylline deaths. *JAMA 123*: 1115.

Miceli, J. N., Bidani, A., and Aronow, R. (1979). Peritoneal dialysis of theophylline. *Clin. Toxicol. 14*: 539-544.

Miceli, J. N., Clay, B., Fleishman, L. E., Sarnak, A. P., Aronow, R., and Done, A. K. (1980). Pharmacokinetics of severe theophylline intoxication managed by peritoneal dialysis. *Dev. Pharmacol. Ther. 1*: 16-25.

Mountain, R. D., and Neff, T. A. (1984). Oral theophylline intoxication: A serious error of patient and physician understanding. *Arch. Intern. Med. 144*: 724-727.

Nakada, T., Kwee, I. L., Lerner, A. M., and Remler, M. P. (1983). Theophylline-induced seizures: Clinical and pathophysiologic aspects. *West. J. Med. 138*: 371-374.

Nicholson, D. P., and Chick, T. W. (1973). A re-evaluation of parenteral aminophylline. *Am. Rev. Respir. Dis. 108*: 241-247.

Nobuyuki, O., Kripke, D. F., and Mullaney, D. J. (1984). Theophylline delays human sleep phase. *Life Sci. 34*: 933-938.

Nolke, A. C. (1956). Severe toxic effects from aminophylline and theophylline suppositories in children. *JAMA 161*: 693-697.

Ogilvie, R. I., Fernandez, P. G., and Winsberg, F. (1977). Cardiovascular response to increasing theophylline concentrations. *Eur. J. Clin. Pharmacol. 12*: 409-414.

Olson, K. R., Benowitz, N. L., Woo, O. F., and Pond, S. M. (1985). Theophylline overdose: acute single ingestion versus chronic repeated over-medication. *Am. J. Emerg. Med. 3*: 386-394.

Owens, G. R., and Tannenbaum, R. (1981). Theophylline-induced urinary retention. *Ann. Intern. Med. 94*: 212-213.

Parfrey, P., and Davies, S. J. (1970). Seizures after aminophylline by suppository. *Lancet 2*: 497-498 (letter).

Park, G. D., Radomski, L., Goldberg, M. J., Spector, R., Johnson, G. F., Quee, C. K. (1983a). Effects of size and frequency of oral doses of charcoal on theophylline clearance. *Clin. Pharmacol. Ther. 34*: 663-666.

Park, G. D., Spector, R., Roberts, R. J., Goldberg, M. J., Weismann, D., Stillerman, A., and Flanigan, J. J. (1983b). Use of hemoperfusion for treatment of theophylline intoxication. *Am. J. Med. 74*: 961-966.

Patel, A. K., Skatrud, J. B., and Thomsen, J. H. (1981). Cardiac arrhythmias due to oral aminophylline in patients with chronic obstructive pulmonary disease. *Chest 80*: 661-665.

Pfeifer, H. J., and Greenblatt, D. J. (1978). Clinical toxicity of theophylline in relation to cigarette smoking. *Chest 73*: 455-459.

Quee, C. K. (1984). Model for theophylline overdose treatment with oral activated charcoal. *Clin. Pharmacol. Ther. 35*: 402-408.

Radomski, L., Park, G. D., Goldberg, M. J., Spector, R., Johnson, G. F., and Quee, C. K. (1984). Model for theophylline overdose treatment with oral activated charcoal. *Clin. Pharmacol. Ther. 35*: 402-408.

Rall, T. W. (1980). The xanthines. In *The Pharmacological Basis of Therapeutics.* Edited by A. G. Gilman, L. S. Goodman, and A. Gilman. New York, Macmillan, pp. 592-607.

Reinhardt, D., Richter, O., Genz, T., and Fuchs, F. (1982). Linear elimination kinetics but non-linear pharmacodynamics in theophylline intoxication in a child. *Int. J. Clin. Pharmacol. Ther. Toxicol. 20*: 171-173.

Rounds, V. J. (1954). Aminophylline poisoning. *Pediatrics 14*: 528-531.

Russo, M. G. (1979). Management of theophylline intoxication with charcoal-column hemoperfusion. *N. Engl. J. Med. 300*: 24-26.

Sahney, S., Abarzua, J., and Sessums, L. (1983). Hemoperfusion in theophylline neurotoxicity. *Pediatrics 71*: 615-619.

Schwartz, M. S., and Scott, D. F. (1974). Aminophylline-induced seizures. *Epilepsia 15*: 501-505.

Shim, C. S., Scher, S. M., and Williams, M. H. (1976). Effect of bronchodilator agents on arrhythmia. *N. Y. State J. Med. 76*: 1973-1976.

Simons, F. E. R., Friesen, F. R., and Simons, K. J. (1980). Theophylline toxicity in term infants. *Am. J. Dis. Child. 134*: 39-41.

Snodgrass, W., Sawyer, D., Conner, C. S., Rumack, B. H., Peterson, R. G., and Sullivan, J. B. (1980). Asymptomatic theophylline overdose. *Drug Intell. Clin. Pharm. 14*: 783-785.

Soifer, H. (1957). Aminophylline toxicity. *J. Pediatr. 50*: 657-669.

Stein, M. R., Towner, T. G., Weber, R. W., Mansfield, L. E., Jacobson, K. W., McDonnell, J. T., and Nelson, H. S. (1980). The effect of theophylline on the lower esophageal sphincter pressure. *Ann. Allergy 45*: 238-241.

True, R. J., Berman, J. M., and Mahutte, C. K. (1984). Treatment of theophylline toxicity with oral activated charcoal. *Crit. Care Med. 12*: 113-114.

Vallner, J. J., Speir, W. A., Kolbeck, R. C., Harrison, G. N., and Bransome, E. D. Jr. (1979). Effect of pH on the binding of theophylline to serum proteins. *Am. Rev. Respir. Dis. 120*: 83-86.

Vaucher, Y., Lightner, G. S., and Walson, P. D. (1977). Theophylline poisoning. *J. Pediatr. 90*: 827-830.

Veum, J., and Schwartz, A. B. (1956). Toxic effects of half-strength aminophylline suppositories in asthmatic children. *J. Pediatr. 49*: 703-707.

Vincent, F. M. (1978). Case report: Fatal theophylline-induced seizures. *Postgrad. Med. 63*: 76-77.

Wasser, W. G., Bronheim, H. G., and Richardson, B. K. (1981). Theophylline madness. *Ann. Intern. Med. 95*: 191.

Wein, A., Gregory, J., Sansone, T., and Schoenberg, H. (1972). The effects of aminophylline on ureteral and bladder contractility. *Invest. Urol. 9*: 290-293.

Weinberger, M. M., and Ginchansky, E. (1977). Dose-dependent kinetics of theophylline disposition in asthmatic children. *J. Pediatr. 91*: 820-824.

Wells, D. H., and Ferlauto, J. J. (1979). Survival after massive aminophylline overdose in a premature infant. *Pediatrics 64*: 252-253.

White, B. H., and Daeschner, C. W. (1956). Aminophylline (theophylline ethylenediamine) poisoning in children. *J. Pediatr. 49*: 262-271.

Winke, C. L., Bricker, J. D., Collom, W. D., and Fochtman, F. W. (1980). Theophylline fatalities. *Forensic Sci. Int. 15*: 233-236.

Winter, M. E. (1980). Basic principles: Desired plasma concentrations. In *Basic Clinical Pharmacokinetics.* Edited by M. E. Winter, B. S. Katcher, and M. A. Koda-Kimble. San Francisco, Applied Therapeutics, pp. 9-16.

Woodcock, A. A., Johnson, M. A., and Geddes, D. M. (1983). Theophylline prescribing, serum concentrations, and toxicity. *Lancet 2*: 610-612.

Yarnell, P. R., and Chu, N. S. (1975). Focal seizures and aminophylline. *Neurology 25*: 819-822.

Zwillich, C. W., Sutton, F. D., Neff, T. A., Cohn, W. M., Matthay, R. A., and Weinberger, M. M. (1975). Theophylline-induced seizures in adults: Correlation with serum concentrations. *Ann. Intern. Med. 82*: 784-787.

26

Toxicity of Beta-Adrenergic Drugs

R. MICHAEL SLY

Children's Hospital National
Medical Center
Washington, D.C.

JOHN W. JENNE

Loyola-Stritch School of
Medicine, Maywood, and
Edward Hines, Jr. Veterans
Administration Hospital
Hines, Illinois

JUDITH COHN

Edward Hines, Jr. Veterans
Administration Hospital
Hines, and Rush-Presbyterian
St. Luke's Medical Center
Chicago, Illinois

I. Historical Overview

Potential adverse effects of beta-adrenergic agonist drugs can involve many systems. The most serious are cardiac arrhythmias, angina, and even myocardial necrosis. Increased airway obstruction following aerosolization has been reported, and transient decreases in arterial PO_2. Some tolerance or subsensitivity can develop on continual treatment. These agents can cause undesirable metabolic effects, muscle tremor, and stimulation of the central nervous system. This abundance of unwelcome effects has restrained intemperate use of these drugs, but uncertainty over the clinical relevance of some of the most serious effects has caused confusion. Some clinicians completely avoid prescribing sympathomimetic metered dose inhalers, although the inhalational route permits optimal response while minimizing adverse effects. Other physicians recommend unlimited use of beta-adrenergic agonists because of their effectiveness as bronchodilators. Prudence demands thoughtful consideration of the posssible adverse effects of both underuse and overuse of these potent drugs.

A gradual increase in mortality from asthma began in England and Wales in 1960. The death rate from asthma increased from 2.60 per 100,000 population in 1960 to 4.35 in 1965 and 4.24 in 1966 (Speizer et al., 1968a). The increase in mortality from asthma affected all age groups, but it was least pronounced in those below 5 and beyond 55 years of age. The rate increased from 0.7 to 2.2 for those 5-34 years of age, a group in which there should be little uncertainty of diagnosis. The greatest increase occurred in children 10-14 years old, among whom the rate increased from 0.33 in 1959 to 2.46 in 1966. After March 1967, the number of deaths from asthma fell in all age groups and remained less than 2.5 from 1974 to 1978 (Sly, 1984). Total annual deaths from asthma declined after the peak in 1965.

Metered dose inhalers that delivered epinephrine or isoproterenol became available in England and Wales in 1961, and a correlation between sales of pressurized bronchodilator aerosols and deaths from asthma suggested the possibility of adverse effects of the drugs (Inman and Adelstein, 1969). Total sales of the metered dose inhalers did not decline until 1967, however, 2 years after the decline in deaths from asthma had begun. Based on data from 174 patients who died during one period of 6 months, an estimated 84% of asthmatics between 5 and 34 years of age who died had used pressurized bronchodilator aerosols, and excessive use was suspected in at least 17% (Speizer et al., 1968a). Isoprenaline Forte, a preparation of isoproterenol in a pressurized cannister delivering 400 μg with each actuation instead of the usual 80 μg, was especially suspect, and accounted for approximately 30% of the nebulizer sales in England and Wales during the epidemic of deaths.

No increases in mortality from asthma occurred between 1959 and 1968 in the United States and Canada among people 5-34 years old, and Isoprenaline Forte was never licensed here (Stolley, 1972). However, estimated sales of bronchodilator aerosol nebulizers did triple from 1962 to 1967 in the United States. Nor did mortality from asthma increase in the Netherlands or Belgium, where Isoprenaline Forte was not marketed until 1966. Slight increases in mortality from asthma did occur in Japan from 1959 to 1967, however, although Isoprenaline Forte was not marketed there.

Publicity about the increasing rate of deaths from asthma began in the English medical literature in August 1965, but manufacturers' instructions for patients were not modified until 1968, and bronchodilator aerosols were not restricted to prescription sales until December 1968, after the epidemic had ended (Inman and Adelstein, 1969). Earlier verbal communication of possible hazards is conceivable.

Mortality from asthma in Australia increased in 1964, declined after 1966, and had returned to the preepidemic baseline by 1968 (Gandevia, 1973). Sales of pressurized bronchodilator aerosols in Australia increased progressively from 1961 to 1970, including sales of Isoprenaline Forte. Data from the four most heavily populated states indicate significant correlations between sales and deaths from 1961 to 1966 but not after 1966 (Campbell, 1976). These data do not implicate use or misuse of aerosolized bronchodilators as a cause of the increase in deaths from asthma in Australia unless there was a tempering of overuse by education, an effect that was not evident in total sales.

The concomitant increase in mortality from asthma in New Zealand did not plateau until 1980 (Jackson et al., 1982; Sly, 1984). Intensive study has failed to identify any single cause, but it may be relevant that the year in which the rate of increase abated was the year in which sales of drugs for the treatment of asthma, including sympathomimetic aerosols, nearly doubled in New Zealand (Wilson et al., 1981; Keating et al., 1984). The previous progressive increases in rates of death from asthma in New Zealand may have been due to undertreatment rather than overtreatment.

Increases in death rates from asthma since 1979 in the United States, associated with rapidly increasing sales of beta-adrenergic agonists delivered by metered dose inhaler as well as sustained-release theophylline preparations, have not been as extensive as those that occurred in England from 1960 to 1966 (Sly, 1984, 1985). Certainly, overreliance on medications that previously had afforded rapid relief may have contributed to delays in seeking other therapy when inhaled beta-agonists were no longer effective, whether because of tolerance or inflammation. The possibility that education of physicians and the public may have terminated the earlier epidemic, and the uncertainty over whether too little or too much drug may have been responsible, established the urgency of resolving these questions.

A. Aerosol Propellants

Young people have died suddenly after inhaling solvents or fluorocarbon aerosol propellants from plastic bags. This suggested the possible induction of cardiac arrhythmias after sensitization to the effects of endogenous catecholamines (Bass, 1970). Induction of arrhythmias by inhalation of fluorocarbon propellants by anesthetized, hypoxic mice reported from one laboratory, however, could not be replicated in others because hypoxia alone caused arrhythmias (Taylor and Harris, 1970; Jack, 1971). Large doses of fluorocarbon propellants can enhance the arrhythmia-inducing effect of large doses of epinephrine in dogs (Jack, 1971; Clark and Tinston, 1972). The combination of inhaled fluorocarbons and intravenous isoproterenol failed to cause cardiac arrhythmias in hypoxic dogs when isoproterenol was administered at dosages of 0.5 μg/kg every 30 sec for 5 min or every 15 sec for 2 min (Clark and Tinston, 1972). Tachycardia did occur. Continual administration of propellant, without access to air, with or without isoproterenol or albuterol administered as one inhalation with each of 40 successive inspirations, was required to cause convulsions in dogs, and all except two dogs that received isoproterenol recovered (Jack, 1971). Permitting a few inhalations of air at intervals of five to eight inhalations of propellant or bronchodilator prevented convulsions and deaths.

The peak arterial plasma concentrations of fluorocarbons that follow two inhalations of albuterol administered at an interval of 30 sec with breath-holding for 10 sec after inhalation are less than 50 μg/ml, occur within 20 sec and dissipate rapidly, leaving little detectable propellant by 2 min in patients treated for acute asthma (Dollery et al., 1974). Inhalation of the drug delivered by an actuation of the metered dose inhaler during each of 12-24 successive breaths would be required to reach concentrations of fluorocarbons in the blood and myocardium shown to sensitize dogs to toxic effects of epinephrine, and even higher concentrations may be necessary for sensitization to effects of isoproterenol or albuterol. Fluorocarbon propellants are not likely to contribute to any adverse cardiac effect of bronchodilator aerosols, except with very extreme overuse.

B. Adverse Interaction of Beta-Agonists with Theophylline

It is not surprising that many deaths from asthma have occurred in patients treated with both beta-agonists by inhalation and oral theophylline, because this is a combination frequently prescribed. Some of the deaths have been sudden, but cardiac abnormalities have rarely been found at postmortem examination, although microscopic examination of the heart often may not have been extensive (Speizer et al., 1968a; Wilson et al., 1981) and should be done with special stains to detect patchy necrosis. Treatment of asthma with intravenous infusions or isoproterenol can cause chest pain and electrocardiographic evidence of myocardial ischemia in both adults and children, however (Winsor et al., 1975; Matson et al., 1978). Multiple areas of myocardial necrosis were found at postmortem examination of an 18-year-old asthmatic woman after she died of sudden cardiorespiratory arrest during treatment of status asthmaticus with aminophylline and isoproterenol by intravenous infusion (Kurland et al., 1979). Serum theophylline concentrations in this woman had been as high as 30 μg/ml.

Subcutaneous administration of aminophylline to fat rats at relatively high blood levels enhances the toxic effect of isoproterenol or terbutaline, increasing the frequency of fatal cardiac arrhythmias (Nicklas et al., 1984). Although the doses of beta-adrenergic agonists may seem excessive, drugs generally must be given in much larger dosages than those used in humans to elicit similar responses in rodents. Myocardial lesions found at postmortem examination consist of localized interstitial edema and residual heart muscle cells intermixed with abundant macrophages and neutrophils. Obesity and increased age predispose rats to the more severe myocardial lesions and to arrhythmias, and there are marked species differences in susceptibility. These experiments will be described in more detail later.

The clinical relevance of these observations remains uncertain except to indicate a need for extreme caution if isoproterenol is administered by intravenous injection. Most clinical studies of treatment of asthma with beta-adrenergic agonists administered by inhalation, subcutaneous injection, or orally with or without oral theophylline or intravenous aminophylline have disclosed no serious toxicity at therapeutic doses, even when prolonged electrocardiographic monitoring has been done (Kemp et al., 1984; Joad et al., 1985).

Patients differ in their susceptibility to common side effects of beta-adrenergic agonists, including tachycardia and palpitations, however. Concurrent treatment with oral theophylline and beta-adrenergic agonists has caused chest pain and electrocardiographic changes in a few asthmatic children (Kravitz et al., 1982). The changes were reversed by discontinuation of the beta-agonist. Nebulized solutions of salbutamol containing 5 mg or more have caused angina in patients with underlying ischemic heart disease, although the same patients could tolerate a dose of 1 mg (Neville et al., 1982). Theophylline can stimulate release of endogenous epinephrine as well as norepinephrine in healthy adults (Higbee et al., 1982). Thus, concurrent treatment with theophylline and a beta-adrenergic agonist might be expected to intensify any adverse effect of the beta-agonist. The stress of acute asthma itself does not cause release of endogenous epinephrine, however, although concentrations of circulating norepinephrine do increase (Ind et al., 1985). The increased frequency with which painless myocardial infarction may occur during acute asthma in patients who have not received excessive doses of beta-agonists or theophylline emphasizes further the urgent need to define effects of these drugs (Chappell, 1984).

II. Cardiovascular Toxicity

A. Clinical Studies

Arrhythmias

Large doses of epinephrine can cause premature ventricular systoles, and inadvertent intravenous administration has caused premature ventricular systoles followed by multifocal ventricular tachycardia (Weiner, 1980). Subsequent atrial tachycardia has also been associated, occasionally with AV block. Cardiac $beta_2$-adrenergic receptors that can mediate tachycardia probably account for some of the tachycardia that may follow administration of a selective $beta_2$-adrenergic drug such as albuterol or terbutaline (Brown et al., 1983b). Radioligand binding studies indicate a $beta_1/beta_2$ adrenergic receptor ratio of approximately 65:35 in human left atrium and left ventricle and 50:50 in human right atrium as determined in different laboratories (Heitz et al., 1983; Robberecht et al., 1983). Activation of cardiac adenylate cyclase in the human heart has been said to be mediated by $beta_2$- rather than $beta_1$-adrenergic receptors (Waelbroeck et al., 1983). However, $beta_2$-selective adrenergic agonists have only a small inotropic action on the left ventricle compared to isoproterenol. The increase in heart rate caused by $beta_2$-selective drugs has been assumed to be predominantly due to a baroreceptor-mediated $beta_1$-sympathetic response to the reduction in afterload from stimulation of vascular $beta_2$-receptors (Sly et al., 1977).

Single doses of oral terbutaline (5 mg) can cause premature ventricular contractions and ventricular tachycardia in susceptible adults with chronic obstructive pulmonary disease (Banner et al., 1979). The mechanism is unknown, but alterations in intracellular potassium concentrations may contribute to the arrhythmias. Hypokalemia can cause changes in conduction, and systemic administration of albuterol or terbutaline can cause significant decreases in serum potassium concentrations (Neville et al., 1977; Kung et al., 1984). Treatment of acute asthma with conventional doses of 1:1,000 aqueous epinephrine by subcutaneous injection and aminophylline by intravenous infusion can elicit cardiac arrhythmias in patients with no history of cardiovascular disease, especially when both drugs are used (Josephson et al., 1980). Treatment with theophylline alone can exaggerate benign multifocal atrial tachycardia in some patients at serum concentrations of 12-20 μg/ml (Levine et al., 1985). Rarely, paroxysmal nodal tachycardia can follow inhalation of 1,500 μg metaproterenol, 700 μg epinephrine acid tartrate, or large doses of isoproterenol (Riding et al., 1970).

Studies in dogs demonstrate the enormous potentiating effect of hypoxemia (12% oxygen) on arrhythmias caused by isoproterenol inhalation (Cullins et al., 1969). These canine studies strongly support the use of oxygen during acute attacks of bronchospasm, whether in the hospital or at home.

Heart Rate

The modest increase of 8-15 beats/min in heart rate that can follow administration of a selective $beta_2$ adrenergic agonists orally or by subcutaneous injection at recommended doses is of little clinical significance (Sly et al., 1977; Banner et al., 1979; Sackner et al., 1974; Tashkin et al., 1975; Kemp et al., 1984).

There are host factor variables in the pulse response. Increase in pulse rate in patients with asthma or chronic obstructive pulmonary disease have been substantially less than those elicited by beta agonists in normal subjects, possibly because of tolerance induced by prior therapy with beta agonists (Sackner et al., 1975; Paterson et al., 1968) and/or inherently less beta-adrenergic responsiveness in asthmatics (Shelhamer et al., 1980). Some investigators have found little evidence of induction of tolerance to cardiovascular effects of $beta_2$ agonists, however (Svedmyr et al., 1976; Wilson et al., 1976).

The increase in heart rate induced by intravenous infusion of albuterol in normal adults can be increased further by hypoxemia and further still by a combination of hypoxemia and hypercapnea induced by breathing decreased concentrations of oxygen and increased concentrations of carbon dioxide (Leitch et al., 1976).

The usually recommended dosage of isoproterenol, 160-200 μg, delivered by metered dose inhaler, causes little or no increase in heart rate in most asthmatic subjects although a mean increase of 10% followed inhalation of 130 μg in one study (Shim and Williams, 1975; Spector and Gomez, 1977). Dosages as large as 520 μg may cause a mean increase of 20% (Spector and Gomez, 1977). When tachycardia occurs it peaks within 5 min and resolves within 1 hr. The usual dose of albuterol, 180 μg, delivered by metered dose inhaler, causes no increase in heart rate in asthmatics; dosages as large as approximately 700 μg caused a mean increase of only 9% within 5 min with return to baseline within 2 hr (Sly et al., 1975; Riding et al., 1970; Mahajan et al., 1977; Spector and Gomez, 1977). Dosages of 800 μg caused a mean increase in heart rate of 26% in one study (Collier et al., 1980). Significant increases in heart rate do not occur after delivery of 180 μg albuterol by inhalation chamber in children as young as 3-6 years of age (Chang et al., 1985).

The few studies in asthmatic subjects that have compared effects of isoproterenol and albuterol by metered dose inhaler on the heart rate at doses that elicit comparable peak bronchodilation have confirmed no increase after albuterol, 200 μg, but increases to 10-13% after isoproterenol, 500 or 1,000 μg (Choo-Kang et al., 1969; Tattersfield and McNicol, 1969). In normal subjects, somewhat greater increases in heart rate followed administration of isoproterenol by metered dose inhaler (increases of 29% after 85 μg and 56% after 680 μg), but albuterol caused no increase in heart rate at dosages as high as 900 μg and a mean increase of only 14% at 1,200 μg (Finch, 1981). Fenoterol, in the recommended dosages of 200-400 μg, one to two puffs, caused no pulse elevation nor ectopic beats in patients with chronic reversible airway obstruction, but seven puffs raised the pulse by eight beats/min with an increase in ectopic beats. Up to 13 puffs of salbutamol had no effect. In contrast to salbutamol, overdoses of fenoterol have been considered to have stimulatory effects on the heart (Tandon, 1980). As many as seven inhalations of terbutaline, 250 μg each, by metered dose inhaler usually caused no increase in heart rate in asthmatic subjects (Weber et al., 1979). Inhalation of metaproterenol, 1,500 μg by metered dose inhaler, caused no significant increase in heart rate in adults with chronic asthma (Choo-Kang et al., 1969).

Administration of solutions of selective beta_2-adrenergic agonists by simple nebulization or by intermittent positive pressure breathing to asthmatic subjects has also caused little if any increase in heart rate except at very large dosages of 10 or 15 mg albuterol (8 or 13% increase in heart rate). However, 12, 26, and 40% increases in heart rate can follow delivery of nebulized isoproterenol 2.5, 5, and 10 mg, respectively (Light et al., 1979; Weber et al., 1979) (Fig. 1). Thus, inhalation of selective beta-adrenergic agonists does cause much less cardiac stimulation than inhalation of isoproterenol even though there are cardiac beta_2 receptors.

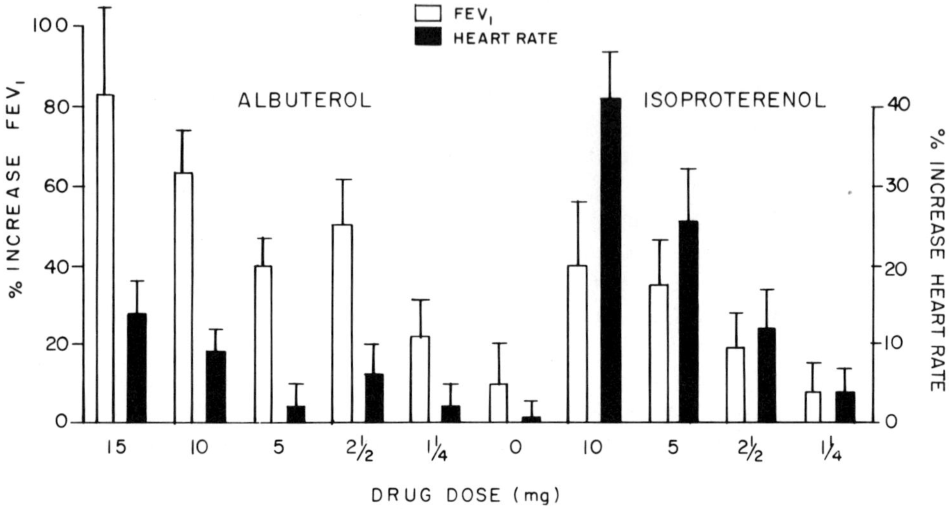

Figure 1 Time-weighted mean percent increases from baseline over 6 hr comparing albuterol and isoproterenol. Forced expiratory volume in 1 sec (FEV_1) and peak mean percent increases from baseline in heart rate are indicated (±SEM). Solutions delivered by IPPB (from Light et al., 1979).

Blood Pressure and Peripheral Vascular Resistance

Changes in cardiac output following the initial dose of a systemic beta agonist are not trivial. In normal adults, subcutaneous injection of 0.5 mg epinephrine caused a peak increase in heart rate of 17 beats/min at 30 min with an increase of 62% in cardiac output and a peak increase of 27% in stroke volume at 15 min (Sackner et al., 1975). Mean systolic blood pressure increased from 124 to 152 mmHg by 30 min and diastolic blood pressure decreased from 79 to 66 by 15 min. Calculated systemic vascular resistance fell 39% by 15 min, while calf blood flow increased. Similar but less extreme changes followed the smaller dosage of 0.25 mg.

Inadvertent intravenous injection of epinephrine, or subcutaneous injection of large doses in older patients, has resulted in cerebral hemorrhage due to a rise in pressure and therefore it is inadvisable in this age group. It is contraindicated in patients with hypertension, hyperthyroidism, ischemic heart disease, and cerebrovascular insufficiency and patients on monoamine oxidase inhibitors.

Subcutaneous injection of only 0.25 mg terbutaline to normal adults elicited changes similar to those caused by 0.5 mg epinephrine, including an increase in heart rate of 17 beats/min at 60 min, increase in cardiac output of 48% at 30-60 min, increase in stroke volume of 14% at 15 min. Systolic blood pressure increased from 130 to 140 at 30 and 60 min; diastolic pressure fell from 81 to 66 mmHg at 15 min. Systemic vascular resistance fell 36% at 30 min with an increase in calf blood flow at 60 min. More extreme changes followed the larger dosage of 0.5 mg terbutaline.

Administration of conventional dosages of terbutaline by subcutaneous injection to asthmatic children and to adults with chronic obstructive pulmonary disease had little if any effect on systolic blood pressure but did cause small but statistically significant decreases of 6-9% in diastolic blood pressure (Sackner et al., 1974; Sly et al., 1977). Following administration of oral terbutaline, 5 mg, to asthmatic subjects, some have reported small but statistically significant increases in systolic blood pressure of 4-9 mmHg and small decreases in diastolic blood pressure of 5 mmHg (Tashkin et al., 1975). Others have reported that oral terbutaline causes no change in blood pressure in patients with chronic obstructive pulmonary disease (Banner et al., 1979).

In normal volunteers inhalation of albuterol by metered dose inhaler at a dosage of 150 μg caused a maximum increase of less than 6% in systolic blood pressure but a decrease of 18% in diastolic pressure (Finch, 1981). Larger dosages had only slightly more effect. Inhalation of isoproterenol, 170 μg, caused an increase of nearly 12% in systolic blood pressure and a decrease of 13% in diastolic pressure, and 1,020 μg caused an increase of 20% in systolic pressure and a decrease of 21% in diastolic pressure.

In patients with reversible obstructive pulmonary disease, inhalation of albuterol or isoproterenol at modest doses apparently has little effect on blood pressure (Zsoter and Epstein, 1973). Inhaled albuterol does cause a more sustained reduction in arterial resistance than isoproterenol and a more sustained increase in forearm blood flow. Others have confirmed that recommended dosages of albuterol and isoproterenol delivered by metered dose inhaler have no significant effect on blood pressure in asthmatic subjects (Mahajan et al., 1977). Nebulized fenoterol, 2.5 mg, caused a small but statistically significant decrease in diastolic blood pressure with no significant effect on systolic blood pressure in asthmatic adults (Ruffin et al., 1979).

Although two puffs, or 400 μg fenoterol, produced only small effects on pulse and blood pressure in normals, mean cardiac output was increased 26% 15 min later, accompanied by an 18% mean drop in peripheral vascular resistance, 16% increase in stroke volume, and an 18% increase in velocity of circumferential shortening of the left ventricle (Chapman et al., 1984). In fact, in one of the eight subjects, cardiac output increased 117%. Surprisingly, there was no demonstrable tolerance to these effects after 2 weeks of regular therapy. The authors make the point that mere observance of pulse rate and blood pressure can underestimate the effects of metered dose inhalers on the cardiovascular system.

Table 1 Effects of Intravenous Isoproterenol and Salbutamol in Man (Mean Values in Six Patients with Mitral Valve Disease, ± S.D.)

	Isoproterenol		Salbutamol	
	Control	0.1 μg/kg	Control	2.0 μg/kg
Heart rate (beats/min)	70 ± 7.8	+10.6 ± 5.0	78 ± 13.0	+25.5 ± 7.5
Cardiac output (liters/min)	2.8 ± 0.5	+1.05 ± 0.35	3.0 ± 0.65	+1.1 ± 7.5
Peripheral resist (units)	38.0 ± 2.0	-12.5 ± 3.8	37.0 ± 7.4	-14.4 ± 4.1
Ejection time (m/sec)	280 ± 250	-48.0 ± 30.0	250 ± 150	-15.0 ± 8.3
Ejection rate (ml/sec)	135 ± 20	+62 ± 27.0	160 ± 24.0	+8.0 ± 11.2
Stroke volume (ml)	39.0 ± 4.5	+7.6 ± 2.6	38.0 ± 5.5	+0.7 ± 2.1

Adapted from Gibson and Coltart, 1971, with permission.

Table 2 Hemodynamic Effects of Terbutaline Given Intramuscularly and by Metered Dose Inhaler (MDI) in Eight Asthmatics

Dosage (mg)	PEPI (msec)	PEP/LVET	Ht. rate	Syst (mm)	Diast (mm)	PP (mm)	PEF (L/min)
placebo IM	126 11	0.338/0.057	75	126	81	44	399
0.125 IM	114 12	0.290/0.056	87	126	76	49	431
0.250 IM	109 9	0.276/0.051	93	131	78	53	455
0.50 IM	102 7	0.245/0.033	97	139	79	61	450
1.0 IM	105 8	0.243/0.034	103	134	76	59	461
2.5 MDI	118 14	0.301/0.070	81	123	79	46	458

PEPI, preinjection period index; PEP, preinjection period; LVET, left ventricular injection time; Sys, Diast, and PP, systolic, diastolic, and pulse pressure; PEF, peak expiratory flow.
From Buch and Bundegaard, *Arch. Pharmacol. Toxicol. 54*: 183-188, 1985, with permission.

Ventricular Contractility

This finally brings us to the question of the acute inotropic effects of beta agonists on the myocardium. The more $beta_2$-selective agonists, such as salbutamol and terbutaline, have minimal inotropism compared to isoproterenol. Graded doses of isoproterenol and salbutamol were administered intravenously to six patients during cardiac catheterization studies of mitral stenosis (Gibson and Coltart, 1971). At the maximum dosages used, the results shown in Table 1 were found.

Both drugs caused an increase in whole body oxygen uptake and central blood volume and a decrease in peripheral resistance. Despite equal effects in lowering peripheral resistance, the minimal increase in ejection rate and stroke volume from salbutamol contrasted sharply with the stimulatory effect of isoproterenol on myocardial contractility.

Hemodynamic dose-response studies have been done in asthmatics comparing various injected doses of terbutaline subcutaneously and metered dose inhalation (MDI) (Buch and Bundgaard, 1984). While most of the increased cardiac output appears to be due to the decreased peripheral vascular resistance, some of it is due to a direct effect of this $beta_2$-selective agonist on the myocardium, albeit much less than from isoproterenol. In one male and seven female asthmatics averaging 38 years in age (15-66) the results shown in Table 2 were obtained. All measurements were made 15 min after the dose. Terbutaline 2.5 mg (10 puffs) by MDI gave even less hemodynamic stimulation than 0.125 mg terbutaline intramuscularly (IM), but as much bronchodilation as 0.25 mg terbutaline IM. In another study, liquid aerosols of salbutamol up to 5 mg had no significant effect on right and left ventricular ejection fraction (Winter et al., 1984).

In severe left ventricular dysfunction studies, $beta_2$-selective agonists have been shown to exert both afterload reduction and positive inotropism without energy cost to the myocardium (Timmis et al., 1981). Thus, in 10 patients with severe arteriosclerotic heart disease, an oral dose of 20 mg pirbuterol was compared to 6 mg salbutamol. These two drugs had indistinguishable effects, consisting of a fall in systemic vascular resistance from 23 to 19 units, a rise in cardiac output from 3.7 to 4.5 liters/min, an increase in left ventricular dp/dt max from 821 to 1,411 mg/Hg sec, but no change in myocardial O_2 uptake or extraction of lactate, glucose, and free fatty acids. The authors concluded that positive inotropism occurred without cost to the myocardium.

In intact dogs, relatively high doses of salbutamol enhanced left ventricular function with increased coronary flow, but, in contrast to metaproterenol and isoproterenol, did not deplete high-energy stores of the myocardium while consuming much less oxygen (Naylor and McInnes, 1972).

A final comment is necessary. The effects of beta-adrenergic drugs on the cardiovascular system are usually described for the initial, acute exposure. Many of the organs involved undergo a degree of tolerance with repeated exposure. An example is the marked loss of effect of pirbuterol on ejection fraction after a week of maintenance dosing (Colucci et al., 1981), possibly more as a result of diminished vasodilator action on $beta_2$ receptors.

B. Animal Models of Myocardial Injury

For years, pharmacologists have studied the occurrence of myocardial necrosis, arrhythmias, and death following administration of beta-adrenergic drugs, particularly isoproterenol, to animals (Rona et al., 1959; Balazs and Bloom, 1962; Kahn et al., 1969; Csapo et al., 1972), and have been aware of similar lesions in humans. In humans, the best documented examples of catecholamine-induced myocardial necrosis (CAT-MN) are seen at autopsy of patients with pheochromocytomas of the adrenal gland and frequent "adrenal storms." These consist of individual focal lesions of myocardial necrosis with a lymphocytic and histiocytic infiltrate, but only rare neutrophils, involving primarily the endocardial zone of the left ventricle (Balazs and Bloom, 1982). It has also been postulated that the high levels of endogenous catecholamines associated with myocardial infarction could contribute to its extension.

Of current concern to toxicologists is the possibility that large doses of isoproterenol and other beta-adrenergic agents used in the treatment of asthma, often combined with theophylline, pose a hazard to the asthmatic. An impetus for this was the epidemic of deaths in the mid-1960s in asthmatics who often used a high-potency isoproterenol inhalant as described above (Speizer et al., 1968a). More recently, the controversy surrounding an apparent excess of deaths in young New Zealand asthmatics using inhaled beta agonists and theophylline has further fueled these concerns (Wilson et al., 1981; Nicklas et al., 1984), although most analysts consider the deaths to be due to delay in treatment (Grant, 1981). The FDA is conducting extensive animal studies exploring interactions of these drugs with the myocardium in an attempt to define this hazard better in humans (Joseph et al., 1981; Whitehurst et al., 1983; Balazs and Bloom, 1982). In the following discussion, we will summarize these studies and discuss some of the hypotheses currently invoked in the literature for the genesis of these lesions.

Pathology

Isoproterenol produces focal myocardial necrosis in various species over a wide dosage range (Fig. 2). The apex and papillary muscle are the sites of the predilection (Rona et al., 1959). Electron microscopic investigations have shown the initial morphologic lesions to be located in the myofibrils, suggesting a direct myofibrillar action of isoproterenol (Csapo et al., 1972). Necrotic lesions can be demonstrated within 2 hr after injection and generally consist of two types,

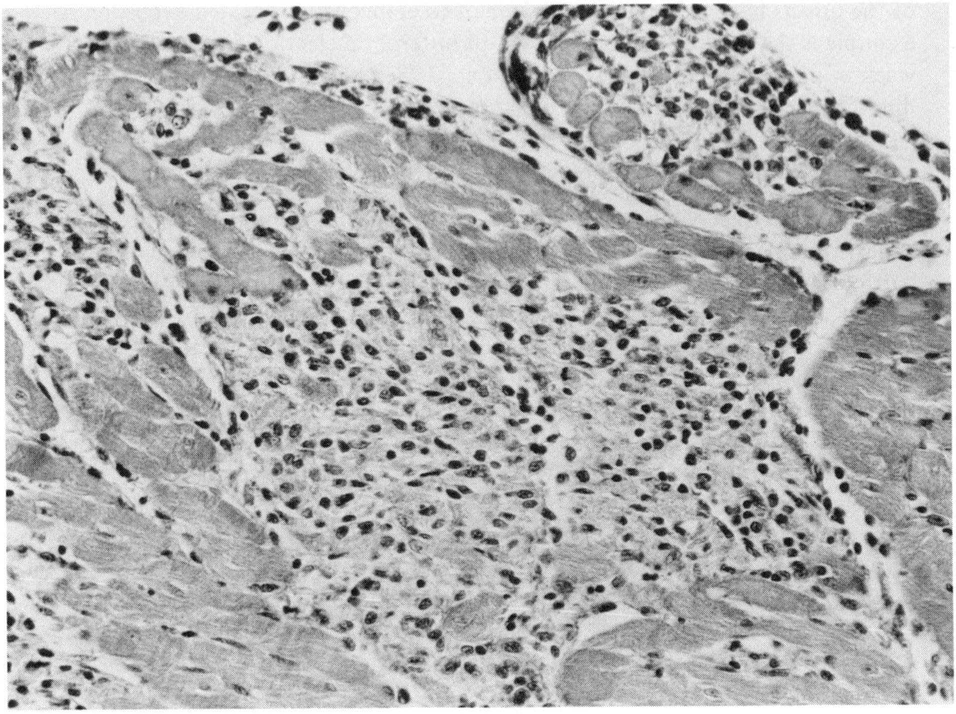

Figure 2 Myocardial necrosis in rats injected with 50 μg/kg isoproterenol subcutaneously. (Courtesy of T. Balazs.)

representing grades of severity: a nonhomogeneous confluent type in the area of gross change (caused by high dosages) and a disseminated focal variety (caused by low dosages) in the papillary muscles and subendocardially in both ventricles and occasionally in the atria. Additional scattered foci may be found throughout the remainder of the ventricular myocardium, occasionally involving the epicardial aspect of the myocardium at the atrioventricular groove. The dosage range for producing these lesions in rats is enormous and depends on weight and age. Dogs are more sensitive than rats (Rona et al., 1959) and rabbits are relatively resistant (Whitehurst et al., 1983).

In 1962, Balazs et al. showed that rats with increased body fat were much more sensitive to the cardiotoxicity of isoproterenol than lean rats, and later studies showed that sensitivity returned to normal with reduction in body weight through caloric restriction (Balazs and Bloom, 1982). The data summarized in Tables 3-5 are combined from two recent studies (Joseph et al., 1981; Whitehurst et al., 1983) and show a 2,000-fold difference in sensitivity between

Table 3 Arrhythmias and Mortality in Heavy (500-600 g) and Small (150-200 g) Rats Treated with Varying Dosages of Isoproterenol, Terbutaline, and Bitolterol With and Without Aminophylline in Groups of 10

Body wt (g)	Pretreatment (mg/kg sc)	Treatment (mg/kg sc)	Arrhythmia	Deaths
500-600	Physiological saline +	Isoproterenol (0.015)	1	0
	Physiological saline +	Isoproterenol (0.1)	2	2
	Physiological saline +	Terbutaline (0.1)	0	0
	Physiological saline +	Terbutaline (5.0)	1	0
	Aminophylline (37.5) +	Physiological saline	0	0
	Aminophylline (37.5) +	Isoproterenol (0.015)	6	0
	Aminophylline (37.5) +	Isoproterenol (0.1)	10	3
	Aminophylline (37.5) +	Terbutaline (0.1)	0	1
	Aminophylline (37.5) +	Terbutaline (5.0)	8	4
	Aminophylline (37.5) +	Bitolterol (0.1)	1	1
	Aminophylline (18.75) +	Isoproterenol (0.1)	8	1
150-200	Physiological saline +	Isoproterenol (700)	1	3
	Aminophylline (75) +	Isoproterenol (700)	1	10

Combined data from Joseph et al., 1981, and Whitehurst et al., 1983.

Table 4 Arrhythmias and Mortality Rates in Rabbits Treated with Isoproterenol and/or Aminophylline Pretreatment (mg/kg IV)

Pretreatment (mg/kg iv)	Treatment (μg/kg/min × 60 min)	Arrhythmia	Deaths
Physiological saline +	Isoproterenol (10)	0	0
Physiological saline +	Isoproterenol (100)	0	0
Physiological saline +	Terbutaline (10)	0	0
Physiological saline +	Terbutaline (100)	0	0
Aminophylline (40) +	Physiological saline	0	0
Aminophylline (40) +	Isoproterenol (100)	3	1
Aminophylline (40) +	Terbutaline	0	0

Combined data from Joseph et al., 1981, and Whitehurst et al., 1983.

Table 5 Degree of Myocardial Lesions in Heavy Rats Treated with Beta-Agonists or Aminophylline Alone and in Combination

Pretreatment (mg/kg)	Compound (mg/kg sc)	Grade lesion (mean)
Saline +	Isoproterenol (0.015)	1.3
Saline +	Isoproterenol (0.1)	2.6
Saline +	Terbutaline (0.1)	0.1
Saline +	Terbutaline (5.0)	1.7
Saline +	Bitolterol (0.1)	0.5
Aminophylline (37.5) +	Saline 0	
Aminophylline (37.5) +	Isoproterenol (0.015)	2.2
Aminophylline (37.5) +	Isoproterenol (0.1)	3.2
Aminophylline (37.5) +	Terbutaline (0.1)	1.44
Aminophylline (37.5) +	Bitolterol (0.1)	2.7
Aminophylline (18.75) +	Terbutaline	3.75

Lesions graded from 0 (none) to 4 (severe).
Data combined from Joseph et al., 1981, and Whitehurst et al., 1983.

Sprague-Dawley male rats weighing 500-600 g (4-5 months) and those weighing 150-200 g (1.5-2 months). In all rat studies, groups of 10 animals were injected subcutaneously with saline, isoproterenol, or the $beta_2$-selective bitolterol and terbutaline. Some rats also received aminophylline subcutaneously. A dosage of 37.5 mg/kg aminophylline produced serum levels of about 40 μg/ml. Electrocardiographic monitoring was done at 5-min intervals for 3 hr after injection. Surviving rats were autopsied at 24 hr.

The apical-most section of myocardium was chosen for grading of lesions in four degrees of severity: 0, no lesions; 1, less than 5%; 2, 5-10%; 3, 10-15%; 4, over 15%. A trichrome stain was used to facilitate grading under low power, staining areas of necrosis blue. Lesions were observed in the apex, left ventricle, and papillary muscles. They were predominantly in a subendocardial location of the wall and septum, and consisted of edema, residual muscle cells, and abundant macrophages with scattered neutrophils. Necrotic muscle cells showed a loss of the normal pattern of cross-striation with prominent "contraction bands" (agglomerated masses of contractile protein) in their cytoplasm. Commonly observed arrhythmias were premature contractions, ventricular tachycardia, and ventricular fibrillation.

Studies comparing salbutamol, terbutaline, and orciprenaline demonstrated that only the latter agent had similar myocardial toxicity to isoproterenol (Poynter and Spirling, 1971; Magnusson and Hansson, 1973). The data suggest that the more $beta_1$-stimulating action a compound has, the more likely it is to cause myocardial necrosis. When myocardial injury is measured by the release of MB-CPK into the blood of 400-500-g Sprague-Dawley rats, it is observed that 45 mg/kg salbutamol produces significantly less damage than 5.25 mg/kg isoproterenol (Brown-Lukacsko and Lukacso, 1982), and significantly less increase in myocardial cyclic AMP and decrease in ATP despite an equal drop in blood pressure and increase in heart rate. The $beta_1$-agonist practolol is able to block all myocardial changes without affecting the drop in blood pressure from either drug, indicating again that the $beta_1$ actions of salbutamol are responsible, its relative $beta_2$-selectivity not withstanding, and that hypoperfusion is not the cause of damage.

Isoproterenol-induced arrhythmia and necrosis are potentiated by corticosteroids and thyroxin (Balasz and Bloom, 1982). Desoxycorticosterone acetate (DOCA) is more effective than hydrocortisone. In fact, DOCA and salt-loading produced a 20,000-fold potentiation of fatal arrhythmias in normal rats. Equally surprising was the fact that epinephrine did not produce arrhythmias (Guidero et al., 1974).

Relative Ischemia

Myocardial necrosis is maximal in the subendocardial region of the left ventricle and interventricular septum. These changes resemble subendocardial lamina necrosis produced by myocardial ischemia in humans (Davies, 1977; Chappel et al., 1959), leading to the suggestion that the inotropic and chronotropic effects of the amine produce relative underperfusion of the subendocardial region (Salisbury et al., 1963; Moir and DeBra, 1967). The disproportion between supply and demand of oxygen with accompanying hypoxia results from the peripheral vasodilation, lowered blood pressure, tachycardia, increased force of myocardial contraction, and general increase in basal metabolism. In addition, it has been reported that even though isoproterenol causes an increase in blood flow to all layers of the heart, the ratio of endocardial to epicardial blood falls such that flow is directed away from the endocardial layer (Pieper et al., 1979). The endocardium shows signs of severe damage within 30 min of isoproterenol injection and the adjacent myocardium after 1 hr (Noronhu-Dutra et al., 1984).

Differential myocardial vasodilation resulting in a maldistribution of blood flow has been implicated in patients with coronary artery disease receiving isoproterenol infusions and has been termed "isoproterenol coronary steal" (Vaisrub, 1974; Row, 1970; Downey et al., 1972).

Platelet Aggregation

Another proposed mechanism for isoproterenol cardiotoxicity is increased platelet aggregation (Haft et al., 1972). However, isoproterenol does not directly aggregate rat platelets, as shown in vitro (Berry and Miller, 1974), and could not be shown to do so in animal models (Moscho et al., 1978; Noronha-Dutra et al., 1984). In the later study platelets were present only where the subendothelium had been exposed, either because of endocardial cell separation or desquamation. Platelets were also present in capillaries but never as aggregates.

Calcium Overload

Still other investigators believe the cardiotoxic effects of sympathomimetics are mediated by changes in the concentration of divalent cations particularly calcium (Bloom and Davis, 1972; Fleckenstein et al., 1971). Beta-agonist selectively increase the transmembrane Ca^{2+} inward current during cardiac excitation. Studies have suggested that the cardiac cell damage might result from reduction of ATP caused by excessive activation of calcium-dependent ATPases as well as the inhibition of ATP production in calcium-overload mitochondria. Calcium uptake may also result from cell membrane damage. Intracellular Ca^{2+} accumulation is associated with enhancement of Mg^{2+} efflux. Because of interference with Mg-dependent enzyme systems concerned with oxidative phosphorylation, the resultant diminution of energy production may then also contribute to the loss of K^+ and the further accumulation of Na^+ and Ca^{2+}.

Ca antagonists, such as verapamil, D600, or prenylamine, by inhibiting excessive Ca uptake, neutralize the cardiotoxic effects of large overdoses of beta-adrenergic catecholamines (Fleckenstein et al., 1975). However, only antioxidants are able to block a second phase of calcium uptake seen with large concentrations of isoproterenol (Ramos et al., 1984). Hypocalcemia produced by hemodialysis in dogs also had a protective effect against the cardiotoxic action of isoproterenol (Darsinos et al., 1984).

Damage to Cell Membranes by Free Fatty Acids

Catecholamines increase plasma free fatty acid (FFA) levels by stimulating lipolysis in depot fat (Gordon and Cherekes, 1956) and the heart takes up plasma FFA in proportion to their concentration (Scott et al., 1962). Thus, another mechanism by which catecholamines might produce myocardial necrosis, as suggested in rats, and particularly in view of the increased susceptibility of fat rats, is the deposition of Ca and FFA as soaps in the plasma membranes of myocardial cells causing permeability changes leading to cell injury (Mallov, 1983). Inhibition of lipolysis has been found to reduce the myocardial ischemia promoted by administration of norepinephrine or isoproterenol (Mjos et al., 1974). Feeding high-fat diets increases sensitivity to isoproterenol (Balazs et al., 1962), feeding aspirin or impairing prostaglandin synthesis with dietary manipulation is protective (Runyon and Shagestek, 1983).

Damage by Catecholamine-Derived Free Radicals

Isoproterenol and epinephrine undergo oxidation with formation of oxygen free radicals that can initiate peroxidation of lipids from circulating lipoprotein (Bors et al., 1978). These peroxidation products may be responsible for the early myocardial changes (Noronha-Dutra and Steen, 1982). The oxidized products of catecholamines, rather than the catecholamines themselves, produce necrotic damage (Yates and Shella, 1975) and are potent inhibitors of mitochondrial oxidative phosphorylation (Park et al., 1956). Damage by isoproterenol to cultured heart cells is obliterated by antioxidants. Free radicals may be acting by inhibiting membrane-bound Na-K ATPase or interacting with cellular sulfhydril groups (Ramos et al., 1983).

Resistance to Isoproterenol-Induced Necrosis

The heart has a curious ability to adapt to insults such as ischemic necrosis produced by isoproterenol. Ligation of the left coronary artery with subsequent necrosis (Dusek et al., 1970), a preconditioning dose of isoproterenol sufficient to produce necrosis and scarring (Balazs et al., 1972), or small daily doses of isoproterenol (Abri and Hecht, 1981) all produce resistance to isoproterenol-induced injury (Joseph et al., 1983). When 50 μg/kg isoproterenol is administered SC to 300-400-g Sprague-Dawley rats, nonlethal necrosis and scarring occur. When rechallenged 5 days later, the rat is still sensitive, but rechallenge beyond this produces much less necrosis, and this resistance persists for 19-20 weeks or more (Joseph et al., 1983). The locus of resistance is beyond the generation of cyclic AMP, since resistant hearts generate as much cyclic AMP as normal hearts (Joseph et al., 1984).

Relevance of Animal Toxicity Studies to Humans

Due to differences in species, body fat, age, previous drug exposure, and mode of administration, it is impossible to translate directly the myocardial toxicity data in experimental animals to the human case. Furthermore, the disparity between fatal dosage and the dosage producing microscopic lesions means that we may be missing damage that is occurring in humans because we do not have a sensitive end-point.

Balazs et al. (1982) and Blood (1982) state that administration of 0.1 mg/kg subcutaneous isoproterenol to the lean rat causes a pulse elevation of 20%. In the obese rat in the presence of theophylline, this dosage would probably produce some fatal arrhythmias (Table 4). Those who use isoproterenol by intravenous infusion in life-threatening pediatric asthma increase the dosage as necessary, using a cut-off point of 180-200 beats/min. If these children are equivalent to fat rats in their sensitivity to myocardial damage, this dosage should be producing some fatal arrhythmias and microscopic damage in the presence of theophylline. The only case report that suggests this was in an 18-year-old girl with theophylline levels of 25-30 μg/ml who received isoproterenol in dosages up to 0.32 μg/kg/min for over 24 hr, and who was improving and receiving a lower dosage when she developed more bronchospasm followed by cardiac arrest (Kurland et al., 1979). We now have more evidence. Elevated cardiac-specific serum creatine phosphokinase MB (CPK-MB) isoenzyme levels indicative of myocardial injury are found in 15 of 19 children treated with IV isoproterenol, methyl prednisolone, and aminophylline for life-threatening asthma (Maguire et al., 1986). In view of the species differences and the unique sensitivity of the fat rat, and the failure to experience this complication more often, we can draw some comfort. Yet the FDA investigators are correct in pointing out the potential danger of these dosages. Our personal preference is to avoid this therapy. If an intravenous isoproterenol infusion is considered necessary, theophylline should probably be discontinued. Otherwise, terbutaline or albuterol would seem to be a better choice.

III. Adverse Pulmonary Effects

A. Rebound Bronchospasm

In 1966, Keighley reported increased airway obstruction following inhalation of isoproterenol, after both liquid nebulization and delivery from metered dose inhalers. This was demonstrated in three asthmatics in whom refractory asthma had not remitted completely until discontinuation of all adrenergic aerosols (Keighley, 1966). Others confirmed that airway obstruction could follow inhalation of isoproterenol or epinephrine (Reisman, 1970; Trautlein et al., 1976; Stanescu and van de Woestijnem, 1972). Decreases in FEV_1 occurred within 15-60 min, sometimes after only a very brief improvement in FEV_1. This phenom-

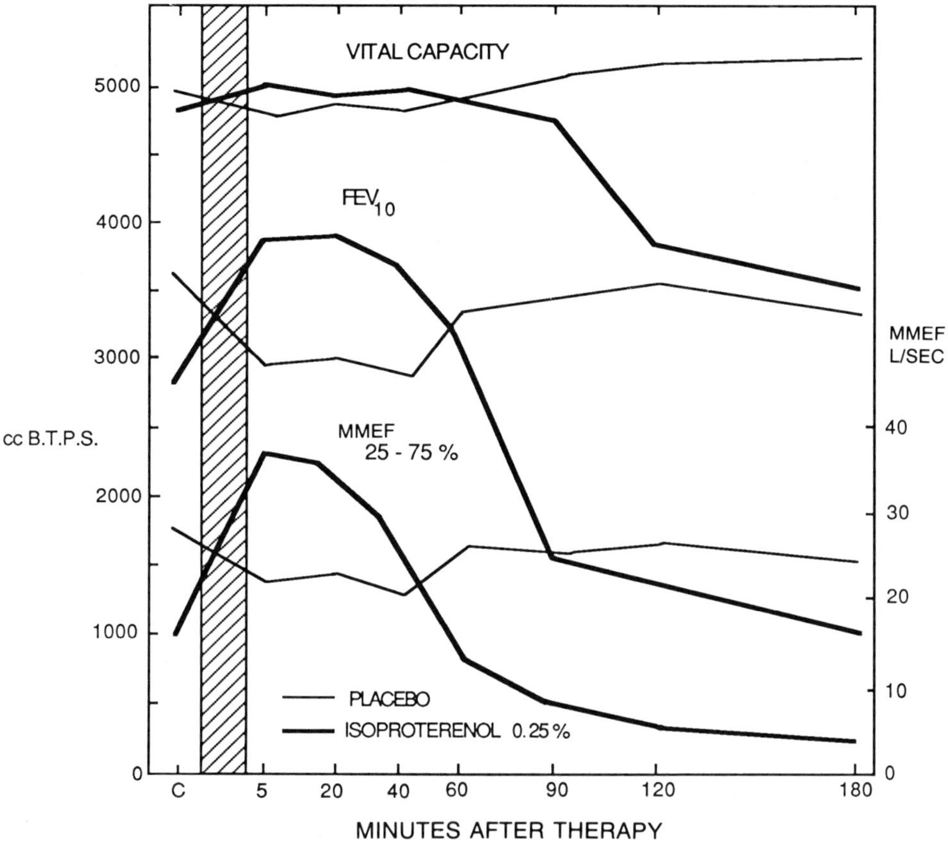

Figure 3 Rebound bronchoconstriction. While stable, the patient obtained transient improvement from 0.25% isoproterenol dissolved in water, delivered from a DeVillbiss 42 nebulizer over the period indicated by the shaded area. On another occasion, he inhaled 25% propylene glycol in water (placebo). He also reacted adversely to isoproterenol by metered dose inhaler (from Keighley, 1966).

enon has been termed rebound bronchoconstriction, as shown in Figure 3. Rebound has not been reported to follow inhalation of aerosolized metaproterenol, albuterol, terbutaline, fenoterol, or bitolterol mesylate.

Paterson and colleagues (1971) found that although doubling doses of intravenous isoproterenol caused bronchoconstriction in severe asthmatics who required continual drug therapy, discontinuation of the infusion was followed by severe airway obstruction in 4 of 15 patients studied. In two of these, the obstruction did not respond to intravenous albuterol, but was quickly reversed with aminophylline along with hydrocortisone.

Many studies of rebound bronchospasm have not controlled for the effects of withholding other bronchodilators for the duration of the study, and this could possibly lead to worsening in some cases. Clinical improvement has followed discontinuation of inhaled beta agonists in some patients who had previously been using them more frequently than recommended (Reisman, 1970; Caplin and Haynes, 1969). However, lack of bronchodilation, or bronchoconstriction, has followed inhalation of isoproterenol in patients who had received none in the previous year (Trautlein et al., 1976).

The mechanism of rebound bronchoconstriction could be the induction of acute and/or chronic tachyphylaxis or tolerance, even by the single administration, in highly susceptible subjects, with temporary failure of subsequent endogenous beta-adrenergic influences on bronchial tone, but this is speculative. Other possibilities are an effect of the weak alpha-adrenergic component in isoproterenol. Sulfite sensitivity to the solution seems to be ruled out, at least in those cases also responding to a metered dose inhaler.

B. Sulfite-Induced Bronchoconstriction

Sulfites used as antioxidants in bronchodilator solutions (racemic epinephrine, isoproterenol, isoetharine, and metaproterenol) can cause bronchoconstriction in some asthmatics within 10 min (Koepke et al., 1983). Sulfur dioxide concentrations generated by nebulization of isoproterenol solutions can vary from 2.6 to 6.0 ppm. Lower concentrations are produced by nebulization of isoetharine, metaproterenol, and racemic epinephrine solutions.

One manifestation of the increased airway reactivity typical of asthma is induction of bronchoconstriction by inhalation of sulfur dioxide in most asthmatics (Sheppard et al., 1980), but some are especially sensitive to the bronchoconstriction effect, possibly because of a deficiency of sulfite oxidase (Stevenson and Simon, 1984). As many as 8% of asthmatics may have some sensitivity to sulfite, but fewer have the extreme sensitivity characterized by sudden, severe airway obstruction after ingestion of food to which sulfites have been added (Simon et al., 1982).

Solutions of terbutaline sulfate and unit dose metaproterenol contain no sulfites, and metered dose inhalers have never contained sulfites.

C. Hypoxemia

Following inhalation of isoproterenol, about 50% of asthmatics will have a drop in arterial PO_2, ranging up to 15 mmHg. This drop reaches a maximum in 5 min, and resolves over the next 15 min (Ingram et al., 1970; Wagner et al., 1978) (Fig. 4). It also occurs with intravenous aminophylline (Tai and Read, 1967) but not with inhaled anticholinergics (Field, 1967). Studies of inhaled

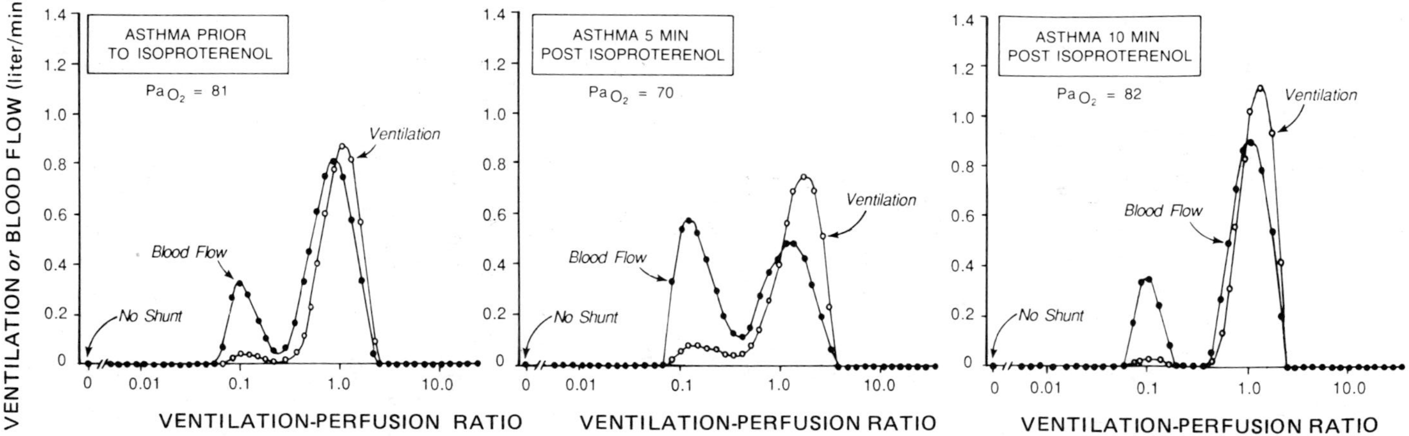

Figure 4 Sequence of $\dot{V}/\dot{Q}$ ratios at baseline, 5, and 10 min postinhalation of isoproterenol determined by the six-inert-gas technique. Note that at 5 min there is nearly twice the perfusion through the low $\dot{V}/\dot{Q}$ mode (adapted from Wagner et al., 1978).

$beta_2$ agonists such as salbutamol (Palmer et al., 1970), and fenoterol (Ashraf et al., 1978) and even intravenous salbutamol (Warrell et al., 1970) have shown small to no effects and the few mmHg drops in PO_2 recorded could as easily by due to experimental error. However, a recent study in acutely asthmatic children employing noninvasive oximetry recorded a fall in S_aO_2 of 5% in half the patients after liquid aerosols of salbutamol corresponding to significant drops in PO_2 (Tal et al., 1984). Therefore, a significant fall appears possible even with selective $beta_2$ agonists in a sufficient dosage. Routine pulmonary function tests are unpredictive of which patients will respond in this manner. In general, the largest drops occur in those patients with initial PO_2s higher on the oxyhemoglobin dissociation curve, and therefore of little consequence. However, during the hypoxemia of a severe attack, any further fall in PO_2 could be deleterious and is an added reason for supplemental oxygen.

The drop has been attributed to increased perfusion of poorly ventilated areas of the lung, in which vessels are constricted to some degree by hypoxemia and/or alveolar overinflation. Part of the increased perfusion may occur from the increase in cardiac output being preferentially distributed to these areas as they open up (Wagner et al., 1978). Since the smooth muscle of pulmonary vessels contains exclusively $beta_2$ receptors (Carstairs et al., 1985) relaxation of vasoconstriction should occur with both isoproterenol and $beta_2$-specific agents.

By dividing the lung into two compartments with Briscoe's nitrogen washout technique, it has been shown that these asthmatics responding to isoproterenol with a drop in PO_2 have a larger initial volume and greater ventilation-perfusion ratio of their poorly ventilated "slow space." After isoproterenol there is an increase in its perfusion and a decreased ventilation-perfusion ratio, just the opposite of those whose PO_2 remains fixed (Chick et al., 1973).

With the multiple inert gas technique, these changes have been studied more precisely (Wagner et al., 1978) (Fig. 4). In six mild asthmatics and one with severe obstruction, there was clearly a bimodal distribution of $\dot{V}/\dot{Q}$ ratios, with the minor mode involving ratios of 0.01:0.1 and containing 20% of the cardiac output but little ventilation. Following isoproterenol, perfusion to this mode doubled, resulting in an average PO_2 drop of 10 mmHg in the mild asthmatics, but no drop in the severely obstructed patient whose PO_2 stayed at 52 mmHg.

D. Pulmonary Edema

A variety of $beta_2$-adrenergic drugs are used orally or intravenously for tocolysis, such as in the attempt to forestall premature delivery by relaxing uterine smooth muscle. Unfortunately, some of these women develop pulmonary edema during the period within 16 hr before and 2 hr after delivery. This occurred in 5% of 120 deliveries in one series (Katz et al., 1981). Analysis of these cases and others reveals that this complication is more likely if saline rather than glucose solutions are used for the intravenous drugs, if glucocorticoids are used (to promote lung maturation), and if multiple fetuses are involved. All of these factors further overload and increase cardiac output, which is already increased. Furthermore, the $beta_2$-agonist action in blood vessels lowers peripheral resistance, increasing cardiac output and sometimes promoting further fluid administration to maintain pressure. Most of the patients in pulmonary edema develop ischemic changes on ECG, and some develop arrhythmias. In one series, patients developing pulmonary edema had a positive fluid balance three to five times greater than those without (Finley et al., 1984). Plasma drug levels are rather higher during tocolysis than chronic asthma therapy. Pulmonary edema has not been observed as a complication of long-term treatment in nonpregnant women.

IV. Metabolic Effects

The diversity of side effects from $beta_2$-adrenergic stimulants reflects the wide distribution of $beta_2$-receptors throughout tissues, including striated muscles, vascular smooth muscle, liver, and pancreas. Of the metabolic responses, the effects on potassium, carbohydrate, and lipid metabolism and plasma and urine cyclic AMP are the best documented. Upon initial beta-agonist administration there are increases in insulin and blood glucose concentrations and a decrease in plasma and urinary potassium (Bengtsson and Fagerstrom, 1982; Peters et al., 1981) and a rise in plasma and urine cyclic AMP and in plasma lactate (Ball et al., 1972). These effects disappear when examined after approximately 2 weeks of daily administration due to tolerance or reduced response of the effector organs (Bengtsson and Fagerstrom, 1982; Jenne et al., 1977b). Tolerance to the hypokalemic effects of oral albuterol has been shown to occur within 48-72 hr with chronic administration (Hartwell and Lambert, 1978).

A. Hypokalemia

A marked fall in serum potassium, averaging 0.82 ± 0.19 ng/ml, occurred within 30 min of the start of an epinephrine infusion, producing a 30-fold increase in plasma epinephrine levels to 1.74 ± 0.65 ng/ml (Brown et al., 1983a). It did not occur during an isoproterenol infusion. Likewise, a 0.25-mg subcutaneous injection of terbutaline caused a mean decrease of 0.6 mEq/liter in serum potassium as shown in Figure 5 (Kung et al., 1984). A constant salbutamol infusion resulted in greater and more prolonged potassium falls than an equivalent dose given intravenous over 1 min (Elegbeye et al., 1978). Normal subjects showed no change in serum potassium after 200 μg albuterol aerosol (Neville et al., 1977), but progressively greater hypokalemia has been reported to occur after 6, 9, and 12 200-μg puffs of fenoterol inhaled over 60 min (Haalboom et al., 1985).

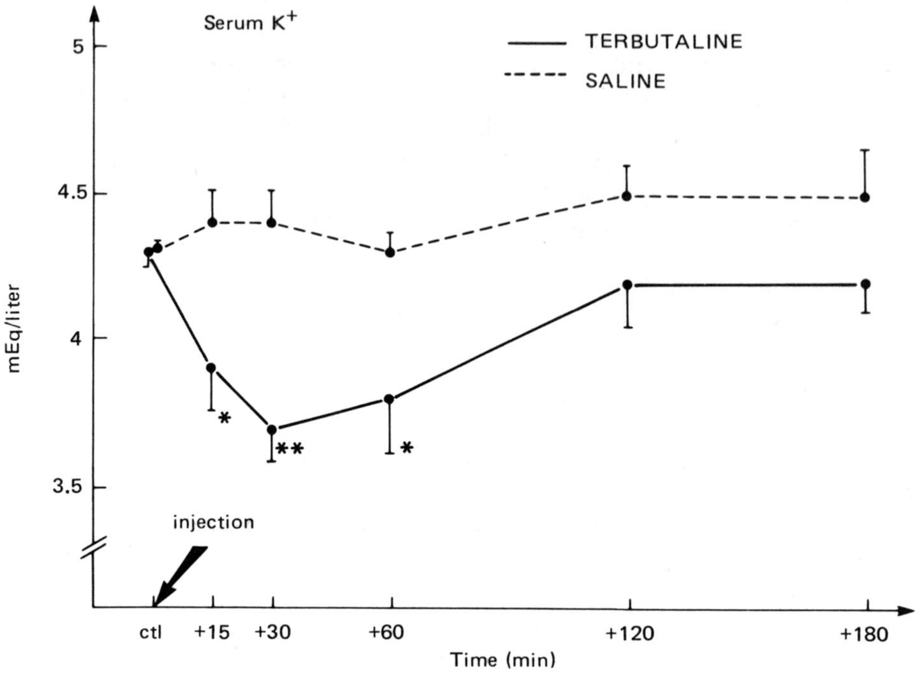

Figure 5 Serum potassium (K^+) in the control state (Ctl) and at various times after subcutaneous injection of 0.25 mg terbutaline sulfate (solid line) or saline (dotted line) in seven subjects. Values are mean ± SEM, and significance is indicated by *(P < 0.05) and **(P < 0.01) (from Kung et al., 1984).

Profound hypokalemia can occur at plasma epinephrine levels found during severe stress such as insulin-induced hypoglycemia and acute myocardial infarction (Cryer, 1980; Rolton et al., 1981). In the latter, hypokalemia is associated with an impaired prognosis (Dykner et al., 1975). It has been shown that plasma supplementation is beneficial to some patients prone to ventricular fibrillation (Harrington et al., 1982). The hypokalemia is due to a shift of potassium from extracellular to intracellular space, probably through stimulation of sodium-potassium ATP-ase in skeletal muscle (Brown et al., 1983a). In humans, this enzyme appears to be linked to beta$_2$-adrenoceptors (Struthers and Reid, 1984) and also this has been shown in cat soleus muscle (Clauson and Flatman, 1980). Timolol, a nonspecific beta-antagonist, blocks epinephrine-induced hypokalemia whereas atenolol, a beta$_1$-specific antagonist, does not (Struthers and Reid, 1984), but the beta$_2$-specific blocker, ICI 118551, still does (Brown et al., 1983).

B. Glycogenolysis

Glycogen breakdown in skeletal muscle can be precipitated by stimulation of $beta_2$ receptors (Stull and Mayer, 1971; Gross and Mayer, 1974; Thomas et al., 1977). With either terbutaline orsalbutamol, elevations in the glucose level of 5-6 nmol/liter can be achieved. In late pregnancy these agents produce hyperglycemia and hyperlactacidemia when used to forestall preterm labor (Smythe and Sakskini, 1981). The rise in glucose levels in such patients is more marked in diabetic patients than nondiabetics. Hyperglycemic ketoacidosis has been reported in previously well-controlled diabetic women following treatment for preterm labor with intravenous salbutamol (Thomas et al., 1977). It would therefore be wise to use these agents cautiously in diabetics in labor.

C. Hyperinsulinemia

In normal individuals and asthmatic or pregnant women, there is a significant and sustained rise in plasma levels of insulin following isoproterenol or salbutamol by various routes (intravenous, subcutaneous, aerosol) as a result of a direct effect on the beta cells of the pancreas (William-Olsson et al., 1978; Leitch et al., 1976; Phillips et al., 1980; Neville et al., 1977). By contrast, epinephrine levels over 400 pg/ml suppress insulin levels due to the alpha-adrenergic stimulation (Clutter et al., 1980).

D. Lipid Derangements

Beta-adrenergic stimulants mobilize free fatty acids from adipose tissue through $beta_1$-receptors. For example, a 4-mg dose of salbutamol causes a significant rise in plasma free fatty acid after 60 min in healthy individuals and a similar rise in glycerol in pregnant women after 90 min (Lunell et al., 1978), while 5 mg terbutaline also causes a small elevation of free fatty acids (Jenne et al., 1977a). These changes are exaggerated in diabetes, as shown with intravenous salbutamol (Gündogdu et al., 1979). On a regimen of 2.5 mg terbutaline four times daily for a 2-week period, there was a significant elevation of HDL cholesterol concentration, which returned to near baseline values 1 week after drug cessation. Total cholesterol, LDL cholesterol, and triglyceride levels did not change significantly (Hooper et al., 1981). The glucose response tends to be affected more readily than the glycerol and free fatty acid responses (Nelson et al., 1976).

The unwanted metabolic responses to therapeutic doses of $beta_2$-stimulants are wide ranging but in the majority of cases do not present a significant risk to the patient and some of them diminish with prolonged treatment (Jenne et al., 1977b).

V. Tremor

Catecholamines increase the amplitude of physiological tremor of the outstretched fingers by stimulating peripheral beta$_2$-adrenergic receptors in skeletal muscle (Marsden et al., 1967). Although human striated muscles contain both fast- and slow-contracting motor units in varying proportions, only the slow-contracting fibers are thought to be sensitive to circulating catecholamines, even at stress levels (Bowman and Nott, 1979). Therefore, the effects of epinephrine on fast fibers (increased twitch tension, increased fusion) are not relevant, whereas the effects on slow fibers (decreased twitch tension, decrease in subtetanic fusion) are (Bowman and Nott, 1979). Beta-adrenergic stimulation decreases the time that the fiber remains contracted because it increases relaxation time. Figure 6 shows the effect in decreasing twitch tension and fusion while increasing the amplitude of tremor of the soleus muscle of the cat when stimulated at 10 Hz (Bowman and Zaimis, 1958). The agonist specificities of the skeletal and bronchial smooth muscle beta$_2$-adrenergic receptors are thus far indistinguishable (Olsson et al., 1979).

Tremor is the limiting side effect when one is administering oral beta$_2$-adrenergic drugs. Although the tremorigenic effect appears to lessen with time, some patients cannot tolerate these agents at all, even at low dosages. There is a considerable range of tremor responses between patients. Figure 7 shows that

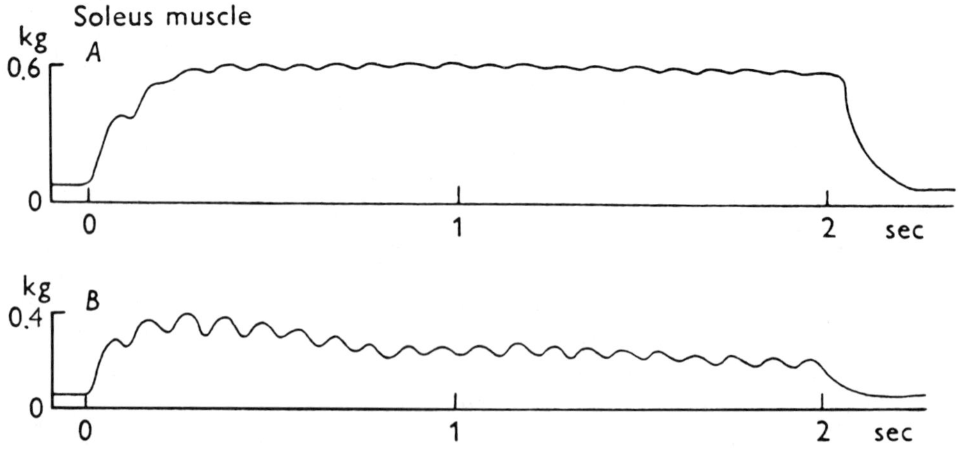

Figure 6 Electrically recorded tetani of the cat soleus muscle in situ, elicited indirectly with supramaximal shocks at a frequency of 10 sec (a). Before epinephrine. (b) 140 sec after intravenous administration of 12 μg epinephrine. Note that the maximum force is reduced and the individual twitches accentuated (from Bowman and Zaimis, 1958).

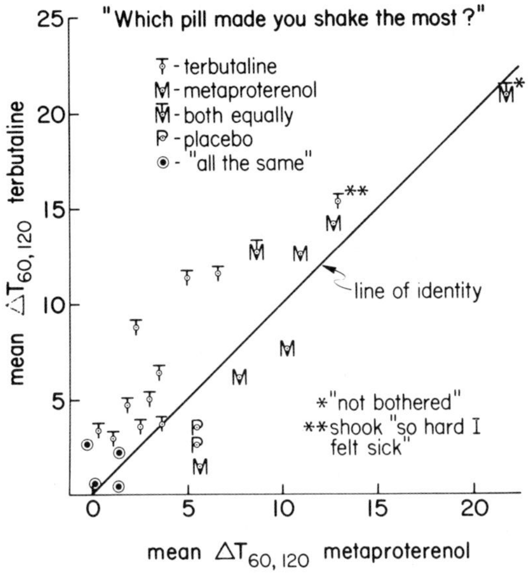

Figure 7 Relationship between tremor responses to 5 mg terbutaline ($T_{60,120}$), and 20 mg metaproterenol and placebo with each subject's selection of the most active preparation in tremor production. Note that the ability to discriminate correctly is still present at relatively low tremor intensities. $T_{60,120}$ is the mean tremor intensity measured by the Grass accelerometer attached to the finger averaged at 60 and 120 min (from Jenne et al., 1982).

the range of responses to the first dose of 5 mg terbutaline and 20 mg metaproterenol in 24 COPD patients varied widely (Jenne et al., 1982). However, the drug response (T_{max}) was significantly correlated with baseline tremor, T_B. The difference in response between patients is therefore a function of the individual sensitivity of the muscle itself and not of drug metabolism differences. Yet patients with even small tremor responses were still able to sense correctly which tablet produced the greatest response, as shown in Figure 7. Thus, it appears that subjective sensitivity is a function of the relative increase in tremor over baseline rather than absolute tremor per se.

In general, tremor becomes uncomfortable when the baseline amplitude approximately doubles (Watson and Richens, 1974) and this condition is just met after 20 mg metaproterenol or 5 mg terbutaline orally as shown in Figure 8. Yet individual patients vary considerably in their discomfort, some being very disturbed while others are oblivious to considerable tremor unless it interferes with their activities (Fig. 7).

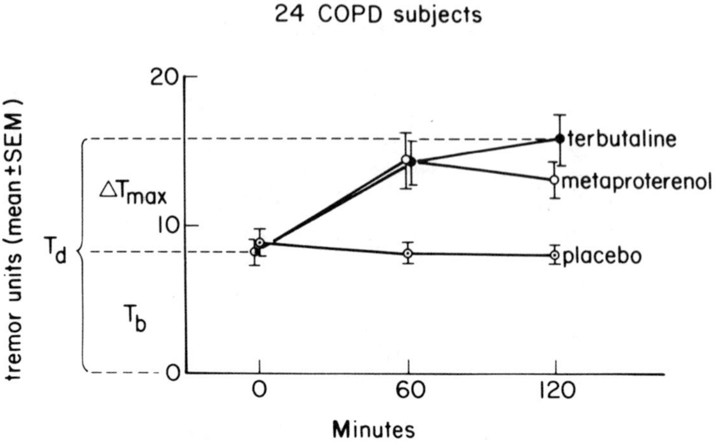

Figure 8 Mean tremor responses to 5 mg terbutaline, 20 mg metaproterenol, and placebo given fasting at 60 and 120 min to 24 COPD subjects. Note that metaproterenol peaks at 60 min, and that the drug-induced tremor (ΔT_{max}) is barely twice the basal tremor (from Jenne et al., 1982).

On a divided dose regimen of either salbutamol or terbutaline, baseline tremor rises over the first 2-3 days, finally plateauing as equilibrium is established between drug intake and elimination (Van den Berg, 1982; Jenne et al., 1986). Thus, patients have continuous tremor that is increased slightly with each tablet. The question of tachyphylaxis, or tolerance, in this situation is complicated. One must consider both the elevated baseline tremor at steady state, and the response to each individual tablet. Tremor production lessens with time, as demonstrated with isoproterenol dose-response curves at various times after commencing oral terbutaline (Thiringer and Svedmyr, 1974). Yet some of the apparent tolerance on a divided dose schedule must be attributed to the fact that individual peak-trough differences in drug levels are smaller at steady state than for the initial dose, purely for pharmacokinetic considerations.

VI. CNS

Epinephrine injections may cause transient fear, anxiety, headache, weakness, and dizziness and patients may require reassurance. Without any ring additions, oral ephedrine easily crosses the blood brain barrier and can produce excitation, nervousness, and insomnia. These side effects are countered with small dosages of barbiturates in combined bronchodilator preparations. Hypertension may develop and urinary retention may occur in patients with prostatic hypertrophy.

Selective $beta_2$-agonists can cause nervousness, weakness, and drowsiness, and the large dosages given for tocolysis may, in addition, produce nausea, vomiting, and headache. Radioautography of terbutaline distribution in the rat shows no uptake by brain after 4 hr, although some may eventually occur (Ryerfeldt and Ramsay, 1984). Assays of these drugs in cerebrospinal fluid are not yet available.

VII. Oncogenesis and Teratogenesis

Rats fed $beta_2$-agonists for 2 years develop benign ovarian or mesovarian leiomyomas in an incidence up to 25% in some strains. No one agent is implicated among this group of drugs. Differences between them are attributable to differences in absorption, potency, and dosage. When albuterol or terbutaline intake was adjusted to provide equal plasma levels, around 20 ng/ml, an equal incidence of tumors was observed (Jack et al., 1983).

This side effect is particularly disturbing because these blood levels are not too dissimilar from plasma levels found with chronic oral dosing in human asthma. But there are species differences since the tumors are not found in mice or hamsters. In women, ovarian leiomyoma is a rare tumor, and no increase in incidence has been observed in long-standing asthmatics.

An increased incidence of pituitary enlargement due to chromophobe adenoma and intermediate cell hyperplasia occurs in male rats (but not female) taking oral albuterol in dosages ranging from 2 to 10 mg/kg per day, fed for 24 months (Schering Corp, data from files). Control rats also develop these abnormalities, but the incidence goes up with the dosage of albuterol. These growths show marked cellular atypism, but lack invasive or metastatic character and so are considered benign.

The *Physician's Desk Reference* states that albuterol is tetratogenic in mice (cleft palate) at 14 times the human oral dose, and metaproterenol at 62 times but not 31 times. In pregnant women, there are no controlled studies. Until more is known, the use of systemic $beta_2$-adrenergic bronchodilators in pregnant women is inadvisable. Ephedrine and theophylline are considered safe, however (Greenberg and Patterson, 1985).

VIII. Summary and Conclusions

Although beta-adrenergic agonists are among the most effective drugs for the treatment of asthma they can have a number of adverse effects, including induction of cardiac arrhythmias and tachycardia. The chronotropic effect is enhanced by hypoxemia and hypercapnea. Experimental evidence suggests the possibility of an adverse interaction on the myocardium when combined with theophylline, at least at large dosages and in the initial stages of treatment. There are known species variation in susceptibility to this damage, and there is no evidence that this occurs in humans using clinical dosages. Effects on blood pressure are negligible.

Rebound bronchoconstriction probably occurs only in rare patients and clinically relevant sensitivity to sulfites probably is relatively rare. Slight subsensitivity occurs in most asthmatics treated for more than a few days with a beta-agonist and this may possibly contribute to status asthmaticus with excessive intake in some patients. The decrease in arterial PO_2 that may follow treatment with a beta-agonist is usually slight, is less frequent with selective $beta_2$-agonists than with isoproterenol, and can be prevented by administration of supplemental oxygen.

Metabolic effects are usually of little clinical relevance except for hypokalemia, which may enhance adverse cardiac effects. Adverse effects of recommended dosages on the central nervous system are usually of little consequence, but in occasional patients may be sufficiently annoying to require a trial with another drug such as theophylline or cromolyn. Tremor due to action on skeletal muscle is usually sufficiently mild to constitute only a minor annoyance except for occupations and avocations that require a steady hand.

Administration of recommended dosages by inhalation rather than by other routes minimizes adverse effects. Administration of supplemental oxygen minimizes adverse cardiac effects as well as the decrease in PO_2 that may follow treatment during severe airway obstruction. Clinicians who prescribe these drugs must be aware of possible adverse effects; continual cardiac monitoring may be necessary when beta-agonists are required in large dosages, especially when intravenous theophylline is also required in large dosages.

Use of bronchodilator solutions for nebulization should be limited to those that contain no sulfites. The possibility of a relationship of the increased frequency of death from asthma to adverse effects of beta-agonists remains open, but any such association with their use is probably better explained by misplaced reliance on a drug that had become ineffective in reversing airway obstruction, thereby delaying medical attention and particularly the use of corticosteroids. However, the possibility of fatal, adverse cardiac effects in a few patients cannot be excluded. Medical supervision of patients using these drugs is necessary to ensure restriction to appropriate indications and use of recommended doses provide necessary instruction in optimal methods of delivery when the inhalational route is employed, advise the patient of possible adverse effects, and facilitate access to medical care in emergencies (Sly et al., 1985).

References

Abri, O., and Hecht, A. (1981). The influence of long-term application of isoproterenol on the results of temporary ischemia of the rat heart muscle. *Exp. Pathol. 20*: 146-152.

Ashraf, M., Sharp, J., Kehoe, T., and Cugell, D. W. (1978). A comparison of the effects of Th 1165a (fenoterenol) and isoproterenol on spirometry and arterial blood gases. *Chest* 73S, 981.

Balazs, T., and Bloom, S. (1982). Cardiotoxicity of adrenergic bronchodilator and vasodilating antihypertensive drugs. In *Cardiovascular Toxicology*. Edited by E. W. Van Stee. New York, Raven Press, pp. 199-219.

Balazs, T., Murphy, J. B., and Grice, H. C. (1962). The influence of environmental changes on the cardiovascular toxicity of isoproterenol. *J. Pharm. Pharmacol. 14*: 750-755.

Balazs, T., Otake, S., and Noble, J. F. (1972). The development of resistance to the ischemic cardiopathic effect of isoproterenol. *Toxicol. Appl. Pharmacol. 21*: 200-213.

Ball, J. A., Kaminsky, N. I., and Hardman, J. G. (1972). Effects of catecholamines and adrenergic-blocking agents on plasma and urinary cyclic nucleotides in man. *J. Clin. Invest. 51*: 2124-2129.

Banner, A. S., Sunderrajan, E. V., Agarwal, M. K., and Addington, W. W. (1979). Arrhythmogenic effects of orally administered bronchodilators. *Arch. Intern. Med. 139*: 434-437.

Bass, M. J. (1970). Sudden sniffing death. *JAMA 212*: 2075-1079.

Bengtsson, B., and Fagerstrom, P. O. (1982). Extrapulmonary effects of terbutaline during prolonged administration. *Clin. Pharmacol. Ther. 31*: 726-732.

Berry, D. G., and Miller, J. W. (1974). The effects of sympathomimetic agents in ADP aggregation of rat platelets in vitro. *Eur. J. Pharmacol. 28*: 17.

Bloom, S., and Davis, D. L. (1972). Calcium as mediator of isoproterenol-induced myocardial necrosis. *Am. J. Pathol. 69*: 459-470.

Bors, W., Mickel, C., Saran, M., and Lengfelder, E. (1978). The involvement of oxygen radicals during autooxidation of adrenalin. *Biochem. Biophys. Acta 548*: 162-172.

Bowman, W. C., and Nott (1964). Actions of sympathomimetic amines and their antagonists on skeletal muscle. *Pharmacol. Rev. 21*: 27-61.

Bowman, W. C., and Zaimis, E. (1958). The effects of adrenaline, noradrenaline and isoprenaline on skeletal muscle contractions in the cat. *J. Physiol. 144*: 92-107.

Brown, M. J., Brown, D. C., and Murphy, M. B. (1983a). Hypokalemia from $beta_2$-receptor stimulation by circulatory epinephrine. *N. Engl. J. Med. 308*: 1414-1419.

Brown, J. E., McLeod, A. A., and Shand, D. G. (1983b). Evidence for cardiac β_2-adrenoceptors in man. *Clin. Pharmacol. Ther. 33*: 424-428.

Brown-Lukacsko, A., and Lukacsko, P. (1982). $Beta_2$-mediated hypotension and myocardial injury. *Can. J. Physiol. Pharmacol. 60*: 1144-1148.

Buch, J., and Bundgaard, A. (1985). Cardiovascular effects of intramuscular or inhaled terbutaline in asthmatics. *Acta Pharmacol. Toxicol. 54*: 183-188.

Campbell, A. H. (1976). Mortality from asthma and bronchodilator aerosols. *Med. J. Aust. 1*: 386-391.

Caplin, I., and Haynes, J. T. (1969). Complications of aerosol therapy in asthma. *Ann. Allergy 27*: 65-69.

Carstairs, J. R., Nimmo, A. J., and Barnes, P. J. (1985). Autoradiographic visualization of beta-adrenergic subtypes in human lung. *Am. Rev. Respir. Dis. 132*: 541-547.

Chang, B., Sly, R. M., Eby, D., and Middleton, H. B. (1985). Delivery of albuterol aerosol by Inhal-Aid to young children. *J. Allergy Clin. Immunol. 75*: 159.

Chapman, K. R., Smith, D. L., Rebuck, A. S., and Leenan, F. H. H. (1974). Hemodynamic effects of an inhaled $beta_2$ agonist. *Clin. Pharmacol. Ther. 35*: 762-767.

Chappel, A. G. (1984). Painless myocardial infarction in asthma. *Br. J. Dis. Chest. 78*: 174-179.

Chappel, C. I., Rona, G., Balazs, T., and Gaudry, R. (1959). Comparison of cardiotoxic actions of certain sympathomimetic amines. *Can. J. Biochem. Physiol. 37*: 35-42.

Chick, T. W., Nicholson, D. P., and Johnson, R. L. Jr. (1973). Effects of isoproterenol on distribution of ventilation and perfusion in asthma. *Am. Rev. Respir. Dis. 107*: 869-873.

Choo-Kang, Y. F. J., Simpson, W. T., and Grant, I. W. B. (1969). Controlled comparison of the bronchodilator effects of three β-adrenergic stimulant drugs administered by inhalation to patients with asthma. *Br. Med. J. 2*: 287-289,

Clark, D. G., and Tinston, D. J. (1972). Cardiac effects of isoproterenol, hypoxia, hypercapnea and fluorocarbon propellants and their use in asthma inhalers. *Ann. Allergy 30*: 536-541.

Clauson, T., and Flatman, J. A. (1980). $Beta_2$ adrenoceptors mediate the stimulating effect of adrenaline on active electrogenic NA-K transport in rat soleus muscle. *Br. J. Pharmacol. 68*: 749-755.

Clutter, W., Bier, D., Shah, S., and Cryer, P. (1980). Epinephrine plasma metabolic clearance rates and physiological thresholds for metabolic and hemodynamic actions in man. *J. Clin. Invest. 66*: 94-101.

Collier, J. G., Dobbs, R. J., and Williams, I. S. (1980). Salbutamol aerosol causes a tachycardia due to the inhaled rather than the swallowed fraction. *Br. J. Clin. Pharmacol. 9*: 273-274.

Colucci, W. S., Alexander, R. W., Williams, G. H., Rude, R. E., Holman, B. L.,

Koonstarns, M. A., Wynne, J., Mudge, G. H., Jr., and Braunwald, E. (1981). Decreased lymphocyte beta adrenergic receptor density in patients with heart failure and tolerance to the beta-agonist pirbuterol. *N. Engl. J. med. 305*: 185-190.

Cryer, P. E. (1980). Physiology and pathology of the human sympathoadrenal neuroendocrine system. *N. Engl. J. Med. 303*: 436-444.

Csapo, Z., Dusek, J., and Rona, G. (1972). Early alterations of the cardial muscle cell in isoproterenol-induced necrosis. *Arch. Pathol. 93*: 356-365.

Cullins, J. M., McDevitt, D. G., Shanks, R. G., and Swanton, J. G. (1969). The cardiotoxicity of isoprenaline during hypoxia. *Br. J. Pharmacol. 36*: 35-45.

Darsinos, J. T., Karli, J. N., Stathaki, S. N., Ziroyannis, P. N., Pistevas, A. C., Levis, G. M., and Moulopoulos, S. D. (1984). Effect of hypocalcemia on isoproterenol induced cardiotoxicity in dogs. *Angiology 35*: 152-162.

Davis, M. J. (1977). The pathology of myocardial ischemia. *J. Clin. Pathol. 30*: (Suppl 11): 45-52.

Dollery, C. T., Williams, F. M., Draffan, G. H., Wise, G., Sahyoun, H., Paterson, J. W., and Walker, S. R. (1974). Arterial blood levels of fluorocarbons in asthmatic patients following use of pressurized aerosols. *Clin. Pharmacol. Ther. 15*: 59-66.

Dusek, J., Rona, G., and Kahn, D. S. (1970). Myocardial resistances. A study of its development against toxic doses of isoproterenol. *Arch. Pathol. 89*: 79-83.

Dyckner, T., Helmers, C., Lundman, T., and Webster, P. O. (1975). Initial serum potassium level in relation to early complications and prognosis in patients with acute myocardial infarction. *Acta Med. Scand. 197*: 207-210.

Elegbeye, O. O., Williams, K. O., and Femi-Pearse, D. (1978). Comparison of the metabolic effects of salbutamol administered in a one minute bolus and a continuous infusion in patients with bronchial asthma. *Israel J. Med. Sci. 14*: 455-458.

Field, G. B. (1967). The effects of posture, oxygen, isoproterenol and atropine on ventilation-perfusion relationships in the lung. *Clin. Sci. 32*: 279-288.

Finch, J. S. (1981). Cardiovascular toxicity: Clinical evaluation of albuterol, isoproterenol and placebo in rising dose tolerance trial. *Ann. Allergy 47*: 402-404.

Finley, J., Katz, M., Rojas-Perez, M., Roberts, J. M., Creasy, R. K., and Schiller, H. B. (1984). Cardiovascular consequences of beta-agonist tocolysis: An echocardiographic study. *Obstet. Gynecol. 64*: 787.

Fleckenstein, A. (1971). Specific inhibitors and promoters of calcium action in the excitation-contraction coupling of heart muscle and their role in the prevention of the production of myocardial lesions. In *Calcium and the Heart.* Edited by P. Harris and L. H. Poie. London, Academic Press, p. 135.

Fleckenstein, A., Janke, J., and Doring, H. J. (1975). Calcium overload as the

determinant factor in the production of catacholamine-induced myocardial lesions. *Rec. Adv. Study Cardiac Struct. Metab. 6*: 21-32.
Gandevia, B. (1973). Pressurized sympathomimetic aerosols and their lack of relationship to asthma mortality in Australia. *Med. J. Austr. 1*: 273-277.
Gibson, D. G., and Coltart, D. J. (1971). Haemodynamic effects of intravenous salbutamol in patients with mitral valve disease: Comparison with isoprenaline and atropine. *Postgrad. Med. J. 40*.
Gordon, R. S., Jr., and Cherkes, A. (1956). Unisterified fatty acid in human blood plasma. *J. Clin. Invest. 35*: 206-212.
Grant, I. W. B. (1981). Has the change to beta-agonist combined with theophylline increased cases of fatal asthma? *Lancet* (letter) *2*: 36-37.
Greenberg, P. A., and Patterson, R. (1985). Management of asthma during pregnancy. *N. Engl. J. Med. 312*: 897-902.
Gross, S. R., and Mayer, S. E. (1974). Regulation of phosphorylase B to A conversion in muscle. *Life Sci. 14*: 401-414.
Guidero, G., Barletta, M. A., and Lehr, D. (1974). Extraordinary potentiation of isoproterenol cardiotoxicity by corticosteroid pretreatment. *Cardiovasc. Res. 8*: 775-786.
Gündogdu, A. S., Brown, D. M., Juul, S., Sachs, L., and Sönksen, P. H. (1979). Comparison of hormonal and metabolic effects on salbutamol infusion in normal subjects and insulin-requiring diabetics. *Lancet 2*: 1317-1320.
Haalboom, J. R. E., Deenstra, M., and Struyvenberg, A. (1985). Hypokalemia induced by inhalation of fenoterol. *Lancet 1*: 1125-1127.
Haft, J. I., Kranz, P. D., Albert, F. J., and Faui, K. (1972). Intravascular platelet aggregation in the heart induced by norepinephrine. *Circulation 46*: 698-708.
Harrington, J. T., Isner, J. M., and Kassirer, J. P. (1982). Our national obsession with potassium. *Am. J. Med. 73*: 155-159.
Hastwell, G., and Lembert, B. E. (1978). The effect or oral salbutamol on serum potassium and blood sugar. *Br. J. Obstet. Gynecol. 85*: 767-769.
Heitz, A., Schwartz, J., and Velly, J. (1983). B-adrenoceptors of the human myocardium: Determination of β_1 and β_2 subtypes of radioligand binding. *Br. J. Pharmacol. 80*: 711-717.
Higbee, M. D., Kumar, M., and Galant, S. P. (1982). Stimulation of endogenous catecholamine release by theophylline: A proposed additional mechanism of action for theophylline effects. *J. Allergy Clin. Immunol. 70*: 377-382.
Hooper, P. L., Woo, W., Visconti, L., and Pathak, D. E. (1981). Terbutaline raises higher density lipoprotein-cholesterol levels. *N. Engl. J. Med. 305*: 1455-1457.
Ind, P. W., Causon, R. C., Brown, M. J., and Barnes, P. J. (1985). Circulating catecholamines in acute asthma. *Br. Med. J. 290*: 267-269.
Ingram, R. H., Jr., Krumpe, P. E., Doffell, G. M., et al. (1970). Ventilation per-

fusion relationships after aerosolized isoproterenol in asthma. *Am. Rev. Respir. Dis. 101*: 364-370.

Inman, W. H. W., and Adelstein, A. M. (1969). Rise and fall of asthma mortality in England and Wales in relation to use of pressurized aerosols. *Lancet 2*: 279-285.

Jack, D. (1971). Sniffing syndrome. *Br. Med. J. 2*: 708-709.

Jack, D., Poynter, D., Spurling, N. W., and Spurling (1983). Beta-adrenoceptor stimulants and mesovarian leiomyomas in the rat. *Toxicology 27*: 315-320.

Jackson, R. T., Beaglehole, R., Rea, H. H., and Sutherland, D. C. (1982). Mortality from asthma: A new epidemic in New Zealand. *Br. Med. J. 285*: 771-774.

Jenne, J. W., Chick, T. W., Strickland, R. D., and Wall, F. J. (1977a). A comparison of beta adrenergic function in asthma and chronic bronchitis. *J. Allergy Clin. Immunol. 60*: 346-356.

Jenne, J. W., Chick, T., Strickland, R. D., and Wall, F. J. (1977b). Subsensitivity of beta responses during therapy with long acting beta-2 preparation. *J. Allergy Clin. Immunol. 59*: 383-390.

Jenne, J. W., Ridley, D. J., Marucci, R. A., Druz, W. J., and Rook, J. C. (1982). Objective and subjective tremor responses to oral $beta_2$ agents on first exposure. *Am. Rev. Respir. Dis. 126*: 607-610.

Jenne, J. W., Valcarenghi, G., Druz, W. S., Starkey, P. W., Yu, C., and Shaughnessy, T. K. (1985). Comparison of tremor responses to oral abuterol and terbutaline. *Am. Rev. Respir. Dis. 134*: 708-713.

Joad, J., Ahrens, R., Lindgren, S., and Weinberger, M. (1985). Physiological and psychological variables during maintenance therapy with inhaled albuterol and theophylline used separately and in combination. *J. Allergy Clin. Immunol. 75*: 113.

Joseph, X., Whitehurst, V. E., Bloom, S., and Balazs, T. (1981). Enhancement of cardiotoxic effects of beta-adrenergic bronchodilators by aminophylline in experimental animals. *Fund. Appl. Toxicol. 1*: 443.447.

Joseph, X., Bloom, S., Pledger, G., and Balazs, T. (1983). Determinants of resistance to the cardiotoxicity of isoproterenol in rats. *Toxicol. Appl. Pharmacol. 69*: 199-205.

Joseph, X., Jordan, A. W., and Balazs, T. (1984). Ventricular fibrillation threshold and myocardial cyclic AMP production in rats sensitive or resistance to isoproterenol. *Res. Commun. Chem. Pathol. Pharmacol. 44*: 239-249.

Joseph, G. W., Kennedy, H. L., MacKenzie, E. J., and Gibson, G. (1980). Cardiac dysrhythmias during the treatment of acute asthma. *Chest 78*: 429-435.

Kahn, D. S., Rona, G., and Chappel, C. I. (1969). Isoproterenol induced cardiac necrosis. *Ann. N.Y. Acad. Sci. 156*: 285-293.

Katz, M., Robertson, P. A., and Creasy, R. K. (1981). Cardiovascular complications associated with terbutaline treatment for preterm labor. *Am. J. Obstet. Gynecol. 139*: 605.

Keating, G., Mitchell, E. A., Jackson, R., Beaglehole, R., and Rea, H. (1984). Trends in sales of drugs for asthma in New Zealand, Australia, and the United Kingdom, 1975-81. *Br. Med. J. 289*: 348-351.

Keighley, J. F. (1966). Iatrogenic asthma associated with adrenergic aerosols. *Ann. Intern. Med. 65*: 985-995.

Kemp, J. P., Chervinsky, P., Orgel, H. A., Meltzer, E. O., Noyes, J. H. M., and Mingto, T. S. (1984). Concomitant bitolterol mesylate aerosol and theophylline for asthma therapy, with 24 hr electrocardiographic monitoring. *J. Allergy Clin. Immunol. 73*: 32-43.

Koepke, J. W., Selner, J. C., and Dunhill, A. L. (1983). Presence of sulfur dioxide in commonly used bronchodilator solutions. *J. Allergy Clin. Immunol. 72*: 504-508.

Kravitz, S., Saccar, C., Sacks, E., Mansmann, H., Jr., McGready, S., and Gentlesk, M. (1982). Electrocardiographic abnormalities in asthmatic children on oral beta-2 agonist therapy. *Ann. Allergy 48*: 261.

Kung, M., White, J. R., and Burki, N. K. (1984). The effect of subcutaneously administered terbutaline on serum potassium in asymptomatic adult asthmatics. *Am. Rev. Respir. Dis. 129*: 329-332.

Kurland, G., Williams, J., and Lewiston, N. W. (1979). Fatal myocardial toxicity during continuous infusion intravenous isoproterenol therapy of asthma. *J. Allergy Clin. Immunol. 63*: 407-411.

Leitch, A. G., Clancy, L. J., Costello, J. F., and Flenley, D. C. (1976). Effect of intravenous infusion of salbutamol on ventilatory response to carbon dioxide and hypoxia on heart rate and plasma potassium in normal men. *Br. Med. J. 1*: 365-367.

Levine, J. H., Michael, J. R., and Guarnieri, T. (1985). Multifocal atrial tachycardia: A toxic effect of theophylline. *Lancet 1*: 12-14.

Light, R. W., Taylor, R. W., and George, R. B. (1979). Albuterol and isoproterenol in bronchial asthma. *Arch. Intern. Med. 139*: 639-643.

Lunell, N. O., Wager, J., Fredholm, B. B., and Persson, B. (1978). Metabolic effects of oral salbutamol in late pregnancy. *Eur. J. Clin. Pharmacol. 14*: 95-99.

Magnusson, G., and Hansson, E. (1973). Myocardial necrosis in the rat: A comparison between isoprenaline, orciprenaline, salbutamol and terbutaline. *Cardiology 58*: 174-180.

Maguire, J. F., Geha, R. S., and Umetsu, D. J. (1986). Myocardial specific creatinine phosphokinase isoenzyme elevation in children with asthma treated with intravenous isoproterenol. *J. Allergy Clin. Immunol. 78*: 631-636.

Mahajan, V. K., Tomashefski, J. F., and Huber, G. L. (1977). Comparative study of acute effects of albuterol and isoproterenol sulfate aerosols in bronchial asthma. *Ann. Allergy 39*: 319-324.

Mallov, S. (1983). Role of calcium and free fatty acids in epinephrine-induced myocardial necrosis. *Toxicol. Appl. Pharmacol. 71*: 280-287.

Marsden, C. D., Foley, T. H., Own, D. A. L., and McAllister, R. G. (1967). Peripheral beta-adrenergic receptors concerned with tremor. *Clin. Sci. 33*: 53-65.

Matson, J. R., Loughlin, G. M., and Strunk, R. C. (1978). Myocardial ischemia complicating the use of isoproterenol in asthmatic children. *J. Pediatr. 92*: 776-778.

McDevitt, D. G., Shanks, R. C., and Swanton, J. C. (1974). Further observations on the cardiotoxicity of isoprenaline during hypoxia. *Br. J. Pharmacol. 50*: 325-344.

Mjøs, D. D., Kjekshaw, J. K., and Lekven, J. (1974). Importance of free fatty acids as a determinant of myocardial oxygen consumption and myocardial injury during norepinephrine infusion in dogs. *J. Clin. Invest. 53*: 1290-1299.

Moir, T. W., and DeBra, I. (1967). Effects of left ventricular hypotension, ischemia and vasoactive drugs on the distribution of coronary flow. *Circ. Res. 21*: 65-74.

Moschos, C. B., Haider, B., Khan, Y., Lyons, M. M., and Regan, T. J. (1978). Relation of platelets to catecholamines induced myocardial injury. *Cardiovasc. Res. 12*: 243-246.

Naylor, W. G., and McInnes, I. (1972). Salbutamol and orciprenaline induced changes in myocardial function. *Cardiovasc. Res. 6*: 725-733.

Nelson, H. S., Raine, D., Branch, B., and Kalisker, A. (1976). Adrenergic subsensitivity induced by chronic administration of terbutaline. *J. Allergy Clin. Immunol. 57*: 259 (abstract).

Neville, A., Palmer, J. B. D., Gaddie, J., May, C. S., Palmer, K. N. V., and Murchison, L. E. (1977). Metabolic effects of salbutamol: Comparison of aerosol and intravenous administration. *Br. Med. J. 1*: 413-414.

Neville, E., Corris, P. A., Vivian, J., Nariman, S., and Gibson, G. J. (1982). Nebulized salbutamol and angina. *Br. Med. J. 258*: 796-797.

Nicklas, R. A., Whitehurst, V. E., Donohoe, R. F., and Balazs, T. (1984). Concomitant use of beta adrenergic agonists and methylxanthines. *J. Allergy Clin. Immunol. 73*: 20-24.

Noronha-Dutra, A. A., and Steen, E. M. (1982). Lipid peroxidation as a mechanism of injury in cardiac myocytes. *Lab. Invest. 47*: 346-353.

Noronha-Dutra, A. A., Steen, E. M., and Woolf, N. (1984). The early changes induced by isoproterenol in the endocardium and adjacent myocardium. *Am. J. Pathol. 114*: 231-239.

Olsson, O. A. T., Swanberg, E., Svedmyr, I., and Waldock, B. (1979). Effects of B-adrenoceptor agonists on airway smooth muscle and on self-contracting skeletal muscle. In vitro and in vivo results compared. *Acta Pharmacol. Toxicol. 44*: 272-276.

Palmer, K. N. V., Legge, J. S., Hamilton, W. F. D., and Diament, M. L. (1970). Comparison of effect of salbutamol and isoprenaline on spirometry, blood gas tensions in bronchial asthma. *Br. Med. J. 2*: 23-24.

Park, J. H., Meriwether, B. P., Park, C. R., Mudd, S. H., and Lipmann, F. (1956). Glutothione and ethylenediamine-tetraacetate antagonism of uncoupling of oxidative phosphorylation. *Biochem. Biophys. Acta 22*: 403-406.

Paterson, J. W., Conolly, M. E., Davies, D. S., and Dollery, C. T. (1968). Isoprenaline resistance and the use of pressurized aerosols in asthma. *Lancet 3*: 426-429.

Paterson, J. W., Evans, R. J. C., and Prime, F. J. (1971). Selectivity of bronchodilator action of salbutamol in asthmatic patients. *Br. J. Dis. Chest 65*: 21-38.

Peters, K. R., Hurlbert, B. J., Edelman, J. D., and Goodlin, R. C. (1981). Potassium supplementation in ritodrine induced hypokalemia. *Am. J. Obstet. Gynecol. 149*: 393-396.

Phillips, P. J., Vedig, A. E., Jones, P. G., Chapman, M. G., Collins, M., Edwards, J. B., Smeaton, T. C., and Ducan, B. M. (1980). Metabolic and cardiovascular side effects of the beta-2 adrenoceptor agonists salbutamol and rimiterol. *Br. J. Clin. Pharmacol. 9*: 483-491.

Pieper, G., Clayton, F., Todd, G., and Eliot, R. (1979). Transmural distribution of metabolites and flow in the canine left ventricle following isoproterenol infusion. *J. Pharmacol. Exp. Ther. 209*: 334-341.

Poynter, D., and Spirling, W. W. (1971). *Postgrad. Med. J. 47*: Suppl. 21-25.

Ramos, K., Combs, A. B., and Acosta, D. (1983). Cytotoxicity of isoproterenol to cultured heart cells. Effect of antioxidants on modifying membrane damage. *Toxicol. Appl. Pharmacol. 70*: 317-323.

Ramos, K., Combs, A. B., and Acosta, D. (1984). Role of calcium in isoproterenol cytotoxicity to cultured myocardial cells. *Biochem. Pharmacol. 33*: 1989-1992.

Reisman, R. E. (1970). Asthma induced by adrenergic aerosols. *J. Allergy 46*: 162-177.

Riding, W. D., Dinda, P., and Chatterjee, S. S. (1970). The bronchodilator and cardiac effects of five pressure-packed aerosols in asthma. *Br. J. Dis. Chest 64*: 37-45.

Robberecht, P., Delhaye, M., Taton, G., et al. (1983). The human heart beta-adrenergic receptors. I. Heterogeneity of the binding sites: presence of 50% $beta_1$- and 50% $beta_2$-adrenergic receptors. *Mol. Pharmacol. 24*: 169-173.

Rolton, H., Simpson, E. J., Donnelly, T., and Rodger, J. C. (1981). Plasma potassium in acute myocardial infarction. *Eur. Heart J.* (Suppl 2A): 21.

Rona, G., Chappel, I. C., Balazs, T., and Gaudry, P. (1959). An infarct like lesion and other toxic manifestations produced by isoproterenol in the rat. *Arch. Pathol. 67*: 443-453.

Ruffin, R. E., Montgomery, J. M., and Newhouse, M. T. (1979). Aerosol fenoterol by intermittent positive pressure breathing in asthmatic patients. *Clin. Pharmacol. Ther. 25*: 821-825.

Runyon, T. J., and Shagestek, M. R. (1983). Isoproterenol-induced mortality and cardiac lipids of aspirin pretreated rats with various fat intakes. *Prostaglandins 25*: 581-590.

Ryerfeldt, A., and Ramsey, C. H. (1984). Distribution of terbutaline. *Eur. J. Respir. Dis. 65,* Suppl. 134: 63-72.

Sackner, M. A., Greenleth, M., Silva, G., and Wanner, A. (1974). Bronchodilator effects of terbutaline and ephedrine in obstructive lung disease. *Clin. Pharmacol. Ther. 16*: 499-506.

Sackner, M. A., Dougherty, R., Watson, H., and Wanner, A. (1975). Hemodynamic effects of epinephrine and terbutaline in normal man. *Chest 68*: 616-624.

Salisbury, P. F., Gross, C. E., and Rieben, P. A. (1963). Acute ischemia of inner layers of ventricular wall. *Am. Heart J. 66*: 650-656.

Scott, J. C., Finkelstein, J., and Spitzer, J. J. (1962). Myocardial removal of free fatty acids under normal and pathological conditions. *Am. J. Physiol. 203*: 482-486.

Shelhamer, J. H., Metcalf, D. D., Smith, L. J., et al. (1980). Abnormal adrenergic responsiveness in allergic subjects: Analysis of isoproterenol-induced cardiovascular and plasma cyclic adenosine monophosphate responses. *J. Allergy Clin. Immunol. 66*: 52.

Sheppard, D., Wong, W. S., Uehara, C. F., Nadel, J. A., and Boushey, H. A. (1980). Lower threshold and greater bronchomotor responsiveness of asthmatic subjects to sulfur dioxide. *Am. Rev. Respir. Dis. 122*: 873-878.

Shim, C., and Williams, M. H., Jr. (1975). Cardiac response to repeated doses of isoproterenol aerosol. *Ann. Intern. Med. 83*: 208-211.

Simon, R. A., Green, L., and Stevenson, D. D. (1982). The incidence of ingested metabisulfite sensitivity in an asthmatic population. *J. Allergy Clin. Immunol. 69*: 118.

Sly, R. M. (1984). Increase in deaths from asthma. *Ann. Allergy 53*: 20-25.

Sly, R. M. (1985). Effects of treatment on mortality from asthma. *Ann. Allergy* (submitted).

Sly, R. M., Puapan, P., Ghazanshahi, S., and Midha, R. (1975). Exercise-induced bronchospasm: Evaluation of albuterol aerosol. *Ann. Allergy 34*: 7-14.

Sly, R. M., Badiei, B., and Faciane, J. (1977). Comparison of subcutaneous terbutaline with epinephrine in the treatment of asthma in children. *J. Allergy Clin. Immunol. 59*: 128-135.

Sly, R. M., Anderson, J. A., Bierman, C. W., et al. (1985). Adverse effects and complications of treatment with beta adrenergic agonist drugs. *J. Allergy Clin. Immunol.* 75 (in press).

Smythe, A. R., and Sakskini, J. Jr. (1981). Maternal metabolic alterations secondary to terbutaline therapy for premature labor. *J. Obstet. Gynecol. 57*: 566-570.

Spector, S. L., and Gomez, M. G. (1977). Dose-response effects of albuterol aerosol compared with isoproterenol and placebo aerosols. *J. Allergy Clin. Immunol. 59*: 280-286.

Speizer, F. E., Doll, R., and Heaf, P. (1968a). Observations on recent increase in mortality from asthma. *Br. Med. J. 1*: 335-339.

Speizer, F. E., Doll, R., Heaf, P., and Strang, L. B. (1968b). Investigation into use of drugs preceding death from asthma. *Br. Med. J. 1*: 339-343.

Stanescu, D. C., and van de Woestijne, K. P. (1972). Asthma attack induced by isoprenaline aerosols. *Respiration 29*: 532-537.

Stevenson, D. D., and Simon, R. A. (1984). Sulfites and asthma. *J. Allergy Clin. Immunol. 74*: 469-472.

Stolley, P. D. (1972). Asthma mortality. Why the United States was spared an epidemic of deaths due to asthma. *Am. Rev. Respir. Dis. 105*: 883-890.

Struthers, A. D., and Reid, J. L. (1984). Adrenaline causes hypokalemia in man by $beta_2$ adrenoceptor stimulation. *Clin. Endocrinol. (Oxf.) 20*: 409-414.

Stull, J. T., and Mayer, S. E. (1971). Regulation of phosphorylase activation in skeletal muscle in vivo. *J. Biol. Chem. 246*: 5716-5723.

Svedmyr, N. L. V., Larsson, S. A., and Thiringer, G. K. (1976). Development of "resistance" in beta-adrenergic receptors of asthmatic patients. *Chest 69*: 479-483.

Tai, E., and Read, J. (1967). Response of blood gas tensions to aminophylline and isoprenaline. *Thorax 22*: 543-549.

Tal, A., Pasterkemp, H., and Leahy, F. (1984). Arterial oxygen desaturation following salbutamol inhalation in acute asthma. *Chest 86*: 868-869.

Tandon, M. K. (1980). Cardiopulmonary effects of fenoterol and salbutamol aerosols. *Chest 77*: 429-431.

Tashkin, D. P., Meth, R., Simmons, D. H., and Lee, Y. E. (1975). Double-blind comparison of acute bronchial and cardiovascular effects of oral terbutaline and ephedrine. *Chest 68*: 155-161.

Tattersfield, A. E., and McNicol, M. W. (1969). Salbutamol and isoproterenol. A double-blind trial to compare bronchodilator and cardiovascular activity. *N. Engl. J. Med. 281*: 1323-1326.

Taylor, G. J. IV, and Harris, W. S. (1970). Cardiac toxicity of aerosol propellants. *JAMA 214*: 81-85.

Timmis, A. D., Bergman, G., Atkinson, L., Monoghan, M., and Jewitt, D. E. (1981). Potential value of oral $beta_2$ adrenoceptor agonists in left ventricular failure. *Am. J. Cardiol. 47*: 427.

Thiringer, G., and Svedmyr, N. (1974). Studies of muscle tremor induced by beta adrenostimulating drugs. *Scand. J. Respir. Dis.* (Suppl) *88*: 5455.

Thomas, D. J. B., Gill, B., Brown, P., and Stults, W. A. (1977). Salbutamol-induced diabetic ketoacidosis. *Br. Med. J. 2*: 438.

Trautlein, J., Allegra, J., Field, J., and Gillin, M. (1976). Paradoxic bronchospasm after inhalation of isoproterenol. *Chest 70*: 711-714.

Van den Berg (1982). Clinical implications of drug-induced desensitization of the beta receptor and the continuous oral use of terbutaline. *J. Allergy Clin. Immunol. 69*: 410.

Waelbroeck, M., Taton, G., Delhaye, M., et al. (1983). The human heart beta-adrenergic receptors. II. Coupling of $beta_2$-adrenergic receptors with the adenylate cyclase system. *Mol. Pharmacol. 24*: 174-182.

Wagner, P. D., Dantzker, D. R., Iacovoni, V. E., Tomlin, W. C., and West, J. B. (1978). Ventilation perfusion inequality in asymptomatic asthma. *Am. Rev. Respir. Dis. 118*: 511-524.

Warrell, D. A., Robertson, D. G., and Howes, J. N. (1970). Comparison of cardiorespiratory effects of isoprenaline and salbutamol in patients with bronchial asthma. *Br. Med. J. 1*: 65-70.

Watson, E. M., and Richens, A. (1974). The effects of salbutamol and terbutaline on physiological tremor, bronchial tone, and heart rate. *Br. J. Clin. Pharmacol. 1*: 223-227.

Weber, R. W., Petty, W. E., and Nelson, H. S. (1979). Aerosolized terbutaline in asthmatics. *J. Allergy Clin. Immunol. 63*: 116-121.

Weiner, N. (1980). Norepinephrine, epinephrine, and the sympathomimetic amines. In *The Pharmacologic Basis of Therapeutics,* 6th ed. Edited by A. G. Gilman, L. S. Goodman, and A. Gilman. New York, Macmillan, pp. 138-175.

Whitehurst, V. E., Joseph, X., Hohmann, J. R., Pledger, G., and Balazs, T. (1983). Cardiotoxic effect in rats and rabbits treated with terbutaline alone and in combination with aminophylline. *J. Am. Coll. Toxicol. 2*: 147-153.

William-Olsson, T., Fellenius, E., Björntorp, P., and Smith, V. (1979). Differences in metabolic responses to beta-adrenergic stimulation after propranolol or metaproterenol administration. *Acta Med. Scand. 205*: 201-206.

Wilson, A. F., Novey, H. S., Cloninger, P., Davis, J., and White, D. (1976). Cardiopulmonary effects of long-term bronchodilator administration. *J. Allergy Clin. Immunol. 58*: 204-212.

Wilson, J. D., Sutherland, D. C., and Thomas, A. C. (1981). Has the change to beta-agonists combined with oral theophylline increased cases of fatal asthma? *Lancet 1*: 1235-1237.

Winsor, T., Mills, B., Winbury, M. M., Howe, B. B., and Berger, H. J. (1975). Intramyocardial diversion of coronary blood flow: Effects of isoproterenol-induced subendocardial ischemia. *Microvasc. Res. 9*: 261.

Winter, R. J. D., Langford, J. A., and Rudd, R. M. (1984). Effects of oral and inhaled salbutamol and oral pirbuterol on right and left ventricular function in chronic bronchitis. *Br. Med. J. 288*: 824-825.

Yates, J. C., and Shella, N. S. (1975). Induction of necrosis and failure in the isolated perfused rat heart with oxidized isoproterenol. *J. Mol. Cell. Cardiol. 7*: 807-816.

Zsoter, T. T., and Epstein, S. W. (1973). Effect of salbutamol on the peripheral circulation in man. *Chest 64*: 465-471.

27

Platelet Activating Factor and the Search for Prophylactic Antiasthma Drugs

JOHN MORLEY

Sandoz AG
Basel, Switzerland

I. Prophylaxis in Asthma

The marked dyspnea of acute asthma is associated with grossly impaired ventilation, as is readily demonstrated by measurement of forced expiratory volume or peak expiratory flow rate. In such circumstances, there is an immediate requirement from the patient to establish improved airflow and hence, the physician is impelled to instigate treatment according to the symptoms. Such predilection for symptomatic therapy is not restricted to thoracic medicine; for it extends into asthma research in both academic and industrial environments, as can be illustrated by the emphasis that has been given in recent years to the proposal that peptidoleukotrienes are central to asthma symptoms (Lewis and Austen, 1981). The discovery of peptidoleukotrienes as constituents of slow-reacting substance of anaphylaxis (SRS-A) was widely considered to be a major advance in asthma research, largely because these substances effect protracted contraction of airway tissue in vitro and are potent airway spasmogens in vivo (Piper, 1980). The high expectations of leukotriene research were ill conceived, for it can easily be shown that beta-adrenoceptor agonists will fully reverse airway obstruction that is produced by these particular spasmogens; hence, if mere contraction of airway smooth muscle were the essence of asthma pathology, bronchodilator drugs would long since have provided an adequate therapy for asthma.

The emphasis that has been given to bronchospasm is underlined by the definitions that have been agreed upon for asthma (Ciba Guest Symposium, 1959; American Thoracic Society, 1962); definitions which focus upon the episodic nature of airway obstruction. Rapid changes in airway resistance are most readily achieved by changing the tone of airway smooth muscle; however, it does not follow that these changes necessarily depend upon contraction of airway smooth muscle, since plasma protein accumulation during increased vascular permeability achieves a maximal value within a few minutes (Morley and Williams, 1971) and glandular secretion in response to nerve stimulation has negligible latency. On the other hand, it must be acknowledged that rapid resolution of edema and rapid elimination of airway mucus are implausible, so that instances of prompt reversal of airway obstruction in asthma implicate smooth muscle as the effector agency of obstruction. It is evident that a rapid reduction of airway obstruction, following inhalation of a beta-adrenoceptor agonist, has been decisive in shaping the opinion, that airway smooth muscle is considered a primary determinant of asthma symptoms.

To contest that changes in airway smooth muscle contractility provide a basis for asthma pathology can be considered a rather narrow viewpoint, although it does have a virtue in that it allows the possibility that contraction of airway smooth muscle may depend upon some mechanism in which formation or action of a particular spasmogen is obligatory. The selection of leukotrienes and other lipoxygenase products as putative mediators of bronchospasm in asthma rather than to other spasmogens might be presumed to have been influenced by such thoughts, but there is unequivocal experimental evidence that peptides, acetylcholine, or histamine can effect contraction of sirway smooth muscle independently of arachidonate metabolism. Such argument can be extended to hyperreacivity, for it is now known that the increased reactivity of airway smooth muscle, as following exposure of the guinea-pig to inhalation or injection of platelet activated factor (PAF) is independent of arachidonate metabolism (Morley et al., 1987a).

Once it is accepted that there is a plurality of endogenous airway spasmogens, the rather obvious conclusion can be made that symptomatic relief in asthma will be achieved more readily by use of nonselective bronchodilator drugs (e.g., beta-adrenoceptor agonists) than by materials which limit the formation or action of a restricted range of mediators. This conclusion is reinforced by consideration of the effects of histamine (H1) antagonists in asthma therapy. Drugs in this category can achieve limited symptomatic relief when allergic bronchospasm is the predominant symptom, yet histamine (H1) antagonists do not produce sustained benefit in clinical asthma (Chai, 1980). Experience of histamine

(H1) antagonists in asthma provides a precedent for leukotriene antagonists or lipoxygenase inhibitors and early clinical experience of Piriprost supports the prediction that this class of drug will be without noteworthy benefit, since piriprost is without influence upon airway obstruction that results from inhalation of allergen (Holgate et al., 1986) or exposure to analgesic drugs (Nizankowska, in press). Such negative outcome is in direct contrast to cromoglycate and ketotifen which are clearly effective in these clinical tests (Pepys et al., 1968; Girard and Cuevas, 1977; Delany, 1976; 1983). Faced with this evidence, there seems little likelihood that sustained clinical benefit will result from use of compounds with the pharmacological profile of leukotriene antagonism or lipoxygenase inhibition.

Examination of a wide range of endogenous materials which produce contraction of airway smooth muscle has revealed that, bronchospasm can be reversed by nonselective bronchodilator drugs in every instance. Hence, it could be advocated that a potent spasmolytic bronchodilator drug would suffice for asthma therapy. Two observations negate this proposition: first, regular therapy of bronchodilators beta-adrenoceptor agonists can be insufficient in many patients including patients with mild childhood asthma (Mueller and von der Hardt, 1985); second, it has been recognized that cromolycate is an effective therapy in asthma, even though this drug lacks bronchodilator or receptor antagonist activities. In conventional screening tests, cromoglycate has a severely restricted pharmacology (Brodgen et al., 1974); consequently, there was a need to establish some property of cromoglycate that might pertain to efficacy in asthma, the evidence that cromoglycate exhibited the (then) unusual property of inhibiting allergic reactions led to an interpretation that "antiallergic" activity accounts for prophylactic efficacy in asthma. Cromoglycate is a potent inhibitor of passive cutaneous anaphylaxis in the rat (Cox, 1967), but has more modest efficacy as an inhibitor of mediator release from chopped human lung fragments (Sheard et al., 1967). These limited observations provided a basis for the claim that mast cell stabilization is a property of cromoglycate that may be decisive for efficacy in asthma, but the interpretation was reinforced strongly by the clinical observation that cromoglycate could inhibit both acute and late-onset airway obstruction in reactions to allergen inhalation (Pepys et al., 1968), thereby extending the interpretation, if not the evidence, to asthma patients. From this tenuous base, emerged the "mast cell concept of asthma," which has preoccupied many investigators over the last two decades. However, within research laboratories of the pharmaceutical industry this concept is now widely disregarded, even though it has engendered a self-sustaining momentum within academic circles. Disenchantment in industry can be readily understood, since effective antiasthma drugs have not been realized using this approach (Buckle, 1984) and deficiencies of the mast cell concept remain unanswered (Morley, 1986).

II. Oral Prophylactic Agents

Irrespective of the merits or limitations of the mast cell concept, cromoglycate therapy rapidly became an established treatment for asthma (Altounyan, 1980). Such success in therapeutic practice attested to the claim of a novel effect that could not be afforded by bronchodilator drugs. In retrospect, acceptance of cromoglycate as an asthma therapy might be considered exceptional, since cromoglycate is not absorbed from the gastrointestinal tract and has to be inhaled as a solid suspension from a special device; moreover, cromoglycate therapy was without immediate benefit, except when special studies were conducted (e.g., inhalation of allergen, ingestion of aspirin, brief periods of exercise, etc.). Furthermore, despite the evidence of prompt and profound effects in acute laboratory and clinical tests, experience of this drug in clinical asthma led to debate as to whether objective benefit could be demonstrated; and large protracted trials, such as the Brompton Hospital/Medical Research council trial (1972), were necessary in order to establish unequivocally that the drug had prophylactic efficacy.

The clinical success of a highly innovative drug of limited solubility and with suboptimal pharmacokinetics (in consequences of inhaled administration). prompted many large pharmaceutical companies to initiate research programs directed toward identifying analogous compounds that could be administered orally. The failure of so many established pharmaceutical companies to achieve their goal, in what appears to be more an exercise in drug development, as opposed to discovery of a novel therapeutic entity, merits close attention.

First, it should be acknowledged that most pharmaceutical companies engaged in the search for successor compounds to cromoglycate achieved a degree of success in that chemicals more potent than cromoglycates were identified by reference to oral absorption and potency in tests such as inhibition of passive cutaneous anaphylaxis in the rat or other species and inhibition of histamine release or SRS-A generation by human lung fragments (Buckle, 1984). In this way, it has proved possible to select compounds with an effect upon mast cell activation that is indistinguishable from cromolgycate, as evidenced by tachyphylaxis or cross-tachyphylaxis with cromoglycate; equally, it was possible to select compounds which lack cross-tachyphylaxis and hence stabilize mast cells by an unrelated mechanism. Notwithstanding differences of mechanism and divergence of chemical structures, clinical experience of these compounds has been consistently disappointing (Stokes and Morley, 1981). The negative outcome of clinical evaluation should have been anticipated for such substances, since it was known that $beta_2$-adrenoceptor agonists have considerable potency as inhibitors of mast cell activation in both animal or human lung (Butchers et al., 1979), yet drugs in this category have proved ineffective as prophylactic agents in asthma.

The recent introduction of tranilast, oxatomide, azalestine, and nedocromil into asthma therapy on the basis of activity in tests of mast cell stabilization does not invalidate this conclusion. First, clinical efficacy in asthma cannot be anticipated for these drugs on the basis of laboratory data. For instance, nedocromil is a modest inhibitor of mast cell activation (Eady et al., 1985), yet appears more effective in clinical asthma than does oxatomide, which combines considerable potency as a mast cell stabilizing agent with potency as a histamine (H1) antagonist (Richards et al., 1984). Indeed, oxatomide proved ineffective in a major clinical trial (Stokes and Darbyshire, 1981) which followed a design that was used to establish efficacy for cromoglycate (Brompton Hospital/Medical Research Council, 1972). It might be argued that administration by inhalation may contribute to the efficacy of nedocromil, but use of this route per se cannot account for clinical efficacy, since more potent mast cell stabilizing agents (including beta-adrenoceptor agonists) can be administered in this manner, yet prove ineffectual in asthma prophylaxis (Stokes and Morley, 1981). Second, the clinical failure of a series of compounds selected by reference to mast cell stabilization requires some explanation, for it is clearly anomalous to claim that a minority have efficacy in clinical asthma, while accepting that the majority, which include more potent inhibitors of mast cell activation, have proved ineffective.

Faced with such evidence, it is not unreasonable to reject the original presumption that cromoglycate is effective in prophylaxis by influencing the activation of mast cells and it must be concluded that there must be some other property of cromoglycate that is central to efficacy in asthma prophylaxis. The evidence that is necessary to substantiate this conclusion has been available for at least a decade (Morley, 1986); however, it has been the emergence of PAF as a potential mediator of asthma (Morley et al., 1984) that has brought these arguments into focus and ketotifen has provided a pivotal linkage between the concept of PAF as a mediator of asthma and the pharmacology of prophylactic antiasthma drugs.

III. Ketotifen and Asthma Prophylaxis

Ketotifen is a benzocycloheptathiophene with a structural affinity to cyproheptadine; it was selected for clinical development because of its potency as a histamine (H1) receptor antagonist (pA_2 9.49) (Craps et al., 1985). Ketotifen is well absorbed from the gastrointestinal tract, so that this drug can be administered orally. It has an extended half-life and a lengthy period is required to achieve steady-state tissue levels. As a histamine (H1) antagonist, ketotifen was introduced as a therapy for allergic conditions in which asthma could be an incidental component; hence, the first evidence of benefit in asthma derived from clinical experience.

Efficacy of a histamine (H1) antagonist in asthma was not to be expected, for although this class of drugs can effect some symptomatic benefit in asthma, especially during exacerbation due to persisting allergen exposure, there has been a long-standing consensus that histamine (H1) antagonists are not an effective therapy for asthma. The opinion that the benefit of ketotifen in asthma does not derive from histamine (H1) antagonism was reinforced by comparison between ketotifen and other histamine (H1) antagonists, which reveals an advantage for ketotifen (Craps, 1980). It would seem reasonable therefore, to conclude that ketotifen must possess some property which confers efficacy in asthma that is additional to histamine (H1) antagonism. An analogous conclusion could be made for urticaria, since ketotifen is markedly more effective than other histamine (H1) antagonists in this condition (Craps, 1985). To search for a novel drug effect in patients would be impractical, hence preclinical studies were initiated in an effort to resolve this issue.

A decade ago, inhibition of mast cell activation was the predominant theory to account for prophylaxis in asthma; hence, initial preclinical investigations concentrated upon investigation of aspects of mast cell function, using techniques that were known to reveal positive effects for cromoglycate. It was possible to demonstrate that ketotifen could diminish reactions of passive cutaneous anaphylaxis in the guinea-pig or rat and to differentiate such effects from histamine (H1) antagonism (Martin and Baggiolini, 1981). These in vivo observations were complemented by in vitro studies which revealed an inhibition of mediator release from human chopped lung (Ross et al., 1979), but as with cromoglycate, neither potency nor efficacy on these tests were impressive when compared to beta-adrenoceptor agonists. Mast cell stabilization by ketotifen does not exhibit tachyphylaxis and is not influenced by prior exposure to cromoglycate; hence any action of ketotifen upon mast cell activation is distinct from that of cromoglycate (Martin and Roemer, 1977). Calcium influx has been shown to be diminished by high concentrations of ketotifen, when using gastrointestinal smooth muscle as an indicator tissue (Lowe and Richardson, 1980). Such a property might account for the capacity of ketotifen to inhibit mediator secretion by inflammatory cells in vitro, since secretion of mediators is regulated by the concentration of calcium within such cells.

When considering whether drugs might effect mediator secretion during an allergic response, it is necessary to differentiate impaired mediator secretion from antagonism of mediator effects. In this context, it is evident that ketotifen not only inhibits the response of airway smooth muscle to histamine, but also inhibits responses to peptidoleukotrienes (Martin et al., 1981). Consequently, inhibitory effects of ketotifen during allergic responses may reflect inhibition of mediator actions as well as reduction of mediator release by inflammatory cells.

As has already been pointed out, the concept of mast cell activation as a primary determinant of airway hyperreactivity was not universally accepted;

thus, as deficiencies of the mast cell theory become evident in the late 1970s, attention was redirected toward the concept that airway hyperreactivity might be a consequence of impaired beta-adrenoceptor function (Szentivanyi, 1980). In this context, it was shown that intravenous injection of ketotifen will reverse tachyphylaxis to isoprenaline, as revealed by allergic reactions in rat skin (Bretz et al., 1983); while in humans, it was reported that administration of ketotifen could pre-empt the loss of beta-adrenoceptor binding sites on peripheral blood lymphocytes that results from repeated exposure to isoprenaline (Brodde et al., 1985). While it can be postulated that ketotifen might modify beta-adrenoceptor responsivity in this way, it should be recognized that other interactions between beta-adrenoceptor agonists and ketotifen may be significant in airway tissue. Thus, it can be shown that an infusion of isoprenaline in the guinea-pig induces airway hyperreactivity even though such doses of isoprenaline are insufficient to diminish beta-adrenergic sensitivity (Mazzoni et al., 1987). Hyperreactivity in response to isoprenaline infusion is greatly diminished in animals pretreated with ketotifen. Since induction of hyperreactivity can be achieved by other catecholamines (Mazzoni et al., 1987), the capacity of ketotifen to inhibit this anomalous action of isoprenaline may extend to other manifestations of hyperreactivity, such as the response to allergen, when release of endogenous catecholamines contributes to the overall response.

Despite identification of a number of properties that could contribute to prophylactic efficacy of ketotifen in asthma, no decisive evidence of a second property emerged; and of particular significance is that compounds that exhibit properties such as SRS-A antagonism, mast cell stabilization, and histamine antagonism have not proved successful in asthma therapy. Consequently, the report that high doses of ketotifen could diminish airway responses to PAF (Medieros et al., 1983) merited further investigation, since PAF had biological properties that made it *unique* among potential mediators of allergic asthma. Since PAF was a product of diverse inflammatory cells, it could account for exacerbation of asthma by both allergic and nonallergic processes (Morley et al., 1984).

IV. PAF and Asthma

Platelet activating factor (PAF) is a mixture of ether-linked phospholipids of closely related structure that are formed by certain inflammatory cells as a result of the concerted action of phospholipase A_2 and acetyl coA:acyltransferase upon ether phospholipids within cell membranes (Fig. 1). Interest in PAF as a mediator of asthma had its origin with the recognition that PAF was a potent spasmogen of airway smooth muscle in laboratory animals (Vargaftig et al., 1980). However, subsequent investigation established that it is the inflammatory properties of PAF that are more impressive (Page et al., 1984). In guinea-

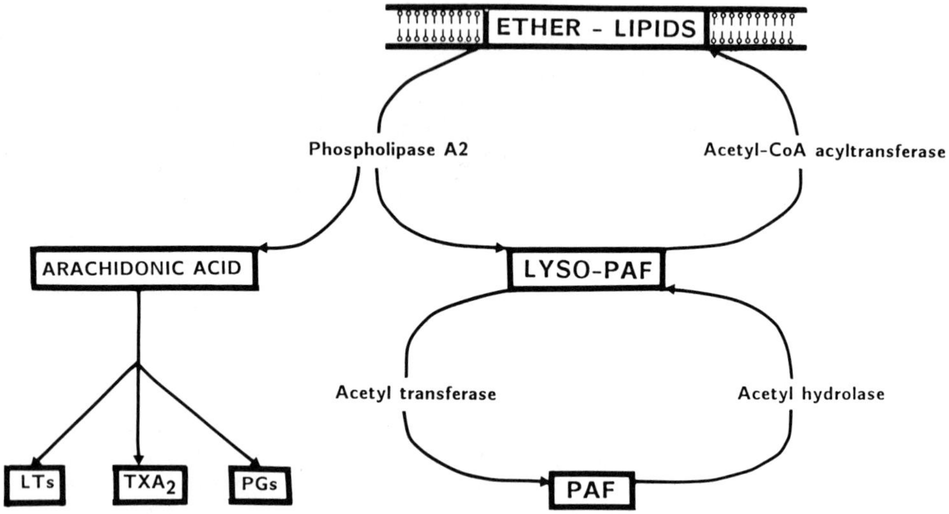

Figure 1 Generation of eicosanoids and PAF from precursor ether phospholipids within cell membrane.

pig skin, PAF induces an intense, but transient, increase of vascular permeability (Morley et al., 1983). This acute reaction is succeeded by a protracted response, as evidenced by an accumulation of inflammatory cells which can persist for days (Dewar et al., 1984). Accumulation of inflammatory cells at sites of PAF application distinguishes the effect of this material from other allergic mediators, none of which can recruit and activate both polymorphonuclear and

---

Figure 2 Eosinophils (activated by IgE or T-cell products), macrophages (activated by IgE, T-cell products or phagocytic stimuli) or neutrophils activated by T-cell products or phagocytic stimuli) are likely sources of PAF in asthma. Two distinct effects are envisaged as contributing to protracted changes of airways: eosinophil-mediated change of airway epithelium due to major basic protein (MBP), eosinophil cationic protein (ECP) release, which contributes to hyperreactivity and also determines impaired mucociliary clearance and cough; platelet-dependent induction of smooth muscle hyperplasia following release of platelet derived growth factor (PDGE), thereby effecting increase reactivity. The capacity of hyperreactive smooth muscle in asthma to respond to diverse chemical stimuli (acetylcholine; histamine, serotonin, adenosine, prostaglandins D_2, F_2 alpha and E_2, thromboxane A_2 neurokinin A, bombesin, bradykinin, leukotriene C_4 and D_4) has been depicted schematically in order to emphasize the futility of selective antagonism.

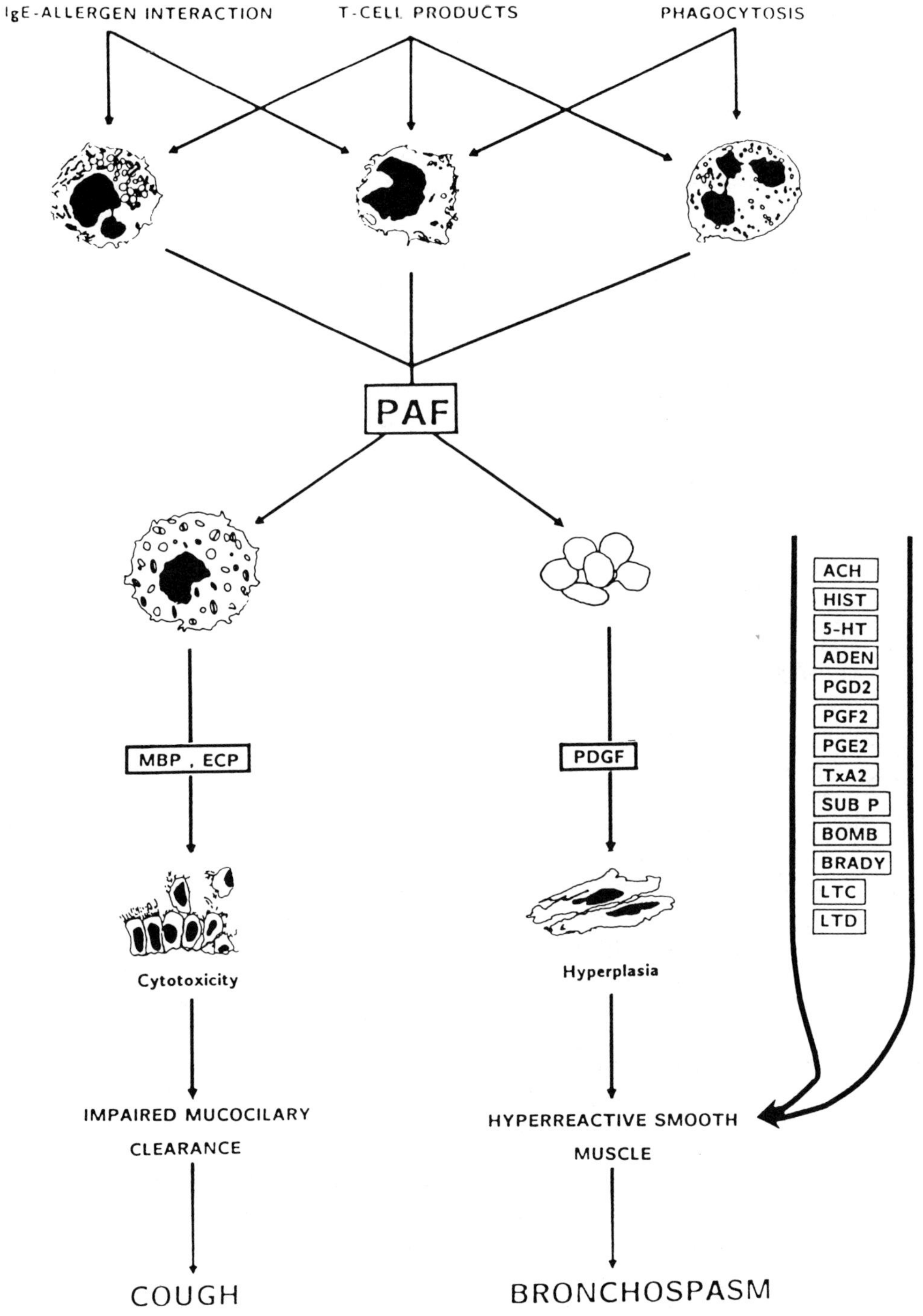
IgE-ALLERGEN INTERACTION
T-CELL PRODUCTS
PHAGOCYTOSIS
PAF
MBP, ECP
PDGF
ACH
HIST
5-HT
ADEN
PGD2
PGF2
PGE2
TxA2
SUB P
BOMB
BRADY
LTC
LTD
Cytotoxicity
Hyperplasia
IMPAIRED MUCOCILARY CLEARANCE
HYPERREACTIVE SMOOTH MUSCLE
COUGH
BRONCHOSPASM

Figure 2

mononuclear cells. It seems likely that this cellular response is secondary to platelet activation, since such a reaction is not evident in the skin of the rat, a species whose platelets lack PAF receptors and hence do not respond to PAF, even though acute plasma protein extravasation in the rat is as intense as that observed in guinea-pig skin (Pirotzky et al., 1984).

In 1985, a general scheme was presented that might account for the exacerbation and perpetuation of asthma by mechanisms in which PAF was a central agency (Morley et al., 1985). At that time, much of the information upon which the hypothesis was based was fragmentary and the purpose of detailing a scheme was to polarize research investigations, so as to test the concept more rigorously. It is worthwhile to reconsider and revise the proposed scheme in light of the information that has since emerged (Fig. 2).

A. Generation of PAF

Selection of the macrophage as a major source of PAF was influenced by the central role of the macrophage in many aspects of the immune reaction and by the evidence that this cell type could generate PAF. It had already been shown that human lung macrophages collected from asthma patients could generate significant quantities of PAF in response to activation by allergen (Arnoux et al., 1982). As a source of asthma symptoms, this type of IgE-dependent response has usually been demoted, or even disregarded, in favor of mast cell or basophil activation; in atopy however, cell activation by this mechanism is probably more relevant to asthma symptoms than is mast cell activation, since the intensity of asthma symptoms can be related to high levels of IgE in plasma (Cockcroft et al., 1979), whereas mast cell and basophil activation are essentially independent of serum levels of IgE.

Secondly, it is now well established that the macrophage is activated by lymphokines in order to serve as an effector cell of cellular immunity. This cell is a major source of lipid-derived mediators (Morley, 1981) as might be anticipated since there are substantial quantities of phospholipase A_2 and arachidonate in the plasmalemma; consequently, macrophages would be favored as a source of PAF during infection or in other circumstances when cells of the airway epithelium are killed, such as exposure to bacterial toxins or airborne pollutants. This concept is strengthened by the experimental evidence that human lung macrophages can generate PAF following exposure to lymphokines or endotoxin in vitro (Beijer and Rylander, 1983). However, other inflammatory cells also serve as sources of PAF within human airways, so that alternative origins of PAF in asthma must now be considered. For instance, neutrophils can generate PAF in response to nonallergic stimuli (O'Flaherty, 1982) and presumably may be activated by lymphokines in like manner to the macrophage. Eosinophils show an even greater capacity for PAF formation (Snyder, 1985) and may be activated by interaction between allergen and cell-bound IgE (Capron et al., 1985) or in response to lymphokines following T-cell activation (Colley, 1973). By way of contrast, activated mast cells release little, if any, PAF.

At present, no particular cell type can be designated as a decisive source of PAF in asthma; however, the unusual capacity of eosinophils to generate PAF and the prevalence of this cell type in asthmatic lung favor the eosinophil as a major source of PAF in asthma, in addition to the macrophage by virtue, which remains the most abundant inflammatory cell within the airway lumen.

B. Airway Obstruction

Two properties of PAF were cited as contributing to increased airway resistance, namely the contraction of airway smooth muscle and the induction of edema in airway mucosa. To these, might now be added increased mucus secretion, although evidence of such an effect of PAF remains slight at present (Hahn et al., 1985). The spasmogenic effects of PAF are poorly understood. PAF-induced bronchospasm is absolutely dependent upon platelets (Morley et al., 1985). Since selective platelet depletion is a most effective inhibitor of the constrictor response of airway smooth muscle to PAF in vivo, this should not be disputed on the basis of studies using high doses of PAF in vitro (Stimler-Gerard, 1986).

The significance of acute spasmogenic actions of PAF in the airways may have been overestimated as a result of the claim that acute bronchospasm to allergen can be fully inhibited by antagonism of the effects of PAF (Braquet et al., 1985). This conclusion is inherently implausible, since it is well established that other mediators are released in acute allergic reactions; hence, since certain of the PAF antagonists do not influence allergic responses in this manner, it must be presumed that if substances such as gingkolide B (Berti et al., 1986) and WEB 2086 (Casals-Stengel, 1986) do diminish acute allergic bronchospasm, then this must represent a property of these materials that is additional to PAF antagonism. Our own experience of gingkolide B and other PAF-antagonists conflict with these reports and indicate a minor role for PAF in acute allergic bronchospasm (Morley et al., 1987).

The capacity of PAF to cause increased vascular permeability in guinea-pig skin is impressive, but it is unlikely that airway edema contributes to the airway obstruction that results from exposure to low doses of PAF (10-32 ng/kg) which cause substantial yet transient, airway obstruction in the guinea-pig. These responses resolve spontaneously to pretreatment levels of airway resistance within minutes and can be fully suppressed by modest doses of isoprenaline, so that any proposal that bronchospasm is in part a consequence of edema appears superfluous. However, edema may be expected to contribute to changed lung function when pharmacological doses of PAF are employed, as by inhalation. Some animals responding to PAF generate substantial airway secretions, although the circumstances that determine this effect of PAF have yet to be defined. Actions of this type may have contributed to the sustained airway obstruction that was observed to follow intratracheal installation of a large dose of PAF in the rabbit (Page et al., 1985).

C. Airway Hyperreactivity

The proposal that PAF might cause airway hyperreactivity was a necessary part of the hypothesis if PAF were to be given a central role in asthma, but it must be admitted that initially this proposal was wholly speculative. It was suggested that two types of mechanism would contribute to relatively protracted airway hyperreactivity, but experimental evidence now implies that at least three agencies may contribute to induction of airway hyperreactivity by PAF.

Initial interpretation of the response pattern of acute bronchospasm in response to intravenous injection of PAF was influenced by the conventional view that airway hyperreactivity would develop over many hours. Consequently, the observation that an acute injection of a small dose of PAF is typically followed by an enhanced response on repetition of the same dose of PAF within a few minutes was not perceived as hyperreactivity. Investigation of this phenomenon revealed that protracted exposure to PAF, by use of infusion or repetitive injection, caused substantial increased reactivity to airway spasmogens (Mazzoni et al., 1985a). This effect of PAF on the airway was nonselective and could be shown to persist for more than 24 hours. Inhalation of PAF is also an effective method for induction of airway hyperreactivity in the guinea-pig (Mazzoni et al., 1985 (Fitzgerald et al., 1987) and such observations have been extended to man with the demonstration that inhalation of PAF causes a nonselective hyperreactivity as gauged by methacholine sensitivity in both normal and asthmatic subjects (Cuss et al., 1986). In man, as in the guinea-pig, the change in sensitivity is modest, but is noteworthy for its very protracted nature.

Investigation into the basis of hyperreactivity in guinea-pig lung has indicated that a number of mechanisms contribute to changed behavior of the airways. The acute change in airway reactivity that follows intravenous infusion of modest quantities of PAF is platelet dependent; interestingly, it is independent of neutrophil accumulation and seems likely to be independent of eosinophil accumulation, although this latter issue has yet to be resolved definitively. The more protracted change in airway sensitivity that results from inhalation of PAF parallels accumulation of eosinophils within the airways (Aoki et al., 1987). In the guinea-pig, this process is compared by damage to airway epithelium and desquamation of ciliated cells into the airway lumen. A role for platelets in the sustained response to PAF has not been established, but equally such a process has yet to be eliminated. An obligatory involvement of platelets in this sustained reaction to PAF is suggested by the observation that cellular inflammation is not a consequence of exposure to PAF in the rat, a species whose platelets lack PAF receptors. Although the role of platelets in the protracted hyperreactivity that follows exposure to PAF is conjectural, the evidence that airway hyperreactivity is paralleled by eosinophil accumulation is unequivocal. It is presumed that the pronounced accumulation of eosinophils is responsible for damage to airway epithelium, which could be expected to result in hyperreactivity as a result of increased activity within local or systemic reflex pathways (Barnes, 1986).

The third type of effect that PAF may have upon airways remains uninvestigated. It was known from studies of vascular smooth muscle in the abdominal aorta of the guinea-pig that repeated exposure to PAF could induce smooth muscle hypertrophy (Handley et al., 1983). The postulate that an analogous effect would occur in the airways was speculative, but had the merits of, for the first time, providing a plausible mechanism to account for this characteristic feature of asthma. Extension of the concept to include airway smooth muscle has not been subject to experimental investigation but it has been reported that inhalation of PAF will promote an emigration of platelets from the pulmonary vessels into lung parenchyma. In these animals, platelets can be observed apposed to airway smooth muscle cells (Lellouch-Tubiana et al., 1985), while in humans it is apparent that platelets are a frequent resident within the airway lumen (Metzger et al., 1987).

The initial concept of PAF as a stimulus to airway hyperreactivity was poorly conceived, for it presumed that airway hyperreactivity in asthma was homogeneous and that a singular entity might account for changes of smooth muscle sensitivity. It has now been established experimentally that agencies can contribute to airway hyperreactivity by mechanisms that are wholly distinct from PAF formation or actions (Morley et al., 1987c). Consequently, it is more reasonable to consider PAF, not as a unique mediator of hyperreactivity in asthma, but rather as an allergic mediator which can contribute to acute manifestation of airway hyperreactivity (within minutes or hours) but that by other mechanisms, involving the attraction and activation of eosinophils, causes a more sustained hyperreactivity (days) and that by a third mechanism, that involves platelets, may modify the response of airway smooth muscle on a relatively permanent basis (weeks or months) as a consequence of increasing the mass of airway smooth muscle. Since several agencies can effect acute transient changes of airway reactivity and since the acute change in airway reactivity that results from an allergic reaction is not diminished by infusion of PAF receptor antagonists, the major significance of PAF must be presumed to lie with the protracted events of an allergic or inflammatory response.

V. The Pharmacology of PAF-Induced Hyperreactivity

The recognition that PAF could cause airway hyperreactivity provided an opportunity to investigate the pharmacology of hyperreactivity; for hitherto, models of hyperreactivity have not proved amenable to extensive pharmacological studies (Morley et al., 1987a). Since ketotifen had proved to be a most potent inhibitor of PAF-induced bronchospasm, it was perhaps not surprising that this drug should inhibit induction of airway hyperreactivity by PAF (Morley et al., 1985). Indeed, more recent analysis of this effect of ketotifen indicate that acute inhibition of bronchial responses to PAF largely represent an inhibition of hyperreactivity. Theophylline, is also a potent inhibitor of PAF-induced bronchospasm, so that similar arguments might apply to this drug; however, such considerations cannot extend to cromoglycate or hydrocortisone, neither of which impair the acute bronchospasm that results from intravenous injection of PAF. Nevertheless, both cromoglycate and hydrocortisone resemble ketotifen and theophylline as inhibitors of the acute increased airway hyperreactivity that results from an infusion of PAF (Mazzoni et al., 1985b).

Thus, for the first time, those drugs known to be effective in asthma prophylaxis have been shown to exhibit a common property and moreover a property that may be related readily to clinical efficacy in asthma prophylaxis. To strengthen such a conclusion, it is necessary to extend these observations to include other drugs which have properties in common with ketotifen, cromoglycate, methylxanthines, and glucocorticosteroids, but which are not necessarily effective in asthma. Such properties include antagonism of histamine, serotonin, SRS-A and PAF, inhibition of lipoxygenase or cyclo-oxygenase enzymes, mast cell stabilization, and bronchodilator activity (Morley et al., 1987a). With the exception of PAF-receptor antagonists, no drug category has revealed the capacity to inhibit PAF-induced hyperreactivity, which may therefore be regarded as a rigorous test of the hypothesis proposed in 1984.

VI. The Cellular Basis of Hyperreactivity

It is worth re-emphasizing that airway hyperreactivity in consequence of autocoid release or generation is not a unitary process. It might be considered that the ability of leukotrienes to induce airway hyperreactivity provides evidence of a form of hyperreactivity that is independent of PAF formation. However, leukotriene responses may be secondary to PAF generation (Voelkel et al., 1982) and vice versa (McIntyre et al., 1986), so that such evidence should be regarded as equivocal. PAF-induced hyperreactivity is not diminished by SRS-A antagonists nor by lipoxygenase inhibition, but it has yet to be determined whether leukotriene-induced hyperreactivity is resistant to PAF antagonists. However, the existence of distinct pathogenic processes which induce airway hyperreactivity has been revealed most clearly by considering the effect of isoprenaline upon responses to PAF. Isoprenaline was evaluated as a potential inhibitor of PAF-induced hyperreactivity, because of its use as an antiasthma drug. Surprisingly, isoprenaline consistently enhanced the hyperreactivity that resulted from an infusion of PAF (Mazzoni et al., 1985b). It was considered initially that this effect might be a consequence of vasodilator, proinflammatory effects of isoprenaline, but a similar phenomenon could not be produced by infusion of PGE_2. The issue lay dormant until the experiment of infusing isoprenaline alone was performed, thereby revealing that isoprenaline per se induces hyperreactivity to an exten that is closely similar to PAF (Morley et al., 1987c). In order to exclude PAF or other platelet-dependent mechanisms as a basis for the effect of isoprenaline, such experiments were repeated using animals depleted of platelets, when there was no diminution of the response. Conversely, vagal section, which does not modify the response to PAF, fully inhibits the hyperreactivity that follows infusion of isoprenaline. As endogenous catecholamines can effect such hyperreactivity, it is reasonable to conclude that acute hyperreactivity, as evidenced in reaction to allergen exposure, involves not only PAF but other, unrelated, pathogenic processes, for which catecholamines provide one example. The inability of PAF antagonists to diminish acute bronchospasm, acute platelet accumulation, and associated airway hyperreactivity, during reactions to allergic stimuli (Morley et al., 1986) accords with this conclusion.

Although mechanisms that induce acute airway hyperreactivity are heterogenous, such a conclusion cannot be extended to eosinophil accumulation and smooth muscle hyperplasia, since at present, other mediators have not been shown to induce these biological effects. A central role for PAF in eosinophil activation might be anticipated on the basis of in vitro studies (Lee et al., 1984), so that it might be proposed that PAF could serve as a link between nonallergic agencies or hyperreactivity, such as bacterial toxins or airborne pollutants and eosinophil activation; in this way, PAF provides an alternative mechanism whereby eosinophils may be activated in addition to IgE-dependent activation in allergy and lymphokine-dependent activation in cellular immune reactions. A role for platelets in these events is a tantalizing possibility; however, the potency of PAF as a stimulus to platelet activation makes it difficult to establish whether platelet activation is central to asthma pathology or whether platelet activation is incidental to PAF generation. In large part, platelets have been disregarded as significant participants during allergic responses in experimental animals or in clinical asthma. Nonetheless, there is both animal and clinical data which implies a role for platelets in acute and protracted forms of hyperreactivity, so that platelet activation in asthma may have greater significance than has been accorded hitherto.

It is important to establish whether platelet activation can determine smooth muscle hyperplasia of airway smooth muscle and hence persistent hyperreactivity. Recognition that a proportion of PAF-induced airway hyperreactivity may be qualitatively different and have a from that is immune to acute therapeutic intervention is an important conclusion, for although the clinical counterpart of drug-resistant hyperreactivity has long been acknowledged, it is frequently disregarded when evaluating drug effects in asthma.

VII. Implications for Asthma Prophylaxis

Investigation of the pharmacology of PAF-induced pulmonary pathology was inspired primarily by the need to investigate the antiasthma action of ketotifen and other prophylactic antiasthma drugs. These studies have been illuminating, but have consequences that extend beyond industrial research, for they help to account for certain clinical phenomena that hitherto have appeared to be anomalous.

Acute benefit as a consequence of acute administration of prophylactic antiasthma drugs can be readily demonstrated by challenge studies, as may be illustrated by the capacity of cromoglycate or ketotifen to inhibit the increased airway obstruction that results from exercise, allergen-inhalation or analgesic-injection. Such acute effects are not disputed, yet the clinical efficacy of these drugs has often been subject to debate, since during formal trials in clinical asthma, striking symptomatic benefits (e.g., diminished nocturnal cough, reduced sleep disturbance) may not be paralleled by acute changes of lung function indices. This has been compounded by a need to treat with prophylactic drugs for some weeks before clinical benefit becomes evident objectively. The effects of PAF upon airways provides a mechanism that could account for these clinical experiences. Prophylactic drugs such as cromoglycate or ketotifen do not reverse existing asthma pathology acutely; hence these drugs may be expected to induce benefit over a protracted period much in the manner of allergen avoidance, when improvement may not be apparent until weeks or months have elapsed (Platts-Mills et al., 1982). The evidence that PAF produces very protracted effects upon the airways after a single exposure in animals (Camussi et al., 1983) or man (Cuss et al., 1986) thus affords a rationale to account for this phenomenon and the recognition that protracted sequelae result from a single exposure to PAF, compounds the problem of noncompliance during clinical trials, especially when neither patient or physician are able to perceive benefit (Reed, 1986). It follows that marked improvement of lung ventilation indices would be a welcome consequence of prophylactic antiasthma therapy, but this should not be considered to be a primary objective of prophylaxis. The preeminence of airflow indices in the clinical evaluation of asthma has led to designation of prophylactic antiasthma drugs as "weak" drugs, which assessment further emphasizes the preoccupation with symptomatic therapy. It should be appreciated that inhibition of eosinophil accumulation would diminish desquamation of epithelial cells; yet such effects need not necessarily be accompanied by notable changes in lung function, since asthmatic patients whose lung function tests lie within normal ranges are categorized as being in remission yet can have marked impairment of mucociliary clearance (Bateman et al., 1983; Pavia et al., 1985), which may in turn be a reflection of the frank damage to airway epithelium that has been observed in biopsy material from mild asthmatics (Laitinen et al., 1985). Consequently, it may be unrealistic to measure the benefit of prophylactic therapy by ketotifen or cromoglycate by use of conventional indicators. Clinical studies will be required to establish appropriate indicators, but there is already evidence that these drugs have inhibitory actions on eosinophil accumulation (Arnoux et al., 1985; Diaz et al., 1984) plasma protein extravasation (Heilpern and Rebuck, 1972) and allergen-induced retardation of mucociliary clearance (Mezey et al., 1978).

PAF research can be expected to have a considerable impact upon the process whereby prophylactic antiasthma drugs are selected. Prior to the use of PAF, no convenient mechanism for induction of hyperreactivity existed other than exposure of normal animals to drugs such as indomethacin or beta-adrenoceptor antagonists (Morley et al., 1987a). PAF has provided a method for induction of hyperreactivity that depends upon the properties of an endogenous material that is released during allergic responses of animal and humans and hence can be related to clinical asthma. Study of drug effects upon the reaction to PAF has extended this analysis by demonstrating that hyperreactivity of comparable magnitude can result from exposure to catecholamines and related compounds, but by mechanisms distinct from PAF formation or action. This observation establishes that hyperreactivity in allergic and other circumstances may be due to a plurality of mediators so that by analogy with acute bronchospasm, selective antagonists might be poorly effective as inhibitors of allergic hyperreactivity, or even ineffectual when confronted with complex endogenous reactions. These considerations may redirect research effort toward in vivo preparations in laboratory animals, rather than chemically oriented research projects (e.g., antagonism of leukotrienes or PAF).

Induction of protracted hyperreactivity is a property that distinguishes PAF from other mediators and leads to consideration as to whether persisting hyperreactivity depends upon structural changes or is the result of an active process. For example, it can be contested that changes of basal airway dimensions may suffice to account for altered hyperreactivity (Moreno et al., 1986); yet equally it might be presumed that protracted hyperreactivity is secondary to sustained recruitment and activation of eosinophils which could preclude regeneration of airway epithelium. Whether these events contribute to persistent hyperreactivity remains an open issue, but if airway smooth muscle hyperplasia can be shown to follow exposure to PAF, the question must be posed as to whether such long lasting airway hyperreactivity is open to pharmacological intervention. The persistent element of hyperreactivity is poorly documented and hence has been infrequently considered by pharmacologists. Since, a return to normal lung function parameters has been reported to follow a three-year period of therapy which included ketotifen (McDonald et al., 1986), sustained hyperreactivity may represent an active process with a much longer half-life than the exacerbation of hyperreactivity than follows exposure to PAF or allergen.

The search for distinctive properties of prophylactic antiasthma drugs has eliminated certain theories for asthma pathophysiology. Mast cell activation and/or leukotriene generation can now be recognized as too limited to account for asthma pathology. The demise of these ideas has been paralleled by an awareness that activation of eosinophils provides a more plausible basis for asthma pathology and that PAF formation is central to certain patterns of eosinophil behavior. However, selective antagonism of this mediator will be an insufficient approach to therapy since it is evident that this would afford only limited symptoms benefit acutely. On the other hand, it is becoming clear that PAF is likely to account for protracted changes in asthma so that antagonism of PAF may remain an obligatory component of the pharmacological profile of prophylactic antiasthma drugs.

References

Altounyan, R. E. C. (1980). Review of clinical activity and mode of action of sodium cromoglycate. *Clin. Allergy* (Suppl.) *10*:481-489.

American Thoracic Society. (1962). Chronic bronchitis, asthma, and pulmonary emphysema. A statement by the committee on diagnostic standards for nontuberculous respiratory diseases. *Am. Rev. Respir. Dis. 85*:762-768.

Aoki, S., Boubekeur, K., Burrows, L., Morley, J., and Sanjar, S. (1987). Recruitment of eosinophils by platelet activating factor in the lung and peritoneum. *J. Physiol.* Proceedings of the University College of London Meeting (in press).

Arnoux, B., Denjean, A., Page, C. P., Morley, J., and Benveniste, J. (1985). Pulmonary effects of platelet activating factor in a primate are inhibited by ketotifen. *Am. Rev. Respir. Dis. 131*:A2.

Arnoux, B., Simoes-Caeiro, M. H., Landes, A., Mathieu, M., Duroux, P., and Benveniste, J. (1982). Alveolar macrophages from asthmatic patients release platelet activating factor (Paf-acether) and lyso Paf-acether when stimulated with the specific allergen. *Am. Rev. Respir. Dis. 125*:A50.

Barnes, P. J. (1986). Asthma as an axon reflex. *Lancet 1*: 242-244.

Bateman, J. R., Pavia, D., Sheahan, N. F., Agnew, J. E., and Clarke, S. W. (1983). Impaired tracheobronchial clearance in patients with mild stable asthma. *Thorax 38*: 463-467.

Beijer, L., and Rylander, R. (1983). Macrophage and neutrophil production of P.A.F. after exposure to endotoxin. *J. Pharmacol.* (Paris) *14*: 55.

Berti, F., Omini, C., Rossoni, G., and Braquet, P. (1986). Protection by two ginkgolides, BN 52020 and BN 52021 against guinea-pig lung anaphylaxis. *Pharmacol. Res. Commun. 18*: 775-793.

Braquet, P., Etienne, A., Touvay, C., Bourgain, R. H., Lefort, J., and Vargaftig, B. B. (1985). Involvement of platelet activating factor in respiratory anaphylaxis, demonstrated by PAF-acether inhibitor BN 52021. *Lancet i*: 1501.

Bretz, U., Martin, U., Mazzoni, L., and Ney, U. (1983). Beta-adrenergic tachyphylaxis in the rat and its reversal and prevention by ketotifen. *Eur. J. Pharmacol. 86*: 321-328.

Brodde, O. E., Drinkmann, M., Schemuth, R., O'Hara, N., and Daul, A. (1985). Terbutaline-induced desensitisation of human lymphocyte beta2 adrenoceptors. Accelerated restoration of beta-adrenoceptor responsiveness by prednisone and ketotifen. *J. Clin. Invest. 76*: 1096-1101.

Brodgen, R. N., Speight, T. M., and Avery, G. (1974). Sodium cromoglycate (cromolyn sodium): A review of its mode of action, pharmacology therapeutic efficacy and use. *Drugs 7*: 164-269.

Brompton Hospital/Medical Research (1972). Long-term study of disodium cromoglycate in treatment of severe extrinsic or intrinsic bronchial asthma in adults. *Br. Med. J. 4*: 383.

Buckle, D. R. (1984). Disodium cromoglycate and compounds with similar activities. In *Development of Anti-Asthma Drugs.* Edited by D. R. Buckle and H. Smith) London, Butterworths, pp. 261-296.

Butchers, P. R., Fullerton, J. R., Skidmore, I. F., Thompson, L. E., Vardey, C. J., and Wheeldon, A. (1979). A comparison of the anti-anaphylactic activities of salbutamol and disodium cromoglycate in the rat, the rat mast cell and in human lung tissue. *Br. J. Pharmacol. 67*: 23-32.

Camussi, G., Pawlowski, I., Tetta, C., Roffirello, C., Alberton, H., Brentjens, J., and Andres, G. (1983). Acute lung inflammation induced in the rabbit by local instillation of 1-o-octadecyl-2-acetyl-syn-glyceryl-3-phosphorylcholine or of a native platelet activating factor. *Am. J. Pathol. 115*: 78-88.

Capron, M., Kusnierz, J. P., Prin, L., Spiegelberg, H. L., Ovlaque, G., Gosset, P., Tonnel, A. B., and Capron, A. (1985). Cytophilic IgE on human blood and tissue eosinophils: detection by flow microfluorometry. *J. Immunol. 134*: 3013-3018.

Casals-Stenzel, J. (1986). Effects of WEB 2086, a novel antagonist of platelet activating factor, in active and passive anaphylaxis. *Immunopharmacology* (in press).

Chai, H. (1980). Antihistamines and asthma. Do they have a role in therapy? *Chest 78*: 420.

Ciba Guest Symposium. (1959). Terminology, definitions and classifications of chronic pulmonary emphysema and related conditions. *Thorax 14*: 286-299.

Cockcroft, D. W., Ruffin, R. E., Frith, P. A., Cartier, A., Juniper, E. J., Dolovich, J., and Hargreaves, F. E. (1979). Determinants of allergen induced asthma: Dose of allergen, circulating IgE concentrations, and bronchial responsiveness to inhaled histamine. *Am. Rev. Respir. Dis. 120*: 1053-1058.

Colley, D. C. (1973). Eosinophils and immune mechanisms I. Eosinophil stimulation factor (ESP): a lymphokine induced by specific antigen or phytohaemagglutinin. *J. Immunol. 110*: 1419-1429.

Cox, J. S. G. (1967). Disodium cromoglycate (FPL 670) (INTAL). Specific inhibitor of reaginic antibody-antigen mechanisms. *Nature 216*: 1328-1329.

Craps, L. (1980). The prophylaxis of bronchial asthma with ketotifen. Five years of clinical investigations. *Acta Therapeutica 6*: 213-225.

Craps, L. (1985). Immunologic and therapeutic aspects of ketotifen. *J. Allergy Clin. Immunol. 76*: 389-393.

Craps, L. P., Greenwood, C., and Ney, U. M. (1985). Ketotifen and asthma. In *Bronchial Asthma: Mechanisms and Therapeutics.* Edited by E. B. Weiss, M. S. Segal, and M. Stein. Boston, Little, Brown and Co., pp. 734-739.

Cuss, F. M., Dixon, C. M. S., and Barnes, P. J. (1986). Effects of inhaled platelet activating factor on pulmonary function and bronchial responsiveness in man. *Lancet ii*: 189-192.

Delaney, J. C. (1976). The effect of sodium cromoglycate on analgesic-induced asthmatic reactions. *Clin. Allergy 6*: 365-368.

Delaney, J. C. (1983). The effect of ketotifen on aspirin-induced asthmatic reactions. *Clin. Allergy 13*: 247-251.

Dewar, A., Archer, C. B., Paul, W., Page, C. P., MacDonald, D. M., and Morley, J. (1984). Cutaneous and pulmonary histopathological responses to platelet activating factor (Paf-acether) in the guinea-pig. *J. Pathol. 144*: 24-34.

Diaz, P., Galleguillos, F. R., Gonzales, M. C., Pantin, F. C. A., and Kay, A. B. (1984). Bronchoalveolar lavage in asthma: the effect of disodium cromoglycate (cromolyn) on leukocyte counts, immunoglobulins, and complement. *J. Allergy Clin. Immunol. 74*: 41-48.

Eady, R. P., Greenwood, B., Jackson, D. M., Orr, T. S. C., and Wells, E. (1985). The effect of nedocromil sodium and sodium cromoglycate on antigen-induced bronchoconstriction in the *Ascaris*-sensitive monkey. *Br. J. Pharmac. 85*: 323-325.

Fitzgerald, M. F., Lees, I. W., Parente, L., and Payne, A. N. (1987). Exposure to PAF-acether aerosol induces airway hyperreactivity in guinea-pigs. *Br. J. Pharmacol.* (in press).

Girard, J. P., and Cuevas, M. (1977). Anti-asthmatic properties of a new peroral drug (HC 20-511). *Acta Allergologica 32*: 27-34.

Hahn, H. L., Purnama, I., Lang, M., Sannwald, U., and Stenzel, H. (1985). Effects of platelet activating factor on release of mucous from tracheal submucosal glands of the ferret. *Am. Rev. Respir. Dis. 131*: A27.

Handley, D. A., Lee, M. L., and Saunders, R. N. (1983). Extravasation and aortic ultrastructural changes accompanying acute and sub-acute intraperitoneal administration of PAF. Platelet Activating Factor; INSERM symposium No. 23. Edited by J. Benveniste, and B. Arnoux. B. V. Amsterdam, Elsevier Science Publishers, pp. 245-250.

Heilpern, S., and Rebuck, A. S. (1972). Effect of disodium cromoglycate (Intal) on sputum protein composition. *Thorax 27*: 726-728.

Holgate, S. T., Hardy, C., Robinson, C., Agius, R. M., and Howarth, P. H. (1986). The mast cell as a primary effector cell in the pathogenesis of asthma. *J. Allergy Clin. Immunol. 77*: 274-282.

Laitinen, L. A., Heino, M., Laitinen, A., Kava, T., and Haahtela, T. (1985). Damage of the airway epithelium and bronchial reactivity in patients with asthma. *Am. Rev. Respir. Dis. 131*: 599-606.

Lee, T. C., Lenihan, D. J., Malone, B., Roddy, L. L., and Wasserman, S. I. (1984). Increased biosynthesis of platelet activating factor in activated human eosinophils. *J. Biol. Chem. 259*: 5526-5530.

Lellouch-Tubiana, A., Lefort, J., Pirotzky, E., Vargaftig, B. B., and Pfister, A. (1985). Ultrastructural evidence for extravascular platelet recruitment in the lung upon intravenous injection of platelet activating factor (Paf-acether) to guinea-pigs. *Br. J. Exper. Pathol. 66*: 345-356.

Lewis, R. A., and Austen, K. F. (1981). Mediation of local homeostasis and inflammation by leukotrienes and other mast cell-dependent compounds. *Nature 293*: 103-108.

Lowe, D. A., and Richardson, B. P. (1980). The effects of cyproheptadine, ketotifen and sodium nitroprusside on mechanical activity and calcium uptake in guinea-pig taenia coli in vitro. *Prog. Respir. Res. 14*: 134-140.

Martin, U., and Baggiolini, M. (1981). Dissociation between the anti-anaphylactic and the anti-histaminic action of ketotifen. *Arch. Pharmacol. 316*: 186-189.

Martin, U., Greenwood, C., Craps, L., and Baggiolini, M. (1981). Ketotifen. In *Pharmacological and Biochemical Properties of Drug Substances.* Edited by M. E. Goldberg. Washington, D. C. Academy of Pharmaceutical Sciences, Volume 3, p. 424.

Martin, U., and Roemer, D. (1977). Ketotifen, a new type of antianaphylactic agent. *Allergology Immunopathol.* (Suppl) *V*, 5.

Mazzoni, L., Morley, J., Page, C. P., and Sanjar, S. (1985). Induction of hyperreactivity by platelet activating factor in the guinea-pig. *J. Physiol. 365*: 107P.

Mazzoni, L., Morley, J., Page, C. P., and Sanjar, S. (1985). Prophylactic anti-asthma drugs impair the airway hyperreactivity that follows exposure to platelet activating factor (PAF). *Br. J. Pharmacol. 86*: 571P.

Mazzoni, L., Morley, J., Sanjar, S., and Schaeublin, E. (1987). An anomalous interaction between propanolol and isoprenaline. *Br. J. Pharmacol.* Proceedings of the Cambridge Meeting.

McDonald, G. F., Plumley, D. L., and Kobric, M. (1986). Normalisation of pulmonary function in bronchial asthma in response to ketotifen prophylaxis: a three year study. *Immunol. Allergy Prac. 8*: 22-28.

McIntyre, T. M., Zimmerman, G. A., and Prescott, S. M. (1986). Leukotrienes C4 and D4 stimulate human endothelial cells to synthesize platelet-activating factor and bind neutrophils. Proceedings of the National Academy of Sciences of the United States of America 83: 2204-2208.

Medieros, M. C., Lefort, J., Joseph, D., and Vargaftig, B. B. (1983). Interferance de l'aminophylline et du dipyridamol avec les effets plaquettaires in vitro et bronchoconstricteurs in vivo du paf-acether chez le cobaye. *J. Pharmacol.* (Paris) *14*: 98.

Metzger, W. J., Sjoerdsma, K., Richerson, H. B., Moseley, P., Zavala, D., Monick, M., and Hunninghake, G. W. (1987). Platelets in bronchoalveolar lavage from asthmatic patients and allergic rabbits with allergen-induced late phase responses. *Agents Actions* (Suppl) (in press).

Mezey, R. J., Cohen, M. A., Fernandez, R. J., Januszkiewicz, A. J., and Wanner, A. (1978). Mucociliary transport in allergic patients with antigen-induced bronchospasm. *Am. Rev. Respir. Dis. 118*: 677-684.

Moreno, R. H., Hogg, J. C., and Pare, P. D. (1986). Mechanics of airway narrowing. *Am. Rev. Respir. Dis. 133*: 1171-1180.

Morley, J., (1981). Role of prostaglandins secreted by macrophages in the inflammatory process. *Lymphokines 4*: 377-394.

Morley, J. (1986). Cromoglicate and Asthma. *Trends Pharmaceutical Sci. 7*: 132-133.

Morley, J., Mazzoni, L., and Sanjar, S. (1987a). Pharmacology of airway hyperreactivity in animals. In *PAF and Asthma.* Edited by J. Morley, and G. Holme. London, Academic Press, (in press).

Morley, J., Mazzoni, L., and Sanjar, S. (1987b). Pharmacology of airway hyperreactivity in animals. In *PAF and Asthma.* Edited by J. Morley, and G. Holme. London, Academic Press, (in press).

Morley, J., Page, C. P., Mazzoni, L., and Sanjar, S. (1985). Anti-allergic drugs in asthma. *Triangle 24*: 59-70.

Morley, J., Page, C. P., and Paul, W. (1983). Inflammatory actions of platelet activating factor (Paf-acether) in guinea-pig skin. *Br. J. Pharmacol. 80*: 503-509.

Morley, J., Page, C. P., and Sanjar, S. (1985). Platelets in asthma. *Lancet ii*: 726-727.

Morley, J., Sanjar, S., and Doran, J. (1987c). The role of arachidonate metabolites in the response of guinea-pig airways to platelet activating factor (PAF). *Agents Actions* (Suppl) in press.

Morley, J., and Williams, T. J. (1971). Increased vascular permeability in allergic inflammation. *J. Physiol. 222*: 95-97P.

Muller, W., and Von Der Hardt, H. (1985). Medikamentoese Langzeittherapie des Asthma bronchiale im Kindesalter. *Monatsschrift Kinderheilkd 133*: 882-886.

Nizankowska, E. (1987). Pharmacological attempts to modulate leukotriene synthesis in aspirin-induced asthma. *Agents Actions* (Suppl) (in press).

O'Flaherty, J. T. (1982). Lipid mediators of inflammation and allergy. *Lab. Invest. 47*: 314-329.

Page, C. P., Archer, C. B., Paul, W., and Morley, J. (1984). Paf-acether: a mediator of inflammation and asthma. *Trends Pharmacol. Sci. 5*: 239-241.

Page, C. P., Tomiak, R. H. H., Sanjar, S., and Morley, J. (1985). Suppression of Paf-acether responses: an anti-inflammatory effect of anti-asthma drugs. *Agents Actions 16*: 33-35.

Pavia, D., Bateman, J. R. M., Sheahan, N. F., Agnew, J. E., and Clarke, S. W. (1985). Tracheobronchial mucociliary clearance in asthma: impairment during remission. *Thorax 40*: 171-175.

Pepys, J., Hargreave, F. E., Chan, M., and McCarthy, D. S. (1968). Inhibitory effects of disodium cromoglycate on allergen-inhalation tests. *Lancet ii*: 134-137.

Piper, P. J. (Ed). (1980). *SRS-A and Leukotrienes.* Chichester, Wiley.

Pirotzky, E., Page, C. P., Roubin, R., Pfifster, A., Paul, W., Bonnet, J., and Benveniste, J. (1984). Paf-acether-induced plasma exudation in rat skin is independent of platelets and neutrophils. *Microcirculation Endothelium Lymphatics 1*: 107-122.

Platts-Mills, T. A. E., Tovey, E. R., Mitchell, E. B., Moszoro, H., Nock, P., and Wilkins, S. R. (1982). Reduction of bronchial hyperreactivity during prolonged allergen avoidance. *Lancet ii*: 675-678.

Reed, C. E. (1986). New therapeutic approaches in asthma. *J. Allergy Clin. Immunol. 77*: 537-543.

Richards, D. M., Brodgen, R. N., Heel, R. C., Speight, T. M., and Avery, G. S. (1984). Oxatomide: A review of its pharmacodynamic properties, and therapeutic efficacy. *Drugs 27*: 210-231.

Ross, W. J., Harrison, R. G., Jolly, M. R. J., Neville, M. C., Todd, A., Verge, J. P., Dawson, W., and Sweatman, W. J. F. (1979). Antianaphylactic agents, 1,2-(acylamino) oxazoles. *J. Med. Chem. 22*: 412.

Sheard, P., Killingback, P. G., and Blair, A. M. J. N. (1967). Antigen induced release of histamine and SRS-A from human lung passively sensitized with reaginic serum. *Nature 216*: 283-284.

Snyder, F. (1985). Chemical and biochemical aspects of platelet activating factor: A novel class of acetylated ether-linked choline-phospholipids. *Med. Res. Rev. 5*: 107-140.

Stimler-Gerard, N. P. (1986). Parasympathetic stimulation as a mechanism for platelet activating factor-induced contractile responses in the lung. *J. Pharmacol. Exp. Ther. 237*: 209-213.

Stokes, T. C., and Darbyshire, J. (1981). A controlled trial of oxatomide in the treatment of asthma with or without perennial rhinitis. *Clin. Allergy 11*: 483-490.

Stokes, T. C., and Morley, J. (1981). Prospects for an oral Intal. *Br. J. Dis. Chest 75*: 1-14.

Szentivanyi, A. (1980). The beta-adrenergic theory of the atopic abnormality in bronchial asthma. *J. Allergy 42*: 203-232.

Vargaftig, B. B., Lefort, J., Chingard, M., and Benveniste, J. (1980). Platelet-activating factor induces a platelet dependent bronchoconstriction unrelated to the formation of prostaglandin derivatives. *Eur. J. Pharmacol. 65*: 185-192.

Voelkel, N. F., Worthen, S., Reeves, J. T., Henson, P. M., and Murphy, R. C. (1982). Non-immunological production of leukotrienes induced by platelet activating factor. *Science 218*: 286-288.

Appendix

H. WILLIAM KELLY and SHIRLEY MURPHY

University of New Mexico
School of Medicine
Albuquerque, New Mexico

JOHN W. JENNE

Loyola-Stritch School of Medicine
Maywood, and Edward Hines, Jr.
Veterans Administration Hospital
Hines, Illinois

I. Structure of Compounds

I. BETA—ADRENERGIC AGONISTS

Epinephrine/Adrenaline

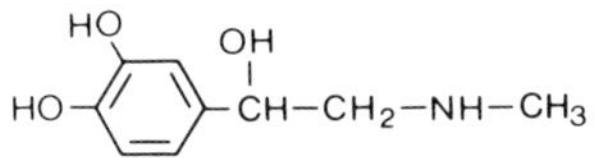

Ephedrine

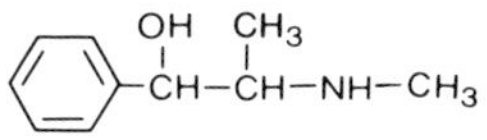

Isoproterenol/Isoprenaline

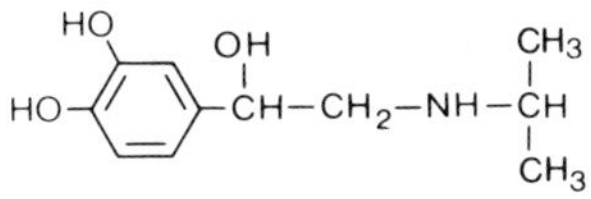

Isoetharine

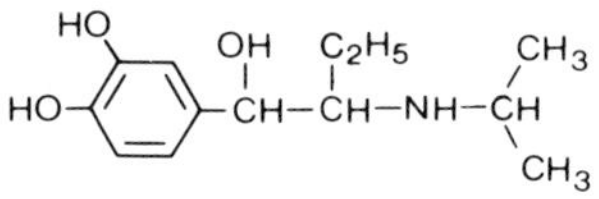

Metaproterenol/Orciprenaline

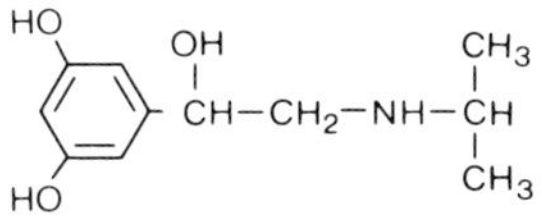

Rimiterol

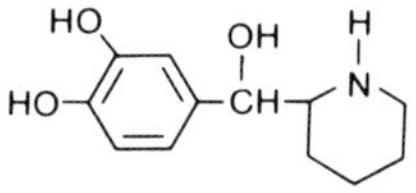

Albuterol / Salbutamol

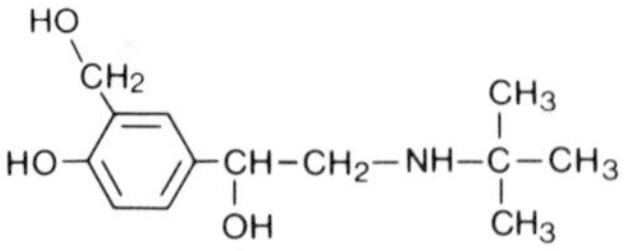

Terbutaline

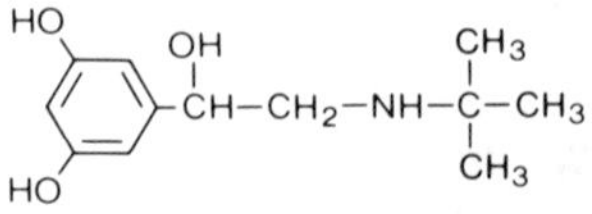

Fenoterol

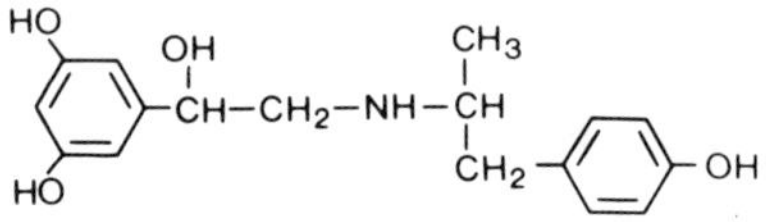

Pirbuterol

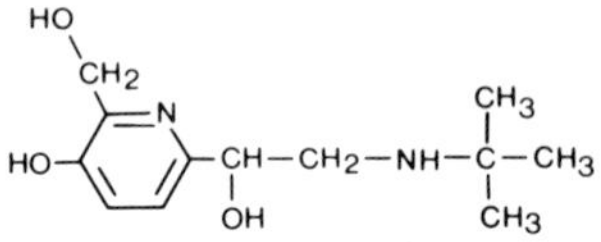

Bitolterol

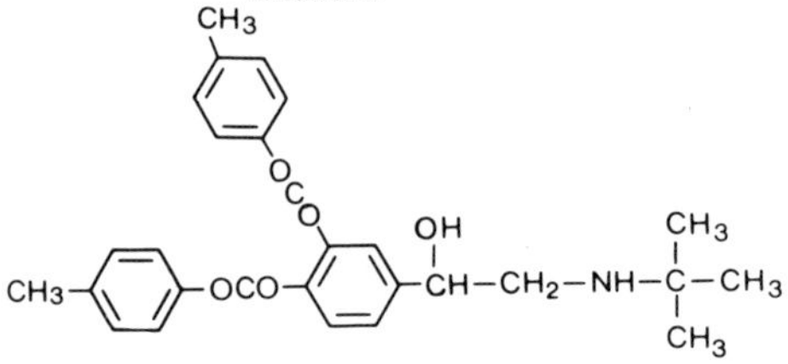

esterase hydrolysis

Colterol

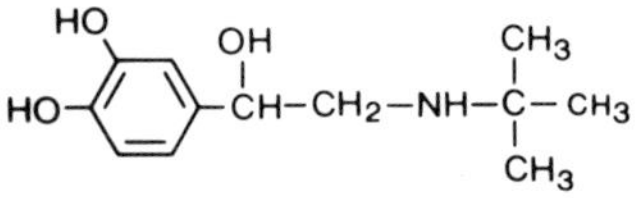

Reproterol

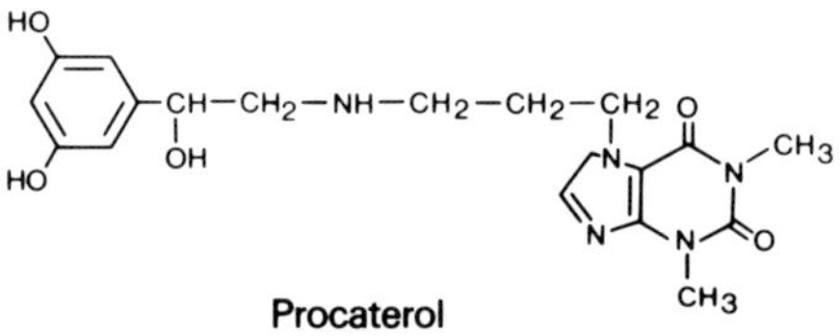

Procaterol

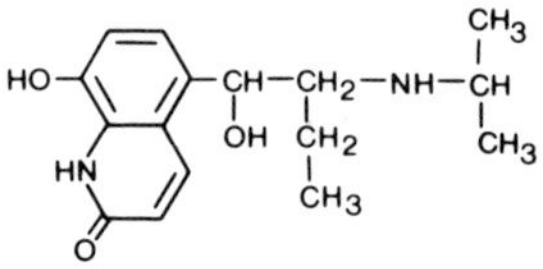

II. XANTHINES:

Theophylline

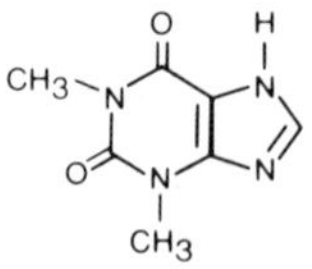

Caffeine

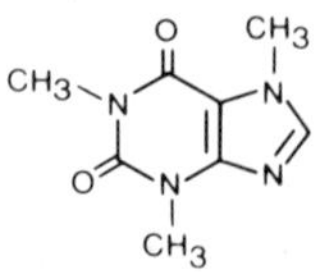

Theobromine

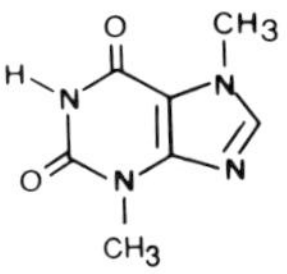

Enprofylline

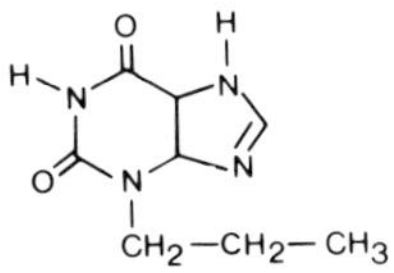

Dyphylline

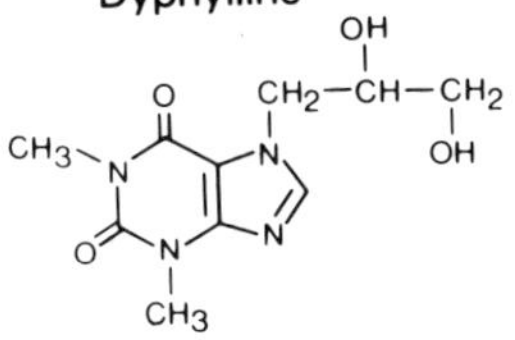

Proxphylline

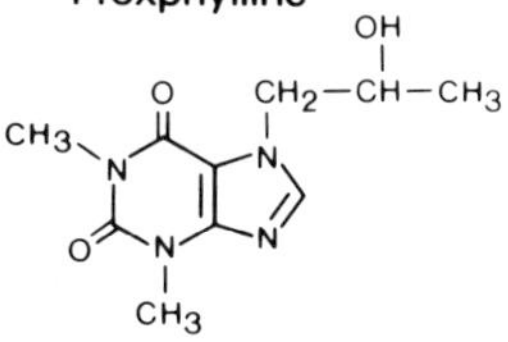

III. ANTICHOLINERGICS

Atropine

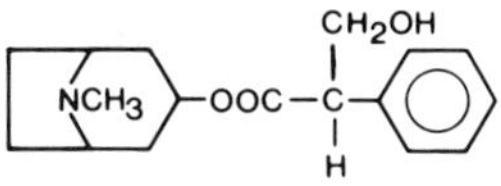

Atropine Methonitrate

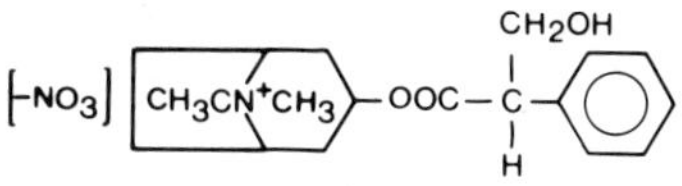

Ipratropium Bromide

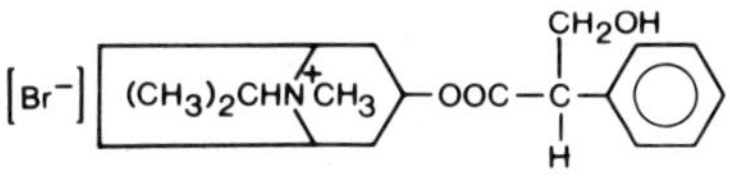

IV. Cromolyn

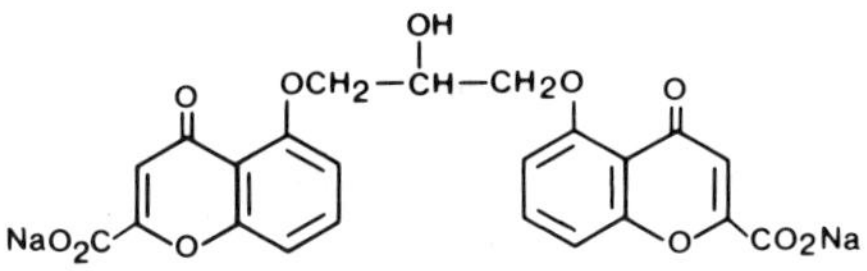

V. CORTICOSTEROIDS:

Hydrocortisone

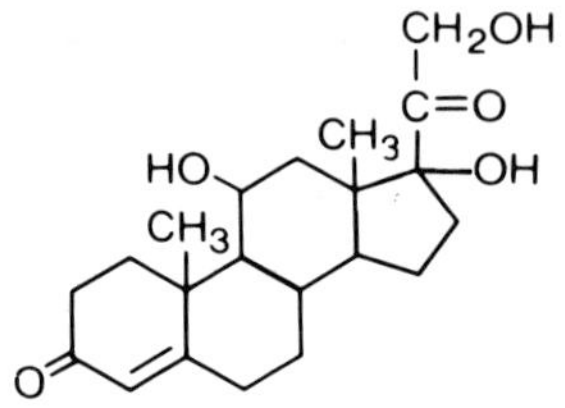

Prednisone

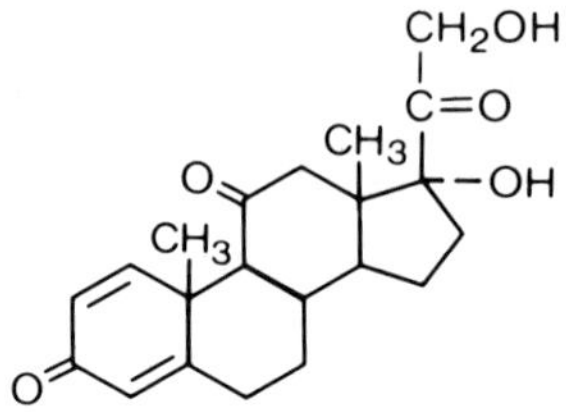

Methylprednisolone

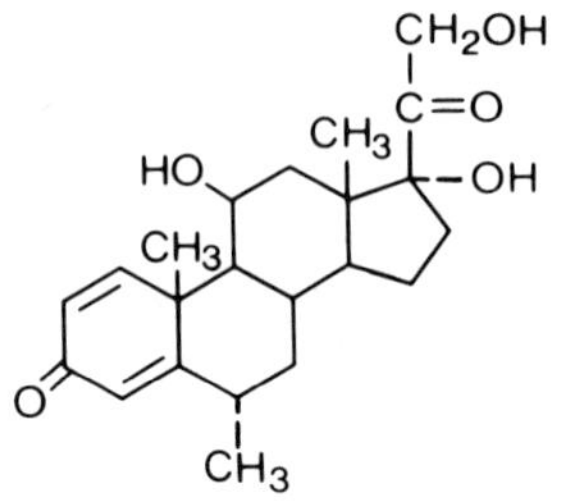

Beclomethasone Dipropionate

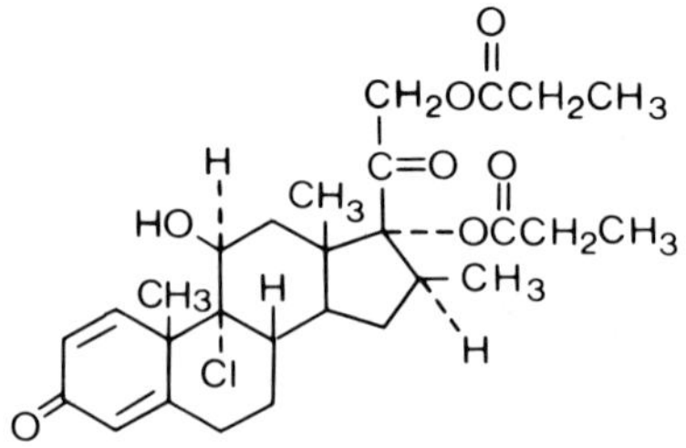

Triamcinolone Acetonide

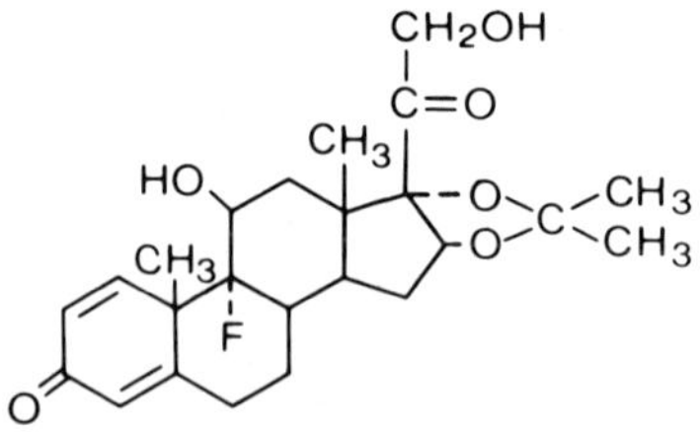

Flunisolide

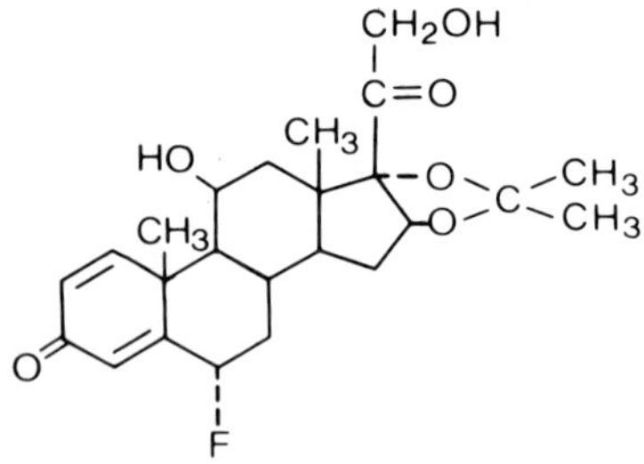

Betamethasone Valerate

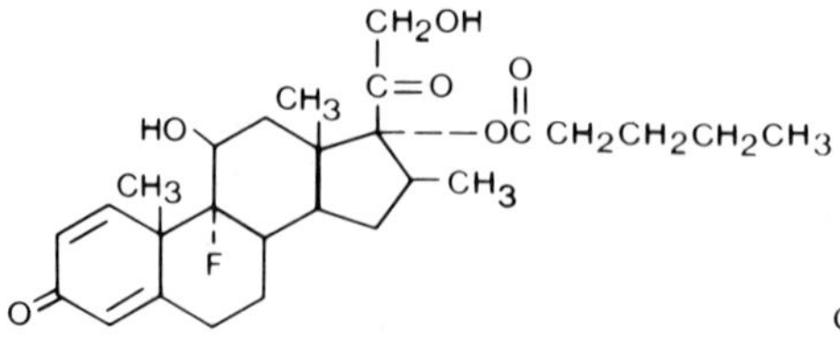

Budesonide

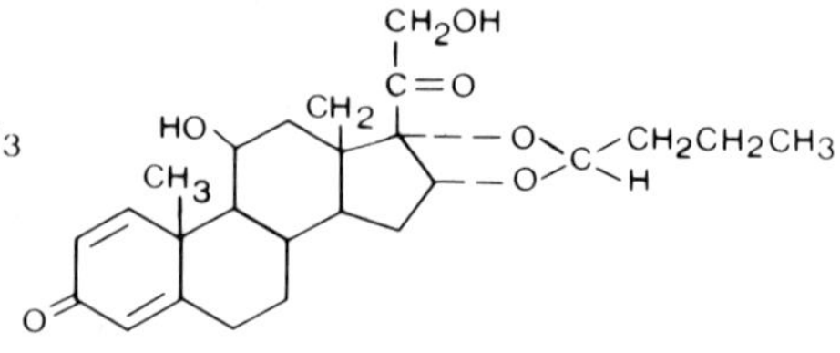

II. Preparations Available in the United States with Dosing Range

A. Beta-Adrenergic Agonists

Product/manufacturer	Available form	Dosages: Pediatrics	Dosages: Adults
Oral:			
Ephedrine sulfate Various manufacturers,	25 and 50 mg tablets and capsules; 11 mg/ 5 ml and 20 mg/5 ml syrups	2-3 mg/kg daily in 4-6 doses	25-50 mg every 3-4 hours
Ectasule, Fleming	15, 30, 60 mg	every 6-8 hr	every 6-8 hrs
Albuterol Ventolin, Glaxo Proventil, Schering	2 and 4 mg tablets 2 mg/5 ml syrup sugar free	0.1-0.2 mg/kg every 6-8 hrs	2-4 mg every 6-8 hrs, may increase as tolerated
Metaproterenol Alupent, Boehringer Metaprel, Dorsey	10 and 20 mg tablets, 10 mg/5 ml syrup sugar free	0.5 mg/kg every 4-6 hours increase by 0.25 mg/kg as tolerated	20 mg every 4-6 hrs, increase as tolerated
Terbutaline Brethine, Geigy Bricanyl, Merrell Dow	2.5 and 5.0 mg tablets	0.075 mg/kg every 6 hrs, may increase by 0.025 mg/kg as tolerated	5 mg every 6-8 hrs, may increase as tolerated
Aerosol:			
Epinephrine HCl	1% (1:100) solution for nebulization; 2.25% racemic epinephrine	0.03 ml (0.3 mg) of solution every 2 hrs	0.03 ml (0.3 mg) every 2 hrs
Primatene Mist, Whitehall Bronkaid Mist, Winthrop	200 μg/spray 270 μg/spray	Not recommended	1-2 sprays every 2 hrs as needed
Epinephrine bitartrate Medihaler Epi, Riker AsthmaHaler, Norcliff Thayer	160 μg/puff	Not recommended	1-2 puffs every 2 hrs as needed
Isoproterenol HCl and sulfate, various manufacturers	Solutions 0.25% (1:400) 2.5 mg/ml 0.50% (1:200) 5 mg/ml 1.0% (1:100) 10 mg/ml	0.05-0.1 mg/kg every 2-4 hrs	1-2 inhalations of 0.25% solution by hand bulb nebulizer 2.5 ml of a 0.05% solution via compressor-driven nebulizer

Product/manufacturer	Available form	Dosages: Pediatrics	Dosages: Adults
Isoproterenol (continued)			
Isuprel Mistometer, Breon	131 μg/spray	1-2 inhalations every 4-6 hrs	1-2 sprays every 2-4 hrs as needed
Norisodrine Aerotrol, Abbott	120 μg/spray		
Medihaler-Iso, Riker	80 μg/spray		
Norisodrine sulfate	45 μg/spray		
Aerohaler, Abbott	110 μg/spray		
Isoetharine			
Isoetharine HCl Inhalation, Roxane	0.1%, 0.125%, 0.2%	0.1-0.2 mg/kg every 2-4 hrs	3-5 mg undiluted via nebulizer on O_2 at 4-6 L/min over 15-20 min
Bronkosol unit dose, Various	0.25% 0.5%, 1%		0.5 and 1% solutions diluted 1:3 with 0.9% sodium chloride
Bronkometer, Breon	340 μg/spray	1-2 puffs every 4-6 hrs, may increase to every hour for acute attacks	1-2 puffs every 4-6 hours may increase to every 1-2 hours for acute attacks
Metaproterenol Alupent, Boehringer Ingelheim Metaprel, Dorsey	5% (50 mg/ml) solution for nebulization 0.6% unit dose vial of 2.5 ml (15 mg)	0.25-0.5 mg/kg every 2-4 hrs maximum 15 mg	5-15 inhalations of 5% undiluted from hand bulb nebulizer. Or 0.3 ml of 5% diluted with 2.5 ml 0.9% sodium chloride in nebulizer every 2-4 hrs
Metered dose inhalers (MDI)	0.65 mg/puff 300 puffs, powder suspension	1-2 puffs every 4-6 hrs and prior to exercise	2-3 puffs every 4-6 hrs and prior to exercise
Albuterol			
Ventolin, Glaxo Proventil, Schering	90 μg/puff 200 puffs powder suspension	1-2 puffs every 4-6 hrs and prior to exercise	1-2 puffs every 4-6 hrs and prior to exercise
	0.5% (5 mg/ml) solution for nebulization	0.05-0.15 mg/kg every 2-6 hrs as needed	2-5 mg every 2-6 hrs as needed
Terbutaline			
Brethaire, Geigy Inhaler	0.2 mg/puff powder suspension 300 puffs	1-2 puffs every 4-6 hrs and prior to exercise	1-2 puffs every 4-6 hrs and prior to exercise

Product/manufacturer	Available form	Dosages: Pediatrics	Dosages: Adults
Terbutaline (continued)			
Brethine, Geigy Bricanyl, Merrell Dow	0.1% (1 mg/ml) solution in 0.9% sodium chloride for injection (not approved for this use)	0.1-0.3 mg/kg every 2-6 hrs as needed	5-7 mg (5-7 ml) undiluted every 4-6 hrs as needed
Bitolterol mesylate Tornalate, Breon	0.37 mg/spray 300 sprays, solution	1-2 puffs every 4-6 hrs	1-3 puffs every 4-6 hrs
Fenoterol HBR Berotec, MDI, Boehringer Ingelheim	0.16 mg/puff, powder suspension, 300 puffs	1-2 puffs every 4-6 hrs	1-2 puffs every 4-6 hrs
Parenteral:			
Epinephrine HCl Various manufacturers	1:1000 (1 mg/ml)	0.01 mg/kg or 0.3 mg/m^2 subcutaneously up to 0.5 mg every 20 min for 3 doses	0.3 to 0.5 mg subcutaneously every 20 min for 3 doses for acute attacks
Sustained action Susphrine, Berlex	1:200 (5 mg/ml)	0.005-0.01 ml/kg not to exceed .15 ml every 6-10 hrs subcutaneously	0.5-0.75 mg (0.1-0.15 ml) subcutaneously every 6-10 hrs
Isoproterenol	1:5000 (0.2 mg/ml)	0.1 μg/kg/min increase at 15 min intervals as necessary or heart rate not greater than 180-200/min	0.08-1.7 μg/kg/min as necessary for response
Terbutaline	1 mg/ml in 0.9% sodium chloride 1 ml/vial	0.01 mg/kg (0.01 ml/kg) up to 0.25 mg every 2-6 hrs as needed	0.25-0.5 mg every 2-6 hrs as necessary

B. Theophylline Preparations

	Theophylline content	Dosing interval: Pediatric	Dosing interval: Adult
Liquids			
Elixophyllin (20% alcohol)	5.3 mg/ml (80 mg/15 ml)	q 4-6 h	q 6-8 h
Bronkodyl (20% alcohol)	5.3 mg/ml	q 4-6 h	q 6-8 h
Slophyllin 80 Syrup, Rorer	5.3 mg/ml (sugar free)	q 4-6 h	q 6-8 h
Choledyl Pediatric Syrup, Parke-Davis	6.4 mg/ml	q 4-6 h	q 6-8 h
Theolair, Riker	5.3 mg/ml	q 4-6 h	q 6-8 h
Theophyl 225, McNeil	7.5 mg/ml (5% alcohol)	q 4-6 h	q 6-8 h
Accurbron, Merrel Dow	10 mg/ml (7.5% alcohol)	q 4-6 h	q 6-8 h
Aerolate, Fleming	10.7 mg/ml (sugar free)	q 4-6 h	q 6-8 h

	Theophylline content	Dosing interval Pediatrics	Adults
Liquids (continued)			
Somophyllin, Fisons	18 mg/ml (sugar free)	q 4-6 h	q 6-8 h
Lixaminol, Ferndale	13.1 mg/ml (20% alcohol)	q 4-6 h	q 6-8 h
Rapid Release Tablets:			
Theophylline, various manufacturers	100, 200 mg	q 4-6 h	q 6-8 h
Aminophylline, various manufacturers	78.9, 157.8 mg	q 4-6 h	q 6-8 h
Theolair, Riker	125 mg	q 4-6 h	q 6-8 h
Theophyl-225	225 mg	q 4-6 h	q 6-8 h
Theophyl Chewable	100 mg	q 4-6 h	q 6-8 h
Quibron-T Dividose, Mead Johnson	300 mg	q 4-6 h	q 6-8 h
Choledyl, Parke-Davis, enteric coated	64, 127 mg	q 4-6 h	q 6-8 h
Sustained Release Tablets			
Phyllocontin, Purdue-Federick	178 mg	q 8 h	q 12 h
Aminodur Duratabs, Berlex	240 mg (scored)	q 8 h	q 12 h
Theo-Time, Major	100, 200, 300 mg	q 8 h	q 12 h
Duraphyl, McNeil	100, 200, 300 mg (scored)	q 8 h	q 8-12 h
Constant-T, Geigy	200, 300 mg (scored)	q 8 h	q 12 h
Choledyl SA, Warner Lambert	256, 364 mg	q 8 h	q 12 h
LaBID, Norwich-Eaton	250 mg (scored)	q 6-8 h	q 8-12 h
Theolair-SR, Riker	250, 500 mg (scored)	q 8 h	q 12 h
Respbid, Boehringer Ingelheim	250, 500 mg (scored)	q 8 h	q 12 h
Theochron, Forest	300 mg	q 8 h	q 12 h
Quibron-T/SR, Mead Johnson	300 mg (multiscored)	q 8-12 h	q 12 h
Sustaire, Roerig	100, 300 mg (scored)	q 12 h	q 12 h
TheoDur, Key	100, 200, 300 mg (scored)	q 12 h	q 12-24 h
Uniphyl, Purdue-Federick	200, 400 mg (scored)		q 12-24 h
Sustained Release Capsules:			
Somophyllin-CRT, Fisons	100, 200, 250, 300 mg	q 8 h	q 12 h
Aerolate, Fleming	65, 130, 260 mg	q 8 h	q 12 h
Slophyllin Gyrocaps, Rorer	60, 125, 250 mg	q 8 h	q 8-12 h
Theophyl-SR, McNeil	125, 250 mg	q 8 h	q 8-12 h
Physpan, Savage	130, 260 mg	q 6-8 h	q 8-12 h
Theoclear LA, Central	130, 260 mg	q 6-8 h	q 8-12 h
Theospan, Laser	130, 260 mg	q 6-8 h	q 8-12 h
Bronkodyl S-R, Breon	300 mg	q 8 h	q 8-12 h
Elixophyllin-SR, Berlex	125, 250 mg	q 8 h	q 8-12 h
Theobid, Glaxo	130, 260 mg	q 8 h	q 12 h
Theovent, Schering	125, 250 mg	q 8 h	q 12 h
Theobron, Upsher-Smith	125, 250 mg	q 8 h	q 12 h
TheoDur Sprinkle, Key	50, 75, 125, 200 mg	q 8-12 h	q 12 h
Slo-Bid Gyrocaps, Rorer	50, 100, 200, 300 mg	q 12 h	q 12 h
Theo-24, Searle	100, 200, 300 mg	q 12 h	q 12-24 h
Rectal:			
Somophyllin, Fisons	51.4 mg/ml	q 6 h	q 6-8 h
Aminophylline suppositories, various manufacturers	125, 250 mg	q 6 h	q 6-8 h

	Theophylline content	Dosing interval: Pediatrics	Adults
Parenteral:			
Aminophylline (25 mg/ml), various manufacturers	20 mg/ml	q 6 h or constant infusions	q 6-8 h
Theophylline and 5% dextrose, Travenol	200 mg/50 and 100 ml 400 mg/100, 250, 500, and 1000 ml 8000 mg/500 and 1000 ml		

C. Dyphilline

		Dosing interval: Pediatric	Adult
Liquid			
Lufyllin Elixer, Wallace	33 mg/5 ml (20% alcohol)	q 6 h	q 6 h
Dilor, Savage	53 mg/5 ml (18% alcohol)	q 6 h	q 6 h
Neothylline, Lemmon	53 mg/5 ml (18% alcohol)	q 6 h	q 6 h
Droxine, Shear-Kershman	100 mg/5 ml (sugar free)	q 6 h	q 6 h
Tablets:			
Dilor, Savage	200, 400 mg (scored)	q 6 h	q 6 h
Dyflex, EconoMed	200, 400 mg (scored)	q 6 h	q 6 h
Lufyllin, Wallace	200, 400 mg	q 6 h	q 6 h
Neothylline, Lemmon	200, 400 mg	q 6 h	q 6 h
Sustained Release Tablets:			
Airlet LA, Norwich Eaton	400 mg (scored)		q 8 h
Droxine LA, Shear-Kershman	400 mg (dye free)		q 8 h
Parenteral:			
Various manufacturers	250 mg/ml (intramuscular)		q 6 h

D. Anticholinergics

		Dosage: Pediatric	Adult
Atropine Sulfate			
Dey-Dose Atropine Sulfate, Dey	0.2% (1 mg), 0.5% (2.5 mg) in 0.5 ml unit dose	0.05-0.075 mg/kg every 6 hr; in 2-3 ml of 0.9% sodium by nebulizer	0.025-0.05 mg/kg every 6 hrs
Atropine Sulfate Ophthalmic, various manufacturers	0.5% (5 mg/ml) 1.0% (10 mg/ml) without methylcellulose	0.05-0.075 mg/kg every 6 hrs	0.025-0.05 mg/kg every 6 hrs
Ipratropium bromide			
Atrovent, Boehringer Ingelheim	20 μg/puff (18 μg reaches patient), 300 puffs/inhaler 0.025% solution	1-2 puffs every 4-6 hrs 250 μg every 6 hrs every 4-6 hrs	2-3 puffs every 4-6 hrs 250 μg-500 μg every 4-6 hrs

E. Cromolyn Sodium

		Dosage: Pediatrics	Dosage: Adults
Cromolyn NA Intal, Fisons	20 mg/capsule for Spinhaler, contains 20 mg lactose	1 capsule 4 times daily initially then reduce as tolerated	1-2 capsules 4 times daily
Intal Nebulizer Solution, Fisons	20 mg/2 ml ampule	1 ampule via power-driven nebulizer 3 to 4 times daily (hand nebulizers are not adequate)	1 ampule 4 times daily
Intal Inhaler, Fisons	800 μg/puff 112 puffs 200 puffs	2 puffs 4 times daily and prior to exercise	2 puffs 4 times daily and prior to exercise

F. Corticosteroids

		Dosage: Pediatrics	Dosage: Adults
Oral:			
Prednisone, USP Various manufacturers	1-50 mg	0.5-2 mg/kg/day or every other day	10-50 mg/day or every other day
Prednisolone, USP	1, 2.5.5 mg	0.5-2 mg/kg/day or every other day	10-50 mg/day or every other day
Parenteral:			
Cortisol Solu-Cortef, Upjohn	100, 250, 500 mg, 1 g sodium succinate powder	4-6 mg/kg every 4-6 hrs until response then 4 mg/kg/day	4 mg/kg every 4-6 hrs until response then 4 mg/kg/day
Methylprednisolone Solu-Medrol, Upjohn	40, 125, 500 mg, 1 g sodium succinate powder	1-2 mg/kg every 4-6 hrs until response then 1-2 mg/kg/day	1-2 mg/kg every 4-6 hrs until response then 1 mg/kg/day
Aerosol:			
Beclomethasone dipropionate Beclovent, Glaxo Vanceril, Schering	42 μg/puff powder suspension, 200 doses/cannister	1-2 puffs 3-4 times daily	2 puffs 3-4 times daily
Dexamethasone Decadron Respihaler, MSD	84 μg/puff, 170 puffs/cannister	2 puffs every 6-8 hours *(Not recommended)*	3 puffs every 6-8 hrs *(Not recommended)*

		Dosage	
		Pediatrics	Adults
Triamcinolone Acetonide Azmacort, Rorer	100 μg/puff, 240 puffs/inhaler powdered suspension	1-2 puffs every 6-8 hrs	2 puffs every 6-8
Flunisolide AeroBid, Key	250 μg/puff, 100 puffs/inhaler	1-2 puffs twice daily	2 puffs twice daily

H. Ketotifen

		Dosage	
		Pediatrics	Adults
Oral:			
Sandoz Zaditen, Zasten	1 mg capsules (not available in U.S.)	1 mg p.o. bid	1 mg p.o. bid

I. Antiasthmatic Preparations Containing Sulfites

Epinephrine	Adrenaline, Parke-Davis Ana-Kit, Hollister-Stier Epi-Pen, Center Micronefrin, Bird (aerosol)
Isoetharine HCl	Bronkosol, Breon Dispos-a-Med, Parke-Davis Isoetharine HCl, Roxane
Isoproterenol	Isuprel, Breon Dispos-a-Med, Parke-Davis
Metaproterenol	Alupent Syrup, Boehringer-Ingelheim Metaprel Syrup, Dorsey Alupent-5% solution, Boehringer-Ingelheim Metaprel-5% solution, Dorsey
Hydrocortisone	Hydrocortone-inj., MSD Hydrocortone Acetate-inj., MSD
Dexamethasone	Decadron LA-inj., MSD Decadron-inj., MSD Dexon LA-inj., Kay
Prednisolone	Hydeltrasol-inj., MSD

Devices for Maximizing Aerosol Delivery, Available in the United States

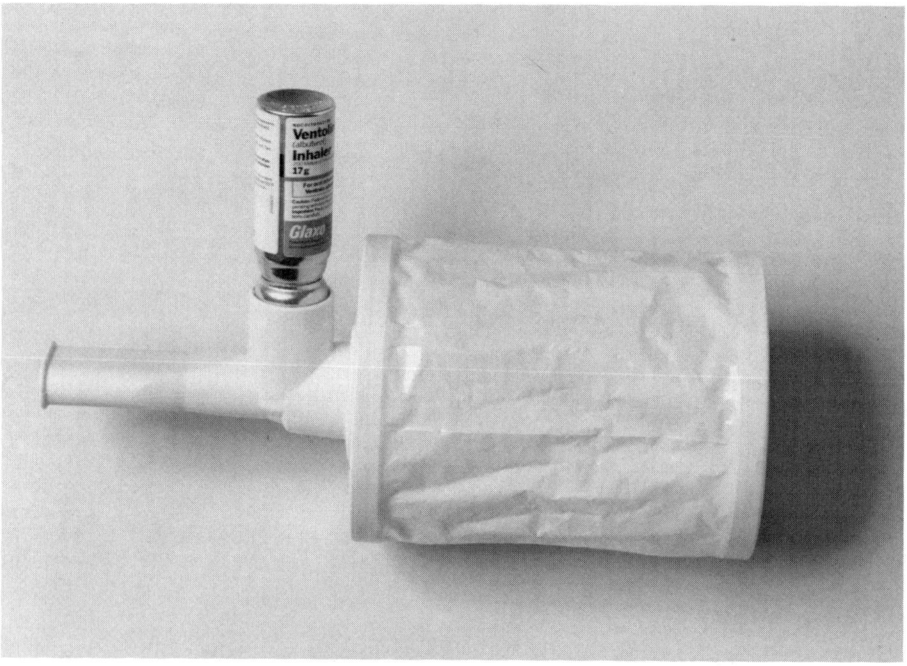

(a)

Figure 1 (a) Inspirease (Key Pharmaceuticals, Inc.). A collapsable bag with a flow indicator whistle. (b) Inhalaid (Key Pharmaceuticals, Inc.). A plastic spherical chamber with a flowmeter and one-way valve. (c) Brethancer (Geigy Pharmaceuticals), 10 cm open-ended telescopic tube. The Aerochamber (Monaghan Medical Co.), a cylinder with a one-way baffle, is not shown.

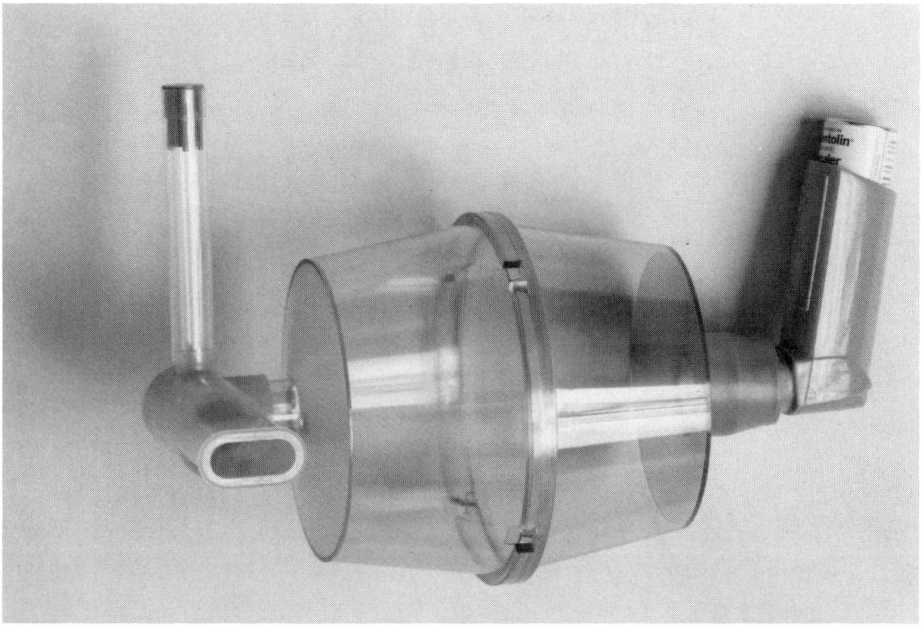

(b)

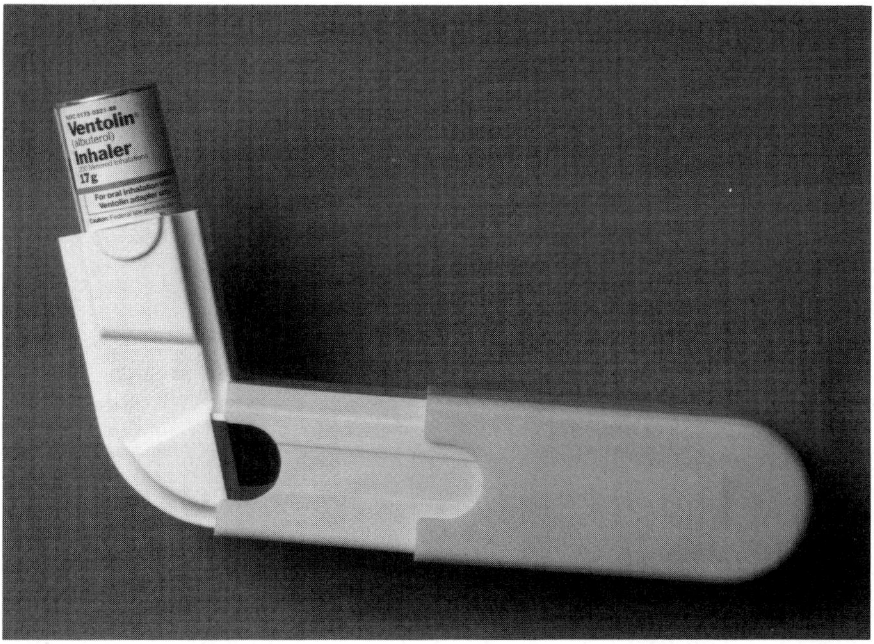

(c)

III. Theophylline Dosing Schedules

A. Pediatric Theophylline Dosing Recommendations

The following theophylline dosage recommendations have been in use at the University of New Mexico Pediatric Pulmonary Center for the past 6 years. Any dosage recommendations must be accompanied by the following caveat: These recommendations are based on the average clearance values reported in the literature for the various age groups. The user should be aware that the theophylline clearance within any age group frequently varies greater than twofold. As a result, serum theophylline concentration monitoring should accompany any dosage recommendations or adjustments.

With this general warning comes this brief explanation of our dosing recommendations. The recommendations are based on the pharmacokinetic variables for theophylline in children and are aimed at achieving mean steady-state theophylline concentrations of *15 μg/ml.* If the clinician is not in a situation with readily available serum theophylline level determinations (s)he may want to use lower dosages that would provide a larger margin of safety. The doses are based on the following relationships:

$$Cp^{o} = D/Vd$$

$$Cpss = D/Cl \cdot \tau$$

Where Cp^{o} is the increase in plasma concentration following a single dose (D) and Vd is the apparent volume of distribution of theophylline, Cpss is the steady-state plasma concentration achieved following continuous administration of a given dose (D) at any given dosing interval (τ). For continuous infusions D/τ = Infusion rate. Cl is the clearance.

Acute Severe Asthma

Loading Dose

Loading doses are used to obtain a desired plasma concentration quickly. A loading dose may be administered intravenously or orally. The apparent volume of distribution of theophylline ranges from 0.3 to 0.7 L/kg with a mean of 0.45 L/kg in children and 0.5 L/kg in adults. The distribution volume is greater in neonates (0.69-0.91 L/kg). Theophylline is 55-70% protein bound in adults and children. For convenience, one can use an apparent Vd for all patients of 0.5 L/kg. This predicts that any 1 mg/kg dose will give an approximate increase in plasma concentration of 2 μg/ml (2 μg/ml = 1 mg/kg ÷ 0.5 L/kg). Therefore one can easily estimate the loading dose required to achieve any given increase in plasma concentration required. The following are general loading dose recommendations when the current theophylline concentration is unknown.

Category	IV Dose (Based on aminophylline which contains 80% anhydrous theophylline) Give intravenous loading doses over 20 minutes	Oral Dose (Based on 100% anhydrous theophylline with complete bioavailability)
Neonates	5-6 mg/kg	4-5 mg/kg
Children and Adults		
No previous theophylline	9 mg/kg	7.5 mg/kg
Previous theophylline[a]		
> 6 hours	6 mg/kg	5 mg/kg
< 6 hours	3 mg/kg	2.5 mg/kg
Previous sustained-release[a]		
> 12 hours	6 mg/kg	5 mg/kg
< 12 hours	3 mg/kg	2.5 mg/kg

[a]It is recommended that any patient with a history of previous theophylline administration have blood drawn for a serum theophylline level determination.

Intravenous Infusion Rates for Acute Severe Asthma

The infusion rates are based on the amount of intravenous aminophylline (80% theophylline) required to achieve a steady-state theophylline concentration of 15 μg/ml.

Category	Mean Clearance (L/hr/kg)	Infusion Rate (mg/kg/hr)
1-6 mo[a]	0.033	0.5
6 mo-1 yr	0.067	1.0
1-9 yrs	0.094	1.5
10-16 yrs	0.077	1.2

[a]This age range has the widest interpatient variability and is based on the fewest number of patients. Caution is advised for this age group.

Due to the frequent occurrence of apparent nonlinear (saturation) pharmacokinetics in children, dosage adjustments are not made in a linear fashion. The authors empirically increase the infusion rate 50 to 75% of what the linear increase would be in order to achieve higher plasma theophylline concentrations.

If the plasma theophylline levels are excessive and associated with toxicity, stopping the infusion for a period of 2-4 hours is recommended prior to reinstituting the new lower infusion rate.

There are numerous methods for monitoring plasma theophylline levels while on an intravenous infusion. Most children will be within 95% of their steady-state level within 12-15 hours on the infusion. Dosages can be adjusted based on one steady-state level. Alternatively, one can obtain a level 30 minutes after the loading dose and then a second level at 8-12 hours. This will give the clinician what the loading dose achieved and an estimate of whether the infusion rate should be increased or decreased based on what direction the second level is from the first (increased or decreased).

Chronic Oral Dosing: Based on Anhydrous Theophylline Content

Category	Dosage (mg/kg/day)
Neonates	3-9
1 mo-6 mo	10
6 mo-1 yr	15
1 yr-8 yrs	24
9 yrs-12 yrs	20
12 yrs-16 yrs	18

These dosages conform to the maximum dosage recommended before theophylline blood levels are necessary, however, due to the wide interpatient variability in the ability to eliminate theophylline, we recommend following blood levels on all patients. Our belief is that while theophylline levels maintained between 10 and 20 μg/ml will provide optimal results in the majority of patients, each patient should be individualized and whatever plasma theophylline concentration provides optimal effect with minimum side effects is the "therapeutic range" for a given individual. There are a large number of theophylline preparations available for chronic oral dosing. We prefer the sustained-release formulations because they improve patient compliance through their ease of administration. In children we prefer the following products: Slo-bid Gyrocaps as a sustained-release capsule and TheoDur as a sustained-release tablet. Neither product is significantly affected by coadministration with food and both are suitable to q12h dosing in most pediatric patients. Suitable alternatives include Somophyllin CRT as a sustained-release capsule and Quibron T/SR as a sustained-release tablet. The disadvantage of Somophyllin CRT is that it is not available in 50 mg in the United States. Quibron T/SR is more rapidly absorbed than TheoDur. The liquid theophylline preparations are the most expensive and least palatable method of administering theophylline. We recommend using a preparation without alcohol, sugar, and dyes.

Our usual method of monitoring patients is to begin them on an average dose based on the patient's age. After at least three days on that dose, have the patient return for a theophylline level determination. If patients are taking a rapid-release product, we obtain a trough (lowest) theophylline level. We attempt to maintain trough levels between 5 and 10 μg/ml. The corresponding peak levels may be roughly estimated from the 1 mg/kg = 2 μg/ml. The peak following rapid-release tablets and liquids occurs anywhere from 30 min to 3 hours following administration and is as easily estimated as obtained.

With sustained-release theophyllines (SRT), the slow absorption provides a lower peak-trough difference so that the peak level is a better estimate of the steady-state plasma level, therefore, we monitor the peak concentrations. If patients are having increased symptoms at the end of a dosing interval, a serum theophylline determination at that time will help guide the decision whether to administer the drug every 8 hours. The slower the release the more inconsistent the time to peak, however the difference in peak and trough concentration are less. TheoDur peaks or plateaus 3-9 hours after a dose. Quibron more consistently (due to slightly more rapid release) peaks between 4 and 6 hours after a dose. Slobid Gyrocaps peak at 4 to 6 hours after a dose while Slophyllin Gyrocaps, a q8h preparation, peak at 4 hours.

B. Adult Theophylline Dosing

Acute

Several published schemes recommend an initial target concentration for theophylline of 10 μg/ml. This virtually assures that levels will not significantly exceed 20 μg/ml if beginning at 0 μg/ml. Subsequent loading and maintenance dose adjustments are based on further measurements. Other authors aim at an initial target concentration of 15 μg/ml.

The following scheme is used at the Hines Veterans Administration Medical Center. It is a simplified version of the FDA recommendations. Note that doses are expressed in aminophylline equivalents, where theophylline 0.8 × aminophylline. We also include some data on approximate theophylline clearances as summarized from the literature (see references below).

Loading Dose

Category	IV Aminophylline
Not already on theophylline	6 mg/kg over 20 min
On theophylline or ?? [a]	3 mg/kg over 20 min

[a] Unless urgency exists, it is possible to obtain a STAT level before further loading.

Maintenance Dose

Category	Initial clearance (ml/kg/hr)	IV aminophylline (mg/kg/hr)
Uncomplicated		
nonsmoking	40 ± 12	0.5
smoking	70 ± 28	0.8
Critically ill, all varieties (Westerfield et al.)	43 ± 16	0.5
Congestive heart failure severe pneumonia (Powell et al.)	25 ± 12	0.2

Any theophylline level, whether obtained before or after loading, will facilitate optimal dosing. As a minimum, however, a level should be obtained 18-24 hours after loading to detect and avoid levels that might be heading into a toxic range. Obviously, critically ill patients with their variable clearance require closer monitoring.

A second approach is that used at the University of Iowa Hospitals for both adults and children (Courtesy of M. W. Weinberger, M.D.). It involves close monitoring. *Note that doses are expressed in theophylline equivalents.*

Chronic

The adult is more likely than the child to encounter dosing complexities for the following reasons: (1) organ failure of the heart or liver can be present, or develop, with reduced theophylline clearance; (2) smoking status is highly significant, smokers having about a 60% increase in theophylline clearance; (3) drugs which alter theophylline clearance may be added, for example, cimetidine or oral contraceptives, often without the knowledge of the physician treating the lung problem; (4) older patients may be unreliable in taking the prescribed medication. Furthermore, the effect of aging on reduction of clearance is still controversial, but may be a factor.

Another problem in the adult is the greater difficulty of close followup. The busy working person or the homebound patient can present problems for close followup and dose adjustment. Often the next appointment is a month or more later after beginning theophylline, so that toxic levels are left uncorrected. For these reasons the authors present a conservative full dose regimen whose mean theophylline level is calculated to be about 10 μg/ml initially instead of 15 μg/ml. Dose adjustment then can be made as desired from the level obtained on the next visit, with peak levels aimed at about 15 μg/ml, and mean levels between 10 and 15 μg/ml. Of course, patients must be instructed to reduce the dose if side effects occur, and warned not to arbitrarily increase the

the dose if symptoms increase. This system is used at Hines VA Medical Center in treating older adults.

Conservative approach with minimal monitoring (Hines VA Medical Center)

Category	Oral Dose
	(aimed at a mean level of 10 μg/ml, with later dose adjustment prn)
Nonsmoking adult, no other organ disease	10 mg/kg (range 500-800 mg for 50-80 kg I.B.W.)
Smoking adult, no other disease	13 mg/kg (range 700-1000 mg for 50-80 kg I.B.W.)

An alternative approach is that used in the University of Iowa Hospital system (Courtesy of M. W. Weinberger, M.D.) in which levels are monitored 48 hours after full dosage is achieved. This approach uses a stepwise incremental dose increase beginning at 400 mg/day in adults to minimize side effects and makes no smoking distinction.

Approaches Used at University of Iowa Hospitals

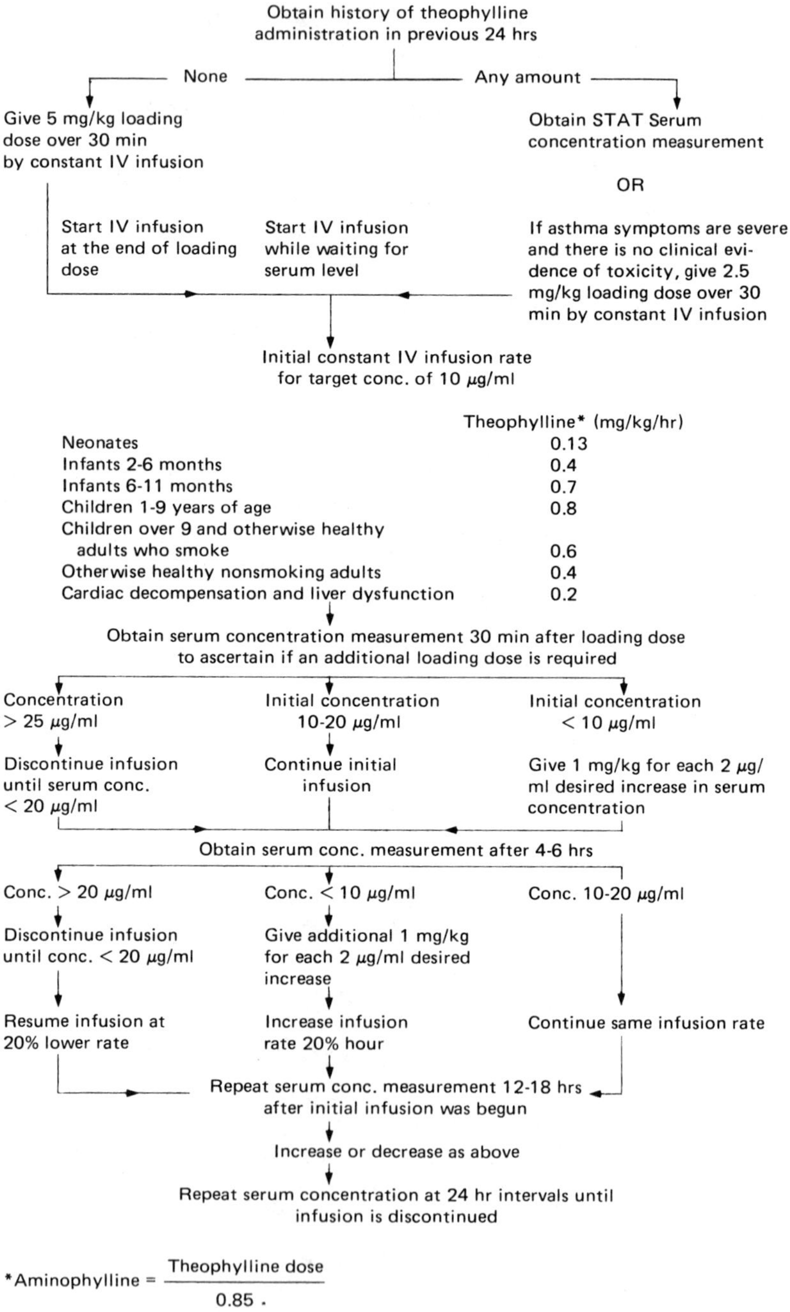

Scheme 1 Algorithm for the use of theophylline to relieve acute symptoms of asthma.

Initial dose

16 mg/kg/day (8 mg/kg/day for infants ages 6 to 24 weeks, *or* 400 mg/day, ***whichever is less.*** Simultaneously, clear nonbronchodilator responsive airway obstruction with short course of high dose prednisone.

↓

Maximum premeasurement dose*

Increase dose *if tolerated* in approximately 25% increments at 3-day intervals, not to exceed the following

Age	Total daily dose (ideal body weight)
Infants 6 to 51 weeks	mg/kg – (0.3) X (age in weeks) + 8
Children 1 to 9 years	24 mg/kg
Children 9 to 12 years	20 mg/kg
Adolescents 12 to 16 years	18 mg/kg
Adults	13 mg/kg or 900 mg *whichever is less*

Do not attempt to maintain any dosage that is not tolerated

↓

Final dose

Measure peak serum theophylline (no missed doses in previous 48 hours, blood drawn at 2 hours after most recent dose for rapidly absorbed preparations or at 4 hours for sustained-release preparations). Adjust as instructed in Table 1.

↓

If final dose not tolerated and resulting serum concentration does not exceed 20 μg/ml and lower dose does not control asthma *then* Try substitute medication.

Medication tolerated *and* asthma controlled *then* Maintain dosage until remission suspected (may be months or years). Recheck serum concentrations at 6- to 12-month intervals. If occasional acute exacerbations occur treat vigorously with additional measures.

Medication tolerated *but* asthma not controlled *then* Add additional therapy as indicated

Scheme 2 Algorithm for the use of theophylline to prevent symptoms of chronic asthma. Doses are expressed as 24 hour total amounts and should be divided into 2 or 3 equal intervals depending on the product and patient. *Note: This schedule has been recently revised to reach a "maximum premeasurement dose" of 800 mg for adults and children ⩾ 45 kg with only one intermediate dosing step.

Dosage adjustment after serum theophylline measurement

If serum theophylline is		Directions
Within normal limits	10 to 20 μg/ml	Maintain dosage if tolerated. Recheck serum theophylline concentration at 6- 12-month intervals.[a]
Too high	25 to 25 μg/ml	Decrease doses by about 10%. Recheck serum theophylline concentration at 6- to 23-month intervals.[a]
	25 to 30 μg/ml	Skip next dose and decrease subsequent doses by about 25%. Recheck serum theophylline.
	Over 30 μg/ml	Skip next 2 doses and decrease subsequent doses by 50%. Recheck serum theophylline.
Too low	7.5 to 10 μg/ml	Increase dose by about 25%.[b] Recheck serum theophylline concentration at 6- to 12-month intervals.[a]
	5 to 7.5 μg/ml	Increase dose by about 25% to the nearest dose increment[b] and recheck serum theophylline for guidance in further dosage adjustment (another increase will probably be needed, but this provides a safety check).

[a]Finer adjustments in dosage may be needed for some patients.
[b]Dividing the daily dose into 3 doses administered at 8-hour intervals may be indicated if symptoms occur repeatedly at the end of a dosing interval.

IV. Inhaled Beta Agonists for Life-Threatening Asthma

The safety and efficacy of inhaled beta-agonists in severe asthma have been demonstrated in numerous trials. Research evaluating the optimal dosing of these agents for life-threatening asthma is ongoing. Presented below are dosage regimens that have been used successfully by various authorities. They generally exceed the usual recommended doses and are not formally approved by the FDA. In all cases the drugs can be administered by compressor-driven nebulization or oxygen at 6 liters min^{-1}. Delivery by IPPB does not improve efficacy. A mouthpiece with nose clips, or facemask are equally efficacious.

A. Albuterol/Salbutamol (As Used in Children by Robertson et al., 1985)

Initially 0.15 mg/kg up to 5 mg in 2 ml saline, then 0.05 mg/kg up to 1.7 mg at 20 minute intervals for a total of 6 doses as needed.

Seventeen patients receiving the above regimen demonstrated a mean improvement in FEV_1 of 84% compared to a 38% improvement for 16 patients receiving 0.15 mg/kg nebulized every hour. Nine patients exhibited a fine tremor and two patients vomited. The salbutamol was diluted with 2 ml of 0.9% saline and nebulized with continuous flow oxygen at 5 to 6 liters min^{-1}.

B. Isoproterenol (As Used by Fanta et al., 1986)

Three doses of 2.5 mg (0.5 ml of a 0.5% solution) in 2.5 ml saline at 20 minute intervals administered by hand-bulb nebulizers.

Forty-one patients receiving this regimen demonstrated greater improvement in FEV_1 (mean 0.72 ± 0.9 liters) than patients receiving aminophylline or subcutaneous epinephrine. Combination therapy was not more effective than isoproterenol. In 22 patients with the most severe obstruction ($FEV_1 < 35\%$ of predicted normal), a significantly greater improvement for aerosol isoproterenol than for subcutaneous epinephrine was demonstrated. There was no significant change in heart rate.

C. Metaproterenol (As Used by Siegel et al., 1985)

Doses of 15 mg in 2.0 ml saline every 60 minutes for 4 doses administered by hand jet nebulizer with 100% oxygen at 8 L/min.

Seventeen patients receiving this regimen demonstrated equivalent response to patients receiving aminophylline plus the above regimen. Mean improvement in FEV_1 for all patients was 53%.

D. Terbutaline

(As used in adults by Nelson et al., 1986): 2 mg of 1 mg/ml injectable solution every 20 minutes until response. (As used in children. Courtesy S. Murphy, M.D. and H.W. Kelly, Pharm. D. Division Pulmonary/Critical Care Medicine, Department of Pediatrics, University of New Mexico Hospital. Albuquerque, New Mexico): 0.1-0.3 mg/kg up to 5 mg of 1 mg/ml injectable terbutaline solution undiluted every 20 minutes or nebulized continuously until response occurs. Dosing interval is then extended to 1-2 hours as patient improves. This regimen has been used in 80 patients over the past 6 years by the pediatric pulmonary division of University of New Mexico Hospital. The injectable solution of 1 mg/ml is packaged dissolved in normal saline so that further dilution is unnecessary.

V. Intravenous Beta Agonist for Life-Threatening Asthma

The following regimens are provided without comment. They are not formally approved by the FDA, but have been used successfully by various authorities when circumstances warranted.

A. Albuterol/Salbutamol (As Used in Children by Bohn et al., 1984)

Loading dose: 10 μg/kg over 10 min (1 μg/kg/min)

Maintenance dose: Continuous infusion of 0.2 μg/kg/min. Increase in 0.1 μg/kg steps every 15 minutes according to response as judged by $PaCO_2$ and bronchospasm. IV bicarbonate is given for pH below 7.20.

In 16 episodes 11 responded and did not require intubation. The mean duration of infusion was 36 hours (range 17 to 64) and the mean infusion rate 1.7 μg/kg/min, with maximum 4 μg/kg/min. In responding patients, the infusion was maintained at least four hours and then decreased gradually over the next 36 hours. Patients who failed to respond were maintained on the infusion while being ventilated.

B. Isoproterenol (As Used in Children by Downes et al., 1973)

Infuse with IVAC at initial rate to provide of 0.1 μg/kg/min. Increase dose by 0.1 μg/kg/min every 15 minutes, until improvement occurs, or until heart rate exceeds 190 beats/min. Stop infusion when $PaCO_2$ remains below 45 torr with a clinical score below 4 (see original reference) at a dose of 0.1 μg/kg/min.

Patients also receive aminophylline, corticosteroids, and bicarbonate prn to keep pH above 7.20.

In 20 episodes, 18 responded with prompt and sustained reduction in $PaCO_2$ after an average of 1.7 hour. The mean peak dose was 0.80 μg/kg/min (range 0.08 to 1.60) and duration of infusion 45 hr. Two patients did not respond.

C. Terbutaline (As Used in Adults and Children. Courtesy of R. Hyatt, M.D., Park Nicollet Medical CTR, Minneapolis, MN)

Loading dose: 10 μg/kg over 10 min (1 μg/kg/min).

Maintenance dose: Continuous infusion of 0.1 μg/kg/min. Increase in 0.1 μg/kg/min steps as necessary to maximum of 0.4 μg/kg/min.

Example, using IVAC and 80 kg patient:

1. Place 4 mg terbutaline (from 4 ampoules) in 100 ml saline.
2. Set IVAC rate/hr at (wt(kg) × 1.5). *Give for 10 minutes.* Example: 80 kg pt = 120 cc/hr = 20 cc/10 min = 0.8 mg
3. Cut back after 10 min to 1/10 this rate. Example: 80 kg pt = 12 cc/hr = 8.0 μg/min.
4. Increase as necessary to maximum of 50 cc/hr.

References

Bohn, D., Kalloghlian, A., Jenkins, J., Edmonds, J., and Barker, G. (1984). Intravenous salbutamol in the treatment of status asthmaticus in children. *Crit. Care Med. 12*: 392-896.

Bukowsky, M., Nakatsu, K., and Munt, P. W. (1984). Theophylline reassessed. *Ann. Intern. Med. 101*: 63-73.

Downes, J. J., Wood, D. W., Harwood, I., Sheinkopf, H. N., and Raphaely, R. C. (1973). Intravenous isoproterenol infusion in children with severe hypercapnia due to status asthmaticus. *Crit. Care Med. 1*: 63-68.

Food and Drug Administration (1980). IV dosage guidelines for theophylline products. *FDA Drug Bull. 10*: 4.

Gardner, M. J., and Jusko, W. J. (1982). Effect of age and sex on theophylline clearance in young subjects. *Pediatr. Pharmacol. 2*: 157-169.

Greenberg, A., Piraino, B. H., Kroboth, P. D., and Weiss, J. (1984). Severe theophylline toxicity-role of conservative measures, antiarrhythmic agents, and charcoal hemoperfusion. *Am. J. Med. 76*: 854-860.

Hendeles, L. (1985). Update on pharmacodynamics and pharmacokinetics of theophylline. *Chest 88* (Suppl 2): 1125-1175.

Hendeles, L., and Weinberger, M. (1983). Theophylline: A 'state the art' review. *Pharmacotherapy 3*: 2-44.

Hendeles, L., Weinberger, M., and Bighley, L. (1978). Disposition of theophylline after a single intravenous infusion of aminophylline. *Am. Rev. Respir. Dis. 118*: 97-103.

Jacobs, M. H., Senior, R. M., and Kessler, G. (1976). Clinical experience with theophylline: relationships between dosage, serum concentration and toxicity. *JAMA 235*: 1983-1986.

Jusko, W. J., Gardner, M. J., Mangione, A., Schentag, J. J., Koup, J. R., and Vance, J. W. (1979). Factors affecting theophylline clearance: Age, tobacco, marijuana, cirrhosis, congestive heart failure, obesity, oral contraceptives, benzodiazepines, barbiturates and ethanol. 68: 1358-1366.

Nelson, H. S. (1986). Adrenergics in asthma: where we stand today. *J. Respir. Dis. 7*(7): 43-49.

Ogilvie, R. I. (1978). Clinical pharmacokinetics of theophylline. *Clin. Pharmacokinetics 3*: 267-293.

Olson, K. R., Benowitz, N. L., Woo, O. F., and Pond, S. M. (1985). Theophylline overdose: Acute single ingestion versus chronic overmedication. *Am. J. Emerg. Med. 3*: 386-394.

Powell, J. R., Voseh, S., Hopewell, P., Costello, J., Sheiner, L. B., and Riegelman, S. (1978). Theophylline disposition in acutely ill hospitalized patients. The effect of smoking, heart failure, severe airways obstruction and pneumonia. *Am. Rev. Respir. Dis. 118*: 229-238.

Robertson, C. F., Smith, F., Beck, R., and Levison, H. (1985). Response to frequent low doses of nebulized salbutamol in acute asthma. *J. Pediatr. 106*: 672-674.

Siegel, D., Sheppard, D., Gelb, A., and Weinberg, P. F. (1985). Aminophylline increases the toxicity but not the efficacy of an inhaled beta-adrenergic agonist in the treatment of acute exacerbations of asthma. *Am. Rev. Respir. Dis. 132*: 283-286.

Uematsu, T., and Vozeh, S. (1985). Update of theophylline pharmacokinetics. *Prac. Cardiol. 11*: 95-106.

Voseh, S., Kewitz, G., Perruchoud, A., Tschan, M., Kopp, C., Heitz, M., and Follath, F. (1982). Theophylline serum concentration and therapeutic effect in severe acute bronchial obstruction: The optimal use of intravenously administered theophylline. *Am. Rev. Respir. Dis. 125*: 181-184.

Westerfield, B. T., Carder, A. J., and Light, R. W. (1981). The relationship between arterial blood gases and serum theophylline clearance in critically ill patients. 12: 17-20.

Zwillich, C. W., Sutton, F. D., Jr., Neff, T. A., Cohn, W. M., Matthay, R. A., and Weinberger, M. W. (1975). Theophylline induced seizures in adults. *Ann. Intern. Med. 82*: 784-787.

AUTHOR INDEX

Numbers in brackets give the page on which the complete reference work is listed.

A

B

C

D

E

F

H

I

J

K

N

O

P

Q

R

S

U

V

Y

SUBJECT INDEX

B

C

H

I

K

L

M

R

V

X